Advanced Practice in Endocrinology Nursing

Sofia Llahana · Cecilia Follin
Christine Yedinak · Ashley Grossman
Editors

Advanced Practice in Endocrinology Nursing

With Paediatric Editors Kate Davies
and Margaret F. Keil

Volume I

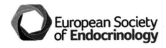
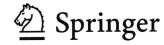

Editors
Sofia Llahana
School of Health Sciences, City
University of London
London
UK

Cecilia Follin
Department of Oncology
Skåne University Hospital
Lund
Sweden

Christine Yedinak
Northwest Pituitary Center
Oregon Health and Sciences University
Portland, OR
USA

Ashley Grossman
Churchill Hospital
University of Oxford
Oxford
UK

ISBN 978-3-319-99815-2   ISBN 978-3-319-99817-6   (eBook)
https://doi.org/10.1007/978-3-319-99817-6

Library of Congress Control Number: 2018968596

This Springer imprint is published by the registered company Springer Nature Switzerland AG
The registered company address is: Gewerbestrasse 11, 6330 Cham, Switzerland

Sofia Llahana
Dedicated to my daughter Elise-Katerina, my husband Richard, and my parents and role models Eirini and Vasilis

Cecilia Follin
Dedicated to Anders, Jesper and Alexander

Christine Yedinak
Dedicated to my husband and cheerleader Marty

Ashley Grossman
Dedicated to my daughters: Emily, Sophie, Annabel, Camilla, Cordelia, and Elizabeth

Foreword

Endocrinology nursing is a fast-developing specialty with nurses performing advanced roles and expanding their practice to cover key roles in the future multidisciplinary centres of excellence like the PTCOE (Pituitary Tumor Centers of Excellence). This book has the merit of providing a comprehensive guide for nurses practising in all areas of endocrinology including bone metabolic diseases, obesity, and lipid disorders. Particularly interesting and modern are the chapters devoted to endocrine emergencies and endocrine abnormalities consequent to cancer treatment. Moreover, the book is suitable for nurses serving in both paediatric and adult endocrine units and at any level of expertise.

The book has been written by an international team of eminent nurses, physicians, surgeons, psychologists, and other healthcare professionals, which makes this book a valuable resource not only for nurses but also for other members of any multidisciplinary team. Patient advocacy groups have also contributed to most chapters with case studies and examples of collaborative working with healthcare professionals to improve patient care.

This is the first book ever published specifically for nurses working in endocrinology, but it is also an excellent resource for nurses working in other specialties such as internal medicine, gynaecology, urology, and rheumatology due to the wide range of topics covered in the book from fertility to osteoporosis and erectile dysfunction. Specialty trainees, general practitioners, students, psychologists, and expert patients wanting in-depth information will also find this book a useful resource.

The editors have led the way in advancing nursing practice, and this book is a reflection of their dedication to developing a solid doctrinal body for the discipline of endocrine nursing worldwide.

Milan, Italy   Andrea Giustina

Preface

We are extremely pleased and proud that our ambitious idea to write the first ever published book for endocrine nurses has finally come to fruition. We wanted this to be a useful resource for endocrine nurses across the globe working at different settings and levels of practice, from novice to expert and from bedside nursing to advanced practice nursing running independent nurse-led services. We recognised that this would be a challenging project to undertake, especially as the endocrinology nursing role varies significantly from country to country. We were, however, overwhelmed by the interest we received from colleagues who wanted to contribute to this book, echoing the great need for such a resource and especially from physicians and other healthcare professionals who recognise the endocrine nurse as a vital member of the multidisciplinary team.

The *European Society of Endocrinology* (ESE) formed our initial working hub and supported this textbook from its inception. We created a strong collaborative European and international network; 118 eminent authors from 15 countries contributed to this book. Most of our authors are nurses, but physicians, surgeons, psychologists, dieticians and geneticists have also contributed, emphasising the multidisciplinary focus of this book.

Built on the growing body of knowledge, expertise and the expanding nature of advanced practice in endocrinology nursing, this book provides a comprehensive resource to support nurses to develop their competence at different levels of their career. The authors in each chapter have done a tremendous job presenting a comprehensive review of anatomy, pathophysiology, diagnosis and treatment of different endocrine conditions supported by the latest evidence and clinical guidelines. Patient stories, case studies and good clinical practice examples are included to illustrate the impact of endocrine conditions on patients and their families, to stimulate the readers' critical thinking and reflection and to make information in this book applicable to their clinical practice. Many patient advocacy groups have contributed with case studies and educational resources, supporting the emphasis this book places on user involvement and shared decision-making in patient care.

Comprising of 13 parts and a total of 69 chapters, this book is a comprehensive resource for paediatric and adult nurses working in endocrinology but should also be useful for specialty trainees, general practitioners, students and expert patients. It also covers endocrine-related topics within other specialties such as fertility, osteoporosis, oncology, urology, gynaecology, obesity and metabolic disorders. Each part covers conditions within a specific endocrine gland (pituitary, adrenal, thyroid, parathyroid and bone disorders and male and female reproduction) and other relevant endocrine conditions such as late effects of cancer treatment, neuroendocrine tumours, endocrine emergencies, obesity and metabolic disorders. There are two paediatric-specific parts (11 chapters); paediatric aspects have also been incorporated in many other chapters, where relevant. The final part focuses on advanced practice nursing (APN) presenting an overview of role development, definition and components of APN, including research, with many useful resources to support career progression within endocrinology nursing. The work by our part editors has been vital as they invited authors and coordinated and edited the chapters in each part; we could not have completed this book without their amazing contribution. We hope and trust this book will assist and advise all our colleagues to ensure the best possible patient care.

London, UK   Sofia Llahana
Lund, Sweden   Cecilia Follin
Portland, OR, USA   Christine Yedinak
Oxford, UK   Ashley Grossman

Acknowledgements

This book is a testament of a successful global collaboration of healthcare professionals, learned societies and patient advocacy groups, and it would not have been possible without the great effort that everyone put into this project.

We express our deep gratitude to our 118 authors who contributed to this book; this was an international multidisciplinary collaboration of nurses, physicians, surgeons, psychologists, geneticists, dieticians and nurse academics from 15 different countries. This book covers adult and paediatric topics; we are indebted to Kate Davies (UK) and Margaret Keil (USA) for editing the paediatric parts and for inviting and supporting authors who contributed with paediatric aspects to many other chapters where relevant in the book. Our gratitude also goes to our part editors who invited contributing authors and edited the chapters in each part: Judith van Eck (the Netherlands), Violet Fazal-Sanderson (UK), Gerard Conway (UK), Andrew Dwyer (Switzerland/USA), Ann Robinson (Australia), Philip Yeoh (UK), Anne Marland (UK) and Michael Tadman (UK). Their names are listed in the respective textbook parts.

The textbook was initiated and developed under the auspices of the European Society of Endocrinology (ESE) and has its full endorsement. We are very grateful to Professor AJ van der Lely, ESE President (2015–2019); Helen Gregson, ESE Chief Executive Officer; Professor Jérôme Bertherat, Chair of ESE Clinical Committee; members of the ESE Executive Committee; and, in particular, Professor Andrea Giustina, incoming ESE President (2019), who has supported this textbook since its inception in 2015.

Special thanks go to Professor Philippe Bouchard, past President of the ESE, and Professors Pia Burman and Richard Ross, past members of the ESE Executive Committee. Their support was instrumental in developing and establishing the ESE Nurses Committee, through which we met and worked together on this book and on other European and international projects.

We are also grateful to the following Nursing Organisations for their support and for approving this textbook as a valuable resource for endocrine nurses:

- The Federation of International Nurses in Endocrinology (FINE)
- The Endocrine Nurses Society (ENS)—USA
- The Endocrine Nurses' Society of Australia (ENSA)—Australasia
- The Pediatric Endocrinology Nursing Society (PENS)—USA, Canada

Representatives from many Patient Advocacy Groups across the globe contributed with case studies and educational resources; we are very grateful and have acknowledged their input in each respective chapter. We would also like to express our gratitude to patients and their families who shared their stories to help our readers understand the impact of endocrine conditions. We all learn so much from our patients and are grateful for the opportunity to be a part of their lives and to support them throughout different stages of living with their condition.

Very special thanks go to Nathalie L'Horset-Poulain, our Senior Publishing Editor, for her amazing guidance throughout this project. We have been very privileged to work with Nathalie and would not have been able to complete this book without her outstanding support. Special thanks also go to Marie-Elia Come-Garry (Associate Editor), Sushil Kumar Sharma (Project Coordinator), Vishal Anand (Project Manager) and all the other members of the Springer Nature Team for their support.

Finally, we would like to express our sincere gratitude to our families, but also the families of all of our authors, for their patience and support during the past 3 years. We sacrificed many weekends and evenings to produce this book and would not have been able to complete it without their unlimited and unconditional support and encouragement.

Sofia Llahana
Cecilia Follin
Christine Yedinak
Ashley Grossman

Contents

About the Editors

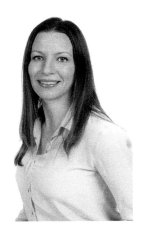

Sofia Llahana, DNSc, MSc, BSc(Hons), RN, INP is a Senior Lecturer, Education and Research, and Programme Director for Advanced Clinical Practice at City, University of London. Dr Llahana was the first consultant nurse in endocrinology in the United Kingdom and worked at University College Hospital in London where she continues to maintain an honorary position. Her clinical and research interest is in pituitary and adrenal conditions, reproductive endocrinology, men's health, self-management, adherence to medication and behavioural medicine. Her current research portfolio includes ongoing and new investigator-led and collaborative national and European studies in adrenal insufficiency, testosterone replacement therapy, male reproduction, growth hormone deficiency, and type 2 diabetes. Dr Llahana is the Chair of the Nurses Committee and a member of the Executive Committee of the European Society of Endocrinology (ESE), a board member of the Federation of International Nurses in Endocrinology (FINE), and the only nurse member in the Scientific Committee for the International Congress in Men's Health. She also holds affiliations with several learned societies and patient advocacy groups in endocrinology.

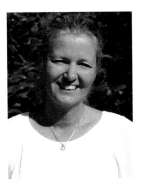

Cecilia Follin graduated as a registered nurse from the Institution of Healthcare Science at the Medical Faculty of Lund University in Sweden. Dr Follin has over 15 years of experience from the field of endocrinology. She holds particular interests in late complications after childhood cancer and pituitary and hypothalamic disorders. Cecilia is initiator and chair of the Nordic Network of Endocrine Nurses. In 2010, Dr. Follin was awarded with a PhD degree in endocrinology. The thesis was titled "Late complications of childhood acute lymphoblastic leukemia (ALL), with special reference to hormone secretion, cardiovascular risk and bone health." In 2010–2012, Cecilia had a postdoc position at the Institution of Clinical Sciences, and currently she has a position as researcher and senior teacher at Lund University. Dr. Follin has published numerous papers.

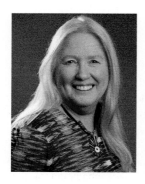

Christine Yedinak, DNP, FNP-BC, MN, Grad DipEd, RN is a doctor of nursing practice and a board-certified family nurse practitioner. She is an assistant professor at the Northwest Pituitary Center, Oregon Health & Sciences University, Portland, Oregon, USA. Dr. Yedinak completed her undergraduate training in Australia and received her postgraduate diploma in tertiary education at the University of Southern Queensland, Toowoomba. She completed her postgraduate and doctoral studies at Oregon Health & Sciences University, Portland, Oregon. Her ongoing research focus is on quality of life and clinical outcomes for patients with pituitary diseases. Dr. Yedinak is president of the Endocrine Nurses Association (USA) and a board member of the European Society of Endocrinology Nurses' Group. She is co-founder and president of the Federation of International Nurses in Endocrinology (FINE).

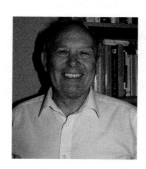

Ashley Grossman, BA, BSc, MD, FRCP, FMedSci initially graduated with a BA in psychology and social anthropology from the University of London, then entered University College Hospital Medical School in London, and received the University Gold Medal in 1975. He also obtained a BSc in neuroscience. Professor Grossman joined the Department of Endocrinology at St. Bartholomew's Hospital where he spent most of his career, eventually as professor of neuroendocrinology, but then moved to become professor of endocrinology at the University of Oxford in the Oxford Centre for Diabetes, Endocrinology and Metabolism. Most recently, he has moved to the Royal Free London where he has specialized in neuroendocrine tumors. In 1999, he was appointed a fellow of the Academy of Medical Sciences, and in 2011, he was made a fellow of Green Templeton College at the University of Oxford. Professor Grossman has published more than 900 research papers and reviews. He has a major interest in tumors of the hypothalamo-pituitary axis, especially Cushing's disease, but his clinical concern and research have expanded increasingly to include broad areas of endocrine oncology, most especially neuroendocrine tumors of all types, including pheochromocytomas, paragangliomas, adrenocortical cancer, medullary thyroid cancer, and hereditary endocrine tumor syndromes. He is past president of the European Neuroendocrine Association (ENEA), past chairman of the UKI Neuroendocrine Tumour Society (UKINETS), and past president of the Society of Endocrinology and the Pituitary Society. He was previously editor of the journal, *Clinical Endocrinology*; is on the editorial board of the major textbook, *Endocrinology*, by De Groot and Jameson; is vice chairman of the major online textbook, *Endotext.org*; and serves on the editorial boards of many journals.

About the Part Editors

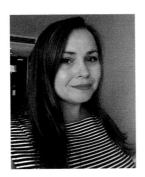

Kate Davies, RN(Child) BSc(Hons) MSc PGDip has over 25 years of experience as a children's nurse, with over 18 years in pediatric endocrinology. She has subspecialized in growth and puberty, Cushing's syndrome, multiple endocrine neoplasia in children, neuroendocrine late effects of childhood brain tumors, adrenal disorders, and disorders of sex development. She is currently a senior lecturer in children's nursing and course director of the PGDip/MSc Children's Advanced Nurse Practitioner program at London South Bank University, UK. She has been chair of the Royal College of Nursing Paediatric Endocrine Special Interest Group (2002–2008), a member of the UK Society of Endocrinology Nurse Committee (2012–2017), and is currently secretary of the European Society of Paediatric Endocrine Nurses Group. She was awarded the BSPED Ipsen Paediatric Endocrine Nurse Award in 2014. Kate is a fellow of the Higher Education Academy, a NMC-registered nurse teacher, and a children's advanced nurse practitioner.

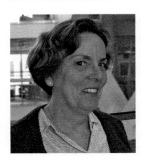

Margaret F. Keil, PhD, CRNP is a board-certified pediatric nurse practitioner with 30+ years of experience in pediatric nursing caring for children with chronic medical conditions in a variety of clinical settings. Dr. Keil received her PhD in nursing from the Uniformed Services University of the Health Sciences and is a graduate of the University of Colorado and Georgetown University. Dr. Keil is a clinical researcher at the National Institutes of Health; her research focuses on biobehavioral outcomes of early life adversity and quality of life and other outcomes associated with chronic endocrine disorders in children. Dr. Keil has authored or co-authored numerous articles published in peer-reviewed journals on pediatric endocrine disorders, including Cushing syndrome, quality of life outcomes, congenital adrenal hyperplasia, obesity, and pituitary tumors. She holds leadership positions in the Pediatric Endocrinology Nurses Society and the Cushing Support and Research Foundation and is a member of the European Society of Endocrinology and the Federation of International Nurses in Endocrinology.

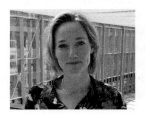

Judith P. van Eck is one of the first advanced practice nurses specialized in endocrinology in the Netherlands. Her career in nursing started in 2004 when she received her bachelor degree in nursing science. Afterward, she worked from 2004 to 2008 as a registered nurse on the clinical department of internal medicine at the Erasmus Medical Center in Rotterdam, the Netherlands. From 2008 to 2010, she followed the Master in Advanced Nursing Practice at Rotterdam University of Applied Sciences. From 2010 until 2018, she worked as a nurse practitioner for the Pituitary Center at the Erasmus Medical Center in Rotterdam, the Netherlands. She was also running a nurse-led clinic for patients with radiation induced hypopituitarism. Currently, she works as a nurse practitioner at the department of Pediatric Endocrinology at Erasmus MC- Children's Hospital in Rotterdam, The Netherlands. She also runs a nurse-led clinic for patients with radiation induced hypopituitarism. She has been a member of the ESE nurses working group from 2013 to 2017, and currently, she is a member of the Dutch Endocrine Nurses Group.

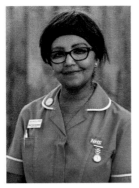

Violet Fazal-Sanderson's, RGN, BSc(Hons), MSc, IP nursing career took off in Oxford where she worked for several years as a staff nurse in the intensive care unit at the Oxford University Hospitals NHS Foundation Trust. She graduated with a BSc (hons) in critical care nursing at Oxford Brookes University. From 2000 to 2016, she worked in the endocrine investigations unit as an advanced nurse practitioner at the Oxford Centre for Diabetes, Endocrinology and Metabolism. She developed an interest in acromegaly and thyroid nurse-led clinics and involved herself in 40 research projects from which emerged several published abstracts and 2 nurse awards.

In 2017, she gained an MSc in endocrinology and now works as a senior endocrine clinical specialist nurse at the Royal Berkshire Hospital NHS Foundation Trust, Reading, and continues to work in endocrinology and thyroid virtual nurse-led clinics. Violet is a member of the British Society for Endocrinology Nurse Committee and the UK TEDct.

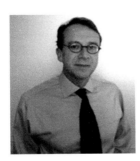

Gerard S. Conway is a consultant endocrinologist at University College London Hospitals and professor of clinical medicine in the Institute for Women's Heath, University College London. His clinical practice covers general endocrinology including pituitary, adrenal, thyroid, and reproductive endocrinology.

His clinical research interests are in the field of reproductive endocrinology particularly polycystic ovary syndrome, ovarian and testicular function, disorders of sexual development, and Turner syndrome. This research has formed the basis of over 160 academic publications.

Professor Conway qualified from the Royal London Hospital in 1981 and trained in diabetes, endocrinology, and general medicine in several centers in Central London. He has been professor of clinical medicine in the Institute for Women's Health UCL since 2012.

With a major interest in teaching, Professor Conway lectures in reproductive endocrinology, for the Society for Endocrinology, the Royal College of Obstetricians and Gynaecologists, and internationally with the endocrine societies in the USA, Sri Lanka, India, New Zealand, Australia, Japan, and throughout Europe.

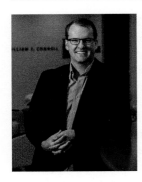

Andrew A. Dwyer, PhD, FNP-BC, FNAP is a board-certified family nurse practitioner with 18+ years of experience in reproductive endocrinology and translational research at the Massachusetts General Hospital (MGH) in Boston (USA) and the University Hospital of Lausanne (CHUV) in Switzerland. Professor Dwyer specializes in genetic disorders of growth/puberty and has helped develop and test structured transitional programs for young adults with chronic endocrine conditions. He presents internationally and has authored/co-authored more than 50 articles on these topics. He holds leadership positions in several organizations including the European Society of Endocrinology, Pediatric Endocrine Nursing Society, European Society of Paediatric Endocrine Nursing, International Society of Nurses in Genetics, and Global Genomic Nursing Alliance. In 2018, Professor Dwyer was inducted into the National Academies of Practice (nursing) as a distinguished fellow.

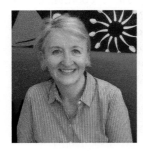

Ann Robinson is an endorsed nurse practitioner (NP) with experience in both public and private sectors. With a background in diabetes and endocrine nursing, her main area of clinical work is now bone health and fracture prevention in high-risk populations. In addition, Ann sits on the governing board of the SOS Fracture Alliance and is past president of the Endocrine Nurses Society of Australasia. Ann works at Gold Coast Health as a nurse practitioner collaborating between hospital and community services to improve osteoporosis awareness and reduce the burden of osteoporotic fractures. She collaborates with the orthopedic teams and has an interest in when to commence treatment, for how long, and when, if ever to stop treatment.

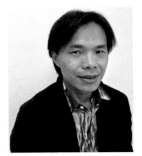

Phillip Yeoh, RN, BSc, MSc, PhD(c) completed registered nurse training in London, BSc from the University of Manchester, and MSc from Brunel University. Philip is currently doing a PhD in Nursing at King's College in London. He is consultant nurse in endocrinology and manager for Endocrine and Diabetes Department within the London Clinic, providing inpatient and outpatient care. His interests in endocrinology focus on adrenal diseases, pituitary conditions, Cushing's disease, acromegaly, neuroendocrine conditions, parathyroid diseases, thyroid cancers, Conn's syndrome, endocrine malignancy such as adrenocortical carcinoma, endocrine testing, endocrine nurse clinical roles, and endocrine nurse educations. He is co-author of *Competency Framework for Adult Endocrine Nursing (Society for Endocrinology)* editions I and II. Currently, he is involved in various research projects looking at dynamic function tests and endocrine nurse role in continuous subcutaneous hydrocortisone infusion pump for patients with adrenal insufficiency. He is coordinator for Federation of International Nurses in Endocrinology. He was a nurse committee member for European Society of Endocrinology and Society for Endocrinology. He is also a trustee for Addison's Disease Self-Help Group UK.

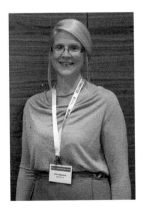

Anne Marland, RGN, INP, BSc, MSc, PhD(c) is advanced nurse practitioner in adult endocrinology and independent nurse prescriber (INP) at the Oxford Centre for Diabetes, Endocrinology and Metabolism (OCDEM) in the UK. Anne worked in the Neuroscience Department in Oxford, and in 1998, she took on a senior research nurse role in OCDEM and, following this, advanced nurse practitioner. Anne has a keen interest in the clinical area of "late effects in endocrinology" and is currently studying for a PhD in this area. She is the patient and public involvement representative for the NIHR for endocrinology and rare disease in the UK. Anne has a keen interest in education and regularly lectures worldwide. She chairs the working party which developed the Society for Endocrinology MSc in Adult Endocrine Nursing in collaboration with Oxford Brookes University in the UK. Anne is the current chair for the British Society for Endocrinology Nurse Committee and member of the Public Engagement Committee.

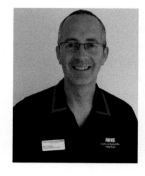

Mike Tadman is a cancer nurse specialist with over 20 years of experience both in practice and education, mainly within Oxford, but has also practiced in Edinburgh and briefly in Melbourne. He set up the Neuroendocrine Tumours Specialist Nursing Service at the Oxford University Hospitals NHS Foundation Trust in 2013. He is an active member of UKINETs and ENETs and has presented regularly at national and international conferences on NETs. He has completed a survey of how centers commence and he has recently published research into the use of somatostatin analogue test dosing and urine 5HIAA testing. He is author of the *OUP Cancer Nursing Handbook*, having just completed editing its 2nd edition.

Contributors

Daphne T. Adelman Division of Endocrinology, Metabolism and Molecular Medicine, Northwestern University, Feinberg School of Medicine, Chicago, IL, USA

Bushra Ahmad Bristol Royal Infirmary, University of Bristol, Bristol, UK

Clare Akers Urology Department, Westmorland Street Hospital, University College London Hospitals NHS Foundation Trust, London, UK

Ahmed Al Sajwani Department of Endocrinology, Tallaght Hospital, Dublin and Trinity College, Dublin, Ireland

Susie Aldiss Faculty of Health and Medical Sciences, University of Surrey, Surrey, UK

Wiebke Arlt Queen Elizabeth Hospital Birmingham, University Hospitals Birmingham NHS Foundation Trust, Birmingham, UK

Miriam Asia Department of Endocrinology, Birmingham University Hospital, Birmingham, UK

Margaret G. Au Department of Pediatrics, Cedars-Sinai Medical Center, Los Angeles, CA, USA

Theingi Aung Centre for Diabetes and Endocrinology, Royal Berkshire Hospital NHS Foundation Trust, Reading, UK

Lesley Baillie School of Health, Wellbeing and Social Care Nursing, The Open University, Milton Keynes, UK

Stephanie E. Baldeweg Department of Diabetes and Endocrinology, University College London Hospitals, London, UK

Kelly Mullholand Behm Orlando, FL, USA

Sarah Benzo Surgical Neurology Branch, National Institute of Neurologic Disorders and Stroke, National Institutes of Health, Bethesda, MD, USA

Jérôme Bertherat Service d'Endocrinologie, Hôpital Cochin, Paris, France

Beth Brillante National Institutes of Health, National Institute of Dental and Craniofacial Research, Craniofacial and Skeletal Diseases Branch, SCSU, Bethesda, MD, USA

Chloe Broughton North Bristol NHS Trust, Bristol, UK

Adrian Brown Imperial College London, London, UK

Debbie Carrick-Sen School of Nursing, Institute of Clinical Sciences, College of Medical and Dental Sciences, University of Birmingham, Birmingham, UK

Paul V. Carroll Department of Endocrinology, Guy's & St. Thomas' NHS Foundation Trust, DEDC 3rd Floor Lambeth Wing, St. Thomas' Hospital, London, UK

Harvinder Chahal Imperial Weight Centre, St. Mary's Hospital, Imperial College Healthcare NHS Trust, London, UK

Yuk Fun Chan Department of Endocrinology and Metabolism, Prince of Wales Hospital, Randwick, NSW, Australia

Kathryn Clark University of Michigan Hospital, Ann Arbor, MI, USA

Sharron Close Emory School of Medicine, Emory University School of Nursing, The eXtraordinarY Clinic at Emory, Atlanta, GA, USA

Arthur D. Conigrave Faculty of Medicine and Health, University of Sydney, Sydney, NSW, Australia

Gerard S. Conway Institute for Women's Health, University College London, London, UK

Sherwin Criseno University Hospitals Birmingham NHS Foundation Trust, Birmingham, UK

Rachel Crowley St. Vincent's University Hospital and University, College Dublin, Dublin, Ireland

Marina Cunha-Silva Disciplina de Endocrinologia e Metabologia do Hospital das Clínicas da Faculdade de Medicina da Universidade de São Paulo, Brazil, São Paulo, Brazil

Christine Davies Children's Hospital for Wales, Cardiff and Vale UHB University Hospital of Wales (UHW), Cardiff, UK

Kate Davies Department of Advanced and Integrated Practice, London South Bank University, London, UK

Philippa Davies NET Unit, Royal Free London NHS Foundation Trust, London, UK

Andrew P. Demidowich National Institutes of Health, Bethesda, MDUSA

Louise Doodson Great Ormond Street Hospital for Children NHS Trust, London, UK

Andrew A. Dwyer William F. Connell School of Nursing, Boston College, Chesnut Hill, MA, USA

Margaret Eckert-Norton SUNY Downstate, Brooklyn, NY, USA

Anne L. Ersig UW-Madison School of Nursing, UW Health American Family Children's Hospital, Madison, WI, USA

Violet Fazal-Sanderson Centre for Diabetes and Endocrinology, Royal Berkshire Hospital NHS Foundation Trust, Reading, UK

Chona Feliciano Queen Elizabeth Hospital Birmingham, University Hospitals Birmingham NHS Foundation Trust, Birmingham, UK

Cecilia Follin Department of Endocrinology, Skane University Hospital, Lund, Sweden

Rebecca Ford Bristol Eye Hospital, University Hospitals Bristol NHS Trust, Bristol, UK

Kirtan Ganda Concord Hospital, Sydney, NSW, Australia

Rhonda Garad Monash Centre for Health Research and Implementation (MCHRI), Monash University, Clayton, VIC, Australia

Claire Gilbert Great Ormond Street Hospital for Children NHS Trust, London, UK

Helena Gleeson Department of Endocrinology, University Hospitals Birmingham NHS Foundation Trust, Birmingham, UK

Clare Grace Relish Nutrition Consultancy, North Yorkshire, UK

Ashley Grossmann Royal Free Hospital, London, UK
Green Templeton College, University of Oxford, Oxford, UK
Barts and the London School of Medicine, London, UK

Lori Guthrie National Institutes of Health, National Institute of Dental and Craniofacial Research, Craniofacial and Skeletal Diseases Branch, SCSU, Bethesda, MD, USA

Saira Hameed Imperial Weight Centre, St. Mary's Hospital, Imperial College Healthcare NHS Trust, London, UK

Geraldine Hamilton Macmillan Support Line, Macmillan Cancer Support, Glasgow, UK

Ingrid Haupt-Schott Velindre NHS Trust, Velindre Cancer Centre, Cardiff, UK

Christina Hayes Surgical Neurology Branch, National Institute of Neurologic Disorders and Stroke, National Institutes of Health, Bethesda, MD, USA

Frances J. Hayes Endocrine Division, Harvard Medical School, Massachusetts General Hospital, Boston, MA, USA

Saundra Hendricks Department of Medicine, Center of Bioenergetics, Houston Methodist Hospital, Houston, TX, USA

Fiona Holden Urology Department, Westmorland Street Hospital, University College London Hospitals NHS Foundation Trust, London, UK

Jürgen Honegger Department of Neurosurgery, University of Tuebingen, Tuebingen, Germany

Irena R. Hozjan Endocrine Program, Department of Pediatrics, The Hospital for Sick Children, Toronto, ON, Canada

Khalid Hussain Great Ormond Street Hospital for Children NHS Trust, London, UK

Sue Jackson Psychology Department, University of the West of England, Bristol, UK

Channa Jayasena Reproductive Endocrinology and Andrology, Imperial College and Hammersmith Hospital, London, UK

Peggy Kalancha Clinical Resource, Pediatric Endocrine and Gynecology Clinics, Alberta Children's Hospital, Calgary, AB, Canada

Niki Karavitaki Institute of Metabolism and Systems Research, University of Birmingham and Queen Elizabeth Hospital, Birmingham, UK

Margaret F. Keil Eunice Kennedy Shriver National Institute of Child Health and Human Development, National Institutes of Health, Bethesda, MD, USA

Dev A. Kevat Monash Health and Western Health, Melbourne, VIC, Australia

Nicole Kirouac St. Amant Inc., Winnipeg, MB, Canada

Kathryn Evans Kreider Duke University School of Nursing and Duke University Medical Center, Durham, NC, USA

Ana Claudia Latronico Disciplina de Endocrinologia e Metabologia do Hospital das Clínicas da Faculdade de Medicina da Universidade de São Paulo, Brazil, São Paulo, Brazil

Megan K. Lessig Division of Endocrinology and Diabetes, Children's Hospital of Philadelphia, Philadelphia, PA, USA

Karen J. P. Liebert Neuroendocrine Unit, Massachusetts General Hospital, Boston, MA, USA

Terri H. Lipman Division of Endocrinology and Diabetes, Children's Hospital of Philadelphia, Philadelphia, PA, USA

Sofia Llahana School of Health Sciences, City, University of London, London, UK

Lucy Mackillop Nuffield Department of Women's and Reproductive Health, University of Oxford, Level 6, Women's Centre, John Radcliffe Hospital, Oxford, UK

Anne Marland Oxford Centre for Diabetes, Endocrinology and Metabolism, Radcliffe Department of Medicine, University of Oxford, Oxford, UK

Lee Martin Barts Health NHS Trust, The Royal London Hospital, London, UK

Raven McGlotten National Institutes of Health, Bethesda, MD, USA

Gisela Michel Department of Health Sciences and Health Policy, University of Lucerne, Luzern, Switzerland

Radu Mihai Department of Endocrine Surgery, Churchill Cancer Centre, Oxford University Hospitals Foundation Trust, Oxford, UK

Kerry-Lee Milner Department of Endocrinology and Metabolism, Prince of Wales Hospital, Randwick, NSW, Australia

Irene Mitchelhil Department of Endocrinology, Sydney Children's Hospital (SCHN), Randwick, NSW, Australia

Bin Moore The Children's Hospital, Westmead, NSW, Australia

Kate Morgan Great Ormond Street Hospital for Children NHS Trust, London, UK

Amy Mundy McGuire Veterans Medical Center, Richmond, VA, USA

Pauline Musson Southampton Children's Hospital, Southampton, UK

Sebastian J.C.M.M. Neggers Department of Medicine, Section Endocrinology, Erasmus Medical Centre, Rotterdam, The Netherlands

Milla Pantovic Department of Neuroendocrinology, Clinic for Endocrinology, Clinical Center Serbia, Belgrade, Serbia

Petro Perros Newcastle upon Tyne Hospitals NHS Foundation Trust and Institute of Genetic Medicine, Newcastle University, Newcastle upon Tyne, UK

Catalina Poiana Department of Endocrinology, "Carol Davila" University of Medicine and Pharmacy, Bucharest, Romania

Vera Popovic Department of Neuroendocrinology, Clinic for Endocrinology, Clinical Center Serbia, Belgrade, Serbia

Alison Pottle Royal Brompton and Harefield NHS Foundation Trust, London, UK

Alessandro Prete Queen Elizabeth Hospital Birmingham, University Hospitals Birmingham NHS Foundation Trust, Birmingham, UK

Eileen Pyra Alberta Children's Hospital, Endocrine Clinic, Calgary, AB, Canada

Marcus Quinkler Department of Medicine for Endocrinology, Diabetes and Nutrition Medicine, Charité Universitätsmedizin Berlin, Berlin, Germany

Richard Quinton Newcastle-upon-Tyne Hospitals Foundation NHS Trust (Royal Victoria Infirmary), Newcastle-upon-Tyne, UK

Rabia Arfan Centre for Diabetes and Endocrinology, Royal Berkshire Hospital NHS Foundation Trust, Reading, UK

Ann Robinson Gold Coast University Hospital, Parkwood, Queensland, Australia

Katharina Roser Department of Health Sciences and Health Policy, University of Lucerne, Luzern, Switzerland

Elisabeth Rutten Department of Endocrinology, Ghent University Hospital, Ghent, Belgium

Katrin Scheinemann Division of Hematology/Oncology, University Children's Hospital Basel (UKBB), Basel, Switzerland

Wendy Schwarz Alberta Children's Hospital, Endocrine Clinic, Calgary, AB, Canada

Mark Sherlock Department of Endocrinology, Tallaght Hospital, Dublin and Trinity College, Dublin, Ireland

Soulmaz Shorakae Monash Centre for Health Research and Implementation (MCHRI), Monash University, Clayton, VIC, Australia

Klaus Sommer Concord Hospital, Sydney, NSW, Australia

Victoria J. Stokes Endocrinology and Metabolism, Oxford Radcliffe Hospitals NHS Foundation Trust, Churchill Hospital, Oxford, UK

Mike Tadman Oxford University Hospitals NHS Foundation Trust, Oxford, UK

Helena Teede Monash Centre for Health Research and Implementation (MCHRI), Monash University, Clayton, VIC, Australia

Raluca-Alexandra Trifanescu Department of Endocrinology, "Carol Davila" University of Medicine and Pharmacy, Bucharest, Romania

Helen E. Turner The Oxford Centre for Diabetes, Endocrinology and Metabolism, Oxford University Hospitals NHS Foundation Trust, The Churchill Hospital, Oxford, UK

Suma Uday University Hospitals Birmingham NHS Foundation Trust, Birmingham, UK

Tanya L. Urquhart Sheffield Hallam University, Sheffield, UK

Judith P. van Eck Department of Medicine, Section Endocrinology, Erasmus Medical Centre, Rotterdam, The Netherlands

Marsha M. van Oostwaard Department of Internal Medicine and Endocrinology, Veldhoven, The Netherlands

Artemis Vogazianou Department of Diabetes and Endocrinology, University College Hospital, London, UK

Jerry K. Wales Lady Cilento Children's Hospital, Brisbane, QLD, Australia

Chris White Department of Endocrinology and Metabolism, Prince of Wales Hospital, Randwick, NSW, Australia

Amanda Whitehead Leeds Children's Hospital, Leeds General Infirmary, Leeds, UK

Tara Whyand NET Unit, Royal Free London NHS Foundation Trust, London, UK

Elizabeth Williamson Reproductive Medicine Unit, University College London Hospitals, London, UK

Christine Yedinak Northwest Pituitary Center, Oregon Health and Sciences University, Portland, OR, USA

Phillip Yeoh Department of Diabetes and Endocrinology, The London Clinic, London, UK

Kathrin Zopf Department of Medicine for Endocrinology, Diabetes and Nutrition Medicine, Charité Universitätsmedizin Berlin, Campus Charité Mitte, Berlin, Germany

Part I

Growth and Development

Kate Davies and Margaret F. Keil

The Importance of Auxology for Growth Assessment

1

Terri H. Lipman and Megan K. Lessig

Contents

Abstract

Auxology is the basis of a proper growth evaluation. It is through the history, physical exam, and auxology that we are able to properly assess a child's growth. Auxology enables us to establish a child's growth patterns and determine if growth is indeed normal. An accurate and reliable measurement, along with appropriate and accurate charting, is critical for a proper growth evaluation.

Keywords

Auxology · Growth chart · Measurement

T. H. Lipman (✉)
University of Pennsylvania School of Nursing, Philadelphia, PA, USA

Division of Endocrinology and Diabetes, Children's Hospital of Philadelphia, Philadelphia, PA, USA
e-mail: lipman@nursing.upenn.edu

M. K. Lessig
Division of Endocrinology and Diabetes, Children's Hospital of Philadelphia, Philadelphia, PA, USA
e-mail: LESSIGM@email.chop.edu

Abbreviations

BMI	Body mass index
CDC	Center for Disease Control
cm	Centimeter
in	Inch
kg	Kilogram
lb	Pound

© Springer Nature Switzerland AG 2019
S. Llahana et al. (eds.), *Advanced Practice in Endocrinology Nursing*,
https://doi.org/10.1007/978-3-319-99817-6_1

LGA	Large for gestational age
m	Meter
MPH	Midparental height
MUC	Mid upper arm circumference
NHANES	National Health and Nutrition Survey
oz	Ounce
SD	Standard deviation
SGA	Small for gestational age
WHO	World Health Organization

Key Terms
- **Auxology:** Science of human growth and development.
- **Accuracy:** A measure of how close the measurement is to the actual measurement.
- **Diurnal variation:** Normal fluctuations that occur over the course of a day.
- **Frankfort plane:** Eye ear plane which is a standard horizontal cephalometric reference.
- **LGA (large for gestational age):** Refers to infants who have birthweights greater than the 90th percentile for babies of the same gestational age.
- **Measurement error:** Difference between a measured quantity (e.g., height) and its true value (e.g., actual height).
- **Reliability:** This is the quality of the measurement. It predicts how likely a repeat measurement will be the same when repeated. Expressed in a percentage.
- **SGA (small for gestational age):** Refers to infants who have birth weights below the 10th percentile for babies of the same gestational age.

Key Points
- Learners will be able to properly identify and obtain proper measurements for a growth evaluation.
- Learners will be able to accurately interpret meaning of these measurements though proper charting.

1.1 Importance of Growth Monitoring

Linear growth is the single most important indication of the health of a child (Tanner 1986). Since healthy infants and children have predictable patterns of linear growth (length/height), normal growth is used as a standard for assessing child health and well-being. Children with growth pattern deviations (e.g., unexplained short or tall stature, growth failure, unexpected growth acceleration) should be evaluated to differentiate between normal growth variants and pathologic conditions. Growth is such a sensitive indicator of health that abnormal growth may be the earliest sign of pathology (Craig et al. 2011; Haymond et al. 2013). Pathological growth may result from nutritional disease, a genetic disorder, an endocrine cause, psychosocial problems, intrauterine growth retardation, or systemic disease and/or disease progression or exacerbation. (Haymond et al. 2013; Rogol and Hayden 2014; Richmond and Rogol 2014).

1.2 Stages of Growth and Growth Rates by Age

From infancy through adolescence, both cell number and cell size increase and body composition changes significantly in terms of absolute and relative changes in the amount of lipid, protein, water, and minerals (Beker 2006). Growth during childhood is tightly regulated and depends on the proper functioning of multiple systems including maternal nutrition and uterine size; genetic growth potential inherited from parents; and nutrition. Growth also is affected by the interaction of multiple hormones, including growth hormone (GH), thyroid hormone, insulin, and sex hormones, all of which effect growth at different points in development.

Child growth generally is divided into six periods: (1) conception to birth, (2) infancy (birth to 1 year of age), (3) toddlerhood (1–3 years of age), (4) early childhood (3–6 years), (5) school-age (6–12 years), and (6) adolescence (12–18 years) (Weintraub 2011).

1.3 Measurements Used in Evaluation of Growth

1.3.1 Growth Parameters

1.3.1.1 Length or Height

Accurate measurement of linear growth is paramount when evaluating pediatric growth. (Foote et al. 2015) A multicenter study in eight cities in the United States demonstrated that only 30% of children in primary care practices were measured accurately (Lipman et al. 2004).

To ensure accuracy, children younger than 24 months must be measured supine and have growth plotted on a length growth chart. When incorrectly obtaining a standing height on a child who is younger than 24 months, the measurement must be plotted on length growth chart—as the height growth chart begins at age 2. A supine measurement is greater than a standing measurement—particularly in children under two who stand with a marked lordosis. Therefore, a child who is measured standing before age 2, and plotted on a length chart, will appear to have linear deceleration which may result in an inappropriate referral for a growth evaluation. Children 24 months and younger should be measured, on a firm platform with a yardstick attached, a fixed head plate, and a moveable footplate (e.g., recumbent measuring board) (Rosenfeld and Arnold 1993; Wales et al. 2003) (Fig. 1.1). Due to slight changes in a child's posture with each

measurement it is recommended that three consecutive linear measurements be obtained on each child. All children must be measured in centimeters rounded to the closest millimeter. The average of the three measurements is considered to be closer to the true height of the child (Voss and Bailey 1994; Foote et al. 2009).

All children older than age 3 should be measured standing. Patients that are between 24 and 36 months can be measured either standing or supine. However, it is important that these children are then plotted on the correct growth chart. When obtaining height, children should be measured while standing against a wall mounted device (e.g., stadiometer) with a fixed right angle at the head (Foote et al. 2009). The child's head, shoulders, buttocks, and heels should be against the wall and feet should be forward facing and together. Gentle traction should be placed under the child's jaw to accurately position the head forward and the head plate should touch the child's scalp, potentially causing hair accessories to be removed or hair styling to be flattened (Foote et al. 2009) (Fig. 1.2). All measurements should be obtained by personnel who have proper and regular training (Foote et al. 2009). Ideally, serial measurements should be taken at the same time of day due to diurnal variation. Studies have shown that there is minimal height loss that can range from 0.47 to 2.8 cm when children are measured in the afternoon versus the morning (Foote et al. 2009).

Fig. 1.1 Measurement of infant length

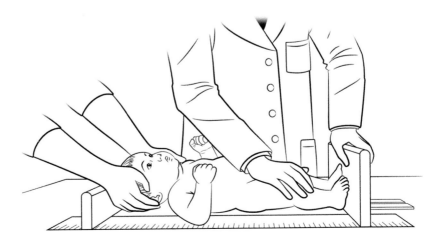

Fig. 1.2 Correct technique for measuring linear height. Reprinted with permission of Nichole Jonas, Graphic Designer. *Eunice Kennedy Shriver* National Institute of Child Health and Human Development, National Institutes of Health, Bethesda, MD USA

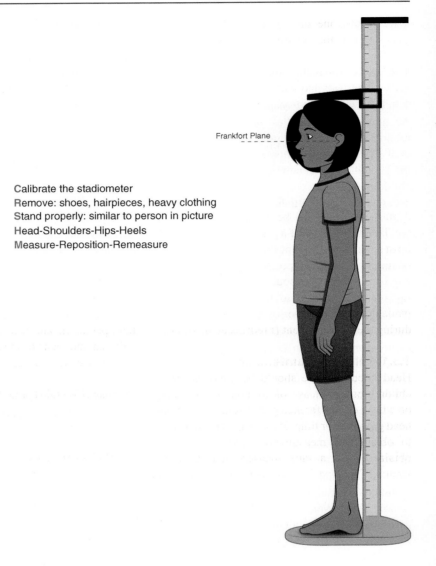

Frankfort Plane

Calibrate the stadiometer
Remove: shoes, hairpieces, heavy clothing
Stand properly: similar to person in picture
Head-Shoulders-Hips-Heels
Measure-Reposition-Remeasure

1.3.1.2 Calibration of Measuring Devices

Instruments must be calibrated at least monthly. Calibration should be more frequent if variance is noted or if recommended by the manufacturer (Voss 2000). A rod of known and fixed height/length can be used to check the calibration of instruments (Foote et al. 2009).

1.3.1.3 Segment Measurements

If full body recumbent length is measured in a child with spasticity, contractures, and/or other musculoskeletal abnormalities, measure the side of the body that is unaffected or less affected and that can be extended the fullest. Record the side measured and the presence of spasticity, joint contractures, and/or other musculoskeletal issues. Alternative measurements, such as arm span, crown-rump length, sitting height, knee height, and other segmental lengths, may be taken to assess growth (Foote et al. 2009).

1.3.1.4 Arm Span

Arm span, after 10 years of age, approximates height in normally proportioned children. It is obtained when it is not possible to obtain a standing height or when a child appears disproportionate. Arm span is the physical measurement of the length from one end of an individual's arms (measured at the fingertips) to the other when raised parallel to the ground at shoulder height at a 90° angle. The patient should be placed with the back to the wall and feet together. The measurer should stretch a measuring tape from the tip of the middle finger on one hand to the tip of the middle finger on the other hand. Measurements of arm span should be obtained in centimeters and rounded to the closest millimeter.

1.3.1.5 Sitting Height

Sitting height should be measured by bringing the fixed right angle of a measuring device to the most superior midline of the head while the child is sitting in an erect position on a flat surface. Arching of the back should be avoided by applying upward pressure to the mastoid processes while the child breathes deeply and holds breath during the measurement (Fredriks et al. 2005).

1.3.1.6 Head Circumference

Head circumference should be measured in all children under the age of 36 months and plotted on a head circumference growth chart to evaluate head growth over time. Two measurers are needed to obtain this measurement and it should be obtained with a tape measure that does not stretch. The tape is positioned across two land marks—the supraorbital ridge and the occiput. Measurements of head circumference should be obtained in centimeters and rounded to the closest millimeter. These measurements are so important in the early months of life, as these measurements are a reflection of intracranial volume and brain growth (Hall et al. 1989). Identification of abnormal growth patterns can lead to early diagnosis of treatable conditions, such as hydrocephalous (Nellhaus 1968).

1.3.1.7 Weight

Younger infants should be weighed nude or in a clean diaper on a calibrated beam or electronic scale. Weigh older infants in a clean, disposable diaper. Position the infant in the center of the scale tray. It is preferable to have two people when weighing an infant. One measurer weighs the infant and protects the child from falling and reads the weight as it is obtained. The other measurer notes the measurement in the infant's chart. Weigh the infant to the nearest 0.01 kilogram (kg) or 1/2 ounce (oz).

A child older than 36 months who can stand without assistance should be weighed using a calibrated beam balance or electronic scale wearing only lightweight clothes or a gown. It is important to stand on the center of the platform of the scale. Children should be weighed to the closed 0.01 kg or ½ oz (Tanski et al. 2007).

1.3.1.8 BMI

The body mass index (BMI) is utilized to quantify the amount of tissue mass in an individual and then categorize that person as underweight, normal weight, overweight, or obese. BMI is used to determine childhood overweight and obesity. Overweight is defined as a BMI at or above the 85th percentile and below the 95th percentile for children and teens of the same age and sex. BMI can be calculated using the following formulas:

$$\text{English} : \left(\text{Weight} \left(\text{pound} \left(\text{lb} \right). \right) \middle/ \left[\text{height inch} \left(\text{in} \right) \times \text{height} \left(\text{in} \right) \right] \right) \times 703$$

$$\text{Metric} : \text{Weight} \left(\text{kg} \right) \middle/ \left[\text{height meter} \left(\text{m} \right) \times \text{height} \left(\text{m} \right) \right]$$

BMI is then plotted on growth chart for age and sex to determine BMI percentile (Tanski et al. 2007).

1.3.1.9 Waist Circumference

Waist circumference is a useful measurement when evaluating a child for obesity or overnutrition. The measurement is obtained by measuring a child between the lower ribs and the ischial ridge at the level of the umbilicus at the end of a normal expiration (Tanski et al. 2007). Skinfold measurements, described in more detail below, can also be used when evaluating a child for weight concerns, as these measurements allow the practitioner to better estimate fat distribution. These measurements become more valuable clinically when used serially to establish a potential improvement from a clinical intervention. To obtain a waist circumference, have the child hold his gown above the waist, cross his arms, and then place hands on opposite shoulders, as if he is giving himself a hug. Next, mark the measurement site. To do this, the measurer should stand on the right side of the child, palpate the hip area to locate the right ilium of the pelvis, and with a cosmetic pencil draw a horizontal line just above the uppermost lateral border of the right ilium. It is important that the measurer ensures that this line crosses the midaxillary line, which is the line that extends from the armpit to the down the side of the torso. To obtain the actual measurement, the measurer should extend the measuring tape around the waist. The measuring tape should be positioned in horizontal plane at the same level as the measurement mark and the zero end of the tape should be positioned below the part of the tape containing the measurement value. The measurement tape should fit snug but should not compress the skin. The measurement should be measured to the nearest 0.1 cm at the end of a normal expiration. The National Health and Nutrition Survey (NHANES) and the Center for Disease Control (CDC) provide a table of ranges of waist circumferences based on age, race, and weight. This enables us to better interpret and use the data (https://www.cdc.gov/nchs/data/series/sr_11/sr11_252.pdf).

1.3.1.10   Skinfolds

Skinfold thickness is another measurement that can be used in conjunction with the waist circumference when evaluating an overweight child. Although four sites can be used, including the triceps, subscapular, biceps and suprailiac, the current National Health and Nutrition Examination Survey (NHANES) anthropology protocol recommends the triceps and subscapular skinfold measurements for patients 2 months of age and older (CDC 2007). In order to accurately obtain this measurement, a skinfold caliper must be used. THE NHANES recommends the Holtain skinfold caliper. Regardless of site, the skinfold measured must contain a double thickness of skin and underlying adipose tissue. To obtain the triceps skinfold, use the thumb and index finger to grasp a fold of skin and subcutaneous tissue at the midpoint of the dorsum of the upper arm. The

tips of the caliper jaws are then placed over the complete skinfold. Release the caliper handle to apply full tension while continuing to hold the skinfold in place so the measurement will register accurately. This should be held for approximately 3 seconds before the measurement is read and recorded. For the subscapular skinfold, the measurement is taken at the inferior angle of the right scapula while arms are in the relaxed position. It is important to not hold the caliper more than 3 seconds or repeat the measurement too frequently at the same spot, as the tissue can be compressed, and ultimately the measurement is falsely low (Hall et al. 1989). Just as in waist circumference, there are charts for normative values for skinfolds (CDC 2007, 2012).

https://www.cdc.gov/nchs/data/series/sr_11/sr11_252.pdf

1.3.1.11   Mid Upper Arm Circumference

A mid upper arm circumference (MUAC) is a measurement that can be utilized when evaluating a child that is undernourished. This measurement is obtained using a flexible nonstretch tape measure. The tape measure is placed mid-way between the elbow and shoulder. The World Health Organization provides standards for arm circumference (http://www.who.int/childgrowth/standards/ac_for_age/en/).

1.4   Growth Charts

To assess if a child's growth pattern is normal, it is crucial that the length or height is plotted on a growth chart with established standards, plotted correctly, and plotted on the correct growth chart. To plot an infant or child, the correct growth chart needs to be identified (i.e., length chart for <36 months and height chart for all children older than 36 months of age). To actually plot the child or infant on the growth chart, the correct age needs to be determined and located on the x-axis of the growth chart. For infants, the age should be calculated to the nearest week. For a child over 36 months of age, the age should be calculated to the nearest month. Once this age is determined, draw a vertical line using a straight edge. Next, on the y-axis, identify the child's height or length. Similarly, a horizontal line should be drawn at this exact measurement. The height or length for age is the intersection of the two lines.

The actual growth charts utilized vary among countries. Internationally, the World Health Organization's growth charts are most frequently used. These growth charts are based on measurements of 8400 infants and children from varying countries of different ethnic backgrounds that were in environments to support optimal growth and were obtained between 1997 and 2003 as part of the Multicentre Growth Reference Study (World Health Organization). The study included two components, longitudinal data for infants to 2 years of age as well as cross-sectional data for those children 18–71 months. The similarities between the data in the six different countries made a case for pooling the data and making an international growth chart (WHO Multicentre Growth Reference Study Group 2006).

The Centers for Disease Control and Prevention's growth charts are most used by practitioners in the United States (Koren and Grimberg 2011). However, for infants to 2 years of age, the CDC recommends utilizing the WHO growth chart, as these charts better illustrate how infants should grow under optimal conditions, rather than how a select group of children in the United States did grow (CDC). The CDC growth charts are based on cross-sectional data provided by the National Center for Health Sciences (NCHS), which is now a part of the CDC (Rosenfeld and Cohen 2002). These charts are particularly helpful for plotting children between the 3rd or 5th, 10th, 25th, 50th, 75th, 90th, and 95th–97th percentile, but unfortunately are limited, as they do not define growth rates for children below the 3rd percentile or above the 97th percentile. The data from these growth charts do, however, allow standard deviation scores (SD) to be calculated. These SD scores (or Z scores) can better describe children's growth rates who are at one spectrum or the other (Rosenfeld and Cohen 2002). For example, a child can be described as having a growth rate that is −4.5 or −2.2 SD from normal. This cross-sectional data is quite helpful during infancy and childhood, but during puberty, when there is a normal variation of the timing of pubertal growth spurts, it may pose a challenge due to the fact that children begin puberty and the increase in growth velocity that accompanies puberty subsequently occurs at varying ages. For this reason, Tanner and colleagues established longitudinal growth charts that take into the consideration the varying ages for the activation of puberty (Rosenfeld and Cohen 2002).

There can be considerable difference in heights of children of the same ages. Because of this, the growth velocity, especially between the age of 2 years and prepubertal years, should be more consistent around 2–3 in per year. When a child crosses percentiles during these ages, further evaluation is warranted.

It is important that children are plotted on the correct growth chart. Because children between the ages of 2 and 3 years can be measured either supine or standing, it is crucial that the type of measurement is then plotted on the appropriate growth chart. Length is the measurement obtained when a child is laying down, as height is obtained while a child is standing. If a 26-month-old child is measured standing up and then plotted on a length growth chart, it will appear that the growth has decelerated. For this reason, the 26-month-old should be plotted on a height chart in order to obtain a true growth trend. Similarly, if this same 26-month-old was measured supine, the measurement should be plotted on a length chart.

In addition to the standard growth charts established by WHO and the CDC, there are specialized growth charts available. For instance, patients with Turner Syndrome, SGA, Russell Silver Syndrome, and Down syndrome have been established in order to better define normative values for these more specialized populations.

The American Academy of Pediatrics recommends that infants and children routinely get measured and weighed as part of their well visit care. The recommended timing of both length/height and weight is as a newborn, 3–5 days, by 1 month, 2 months, 4 months, 6 months, 9 months, 12 months, 15 months, 18 months, 24 months, 30 months, 3 years, and then annually for subsequent years at well child visits (AAP

2017). Insofar as children may only visit the primary care practitioner when ill, and that children with chronic disorders are most often seen at specialty visits, it is critical that children also be measured at sick visits and during evaluation by specialty care (Lipman et al. 2000).

## 1.5	Tools for Adult Height Prediction

### 1.5.1	Bone Age X-Ray

A bone age is a radiograph of the left wrist and hand. As a child ages, the ossification centers in the skeleton appear and progress in predictable fashion. When compared with normal age related standards, a child's bone age can be determined. Gruelich and Pyle established such standards for a child's left hand and wrist to determine a child's bone age (Brook and Dattani 2012; Greulich and Pyle 1999). A bone age is the only quantitative indicator of somatic maturation, and allows the practitioner to assess the remaining growth potential of a child (Koren and Grimberg 2011). The bone age can then be utilized to predict a child's adult height. The classic method for predicting adult height is based on Greulich and Pyle's Radiographic Atlas of Skeletal Development, and was developed by Bayley and Pinneau (Greulich and Pyle 1999). This method uses a child's bone age and height at the time bone age was completed (Rosenfeld and Cohen 2002). Using the bone age, a height prediction can be made. Since Bayley and Pinneau, there have been other variations of this height prediction formula that includes further information such as midparental height, and weight. It is important to note that all of these methods for predicting adult height are based on normal children and would not be applicable to children with growth abnormalities, such as achondroplasia.

### 1.5.2	Midparental Height

When completing a growth evaluation, it is important to determine one's height potential based on his family's genetics. A child's parental

target height is within 2 SD (approximately ±10 cm) of the child's midparental height (MPH). MPH is a simple calculation that is gender adjusted and utilizes the heights of the child's parents. A gender adjusted midparental height for a boy can be calculated by adding the father's height and the mother's height plus 5 in (or 13 cm) divided by 2. Similarly for a girl, this can be calculated by adding the mother's height and the father's height minus 5 in (or 13 cm) divided by 2. As more practices move toward electronic health records (EHR), it is imperative that these EHR in pediatric practices support pediatric functions, such as midparental height. A study completed in 2015 that implemented a midparental height auto-calculator in electronic health records in pediatric practices proved to change PCP decision making, both prompting and preventing unnecessary endocrine referrals (Lipman et al. 2016). Therefore, when a child's current height deviates more than 2 SD from their midparental height, one must consider a pathologic process and consider referral.

## 1.6	Conclusions

Linear growth is the single most important indication of the health of a child (Tanner 1986).

Determination of proper linear growth requires a trained clinician to not only properly obtain the various growth measurements, but also to document and interpret these measurements correctly. It is essential for pediatric health care providers to understand basic auxology of growth. The understanding of normal growth patterns leads to better care of a child and ultimately appropriate endocrine referrals.

References

AAP. Recommendations for preventive pediatric care. bright futures: guidelines for health supervision of infants, children, and adolescents. 4th ed. Elk Grove Village, IL: American Academy of Pediatrics; 2017.
Beker L. Principles of growth assessment. Pediatr Rev. 2006;27(5):196.
Brook CGD, Dattani MT. Handbook of clinical pediatric endocrinology. 2nd ed. West Sussex: Wiley Blackwell; 2012.

CDC. Safer healthier people. National Health and Nutrition Examination Survery. Anthropology procedures manual. 2007.

CDC. Anthropometric reference data for children and adults: United States, 2007–2010. 2012.

Craig D, Fayter D, Stirk L, Crott R. Growth monitoring for short stature: Update of a systematic review and economic model. Health Technol Assess. 2011;15(11):1–64. https://doi.org/10.3310/hta15110.

Foote J, Brady LH, Burke AL, Cook JS, Dutcher ME, Gradoville K M, et al. Evidence based clinical practice guideline on linear growth measurement of children. 2009.

Foote JM, Kirouac N, Lipman TH. PENS position statement on linear growth measurement of children. J Pediatr Nurs. 2015;30(2):425–6.

Fredriks A, van Buuren S, Dijkman-Neerinex RHM, Verloove-Vanjorick SP, Wit JM. Nationwide age references for sitting height, leg length, and sitting height/height ratio, and their diagnostic value for disproportionate growth disorders. Arch Dis Child. 2005;90(8):807–12. https://doi.org/10.1136/adc.2004.050799.

Greulich W, Pyle SI. Radiographic atlas of skeletal development of the hand and wrist. Palo Alto, CA: Stanford University Press; 1999.

Hall J, Froster-Iskenius UG, Allanson JE. Handbook of normal physical measurements. Oxford: Oxford University Press; 1989.

Haymond M, Kappelgaard A, Czernichow P, Biller BMK, Takano K, Kiess W. Early recognition of growth abnormalities permitting early intervention. Acta Paediatr. 2013;102:787–96. https://doi.org/10.1111/apa.12266.

Koren D, Grimberg A. Disorders of the endocrine system: disorders of growth. In: Florin T, Ludwig S, editors. Netter's pediatrics. Philadelphia, PA: Elsevier Saunders; 2011. p. 457–64.

Lipman TH, Hench K, Logan JD, DiFazio DA, Hale PM, Singer-Granick C. Assessment of growth by primary health care providers. J Pediatr Health Care. 2000;14:166–71. https://doi.org/10.1067/mph.2000.104538.

Lipman TH, Hench KD, Benyi T, Delaune J, Gilluly K, Johnson L, Johnson MG, McKnight-Menci H, Shorkey D, Shults J, Waite FL, Weber C. A multicentre randomized controlled trial of an intervention to improve the accuracy of linear growth assessment. Arch Dis Child. 2004;89:342–6.

Lipman TH, Cousounis P, Grundmeier RW, Massey J, Cucchiara AJ, Stallings VA, Grimberg A. Electronic health record mid-parental height auto-calculator for growth assessment in primary care. Clin Pediatr. 2016;55(12):1100–6. https://doi.org/10.1177/0009922815614352.

Nellhaus G. Head circumference from birth to eighteen years: Practical composite international and interracial graphs. Pediatrics. 1968;41:106–14.

Richmond EJ, Rogol AD. The child with tall stature and/or abnormally rapid growth. The child with tall stature and or abnormally rapid growth? [Internet]. 2014. https://www.uptodate.com/contents/search?search=the&sp=&searchType=PLAIN_TEXT&source=USER_INPUT&searchControl=TOP_PULLDOWN&searchOffset=1&autoComplete=false&language=&max=0&index=&autoCompleteTerm=

Rogol AD, Hayden GF. Etiologies and early diagnosis of short stature and growth failure in children and adolescents. J Pediatr. 2014;164:S1–S14. https://doi.org/10.1016/j.jpeds.2014.02.027.

Rosenfeld R, Cohen P. Disorders of growth hormone/insulin-like growth factor secretion and action. In: Sperling M, editor. Pediatric endocrinology. Philadelphia, PA: Saunders; 2002. p. 212–7.

Rosenfeld RG, Conte F, Arnold M. Diagnosis and monitoring of growth disorders. Califon, NJ: Gardiner-Caldwell SynerMed; 1993.

Tanner J. Normal growth and techniques of growth assessment. Clin Endocrinol Metab. 1986;15:411–51. https://doi.org/10.1016/S0300-595X(86)80005-6.

Tanski S, Lynn C, Garfunkel LC. Assessing growth and nutrition in bright futures. Performing preventive services: A bright futures handbook; 2007. p. 51–6.

Voss L. Standardised technique for height measurement. Arch Dis Child. 2000;82(1):14–5.

Voss LD, Bailey BJR. Equipping the community to measure children's height: the reliability of portable instruments. Arch Dis Chad. 1994;70:469–71.

Wales JKH, Wit JM, Rogol AD. Pediatric endocrinology and growth. 2nd ed. Philadelphia, PA: Saunders Elsevier; 2003. p. 1–7.

Weintraub B. Growth. Pediatr Rev. 2011;32(9):404. https://doi.org/10.1542/pir.32-9-404.

WHO Multicentre Growth Reference Study Group. Assessment of difference in linear growth among populations in the WHO Multicentre Growth Reference Study. Acta Pediatr Suppl. 2006;450:56–65.

Short Stature, Growth Hormone Deficiency, and Primary IGF-1 Deficiency

2

Bin Moore, Amanda Whitehead, and Kate Davies

Contents

B. Moore
The Children's Hospital, Westmead, NSW, Australia
e-mail: bin.moore@health.nsw.gov.au

A. Whitehead
Leeds Children's Hospital, Leeds General Infirmary,
Leeds, UK
e-mail: Amanda.whitehead3@nhs.net

K. Davies (✉)
Department of Advanced and Integrated Practice,
London South Bank University, London, UK
e-mail: kate.davies@lsbu.ac.uk

© Springer Nature Switzerland AG 2019
S. Llahana et al. (eds.), *Advanced Practice in Endocrinology Nursing*,
https://doi.org/10.1007/978-3-319-99817-6_2

Abstract

Regular monitoring of a child's growth, using height and weight measurements, is an essential part of the nursing role, as outlined in a previous chapter.

Sequential measurements provide information regarding a child's general health and are invaluable in assessing whether there is a concern regarding their growth pattern. Body proportions, general health, and parental heights will give an indication as to whether the child fits their family pattern or has a growth problem. Review of sequential measurements can help establish whether they have familial or idiopathic short stature, or if they may have a growth and/or other hormone deficiencies.

Growth hormone deficiency (GHD) affects approximately 1:4000 children (Davies, Assessment of growth failure in children: MIMS for Nurses Pocket Guide, 2004).

It can be classified into congenital or genetically associated conditions, or may be acquired due to insult or injury. It may be an isolated deficiency or part of a more complex condition of multiple pituitary hormone deficiencies. Isolated growth hormone deficiency (GHD) is primarily a clinical diagnosis, based upon auxological features, and confirmed by biochemical testing. Once a cause for short stature or GHD is established, treatment can be initiated, which requires daily injections of growth hormone. Growth hormone insensitivity syndrome (GHIS) is rare and requires twice daily injections of insulin-like growth factor 1 (IGF-1).

A long-term commitment to treatment is required by both the patient and their family for best results. A good understanding of the condition and ongoing education is essential to ensure the maximum benefits of treatment are attained.

Growth is a slow process, and often it is easy for families to become complacent or discouraged with treatment regimes. By examining patient behaviour and any concerns they may have regarding their stature, we are in a position to encourage compliance with treatment by recognising that short-term pain (of injections) leads to long-term gain, once final height is reached.

This chapter explores the pathophysiology, clinical characteristics, investigations, and management of children with growth hormone deficiency and growth hormone insensitivity, the treatment required, and nursing considerations needed to manage these children through the ages. The role of the multidisciplinary team will be discussed with emphasis on the role of the Paediatric Endocrine Nurse Specialist in supporting these children and families through many years of treatment.

Keywords

Short stature · Growth hormone deficiency
Multiple pituitary hormone deficiencies
Hypoglycaemia · Growth hormone insensitiv-
ity syndrome · Insulin-like growth factor 1

Abbreviations

BG	Blood glucose
BSPED	British Society for Paediatric Endocrinology and Diabetes
CDGP	Constitutional delay of growth and puberty
CPG	Capillary blood glucose
ENT	Ear, nose, and throat
EU	European Union
GH	Growth hormone
GHD	Growth hormone deficiency
GHIS	Growth hormone insensitivity syndrome
GHR	Growth hormone receptor
GHRH	Growth hormone-releasing hormone
IGF-1	Insulin-like growth factor 1
IGHD	Isolated growth hormone deficiency
MDT	Multidisciplinary team
MPHD	Multiple pituitary hormone deficiencies
PENS	Paediatric Endocrine Nurse Specialist
rhGH	Recombinant human growth hormone
rhIGF-1	Recombinant insulin-like growth factor 1
SPIGFD	Severe primary IGF-1 deficiency
SS	Short stature
STAT5b	Signal transducer and activator of transcription 5b
UK	United Kingdom
USA	United States of America

Key Terms
- **Short Stature:** When a child is considered to be shorter than appropriate for their age, sex and genetic background.
- **Diagnostic pathway:** A series of growth measurements, bone age assessment, physical examination, and dynamic GH testing that

leads to a diagnosis of growth hormone deficiency or (more rarely) GH insensitivity syndrome.
- **GH therapy treatment indications:** A group of diagnosis where children are eligible to be prescribed GH therapy or IGF-1 treatment.
- **GH devices:** A group of medical injection devices for administering GH injections.

Key Points
- Ongoing monitoring of a child's growth is essential if determination of a growth problem is to be identified.
- Growth hormone deficiency (GHD) is a rare condition: Growth hormone insensitivity syndrome (GHIS) is even more rare.
- Treatment involves daily growth hormone injections, twice daily for GHIS.
- The psychosocial aspects of extreme short stature need to be considered.
- Children should always be treated according to their age, not height.

2.1   Short Stature: Definition of Short Stature

Short stature is defined as a height less than −2.0 SDS or more below the mean height for children of the same chronological age and sex (below the 2.3 centile) and with a height velocity of less than −1 SDS.

2.1.1   Short Stature or Slow Growth

At any age, there can be a number of reasons for short stature (SS) or slow growth, and sometimes a cause is never found.

2.1.2   Why Might a Child Be Short?

The causes of short stature can be many and varied. They can range from *normal variants* to *pathological conditions*.

Familial short stature is one of the commonest reasons in otherwise healthy children, meaning that if the child's parents are short, then it is more likely for the child to be short also. However, this may not indicate that the family's short stature is considered to be "normal": (1) there may be an identified growth disorder that runs in the family (2) ethnic and racial growth patterns also need to be considered.

Delayed growth can present at any age and is often seen in teenagers with a delayed puberty and/or growth spurt. *Constitutional delay of growth and puberty* (CDGP) is more commonly seen in boys in comparison to girls and may require endocrine intervention. Criteria for this would include short stature, delayed secondary sexual characteristics, and psychological distress. Psychological distress should not be discounted and can cover a multitude of representations, such as depression, school refusal due to bullying, poor self-image, and the difficulty in being admitted to age appropriate past times (i.e. the cinema or fairground rides) (Raine et al. 2011).

Intrauterine growth retardation or babies born small for gestational age can cause abnormal programming of growth from birth, resulting in babies weighing at least 2 standard deviations (SD) below the mean for the infant's gestational age (Lee et al. 2003).

Genetic conditions can also cause abnormal growth patterns and a karyotype should be done in all children suspected of any genetic condition or if there is no known cause for the abnormal growth pattern. Such conditions can include Turner syndrome (see Chap. 40), Prader-Willi syndrome (see Chap. 9), Down syndrome, or Noonan syndrome (Romano et al. 2010), or if a child appears to have a skeletal dysplasia.

In children with Noonan syndrome, the diagnosis is not usually confirmed with a genetic diagnosis, but on clinical grounds, although there are some defined gene mutations. The condition is characterised by distinctive facial features, such as hypertelorism (where the distance between the inner eye corners is greater than normal), ptosis, and low set prominent ears. The child will often have a cardiac defect, usually pulmonary stenosis, and also have skeletal problems, including short stature, scoliosis, pectus excavatum, and cubitus valgus.

Other endocrine factors to consider would be gonadal problems: most boys have cryptorchidism and also delayed puberty. There may also be a degree of mild learning difficulty (Lee et al. 2003; Skuse et al. 1996).

Nutritional problems, chronic illness or unexplained (idiopathic) reasons despite investigation, are also reasons for concern in families. It is well documented in the literature that chronic illness has an impact on linear growth (Raine et al. 2011) due to the disease process, or its treatment (e.g. systemic corticosteroids)—this is commonly seen in children with asthma, inflammatory bowel disease, renal failure, and children with a decrease in calorie intake, such as cystic fibrosis, coeliac, and Crohn's disease.

2.1.2.1 Psychosocial Short Stature

Although seen less often, another cause for isolated GHD may be due to social deprivation (Skuse et al. 1996; Albanese et al. 1994). Growth failure observed without organic aetiology, but associated with behavioural disturbance and psychosocial stress, has been termed psychosocial short stature.

Children exposed to social deprivation, abuse or neglect, may exhibit signs of social withdrawal, bizarre eating habits, hyperphagia compulsive eating disorders, vomiting, and polydipsia. It has long been recognised that children who are exposed to psychological or physical abuse may present with signs similar to those of a child with isolated GHD. This condition encompasses failure to thrive, stunting secondary to chronic malnutrition, and idiopathic hypopituitarism.

Some children show spontaneous catch-up growth when removed from the source of stress without further treatment, but for some, GHD persists and there are some indications that a possible genetic predisposition may exist. These tend to resolve when the situation is addressed.

2.1.2.2 Idiopathic Short Stature

This is defined as short stature due to an unknown diagnosis or physiological variants. Height is below −2 SDS but the children have a normal birth weight and are GH sufficient. They usually have no finding of any disease when examined by a paediatric endocrinologist, and no identified

Table 2.1 Causes of short stature (Maguire et al. 2013)

Normal Variants	Maturational delay Familial short stature Idiopathic short stature	
Pathological Conditions	**Dysmorphic Syndromes** Chromosomal Other syndromes Non-specific conditions	Turner and Down Syndrome Noonan's or Russell-Silver syndrome Those associated with birth defects/mental retardation
	Intrauterine growth retardation (IUGR)	
	Skeletal disorders	Achondroplasia/hypochondroplasia Chondrodystrophies e.g. Leri-Weill SHOX Rickets/vitamin D deficiency
	Psychosocial deprivation	
	Medication side effects	Glucocorticoids High dose oestrogen or androgens Methylphenidate Dexamphetamines
	Nutritional	Insufficient caloric intake Malabsorption Chronic inflammatory bowel disease Coeliac disease
Endocrine	Isolated GHD Multiple pituitary hormone deficiencies Hypothyroidism Cushing syndrome Consequences of untreated precocious puberty Consequences of childhood cancer treatments—radiotherapy/chemotherapy	

cause for their short stature. Familial short stature and CDGP are commonly included under the umbrella of idiopathic short stature (Cohen et al. 2008).

Hormonal deficiencies, particularly those with thyroid and growth hormone deficiency can present during infancy or at any age, and can have an impact on linear growth. Ongoing monitoring of a child's growth using height and weight measurements is essential if determination of a growth problem is to be identified. Regular sequential measurements provide information regarding a child's general health and are essential in assessing a child's growth pattern (See Chap. 1) (See Table 2.1 (Maguire et al. 2013)).

2.1.3   Why Should Short Stature Be Investigated?

Although short stature is the most common reason why a child is referred to a paediatric endocrine clinic, it is essential that it should be investigated, as there is a multitude of aetiologies that can be the cause (Maghnie et al. 2017). As well as the obvious psychological impact short stature has on the child or young person, it is important to determine the reason, if any, as the pathological cause could be masking other underlying disease. Therefore, once idiopathic, clinical, or other endocrine causes for short stature have been eliminated, then the diagnosis of growth hormone deficiency needs to be considered.

2.2   Growth Hormone Deficiency? (GHD)

See Table 2.2 for causes for GHD (Davies 2004; Raine et al. 2011).

GH deficiency occurs when the pituitary gland fails to produce sufficient levels of hormones, the chemical signals that regulate important biological functions, including growth. It may be an isolated deficiency or part of a condition known as multiple pituitary hormone deficiencies (MPHD). It is rare to have a complete lack of growth hormone but insufficient amounts will lead to poor growth.

The diagnosis of isolated growth hormone deficiency can often be missed in early childhood as the child may be healthy, apart from being smaller than other children their age. It may not be until a child starts school (or prior to starting at senior school) that the diagnosis is made as the size difference is noticeable compared to peers.

Table 2.2 Causes of growth hormone deficiency

Congenital	– Intrauterine infections – Pituitary absence or hypoplasia – Structural abnormality such as septo-optic dysplasia – GHRH deficiency
Acquired	– Central nervous system tumours such as craniopharyngiomas or optic gliomas – Cranial irradiation or total body irradiation – Chemotherapy – Langerhans cell histiocytosis – Traumatic head injury – Inflammatory disease
Transient	– Hypothyroidism – Delayed puberty – Psychosocial deprivation – Prepubertal
Genetic	– GH-1 mutations – GHRH receptor mutations – Pit-1/Prop-1 mutations

2.3 Pathophysiology of GHD

The pituitary gland includes the anterior and intermediate lobes (adenohypophysis) and a posterior lobe (neurohypophysis) and produces a number of hormones, including GH. The release of GH-releasing hormone (GHRH) from the hypothalamus stimulates the release of GH, and somatostatin inhibits the release of GH.

Growth hormone (GH) is secreted from the pituitary gland in a pulsatile fashion, with an increase in the frequency and amplitude of pulses at night (See Fig. 2.1) (Brook et al. 2008).

Its secretion is controlled by the hypothalamus through an interaction between releasing hormones (GHRH and ghrelin) and the inhibitory hormone somatostatin. It binds to receptors and activates the production of insulin-like growth factor 1 (IGF-1). This in turn mediates the various growth-promoting actions of GH.

Concentrations of IGF-1 correlate well with those of GH, but, low IGF-1 levels may also be observed in many conditions (hypothyroidism, malnutrition, poorly controlled diabetes) and chronic disease.

The vascular network of the hypothalamus and pituitary and the structure of the pituitary stalk make them susceptible to the effects of trauma or any other insult to the hypothalamic-pituitary region. Tumours in the hypothalamic-pituitary area may cause endocrine disturbance, either directly or secondary to treatment (surgery,

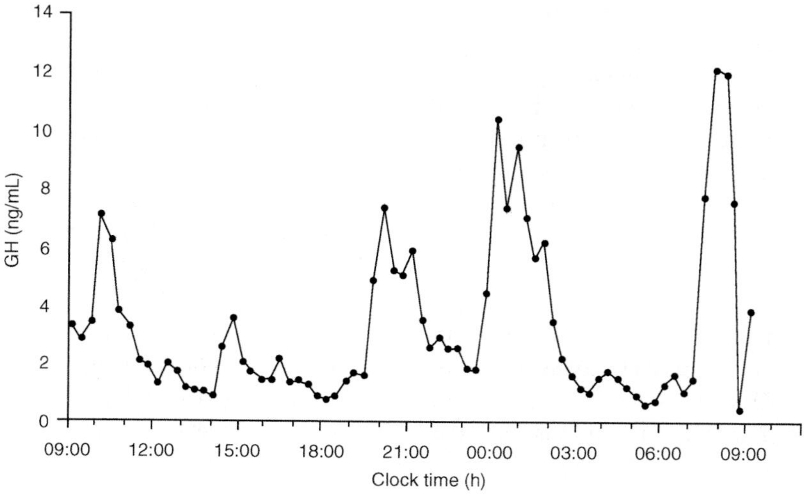

Fig. 2.1 Growth hormone pulsatile secretion (Brook et al. 2008)

radiotherapy), and early signs of endocrine dysfunction or GHD can be seen if there is growth failure.

Therefore, GHD can be classified into *congenital or genetically associated* familial conditions or may be *acquired* due to an insult or injury.

It may be an *isolated deficiency*, or part of a more complex condition of *multiple pituitary hormone deficiencies*.

The single most important clinical indicator of GHD is growth failure. Multiple pituitary deficiencies (MPHD or pan-hypopituitarism) tend to be identified earlier in life, especially if hypoglycaemia is present, but in some cases of congenital isolated GHD, the growth failure may not be established until later in childhood.

Most commonly, patients with IGHD present in late infancy or early childhood, typically with a low growth velocity and short stature. Most cases are idiopathic in origin (See case study 1 in Box 2.1).

Box 2.1 Case Study 1

A young male presents at the age of 4.3 years with a history of slow growth since the age of 2 years. Born at 42 weeks gestation at a birth weight of 3700 g, he had the cord around his neck, but no other neonatal issues. It was noted that he had had an undescended testis, and an inguinal hernia, but the rest of his development was normal.

At presentation parents' height was obtained with mum being 168.4 cm (72 centile) and dad measuring 181 cm (78th centile). This gave him a mid-parental height (MPH) of 181.2 cm (approximately 73rd centile).

On examination, it was noted that he was a small, healthy, non-dysmorphic, proportionate male with a height of 97.0 cm (fourth percentile) and a weight of 14.6 kg (10th percentile) (See Fig. 2.2). He had 2 ml testes, now descended, and normal genitalia. Neurological and thyroid examination were normal, and no other body system abnormalities were detected on examination.

Baseline investigations included FBC, ESR, biochemistry—all normal, a coeliac screen which was negative, TSH 2.3 mIU/l (0.4–5), FT4: 14.6 pmol/l (10–20), IGF-1: 1.5 nmol/l (6–25), prolactin normal. Parents were provided with information regarding GH stimulation tests and had the opportunity to ask questions before proceeding with the glucagon/arginine stimulation test. GH peaks to both stimulation tests showed a blunted response of 3.9 and 4.1 mIU/l (N > 20). An appropriate cortisol peak of 621 nmol/l (>500) was obtained. Bone age was delayed, being 3.5 years at a chronological age of 4.5 years.

A diagnosis of isolated GH deficiency was declared and treatment with GH commenced at a dose of 4.5–6 mg/m^2/week. This dose was reviewed 6 monthly (as per Australian guidelines) and adjusted according to increasing body surface area (BSA).

Long-term progress has shown that no other pituitary deficiencies have evolved. At age 12.9 years, he had 4 ml testes and by 14.1 years has 8 ml testes, PH3, G3, and will continue on GH therapy until he reaches a bone age of 15.5 years or his growth has slowed down to be <2 cms/year.

This will indicate that he has completed approximately 97% of his childhood growth.

Key points to consider when assessing a child with short stature include considering a child's height and EMH in the family context. Any child tracking below, or with EMH below target height range, warrants investigation. Evaluating growth velocity is a valuable indicator and doesn't even require plotting on a growth velocity chart, as a falling height percentile or SD is the same.

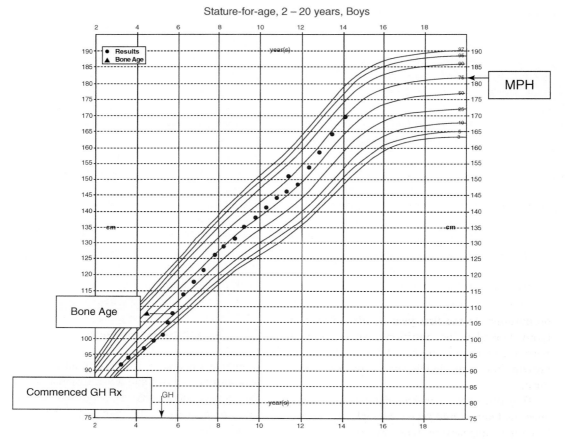

Stature-for-age, 2 – 20 years, Boys

Fig. 2.2 Case study growth chart

Untreated, children with GHD will be short and have delayed puberty, decreased pubertal growth spurt, and a final height standard deviation score (SDS) of −4 to −6, much lower than the general population (Ranke et al. 1997; Wit et al. 1996)

2.3.1 Signs and Symptoms

Hypopituitarism or multiple pituitary insufficiencies can cause a range of symptoms. Abnormalities in the development of the hypothalamus/pituitary access mean that presentation in the neonatal or early infancy period is common.

- Hypoglycaemia
- Prolonged jaundice
- Micro phallus (in boys)
- Impaired vision

- Facial or midline defects such as cleft lip or palate or single central incisor
- Defects in genes associated with the development and function of the pituitary gland can also lead to a diagnosis of isolated GHD (Alatzoglou et al. 2014).

These signs are more common in children with multiple pituitary hormone deficiencies diagnosed in the neonatal period, but may be present as isolated GHD with other deficiencies evolving over time. Recent data suggest that childhood IGHD may have a wider impact on the health and neurodevelopment of children, but it is yet unknown to what extent treatment with recombinant human growth hormone can reverse this effect (Rosenfeld et al. 1995)

Acquired GHD can be due to a variety of causes including tumours in the hypothalamic-pituitary region. These may be benign or malignant, cystic or solid, and may present as a craniopharyngioma, germinoma, or teratoma. GHD may arise due to the tumour, as a result of surgery, or, more commonly, after radiotherapy. If cranial irradiation of the pituitary gland has been indicated for a condition such as leukaemia, medulloblastoma, glioma/astrocytoma, or rhabdomyosarcoma, this can also result in impaired function of growth hormone and other hormones further along in life (See Chaps. 58 and 59).

Whatever the cause of GHD, abnormalities in the growth pattern should be investigated.

2.4 Clinical Characteristics

Children with GHD are small compared to other children of their age but they will have normal proportions. In the first year of life, growth is more dependent on nutrition than on growth hormone secretion, and may be normal, even if growth hormone deficiency is present from birth.

They often have a characteristic facial appearance including, mid-facial hypoplasia, classic "cherubic" appearance, with chubby cheeks and increased truncal adiposity with dimpling of fat. Delayed dentition, single central incisor, and frontal bossing may also be present. Both puberty and bone age may be delayed.

It is worth noting that the condition is highly variable in its clinical presentation so evaluation in reference to other family members, including siblings should also be included.

In acquired GHD, there can be a variety of presentations. Growth failure or a decline in height velocity is sometimes only noticed when shoe or clothing size does not increase over a period of time. Increasing lethargy, vomiting, visual impairment, or photophobia may all be reasons for initial presentation. Continuing visual impairment (of varying severity) can often be seen in patients after the removal of a suprasellar tumour (e.g. craniopharyngioma or optic glioma).

Any child with a history of cranial irradiation, with decelerating growth, even if the height is within the normal range, should be evaluated (Urquhart and Collin 2016) (See Chap. 58).

2.4.1 Clinical Investigations

Any child with severe short stature (3 standard deviation scores [SDS] below mean for population) should be referred to an endocrinologist for evaluation to establish a cause.

The diagnosis of GHD is a stepped process. It is based on a combination of auxological data, the clinical phenotype, dynamic GH testing (See Chap. 64), insulin-like growth factor 1 (IGF-1) and IGF binding protein 3 (IGFBP3) levels, bone age X-ray, and other radiological findings including an MRI of the hypothalamic-pituitary area.

2.4.2 Bone Age Assessment

The bone age is assessed by taking an X-ray of the non-dominant hand and wrist. Comparison is made to a photographic standardised set of X-rays for a child of the same age using the Greulich and Pyle, or Tanner-Whitehouse methods.

This provides an estimation of the skeletal maturation of the bones (Greulich and Pyle 1959; Tanner et al. 2001; Satoh 2015).

A bone age assessment (See Fig. 2.3) can help determine the amount of growth left and give an estimation of what final height will be achieved.

In girls, the epiphyses usually close around the age of 13.5 years, whereas in boys their epiphyses close around the age of 15.5 years. The further behind the bone age is delayed behind the chronological age, the longer the growing period. As long as the growth plates remain open, there is potential for continued growth. Once the bones reach the ages noted above, most of a child's growth is complete.

A thorough medical history should be taken and physical examination done to assess if there is any other cause for growth failure. See Table 2.3 for the diagnostic approach to short stature (Savage et al. 2016)

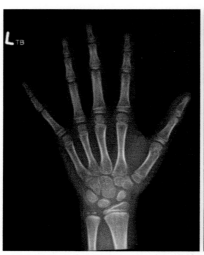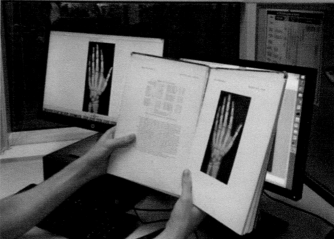

Fig. 2.3 Bone age assessment—Photo from authors collection

Table 2.3 Diagnostic approach to short stature

Take a full history:
- Birth history including weight length gestation
- Heights of parents, siblings, and any other relevant family members
- Parental consanguinity?
- Origin of short stature, nutrition, psychological disturbance
- Appetite, gastrointestinal symptoms, stool frequency/features, abdominal pain, mouth ulcers
- Hypoglycaemia, chronic infections
- Respiratory symptoms, urological symptoms
- Motor skills, intellectual development, milestones, school performance, learning difficulties
- Headache, visual disturbances

Examine the patient standing in front of you:
- Look directly face to face, and look at the head, limbs, hands, fingers, and toes.
- Full systemic examination: Neurological, musculoskeletal, abdominal, respiratory, cardiac, dermatology, and pubertal examination
- Exclude any dysmorphic features
  Dysmorphic features are a difference of body structure. They can be an isolated finding in an otherwise normal individual or can be related to a congenital disorder, genetic syndrome, or birth defect
- General baseline investigations
- Endocrine-specific investigations

Family history should be taken to determine if there is any heritable condition or any other systemic concern. Parental heights should be plotted on the growth chart to determine the mid-parental height (MPH) (or target height) and establish if the child's growth is out of keeping with other family member's stature.

Pituitary hormone deficiencies can evolve with time, so regular monitoring of clinical as well as biochemical investigations is considered good practice.

Height more than 2 SDs below the mean and a growth velocity over 1 year of more than 1 SDs below the mean should be investigated.

A decreasing height velocity in the absence of short stature should also be evaluated if:

- There is a decrease in the height SDS of more than 0.5 SDS over 1 year in children over 2 years,
- There is a decrease in height velocity of more than 1 SDS over the year in children aged over 2 years,
- The height SDS is more than 1.5 SDS below target height SDS,
  The height velocity is >2 SDS below the mean over 1 year or more than 1.5 SDS over a 2-year period. All of these variations should be evaluated when assessing a child's growth pattern (Growth Hormone Research Society 2000; Cook et al. 2009).

2.5 Investigations and Diagnosis

Baseline investigations will help determine the likelihood of GHD which can effectively be excluded in children with a normal bone age and height velocity.

Baseline investigations should include (Cook et al. 2009):

- A full blood count
- Blood chemistry, including thyroid stimulating hormone and free thyroxine level
- Coeliac screen and IgA (Immunoglobulin A) levels
- 25-OH Vitamin D level
- Karyotype in all girls and boys with dysmorphism
- IGF-1

More detailed laboratory evaluation for causes of growth failure may be carried out by a specialist once the initial evaluation is complete. IGF binding protein, hormones to evaluate puberty including luteinising hormone, follicle stimulating hormone, oestradiol, testosterone, and prolactin levels if concerned about pubertal delay should all be measured. Molecular testing or comparative genomic microarray for various genetic conditions may be considered.

GH stimulation testing should be considered if the clinical criteria is insufficient to make the diagnosis of GHD (Chesover and Dattani 2016). Those with a known pituitary abnormality or deficiency of at least one other pituitary hormone, and with obvious growth failure, may not need testing. If there is enough information to determine the cause of growth failure, provocative testing for GHD may not be required (Grimberg et al. 2016).

The most common test to assess GHD is a dynamic GH stimulation test (See Chap. 15). As GH is produced in a pulsatile fashion, it is able to be stimulated to assess pituitary function. A variety of tests are available using pharmacological stimuli and two stimuli are best used to capture the peak levels of GH produced. Provocative agents such as insulin, glucagon, arginine, and clonidine can all be used to assess GH levels. Various cut-off levels have been used, but GHD is generally defined as a value of <10 μg/L (or 3 ng/mL) on two occasions (Butler and Kirk 2011).

Testing should be done after an overnight fast, and in older children (girls>10 years and boys >11 years) is often done after priming with sex steroids for a few days prior to testing. This is done to lessen the chance of a false diagnosis, but there is still some discussion as to whether this is necessary and so is not mandatory (Chesover and Dattani 2016; Rosenbloom 2011).

Testing should be in a recognised testing facility by trained nurses due to the risk of hypoglycaemia associated with many of the stimulation tests.

Finally, an MRI of the brain/pituitary gland will establish if there are any midline defects, structural abnormalities, or evidence of a tumour or cystic mass.

2.6   Treatment

Children with GHD are unlikely to reach their adult potential without treatment. Recombinant human growth hormone is the only treatment that can improve final height but can only influence the active growth phase whilst the bone epiphyses remain open.

In many countries, GH treatment is commonly approved for those not only with GHD but other conditions of short stature as well, such as:

- TS—Turner syndrome
- SGA—Small for gestational age
- PWS—Prader-Willi syndrome
- CRI—Chronic renal insufficiency
- SHOX—Short stature homeobox-containing gene deficiency disorder
- AGHD—Adult growth hormone deficiency
- ISS—Idiopathic short stature (Raine et al. 2011)

More recently, GH has become available in some countries for use in adults with established GHD.

Treatment involves daily subcutaneous injections of recombinant human growth hormone (rhGH), also known as somatropin. Prior to 1985 hGH (human growth hormone) was only used in those with severe GHD, but was withdrawn when concerns regarding its association with Creutzfeldt-Jakob disease (CJD) arose (Buchanan et al. 1991; Boyd et al. 2010).

Treatment today uses a variety of recombinant human growth hormone products. Some products are a liquid formulation, whilst others require powder and diluent to be mixed to maintain product stability. Doses are based on either patient's weight or body surface area depending on which country they reside in, and the clinical indication they are being prescribed for. There are a number of different devices designed for giving injections, with some that can actually hide the needle tip, but as the needles used are small, they are in most cases well tolerated. Each company has a device designed specifically for their product, so they are not interchangeable.

Subcutaneous injections are given daily usually in the evening prior to bed as GH is released in pulses during the night (See Fig. 2.1) and at a similar time each day where possible. Arms, legs, abdomen, and buttocks are used as injection sites, and the 4–6 mm needles used can usually be accommodated in most of these spots.

Current practice is to use each area for approximately one week, rotating on a regular cycle.

Families, parents, and older children are instructed on injection technique at the time GH injections are commenced, but regular review of technique should be encouraged to uncover any problems parents may be having that may impact on compliance.

Adolescents giving their own injections should *always* be supervised by a parent.

Assessment of the families understanding of *why* the treatment is being given should be part of the ongoing review at appointments.

It is sometimes worthwhile reminding families that if injections are regularly missed the benefits of treatment may be compromised.

Side effects with rhGH are uncommon but should be clearly explained at the time of commencement of injections. Usually, rhGH is safe and well tolerated (Quigley et al. 2005; Quigley et al. 2017; Carel et al. 2012). Minor adverse effects such as bruising at injection sites usually diminish once treatment is established and parents become more confident at injecting their child.

Occasionally, in the early stages of treatment some children may retain excess fluid and salt,

causing headaches with some blurring of vision (benign intracranial hypertension). It is not commonly seen and usually disappears when the GH is ceased for a few days, and reintroduced at a lower dose, gradually increasing over time. If it does occur, referral to an ophthalmologist should be made for ongoing assessment in the first few months of treatment.

Slipped capital femoral epiphysis (SCFE) has also been reported to be slightly more common in children receiving GH treatment (Rappaport and Fife 1985). This may cause pain in the hip and knee joints and appears to mostly occur in those with other risk factors such as obesity, trauma, other endocrine conditions, or those who have had previous radiation therapy, or very rapid growth.

Scoliosis has also been observed in some children treated (Clayton and Cowell 2000), but is more the result of an increase in height velocity unmasking the tendency to a curved spine, than the GH itself.

Depending on family history, there may be an increased risk of developing type 2 diabetes mellitus, but as the doses of GH prescribed are mostly physiological the risk is relatively low.

Markedly elevated IGF-1 concentrations have been associated with colon, breast, and prostatic cancer: However, there is no evidence to suggest an increased risk of malignancies using the current dosage recommendations for rhGH. In general, GH should not be given with an active malignant condition. The absence of tumour growth or recurrence should be documented for 12 months before commencing treatment. The long-term safety of GH treatment is, however, uncertain.

The most common questions asked by patients and parents alike when starting treatment is, how much will I grow, and how long will I need to take GH for?

Rapid short-term growth is usually followed by normalisation of long-term growth.

Treatment should be continued until final height or epiphyseal closure is achieved (Clayton et al. 2005). For girls this is when the bone age is around 13.5 years and for boys around 15.5 years.

A good predictor of response to treatment is the height gain attained in the first year of treatment. Other factors that can impact on the response to treatment include age and height at the start of treatment, duration of treatment, and, in patients with isolated GHD, the pre-pubertal growth available when receiving treatment.

Long-term monitoring of treatment is essential and should include:

- Regular measurements, plotted on an age- and sex-appropriate growth chart.

On average, puberty contributes 20–25 cm of height in females and 25–30 cm in males, and this is dependent on adequate GH and insulin-like growth factor 1 (IGF-1) concentrations.

- Frequency of monitoring patients with an acquired cause of GHD (e.g. tumours, radiation) will depend on the individual condition.
- All patients on GH should continue receiving treatment until final height or epiphyseal closure is achieved.
- Prior to transition to an adult endocrinologist, reassessment of IGF-1 levels and possibly of GH levels should be undertaken.
- If after ceasing treatment the IGF-1 level remains in the normal range, GH stimulation testing should be undertaken to establish if the young persons' GH levels have normalised or remain low.

This will assist in determining whether after completion of growth and puberty patients with idiopathic isolated GHD are at risk of ongoing GHD and will ascertain the need for adult GH replacement (See Chap. 6).

In many patients (25–75%), when testing is repeated, the GH response is in the normal range (Cook et al. 2009). The reason for this reversal of GHD is unclear. Pituitary hormone deficiencies can evolve with time, so regular monitoring, both clinically and with regular biochemical investigations, is recommended.

2.6.1 Compliance and Growth Hormone Device Choice

Growth hormone treatment involves a daily injection. For some families, the thought of injecting their child on a daily basis is confronting, and the emotional factors and anxiety around administration can overwhelm them (or their child). There are a number of devices for giving GH available but nearly all require a needle to be inserted into the subcutaneous fat. Many devices can hide the site of the actual needle if required, and for most children the procedure becomes easier over time. In some countries, allowing families some choice in the decision-making around which device to use, compliance can be shown to be improved. Compliance often waivers especially in the adolescent years, as growth is slow, an immediate response cannot be seen, and the idea of having to remember to give an injection each night does not always sit easily in an adolescents life! Feedback regarding the devices assists in compliance as the family or young person feels they have contributed to their treatment in some way. This along with ongoing positive support from nursing staff assists in improving the patient experience (Gau and Takasawa 2017).

2.7 Nursing Considerations

When evaluating a child with short stature, it is important to think about the following questions. Although the causes and clinical presentation of short stature vary by age group, the same questions are relevant for children of any age:

- How short is the child?
- Is the child's height velocity (HV) impaired?
- Are they in keeping with their family pattern?
- What is the child's likely adult height?

By using these questions as a baseline for assessment, the health care professional can determine if there is a growth problem and evaluate how concerned are they about their height.

When assessing a child's growth, there are four main aims:

- To determine if the growth pattern is normal or as expected for the child's family background.
- To attempt to predict future growth and final adult height.
- To determine if there are any modifiable medical or other issues that will improve growth.
- To consider if there are any specific treatments that are possible and appropriate to improve growth.

The most important assessment of growth is reliable, reproducible, and regular measurements, done at 3–6 monthly intervals, and plotted on an appropriate growth chart.

Children under the age of 2 years should have their length measured, and between the ages of 2–3 years all children should be assessed in a lying and standing position, as this is the age that they are usually least cooperative.

This will provide the most accurate assessment, as long as that the same piece of equipment is used, it is calibrated regularly, the same the observer takes the measurement, and the growth is plotted on the same growth percentile chart, and once plotted the growth velocity can be calculated.

Growth velocity is one of the most useful parameters when assessing growth as it determines the change in height over time. It should be calculated over *at least* a 6-month period as any less can lead to inaccuracy or misleading results. It is calculated as the difference in height on two different occasions annualised over 1 year and is age and pubertal status dependent.

Height that plots along a given percentile on the growth chart reflects normal growth velocity. Crossing percentiles or a decreasing velocity reflects poor growth velocity.

Plotting the growth is helpful in establishing if a child is just short (compared to his peers) but growing at a consistent rate, or if are they growing at a slower rate than their peers over time.

Any child with a growth velocity under the third centile at any time should have further evaluation no matter where they sit on the growth chart.

One of the most important things to remember however is that all children should be treated according to their **AGE** and **NOT** their **SIZE**. It is very common when assessing a child who may look younger and be much smaller than their peers, to speak down to them, or treat them inappropriately for their age, and there is nothing worse for a child. Often on further questioning, or once a relationship begins to develop, you may be able to determine if they are being bullied at school or in the playground, and if this is of concern to them. The issues that children with endocrine conditions may encounter, particularly if they do not fit into the social and emotional norms of their peers, can add to the distress of "being different" and isolate them even further. Children who are shorter than most of their peers may find themselves being excluded from sporting teams or even just play dates as younger children. Some may find that they don't have the energy to keep up with their friends particularly if they are severely growth hormone deficient, making interaction even more difficult. Online or cyber bullying and social media has created a whole new set of issues for those with body image and self-esteem concerns (Cohen and Dwyer 2018). A full social history should always be undertaken in all patients, particularly those who present with poor weight gain and failure to thrive.

If growth hormone production is being assessed using a stimulation test, it is important that both the family and the child have an understanding of what the testing involves and what to expect both during and after the evaluation.

Information sheets regarding the tests should be provided (see Appendix), and the opportunity to ask questions prior to testing, must be considered.

The goal of growth hormone (GH) treatment should be to restore hormone levels as close to healthy levels as possible and allow the child to reach their target adult height potential.

During the initial assessment and monitoring phase, it is important to establish a good relationship with the child and family. This allows time for consideration of the likelihood of managing daily GH injections when started on treatment, ongoing compliance with treatment, and also gives the opportunity to evaluate if height is of concern to them as an individual, or if it is more of a parental concern.

Results of any tests done should be clearly explained in language that the family will understand to ensure they have a good comprehension of why GH is required.

Once treatment is approved, the family and child should be educated in the day-to-day management of injections, the storage of medication and general information about expectations of treatment, and the importance of compliance.

2.7.1 Emotional and Social Elements

It is important to provide emotional support for the child with GH deficiency and to emphasise the child's many good and valuable characteristics, so that the child's stature does not limit his opportunities. Society (unfortunately) still places an emphasis on height, and children who are short for their age can initially have problems because friends and teachers treat them as though they are *younger* rather than just *smaller*. Parental expectations are often decreased as they feel their child is unable to do the same tasks as other children their age, and in turn children may then not act their age because it is not expected of them. Schools are sometimes unaware of the problems that children who are very small for their age have to deal with such as practical difficulties of being unable to reach a peg or desk or sit on the toilet. Teasing and/or being called names such as "shorty" or "shrimp" or being carried around the playground because they are "cute and doll like" is not helpful in allowing the child to develop to their full potential. Sometimes a frank and open discussion with teachers and classmates may help alleviate some of the problems. Positive role modelling by parents is essential and as with all parenting issues, there must be consistency. Parents must agree on a unified approach to handling any problems. Discussing and role playing

hypothetical situations and encouraging practice of these role plays can help children anticipate situations that may develop.

Comments when out shopping or on the sporting field cannot be monitored, but the child can work to control their responses. A "toolkit" of responses is one of the best support mechanisms that can be given to parents and children, and the nurse can suggest that families work with their child to practise responses. The best responses are ones that are polite yet assertive, never rude, easy to remember (even in situations of high anxiety), and comfortable for a child to use. Work with the child and family to come up with a short list of responses that he or she can use in social situations when comments are made about stature.

When commencing GH treatment, it is important that the child and family have realistic expectations. It is important to emphasise that growth takes time and that they are not going to grow overnight. Ongoing reassurance may be needed when the child is not growing as expected. Once there has been an initial response to treatment the possible benefit may include a general increased self-esteem and overall happiness that is gained with the increase in height.

2.8 Primary IGF-1 Deficiency/ Growth Hormone Insensitivity Syndrome

Growth hormone insensitivity syndrome (GHIS) is a rare condition (<1:100,000) whereby the action of growth hormone (GH) is either absent or reduced resulting in extreme short stature (Backeljauw and Underwood 2001).

2.9 Pathophysiology

Childhood growth is regulated via the GH/insulin-like growth factor 1 (IGF-1) axis. Primary insulin-like growth factor 1 (IGF-1) deficiency is characterised by an inadequate production of IGF-1, despite sufficient secretion of growth hormone (Mushtaq 2015). Pituitary-

Fig. 2.4 GH-IGF-1 Axis. Courtesy of Professor Martin Savage, Dr. Helen Storr and Dr. Sumana Chatterjee, 2018

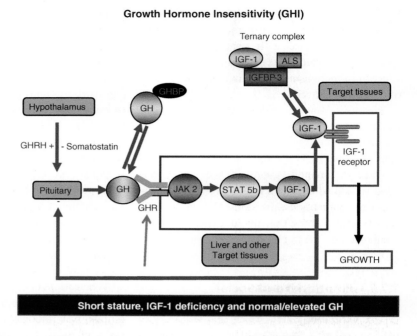

derived GH stimulates both the liver production of IGF-1 and augments the actions of locally produced IGF-1, which result in longitudinal growth. Binding of the GH to its receptor results in activation of downstream signalling molecules which ultimately lead to IGF-1 production. Thus, abnormalities along this signalling cascade can cause GH insensitivity. These may include defects in the GH receptor which inhibit GH binding, post-receptor signalling defects such as signal transducer activator of transcription (STAT)-5b or primary defects of IGF-1 synthesis (See Fig. 2.4).

2.10 Clinical Characteristics

The clinical phenotype of primary GH insensitivity in its classic form is identical to severe GH deficiency and was first described by Laron and colleagues in 1966 (Laron 1966). The clinical characteristics include severe post-natal growth failure, mid-facial hypoplasia, adiposity, and hypoglycaemia. It is therefore important to exclude growth hormone deficiency as a cause for these features. Other features associated with the condition may include reduced muscle strength, dental abnormalities including delayed eruption of teeth and reduced number of teeth, distinctive facial features (protruding forehead, a sunken bridge of the nose, and blue sclera) and thin, fragile hair; however, it should be noted that the phenotype can vary even within the same family. Figures 2.5 and 2.6 demonstrate a child with Laron syndrome.

Abnormalities further downstream the GH/IGF-1 axis such as with (STAT)-5b signalling are associated with immune deficiency, whereas IGF-1 mutations have severe intrauterine growth retardation and intellectual delay. The biochemistry shows elevated serum concentrations of GH with low IGF-1 levels due to an abnormal GH receptor.

Recombinant IGF-1 (rhIGF-1) is licenced for use in the United Kingdom (UK), the European Union (EU), the United States (USA), and Canada for children with severe primary IGF-1 deficiency (SPIGFD). This is defined in children as a height less than −3 SDS, low IGF-1 levels (<2.5th percentile for age and gender), and normal GH levels. Secondary forms of IGF-1 deficiency such as malnutrition, hypothyroidism, and use of pharmacological doses of glucocorticoids need to be excluded

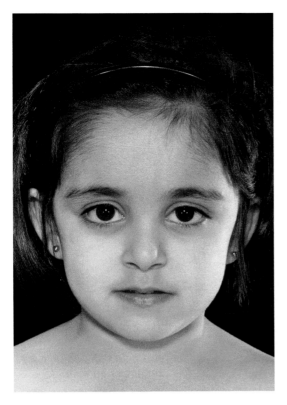

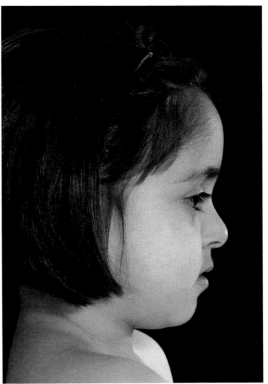

Fig. 2.5 Photo of child with Laron Syndrome (front view); note the eyes and orbits characteristic in patients with Laron Syndrome. (Written consent was obtained from the child's parents to use her photo in the book)

Fig. 2.6 Photo of child with Laron Syndrome (side view); note the eyes and orbits characteristic in patients with Laron Syndrome. (Written consent was obtained from the child's parents to use her photo in the book)

(Grimberg et al. 2016; Mushtaq 2015). It should be borne in mind that although the term GHIS and SPIGFD may be used interchangeably they are distinct entities as the classical Laron's phenotype is not required for the licenced indications.

2.11   Diagnosis

The UK has guidelines formulated by an IGF-1 user's group and endorsed by the British Society for Paediatric Endocrinology and Diabetes (Mushtaq 2015). These state that diagnosis of primary IGF-1 deficiency does not necessarily require either a GH stimulation test or IGF-1 generation test when the presentation is classical. It is recommended that these children have genetic analysis of the growth hormone receptor (GHR)

for understanding the condition and to confirm the clinical diagnosis. Those children who do not have the classical features but have abnormal auxology and features of growth failure may need detailed evaluation which should include assessment of the GH-IGF-1 axis. This evaluation should include a GH stimulation test (See Chap. 15).

The guidelines also state that whilst an IGF-1 generation test may also be included in the evaluation, the clinical value of the test in reaching a diagnosis of SPIGFD is unclear. The protocol for the IGF-1 generation test is illustrated in Box 2.2 below (Butler and Kirk 2011) (See Chap. 15).

It is worth noting that some children with classical SPIGFD may present late as the extreme short stature may have previously been diagnosed as failure to thrive or familial short stature.

Box 2.2 Protocol for the IGF-1 Generation Test

Dose:

– 0.033 mg/kg growth hormone daily × 4

Procedure:

– Day 1—Blood sample for IGF-1 (± IGFBP-3) before first injection of GH
  • GH injection
– Day 2—GH injection
– Day 3—GH injection
– Day 4—GH injection
– Day 5—Blood sample for IGF-1 (± IGFBP-3) 12 h after the fourth injection of GH

Table 2.4 Baseline assessment (Storr 2015)

Baseline Assessment	Standard	Optional
Enter patient on registry	+	
Physical examination: height, weight, sitting height, pubertal stage, blood pressure, fundoscopy, tonsils	+	
Echocardiography	+	
Bone age	+	
Facial photograph (frontal and lateral)	+	
Dietary advice	+	
First injection as an in-patient		+
Fasting cholesterol (HDL, LDL, and total triglycerides)		+
DXA—whole body and lumbar spine		+
Arrange homecare and nurse support		+

BSPED Guidelines (2015) (Cohen et al. 2008).

2.12 Treatment

Once a diagnosis has been determined the treatment options can then be discussed with the family. The current recommended treatment for SPIGFD in the EU, the UK, the USA and Canada is twice daily injections with recombinant IGF-1 (rhIGF-1) therapy (Grimberg et al. 2016; Mushtaq 2015), and the treatment objective is the long-term improvement of adult height.

2.12.1 Initiating Therapy

Both the UK and US and Canada guidelines advocate these patients be managed by a paediatric endocrinologist with experience of managing children with complex growth disorders. Table 2.4 details baseline procedures and checks both standard and optional that should be considered prior to commencing treatment as advised by the IGF-1 users group in the UK.

The UK guidelines recommend a short admission may be needed, particularly in younger children due to the potential risk of hypoglycaemia following the injection. This may not always be possible but the Paediatric Endocrine Nurse Specialist (PENS) plays a vital role in supporting the family at this time to ensure safe initiation of therapy whether in the hospital setting or at home.

The starting dose of rhIGF-1 as recommended by the manufacturer should be 40 µg/kg (micrograms per kilogram) twice daily. The dose should then be increased at regular intervals with the aim of reaching a maintenance dose of 120 µg/kg twice daily approximately three months after starting treatment (Pharmaceuticals I 2007).

As with GH injections, the family are advised to rotate the injection sites with each injection to prevent lipohypotrophy.

One of the most common side effects of the medication is hypoglycaemia. It is therefore advised that the injection should be given after a meal or snack and if the child has not eaten then the dose should be omitted. An important part of the PENS role is to ensure the family are educated to recognise the signs, symptoms, and treatment of hypoglycaemia.

It is also recommended that with initiation of treatment the capillary blood glucose (CBG) should be measured both prior to the injection and post injection. Subsequently, the family is advised to check pre- and post-dose CBG following any dose increase for at least two days and inform the PENS of any problems. Hypoglycaemia is defined in the UK guidelines as a CBG of less than 3.5 mmol/L (Butler and Kirk 2011).

All patients in the UK are asked to give consent for a web-based surveillance registry.

2.12.2 Maintenance of Therapy

Once the young person has been established on treatment it is important they are monitored at regular intervals. Clinic visits are recommended 3–4 monthly and every patient should have an annual review. Table 2.5 details procedures and checks both standard and optional that should be

Table 2.5 Maintenance of therapy (Storr 2015)

Assessment	Every clinic visit	Annually
Enter data on registry	+	
Physical examination: height, weight, sitting height, pubertal stage, blood pressure, fundoscopy, tonsils	+	
Echocardiography		+
Bone age		+
Facial photograph (frontal and lateral)		+
Examination of injection sites		+
DXA—whole body and lumbar spine[a]		+
Audiology[a]		+

BSPED Guidelines (2015) (Cohen et al. 2008).
[a]These investigations are not considered to be standard but may provide objective data on changes in hearing and body composition.

considered during treatment as advised by the IGF-1 users group in the UK.

Each clinic visit should consist of auxology, discussion regarding injections and examination of injection sites. Targeted adverse events should also be discussed at each visit and any positive clinical history may require more detailed assessment, e.g. history of sleep disordered breathing may require oximetry/sleep studies and referral to ear, nose, and throat (ENT) services. See Table 2.6 (Storr 2015) for some of the more common adverse events as per the UK guidelines.

As previously discussed, hypoglycaemia is the most common side effect of treatment. It is therefore important to continue to discuss this at clinic visits and check the families understanding of signs, symptoms, and treatment of hypoglycaemia.

Treatment should be reconsidered if the patient has an increase in height velocity of less than 30% of baseline or a change in height SDS score of <0.3 over a 12-month period although there should be documented good compliance over this time period.

UK guidelines state treatment with a Gonadotrophin-releasing hormone (*GnRH*) agonist may be indicated in pubertal children who are extremely short and have not received IGF-1 for a sufficiently long period (Mushtaq 2015).

Table 2.6 Targeted adverse events

Potential adverse event	Monitoring	Actions
Hypoglycaemia	Monitor BG	Give injections after food
Lymphoid hyperplasia	Check at clinic visits for snoring, apnoea	Refer to ENT
Intracranial hypertension	Headaches, visual disturbance, papilloedema.	Discontinue treatment. Recommence once resolved at low dose and gradually increase
Slipped capital femoral epiphysis(SCFE)/scoliosis	Physical examination. Pain/limp	Refer to orthopaedics
Coarsening of facies	Physical examination. Photographs	Resolves once treatment discontinued at end of growth
Allergic reaction	Check injection sites for hypersensitivity, urticaria, pruritus, and erythema	Discontinue treatment. Consider giving anti-histamines. Allergy specialist
Hypoacusis (Hearing loss)	Check at clinic visits	Send to audiology for hearing test
Cardiac hypertrophy	Echocardiography	Refer to cardiology. Consider stopping treatment

2.13   The Multidisciplinary Team (MDT)

Although these children are primarily managed by a Paediatric Endocrinologist and PENS, both their extreme short stature and treatment requiring twice daily injections are challenging for these families. Therefore, the involvement of other services and local teams is vital to their overall well-being.

2.13.1 Psychology

As these children have extreme short stature, they may benefit from input from psychology services. Although the aim of treatment is to improve their adult height, they may still remain below the normal centiles once the treatment has completed, and some of these young people will remain significantly smaller than their peers. Psychology may therefore be a useful service to help the young people discuss their feelings and adapt to the adult world.

2.13.2 School

Due to their extreme short stature, these children face a number of difficulties at school. It is important for the PENS to offer information, advice, and support both the family and school to enable the child to fully participate in school activities. As discussed earlier, issues may arise with bullying (Cohen and Dwyer 2018). Information should also include being aware of the signs and symptoms of hypoglycaemia and how to respond if the child were to become hypoglycaemic. The school nursing service should be approached to assist with supporting the child. This may also require liaison with occupational therapists to discuss any adaptations/equipment which may be needed.

2.13.3 Community/Home Support Nurses

Support nurses where available are a useful addition to the package of care for these families. In the UK, they are able to offer home visits and phone calls over the duration of the treatment. This not only supports the family thereby helping them adhere better to long-term treatment but also offers an adjunct to the service the PENS is able to provide.

2.13.4 PENS

The role of the PENS is extremely important with these children and families. They play a key role in supporting the families through diagnosis and lengthy treatment.

They can act as liaison between the different members of the MDT and are usually the main point of contact for the families.

2.14   Nursing Considerations

The PENS is likely to have been involved with the family during the monitoring and investigations of their short stature.

As with GH therapy, the rhIGF-1 injections are likely to continue for many years until final height is reached. This requires support for the families undertaking this treatment to maximise adherence in order to gain the greatest benefit.

The role of the PENS is multi-faceted and includes acting as an educator, support service, advocate, and liaison for the family throughout the period of both diagnosis and treatment.

It is important from the outset that the PENS is able to assess the family's understanding of the condition and the ability to undertake the treatment in order to individualise the care package to their needs.

Good written information is extremely important but as the family are also learning how to give injections, check CBG, and monitor their child, this needs to be discussed, demonstrated, and taught effectively.

If the child is to be admitted to start treatment, the PENS role is to ensure this is a smooth process thereby reducing the stress on the family. This offers an opportunity for the PENS to meet with the family and teach them all the practicalities around administration, storage, side effects, omitting doses and checking CBG. All the equipment the family will need to give the injections and check CBG can be available on the ward on the day of admission. The PENS can also support the family through the first few injections until they become more accustomed to the procedure. Unlike GH, there is currently no pen device for the rhIGF-1 injections; therefore, the family need to be taught how to draw up and administer the injections using needles and syringes. This can be a daunting prospect for some families. It is therefore extremely important to give the family clear instructions and the time needed for them to become confident with the technique.

This face-to-face interaction and support can be invaluable to the family whilst they are learning and can help to build a trusting relationship between the family and PENS. It is also important to give supporting literature when they are discharged home including all necessary contact details.

If the treatment is to be started at home by a homecare nursing service, it is important that there has been liaison between the homecare nurse and the PENS beforehand.

Over the course of treatment, the PENS continues to play an important role. They will see the family regularly at clinic visits and give ongoing support. Any concerns or problems they may be having can be discussed. Injection sites can be checked and ensuring continuing education and understanding regarding treatment and side effects should be a routine part of the appointment.

2.15 Patient Support Groups and Useful Websites

Patient support groups have been shown to be a highly valuable resource for patients and their families (Bartlett and Coulson 2011), not just as a clinical and supportive tool, but by also enabling empowerment and enriching the relationship between the child and family and their caregivers (van Uden-Kraan et al. 2009). The advent of social media, with websites and online support groups can add to this, although children and families are advised on which are the more useful. Box 2.3 details the American support group MAGIC: **M**ajor **A**spects of **G**rowth **I**n **C**hildren, with a description of how it as set up. Further useful websites are listed below.

Box 2.3 Patient Support Groups

The MAGIC Foundation
4200 Cantera Drive, Suite 106, Warrenville, IL 60555
    630–836-8200 / fax 630–836-8181 toll free 800–3 MAGIC 3
    www.magicfoundation.org * contactus@magicfoundation.org
    It is hard to remember days without the internet, cell phones, and costly long distance calls. I was heartbroken when my son was diagnosed with growth hormone deficiency in 1978. No way to communicate with others, no internet for information, no Facebook to network with others, just lost and alone. Ten years later, I was blessed with meeting two other mothers facing the same challenges I did. We talked about how difficult our journey was and how we could make a difference for new families entering the world of endocrine disorders. We decided to take on the challenge of a non-profit organisation and The MAGIC Foundation was established in 1989. MAGIC (**M**ajor **A**spects of **G**rowth **I**n **C**hildren) was initiated to help support families of children with "Growth" disorders but little did we know how many disorders were out there affecting a child's growth.

    Since 1989 MAGIC has grown to 11 divisions, supporting specific disorders, so parents would have the opportunity to network with others facing similar situations affecting their child. Currently, our divisions include growth hormone deficiency, panhypopituitarism, septo optic dysplasia/optic nerve hypoplasia, Russell

(continued)

Box 2.3 (continued)

Silver syndrome, small for gestational age, congenital adrenal hyperplasia, precocious puberty, McCune-Albright syndrome/fibrous dysplasia, hypophosphatasia, Cushings, and adult growth hormone deficiency. Facebook groups for all these disorders, both children and adults, are available for networking.

In 2014, MAGIC received a Congressional Resolution for "Growth Awareness Week", the third week of September each year, to increase awareness of growth in children. MAGIC has actively participated in summits and roundtables with Endocrine Societies and Pharmaceutical Companies to provide input to the needs and support of affected families, including educational materials that would be beneficial to those families.

Areas of support have grown over the years to include:

- Quarterly Newsletters (children and adult).
- Annual Educational Convention (attendance approx. 1000+ annually) with over 30 medical professionals providing educational segments.
- 30+ Facebook Accounts
- Friday Email (updating families on research and educational articles).
- Division Consultants for each Division (parent of affected child or affected adult).
- Insurance Appeal Program (provide external appeals when denied therapy).
- International Division, "ICOSEP" (a coalition of support organisations to communicate and network worldwide).

- Web Site—www.magicfoundation.org (all educational brochures and personal stories).
- 30+ Educational Brochures (free to families, medical professionals, and health care professionals, written by medical professionals)
- Physician Referrals (both paediatric and adult endocrinologists).
- Challenge Legislative Issues/Laws affecting the health care of our families.

Annually, MAGIC continues to grow, implement new programs and support systems, continues to build awareness regarding children's growth and so much more. We continue to communicate with the medical community and all health care professionals and hope our services have provided the support and continued education families warrant. Referring families to MAGIC alleviates the feeling of being alone and connects them with others facing similar situations. We help them understand and support them from initial testing right through the years of treatment. You can help your families by simply telling them, "Contact MAGIC and you will not be alone".

Mary Andrews
CEO/Co-Founder
The MAGIC Foundation
mandrews@magicfoundation.org
cell 708-473-9596
contactus@magicfoundation.org

2.16 Useful Websites

https://apeg.org.au/patient-resources/hormones-me-booklet-series/
https://www.bsped.org.uk/clinical-resources/patient-information/patient-resources/
http://magicfoundation.org
http://pituitary.asn.au
www.childgrowthfoundation.org.uk

http://hgfound.org/
http://www.saynobullying.org/
www.noonansyndrome.org.uk
https://noonansyndrome.com.au
https://www.teamnoonan.org/#!
http://www.geneticalliance.org.au/...detail.php?Russell-Silver-Syndrome
https://magicfoundation.org/Growth-Disorders/Russell-Silver-Syndrome

https://dwarfismawarenessaustralia.com
www.lpaonline.org
www.skeletaldysplasiagroup.org.uk
www.bsped.org.uk

2.17 Conclusions

Short stature is a common presenting problem to a general practitioner, and is one of the most common reasons a child is seen in a paediatric endocrine clinic (Davies 2017). Any child presenting with a height outside of their expected potential for no known reason should be evaluated, and all girls being investigated should have a karyotype performed to assess for Turner syndrome.

Regular monitoring of growth using the same piece of equipment, the same technique, and where possible, the same observer, is essential to establish a child's growth pattern. If the growth pattern alters, or growth velocity remains low, further investigation should be undertaken by a paediatrician or endocrinologist to establish whether there is cause for concern or not. Early detection allows for maximal response if treatment is undertaken.

Treatment should always be discussed in consultation with the family as it has been shown that compliance is improved if families have some input into the decision-making. Commitment from the child / young person and family is imperative with regards to treatment compliance: treatment with GH is a once daily injection until final height is achieved, and a diagnosis of SPIGFD and treatment requires twice daily injections, both requiring long-term commitment.

Paediatric endocrine nurses occupy a unique position in the evaluation of short stature and the ongoing management of those receiving GH treatment or IGF-1 therapy. Regular review of the child's progress and ongoing support with treatment with the PENS are key to the child achieving the best possible outcomes. An important part of the PENS role is to understand both the clinical aspects of diagnosis and treatment and the effect this can have on the child and family and support them throughout this in order to achieve the best outcome.

Acknowledgments With special thanks to Mary Andrews, CEO/Co-Founder of the MAGIC Foundation, (MAGIC: **M**ajor **A**spects of **G**rowth **in** **C**hildren) www.magicfoundation.org for her contribution to this chapter with a case study and information on the Patient Advocacy Group.

Appendix: GH Stimulation Test Information Sheet

GLUCAGON/ARGININE STIMULATION TEST INFORMATION SHEET

What is this test?

This test is carried out to assess hormones that the pituitary gland produces. **Glucagon** causes a number of temporary hormonal signals resulting in the release of growth hormone from the pituitary gland and stimulation of cortisol production. These levels are then measured in a series of blood tests. **Arginine** is an amino acid which also stimulates growth hormone secretion in the hypothalamus and pituitary gland. Some older children may need to take low doses of priming hormones before the test if they have delayed puberty so that the testing is accurate; your doctor will have advised if this is needed.

When is this test?

Your child is booked to attend for a glucagon/arginine stimulation test on.

How should I prepare my child?

- Your child will need to be admitted to the hospital for the day (approximately 5 h).
- **Your child should have <u>nothing to eat or drink</u>, except water, <u>from 12 midnight the night before the test.</u>** Babies less than 12 months or children under 10 kg need to fast for 4 h, so should have an early morning feed.
- **Please call to confirm with the endocrine testing nurse, the day before the test.**
- If your child is unwell, please contact us as the test may need to be rescheduled.
- Bring a favourite toy, activity, DVD, or book on the day to keep your child occupied.
- You will be admitted by the clerk and directed to the endocrine testing area.

What happens next?

- The nurse will record your child's height, weight, temperature, pulse and blood pressure, and oxygen saturations.
- Before we insert a cannula (a small needle with a plastic tube attached) into the vein, and so that we cause as little discomfort as possible, anaesthetic cream or an ice stick can be used to anesthetise the area. We will need to take multiple blood samples during the test, and the cannula allows all the samples to be taken from the same site.
- At the beginning of the test, a blood sample is taken and then an injection of glucagon is given into the thigh muscle.
- Another blood sample is collected **one hour later, and further samples are then taken at ½ hourly intervals for another 2 h.**
- The arginine solution is then given via an intravenous drip into the cannula over 30 min.
- **Four more blood samples are then taken every 15 min once the infusion is completed.**
- Some children may feel nauseated or complain of abdominal pain during the test, but this is usually temporary. Occasionally, a child may vomit. We can give medication to ease this.
- Your child's blood glucose level is checked during the test because low values sometimes occur and may need to be treated.

And finally…. after the test?

At the end of the test your child may eat, the cannula is removed and you will be discharged home.

Results are usually available after 2 weeks, so **before leaving make sure that you have details of the follow-up appointment.** If you have any questions following the test, contact your child's doctor or endocrine clinic.

References

Alatzoglou KS, Webb EA, Le Tissier P, Dattani MT. Isolated growth hormone deficiency (GHD) in childhood and adolescence: recent advances. Endocr Rev. 2014;35(3):376–432.

Albanese A, Hamill G, Jones J, Skuse D, Matthews DR, Stanhope R. Reversibility of physiological growth hormone secretion in children with psychosocial dwarfism. Clin Endocrinol. 1994;40(5):687–92.

Backeljauw PF, Underwood LE. Therapy for 6.5 - 7.5 years with recombinant Insulin-Like Growth Factor 1 in children with growth hormone insensitivity syndrome. J Clin Endocrinol Metab. 2001;86:1504–10.

Bartlett YK, Coulson NS. An investigation into the empowerment effects of using online support groups and how this affects health professional/patient communication. Patient Educ Couns. 2011;83(1):113–9.

Boyd A, Klug GM, Schonberger LB, McGlade A, Brandel JP, Masters CL, et al. Iatrogenic Creutzfeldt-Jakob disease in Australia: time to amend infection control measures for pituitary hormone recipients? Med J Aust. 2010;193(6):366–9.

Brook CGD, Clayton PE, Brown R. Brook's clinical paediatric endocrinology. 5th ed. Oxford: Wiley Blackwell; 2008.

Buchanan CR, Preece MA, Milner RDG. Mortality, neoplasia and Creutzfeldt-Jakob disease in patients treated with human pituitary growth hormone in the United Kingdom. BMJ. 1991;302(6780):824–8.

Butler G. Indications for growth hormone therapy. Paediatr Child Health. 2007;17(9):356–60.

Butler G, Kirk J. Paediatric endocrinology and diabetes. Oxford: OUP Press; 2011.

Carel JC, Ecosse E, Landier F, Meguellati-Hakkas D, Kaguelidou F, Rey G, et al. Long-term mortality after recombinant growth hormone treatment for isolated growth hormone deficiency or childhood short stature: preliminary report of the French SAGhE study. J Clin Endocrinol Metab. 2012;97(2):416–25.

Chesover AD, Dattani MT. Evaluation of growth hormone stimulation testing in children. Clin Endocrinol. 2016;84(5):708–14.

Clayton PE, Cowell CT. Safety issues in children and adolescents during growth hormone therapy--a review. Growth Hormon IGF Res. 2000;10(6):306–17.

Clayton PE, Cuneo RC, Juul A, Monson JP, Shalet SM, Tauber M. Consensus statement on the management of the GH treated adolescent in the transition to adult care. Eur J Endocrinol. 2005;152:165–70.

Cohen SS, Dwyer A. PENS position statement on bullying prevention. J Pediatr Nurs. 2018;39:91–3.

Cohen P, Rogol AD, Deal CL, Saenger P, Reiter EO, Ross JL, et al. Consensus statement on the diagnosis and treatment of children with idiopathic short stature: a summary of the Growth Hormone Research Society, the Lawson Wilkins Pediatric Endocrine Society, and the European Society for Paediatric Endocrinology Workshop. J Clin Endocrinol Metab. 2008;93(11):4210–7.

Cook DM, Yuen KC, Biller BM, Kemp SF, Vance ML, American Association of Clinical Endocrinologists. American Association of Clinical Endocrinologists medical guidelines for clinical practice for growth hormone use in growth hormone-deficient adults and transition patients - 2009 update: executive summary of recommendations. Endocr Pract. 2009;15(6):580–6.

Davies K. Assessment of growth failure in children: MIMS for Nurses Pocket Guide. London: Haymarket Publishing; 2004.

Davies K. Care of the child and young person with endocrine problems. In: Pryce J, McAlinden O, editors. Essentials of nursing children and young people. 1st ed. London: Sage; 2017.

Gau M, Takasawa K. Initial patient choice of a growth hormone device improves child and adolescent adherence to and therapeutic effects of growth hormone replacement therapy. J Pediatr Endocrinol Metab. 2017;30(9):989–93.

Greulich WW, Pyle SI. Radiographic atlas of skeletal development of the hand and wrist. 2nd ed. Stanford: Stanford University Press; 1959.

Grimberg A, DiVall SA, Polychronakos C, Allen DB, Cohen LE, Quintos JB, et al. Guidelines for growth hormone and insulin-like growth factor-I treatment in children and adolescents: growth hormone deficiency, idiopathic short stature, and primary insulin-like growth factor-I deficiency. Horm Res Paediatr. 2016;86(6):361–97.

Growth Hormone Research Society. Consensus guidelines for the diagnosis and treatment of growth hormone (GH) deficiency in childhood and adolescence: summary statement of the GH Research Society. GH Research Society. J Clin Endocrinol Metab. 2000;85(11):3990–3.

Laron Z. Genetic pituitary dwarfism with high serum concentration of growth hormone - a new inborn error of metabolism? Isr J Med Sci. 1966;2:152–5.

Lee PA, Chernausek SD, Hokken-Koelga ACS, Czernichow P. Management of short children born small for gestational age. Pediatrics. 2003;111:1253–61.

Maghnie M, Labarta JI, Koledova E, Rohrer TR. Short Stature Diagnosis and Referral. Front Endocrinol (Lausanne). 2017;8:374.

Maguire A, Ambler G, Craig ME. Short stature in children: when is further evaluation and referral requried? Endocrinology Today. 2013;2(1).

Mushtaq T. Recombinant IGF-1 therapy in children with severe prmary IGF-1 deficiency (SPIGFD). BSPED; 2015.

Pharmaceuticals I. Increlex. Ipsen Pharmaceuticals; 2007.

Quigley CA, Gill AM, Crowe BJ, Robling K, Chipman JJ, Rose SR, et al. Safety of growth hormone treatment in pediatric patients with idiopathic short stature. J Clin Endocrinol Metab. 2005;90(9):5188–96.

Quigley CA, Child CJ, Zimmermann AG, Rosenfeld RG, Robison LL, Blum WF. Mortality in children receiving growth hormone treatment of growth disorders: data from the genetics and neuroendocrinology of Short Stature International Study. J Clin Endocrinol Metab. 2017;102(9):3195–205.

Raine JE, Donaldson MDC, Gregory JW, van Vliet G, editors. Practical endocrinology and diabetes in children. 3rd ed. Chichester: Wiley - Blackwell; 2011.

Ranke MB, Price DA, Albertsson-Wikland K, Maes M, Lindberg A. Factors determining pubertal growth and final height in growth hormone treatment of idiopathic growth hormone deficiency. Analysis of 195 patients of the Kabi Pharmacia International Growth Study. Horm Res. 1997;48(2):62–71.

Rappaport EB, Fife D. Slipped capital femoral epiphysis in growth hormone deficient patients. Am J Dis Child. 1985;139(4):396–9.

Romano AA, Allanson JE, Dahlgren J, Gelb BD, Hall B, Pierpont ME, et al. Noonan syndrome: clinical features, diagnosis, and management guidelines. Pediatrics. 2010;126(4):746–59.

Rosenbloom AL. Sex hormone priming for growth hormone stimulation testing in pre- and early adolescent children is evidence based. Horm Res Paediatr. 2011;75(1):78–80.

Rosenfeld RG, Albertsson-Wikland K, Cassorla F, Frasier SD, Hasegawa Y, Hintz RL, et al. Diagnostic controversy: the diagnosis of childhood growth hormone deficiency revisited. J Clin Endocrinol Metab. 1995;80(5):1532–40.

Satoh M. Bone age: assessment methods and clinical applications. Clin Pediatr Endocrinol. 2015;24(4):143–52.

Savage MO, Backeljauw PF, Calzada R, Cianfarani S, Dunkel L, Koledova E, et al. Early detection, referral, investigation, and diagnosis of children with growth disorders. Horm Res Paediatr. 2016;85(5):325–32.

Skuse D, Albanese A, Stanhope R, Gilmour J, Voss L. A new stress-related syndrome of growth failure and hyperphagia in children, associated with reversibility of growth-hormone insufficiency. Lancet. 1996;348(9024):353–8.

Storr HL. Recombinant IGF-1 therapy in children with severe primary IGF-1 deficiency (SPIGFD). BSPED: UK IGF-1User's Group; 2015.

Tanner JM, Healy MJR, Goldstein H, Cameron N. Assessment of skeletal maturity and prediction of adult height (TW3 method): WB Saunders; 2001.

Urquhart T, Collin J. Understanding the endocrinopathies associated with the treatment of childhood cancer: part 2. Nurs Child Young People. 2016;28(9):36–43.

van Uden-Kraan CF, Drossaert CH, Taal E, Seydel ER, van de Laar MA. Participation in online patient support groups endorses patients' empowerment. Patient Educ Couns. 2009;74(1):61–9.

Wit JM, Kamp GA, Rikken B. Spontaneous growth and response to growth hormone treatment in children with growth hormone deficiency and idiopathic short stature. Pediatr Res. 1996;39(2):295–302.

Disorders of Sex Development (DSD)

3

Kate Davies

Contents

K. Davies (✉)
Department of Advanced and Integrated Practice,
London South Bank University, London, UK
e-mail: kate.davies@lsbu.ac.uk

© Springer Nature Switzerland AG 2019
S. Llahana et al. (eds.), *Advanced Practice in Endocrinology Nursing*,
https://doi.org/10.1007/978-3-319-99817-6_3

Abstract

The diagnosis of a DSD—a disorder of sex development—whether made in infancy or as a young person—involves a full multidisciplinary team. Progress has been made in recent years with the advances of nomenclature, treatment, and psychological approaches and the disorders have been categorized into more patient-friendly terminology, leaving behind confusing and upsetting labels and stigma. These predominant DSD will be discussed in accordance with the new categories, detailing clinical presentation, management and nursing considerations in order to implement best practice. Emphasis here is placed on a fully co-operative multidisciplinary team, but also the nurses' role, who can offer continued support and guidance to the child/young person and their families.

Keywords

Ambiguous genitalia · Chromosome · DSD
Gonads · Karyotype

Abbreviations

11-DOC	11-deoxycortisol
17-OHP	17 alpha-hydroxyprogesterone
21-OHD	21-hydroxylase deficiency
5αRD	5 alpha reductase deficiency
A4	Androstenedione
ACTH	Adrenocorticotropic hormone
AIS	Androgen insensitivity syndrome
AMH	Anti-Mullerian hormone
CAH	Congenital adrenal hyperplasia
CAIS	Complete androgen insensitivity syndrome
CNS	Clinical nurse specialist
DHEA	Dehydroepiandrosterone
DHT	Dihydrotestosterone
DSD	Disorder of sex development
FISH	Fluorescence in situ hybridization
FSH	Follicle stimulating hormone
GnRH	Gonadotrophin releasing hormone
GP	General practitioner
HCG	Human chorionic Gonadotrophin
LH	Luteinizing hormone
MDT	Multidisciplinary team

MIS	Mullerian-inhibiting substance
MRKH	Mayer-Rokitansky-Küster-Hauser syndrome
MURCS	Mullerian, renal, cervicothoracic somite abnormalities
NICU	Neonatal intensive care unit
PAIS	Partial androgen insensitivity syndrome
PCOS	Polycystic ovarian syndrome
PENS	Paediatric endocrine nurse specialist
TS	Turner syndrome
UK	United Kingdom

Key Terms

- **Disorder of sex development:** An umbrella term used to describe a group of conditions that involve the internal reproductive system and/or external genitalia (previously known as *Intersex*).
- **Ambiguous genitalia:** Where the genitals do not appear to be clear either male or female.
- **Diagnostic pathway:** This is a kind of clinical tool, or map, to enable quality in the healthcare that is delivered, based on evidence-based practice.
- **Gonadal dysgenesis:** Where the gonads (ovaries or testes) are made of mainly fibrous tissue, are undeveloped, and do not function.
- **Multidisciplinary team:** A group of healthcare professionals from different professions, all providing their specific services for one patient.

Key Points
- Healthcare professionals involved in DSD care should follow the international consensus guidelines in order to offer optimum care.
- A diagnostic pathway should be followed, whether the child is presenting in infancy or in adolescence.
- A full multidisciplinary team should be in place in order to fully support and guide the family in the treatment needed.

- Paediatric endocrine nurses are in prime position to be the key advocate and liaison for the child/young person and their family.

3.1 What Is a DSD?

Disorders or differences of sex development (DSD) is a phrase used to describe a multitude of congenital conditions in which the physical development of either the chromosomes, the gonads, (i.e. the ovaries or the testes), or anatomy is unusual or atypical (Rothkopf and John 2014). It can also be described as where there is a difference between someone's 'genetic sex' to how their internal or external reproductive systems appear (Wisniewski et al. 2012). Many people use the term 'disorder', but that can lead some people to think of 'ill' children, so 'differences' is sometimes used instead. The incidence of actual ambiguous genitalia can occur in 1 in every 5000 live births (Rothkopf and John 2014), and is relatively rare. However, if all genital anomalies are to be considered, then a DSD can occur in approximately 1 in every 300 births (Rothkopf and John 2014). It is difficult to estimate exactly how many conditions come under the DSD umbrella: as the cause of a DSD is quite often a gene regulation breakdown (White and Sinclair 2012) which is responsible for gonadal development, there is the potential for more genetic variants yet to be identified, plus there are also a number of rare multiple malformation syndromes associated with DSD. However, a recent international consensus statement (Lee et al. 2006) has identified a useful classification tool for DSD.

3.2 Nomenclature

Previously to this consensus statement, various terms were used to describe different DSD conditions. Due to further developments in genetics, ethical considerations, patient advocacy voices, as well as patients from affected families, plus also specialists working in the field (Pasterski et al. 2010) it was deemed necessary to replace these terms. Such terms that were used were intersex, hermaphroditism, and pseudohermaphroditism (Woodward and Patwardhan 2010) (See Table 3.1). 'Intersex' was used as a broad term to describe a clinical picture of a child with ambiguous genitalia, whereas hermaphroditism was used to describe an individual with both testicular and ovarian tissue (Raine et al. 2011) and pseudohermaphrodites were either male with testicular tissue or female, with ovarian tissue. Such terminology was confusing and often stigmatized patients and their families (Woodward and Patwardhan 2010). The new classification can be seen in Table 3.2.

3.2.1   46, XX DSD

This category describes individuals who possess the usual number of chromosomes (Crissman et al. 2011) and two X chromosomes (female), but the external and/or internal sex ducts have not developed in the expected female way (Wisniewski et al. 2012). For example, the baby may be born with a womb and fallopian tubes, but their clitoris may look like a small penis. The most common form is congenital adrenal hyperplasia (CAH) and 21-hydroxylase deficiency (21-OHD) (*see Chap. 35*). However, other conditions also fall under this category, but can depend on disorders of ovarian development or androgen excess.

3.2.2   46, XY DSD

This is where the individual is born with a 46, XY (typically male) chromosomal make-up, but like the female 46, XX DSD, their internal or external structures have not developed in what should be

Table 3.1 Proposed revised nomenclature

Previous	Proposed
Intersex	DSD
Male pseudohermaphrodite Undervirilization of an XY male Undermasculinization of an XY male	46, XY DSD
Female pseudohermaphrodite Overvirilization of an XX female Masculinization of an XX female	46, XX DSD
True hermaphrodite	Ovotesticular DSD
XX male or XY female	46, testicular DSD
XY sex reversal	46, XY complete gonadal dysgenesis

Taken from: Hughes, I. A. (2008) Disorders of Sex development: a new definition and classification *Best Prac Res Clin Endocrinol Metab* 22 (1) p.119–34

Table 3.2 DSD Classification table

46, XY DSD	46, XX DSD	Sex chromosome DSD
1. Disorders of gonadal (testicular) development: (a) Complete gonadal dysgenesis (Swyer syndrome) (b) Partial gonadal dysgenesis (c) Gonadal regression (d) Ovotesticular DSD 2. Disorders in androgen synthesis or action: (a) Androgen biosynthesis defect (e.g. 5αRD) (b) Defect in androgen action (e.g. CAIS, PAIS) (c) LH receptor defects (d) Disorders of AMH/AMH receptors	1. Disorders of gonadal (ovarian) development: (a) Ovotesticular DSD (b) Testicular DSD (c) Gonadal dysgenesis 2. Androgen excess (a) Foetal (e.g. 21-OHD) (b) Foetoplacental (e.g. aromatase deficiency) (c) Maternal (e.g. exogenous) 3. Other (e.g. cloacal exstrophy, vaginal atresia, MURCS, other syndromes	1. 45, X (Turner syndrome and variants) 2. 47, XXY (Klinefelter syndrome and variants) 3. 45, X/46, XY (MGD, ovotesticular DSD) 4. 46, XX/46, XY (chimeric, ovotesticular DSD)

Adapted from: Lee, P.A et al. (2006) *Consensus Statement on Management of Intersex Disorders* Pediatrics 118 (2) p. e489–e500

expected for a male. The reasons for a 46, XY DSD are more varied and complex in comparison to a 46, XX DSD, but are usually attributed to the foetus being unable to produce or respond to testicular hormones (Wisniewski et al. 2012)

3.2.3 Sex Chromosome DSD

The sex chromosome DSD is where there is sex chromosome aneuploidy—where there is an abnormal number of X or Y chromosomes (Hewitt and Warne 2012a)—with either an extra or missing chromosome. Here the gonad is affected, and therefore ambiguous genitalia may be present, with also puberty and perhaps fertility also affected.

3.3 Chromosomes and Embryology

It is important to comprehend the principles of sexual differentiation when discussing the foundations of any DSD, and there are three sequential stages: (See Box 3.1).

Specific genes around gestational age week 3 lead to the differentiation of the gonads (Biason-Lauber 2010), but it is now widely known that the SRY gene, which resides on the p arm of the Y chromosome, sends signals to 'sex neutral' tissue to develop into testes (Wisniewski et al. 2012). If this gene is missing, or does not work properly, then healthy testes will not develop. Gonads and internal (Wolffian and Mullerian ducts) and

---

Box 3.1 The Stages of Embryological Differentiation (Rey and Grinspon 2011)
1. An 'undifferentiated' stage, where embryonic structures are identical and start to develop into XY (male) and XX (female) embryos
2. The gonadal stage, where testes or ovaries develop
3. The differentiated development of internal and external genitalia

---

external genitalia will have similar appearance around this time (Raine et al. 2011).

However, around gestational ages week 6–7, these undifferentiated gonads begin to separate: if a Y chromosome is present, the gonad will develop into a testis, and gonadal cells will segregate into testicular cords and interstitial tissue (Rey and Grinspon 2011). The testicular cords are made up of somatic sertoli cells and germ cells, and it is these sertoli cells that produce anti-Mullerian hormone (AMH) or Mullerian-inhibiting substance (MIS). AMH is responsible for the regression of the Mullerian ducts. Testosterone is also made by the testes. In the *absence* of these two hormones, female anatomy is formed—as the Mullerian ducts have not regressed—EVEN if a Y chromosome is present.

As seen in Fig. 3.1 (Kobayashi and Behringer 2003), Mullerian ducts in an XX female that will develop into female reproductive structures (except ovaries), and they grow because there is no AMH to block their development. Therefore no exposure to AMH will enable the internal structures to develop into the upper end of the vagina, the cervix, the womb, and the fallopian tubes (Wisniewski et al. 2012). Conversely, the Wolffian ducts will develop into the epididymides, the two vas deferens, and the seminal vesicles, for the male reproductive system.

There are further hormonal influences that will have an impact on the development of the external genitalia. From around 8 weeks gestation, the male embryo will develop a penis from the genital tubercle, urethral folds will develop into the corpus spongiosum that surrounds the urethra, and the genital folds will also fuse to form the scrotum (Raine et al. 2011). This happens under the influence of a hormone called dihydrotestosterone (DHT), which is converted from testosterone. DHT is made when an enzyme called 5 alpha reductase is available (Wisniewski et al. 2012). If a baby does *not* make DHT, then a vulva will form, involving a clitoris, and the labia minora and majora. It is interesting to note, however, that there is no difference between the size of the clitoris and penis before the 14th week gestation: phalli growth usually peaks in the third

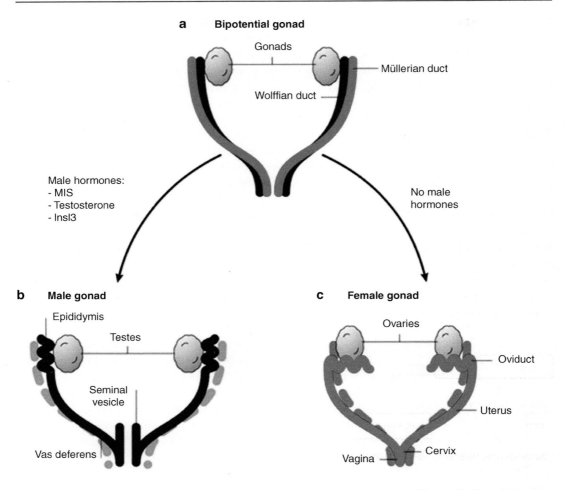

Fig. 3.1 Formation of internal reproductive structures. From: Akio Kobayashi & Richard R. Behringer. <u>Developmental genetics of the female reproductive tract in mammals</u> *Nature Reviews Genetics* 4, 969–980 (December 2003)

trimester, usually from around 28 weeks gestation (Rey and Grinspon 2011).

This is now apparent to see how ambiguous genitalia can occur: why some children who are XY may have female external genitalia, or why XX females may appear male (Wisniewski et al. 2012). It is, therefore, this presentation of a baby with ambiguous genitalia which will initiate a cascade of investigations and support for the child and family.

3.4   Diagnostic Pathway

New guidance (Ahmed et al. 2015) was formed by the United Kingdom (UK) Society of Endocrinology advising on the evaluation of infants and adolescents presenting with a suspected DSD. This guidance principally focuses on the diagnostic approach rather than lifelong management, and it is from this guidance that UK DSD centres follow.

3.5   Infants

Any baby where the appearance of their genitalia provokes questioning surrounding sex assignment needs to be investigated. Careful and sensitive management is needed, and a suggested diagnostic pathway (Kinsman et al. 2010) is seen in Fig. 3.2.

3.5.1   Identification

This is the first step where a suspected DSD in an infant is identified, usually by a midwife, or a paediatrician/obstetrician shortly after birth. It is essential that the baby is referred to a centre which has experience in DSD, and the referring personnel must contact the appropriate team with as much detail as possible, including:

3.5.1.1 Clinical Status

The referring team must describe if the baby is clinically well, for example, if they are ventilated, in an incubator, on antibiotics or intravenous fluids, or having problems with serum sodium or blood glucose levels.

3.5.1.2 Clinical History

A detailed description of the genitalia is needed, such as any hyperpigmentation, labial fusion, urethral meatus position, hypospadias, or chordee (where the head of the penis can curve upwards or downwards), and if the gonads are palpable. The Prader staging of external genitalia (Fig. 3.3) is used to classify the degree of virilization in external genitalia. Hypospadias can be classified by using the hypospadias diagram (Fig. 3.4), and the external masculinization score is used to describe states of labial

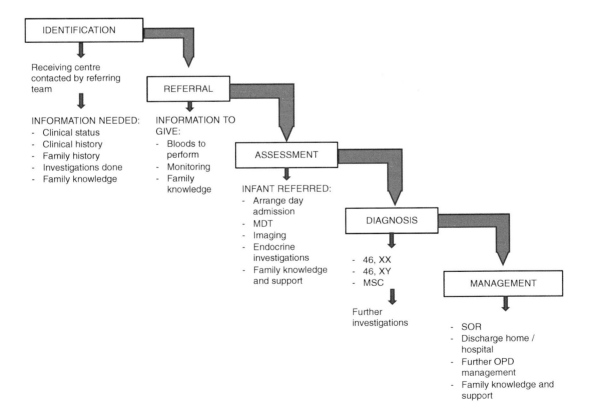

Fig. 3.2 Diagnostic pathway for an infant with a suspected DSD

Prader Stage

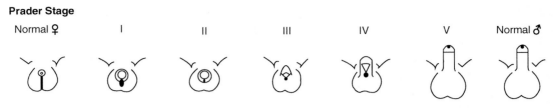

Fig. 3.3 The Prader staging of external genitalia. From: Hewitt, J.K. & Warne, G. L. (2012) 46, XY DSD *in Disorders of Sex Development: An Integrated Approach to Management* p. 65 Springer, Wurzburg

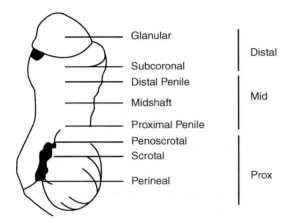

Fig. 3.4 Hypospadias descriptions. From: Hewitt, J.K. & Warne, G. L. (2012) 46, XY DSD *in Disorders of Sex Development: An Integrated Approach to Management* p. 65 Springer, Wurzburg

fusion and if and where the gonads are palpable (Fig. 3.5).

3.5.1.3 Family History

Details from the family are needed, such as antenatal scans and results of prenatal testing, and if there is any maternal history, such as exposure to any medications or other environmental factors (Hughes et al. 2012a), or whether any assisted techniques for conception were used (Ahmed and Rodie 2010). Sensitive questioning is also needed enquiring of ethnicity, any parental consanguinity, or any history of unexplained infant deaths in the family or any other noted cases of DSD.

3.5.1.4 Family Knowledge

Finally, this information needs to be treated with caution, and it is hoped that if the referral centre

is unsure, then no definite sex or rearing has already been given.

3.5.2 Referral

Once it is determined that the infant needs to be referred, the receiving team can advise on the next steps to undertake before the baby can physically arrive at their hospital. An urgent karyotype needs to be performed (Rodie et al. 2011) marked urgent, but blood can also be sent for FISH analysis (fluorescence in situ hybridization); this is a test that can look for specific genetic material and, in this case, X- and Y-specific DNA (Hughes et al. 2007). The results of these can usually be received relatively quickly and can indicate if there is Y-specific material present. Daily monitoring of the baby is advised for serum urea and electrolytes and blood glucose. After the baby is 3 days old, then cortisol and ACTH levels can be recorded, plus also 17-hydroxyprogesterone (17-OHP). Samples taken before this can potentially be abnormal (Raine et al. 2011). 17-OHP is a steroid hormone which would be raised in cases of CAH (congenital adrenal hyperplasia) (*See Chap. 35*).

3.5.3 Assessment

Next, the baby should be admitted to the specialist centre, for a full-day admission. This would include meeting members of the multidisciplinary team (MDT) who could be involved.

External Masculinisation Score

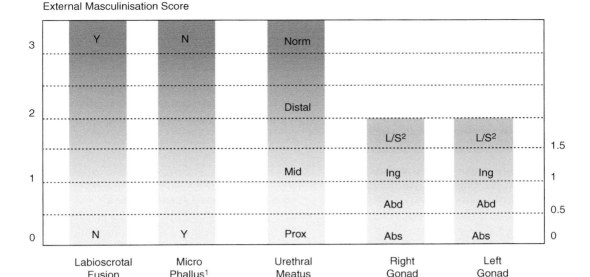

Fig. 3.5 The External Masculinization Score. From: Hewitt, J.K. & Warne, G. L. (2012) 46, XY DSD *in Disorders of Sex Development: An Integrated Approach to Management* p. 65 Springer, Wurzburg

Further clinical assessment would need to take place, including further endocrine investigations, possibly further and more detailed imaging, such as a pelvic and abdominal ultrasound to explore internal structures, and further blood tests looking at testosterone levels, anti-Mullerian hormone (AMH) (or Mullerian-inhibiting substance—MIS), inhibin B, gonadotrophins, and also urinalysis. AMH is detected in boys and is expressed in the sertoli cells in the embryological phases of testicular differentiation (Ahmed et al. 2015), and inhibin B also is produced in the testes.

Including the MDT is paramount, and the family should meet the paediatric endocrine nurse specialist (PENS), the paediatric endocrinologist, the paediatric urologist, and the psychologist, for optimum and sensitive management on this first day of meeting. The team need to work together to develop a plan for immediate clinical assessment and management, exploring differential diagnoses, sex of rearing/gender assignment, and treatment, ensuring that the family have a good understanding. Information leaflets should be available from support groups, and it is recommended to offer them with full explanations.

3.5.4 Diagnosis

Further investigations may need to be undertaken once the karyotype is confirmed to confirm the actual diagnosis. If 46, XX, a short synacthen test and a urine steroid profile are needed to be performed to confirm CAH (Butler and Kirk 2011). If 46, XY, an HCG (human chorionic gonadotropin) stimulation test should be performed, which is used to test the ability of any testes present to produce testosterone (Ishii et al. 2015) (see Box 3.2 below (Butler and Kirk 2011)) Good testicular function is indicated if testosterone rises above 5 nmol/L.

If the chromosomes are 'mixed sex', or 45, X/46, XY, then further investigations similar for Turner syndrome (*See Chap. 40*) need to be carried out, such as thyroid function, a cardiac echocardiograph, audiology, and Turner screening. In cases of 46, XX and 45, X/46, XY, early examinations under anaesthetic and/or laparoscopy for

inspection of internal structures may be necessary, or genitograms to determine any merging
between the vagina and urethra (Raine et al.
2011), although these investigations are only
needed if the diagnosis is proving difficult
(Ahmed et al. 2015).

3.5.5 Management

The decision of sex or rearing/gender assignment
can, usually, be made at the end of the day of the
admission, which is important for parents, as the
need and desire to want to register the baby's
birth with the 'correct' sex is important. The baby
can be discharged either back to the referring
hospital or home if appropriate. Full details have
to be given for any immediate medical management, and education on any sick day and emergency management if the baby is 46, XX CAH,
and the PENS' role here is paramount (*See
Chaps. 37 and 62*). Further management and
support is given, follow-up clinic appointments
for the appropriate members of the MDT should
be made and details of support groups given and
explained (Ahmed et al. 2015).

3.6 Adolescents

A small group of DSD can present in adolescence
and can present in one of three ways:

1. A girl presenting with primary amenorrhea
   (where menstruation has not yet commenced),
   with or without any breast development.
2. A girl who begins to virilize at puberty.
3. A boy with delayed puberty.

3.6.1 Primary Amenorrhea

A full history needs to be taken, including a family history, and full pubertal assessment (*See
Chap. 4*). Further investigations are detailed in
the UK guidance (Ahmed et al. 2015) but are also
outlined in Fig. 3.6. A 46, XX disorder of
Mullerian development would include Mayer-
Rokitansky-Küster-Hauser (MRKH) syndrome,
as this is where the vagina and womb may be
underdeveloped or absent (*See Sect. 6*).
Whichever cause, the management of girls presenting with primary amenorrhea should be
referred to the gynaecology team.

3.6.2 Girls with Virilization

Girls presenting with hirsutism and cliteromeg-
aly is usually indicative of two possible DSD: 5
alpha reductase deficiency (5αRD), and 17β
hydroxysteroid dehydrogenase type 3 deficiency,
which is a condition where testosterone is not
synthesized properly.

3.6.3 Boys with Delayed Puberty

Most boys presenting with delayed puberty are
classified as having 'constitutional delay' (Raine
et al. 2011), but other avenues need to be
explored and investigated. Testosterone and
gonadotrophins need to be measured; if the
gonadotrophins are raised, a karyotype should
be taken to exclude Klinefelter syndrome (47,

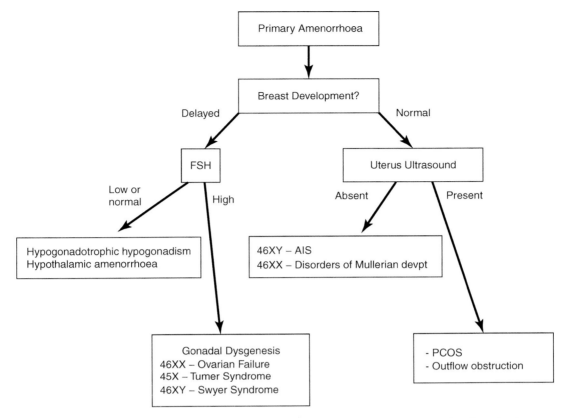

Fig. 3.6 Primary amenorrhoea investigations. From: Ahmed, S.F et al. (2015) Society for Endocrinology UK guidance on the initial evaluation of an infant or an adolescent with a suspected disorder of sex development (Revised 2015) *Clinical Endocrinology* 0, 1–18

XXY) (*See Chap. 10*) and 45,X/46, XY mosaicism (Ahmed et al. 2015).

3.7 46, XX DSD

As seen in the initial classification system (Lee et al. 2006), 46, XX DSD can encompass disorders of ovarian development, androgen excess, and other disorders.

3.7.1 Androgen Excess

More than 50% of all babies born with ambiguous genitalia are 46,XX (Warne and Hewitt 2012a), and this is due to the female foetus being exposed to too many male androgens (Davies 2016). The appearance of the external genitalia can vary in degrees of virilization, and this can be seen in the Prader virilization rating scale (Fig. 3.3). The source of the androgens can be testicular (Warne and Hewitt 2012a): 1 in every 20,000 men has a 46, XX karyotype, and this is due to a translocation of the SRY gene off the tip of the Y chromosome onto one of the X chromosomes. Phenotypically, these men may be similar to men with Klinefelter syndrome. However, the cause of the androgens is usually adrenal, and CAH is the most common cause for this (Woodward and Patwardhan 2010). The majority of these children are assigned as female when they present in the newborn era. (Rothkopf and John 2014) (*See Chap. 35*).

Aromatase deficiencies are also a less common type of enzyme defect, and sometimes the cause may be due to something the mother has ingested, or maternal androgen-secreting tumours. (Warne and Hewitt 2012a)

3.7.2 Disorders of Ovarian Development

This can include 46, XX ovotesticular DSD, which used to be classified as 'true hermaphroditism' (Woodward and Patwardhan 2010). These individuals have both ovarian and testicular tissue present and will present in the neonatal period with ambiguous genitalia, and continue with virilization at puberty. If female sex was assigned, then they may need an orchidectomy, whilst a male may need an orchidopexy. (Woodward and Patwardhan 2010) The phenotype can vary, however, but often the testis is on one side (usually the right), and the ovotestis or ovary would tend to be on the left, and it is the ovary that is more likely to function (Hewitt and Warne 2012a).

3.7.3 Other Causes

Other causes for 46, XX DSD exist, such as disorders of Mullerian development; ovarian function is usually normal (Ahmed et al. 2015), but other physical presentations may manifest, including cloacal dystrophy, vaginal atresia, or MURCS (Mullerian duct aplasia renal agenesis cervicothoracic somite dysplasia) (Lee et al. 2006)

3.8 46, XY DSD

Conversely, 46, XY DSD is where the child has 46, XY chromosomes, but the internal and/or external reproductive system has not developed properly in what should be expected as male. (Wisniewski et al. 2012) It can be due to an interruption in any part of testicular development, abnormal androgen action, or other reasons.

3.8.1 Clinical Presentation

There is a varying amount of possible ways a child with 46, XY DSD can present. They may possess male internal organs (such as epididymides or vas deferens) but external genitalia may be under-masculinized, which can include a small penis resembling a clitoris, or unfused scrotum, which can look like labia. Testes may not have descended into the scrotum (See Fig. 3.5 on how to clinically assess), and the urinary opening may be at the base of the phallus instead of expected at the tip, which could indicate, for example, severe hypospadias (see Fig. 3.4) (Wisniewski et al. 2012). Children can therefore present with ambiguous genitalia at birth, no development of secondary sex characteristics in a boy, or primary amenorrhea in an adolescent girl (Hewitt and Warne 2012b). The reasons why the clinical presentation can vary so much is due to how much androgen production is affected, and also where this specifically occurs within the stages of testicular development.

3.8.2 Incidence

Due to the varying clinical presentations, the actual incidence is unknown, although it is estimated that hypospadias occurs in approximately 1 in every 125 male births (Hewitt and Warne 2012b), and complete androgen insensitivity syndrome (CAIS) is known to occur in 1 in every 20,000 births.

3.8.3 Tumour Risk

There is a risk of gonadal germ cell cancer in children with 46, XY DSD, and this needs to be explored sensitively. This can occur because there is a higher incidence of germ cell tumours in testes that have not developed properly, and Y chromosome material is present. (Hewitt and Warne 2012b) The risk varies in the specific 46, XY DSD condition, (Lee et al. 2006) and management can vary, whether it is close observation with regular endocrine clinic follow-up, biopsy, irradiation, or even a full gonadectomy (Lee et al. 2006). This remains controversial, and recent guidelines state that gonadectomy is not necessary before puberty for children with androgen insensitivity syndrome (Hughes et al. 2007). Gonadectomy, however, in partial androgen insensitivity syndrome (PAIS), is dependent on the sex of rearing.

3.8.4 Disorders of Testicular Development

In complete gonadal dysgenesis (or Swyer syndrome), children will look typically female, but have intra-abdominal 'streak' gonads, and will have some risk of potential tumour development. Streak gonads mean that the gonads (either testes or ovaries) are underdeveloped and do not function and are mainly made from fibrous tissue. In this instance, testes have not formed at all, or were 'lost' in early foetal development. Due to the lack of testes, there is therefore a lack of AMH, thereby resulting in external female looking genitalia, and also internal female reproductive structures (womb and fallopian tubes), but no ovaries (Wisniewski et al. 2012). The child with complex gonadal dysgenesis may be diagnosed if a girl presents with delayed puberty, and a routine karyotype has been performed. (Hewitt and Warne 2012b)

In contrast, in 46, XY partial or mixed gonadal dysgenesis, clinical presentation can vary, as there has been some degree of testicular development, so clitoromegaly may occur, ambiguous genitalia, or a very severe hypospadias (Ahmed et al. 2011). The internal Mullerian structures may or may not be present, and the testes can also vary in size and positioning. (Mendonca et al. 2009) Mixed gonadal dysgenesis signifies some degree of asymmetry in gonadal development, where there may be a 'dysgenetic' testis on one side, and a streak gonad on the other (Hewitt and Warne 2012b).

3.8.5 46, XY DSD Due to Defects in Androgen Synthesis or Action

There are four sub-categories that come under this specific classification: disorders of AMH and AMH receptors, luteinizing hormone (LH) receptor defects, androgen biosynthesis defects, and defects in androgen action.

3.8.5.1 Disorders of AMH and AMH Receptors

Gene mutations can occur which encode AMH or its receptor and can lead to persistent Mullerian duct syndrome (Hewitt and Warne 2012b), which means that Mullerian duct derivatives (i.e. a small womb and/or upper part of the vagina and fallopian tubes) are present because of the lack of action of AMH in foetal development. Phenotypically, the children will look male, but with cryptorchidism (absence of testes in the scrotum) and can present with herniation of the womb in the inguinal canal. A laparoscopic hysterectomy may need to be performed, as well as orchidopexy (surgery to bring the testes down into the scrotum.)

3.8.5.2 LH Receptor Defects

These conditions are more rare and consist of where LH receptor gene mutations have been identified that have an effect on LH receptor proteins, leading to Leydig cell hypoplasia (Ahmed et al. 2015), which means the Leydig cells in the testes (which make testosterone if LH is present), are underdeveloped. Children may present with micropenis, hypospadias, and a bifid scrotum (a deep cleft in the middle of the scrotum caused by incomplete labioscrotal fusion), leading to external genitalia to resemble a phenotypical female.

3.8.5.3 Androgen Biosynthesis Defects

Testosterone is metabolized by DHT, by an enzyme called 5 alpha reductase. If a child does not have enough of this enzyme, then DHT is not produced, therefore having an overall effect on male development, resulting in a condition called 5 alpha reductase deficiency (5αRD). Phenotypically, children present with external female genitalia at birth, but will also have testes in the inguinal region, and internal male reproductive structures (Odame et al. 1992). Most children are reared as females and may undergo gonadectomy. However, if they have not had the surgery by the time they reach puberty, they will begin to virilize: their voices deepen, their phalluses enlarge, but they do not develop any facial or body hair, or acne. At puberty, these children may change their gender to male (Mendonca et al. 2010), and undergo testosterone replacement therapy, or use DHT cream (Odame et al. 1992). However, some may remain as females and subsequently undergo gonadectomy, vaginoplasty, and treatment with oestrogen therapy (Mendonca et al. 1996).

3.8.5.4 Defects in Androgen Action

If androgen receptors do not function properly, then the result may be varying degrees of androgen insensitivity, i.e. a lack of androgen response, and therefore incomplete virilization in a person with 46, XY make-up.

3.8.5.4.1 Complete Androgen Insensitivity Syndrome (CAIS)

CAIS is where a child is 46, XY, but is completely phenotypically female, and has intact testes. Clinical presentation may manifest in infancy, with inguinal hernia or labial swelling (containing the testes), which is rare (Hughes et al. 2012b), or in adolescence, when the adolescent presents to clinic with primary amenorrhea. She will have developed breasts, with a female body shape, which is due to increased oestrogen production by the aromatization of androgens. The testes in the inguinal area, if they have not been removed, may be uncomfortable (Hewitt and Warne 2009), but the risk of malignancy is significantly lower after puberty although lifelong surveillance is advised. To date, the topic of prophylactic gonadectomy in girls with CAIS is still very controversial (Mendonca et al. 2009)

Sex of rearing in CAIS is female, and the girls retain a female gender identity (Tadokoro-Cuccaro and Hughes 2014), with the girls tending to be satisfied with their sexual functioning in adult life, although this is dependent upon vaginal lengths and any previous surgeries (Wisniewski et al. 2000).

3.8.5.4.2 Partial Androgen Insensitivity Syndrome

Whereas gene mutations in androgen receptors are identified in more than 95% of women with CAIS, mutations are less common in PAIS (Mongan et al. 2015), and the phenotype depends on the severity of the androgen receptor dysfunction, and amount of androgen insensitivity. (Tadokoro-Cuccaro and Hughes 2014) However, there is usually some degree of genital ambiguity, and underdevelopment of the penis, severe hypospadias, and a bifid scrotum, which may contain gonads (Hughes et al. 2012b). Parental decisions on sex of rearing can be either as a boy or a girl, depending on the size of the phallus. If female, the testes may be removed to remove the possibility of changes due to testosterone, and again, the risk of germ cell tumours (Hewitt and Warne 2009), and the malignancy risk varies, depending on the location of the testes. If raised as male, then regular surveillance of the testes is essential, and recent data has shown that children with PAIS are raised as male (Tadokoro-Cuccaro and Hughes 2014) although breast development can occur at puberty. There may be a degree of gender dysphoria in adulthood, but again, this is dependent on phallus size and sex assignment at birth. (Mendonca et al. 2009)

3.9 Mixed Sex Chromosome DSD

Mixed sex chromosome DSD occurs when there is aneuploidy—i.e. an abnormal number of chromosomes and can be relatively common (47, XXX, 47, XXY, 45, X, or 47, XYY) or part of a mosaic karyotype (Hewitt and Warne 2012a). This is where one kind of karyotype is present in some cells, and a different karyotype in other cells, for example, 45, X/46, XY.

3.9.1   45, X/46, XY

This is the most common karyotype which is linked with ambiguous genitalia, with CAH and AIS. The anatomy in affected children can result from gonadal dysgenesis, i.e. maldeveloped gonads. Where one gonad is *streak*, and the other is *dysgenetic*, the child is said to have *mixed gonadal dysgenesis*, so asymmetrical gonadal development (Biason-Lauber 2010; Hewitt and Warne 2009).

Children can present differently and have a varied phenotype, but those presenting with a male phenotype tend to be shorted and have dysgenetic testes (Hewitt and Warne 2012a). However, individuals with a female phenotype may have features similar to Turner syndrome, and most have short stature. They can present antenatally, at birth with ambiguous genitalia, or later in adolescence with short stature or delayed puberty, or even in the oncology setting with a germ cell tumour (Hewitt and Warne 2009). Due to this, it has been argued that gonadectomy should be performed in infancy if the child is to be reared as a female. If male, the testes need to be observed regularly with serum tumour markers, and potentially biopsy after puberty. Sex of rearing is dependent on the external genitalia phenotype.

3.9.2   46, XX/46, XY DSD

This is a chimeric genetic disorder, i.e. where a cell can be made up of different zygotes and can be referred to as chromosomal ovotesticular DSD. Because of this mixed sex chromosome, both ovarian and testicular tissues are found in either the same gonad, or the opposite gonad, just as in 46, XX ovotesticular DSD, or 46, XY ovotesticular DSD. The distribution amongst the gonads vary, but both ovarian follicles and seminiferous tubules are present.

Some women with ovotesticular DSD have become mothers, but no ovotesticular DSD males have become fathers (Hewitt and Warne 2012a), so it is clear that the ovary is dominant. If testicular tissue is not removed, then re-evaluation of endocrine status is essential at the time of puberty.

3.9.3   Klinefelter Syndrome: 47, XXY
(See Chap. 10)

Klinefelter syndrome results from two or more X chromosomes in males. Symptoms can vary, and sometimes diagnosis is made when the adult male has investigations into infertility, due to high FSH and LH levels (Hewitt and Warne 2012a). There is decreased testicular function in most affected individuals, so smaller testes are present, and sometimes there may be some degree of learning difficulty (Biason-Lauber 2010).

3.9.4   Turner Syndrome: Monosomy X or 45, X or 45, XO (See Chap. 40)

Part or all of one of the X chromosomes is missing in Turner syndrome (TS). Girls with TS do not tend to come under the 'DSD' classification in clinical practice, but it sits within the consensus nomenclature, and many endocrine centres internationally will have their own TS clinics. There is a characteristic phenotype for girls with TS, including short stature and gonadal dysgenesis. Phenotypically, the girl with TS will also have female external genitalia. Diagnosis can be made antenatally, in infancy, in childhood where slow growth is noted, or adolescence, where the girl presents with delayed puberty and amenorrhea.

3.10 Management

3.10.1 Medical Management

It is common sense that the baby born with ambiguous genitalia needs urgent medical evaluation, including a thorough newborn physical examination (Devlin and Wilkinson 2008), specifically looking for any dysmorphic features (Warne and Hewitt 2012b). Urgent blood samples, as previously stated, need to be performed, as well as clinical monitoring in the immediate newborn period. If a diagnosis of salt wasting CAH is made, then commencing hydrocortisone and fludrocortisone is paramount, as well as salt replacement, (*See Chap. 35*) in order to prevent an adrenal crisis.

Hormone replacement therapy is needed in all females with mixed gonadal dysgenesis, or in genotypic males who have either had their testes removed, or where they experience testicular failure. (Warne and Hewitt 2012b)

3.10.2 Surgical Management

Surgical management of the child with a DSD remains controversial. Reconstructive surgery is performed for cosmetic reasons, to allow vaginal-penile intercourse, and to be able to achieve a 'sex-typical' manner for urination (i.e. for males to be able to stand whilst urinating) (Creighton et al. 2012). The controversy lies behind *if* to perform surgery, and *when*. Early infancy surgery is advocated by some as the procedure is easier, and that there is also less stigma for the family. However, some adults who have undergone surgery in this period are not happy with sexual function and satisfaction. (Creighton et al. 2012) Feminizing genitoplasty (clitoroplasty, vaginoplasty, and sometimes labiaplasty) is only performed in the most severe cases of virilization (Prader 3–5) (Lee et al. 2016), with an emphasis on preservation of erectile function and not cosmetic appearance being of utmost importance. The whole multidisciplinary team, alongside the parents, must be involved in decision-making for this aspect of care although guidelines do state to leave or delay as long as possible (Hughes et al. 2007).

Gonadectomies in under-virilized 46, XY DSD males also remain controversial as stated, and also in individuals with mixed sex chromosome DSD, where the gender identity may vary. (Vidal et al. 2010)

3.10.3 Psychosocial Management

Whilst it is important to focus on the physical aspects of a DSD, it cannot be underestimated that a vast input from psychological services is paramount. (Hughes et al. 2007) Support for the parents with a newborn with ambiguous genitalia is essential, as is support for the child and adolescent, irrespective of when a diagnosis is made. A psychologist can help the family with decisions regarding sex of rearing, timing of any surgery, and possible sex hormone replacement (Lee et al. 2012). Assistance can also be given in how best to tell friends and family on their child's diagnosis, and possible change of sex, especially if they were told something different antenatally (Loughlin 2012).

Support and guidance should be maintained as the child grows and develops, with caution given if there are any questions regarding gender identity. Gender role behaviour can be atypical in children with a DSD, but this is not necessarily an indicator for definitive gender re-assignment (Lee et al. 2016). Nevertheless, gender dysphoria can remain an issue (Hewitt and Warne 2009), especially in adults who may have had surgery as an infant/child, with an unsatisfactory outcome.

Psychological input is also necessary when contemplating diagnosis disclosure to the child or young person, regarding karyotype, gonadal status, and possible future fertility, and it is advised that acceptability and psychosocial adaptation is helped with honest disclosure (Hughes et al. 2007). The psychologist can work closely with the family on this, helping the child and family with counselling and guidance for an optimum quality of life.

3.11   The Multidisciplinary Team (MDT)

It is clear that the management of the child with a DSD, and their family, must take a full multidisciplinary approach (Hughes et al. 2007). Children with a DSD must be able to access centres of excellence which are fully equipped, manned, and experienced in dealing with DSD, and have a full team ready. An integrated team approach can be seen in Fig. 3.7. (Lee et al. 2016; Brain et al. 2010)

3.11.1   The Psychologist

This team member is so important and must be available to the child/young person and family from the very beginning (Moshiri et al. 2012). The diagnosis of a DSD can be unexpected and

overwhelming, and, as discussed, advice and guidance can be given on how to verbalize concerns, how to deal with emerging emotions, and how to guide their child/young person in how to develop alongside their peers. Some families express the need to be in touch with other families experiencing the same, or similar, diagnosis (Boyse et al. 2014). Feelings of isolation or stigmatization can be reduced if the family feels they are not alone. Patient support groups can provide a valuable service to families, providing clear guidance and advice from other families (*See* Sect. 3.12).

3.11.2   The Paediatric Endocrinologist

The paediatric endocrinologist will play a major role in the child's management and

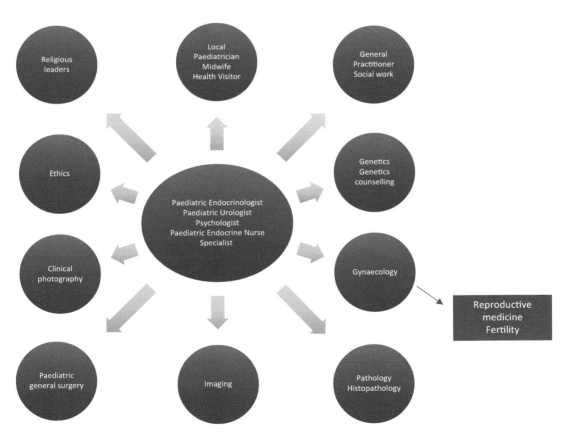

Fig. 3.7 An integrated approach

decision-making of any clinical investigations to be performed (Brain et al. 2010). They are often the first port of call when receiving a baby with ambiguous genitalia. As 46, XX CAH is the most common DSD (Hewitt and Warne 2009), management and education on adrenal crises, replacement, and other medication needs to be co-ordinated by a paediatric endocrine team. Further on, as the child grows, clinical monitoring may be necessary, with regard to hydrocortisone replacement and compliance, mineralocorticoid dosing and salt supplementation (Schaeffer et al. 2010), as well as growth monitoring and pubertal management, especially in individuals with non-functioning gonads (Lee et al. 2016). In addition, gonadotropin releasing hormone (GnRH) therapy may be required in young people where gender identity is uncertain, and also growth hormone therapy and oestrogen in girls with Turner syndrome.

3.11.3 The Paediatric Urologist/ Surgeon

The paediatric urologist also plays a key role. A joint meeting with the paediatric endocrinologist and family is ideal, so as to physically assess and clinically examine the baby with ambiguous genitalia together. As well as the external genitalia, the urologist should be able to palpate/locate the gonads. If any cosmetic surgery is to occur, it should be this experienced surgeon who deems it necessary and is confident in the eventual function and acceptable cosmetic appearance. Hypospadias repair also comes under their remit and also the need for gonadectomy if the risk of malignancy is high (Brain et al. 2010).

3.11.4 The Paediatric Endocrine Nurse Specialist (PENS)

The role of the nurse specialist has been advancing in specialist DSD services (Sanders et al. 2017). The PENS is key in just as a support for the child and family, but for liaising with the MDT, organizing investigations (Ahmed et al. 2015), and ensuring smooth running and organization of MDT clinical meetings. Much has been written on the role of the clinical nurse specialist *(See Sect. 13)* but the PENS multifaceted role can be seen in Fig. 3.8. It can be highlighted here that the role of the patient advocate is at the forefront of the multifaceted role. Families will often have the PENS' contact details and contact them directly with any queries or concerns, rather than waiting for their clinic appointment.

3.11.5 Other MDT Members

Although the healthcare professionals discussed are key (See Box 3.3), other team members play an important role in the care and management of a child with a DSD.

Gynaecologists can be available when the child is an infant to advise on potential outcome of any interventions and advise on pubertal management in girls (Brain et al. 2010). Biochemists can ensure swift management of expedited samples arriving in the laboratory and provide guidance on the investigation to be performed (Ahmed et al. 2015), likewise with genetics services. Ethicists, cultural and religious leaders can also not be discounted and conflicts may arise, and

---

Box 3.3 The MDT

"The Clinical Nurse Specialist (CNS) with specialist skills, knowledge and expertise, plays an essential role within the MDT in caring for children with a DSD condition, and their families. Providing psychological support is extremely important and requires the CNS to work in close liaison with the Clinical Psychologist to support these children from diagnosis throughout childhood into adolescence and adult life."

Nicky Nicoll, Clinical Nurse Specialist in Paediatric Endocrinology

Bristol Royal Hospital for Children, United Kingdom

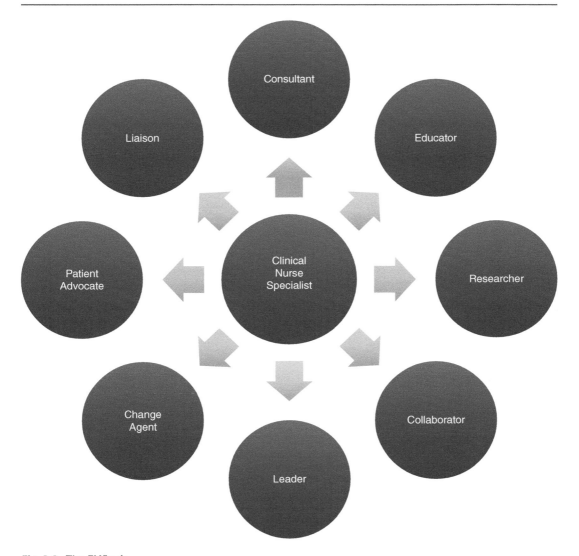

Fig. 3.8 The CNS role

ultimately clinical experts need to act in the best interests for the child (Brain et al. 2010). Ethical principles need to focus on the following: (Moshiri et al. 2012)

1. Minimizing physical risks
2. Minimizing psychological risks
3. Preserving potential fertility
4. Preserving the ability to have satisfactory sexual relationships
5. Respecting parental desires and beliefs

Respecting parental beliefs do need to be considered: for some, a DSD may still have a stigma, and social, religious, and cultural factors may play an important role when deciding on gender roles and gender assignment, especially in 5αRD. Religious leaders may also be able to offer the family continuing support.

Local teams need to be included, such as the local paediatrician, General practitioner (GP), or health visitors, who again can provide ongoing support to families. Links must be made with the GP who may be responsible for repeat medical prescriptions and arrangements to be made with the local paediatrician for immediate paediatric ward access if the child suffers an adrenal crisis. Community nursing teams can also offer assistance in obtaining serum sodium samples in infancy if need be, plus GnRH analogue therapy or testosterone injections where necessary during adolescence. Multidisciplinary teamwork is essential all round to achieve the desired goals for the child and their family.

3.12 Nursing Considerations

3.12.1 At Diagnosis

PENS need to be aware from the beginning how to approach families who's child has been diagnosed with a DSD. Using 'medicalized' language can be daunting and confusing for parents (Sanders et al. 2011), so great care needs to be taken in using understanding terminology. Supporting literature is paramount, especially regarding how and when to administer hydrocortisone medication, or administering salt supplements, if the child has 46, XX CAH, plus also sick day and emergency management advice (*See Chap. 35*). Practicalities to consider for the initial meeting with the MDT during the first admission need to be considered and can be seen in Box 3.4.

The PENS can make contact with the family prior to the admission and explain the need for the practicalities outlined. Babies with ambiguous genitalia should begin their diagnostic pathway as soon as possible, usually within the first 5 days of life, so the PENS must be sensitive with the family who are going through an emotional upheaval regarding a potential diagnosis, notwithstanding having just given birth. The day of admission can be lengthy; as arrangements are usually made at short notice, the need for waiting times between visits from the MDT need to be explained, as they may be holding a clinic or in surgery, so their times need to be co-ordinated carefully. The PENS can act as an advocate and liaison for the family during the admission, enabling potential stressful situations to be eased,

Box 3.4 Admission Practicalities to Consider

For the ward:

- Is the baby ventilated/incubator dependent? (May need to go to NICU)
- Will the referring nurse stay? Does return transport need to be arranged?
- Is a private, comfortable area available for the baby and family?
- Ensure dynamic investigation medication is in stock on the ward (GnRH, synacthen, HCG).
- Arrange interpreter if needed
- Is there baby milk/bottles/teats/sterilizer/breast pump/fridge/freezer facilities available on the ward?
- Has the MDT been informed? Appointments may need to be made throughout the day.

For the parents:

- Bring maternal case notes/scans/reports
- Bring nappies, changes of baby clothes, milk, dummies, etc.
- Money for car parking
- Mobile phone charger/money for pay phone
- Advise that there may be long waits between MDT visits, so bring magazines/books, and also food and drink
- Bring a list of questions

and being able to answer questions with non-medical jargon (Crissman et al. 2011).

3.12.2 Ongoing Management

Prior to discharge, the PENS needs to ensure that the family have a full understanding of the condition, and can offer further, less formal appointments with him/herself to continue with education and support. Again, the role of support groups and perhaps local families cannot be underestimated. Ongoing management in outpatient clinics will be dependent on the specific DSD, but the PENS is the ideal healthcare professional to offer continuing support. Regular MDT meetings can be held monthly and provide updates to healthcare professionals on any emerging issues seen in the outpatient clinic.

3.12.3 Transition and Beyond

Management in adult services is very different to the paediatric world, and it is essential that a seamless transition, and not a simple transfer of care, is enabled (*See Chap. 6*) Long-term studies and data in young adults with DSD is still lacking (Crouch and Creighton 2014), but continued engagement with members of the MDT should be encouraged when meeting with adult services. Continued attendance can also provide healthcare professionals with valuable long-term data in order to be able to provide the best care in future generations of young people with a DSD.

For those young people with a DSD, if not diagnosed in infancy, the diagnosis may have been made recently, so their relationship with paediatric services may have been relatively short, if at all. Issues concerning genital examinations, gonadectomy, disclosure, and psychological issues need to be fully explored and appreciated (Crouch and Creighton 2014), with full realization that 'the patient' is now 'the adult', and all decisions to be made will now transfer to them (Schober et al. 2012). The MDT relationship, however, must not stop, and the journey should continue.

3.13 Conclusions

For children and young people with a DSD, and their families, diagnosis and further management can conjure up a great deal of uncertainty and confusion. Paediatric endocrine nurses need to have a good understanding regarding not just the aetiology and clinical aspects of the different DSD, but also the emotional and psychological impact that a diagnosis of a DSD can have. International consensus guidelines (Lee et al.

2006) have been formulated, and a new classification system has been formed, which has formed the framework of this chapter. Whilst the most common DSD have been discussed, the umbrella of DSD is vast, and not all conditions have been covered here. The emphasis, however, is on the full MDT working with and alongside the child and their family. The PENS needs to consider their multifaceted role and engage in the roles of not just 'clinical expert', but also as 'patient advocate' and 'liaison'. Parents want their child to live as 'normal' a life as possible (Crissman et al. 2011), and it is with the information and guidance from the PENS and the MDT that can hopefully enable seamless transition from diagnosis and beyond.

3.14 Useful Websites

www.dsdfamilies.org UK DSD support group

www.dsdteens.org UK DSD young persons support group

www.aissg.org UK Androgen Insensitivity Syndrome support group

www.aisdsd.org USA AIS support group for women and families

www.accordalliance.org International information page for healthcare professionals and families

www.heainfo.org USA Hypospadias and Epispadias Association

www.hypospadiasuk.co.uk UK Hypospadias support group

www.livingwithcah.com UK CAH support group

www.tss.org.uk UK Turner Syndrome support group

www.turnersyndrome.org USA Turner Syndrome support group

www.ksa-uk.co.uk. UK Klinefelter Syndrome support group

www.genetic.org USA Klinefelter Syndrome support group

www.livingmrkh.org.uk UK MRKH support group

www.MRKH.orgUSA MRKH support group

www.verity-pcos.org.uk UK PCOS support group

www.isna.org USA Intersex Society of North America

References

Ahmed SF, Rodie M. Investigation and initial management of ambiguous genitalia. Best Pract Res Clin Endocrinol Metab. 2010;24(2):197–218.

Ahmed SF, Achermann JC, Arlt W, Balen AH, Conway G, Edwards ZL, et al. UK guidance on the initial evaluation of an infant or an adolescent with a suspected disorder of sex development. Clin Endocrinol. 2011;75(1):12–26.

Ahmed SF, Achermann JC, Arlt W, Balen AH, Conway G, Edwards ZL, et al. Society for Endocrinology UK guidance on the initial evaluation of an infant or an adolescent with a suspected disorder of sex development (Revised 2015). Clin Endocrinol. 2015;0:1–18.

Biason-Lauber A. Control of sex development. Best Pract Res Clin Endocrinol Metab. 2010;24(2):163–86.

Boyse KL, Gardner M, Marvicsin DJ, Sandberg DE. "It was an overwhelming thing": parents' needs after infant diagnosis of CAH. J Pediatr Nurs. 2014;29(5):436–41.

Brain CE, Creighton SM, Mushtaq I, Carmichael PA, Barnicoat A, Honour JW, et al. Holistic management of DSD. Best Pract Res Clin Endocrinol Metab. 2010;24(2):335–54.

Butler G, Kirk J. Paediatric endocrinology and diabetes. Oxford: OUP Press; 2011.

Creighton S, Chernausek SD, Romao R, Ransley P, Salle JP. Timing and nature of reconstructive surgery for disorders of sex development - introduction. J Pediatr Urol. 2012;8(6):602–10.

Crissman HP, Warner L, Gardner M, Carr M, Schast A, Quittner AL, et al. Children with disorders of sex development: a qualitative study of early parental experience. Int J Pediatr Endocrinol. 2011;2011(1):10.

Crouch NS, Creighton SM. Transition of care for adolescents with disorders of sex development. Nat Rev Endocrinol. 2014;10(7):436–42.

Davies K. Disorders of sex development–ambiguous genitalia. J Pediatr Nurs. 2016;31(4):463–6.

Devlin JK, Wilkinson A. Routine examination of the neonate. J Clin Examination. 2008;5:16–21.

Hewitt J, Warne GL. Management of disorders of sex development. Pediatr Health. 2009;3(1):1–65.

Hewitt JK, Warne GL. Mixed sex chromosome and ovotestiular DSD. In: Hutson JM, Warne GL, Grover SR, editors. Disorders of sex development: an integrated approach to management. Wurzberg: Springer; 2012a. p. 81–7.

Hewitt JK, Warne GL. 46, XY DSD. In: Hutson JM, Warne GL, Grover SR, editors. Disorders of sex development: an integrated approach to management. Wurzberg: Springer; 2012b. p. 63–80.

Hughes IA, Nihoul-Fekete C, Thomas B, Cohen-Kettenis PT. Consequences of the ESPE/LWPES guidelines for diagnosis and treatment of disorders of sex development. Best Pract Res Clin Endocrinol Metab. 2007;21(3):351–65.

Hughes IA, Morel Y, McElreavey K, Rogol A. Biological assessment of abnormal genitalia. J Pediatr Urol. 2012a;8(6):592–6.

Hughes IA, Davies JD, Bunch TI, Pasterski V, Mastroyannopoulou K, MacDougall J. Androgen insensitivity syndrome. Lancet. 2012b;380(9851):1419–28.

Ishii T, Matsuo N, Sato S, Ogata T, Tamai S, Anzo M, et al. Human chorionic gonadotropin stimulation test in prepubertal children with micropenis can accurately predict Leydig Cell function in pubertal or postpubertal adolescents. Horm Res Paediatr. 2015;84(5):305–10.

Kinsman L, Rotter T, James E, Snow P, Willis J. What is a clinical pathway? Development of a definition to inform the debate. BMC Med. 2010;8:31.

Kobayashi A, Behringer RR. Developmental genetics of the female reproductive tract in mammals. Nat Rev Genet. 2003;4(12):969–80.

Lee PA, Houk CP, Ahmed SF, Hughes IA. Society icwtpitICCoIobtLWPE, Endocrinology tESfP. Consensus statement on management of intersex disorders. Pediatrics. 2006;118(2):e488–500.

Lee P, Schober J, Nordenstrom A, Hoebeke P, Houk C, Looijenga L, et al. Review of recent outcome data of disorders of sex development (DSD): emphasis on surgical and sexual outcomes. J Pediatr Urol. 2012;8(6):611–5.

Lee PA, Nordenstrom A, Houk CP, Ahmed SF, Auchus R, Baratz A, et al. Global disorders of sex development update since 2006: perceptions, approach and care. Horm Res Paediatr. 2016;85(3):158–80.

Loughlin E. The family. In: Hutson JM, Warne GL, Grover SR, editors. Disorders of sex development: an integrated approach to management. Wurzberg: Springer; 2012. p. 193–201.

Mendonca BB, Inacio M, Costa EMF, Arnhold IJP, Silva FAQ, Nicolau W, et al. Male pseudohermaphroditism due to steroid 5 alpha reductase deficiency: diagnosis, psychological evaluation and management. Medicine. 1996;75(2):64–76.

Mendonca BB, Domenice S, Arnhold IJ, Costa EM. 46,XY disorders of sex development (DSD). Clin Endocrinol. 2009;70(2):173–87.

Mendonca BB, Costa EM, Belgorosky A, Rivarola MA, Domenice S. 46,XY DSD due to impaired androgen production. Best Pract Res Clin Endocrinol Metab. 2010;24(2):243–62.

Mongan NP, Tadokoro-Cuccaro R, Bunch T, Hughes IA. Androgen insensitivity syndrome. Best Pract Res Clin Endocrinol Metab. 2015;29(4):569–80.

Moshiri M, Chapman T, Fechner PY, Dubinsky TJ, Shnorhavorian M, Osman S, et al. Evaluation and management of disorders of sex development: multidisciplinary approach to a complex diagnosis. Radiographics. 2012;32(6):1599–618.

Odame I, Donaldson MD, Wallace AM, Cochran W, Smith PJ. Early diagnosis and management of 5a-reductase deficiency. Arch Dis Child. 1992;67:720–3.

Pasterski V, Prentice P, Hughes IA. Consequences of the Chicago consensus on disorders of sex development (DSD): current practices in Europe. Arch Dis Child. 2010;95(8):618–23.

Raine JE, Donaldson MDC, Gregory JW, van Vliet G, editors. Practical endocrinology and diabetes in children. 3rd ed. Chichester: Wiley - Blackwell; 2011.

Rey RA, Grinspon RP. Normal male sexual differentiation and aetiology of disorders of sex development. Best Pract Res Clin Endocrinol Metab. 2011;25(2):221–38.

Rodie M, McGowan R, Mayo A, Midgley P, Driver CP, Kinney M, et al. Factors that influence the decision to perform a karyotype in suspected disorders of sex development: lessons from the Scottish genital anomaly network register. Sex Dev. 2011;5(3):103–8.

Rothkopf AC, John RM. Understanding Disorders of Sexual Development. J Pediatr Nurs. 2014;29(5):e23–34.

Sanders C, Carter B, Goodacre L. Searching for harmony: parents' narratives about their child's genital ambiguity and reconstructive genital surgeries in childhood. J Adv Nurs. 2011;67(10):2220–30.

Sanders C, Edwards Z, Keegan K. Exploring stakeholder experiences of interprofessional teamwork in sex development outpatient clinics. J Interprof Care. 2017;31(3):376–85.

Schaeffer TL, Tryggestad JB, Mallappa A, Hanna AE, Krishnan S, Chernausek SD, et al. An evidence-based model of multidisciplinary care for patients and families affected by classical congenital adrenal hyperplasia due to 21-hydroxylase deficiency. Int J Pediatr Endocrinol. 2010;2010:692439.

Schober J, Nordenstrom A, Hoebeke P, Lee P, Houk C, Looijenga L, et al. Disorders of sex development: summaries of long-term outcome studies. J Pediatr Urol. 2012;8(6):616–23.

Tadokoro-Cuccaro R, Hughes IA. Androgen insensitivity syndrome. Curr Opin Endocrinol Diabetes Obes. 2014;21(6):499–503.

Vidal I, Gorduza DB, Haraux E, Gay CL, Chatelain P, Nicolino M, et al. Surgical options in disorders of sex development (dsd) with ambiguous genitalia. Best Pract Res Clin Endocrinol Metab. 2010;24(2):311–24.

Warne GL, Hewitt JK. 46,XX disorders of sex development. In: Hutson JM, Warne GL, Grover SR, editors. Disorders of sex development: an integrated approach to management. Wurzberg: Springer; 2012a. p. 53–61.

Warne GL, Hewitt JK. The medical management of disorders of sex development. In: Hutson JM, Warne GL, Grover SR, editors. Disorders of sex development: an integrated approach to management. Wurzberg: Springer; 2012b. p. 159–72.

White S, Sinclair A. The molecular basis of gonadal development and disorders of sex development. In: Hutson JM, Warne GL, Grover SR, editors. Disorders of sex development: an integrated approach to management. Wurzberg: Springer; 2012. p. 1–9.

Wisniewski AB, Migeon CJ, HFL M-B, Gearhart JP, Berkovitz GD, Brown TR, et al. Complete androgen insensitivity syndrome: long-term medical, surgical, and psychosexual outcome. J Clin Endocrinol Metab. 2000;85(8):2664–9.

Wisniewski AB, Chernausek SD, Kropp BP. Disorders of sex development: A guide for parents and physicians. Baltimore, MD: Johns Hopkins University Press; 2012.

Woodward M, Patwardhan N. Disorders of sex development. Surgery (Oxford). 2010;28(8):396–401.

Puberty: Normal, Delayed, and Precocious

4

Eileen Pyra and Wendy Schwarz

Contents

Abstract

Puberty is an important developmental stage for transition from childhood to adulthood. The process of puberty involves hormonal, physical, and psychological changes. Puberty is influenced by genetic and environmental aspects. The timing of puberty varies greatly between ethnicity, geography, and healthy individuals. Within the scope of puberty, it is considered precocious if the female is less than 8 years of age, and the male less than 9 years of age. Puberty is considered delayed if the female is 13 years of age and the male is 14 years of age with no pubertal development. Nurses' understanding of normal puberty and its variants during this time is crucial for helping support children and their families. Whether that be support for when normal puberty occurs or if it's occurring too early or too late. The diagnosis, treatment, and nursing implications of either precocious or delayed puberty will be discussed in this chapter.

Keywords

Puberty · Delayed puberty · Precocious puberty · Adolescent

E. Pyra · W. Schwarz (✉)
Alberta Children's Hospital, Endocrine Clinic,
Calgary, AB, Canada
e-mail: eileen.pyra@ahs.ca;
wendy.schwarz@ahs.ca

© Springer Nature Switzerland AG 2019
S. Llahana et al. (eds.), *Advanced Practice in Endocrinology Nursing*,
https://doi.org/10.1007/978-3-319-99817-6_4

Abbreviations

BA	Bone age
BMI	Body mass index
CA	Chronologic age
CAH	Congenital adrenal hyperplasia
CPP	Central precocious puberty
DHEA	Dehydroepiandrosterone
DHEA-S	Dehydroepiandrosterone sulphate
FSH	Follicle stimulating hormone
GnRH	Gonadotropin releasing hormone
HH	Hypogonadotropic hypogonadism
HPG	Hypothalamic pituitary gonad
HPO	Hypothalamic pituitary ovarian
IGF-1	Insulin-like growth factor 1
IM	Intramuscular
IPP	Incomplete precocious puberty
IU/L	International units/L
LH	Luteinizing hormone
MAS	McCune Albright syndrome
mg	Milligram
mL	Milliliter
MRI	Magnetic resonance imaging
NHANES-III	National Health and Nutrition Examination Survey
OCP	Oral contraceptive pills
PA	Premature adrenarche
PDS	Pubertal Development Scale
PPP	Peripheral precocious puberty
PROS	Paediatric Research in Office Settings
PT	Premature thelarche
PWS	Prader-Willi syndrome
SC	Subcutaneous

Key Terms

- **Adrenarche:** increases in the secretion of adrenal androgen precursors, mainly dehydroepiandrosterone (DHEA) facilitate the appearance of pubic/axillary hair.
- **Androgen:** is responsible for sexual development in males and is produced by the testes. Women have smaller amounts of androgens that are produced in the ovaries. The most

well-known androgen is testosterone, which is responsible for developing the secondary sex characteristics in men.

- **Estradiol:** is a steroid hormone made from cholesterol. The main function is to mature and maintain the female reproductive system. Estradiol also promotes development of breast tissue and increases bone and cartilage thickness.
- **Follicle Stimulating Hormone (FSH):** is released by the anterior pituitary, for pubertal development and function of the ovaries and testes. In females, this hormone stimulates the growth of ovarian follicles. In males, follicle stimulating hormone acts on the Sertoli cells of the testes to stimulate sperm production (spermatogenesis).
- **Gonadotropin Releasing Hormone (GnRH):** is produced and secreted by the hypothalamus to the anterior pituitary, where it stimulates the production of Follicle Stimulating Hormone (FSH) and Luteinizing Hormone (LH).
- **Hypothalamic-Pituitary-Gonadal Axis (HPG):** is the coordinated production of GnRH, LH, FSH, and sex steroids (testosterone and estrogen). The hypothalamus releases gonadotropin-releasing hormone (GnRH) in a pulsatile fashion. In response, the pituitary releases follicle stimulating hormone (FSH) and luteinizing hormone (LH), both of which ultimately control gonadal function.
- **Luteinizing Hormone (LH):** is a gonadotropic hormone produced in the anterior pituitary. In males, LH stimulates Leydig cells in the testes to produce testosterone. In females, LH binds to receptors in ovaries to regulate the production eggs.
- **Pubarche:** is the appearance of pubic hair as the results of rising levels of androgens secreted by the adrenal glands.
- **Spermarche:** is sperm development in boys, at puberty. Spermarche typically occurs between ages 11–15. It starts with the beginning of the development of secondary sexual characteristics, which in boys includes facial hair, voice deepening, and body growth.
- **Testosterone:** Testosterone also exerts effects all around the body to generate male

characteristics such as increased muscle mass, enlargement of the larynx to generate a deep voice, and the growth of facial and body hair.

- **Thelarche:** is the onset of female breast development. Isolated breast development in girls younger than 8 years of age is considered premature thelarche. It usually is benign but may signify a more complicated condition.

> **Key Points**
> - Puberty is an important developmental stage for transition from childhood to adulthood that involves hormonal, physical, and psychological changes.
> - There is increasing evidence of the impact of genetic and environmental influences on puberty. Recent advances have helped to elucidate the genetic determinants of pubertal timing.
> - Delayed puberty can be sorted into three main categories: hypergonadotropic hypogonadism, hypogonadotropic hypogonadism, and functional (or transient) hypogonadotropic hypogonadism.
> - The main goal for the management of precocious puberty is to prevent early fusion of the epiphyseal growth plate allowing for the attainment of adult height within the individual's genetic potential.
> - Nurses have a key role in early identification of abnormalities in pubertal development and referral to pediatric endocrinologist for evaluation.

4.1 Pubertal Development

4.1.1 Introduction

Puberty is a developmental phase that is the result of a process of complex transformations involving both physical and psychological maturation. This process involves a period of rapid growth, development of secondary sexual characteristics,

maturation of reproductive functions, bone mass accrual, as well as psychological and cognitive development. Genetics, hormones, health status, and environmental factors can influence this process (Lifshitz 2006). Although puberty usually occurs in a predictable pattern, it can be variable. Concerns about puberty and the changes that occur during puberty are some of the most common questions for nurses caring for children.

4.1.2 Regulation of Puberty

4.1.2.1 Neuroendocrine Regulation of Puberty

Activation of the hypothalamic-pituitary-gonadal (HPG) axis by gonadotropin releasing hormone (GnRH) results in the anterior pituitary releasing luteinizing hormone (LH) and follicle stimulating hormone (FSH). LH primarily acts on the interstitial cells of the gonads stimulating the production of androgens, while FSH primarily stimulates the ovarian follicles to produce estradiol, inhibin, and gametes (egg and sperm), GnRH release is pulsatile in nature and occurs mostly at night in early puberty. As puberty progresses, the GnRH develops into an adult pattern throughout the day (Wolf and Long 2016).

4.1.2.2 Genetics

A large number of genes are involved in the complex process of initiating puberty. The discovery of Kisspeptins and G-protein has increased our understanding of the GnRH control mechanisms. Kisspeptins are series of peptides that are required for the activation of the hypothalamic-pituitary-gonadal (HPG) axis. During puberty, the *KISS1* is activated and generates the pulsatile GnRH to activate the HPG-axis (Kaur et al. 2012).

4.1.2.3 Timing of Puberty

The timing of puberty varies widely between individuals but tends to run closely within families. The first activation of the HPG system occurs in mid gestation. This is followed by a second activation in early postnatal life, sometimes referred to as "mini-puberty". The third activation occurs at the time of puberty. The onset of puberty could either be the result of the disappearance of inhibitory factors, or the occurrence of stimulatory inputs, or both (Gajdos et al. 2010). Timing varies in the general population and is influenced by genetic and environmental factors Palmert and Hirschhorn (2003) suggest that 50–80% of the variations seen in pubertal timing is caused by genetic factors. Even taking into account the environmental factors, genetic factors are thought to play a more pivotal role.

Timing also varies within different population groups. From the National Health and Nutrition Examination Survey (NHANES III), the difference in Caucasian girls' age of puberty is 10.65–12.55 years, African American 9.7–12.6 years, and Mexican American 10.05–12.25 years. The timing of puberty in boys has not been as well documented. From the NHANES III study, it was found that Caucasian boys reached Tanner II pubic hair at median age of 12 years, African American at 11.2 years, and Hispanic at 12.3 years (Krieger et al. 2015). Despite ongoing discussion, data remains inconsistent on whether there is a trend toward earlier puberty. However, if there is a change in socioeconomic status, it may shift the age of puberty (Lahoti and Sills 2015).

4.1.2.4 Nutrition

Nutritional factors have been known to have an influence on pubertal timing. Nutrition during fetal life and early postnatal life has shown to have effects on physiologic development throughout life (Lifshitz 2006). Body mass index (BMI) is an important factor in the timing of puberty. A higher BMI is associated with early maturation; lower BMI is associated with delayed pubertal development.

4.1.2.5 Endocrine Disruptors

Endocrine disruptors are natural or synthetic environmental chemicals or pollutants that can alter or affect the normal physiologic endocrine process. Endocrine disruptors bind to hormone receptors and impede their function, by way of suppressing or activating the hormonal activity. These chemicals and pollutants are found in agriculture, cleaning products, cosmetics, plastic compounds, and are stored in fat tissue (Lahoti and Sills 2015).

4.1.3 Physical Changes During Puberty

4.1.3.1 Growth

The pubertal growth spurt accounts for 15–18% of final adult height. It is the fastest period of growth after the first 2 years of life (Lifshitz 2006). Estrogen, produced in the ovaries of girls and the aromatization of androgens in boys, accounts for the accelerated growth during puberty. The pubertal growth spurt is also the result of gonadal sex steroids, growth hormone, and insulin-like growth factor 1 (IGF-1). The growth spurt in girls coincides with the start of breast development (Tanner II). In boys, the growth spurt starts with a testicular volume of 10–12 mL (Tanner III). Thus, the growth spurt is a later pubertal development for boys, occurring an average of 2 years later than girls. Along with increase in linear growth, there is an increase in weight and percentage of body fat. Leptin regulates the amount of body fat. Leptin is considered the link between adipose tissue and growth (Wolf and Long 2016).

4.1.3.2 Bone Maturation

During puberty, bone maturation accelerates and epiphysis becomes fused. This maturation appears to parallel pubertal development (Lazar and Phillip 2012). Bone age is assessed based on the changes in the width of the epiphysis, the appearance of ossification centers, capping of the epiphysis and the fusion of the epiphysis (Weise et al. 2001). Bone age X-rays are universally accepted as a diagnostic tool, due to the minimal radiation to the bone and gonads. The most commonly used method for determining bone age is Greulich and Pyle Atlas (1959). This is a simple way of comparing the patient's X-ray of the left hand and wrist to that of the corresponding age and gender of the patient. It should be kept in mind that this is a subjective analysis. Greulich and Pyle are also based on Caucasian children in upper middle class in 1931–1942 and thus may be inaccurate assessment of other ethnicities.

4.1.3.3 Body Composition

In females during puberty, there is an overall increase in lean body mass; however, the percentage of lean body mass decreases due to the increase in adipose mass. The percentage of body fat is related to menstrual function. In males, lean body mass increases during puberty, which reflects increasing muscle mass and decreasing adiposity (Freedman et al. 2002).

4.1.4 Development of Secondary Sexual Characteristics

4.1.4.1 Female

Puberty onset for girls is generally within the range of age 8–13 years. Euling et al. have reported a decline in the age of onset of puberty since 1940. This has been linked to increasing rates of obesity (Krieger et al. 2015; Freedman et al. 2002).

Acceleration in growth is typically the first manifestation of puberty in girls. The second sign of puberty is breast budding, known as thelarche. Menarche typically occurs 2–2.5 years after thelarche. At the same time, pubic hair, known as pubarche, occurs as the result of increased adrenal androgen secretion. However, in as many as 20% of girls pubarche may precede thelarche (Lifshitz 2006).

The hormonal changes are initiated by the process of releasing gonadotropin-releasing hormone (GnRH) from the hypothalamus. LH, FSH, and estradiol levels will increase before any physical changes are seen. The levels of these hormones will further increase throughout puberty resulting in the physical changes that characterize puberty. These changes include breast maturity, genital growth (labia majora), maturation of the vaginal/uterus/endometrium, and change in body composition (female fat pattern). Growth of the uterus and elongation of the vagina occur at the same time that multiple follicles are developing in the ovaries. FSH promotes the growth of ovarian

follicles and LH promotes the ovary to produce estradiol (Lifshitz 2006).

Menarche refers to the first menstrual bleed and typically occurs at Tanner stage IV breast and is rare before Tanner stage III (Lahoti and Sills 2015). The timing of menarche is influenced by genetic and environmental factors. With estradiol production, the vaginal mucosa is stimulated resulting in a thin white vaginal discharge. This process called leucorrhea is typically seen 6–12 months before menarche. The first menarche is often not associated with ovulation. In the first 1–2 years, the cycles are anovulatory and irregular. Cycles typically last 2–7 days and the average blood loss is 30 mL, ranging from 20 to 60 mL. There is international variation on the age of menarche related to socioeconomic conditions, nutrition, and access to health care (Gajdos et al. 2010). On average, girls may gain 4–6 cm of height after menarche (Fig. 4.1) (Lifshitz 2006).

Breast development is estrogen driven and may be asymmetrical and can be tender to palpation. The NHANES III study as well as the US Paediatric Research in Office Settings (PROS) have reported that breast development in girls occurs earlier than previously reported. Both studies reported earlier breast development; however, they did not find any decrease in the age of menarche. Other studies, from Denmark, China, and Europe have also shown a decrease in the age of breast development (Wolf and Long 2016; Lahoti and Sills 2015).

4.1.4.2 Male

Boys typically begin puberty between 9 and 14 years of age. Puberty is marked by testicular enlargement, penile length increase, and pubic hair growth (pubarche). There is a progressive rise in LH, FSH, and testosterone as a result of the upregulating of the hypothalamic-pituitary-testicular axis (Freedman et al. 2002). Boys typically identify pubic hair growth as the first identified sign of puberty. However, an increase in testicular size/volume, >3 mL, is the first physical sign of puberty. There can be an asymmetrical development of the testes. Axillary hair begins at mid-puberty due to the increase in androgen secretion. Other androgen-sensitive

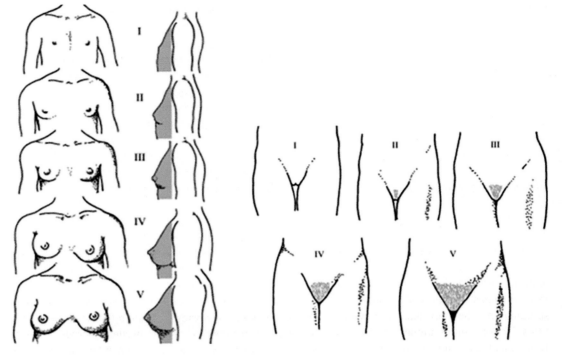

Fig. 4.1 Tanner stage of pubertal development

areas, including face, chest, back, arms, and legs, will then begin showing signs of hair development. Spermarche is the onset of sperm production. The average age of spermarche is 14 years and Tanner III for testes and pubic hair development (Lifshitz 2006; Wolf and Long 2016).

Normal variations in androgen and estrogen ratios can lead to pubertal gynecomastia. This can occur in approximately 50% of boys and typically resolves within 2 years (Lahoti and Sills 2015). It has also been speculated that it may occur in up to two-thirds of pubertal boys. It generally occurs in early or mid-puberty and will plateau at approximately 1 year with regression by 18 months. This is a common variant in normal pubertal development and does not usually indicate underlying abnormalities. However, pathologic causes should be considered (Lifshitz 2006).

4.1.5 Nursing Considerations

Assessment of sexual development or Tanner staging (or "sexual maturity rating" is becoming

a more accepted term) provides a consistent tool to evaluate the progression of puberty (Marshall and Tanner 1969). Historically, puberty has been assessed by a physical exam, with the adolescent undressed. With the perceived intrusiveness of this examination, the Pubertal Development Scale (PDS) has been developed (Wolf and Long 2016). This tool focuses on the development of secondary sexual characteristics including: body hair, skin changes, growth spurt, facial hair, deepening of the voice in boys, and breast development and menarche in girls. The characteristics are rated on a 4-point scale. However, concerns have been raised with this form of assessment over the possibility of inaccurate reporting by the teen and the possible regression of the teen's self-reporting.

Teaching about testicular self-examination should be initiated during puberty. Testicular examination is helpful to identify testicular anomalies, as well as assessing pubertal progression.

It is important to properly examine breast tissue to distinguish actual breast tissue versus adipose tissue in the moderately to severely obese pubertal female or male. For male gynecomastia, a thorough history should include whether there is drug use. Marijuana has been documented to cause gynecomastia in boys (Lahoti and Sills 2015).

Growth velocity is important to monitor in all children during puberty. Variation, or deviation, from the expected growth pattern may lead to detection of medical issues. Systemic illness may first present with poor growth before the onset of symptoms (i.e., inflammatory bowel disease, Celiac). The normal variation of growth between the sexes may cause concern for parents. These parents may be unaware of the different timing of the pubertal growth spurt between males and females (Lifshitz 2006).

Menses is often referred to as the fourth vital sign. What is a normal menstrual period? Talk to your patient to assess the frequency or regularity of their cycles, as well as the adolescent's understanding of their cycles. The World Health Organization international multicenter study found that the timing between first cycle was longer than 40 days in 38% of the girls, with the median being 34 days (Adams Hillard 2014; Bourguignon and Juul 2012). Cycles should increase in regularity with time. If they do not, then other pathology should be investigated, i.e., polycystic ovarian syndrome, eating disorders, thyroid disease or primary ovarian insufficiency. Chronic menstrual abnormalities may be associated with future health risks such as anemia, low bone density, and metabolic and cardiovascular risk (Fig. 4.2) (Wolf and Long 2016).

WHAT IS A NORMAL PERIOD?

- Start before age 15
- Last one week or less
- Are between 21–45 days from the first day of one period to the first day of the next period
- When bleeding, you fill less than one pad per hour

If your periods are not "normal" talk with your clinician

Fig. 4.2 Questions to assess menses

4.1.6 Behavior Changes Associated with Puberty

Biologic as well as social processes influence the behavior changes that occur during puberty. For the purpose of this chapter, we will focus on the biologic process. Hormonal changes affect anatomy and physiology as well as psychological changes through changes in the brain structure and function (Bourguignon and Juul 2012; Berenbaum et al. 2015; Giedd 2015). Adolescent psychological development is influenced by different aspects of puberty. Hormone-behavior links depend on context. As an example, a boy with high salivary testosterone levels may have genetic reasons or may have recently participated in an activity that increases testosterone (i.e., sexual activity or high intensity sports) (Duke et al. 2014). Studies suggest a relationship between testosterone and aggressive behavior, but results are not consistent across studies. Similarly, studies report a correlational relationship between estrogen and depression or aggressive tendencies in girls, but more research is also needed (Susman et al. 2003, 2010).

4.1.7 Delayed Puberty

Delayed puberty is defined as the lack of pubertal development by an age that is 2–2.5 standard deviations beyond the population mean (Abitbol et al. 2016). Delayed puberty affects approximately 2% of adolescents and can be a source of anxiety for the adolescent and their family. The accepted norms for delayed puberty are a chronological age of 13 for girls and 14 for boys. A delay in progression from onset of menarche of >4–5 years is considered prolonged. Delayed puberty may result from the dysfunction of the HPG or from secondary causes such as chronic illness or malnutrition (Palmert and Dunkel 2012).

4.1.7.1 Etiology of Pubertal Delay
Although the differential diagnosis for delayed puberty is varied, the most common cause is constitutional delay for both girls and boys.

Constitutional delay is seen when the HPG axis is delayed and the puberty starts at the far end of the normal spectrum. Constitutional delay should be a diagnosis of exclusion after other causes have been ruled out (Palmert and Dunkel 2012).

There is increasing evidence of the impact of genetic and environmental influences on puberty. Several genes have recently been identified as sources for hypothalamic dysfunction. These include, but are not limited to: leptin receptor deficiency mutations, kisspeptins, kisspeptin receptor *GPR54*, *GNRHR* gene mutations, X-linked Kallman syndrome, and transcription factor mutations (i.e., *PROP1*, *HESX1*) (Fenichel 2012).

Leptin receptor deficiency mutations are associated with delayed puberty. Leptin receptors are present in the hypothalamic region and act as a bridge between reproductive function and energy balance. Replacement of leptin can induce puberty if given at the correct timing in puberty (Farooqi et al. 1999).

Kisspeptins (*KISS1*) are series of peptides that are activated and generate pulsatile GnRH and enable the HPG-axis activation (recent advances in understanding and management). With the *KISS1* receptor mutation primary hypogonadotropic hypogonadism occurs (Kaur et al. 2012).

Environmental exposures such as chemicals (natural or synthetic) can alter normal physiologic endocrine processes. This alteration is often referred to as endocrine disruptors. The chemicals and pollutants accumulate in the environment and are introduced into the body through a variety of ways (e.g., through water, air, foods). These endocrine disruptors bind to hormone receptor and affect the signalling, resulting in suppression (or activation) of that hormone (Howell and Shalet 1998).

4.1.7.2 Categories of Pubertal Delay

Delayed puberty can be sorted into three main categories: *hypergonadotropic* hypogonadism, *hypogonadotropic* hypogonadism, and *functional* (or transient) hypogonadotropic hypogonadism.

Hypergonadotropic hypogonadism is characterized by elevated levels of LH and FSH due to lack of negative feedback from the gonads, while hypogonadotropic hypogonadism is characterized by low levels of LH and FSH due to pituitary or hypothalamic disorders. Functional hypogonadotropic hypogonadism is characterized by delayed maturation of the HPG axis due to an underlying medical condition (Palmert and Dunkel 2012).

Hypergonadotropic hypogonadism may be genetic or acquired. It is categorized by elevated FSH and LH, due to gonadal failure. This failure is caused by the HPG axis being activated and the feedback loop from the sex steroids to the hypothalamus is not present, resulting in elevated LH and FSH. Genetic causes include: Turner syndrome, gonadal dysgenesis, or androgen receptor mutations. Acquired causes include: exposure to chemotherapy or radiation, presence of antibodies (ovarian or gonadotropin), as well as infectious disease such as mumps, shigella, malaria, and varicella (Lifshitz 2006).

Hypogonadotropic hypogonadism (HH) is usually due to hypothalamic dysfunction. This dysfunction may be a delay in the HPG axis maturation resulting in the impaired secretion of GnRH and low levels of gonadotropins (LH and FSH). Causes of HH range from treatable underlying conditions such as a lack of GnRH synthesis (i.e., Kallman syndrome), a defect in the release of GnRH (i.e., leptin or *DAX-1* gene mutations), chronic illness, hypopituitarism (i.e., congenital or acquired from pituitary or hypothalamic lesions and tumors), syndromes (i.e., Prader-Willi, Noonan, cystic fibrosis), or under nutrition: intentional (anorexia, elite athlete) or unintentional. Some medications can also disrupt the HPG axis, such as antipsychotic drugs. Adverse events with stress can also interrupt pubertal development (Palmert and Dunkel 2012; Howell and Shalet 1998; Wei and Crowne 2016).

Kallman syndrome is the most common form of HH. The occurrence is 1:50000 in females and 1:10000 in males. It is usually characterized with anosmia (lack of sense of smell). Most cases are sporadic; however, 5% have a mutation of the *Kal1* gene. Midline defects, (i.e., cleft lip/palate) are also associated with Kallman syndrome. Defect in the release of GnRH–DAX-1 plays a role in sexual differentiation and development of the adrenal gland, hypothalamus, hypophysis, and gonads. Leptin gene deficiency can lead to obesity which is known to cause delayed puberty due to hypogonadotropic hypogonadism.

Hypopituitarism (congenital), septo-optic dysplasia, absent septum pellucidum, or any midline defect can be a cause of hypogonadotropic hypogonadism. Craniopharyngioma is the most common childhood cranial lesion and surgery may lead to hypogonadotropic hypogonadism. Any cranial trauma such as head injury, or infections, infiltrative disease may also cause hypogonadotropic hypogonadism.

Prader-Willi Syndrome (PWS) is characterized by massive obesity which leads to hypothalamic dysfunction. Hypogonadism is a consistent feature of both males and females with PWS. Clinical presentation includes genital hypoplasia, delayed or incomplete puberty, and infertility in the clear majority.

Females with Noonan syndrome have normal pubertal development and ovarian function. Affected boys typically have undescended testes and abnormal Leydig cell function.

Functional hypogonadotropic hypogonadism is typically due to underlying chronic illness, such as inflammatory illness (i.e., celiac disease), thyroid disease, anorexia, bulimia, or excessive exercise that can cause poor growth and delay in puberty (Lifshitz 2006; Harrington and Palmert 2012).

4.1.7.3 Delayed Puberty in Girls

The current average age for a diagnosis of delayed puberty in girls in the United States is 13 years for breast development and 15 years for menarche (Lee 1980). Hypogonadotropic hypogonadism, also referred to as ovarian failure, is a common cause of delayed puberty in girls (i.e., Turner syndrome) (Refer to Chap. 40). Ovarian failure is also seen with autoimmune syndromes such as Addison's disease, type 1 diabetes, hyperparathyroidism, and others (Lifshitz 2006). Approximately 50% of girls who have pelvic radiation will develop primary ovarian failure (Howell and Shalet 1998).

HH as a cause of pubertal delay in girls is most commonly due to constitutional delay. In this population of girls, puberty will start spontaneously and will be maintained. There is often a family history of delayed puberty. Permanent hypogonadotropic hypogonadism is seen with defects in the GnRH secretion (i.e., Kallman syndrome) (Harrington and Palmert 2012).

Girls with normal development of secondary sexual characteristic who have a delay or absence of menarche should be worked up for an anatomical defect (e.g., Mayer-Rokitansky-Küster-Hauser), anovulatory state, or disorders of intersex (i.e., androgen insensitivity).

Primary amenorrhea is defined as no menses by age 16. However, any girl who has not had menses by age 15 should have an evaluation for causes. Primary amenorrhea implies a more permanent dysfunction of the hypothalamic pituitary ovarian (HPO) axis (Lifshitz 2006; Palmert and Dunkel 2012; Harrington and Palmert 2012).

It is well documented that chronic or severe illness will impede the HPG function. For example, the female athlete triad is a syndrome characterized by the coexisting diagnosis of an eating disorder, amenorrhoea, decreased bone density that is associated with morbidity and increased mortality. Figure 4.3 depicts the interaction between the eating disorders, HPG axis, and bone.

4.1.7.4 Delayed Puberty in Boys

Hypogonadotropic hypogonadism, also referred to as testicular failure, may cause pubertal delay in boys. The most common cause is Klinefelter syndrome. Other causes may be diminished testicular function (i.e., anorchia or vanishing testes syndrome), atrophic testes, Leydig cell aplasia, torsion, trauma, infection (mumps, coxsackie), chemotherapy, and radiation. Elevated gonadotropins are also seen in hepatic and renal disease (Lifshitz 2006; Palmert and Dunkel 2012).

Klinefelter syndrome occurs in about 1:500–1000 males. It is typically diagnosed in amniocentesis or during childhood. In some instances,

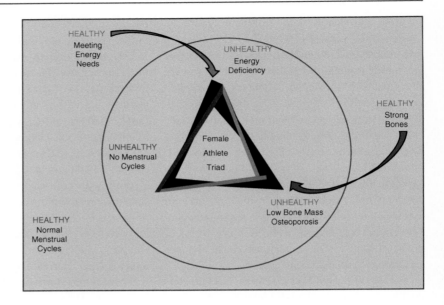

Fig. 4.3 Female athlete triad

delayed puberty and its subsequent work up may lead to the diagnosis. A delayed diagnosis may be made when infertility is an issue. Typical features are tall stature, disproportionate limb length, poor muscular development, micropenis, small firm testes, borderline IQ, poor social skills, and gynecomastia. The pubertal delay is caused by progressive hyalinization of testicular tissue and the seminiferous tubules (Lifshitz 2006; Palmert and Dunkel 2012). (Refer to Chap. 10).

In Leydig cell aplasia, the degree of masculinization is dependent on the mutation, ranging from micropenis to genital ambiguity. Testes may be small to normal size, FSH is typically normal, testosterone is low, and LH is elevated due to the inability to respond to LH or insensitivity (Lifshitz 2006; Palmert and Dunkel 2012).

Hypogonadotropic hypogonadism as a cause of pubertal delay in boys is most commonly due to constitutional delay. The cause however, could be transient or permanent. Transient causes include constitutional delay or chronic/systemic illness (i.e., inflammatory disease such as Crohn's). Permanent causes could be the result of genetic mutations, defects in the HPG—axis, hypopituitarism, or genetic syndromes (i.e.,

Kallman syndrome (see above) (Harrington and Palmert 2012).

Refer to Table 4.1 for a summary of common causes of delayed puberty.

4.1.7.5 Evaluation of Delayed Puberty

A detailed history and physical exam must be obtained with any child presenting with pubertal delay. The detailed history should include family history with timing of puberty (of parents, siblings, and extended family), parental heights (to calculate mid-parental height), birth and pregnancy details, childhood growth patterns, height velocity, consanguinity with the parents, previous illnesses, nutritional and exercise habits, psychological stressors, use of medications, exposure to chemotherapy or radiation, any syndromes diagnosed with the patient or relatives. A complete review of systems to assess for possible metabolic or hormonal causes, neurological symptoms (i.e., headaches, seizures, fundoscopic exam for papilledema), or developmental delay. Physical exam should include accurate height and weight (and plotting on growth chart), standing and sitting height, arm span, upper and lower segment ratio, Tanner staging, testing of smell, size and location of testes, and neurological assessment.

Table 4.1 Common causes for delayed puberty

Hypogonadotropic hypogonadism or HH		
Functional HH	Permanent HH	*Girls*
Hypothyroidism	*Genetic:*	Turner syndrome
Diabetes mellitus	Congenital or isolated/idiopathic HH	XX and XY gonadal dysgenesis
Growth hormone deficiency	Kallman syndrome	Primary ovarian failure
Cystic fibrosis	Septo-optic dysplasia	Oophoritis
Inflammatory bowel disease	Prader-Willi syndrome	*Boys*
Celiac disease	Laurence-Moon and Barder-Biedl syndromes	Gonadal dysgenesis
Systemic lupus	CHARGE syndrome	Vanishing testes syndrome
Juvenile rheumatoid arthritis	*Acquired:*	Testicular biosynthetic defects
Sickle cell disease	CNS tumors (astrocytoma, craniopharyngioma, germinoma, pituitary tumor	Orchitis
Thalassemia	Langerhans' histocytosis	*Both sexes*
Chronic renal disease	Granulomatous or post-infection lesions of the CNS	Chemotherapy
Anorexia nervosa	CNS trauma, surgery, or radiation	Radiation
Malnutrition		Trauma
Intense exercise		Other syndromes (Noonan)

Baseline laboratory assessment of the child presenting with delayed puberty may include: complete blood count, thyroid function tests, electrolytes, albumin, creatinine, liver function tests, sedimentation rate, prolactin, morning serum cortisol, insulin-like growth factor 1 (IGF-1), FSH, LH, estradiol, testosterone, dehydroepi-androsterone sulfate (DHEA-S), sex hormone-binding globulin, and karyotype. As a second line of testing, a GnRH stimulation test would be beneficial in evaluation of hypogonadotropic hypogonadism. Other testing may be indicated based on patient's symptoms and signs as well as family history (Palmert and Dunkel 2012).

Baseline radiologic assessment includes bone age (BA), which is helpful to distinguish between functional and permanent hypogonadism and is useful for adult height prediction. Although BA readings are qualitative rather than quantitative, it helps to round out the clinical picture that can lead to diagnosis and treatment options.

A pituitary or brain magnetic resonance imaging (MRI) is indicated only if there is a suspicion of intracranial lesion or defects, based on the physical exam and history. Ultrasound is useful in phenotypical males with cryptorchidism or phenotypical females suspected of androgen insensitivity; a pelvic ultrasound may be part of the initial assessment. However, in most cases of delayed puberty, this would be deferred or not done at all. Table 4.2 lists common tests utilized in the assessment of delayed puberty (Lifshitz 2006; Palmert and Dunkel 2012).

4.1.7.6 Treatment/Management of Delayed Puberty

Constitutional delay, in some cases, causes significant psychological stress, for the patient and the parents. If there is clinical or biochemical evidence that puberty has started, and the calculated adult height is appropriate, reassurance is often sufficient. However, induction of a pubertal growth spurt can be managed with a variety of medications. If the cause of delayed puberty that is due to a chronic illness, then the illness must be appropriately managed as much as possible to promote physiological puberty.

For girls, a low dose estrogen may be used to induce breast development. A starting dose of ethinylestradiol (a synthetic estrogen) at 2 micrograms/day, with a gradual increase to 20 µg/day, will allow for pubertal growth and gradual breast development. Natural estrogen (17β-estradiol) has much less metabolic effect and is prescribed in 0.2–2 mg/day either orally or by transdermal

Table 4.2 Assessment of delayed puberty

History	Examination	Investigations
Short stature	Serial accurate heights/weights	Baseline pituitary function TSH/FT4, prolactin, cortisol, IGF-1, electrolytes, karyotype
Parental history—age of puberty	Pubertal staging—Tanner	LH, FSH, DHEA-S, SHBG, testosterone/estradiaol
History of chronic illness or prolonged medication	Evidence of underlying chronic disease	CBC, ESR or sed rate, creatinine
Visual disturbances, headaches	Fundoscopy for signs of papilloedema	MRI
History of cranial or gonadal radiation or chemotherapy	Visual field	
Primary Amenorrhea		Pelvic ultrasound
Anosmia	Testing for sense of smell	
Learning difficulties	Inquire about problems with school or if an educational plan is implemented	
Behavior problems	Screen for behavioral concerns	Refer to psychologist for evaluation
Dietary history—evidence of malnutrition	Evidence of malnutrition	Albumin, calcium, magnesium
Exercise history	Inquire about amount and type of physical exercise	

Table 4.3 Treatment options for pubertal induction

Male		
Injection	Testosterone enantate	Start at 25–50 mg every 4 weeks for 3–6 months
IM or SC		Increase gradually every 6 months to 100–150 mg every 4 weeks
Transdermal	Metered dose 2%	Start at 10–20 mg (1–2 metered applications) daily
		Increase by 10 mg every 6 months to 60–80 mg
Female		
Oral	Ethinyl osstradiol Norethisterone 5 mg or medroxyprogesterone acetate 5 mg	Year 1–2 µg daily Year 2–4 µg daily Year 2.5–6 µg daily Year 3–8 µg daily Year 3.5–10 µg daily Year 4–20–30 µg daily—adult dose, with the addition of progesterone
	17β-estradiol	Initial dose 5 µg/kg daily Increase every 6–12 months to 10 µg/kg daily
Transdermal	17β-estradiol	Year 1—¼ patch twice a week Year 2—½ patch twice a week Year 2.5—alternate ½ and whole patch twice per week Year 3—whole patch twice per week

Adapted from Wei and Crowne (2016)

patch. Transdermal patches for girls are available in weekly patches. Once the full dose, of estrogen, is attained progesterone is added. Refer to Table 4.3 for dosing information. This can be done with as oral contraceptive pills (OCP). Some clinicians may prefer two separate compounds of; estrogen and progesterone. However, this may pose difficulties since the girl and her parent need to remember when to take the progesterone in combination with the estrogen. This increases the risk of issues with compliance and efficacy (Palmert and Dunkel 2012).

For boys, a low dose testosterone can be initiated to treat pubertal delay. See Table 4.3 for dosing information. Traditionally, testosterone has been given as an intramuscular (IM) injection. However, more recent data has shown that it can be given subcutaneously (SC) (Fraser et al. 2017). This can lead to patients and their families being taught self-administration. Transdermal patches of testosterone are also available and recommended areas of application are shoulders, upper arms, and abdomen. Testosterone is also available in a gel, supplied in a pump dispenser. Patients should be cautioned about contact with others and transference of the gel to other people. Side effects of androgen replacement therapy are associated with their physiologic effects (i.e., acne, oily skin, gynecomastia) consistent with puberty-related changes. Aromatase inhibitors that block the conversion of androgens to estrogens (and delay epiphyseal closure) are being investigated in clinical trials as a potential therapeutic approach for delayed puberty. Girls and boys with permanent hypogonadism are treated with initial sex-steroid therapy, like patients with constitutional delay, and doses are gradually increased to adult replacement levels. When fertility is desired, induction requires treatment with pulsatile GnRH or exogenous gonadotropins (Palmert and Dunkel 2012).

4.1.7.7 Psychological Issues Related to Delayed Puberty

Few studies have been done to look at the short- and long-term psychological impact of delayed puberty. In the limited studies that have been done, there are reports that delayed puberty in girls has more successful outcomes with regard to academic achievement and depressive symptoms, but late maturing boys had negative impact on school achievement. Among boys, delayed puberty has been linked to elevated depressive symptoms, externalizing behaviors (e.g., disruptive behavior, substance abuse) (Graber 2013). Boys may express concern about lagging in sports due to height and less muscular than peers. Girls may feel different from their peers due to lack of breast development and delayed menarche. It is important to remind adolescents and their parents that the hormonal and psychosocial experiences of puberty show significant individual differences, and one can expect the same with delayed puberty (Baams et al. 2015).

4.1.7.8 Nursing Considerations

Nurses have a key role in early identification of abnormalities in pubertal development and referral to pediatric endocrinologist for evaluation. Accurate anthropometric measurements and plotting on growth charts is critical for early recognition of abnormalities in development and growth.

The nurse has a key role as a member of the health care team to help improve the pediatric patient and family's experiences. Important aspects of the nurse's role include acknowledging the child or adolescent's vulnerability and lack of the experience with the health care system, their need for respect, privacy and confidentiality, communicating at an appropriate developmental level, and acknowledging their developing need for independence.

When the child/adolescent is diagnosed with an endocrine disorder, they may feel vulnerable. As with any new diagnosis, the patient and family should be made aware of any resources that may be available for them. These resources may include support groups, measures to help them attend appointments or access to treatments, and ways to deal with obstacles preventing them from obtaining the health care they need (e.g., school restrictions, travel, and other commitments).

The attitude of the health care staff should be respectful, supportive, and honest. Adolescents are particularly sensitive to the behavior of others and coping with a new medical diagnosis, such as delayed puberty, may heighten that sensitivity. The staff should be empathetic and non-judgmental.

During adolescence, privacy is a very important aspect of their interactions with the health care system. A routine genital examination may be a source of embarrassment and may be very stressful for the adolescent. The nurse should explain the need for the examination and offer privacy for undressing (behind a curtain, or alone in the examination room) and a gown to cover themselves. Often adolescents do not want their parents present during the examination, however, this should still be discussed with the adolescent and parent. Alternatively, a chaperone may be offered (another nurse). This also safeguards the clinician against false accusations of impropriety.

The nurse should speak to the adolescent with respect, as well as with clarity and honesty. It is important to use active listening skills to see what is important to the adolescent. The nurse should avoid a "lecture-like" tone and avoid sounding confrontational, superior, or condescending. Make sure that the discussion is age appropriate which gives the adolescent the opportunity to ask questions. The individual adolescent should have the opportunity to be involved in the decision-making, regarding clinical investigations and treatment options. Explanations and information about hormonal replacement must be given to the patient and family. A discussion about future fertility and options available should also be discussed.

4.1.8 Precocious Puberty

This section will explore precocious puberty in terms of the clinical definition, the causes, how it presents, how it is diagnosed, the treatment options, as well as the expected outcomes and nursing implications related to the care of the child and family.

4.1.8.1 Definition

While there have been epidemiological studies published that document a trend toward an earlier initiation of puberty (Tena-Sempere 2013; Lee and Styne 2013), the classical and currently accepted definition of early or precocious puberty is the presence of secondary sexual characteristics of Tanner II breast development in girls before the age of 8 years and the presence of Tanner II genital development or testicular volume greater than or equal to 4 mL in boys prior to the age of 9 years. These clinical findings along with accelerated linear growth and advanced bone maturation constitutes the definition of pre-

cocious puberty (Lee 1980; Chirico et al. 2014; Radovick and Madhusmita 2018a).

4.1.8.2 Implications for Health and Development

The early production of sex steroids causes advanced bone maturation that decreases the linear growth potential and results in adult short stature due to early fusion of the growth plates (Thornton et al. 2014). As well, early age of menarche has been associated with increased risks of obesity, hypertension, type 2 diabetes, ischemic heart disease, stroke, estrogen-dependent cancer and cardiovascular mortality and development of breast cancer (Pienkowski and Tauber 2016). Some studies report that early puberty can be associated with an increase in adult sexual and delinquent behaviors and more psychological disturbances above general trends (Pienkowski and Tauber 2016).

4.1.8.3 Etiology and Presentation

Physical signs of early puberty can be a result of different causes that have been divided into three categories: central, peripheral, and incomplete precocious puberty (Latronico et al. 2016; Radovick and Madhusmita 2018b).

4.1.8.4 Central Precocious Puberty (CPP)

CPP or GnRH-dependent precocious puberty occurs when there is early activation and maturation of the hypothalamic-pituitary-gonadal axis leading to stimulation of the ovaries in girls and the testes in boys. The early production of GnRH by the pituitary stimulates the ovaries to produce estrogen and the testes to produce testosterone that results in the increase in breast tissue in girls and increased testicular volume in boys (Latronico et al. 2016; Chauhan and Grissom 2013; Macedo et al. 2016). CPP affects 1:5000–10,000 children (Lifshitz 2006; Chirico et al. 2014) and the prevalence is much higher in girls with at least 10:1 occurrence in females compared to males (Pienkowski and Tauber 2016; Macedo et al. 2016). CPP can result from organic, genetic, or idiopathic causes (Chirico et al. 2014; Macedo et al. 2016; Sultan et al. 2012).

Organic causes of CPP include lesions of the central nervous system such as benign hamartomas and malignant tumors usually found in the pineal region, or the optic pathway, such as hypothalamic gliomas (Wendt et al. 2014). Hydrocephalus, infection, trauma, and radiation can also impact the hypothalamus and pituitary and result in early production of GnRH with subsequent production of the relevant gonadal hormone (Bertelloni and Baroncelli 2013).

Genetics is the basis for a diagnosis of familial CPP. Inactivating mutations of the imprinted gene *MKRN3* is responsible for early onset of puberty that presents in certain families across generations (Sultan et al. 2012; Biro and Kiess 2016). This gene is found on chromosome 15q11.2. Inheritance occurs from fathers, so the phenotype can skip one or more generations and both sexes can be affected (Macedo et al. 2016). A very rare genetic cause of CPP involves activating mutations of the genes that encode the kisspeptin system, the major gatekeeper of pubertal onset through activation of the GnRH neurons (Tena-Sempere 2013; Macedo et al. 2016). Overexpression of kisspeptin leads to precocious puberty (Lee and Styne 2013).

Idiopathic CPP is when no lesion or genetic cause can be identified. This accounts for 70–90% of cases of CPP diagnosed in girls and rarely occurs in boys (Chirico et al. 2014; Pienkowski and Tauber 2016; Sultan et al. 2012). There is a slow progressive variant of CPP described in both sexes and is associated with adult height comparable to target height without intervention (Bertelloni and Baroncelli 2013). This form needs to be monitored closely, as the child may switch to rapid progression of puberty and acceleration of skeletal maturation and thus require intervention (Bertelloni and Baroncelli 2013).

The treatment options for CPP can involve close monitoring or intervention with a GnRH analog and will be discussed later in this section.

4.1.8.5 Peripheral Precocious Puberty (PPP)

PPP, or GnRH-independent precocious puberty, occurs when there is increase in the sex steroid, estrogen. or testosterone, and there is no evidence of activation of the hypothalamic-pituitary-gonadal axis, as GnRH is not stimulating the gonads to produce their respective hormones (Chirico et al. 2014). Causes include genetic, neoplasms, hypothyroidism and exposure to exogenous sex steroids (Macedo et al. 2016; Brown et al. 2013; Schoelwer and Eugster 2016). The treatments will be discussed along with the specific causes.

Genetic causes of PPP include congenital adrenal hyperplasia (CAH), McCune-Albright Syndrome (MAS), and familial male-limited precocious puberty (testotoxicosis).

- In CAH, if treatment is inadequate, there can be increased androgen levels secreted by the adrenal gland. This can lead to increased testosterone levels in boys and girls (Brown et al. 2013). (Refer to Chap. 34).

- MAS results from mutations in the *GNAS* gene that is located on chromosome 20q13.32 (Macedo et al. 2016; Brown et al. 2013). It is characterized by the presence of fibrous dysplasia, café-au-lait macules, and precocious puberty. Gonadotropin independent PP occurs in 15–20% of boys and 85% of girls affected with MAS. It is an uncommon condition & substitute: Gonadotropin independent PP occurs in 15–20% of boys and 85% of girls affected with MAS (Brown et al. 2013; Schoelwer and Eugster 2016). In girls, estrogen is secreted autonomously from functioning ovarian cysts and causes breast development, menstrual bleeding, increased linear growth, and advanced bone age (Schoelwer and Eugster 2016). Estrogen receptor modulators have been used to reduce the effects of elevated estrogen levels, such as ketoconazole that inhibits steroid biosynthesis and letrozole, an aromatase inhibitor, but there are concerns over long-term safety and efficacy. (Schoelwer and Eugster 2016). (Refer to Chap. 11).

- Familial male-limited precocious puberty or testotoxicosis is a rare disorder caused by activation of mutations in the gene, located on chromosome 2p21e, that encodes the luteinizing hormone and choriogonadotropin receptor (Latronico et al. 2016; Macedo et al. 2016; Schoelwer and Eugster 2016). It can occur de novo or it can be inherited through autosomal dominance, and is limited to males. Females can be asymptomatic carriers (Latronico et al. 2016). It presents in boys, usually before the age of 4 years, with tall stature, rapid growth, enlarged penis but little testicular enlargement or pubic hair.

Neoplasms such as adrenocortical carcinoma, hepatoblastoma, or gonadal tumors lead to increased production of sex steroids independent of GnRH and cause PPP. These lesions need to be removed and treated as per oncology protocols (Wendt et al. 2014). Hypothyroidism may have associated sexual precocity in both boys and girls. The precise mechanism is unknown but may be related to increase levels of thyrotropin-releasing hormone in the hypothalamus and elevated levels of thyroid stimulating hormone in the pituitary that can act on the FSH receptor. The stimulation of FSH levels can result in production of gonadal sex steroids in the hypothyroid child (Wendt et al. 2014).

Exposure to exogenous sex steroid occurs when users of topical testosterone preparations fail to follow the recommended contact precautions. The increasing use of topical androgens in males with hypogonadism or for increased muscle accretion or enhanced libido has resulted in increased cases of PPP secondary to inadvertent exposure in prepubertal children. Case reports show a return to prepubertal testosterone levels for most children after 4–5 months from the exposure cessation (Martinez-Pajares et al. 2012).

4.1.8.6 Incomplete Precocious Puberty (IPP)

Conditions of incomplete precocious puberty are considered variants of normal puberty and include premature thelarche, premature adrenarche, and isolated metrorrhagia (Chauhan and Grissom 2013; Sultan et al. 2012).

Premature thelarche (PT) is the presence of breast tissue without other signs of secondary sexual characteristics. Breast development is bilateral 50% of the time while the rest are unilateral or asymmetrical. Most are breast Tanner

stage II but breast volumes can be up to Tanner stage IV (Sultan et al. 2012). The breast enlargement usually regresses within months of appearing, but it can fluctuate over time and remain until other pubertal development occurs at an expected age. This usually occurs in children younger than 2 years old but can happen in children up to 7 years old as well (Lazar and Phillip 2012; Sultan et al. 2012; Brown et al. 2013). The cause is likely secondary to aromatization of adrenal androgens (Chauhan and Grissom 2013); however, the role of environmental impact in relation to endocrine disruptors is also considered relevant as the frequency of PT is increasing (Sultan et al. 2012). Many studies with girls report that higher adiposity is associated with thelarche prior to age 8 years, but there is no proven causal link to date (Lee and Styne 2013). Increased adiposity can decrease levels of sex hormone-binding globulin that leads to greater availability of circulating sex steroids (Chauhan and Grissom 2013; Biro and Kiess 2016). As well, the storage of estrogen and aromatization of estrogen precursors are increased with increased adiposity that can result in higher levels of estrogen independent of the HPG axis (Chauhan and Grissom 2013; Biro and Kiess 2016). Bone maturation is normal or may be slightly advanced (Lazar and Phillip 2012; Eksioglu et al. 2013). The enlarged breast tissue may be tender or painful, but there is no discharge and this self-limiting condition requires no treatment other than monitoring (Sultan et al. 2012; Brown et al. 2013).

Premature adrenarche (PA) is the presence of signs of androgen action before age of 8 years in girls and 9 years in boys (Lazar and Phillip 2012; Voutilainen and Jaaskelainen 2015). Pubic hair and/or axillary hair is present in about 50% of the cases. Adult body odor is a very common early sign of PA (Voutilainen and Jaaskelainen 2015) and oily hair or skin, comedones, acne, slightly increased linear growth, mood swings, and behavioral changes may occur (Voutilainen and Jaaskelainen 2015; Williams et al. 2012). It is more typically found in children older than 6 years and 8–9 times more frequently in girls compared to boys

(Sultan et al. 2012; Brown et al. 2013; Williams et al. 2012). There is an elevation of adrenal androgen precursors, dehydroepiandrosterone (DHEA), DHEA-S, and androstenedione; therefore, other causes of excess androgen levels must be excluded (Voutilainen and Jaaskelainen 2015). PA has been associated with preterm birth and SGA, as well as progression to overweight, obesity, and hyperinsulinism. These conditions may increase the risk of adrenal hyperandrogenism in some cohorts, but this is not conclusive in all populations (Sultan et al. 2012; Voutilainen and Jaaskelainen 2015). The BA can be advanced and linear growth increased before puberty, but individuals do reach their genetic potential for adult height (Lazar and Phillip 2012; Voutilainen and Jaaskelainen 2015). There is a wide variability in the presentation of PA but regardless of signs of androgen effect, once other causes of excess androgens are excluded this is considered a benign condition and there is no treatment (Williams et al. 2012).

Isolated metrorrhagia is bleeding from the uterus at irregular intervals. When this occurs in the prepubertal girl, it may be due to transient rises in estrogen from a functional ovarian cyst that is rarely treated but monitored closely. It may also be related to endocrine disruptors such as phthalates, phytoestrogens, and bisphenol A that may have the capacity to mimic estrogen and so result in activation of its hormonal activity (Chauhan and Grissom 2013; Sultan et al. 2012).

4.1.8.7 Diagnostic Evaluation

The gold standard in differentiating and diagnosing precocious puberty is the determination of a lab value of the LH and FSH response to purposeful stimulation of GnRH (Chirico et al. 2014). An LH response above 5–6 international units/L (IU/L) and/or a stimulated peak LH/FSH ratio above 0.66–1.0 is considered a centrally driven pubertal response and the child has CPP. If there is no stimulated LH or FSH response, then elevated levels of estrogen or testosterone are considered from a peripheral source and the child has PPP (Thornton et al. 2014).

A pelvic ultrasound for girls can detect ovarian masses and provide measurements of the uterus and ovaries. Measurements reported as significantly higher than normal in girls aged 0–8 years old supports the diagnosis of CPP. Ultrasound can also assess the progressive maturation of the uterus and ovaries and may assist in monitoring effectiveness of treatment (Sultan et al. 2012; Eksioglu et al. 2013).

BA X-ray of the left hand and wrist can provide information about the maturation stage of the bones as compared to the child's chronological age (CA). In a rapidly progressing CPP, the BA is greater than 2 SD above the CA and the concern is for loss of pubertal growth potential to occur at a usual time of development and a lessening of final adult height. The BA can be helpful in determining whether treatment is needed or if careful monitoring is adequate. A brain MRI is needed to identify or rule out the presence of CNS lesions (Lazar and Phillip 2012). Tumor markers (i.e. alpha fetoprotein, beta HCG) and adrenal DHEA and androstenedione are blood levels that help differentiate the etiology of PPP and IPP (Wendt et al. 2014).

4.1.8.8 Management

The main goals for the management of precocious puberty is to prevent early fusion of the epiphyseal growth plates (Chauhan and Grissom 2013), thus allowing for the attainment of adult height within the individual's genetic potential (Bertelloni and Baroncelli 2013). As well, it is desirable to stop premature sexual maturation at an age that is early with respect to other social development of the child in order to prevent potentially negative somatic and psychological outcomes (Bertelloni and Baroncelli 2013).

Onset of puberty in 6–8-year-old girls is controversial and when puberty starts at 8–9 years old in girls there is no benefit achieved by treating (Chauhan and Grissom 2013; Bertelloni and Baroncelli 2013). Another study reported that boys and girls older than 6 years at onset of puberty and treated with GnRH had a less than expected actual improvement in height prognosis (Lazar and Phillip 2012).

The decision to intervene depends on the etiology, the child's age at presentation, the rapid rate of pubertal progression, the accelerated height velocity, and a BA advancement greater than 2 SD for girls. As boys have acceleration of bone maturation and growth rate later in puberty, rather than using the BA, an increase in testicular volume and secondary sexual characteristics associated with increased testosterone levels are better indicators (Lazar and Phillip 2012).

Surgery and radiation therapy of the CNS lesion are used for a minority of patients with organic causes of CPP (Bertelloni and Baroncelli 2013) and hypothalamic hamartomas should not be treated by surgery (Latronico et al. 2016).

4.1.8.9 Medical Treatment

The treatment of choice for idiopathic and non-treatable organic causes of CPP are synthetic analogs of GnRH (Bertelloni and Baroncelli 2013). The analog has a highly specific binding to the GnRH receptor (Bertelloni and Baroncelli 2013) and after an initial brief stimulation of gonadotropin release there is a desensitization of the gonadotropin-secreting cells to native GnRH that results in suppression of LH and FSH production and subsequent return of the sex steroid to prepubertal levels (Bertelloni and Baroncelli 2013; Brown et al. 2013).

The optimal dose needed to achieve pituitary desensitization continues to be debated. It is important to note that if suppression is incomplete during treatment, GnRH analog may actually stimulate pubertal progression and bone age advancement, thus impairing desired outcome of treatment (Bertelloni and Baroncelli 2013).

The forms of GnRH analog available are daily SC, monthly depots given by IM injection, depots lasting up to 12 weeks given by IM injections, and implants that last up to 24 months (Bertelloni and Baroncelli 2013). Another medication that comes as a nasal spray is currently not commonly used and will not be discussed.

Leuprolide and triptorelin provide GnRH analog most commonly as formulations of 3.75 mg or 7.5 mg strength given every 4 weeks or 11.25 mg or 22.5 mg strength given every 12 weeks, while Goserelin has a 3.6 mg every

4 weeks and a 10.8 mg every 12 weeks formulation (Bertelloni and Baroncelli 2013). If hormonal or clinical criteria warrant, these products may require shorter intervals between injections to achieve adequate gonadotropin suppression (Bertelloni and Baroncelli 2013). From personal practice when a dose of 7.5 mg given every 3 weeks was not sufficient for suppression, a combination of 7.5 mg and 3.75 mg monthly formulation were combined in one syringe to provide 11.25 mg every 3 weeks, as there is no 11.25 mg monthly formulation. The option of using a product that has a longer interval, so that injections are given every 12 weeks instead of every 4 weeks, can improve compliance and quality of life for the child and family (Bertelloni and Baroncelli 2013). The every 12-week formulation has a larger volume per injection, 1.8 mL versus 1.0 mL for the 4-week formulation, so for smaller children this would need to be a consideration. As well, the longer interval product is thicker, and children find that it is more painful albeit it requires less injections.

Yearly histrelin implants seem to provide adequate suppression; however, the clinical experience is limited (Bertelloni and Baroncelli 2013). This involves a surgical subcutaneous implant that suppresses gonadotropins for 12–24 months (Latronico et al. 2016).

Adverse effects such as headaches, rash, gastrointestinal complaints, or hot flashes have been reported in 3–13% of children receiving GnRH analog but are usually transient and resolve spontaneously or with treatment of the symptoms (Latronico et al. 2016). Local complications, such as sterile abscess, has been reported in 1.5–5% of children and are thought to be due to reactions to a variety of polymers used in slowing down the release of the medication in the depot and implant formulations (Chirico et al. 2014; Thornton et al. 2014; Bertelloni and Baroncelli 2013). If these forms of GnRH are not tolerated, the daily subcutaneous formulation can be used.

Efficacy of GnRH analog treatment can be done with a single LH sample taken 30–120 min after the injection of every 4 week or 12-week

GnRH analog formulation. Suppression of the LH level to less than 4.5 IU/L indicates adequate suppression (Latronico et al. 2016). BA can also determine effectiveness of treatment and can be measured every 6–12 months. Initially, skeletal advancement slows to 6–12 months per year and later may show no advancement in both girls and boys receiving GnRH analog (Lazar and Phillip 2012).

In some children, there is an excessive growth velocity deceleration that occurs during treatment and for which there is no known mechanism (Bertelloni and Baroncelli 2013). These children may benefit from adjunctive treatment with GH or very low doses of 17B-estradiol (Bertelloni and Baroncelli 2013) or oxandrolone to optimize growth velocity and adult height; however, very few studies have been reported on this (Latronico et al. 2016).

4.1.8.10 Discontinuation of Medical Treatment

Factors to consider when deciding to discontinue GnRH analog treatment include the family's perspective, psychological, and social issues, as well as the child's response to treatment and the current bone age (Bertelloni and Baroncelli 2013) (G). In most instances, stopping treatment when the BA is close to the physiological age for pubertal onset for girls, which would be 11.5–12.5 years and a similar corresponding BA; for boys a BA of 13.5–14 years, which is close to male peak height velocity (Lazar and Phillip 2012; Latronico et al. 2016; Bertelloni and Baroncelli 2013; Brown et al. 2013).

Following discontinuation of GnRH analog, female menstrual cycle resumes 12–16 months later; however, a wide range of 2–61 months has been reported (Chirico et al. 2014; Latronico et al. 2016; Chauhan and Grissom 2013). Typically, the HPG axis returns to normal within 12 months after stopping treatment (Williams et al. 2012).

Following removal of the final implant of histrelin, recovery of the hypothalamic-pituitary axis has been reported at 6 months (Latronico et al. 2016).

Long-term implications from receiving GnRH analog treatment have been studied. Data suggests that this treatment does not cause or aggravate obesity and does not affect body composition (Thornton et al. 2014; Latronico et al. 2016; Bertelloni and Baroncelli 2013). As well, bone mineral density may decrease during GnRH analog treatment, but subsequent bone mass accrual is usually preserved, and peak bone mass is not negatively affected in either sex (Latronico et al. 2016; Bertelloni and Baroncelli 2013). Long-term data indicates that there is no adverse effects related to normal reproduction function and reproductive potential in both sexes and gonadal function is reactivated once treatment is stopped (Chirico et al. 2014; Latronico et al. 2016). There is no evidence that GnRH analog treatment predisposes females to PCOS or menstrual irregularities (Bertelloni and Baroncelli 2013).

4.1.8.11 Psychosocial Implications

Boys with early pubertal development can be perceived as more mature and smart, while girls have been found to have more difficulty in academic and social environments. As well, girls with early signs of puberty may attract the attention of older boys, thus putting them at risk for exploitation or abuse, as they are not mentally mature enough to handle these situations. Studies have shown that both sexes who mature earlier are at increased risk of participating in risk-taking behaviors at an earlier age (Brown et al. 2013).

4.1.8.12 Nursing Implications

1. Respecting patient and parent needs.
   - The time of diagnosis can be overwhelming for families and nurses can offer vital support in helping the families to understand the medical diagnosis and what is involved with treatment. Written material is valued as many parents are not able to take in all the information that is frequently given at the time of diagnosis. Parents may feel that their child is socially vulnerable when going through puberty too early. They may feel overprotective and fearful that their child may be teased or exploited

by others as they have sexually developed too soon compared to their peers.

2. Coordinating and integrating care that considers the needs and perceptions of patients and their families.

   • Treatment for CPP usually involves scheduled injections, ongoing monitoring with blood tests and medical examinations, which takes time away from parent's work and children's school. Parents may feel unsure of how to explain the need for these absences to school personnel and may need support such as letters of confirmation of appointments. Children may feel embarrassed at having to leave school to attend medical appointments. Costs related to missed work, travel expenses, and parking may be too much for families. The nurse can endeavor to schedule injections and physician assessments at the same time to reduce visits to the medical center.

3. Providing information, communication, and education throughout the care continuum.

   • Families may not know how to discuss their child's early body development with the child. Most young children will ask questions if they want to know something so parents need to be prepared to give them answers tailored to their child's developmental level, so they can understand. As these children are often tall for their actual age, others may expect more from them or treat them as if they were older. Parents may need help to know how to handle these situations. A "buddy" family may be helpful to the parent and child, so they can talk with someone who has had a similar experience.

4. Providing for timely and effective means of pain management.

   • Offer a child friendly space that is inviting and not scary.
   • Have a discussion with parents to help them understand their role in supporting their child during a painful or fear inducing procedure. Allow the child and parent to express their feelings so that they feel heard and understood and be honest about

what to expect. If the child or parent has a fear of needles, more specialized help from child life specialists or child psychologists may be helpful.

   • Use principles of lessening pain of injections and blood tests such as topical numbing medication, skin vibration placed between the injection site and the nerve pathway to the brain, distraction technics, and deep breathing are a few examples of the guidelines suggested by Taddio et al. (2010) (Also see Chap. 5).

5. Include parents and families as partners in the health care team.

   • Extended family members may have questions or concerns that the parents are not able to answer. The parents may feel precocious puberty is an awkward social situation and may need help discussing with family, friends, or those providing child care when parents feel this information needs to be shared.
   • The discussion about stopping treatment for CPP is a time that families need to have information and support about what to expect in terms of progressing through puberty and future implications for normal progression and fertility aspects.

Case Study

4-year-old girl, MG, with Tanner stage 3 breasts and increased height velocity.

GnRH stimulation test shows LH = 60 IU/L, FSH = 20 IU/L, estradiol = 277 pmol/L.

Bone age = 7 years.

MRI of head is normal.

No history of other medical conditions or head trauma.

Mom is fearful that her little girl has lost her childhood and is vulnerable to other children's teasing and even exploitation. MG is terrified of needles and doesn't know why she has to be poked and have the private parts of her body examined.

The pediatric endocrinologist and pediatric endocrine nurse meet with the family to discuss the diagnosis of CPP and prescribes Lupron

Depot (leuprolide) 7.5 mg IM monthly with follow-up labs 40 min post third injection to check for suppression of LH, FSH, and estradiol.

What do you think is important to discuss with the parents?

How could you support MG with the treatment regime in the coming months?

4.1.9 Conclusions

Puberty is not a single process that follows a definitive road map. Time of onset, tempo, and completion of puberty are all variable. It is imperative that a thorough history and physical examination are done to assess the status of puberty. An understanding of pubertal development, including typical or abnormal variations is essential for nurses to provide patient or parent education and guidance.

The timing of puberty varies greatly between individuals, ethnicities, geographical area, environmental, socioeconomic, and nutritional states. The approach to delayed puberty is dependent on the cause of the delay. There is ongoing research into the causes and treatment options for delayed or precocious puberty. It is important for the nurse to be cognizant that the child who presents with delayed or precocious puberty is dealing with physiological as well as psychological issues, both of which need to be addressed. The goal of treatment is to preserve final adult height potential and to support children and their families throughout the process.

References

Abitbol L, Zborovski S, Palmert MR. Evaluation of delayed puberty: what diagnostic tests should be performed in the seemingly otherwise well adolescent? Arch Dis Child. 2016;101(8):767–71.

Adams Hillard PJ. Menstruation in adolescents: what do we know? And what do we do with the information? J Pediatr Adolesc Gynecol. 2014;27(6):309–19.

Baams L, Dubas JS, Overbeek G, van Aken MA. Transitions in body and behavior: a meta-analytic study on the relationship between pubertal development and adolescent sexual behavior. J Adolesc Health. 2015;56(6):586–98.

Berenbaum SA, Beltz AM, Corley R. The importance of puberty for adolescent development: conceptualization and measurement. Adv Child Dev Behav. 2015;48:53–92.

Bertelloni S, Baroncelli GI. Current pharmacotherapy of central precocious puberty by GnRH analogs: certainties and uncertainties. Expert Opin Pharmacother. 2013;14(12):1627–39.

Biro FM, Kiess W. Contemporary trends in onset and completion of puberty, gain in height and adiposity. Endocr Dev. 2016;29:122–33.

Bourguignon JP, Juul A. Normal female puberty in a developmental perspective. Endocr Dev. 2012;22:11–23.

Brown DB, Loomba-Albrecht LA, Bremer AA. Sexual precocity and its treatment. World J Pediatr. 2013;9(2):103–11.

Chauhan A, Grissom M. Disorders of childhood growth and development: precocious puberty. FP Essent. 2013;410:25–31.

Chirico V, Lacquaniti A, Salpietro V, Buemi M, Salpietro C, Arrigo T. Central precocious puberty: from physiopathological mechanisms to treatment. J Biol Regul Homeost Agents. 2014;28(3):367–75.

Duke SA, Balzer BW, Steinbeck KS. Testosterone and its effects on human male adolescent mood and behavior: a systematic review. J Adolesc Health. 2014;55(3):315–22.

Eksioglu AS, Yilmaz S, Cetinkaya S, Cinar G, Yildiz YT, Aycan Z. Value of pelvic sonography in the diagnosis of various forms of precocious puberty in girls. J Clin Ultrasound. 2013;41(2):84–93.

Farooqi IS, Jebb SA, Langmack G, Lawrence E, Cheetham CH, Prentice AM, et al. Effects of recombinant leptin therapy in a child with congenital leptin deficiency. N Engl J Med. 1999;341(12):879–84.

Fenichel P. Delayed puberty. Endocr Dev. 2012;22:138–59.

Fraser B, Jacob J, Kirouac N, editors. SubQ T…is it for me? Reviewing the increasing use of subcutaneous testosterone injections. International Pediatric Endocrine Nurses Summit; 2015; Washington DC. J Pediatr Nurs. 2017.

Freedman DS, Khan LK, Serdula MK, Dietz WH, Srinivasan SR, Berenson GS. Relation of age at menarche to race, time period, and anthropometric dimensions: the Bogalusa Heart Study. Pediatrics. 2002;110(4):e43.

Gajdos ZK, Henderson KD, Hirschhorn JN, Palmert MR. Genetic determinants of pubertal timing in the general population. Mol Cell Endocrinol. 2010;324(1–2):21–9.

Giedd JN. The amazing teen brain. Sci Am. 2015;312(6):32–7.

Graber JA. Pubertal timing and the development of psychopathology in adolescence and beyond. Horm Behav. 2013;64(2):262–9.

Greulich WW, Pyle SI. Radiographic atlas of skeletal development of the hand and wrist. 2nd ed. Stanford, CA: Stanford University Press; 1959.

Harrington J, Palmert MR. Clinical review: Distinguishing constitutional delay of growth and puberty from isolated hypogonadotropic hypogonadism: critical appraisal of available diagnostic tests. J Clin Endocrinol Metab. 2012;97(9):3056–67.

Howell S, Shalet S. Gonadal damage from chemotherapy and radiotherapy. Endocrinol Metab Clin N Am. 1998;27(4):927–43.

Kaur KK, Allahbadia G, Singh M. Kisspeptins in human reproduction—future therapeutic potential. J Assist Reprod Genet. 2012;29(10):999–1011.

Krieger N, Kiang MV, Kosheleva A, Waterman PD, Chen JT, Beckfield J. Age at menarche: 50-year socioeconomic trends among US-born black and white women. Am J Public Health. 2015;105(2):388–97.

Lahoti A, Sills I. Update on puberty and its disorders in adolescents. Adolesc Med State Art Rev. 2015;26(2):269–90.

Latronico AC, Brito VN, Carel JC. Causes, diagnosis, and treatment of central precocious puberty. Lancet Diabetes Endocrinol. 2016;4(3):265–74.

Lazar L, Phillip M. Pubertal disorders and bone maturation. Endocrinol Metab Clin N Am. 2012;41(4):805–25.

Lee PA. Normal ages of pubertal events among American males and females. J Adolesc Health Care. 1980;1(1):26–9.

Lee Y, Styne D. Influences on the onset and tempo of puberty in human beings and implications for adolescent psychological development. Horm Behav. 2013;64(2):250–61.

Lifshitz FE. In: Lifshitz F, editor. Pediatric endocrinology. 5th ed. New York: Marcel Dekker; 2006.

Macedo DB, Silveira LF, Bessa DS, Brito VN, Latronico AC. Sexual precocity—genetic bases of central precocious puberty and autonomous gonadal activation. Endocr Dev. 2016;29:50–71.

Marshall WA, Tanner JM. Variations in pattern of pubertal changes in girls. Arch Dis Child. 1969;44(235):291–303.

Martinez-Pajares JD, Diaz-Morales O, Ramos-Diaz JC, Gomez-Fernandez E. Peripheral precocious puberty due to inadvertent exposure to testosterone: case report and review of the literature. J Pediatr Endocrinol Metab. 2012;25(9–10):1007–12.

Palmert MR, Dunkel L. Clinical practice. Delayed puberty. N Engl J Med. 2012;366(5):443–53.

Palmert MR, Hirschhorn JN. Genetic approaches to stature, pubertal timing, and other complex traits. Mol Genet Metab. 2003;80(1–2):1–10.

Pienkowski C, Tauber M. Gonadotropin-releasing hormone agonist treatment in sexual precocity. Endocr Dev. 2016;29:214–29.

Radovick SM, Madhusmita M, editors. Pediatric endocrinology. Cham: Springer International; 2018a.

Radovick SM, Madhusmita M, editors. Pediatric endocrinology: a practical clinical guide. Cham: Springer International; 2018b.

Schoelwer M, Eugster EA. Treatment of peripheral precocious puberty. Endocr Dev. 2016;29:230–9.

Sultan C, Gaspari L, Kalfa N, Paris F. Clinical expression of precocious puberty in girls. Endocr Dev. 2012;22:84–100.

Susman EJ, Dorn LD, Schiefelbein VL. In: Weiner IB, editor. Puberty, sexuality, and health. New York: Wiley; 2003.

Susman EJ, Dockray S, Granger DA, Blades KT, Randazzo W, Heaton JA, et al. Cortisol and alpha amylase reactivity and timing of puberty: vulnerabilities for antisocial behaviour in young adolescents. Psychoneuroendocrinology. 2010;35(4):557–69.

Taddio A, Appleton M, Bortolussi R, Chambers C, Dubey V, Halperin S, et al. Reducing the pain of childhood vaccination: an evidence-based clinical practice guideline (summary). CMAJ. 2010;182(18):1989–95.

Tena-Sempere M. Keeping puberty on time: novel signals and mechanisms involved. Curr Top Dev Biol. 2013;105:299–329.

Thornton P, Silverman LA, Geffner ME, Neely EK, Gould E, Danoff TM. Review of outcomes after cessation of gonadotropin-releasing hormone agonist treatment of girls with precocious puberty. Pediatr Endocrinol Rev. 2014;11(3):306–17.

Voutilainen R, Jaaskelainen J. Premature adrenarche: etiology, clinical findings, and consequences. J Steroid Biochem Mol Biol. 2015;145:226–36.

Wei C, Crowne EC. Recent advances in the understanding and management of delayed puberty. Arch Dis Child. 2016;101(5):481–8.

Weise M, De-Levi S, Barnes KM, Gafni RI, Abad V, Baron J. Effects of estrogen on growth plate senescence and epiphyseal fusion. Proc Natl Acad Sci U S A. 2001;98(12):6871–6.

Wendt S, Shelso J, Wright K, Furman W. Neoplastic causes of abnormal puberty. Pediatr Blood Cancer. 2014;61(4):664–71.

Williams RM, Ward CE, Hughes IA. Premature adrenarche. Arch Dis Child. 2012;97(3):250–4.

Wolf RM, Long D. Pubertal development. Pediatr Rev. 2016;37(7):292–300.

Treatment Issues in the Care of Pediatric Patients with Endocrine Conditions

5

Peggy Kalancha, Nicole Kirouac, and Eileen Pyra

Contents

P. Kalancha
Clinical Resource, Pediatric Endocrine and
Gynecology Clinics, Alberta Children's Hospital,
Calgary, AB, Canada
e-mail: peggy.kalancha@ahs.ca

N. Kirouac
St. Amant Inc., Winnipeg, MB, Canada
e-mail: nkirouac@stamant.ca

E. Pyra (✉)
Pediatric Endocrine Clinic, Alberta Children's
Hospital, Calgary, AB, Canada
e-mail: eileen.pyra@ahs.ca

Abstract

Treatment issues commonly encountered in pediatric endocrine practice include: preparing children for painful procedures, care of transgender youth, and pubertal issues of girls with developmental disabilities. This chapter provides an overview of these topics.

Pediatric endocrine nurses frequently request blood testing of their patients. Also, nurses teach parents to provide blood sugar

© Springer Nature Switzerland AG 2019
S. Llahana et al. (eds.), *Advanced Practice in Endocrinology Nursing*,
https://doi.org/10.1007/978-3-319-99817-6_5

testing or injections to their children. Selection of the correct needle length is important to ensure correct distribution of medication. Injections and finger sticks are painful or anxiety producing for infants, children, adolescents, and their parents. Many people develop long-term fear or avoidance of needles because of negative childhood experiences. As patient advocates, nurses can ensure that parents and children are prepared for potentially painful experiences by utilizing evidence-based strategies to decrease pain and anxiety. Recognizing that memories of painful experiences can impact current treatment or future experiences allows nurses to intervene to improve upon these. Knowing the guidelines for reducing pain from procedures and practicing these can significantly impact a child's life.

Children who present as gender creative or transgender may be diagnosed with gender dysphoria and require treatment in a pediatric endocrine environment. Following a diagnosis of gender dysphoria by a qualified mental health practitioner, pediatric endocrine nurses can assist with education and support as well as treatment for the youth. Endocrine treatments should be provided following guidelines and standards of care and may include the use of puberty blocking pharmacologic agents or prescribing cross hormone therapy to support transition. Pediatric endocrine nurses can advocate for the best possible hormone treatment for transgender youth to encourage optimal outcomes.

Providing gynecologic care for young women affected with physical or developmental disability during puberty can be complex. Parents of these youth are very concerned as their young person starts to grow and change. This chapter reviews the complex needs of this group of children/adolescents and reviews available medical treatment options. We will also review a number of strategies that nurses can implement to help families to improve quality of life and patient reported outcomes.

Keywords

Cerebral palsy · Contraception · Developmental disabilities · Gender dysphoria · Menstruation Needle fear · Pediatric · Pain reduction Procedural pain · Transgender youth

Abbreviations

ADHD	Attention deficit hyperactivity disorder
ASD	Autism spectrum disorder
cm	Centimeter
CP	Cerebral palsy
DD	Developmental disabilities
DSM-5	American Psychiatric Association Diagnostic and Statistical Manual Version 5
FSH	Follicle stimulating hormone
GAT	Growth attenuation therapy
GD	Gender dysphoria
GnRH	Gonadotropin releasing hormone
HELP-in KIDS	Help Eliminate Pain in KIDS Team
IM	Intramuscular
IUD	Intrauterine device
kg	Kilogram
LARC	Levonorgestrel IUD implants
LGBTQ	Lesbian, gay, bisexual, transgender, queer
LH	Luteinizing hormone
mm	Millimeter
NSAIDS	Non-steroidal anti-inflammatory drugs
OCP	Oral contraceptive pills
PENS	Pediatric Endocrinology Nursing Society
SC	Subcutaneous
SOC	Standards of care
TG	Transgender
WPATH	World Professional Association for Transgender Health

Key Terms
- **Needle phobia:** Extreme fear of medical procedures involving injections or blood draw.
- **Gender dysphoria:** Conflict between a person's physical or assigned gender and a person's emotional or psychological identity.
- **Developmental disabilities:** Diverse group of conditions due to impairment in physical, psychological, language, or behavior that arise before adulthood.

Key Points
- Understand best practices for subcutaneous and intramuscular injections in children. Know the recommendations for injection depth for infants, children, and teens.
- Recognize the benefit of knowing and using pain reduction guidelines for all procedures that break the skin in infants, children, and teens.
- Know the diagnostic criteria and treatment guidelines for transgender children and teens as it relates to endocrinology.
- Puberty is a normal developmental process for all children with many physical, psychological, and cognitive changes. Teens with developmental disabilities gain these benefits as well.
- Teens with developmental disabilities often process through puberty smoothly, and it can be less traumatic than families expect.

5.1   Injections and Pain Reduction Strategies

Children and adolescents who are being evaluated for potential endocrine conditions typically require venipuncture and treatments may often involve years of injections. Carefully choosing the size and length of needles used for injections helps to reduce pain and ensure that medications are administered either subcutaneous (SC) or intramuscular (IM) as prescribed. Ensuring age-appropriate pain-free strategies are used for such procedures from the start should be a priority for all health care providers. Finally, it is now known that memories of negative painful procedures in children lead to decreased compliance of treatment regimens and long-term avoidance of medical care as adults as well as a higher risk of chronic pain development (Noel et al. 2017; McMurtry et al. 2015; Thrane et al. 2017).

5.1.1   Defining Subcutaneous vs. Intramuscular Injections and Best Practice

Needle injection depth recommendations and availability have changed over time. Choosing the right needle length for the prescribed type of injection can help decrease anxiety and pain in the child or adolescent. Ultrasound studies now demonstrate that in order to achieve a subcutaneous injection depth on anyone the needle should be of a 6-mm length or shorter (Hofman et al. 2007; Koster et al. 2009). Most insulin and growth hormone delivery devices are compatible with needle lengths of 4–6 mm to ensure SC injection depth is maintained. A 6-mm needle is recommended to be given at an angled insertion with a pinched skin fold technique to ensure SC depth. Intramuscular injections are reached with a needle length of 8 mm or longer for children up to 60 kg. For those over 60 kg a 1 in (2.5 cm). length needle is recommended to achieve intramuscular depth. This is helpful when considering the change of medication administration routes for testosterone, for example, to change from biweekly or monthly intramuscular to weekly subcutaneous. Recent studies provide support that SC testosterone injections may allow for increased independence and much improved comfort and compliance of this necessary medication.

5.1.2 Pain Reduction and Distraction Techniques Based on Evidence and Best Practice

In 2010, a cross-Canada-independent national multidisciplinary group titled the Help Eliminate Pain in KIDS Team (HELP-in KIDS) developed clinical practice guidelines for vaccination injections in children. Dozens of studies involving thousands of children were reviewed in the development of these guidelines. This helps health care providers and parents identify strategies for injection pain prevention and reduction in infants and children. In 2015, those guidelines were updated to include adults and renamed the Help in Kids & Adults Team (Taddio et al. 2015). The development of the guidelines included examinations of over 130 studies looking at the management of pain across the lifespan. Key components of the guidelines include the following five domains of pain management interventions: (1) Procedural (2) Physical (3) Pharmacologic (4) Psychological (5) Process. The important highlights of these domains for endocrine nurses are summarized in Table 5.1.

High levels of needle fear can be described as a persistent, intense apprehension of or fear in response to a needle procedure and that a person may endure needles with intense distress or avoidance (Taddio et al. 2015). Should you suspect an individual has high levels of needle fear, the person should be referred to a mental health professional with knowledge and skills in needle fear as soon as possible.

One needs to consider a child or adolescents' past experiences of painful procedures before planning new procedures. It is well known that negative experiences with needles or blood draws (venipuncture) can lead to avoidance of medical care as adults (Noel et al. 2012). These negative experiences can start as early as infancy. Reframing memories of pain has been well described by child psychologist, Melanie Noel, from Calgary, Alberta, Canada (Noel et al. 2012). She describes how a child's memory of pain intensity is a better predictor of future pain perceptions than their actual reported pain intensity. Fear contributes to the memory of the event as

Table 5.1 HELP in Kids and Adults Guideline summary for Endocrine Nurses

Procedural interventions (injection techniques)	Age group
Rapid injection with no aspiration for all intramuscular injections	ALL
Inject the most painful medication last for multiple injections	ALL
Use the Vastus Lateralis injection site for intramuscular injections	<1 year especially
Physical interventions (body position and activity)	*Age group*
Breastfeeding during injections (if unable, use non-nutritive sucking)	<2 years
Skin to skin contact during injections	<1 month
Holding child during injections (upright in a bear hug or on the lap)	<3 years
Child/youth sitting up (not lying down)	>3 years
Vibrating device with cold (apply on and then just above injection site)	>3 years
Rub/stroke proximal to the injection site vigorously prior to and during injections (helpful to do in the palm of the hand for finger pokes)	>4 years
Pharmacologic interventions	*Age group*
Topical anesthetics (apply up to 1 h before the procedure)	ALL
Breastfeeding or sucrose +/or glucose solution (2 mL of 24–50% strength solution given 1–2 min prior to injection) with non-nutritive sucking	< 2 years
Oral analgesics prior to injections are not proven to be helpful	ALL
Psychological interventions	*Age group*
Distraction techniques (toys, bubbles, electronic devices)	ALL
DO NOT TELL them "it won't hurt"	ALL
Encourage them to take slow deep breaths (use bubbles or pinwheels)	>3 years
Praise the child/youth for engaging in distraction methods	ALL
Process interventions	*Age group*
Education of clinicians in pain management for injections	ALL
Education of parents before (preferred) or on the day of the injection	0–17 years
Education of the individual having the injection	>3 years
Parent presence for injections	<10 years

Adapted for finger pokes, subcutaneous and intramuscular injections, venipuncture
Adapted from Taddio et al. (2015)

fear is better remembered than the actual pain sensation. Through reframing memories of pain, one can lessen anticipatory fear and help the child manage the painful experience (Noel et al. 2012).

Table 5.2 Resources for nurses to help make procedures pain free

Help **EL**iminate **P**ain in Kids & Adults Guidelines http://phm.utoronto.ca/helpinkids/
Children's Comfort Promise from Children's Minnesota www.childrensmn.org/services/care-specialties www.noneedlesspain.org
"It doesn't have to hurt" is an initiative led by the Centre for Pediatric Pain Research to get research evidence about children's pain directly into the hands of parents who can use it www.itdoesnthavetohurt.ca
International Forum for Injection Technique (FIT) www.fit4diabetes.com
Procedural pain management: A position statement with clinical practice recommendations by the American Society for Pain Management Nursing www.aspmn.org http://www.aspmn.org/documents/Czarnecki_ProcPainPositionStatement_2011.pdf
Distraction in Action Tool: predictive model and individualized coaching information https://webapps1.healthcare.uiowa.edu/CPadApp

Adults, in particular parents, can have a powerful influence before, during, and after the painful procedure by talking to children to help them reframe their memories in a more positive light. Talk about what the child thought went well and focus on what they did that was helpful such as taking deep breaths, blowing bubbles, being brave, and holding still. Praise them for what they did well even if it was the smallest thing so that the focus is positive. You can use "pain denying" talk such as "You were really brave. You didn't even cry, it was _like_ it didn't hurt" (Noel et al. 2012). Tell children that their memory matters and suggest to the child that they focus on the helpful things the next time they have a painful experience, so they learn that they can control how they feel about the situation. Pain-relieving strategies and reframing memories of pain need to involve the nurse, the parent, and the child. Recent research highlights the efficacy of the use of distraction as a cognitive-behavioral intervention to assist children with painful procedures. Nurse researchers at the University of Iowa developed a web-based tool, "Distraction in Action," which is a predictive model that identifies a child's risk for distress with painful procedures and provides instructions for coaching and the use of distraction techniques based on the individual child's characteristics (McCarthy et al. 2010). A list of resources for nurses to help make procedures less painful can be found in Table 5.2.

Case Scenario 1

Finger poke fear

A 6-year-old boy presents to the endocrine clinic with a history of query hypoglycemia. It is decided that he should have a random blood sugar today with a personal blood glucose monitor and take this home to monitor during times of symptoms. He immediately retreats to the corner of the room at the mention of a finger poke. He hides his hands behind his back and says, "no way." The pediatric endocrine nurse gathers supplies for blood sugar testing including a battery operated "vibrating massage tool" that fits in the palm of the hand. She proceeds to show the family the blood glucose testing procedure and asks the father if the boy can help to assess his blood sugar first to test it out. The father agrees. The nurse shows the child how to have the father hold the vibrating massage tool in the palm of his hand and explains how this tool will tell his brain to focus on the vibration so that the finger poke won't hurt so much. After further direction from the nurse the child proceeds to test his father's blood sugar—with great success! Minutes later with a new lancet in the lancing device and new strip in the machine the 6-year-old boy holds the massage tool in the palm of his own hand. As the nurse speaks with parents to not draw too much attention, the boy pokes his own finger and smiles saying, "I hardly felt anything" as he reaches for the glucometer to bring it to the drop of blood. His parents were amazed that he actually did this on his own, considering how afraid he was just 10 min. earlier. The time taken by the nurse to acknowledge the child's anxiety about the finger poke and find strategies to help decrease pain allowed for this first encounter to have a positive outcome for this child and his parents. Praising the child and talking about how he was able to do his own finger poke will help reframe the memory of this experience so that he remembers the positive parts. This will allow him to feel more in control the next time he has to face a painful experience.

Case Scenario 2

Infant and venipuncture

A 1-year-old girl with a diagnosis of congenital adrenal hyperplasia is being seen at the endocrine clinic for a follow-up appointment. Upon checking in, her mother is looking anxious and asks if her daughter really needs to have a blood test today. The nurse answers *"yes"* and explains how the test results are needed to make adjustments in medications in order to ensure adequate treatment. The mother proceeds to say that this is too distressing for her and her daughter; she had to hold her down last time and they were both crying. The nurse recognizes that the past experiences with venipuncture have not been positive for this child or her mother and aims to improve this. The nurse offers an analgesic cream for the venipuncture site. Options of breast or bottle-feeding during the procedure are reviewed, explaining how this helps to decrease the painful sensation for the infant. Further time is taken to explain the importance of making the venipuncture as pain and stress free for both the girl and her family. The mother agrees to the analgesic cream and this is applied by the nurse to two sites on the infant, in case one venipuncture attempt is unsuccessful. The infant's mother explains that she is breastfeeding; therefore, she would like to choose this option when it is time for the venipuncture. With the support of the nurse, the mother holds her child in a comfortable breastfeeding position allowing for her infant's arm to be accessible. The infant fusses with the tourniquet application but continues to breastfeed. The venipuncture proceeds with success. She does not react at all when the needle is inserted. Her mother is able to comfort her quickly after the blood is taken. The nurse supports both the baby and her mother during and after the venipuncture with positive words. The mother comments that she wished she had known these tips months ago and plans on using them moving forward. The nurse explains to the mother that in the future she can ask for help to make needles less painful for her child, especially if options are not offered ahead of time. The nurse follows with explaining that as the child grows new options would be made available to ensure less painful procedures and create positive experiences, including reshaping memories of pain as needed.

5.2 Gender Creative and Transgender Youth (Gender Dysphoria)

Endocrine nurses in a pediatric or adult setting one day will very likely encounter an individual who presents themselves somewhere on a non-typical gender spectrum. Gaining knowledge and developing an understanding and respect for each person's gender expression or presentation is every health care provider's duty in order to provide appropriate support and health care. Not all nursing education programs provide thorough training for students in gender diversity. There are thousands of nurses in the workforce currently who trained over 10, 20, and 30 years ago prior to any cultural or gender awareness programs. Personal beliefs and bias of nurses can significantly impact the health and access to timely care for transgender (TG) individuals (Dorsen 2012; Strong and Folse 2015; Zunner and Grace 2012). Knowing the diagnostic criteria, standards of care, clinical practice guidelines, and supports for TG people can help endocrine nurses make a very important impact in their lives.

The Pediatric Endocrinology Nursing Society (PENS) has a position statement on transgender youth. This document is an excellent resource for all nurses involved with transgender individuals. PENS recommends that all health care professionals receive "gender inclusive and awareness training during both their professional education programs and their workplace orientation for the protection and inclusivity of children, youth and adults who fall under the transgender umbrella" (Kirouac 2015).

5.2.1 Definitions

Gender can be described as how one "feels" as either masculine, feminine, somewhere in between or neither (Veale et al. 2017; Bonifacio and Rosenthal 2015). This gender feeling is sometimes different than one's assigned sex at birth that is typically based on external genitalia. Gender dysphoria (GD) has been described as "Discomfort or distress that is caused by a discrepancy between a person's gender identity and that person's sex assigned at birth (and the associated gender role and/or primary and secondary characteristics)" (World Professional Association for Transgender Health 2017). Children of all ages may present with gender dysphoria. Most very young prepubertal children who may show some signs of cross gender curiosity, expression, and potential dysphoria over time are more likely to identify as gay or lesbian and not persist to be transgender. Young children who very strongly persist with their gender dysphoria into puberty are more likely to continue through to adulthood identifying as transgender (Bonifacio and Rosenthal 2015).

5.2.2 Diagnostic Criteria

For years, those identifying as transgender had been labelled as having gender identity disorder. The last edition of the American Psychiatric Association's Diagnostic and Statistical Manual (DSM-5) published in 2013 renamed the clinical description as gender dysphoria—removing "disorder" (American Psychiatric Association 2013). A qualified mental health practitioner should assess and diagnose all children and adolescents prior to any initiation of feminizing or masculinizing cross hormone therapy.

The increasing body of literature supporting gender expression and acceptance over the past 10 years exceeds the archaic methods of some recommendations that transgender individuals be "repaired" as if they were broken. Reparative or conversion therapy is now banned in some countries and goes against one's human right of gender expression (Bonifacio and Rosenthal 2015).

5.2.3 Treatment Guidelines

The inter-professional World Professional Association for Transgender Health (WPATH), formerly known as the Harry Benjamin International Gender Dysphoria Association, which originated in 1979, developed and updated the "Standards of Care" (SOC) for the treatment of transgender individuals. These standards are supported worldwide and can help to ensure transgender individuals have access to equitable care no matter where they live. This 120-page standards of care was last updated in 2011 making it the 7th version (World Professional Association for Transgender Health 2017).

The Endocrine Society has released a 2017 update to their previous 2009 Clinical Practice Guidelines for the Treatment of Transsexual Individuals, now titled "Endocrine Treatment of Gender-Dysphoric/Gender-Incongruent Persons: An Endocrine Society* Clinical Practice Guideline" (Hembree et al. 2017). Following the WPATH and Endocrine Society Clinical Practice Guidelines will help inter-professional clinics provide competent, sensitive, and timely care for gender creative and transgender youth (Hembree et al. 2017). A summary of current clinical guidelines in the care of Transgender Youth for Endocrine Nurses is summarized by Kirouac and Tan (2017), with permission this can be found in Table 5.3.

5.2.4 Public Education and Support

Health care, school, and social experiences of self-identified transgender youth and young adults have not been very positive. A Canadian Trans Youth Health Survey was performed by an inter-professional team across Canada for 14–25 year olds. Responses from over 900 peo-

Table 5.3 Assessments, hormone therapy, and monitoring for transgender youth

Tanner staging examination for puberty status			
Puberty blocking <u>if</u> Tanner stage 2 or higher <u>and</u> desired by the youth			
Ensure there is no interfering untreated psychiatric comorbidity, youth has the ability to consent, parents/guardian offering support			
*Use an injectable gonadotropin releasing hormone (GnRH) agonist**			
3.75–7.5 mg intramuscularly q 4 weeks OR 11.25–20 mg intramuscularly q 12 weeks			
*Every 3 months monitor**: height, weight, sitting height, tanner stage, LH, FSH, estradiol, and/or testosterone as appropriate. *Every year**: renal and liver functions, lipids, glucose, insulin, HgA1C. Bone density if warranted (deemed high risk) and bone age of left hand			
Male to female (MTF)[a]		Female to male (FTM)	
*Antiandrogens**:		*Menses cessation if not using GnRH*	
Spironolactone (monitor Se. Na + q 2–3 months in year 1)	50 mg/day, increase q 2–4 weeks by 50 mg (max 200 mg/day)	Consider using oral or injectable contraceptive methods that could stop menses	
Cyproterone acetate[b]	50–100 mg/day	or	
		Intrauterine device (e.g., Mirena, by Adol. Gynecology)	
Discuss desire for and potential availability of fertility preservation options			
Refer to fertility specialist prior to cross hormone therapy treatment if desired			
Once there is a gender dysphoria diagnosis per DSM-5 by a qualified mental health practitioner and desire for cross hormone therapy			
Age 16 years and after baseline bloodwork (below*):		Age 16 years and after baseline bloodwork (below*):	
Informed consent for induction of female puberty		Informed consent for induction of male puberty	
Using oral 17-Beta estradiol,		Using intramuscular testosterone esters:	
Increasing the dose every 6 months:		Enanthate (200 mg/mL) or, cypionate (100 mg/mL)	
5 μg/kg/day, 10 μg/kg/day, 15 μg/kg/day, 20 μg/kg/day		Increasing the dose every 6 months:	
Adult dose = 2 mg/day		25 mg/m^2 per 2 weeks IM, 50 mg/m^2 per 2 weeks IM	
		75 mg/m^2 per 2 weeks IM, 100 mg/m^2 per 2 weeks IM	
		Can be divided into weekly subcutaneous (SC) doses for increased independence, <pain[c]	
See every 2–3 months in first year on cross hormone tx., then 1–2 times per year, monitor blood pressure			
*Baseline and q 3 months fasting labs: CBC, liver Fcn, lipids, Gluc, BHCG (FTM), Prl, Testo, estrogen			
		Discuss desire for top surgery and send referral if needed (age of consent is center dependent)	

Reproduced with permission from Kirouac and Tan (2017)
*Adapted from the Endocrine Society Clinical Practice Guidelines (Hembree et al. 2017)
[a]Estrogens used with or without antiandrogens or GnRH agonist
[b]Not available in the United States
[c]Personal communication, Canadian Pediatric Endocrine Nurses Group, Toronto, November 2016

ple showed prominent themes such as the lack of awareness, understanding, and practical knowledge of health care practitioners (Veale et al. 2017). Many individuals do not feel safe talking about gender preference especially with health care providers that have cared for them since birth.

A joint United States and Canada Qualitative Study of Community Resources and Supports for LGBTQ Adolescents found that critical support is found from inclusive education, gay-straight alliances (GSAs), and anti-bullying policies in schools (Eisenberg et al. 2018). Nurses are in a very good position to ask students and parents about access to such resources and encourage participation. There continues to be publications set out by this prominent research group through www.saravyc.ubc.ca.

Nurses are in a unique position to advocate for individuals who present somewhere on the gender spectrum, especially transgender and gender creative youth. A summary of ways to create gender inclusive clinical spaces are outlined in Table 5.4 (Kirouac and Tan 2017). The opportunity to make a positive impact in the life of a gender creative or transgender youth is always there—stay well informed and always listen carefully.

Table 5.4 Creating clinical spaces that are gender inclusive

Know the resources for nurses and families: These are always current from www.bcchildrens.ca/health-info/coping-support/transgender-resources
Have "rainbow" (LGBTQ friendly) signage and handouts and/or resources put on: doors/windows/bathrooms/clinic counters/pamphlet racks/websites
Ensure you have toys in the waiting area that are gender inclusive
Acknowledge and affirm at time of contact with patients their expressed gender variance
Negotiate preferred names and pronouns directly with patients and ensure these are visible on the chart or electronic medical record as "preferred" until legal changes exist
Negotiate safety and confidentiality with your patient before speaking with their parents, primary care practitioners or their school
Explore psychosocial, mental health, and wellness with all patients. Consider accessing validated gender assessment tools such as the Utrecht and body image scales
Obtain a sexual history asking about the use of protection (condoms/contraceptives) and rather than "boyfriend or girlfriend" ask about a partner
Ask the patient what names they prefer for their body parts and be sensitive to their comfort during any physical examinations
Negotiate support systems and encourage patients to use them
Know the resources and referral sources for general mental health (MH) access, specific gender MH assessments and gender specialty care like surgery, electrolysis in your area
Advocate for the child/youth/family within the health care system and community through participating in community/school education, media interviews, government relations

Reproduced with permission by Kirouac and Tan (2017)

Online resources for nurses regarding Gender Creative and Transgender Youth:

The Endocrine Society Clinical Practice Guidelines for the Endocrine treatment of Gender-Dysphoric/Gender-Incongruent Persons (2017)

https://www.endocrine.org/guidelines-and-clinical-practice/clinical-practice-guidelines

The Paediatric Endocrinology Nursing Society Position Statement for Transgender Youth

www.pens.org

Gender Creative Kids CANADA: Resources for gender creative kids and their families, schools and communities

www.gendercreativekids.ca

Gender Spectrum: helping to create gender sensitive and inclusive environments for all children and teens

www.genderspectrum.org

National Centre for Transgender Equality (US)

www.transequality.org

The World Professional Association for Transgender Health: access to Standards of Care

www.wpath.org

Links to the Canadian Trans Youth Health Survey Reports and the USA/Canada Joint Study of Community Resources and Supports through the Stigma and Resilience Among Vulnerable Youth Centre (SARAVYC). Researchers with a focus on youth health equity

www.saravyc.ubc.ca

Case Scenario 3

Gender Creative and Transgender Youth

A 10-year-old natal male child is referred to the pediatric endocrine clinic by the child psychologist with a diagnosis of gender dysphoria. Upon arrival to the clinic, this child appears female with long curly hair and is wearing pink tights and a flower covered t-shirt. Parents are greeted by the receptionist who asks the family name and the child's preferred name. After a few minutes in the waiting room, the child and family are invited to the clinic room where the nurse proceeds to weigh and measure the child. These measurements are plotted on a "male" growth chart that has been photocopied to take out the color. Time is spent with parents and the child to learn the child's medical history, family history, and more specifically their gender preferences and desires for their future self. The nurse explains to the child that there will be a physical exam to help assess the level of puberty they are currently in. The child expresses that they identify as female and prefer female pronouns. Parents confirm that the child is presenting as female at school and in their community. The nurse assesses the child and learns that she is at Tanner stage 2 for testicular development. The child is upset about the examination and tells the nurse she does not want any further puberty development as she is a girl. Time is spent explaining to parents and the child the role of a gonadotropin releasing hormone treatment to put puberty on hold and prevent further masculinization. The child is afraid of needles but is willing to try the treatment to prevent further puberty changes. The nurse reviews options of using analgesic creams, a vibrating device at and above the injection location, as well as distraction techniques at the time of injection. Parents and the child agree to try the gonadotropin releasing hormone treatment and plan an appointment in the upcoming weeks for the first injection. Upon return to the clinic following the successful first injection of the GnRH analogue, routine every three-month bloodwork is ordered for LH, FSH, and testosterone as well as physical examinations to ensure no further testicular growth. The option of an antiandrogen therapy such as spironolactone is offered to parents and the child. At this time, the family and the child would like to continue monitoring with the endocrine clinic every 3 months. The child has shared that she is looking forward to going through puberty like her friends, especially having breast development. The nurse explains that over the coming years the options of cross hormone therapy with estrogen will be further explored. The nurse reinforces that they are following treatment guidelines that are used across the world. The child and family appear reassured that the treatment approach is one that is used worldwide.

5.2.5 Conclusions

Infants, children, and teens attending any endocrine appointment or testing facility are likely to encounter the need for blood testing or injections. Many have not been offered any pre-treatment for these painful procedures to decrease the pain and anxiety they trigger. It is well known that these painful experiences can stay into adulthood, significantly affecting future encounters and access to health care as well as risk of chronic pain. Nurses are urged to consider all options to decrease the painful experiences of procedures in infants, children, and teens while assisting in reshaping their memories of pain to improve their quality of life.

Children and youth identifying as transgender face many challenges with mental health and acceptance by health care providers. Guidelines have been well developed to support transgender youth through an experienced multidisciplinary team as they transition to their preferred gender. All nurses should be familiar with the risks of this population and how to create gender friendly environments. Endocrine nurses can be instrumental in ensuring access to puberty blocking and cross hormone therapy for transgender youth while encouraging family and community supports.

5.3 Girls with Developmental Disability and Puberty

Puberty is a complex developmental period involving both physical and psychological maturation. This includes rapid growth, development of secondary sexual characteristics, maturation of reproductive functions, and bone mass accrual, as well as cognitive and psychological development. This process is the same for children with developmental/physical disabilities but raises a number of associated concerns for the girls with developmental disabilities (DD) and particularly for their families (Wolf and Long 2016; Kirkham et al. 2013).

Puberty and approaching menses can be very stressful for parents. They may share concerns about their daughters who are affected with DD as they increase in size and weight. How will their daughters manage the bleeding and hygiene measures required? How will the family cope with management of menstruation and related hygiene issues if their daughter isn't capable of independent self-care? Issues such as behavioral changes related to the pre-menstrual period, how to manage the pain of menstrual cramps, the risk of pregnancy, or whether puberty will affect their other medical issues (e.g., seizures) are typical concerns of parents of girls with DD (Tracy et al. 2016). Families sometimes may ask the health care team if going through puberty is necessary.

For the purpose of this chapter, "developmental disabilities" (DD) will include girls with moderate to severe global developmental delay, autism spectrum disorder (ASD), moderate to severe cerebral palsy (CP) and neuromuscular conditions, and complex seizure disorders. When there are concerns specific to these diagnosis, these will be pointed out.

5.3.1 Pubertal Benefits

Families may be distressed with the onset of puberty in their child with DD and will ask the health care team if puberty is really necessary, or if it can be stopped entirely. There are many positive outcomes associated with puberty and it is important to review them (Zacharin et al. 2010).

First of all, there are structural and functional changes occurring in the brain including an increased ability to communicate and a greater desire to be independent (Fima 2006; Bourguignon and Juul 2012). Even for non-verbal, severely delayed children changes in cooperation and minimal understanding are reported by families. Physical strength also improves, and the girls may be able to help more with their own position changes. Overall mood is also reported to improve with the onset of puberty (Quint 2008).

Another important factor is the structural changes in bone formation during puberty. This bone formation becomes the base of children's bone mineral density for life. Puberty has been shown to increase bone mass by 40–50% (Lazar and Phillip 2012). Estrogen elevation associated with puberty is also important to the maturity of the cardiovascular system (Fima 2006; Freedman et al. 2002).

However, there are also many difficulties associated with puberty to consider, including hygiene management, comprehension of the physical changes, and the burden of physical care on parents, caregivers, and school support staff to consider. When parents are asked about their experiences in hindsight, they almost always report that their daughters tolerated the onset of menses better than was expected (Zacharin et al. 2010).

5.3.2 Pubertal Onset Differences

In general, girls with DD experience similar onset of puberty similar to non-affected girls. However, there are a few exceptions. Children with cerebral palsy tend to begin puberty earlier, but the timing of menarche is later than non-affected children. The median onset of menses for girls with cerebral palsy is 14 years compared to the typical onset at 12.8 years (Siddiqi et al. 1999). Children with neurodevelopmental disabilities are 20 times more likely to experience early pubertal change. It is not clearly understood why this happens, but it is generally believed to be related to the malformation of the central nervous system and its effect on the hypothalamic-pituitary-ovarian axis (Siddiqi et al. 1999).

Late puberty may also be more common in children with disabilities (Quint 2008) and girls with compromised nutrition (Wei and Crowne 2016). If early onset puberty causes concerns for self-esteem, self-care and hygiene, or risk of sexual abuse, then treatment with a gonadotropin releasing hormone (GNRH) agonist may be an option.

5.3.3 Assessment of Patients

There are many factors for the nurse to take into consideration when obtaining a medical history from DD girls and their families. The young woman should be included in the discussion as much as possible, while taking into consideration her cognitive and developmental level. As well as a typical medical history, the following special concerns need to be assessed (Kirkham et al. 2013; Tracy et al. 2016; Quint 2008):

Medications
- How does the child take her medications? Can she swallow pills? Does she have a feeding tube? It is important to remember that oral contraceptive pills (OCP) need to be swallowed unless access to chewable versions is available, and then they can be crushed and given in a g-tube.
- For children with a seizure disorder, it is important to consider what kind of anticonvulsant they are taking since some anticonvulsant

medications may not be compatible with OCP use due to increased liver clearance of estrogen.

- It is important to assess if the child is taking antipsychotic medication since some antipsychotic medications cause elevated prolactin levels, resulting in irregular periods and lactation.
- The nurse should also inquire whether the girl will be taking her own medication or will be supervised by the parent. For girls with a diagnosis of fetal alcohol syndrome, severe attention deficit hyperactivity disorder (ADHD), or mild-moderate cognitive impairment, impulsivity and poor memory, parents should be counseled to carefully supervise medication management.

Other specific concerns to address in medical history:

- History of previous surgeries since anatomic changes may effect periods (e.g., gastroschisis repair).
- Are they ambulatory, partially or totally wheelchair bound? For non-weight bearing children, bone accrual is very important to consider and any treatment that does not support good bone health is not recommended.
- Can the girl physically manage her own self-care related to hygiene? This may be a concern for girls with severe CP or severe cognitive delay. Studies show that girls who can independently manage toileting needs will learn to manage menses hygiene.
- Do they have issues with increased skin sensitivity (typical with autisn spectrum disorder)? A diagnosis of ASD raises a few concerns including increased skin sensitivity and sensitivity to color. For example, some teens will be very uncomfortable wearing menstrual pads and may remove them or be upset by the sight of blood.
- Other underlying medical concerns, such as chromosomal disorders, being significantly underweight, thyroid disorders, and epilepsy (found in 20–40% of people with intellectual disabilities (Bowley and Kerr 2000)).
- Is the girl verbal or non-verbal?

- Is bowel and bladder incontinence an issue since this can further complicate self-care (Tracy et al. 2016; Quint 2008).

Menses-related medical history assessment (Wolf and Long 2016; Quint 2008):

- Does the girl have pain with periods or if non-verbal, are there behaviors that might indicate this?
- How regular is the period? (every 21–45 days is within normal range for all girls).
- How long does the period last? (4–7 days is within normal range).
- How heavy is the bleeding? heavy bleeding would be changing pads every 1–2 h, clots bigger than 1 cm, gushing with standing up or overflowing pads at night in bed.

Social experiences:

- Does the child/adolescent require periodic or constant adult supervision?
- Is there a risk of abuse or pregnancy due to school or living arrangements?
- Is there a social group this girl can be exposed to? Social experiences play an important role in psychosexual development. Typical teens often get at least some of their information regarding puberty or menses through peers and social contacts. Girls with disabilities are known to have reduced social contacts and therefore may not gain as much knowledge (e.g., STIs) (Quint 2008; Murphy and Elias 2006; Grover 2011).

What are the primary concerns of the child/ adolescent and parent(s)?

- Does regularity and predictability of periods matter or is the actual bleeding the biggest concern? Is treatment aimed towards pain control, bleeding control, hygiene concerns, behavior management, or birth control? There are many options for managing menses in this population. It is important to assess what the family and girl want to "control" and target your treatment recommendation(s).
- Reassure the adolescent and parent that the health care team will address specific concerns

related to menses management when the girl is assessed at Tanner 3. Once menarche has occurred, the medical options can be discussed.

- It is important to remember that many girls with severe physical and developmental issues manage menses well with little to no intervention, particularly if the periods are predictable and manageable.

5.3.4 Medical Treatment Options

5.3.4.1 LARC (Levonorgestrel IUD Implant)

LARC is an intrauterine device (IUD) placed within the uterus that contains progesterone. Progesterone is a naturally occurring hormone that prevents the buildup of the lining of the uterus. Overtime this may cause partial or total amenorrhea. About 65% of patients experience total amenorrhea while the remainder experience periods that are much lighter and typically without cramping. In the special needs patient, this device will be implanted under a brief anesthesia in the operating room (Savasi et al. 2009; Albanese and Hopper 2007).

The patient with a LARC will continue going through the hormonal cycle of menses, so this is sometimes not the best choice for patients with behavioral hormonal issues or seizures proven to be affected by hormones (catamenial) (Quint 2008).

Benefits of LARC:
- Reduced bleeding to complete amenorrhea
- Almost complete reduction of dysmenorrhea
- Little risk for bone depletion
- No risk for blood clots
- Lasts for 3–5 years
- Highest success for birth control

Stated side effects of the LARC:
- Cramping for short term after insertion
- Small amounts of vaginal bleeding (spotting) after insertion for up to 6 months
- Headache
- Mood changes
- Weight gain

LARC is a good choice for patients with:
- Seizure disorders
- Bone health concerns
- Very heavy menstrual bleeding or a bleeding disorder (Savasi et al. 2009; Albanese and Hopper 2007; Dizon et al. 2005)

5.3.4.2 Oral Contraceptive Control Pill or Patch

Oral contraceptive pill (OCP) or patch is a combination medication that contains estrogen and progesterone, which overrides the pituitary ovarian axis and results in anovulation. A low-dose monophasic pill can be used continuously, which may be useful for some patients (Grover 2011).

Benefits of OCP:
- Reduced blood flow with periods
- Reduced pain with periods
- Regular predictable periods
- Contraception
- Acne improvement
- Moods may be more stable

Possible side effects of OCP:
- Slightly increased risk of blood clots may even be higher for wheelchair bound teens
- Break through bleeding
- Nausea
- Headaches
- Mood changes
- Special consideration for those on anticonvulsants due to increased activation of cytochrome P450, which results in higher excretion of estrogen through the liver, that may require a higher dose of OCP (Quint 2008; Savasi et al. 2009; Albanese and Hopper 2007; Dizon et al. 2005)

Continuous use of OCP or patch:
- Once the pill or patch has been successfully introduced with a withdrawal bleed every 3 weeks, the adolescent may transition to continuous use. For example, 9 weeks of OCP back to back without taking a break or placebo pills. This will result in a planned withdrawal bleed every 10 weeks. Using the patch, you

may continue to put a new patch on weekly for 10 weeks and then take it off for the withdrawal bleed.

5.3.4.3 Depo Provera Injections

Depo Provera is an intramuscular injection of progesterone that is given every 12 weeks or more frequently. It reduces buildup of the lining of the uterus and eventually results in anovulation.

Benefits of depo provera:
- Reduced blood flow with periods
- Reduced pain with periods
- Contraception
- Eventual very light periods or none
- Treatment only every 12 weeks

Possible side effects of depo Provera:
- Weight gain
- Suppression of the hypothalamic-pituitary-ovarian axis results in depletion of estrogen and therefore reduction in the accrual of bone; therefore, it is not recommended for those at risk for reduced bone health because of decreased mobility
- Headache
- Breakthrough bleeding (Veale et al. 2017; Bonifacio and Rosenthal 2015; (World Professional Association for Transgender Health 2017))

5.3.5 Permanent Surgical Treatment

The option of surgical treatment as an intervention to manage menstruation varies from country to country. In general, hysterectomy or other forms of permanent sterilization is considered illegal, and possibly unethical. If all other strategies for menses management fail and the girl is experiencing significant distress, surgery may be considered after review with a specialist gynecologist and an appropriate ethics review (American College of Obstetricians and Gynecologists 2017).

- In recent years, there has been a movement towards a treatment referred to as growth attenuation therapy (GAT). Physicians may be asked about growth attenuation, which uses very high dose estrogen therapy and/or hysterectomy/sterilization and mastectomy. The goal of this therapy is to retain a girl in a "child-like state." Supporters of this approach propose that the outcomes of a smaller adult size will allow easier physical care of the adolescent/adult for the caregivers and therefore reduce hygiene concerns, and possibly reduce the possible risk of sexual abuse. However, at this time there is insufficient evidence to support this approach (Quint 2008; Savasi et al. 2009; Albanese and Hopper 2007; Dizon et al. 2005).

5.3.5.1 Pain Control

Painful menstrual periods are experienced by 10–45% of teens (Albanese and Hopper 2007; Dizon et al. 2005). For non-verbal girls, a change in behavior may be the only clue to whether they are experiencing period pain.

Non-steroidal anti-inflammatory drugs (NSAIDS) should be the first line of treatment, started the day before or the first day of bleeding, and given on a regular schedule during the onset of menses. Regular use of NSAIDS may reduce period flow by 30–50% (Quint 2008; Savasi et al. 2009; Albanese and Hopper 2007; Dizon et al. 2005).

At the start of menstrual period:
- Administer NSAIDs to prevent period cramps
- If periods are predictable, can start NSAIDs just before the onset of period and take regularly for the first few days.
- For period cramps due to prostaglandins, NSAIDs can suppress prostaglandins if taken consistently.
- For girls with period-related behavior concerns, treatment with NSAIDs has been shown to be helpful.

5.3.6 Nursing Strategies

The nurse should counsel the parent of a child with DD child regarding strategies to promote adjustment to puberty and menstruation (Kirkham et al. 2013; Zacharin et al. 2010; Quint 2008; Grover 2011).

Prior to the onset of puberty:

- To start adjusting to the texture and sensation of pads, use mini-pads inside of panties for a brief time and gradually increase the time until they are comfortable with the sensation. Then, gradually work up to wearing larger size pads. Buy a few different brands and styles and be aware of perfumes and fragrances if the child has sensitivity to new smells or textures. If the texture causes a concern, try natural fiber or reusable pads (often available at health food stores).
- Mark the place on panties where the pad is to be stuck.
- Once the girl is comfortable wearing a pad, add a few spots of red food color to the pad; if the color causes distress sometimes describing the pad as a "bandage" can help.
- Girls wearing diapers often may want to use pads inside of the diaper. This provides some "normality" to their experience and also saves on the amount of diapers that are used.
- Allowing the girl in the bathroom to observe the mother or sister model the changing of pads may help them realize that this is normal for all women.

After the onset of puberty:

- Parents often describe behavior and mood changes around the time of periods. While this is possible, it may not always be an accurate interpretation. Emotional swings may also be a part of puberty or related to pain with periods. The best way to clarify this is to have parents, girls, or caregivers keep a calendar that includes period days, amount of bleeding, possible pain behaviors, as well as mood. Over a few months, a pattern may often become apparent. If seizures are a concern, they should also be reported in conjunction with periods on the calendar.
- Make a schedule for pad changes at school.

- Make a hygiene pack that can go to school or out with the girls including a change of bottoms, extra pads, and hygiene wipes.

5.4   Conclusions

The key to providing the right support during puberty to children with DD is to take a detailed and specific medical history. There is no method that is perfect for everyone. Different treatment options have different side effects and must be chosen carefully. It is also critical to listen to the family and the girls! They will tell you what they need help with the most and it may not always be what you assume. This is an area of practice that would greatly benefit from more outcome research, so that our practice can be more evidence based.

References

Albanese A, Hopper NW. Suppression of menstruation in adolescents with severe learning disabilities. Arch Dis Child. 2007;92(7):629–32.

American College of Obstetricians and Gynecologists. Sterilization of women: ethical issues and considerations. The American College of Obstetricians and Gynecologists [Internet]. 2017.

American Psychiatric Association. Diagnostic and statistical manual of mental disorders (DSM-5). 5th ed. Arlington, VA: American Psychiatric Association; 2013.

Bonifacio HJ, Rosenthal SM. Gender variance and dysphoria in children and adolescents. Pediatr Clin N Am. 2015;62(4):1001–16.

Bourguignon JP, Juul A. Normal female puberty in a developmental perspective. Endocr Dev. 2012;22:11–23.

Bowley C, Kerr M. Epilepsy and intellectual disability. J Intellect Disabil Res. 2000;44(Pt 5):529–43.

Dizon CD, Allen LM, Ornstein MP. Menstrual and contraceptive issues among young women with developmental delay: a retrospective review of cases at the Hospital for Sick Children, Toronto. J Pediatr Adolesc Gynecol. 2005;18(3):157–62.

Dorsen C. An integrative review of nurse attitudes towards lesbian, gay, bisexual, and transgender patients. Can J Nurs Res. 2012;44(3):18–43.

Eisenberg ME, Mehus CJ, Saewyc EM, Corliss HL, Gower AL, Sullivan R, et al. Helping young people stay afloat: a qualitative study of community resources and supports for LGBTQ adolescents in the United States and Canada. J Homosex. 2018;65(8):969–89.

Fima L. In: Fima L, editor. Pediatric endocrinology. 5th ed. New York: Marcel Dekker; 2006.

Freedman DS, Khan LK, Serdula MK, Dietz WH, Srinivasan SR, Berenson GS. Relation of age at menarche to race, time period, and anthropometric dimensions: the Bogalusa Heart Study. Pediatrics. 2002;110(4):e43.

Grover SR. Gynaecological issues in adolescents with disability. J Paediatr Child Health. 2011;47(9):610–3.

Hembree WC, Cohen-Kettenis PT, Gooren L, Hannema SE, Meyer WJ, Murad MH, et al. Endocrine treatment of gender-dysphoric/gender-incongruent persons: an Endocrine Society clinical practice guideline. J Clin Endocrinol Metab. 2017;102(11):3869–903.

Hofman PL, Lawton SA, Peart JM, Holt JA, Jefferies CA, Robinson E, et al. An angled insertion technique using 6-mm needles markedly reduces the risk of intramuscular injections in children and adolescents. Diabet Med. 2007;24(12):1400–5.

Kirkham YA, Allen L, Kives S, Caccia N, Spitzer RF, Ornstein MP. Trends in menstrual concerns and suppression in adolescents with developmental disabilities. J Adolesc Health. 2013;53(3):407–12.

Kirouac N. PENS position statement on transgender youth. J Pediatr Nurs. 2015;31:230–1.

Kirouac N, Tan M. Gender creative or transgender youth and advanced nursing practice. Pediatr Endocrinol Rev. 2017;14(Suppl 2):441–7.

Koster MP, Stellato N, Kohn N, Rubin LG. Needle length for immunization of early adolescents as determined by ultrasound. Pediatrics. 2009;124(2):667–72.

Lazar L, Phillip M. Pubertal disorders and bone maturation. Endocrinol Metab Clin N Am. 2012;41(4):805–25.

McCarthy AM, Kleiber C, Hanrahan K, Zimmerman MB, Westhus N, Allen S. Factors explaining children's responses to intravenous needle insertions. Nurs Res. 2010;59(6):407–16.

McMurtry CM, Riddell RP, Taddio A, Racine N, Gordon MA, Asmundson JG, Noel M, Chambers CT, Shah V. Far from "just a poke": common painful needle procedures and the development of needle fear. Clin J Pain. 2015;31(10S):S3–7.

Murphy NA, Elias ER. Sexuality of children and adolescents with developmental disabilities. Pediatrics. 2006;118(1):398–403.

Noel M, Chambers CT, McGrath PJ, Klein RM, Stewart SH. The influence of children's pain memories on subsequent pain experience. Pain. 2012;153(8):1563–72.

Noel M, Pavlova M, McCallum L, Vinall J. Remembering the hurt of childhood: a psychological review and call for future research. Can Psychol. 2017;58(1):58–68.

Quint EH. Menstrual issues in adolescents with physical and developmental disabilities. Ann N Y Acad Sci. 2008;1135:230–6.

Savasi I, Spitzer RF, Allen LM, Ornstein MP. Menstrual suppression for adolescents with developmental disabilities. J Pediatr Adolesc Gynecol. 2009;22(3):143–9.

Siddiqi SU, Van Dyke DC, Donohoue P, McBrien DM. Premature sexual development in individuals with neurodevelopmental disabilities. Dev Med Child Neurol. 1999;41(6):392–5.

Strong KL, Folse VN. Assessing undergraduate nursing students' knowledge, attitudes, and cultural competence in caring for lesbian, gay, bisexual, and transgender patients. J Nurs Educ. 2015;54(1):45–9.

Taddio A, McMurtry CM, Shah V, Riddell RP, Chambers CT, Noel M, et al. Reducing pain during vaccine injections: clinical practice guideline. CMAJ. 2015;187(13):975–82.

Thrane SE, Wanless S, Cohen SM, Danford CA. The assessment and non-pharmacologic treatment of procedural pain from infancy to school age through a developmental Lens: a synthesis of evidence with recommendations. J Pediatr Nurs. 2017;31:e23–32.

Tracy J, Grover S, Macgibbon S. Menstrual issues for women with intellectual disability. Aust Prescr. 2016;39(2):54–7.

Veale JF, Watson RJ, Peter T, Saewyc EM. Mental health disparities among Canadian transgender youth. J Adolesc Health. 2017;60(1):44–9.

Wei C, Crowne EC. Recent advances in the understanding and management of delayed puberty. Arch Dis Child. 2016;101(5):481–8.

Wolf RM, Long D. Pubertal development. Pediatr Rev. 2016;37(7):292–300.

World Professional Association for Transgender Health (WPATH). The standards of care for the health of transsexual, transgender, and gender non-conforming people. 2017. www.wpath.org.

Zacharin M, Savasi I, Grover S. The impact of menstruation in adolescents with disabilities related to cerebral palsy. Arch Dis Child. 2010;95(7):526–30.

Zunner BP, Grace PJ. The ethical nursing care of transgender patients: an exploration of bias in health care and how it affects this population. Am J Nurs. 2012;112(12):61–4.

Transition from Paediatric to Adult Services

Susie Aldiss

Contents

S. Aldiss (✉)
School of Health Sciences, University of Surrey,
Surrey, UK
e-mail: s.aldiss@surrey.ac.uk

© Springer Nature Switzerland AG 2019
S. Llahana et al. (eds.), *Advanced Practice in Endocrinology Nursing*,
https://doi.org/10.1007/978-3-319-99817-6_6

Abstract

The transition from child to adult services is a crucial time in the health of young people who may potentially fall into what has been described as a poorly managed 'care gap'. Health service provision, which fails to meet the needs of young people and families at this time of significant change, may result in deterioration in health or disengagement with services, which can have negative long-term consequences. There are two main challenges to providing transitional care: how care is organised and the impact this has on the continuing delivery of care to young people. In this chapter, the issues with transitional care are discussed along with the key principles of transition. Interventions to improve transition are presented along with examples from the literature which include: transition clinics, enhanced support/follow-up, transition coordinator, skills training/education for young people, and technology-based interventions. Endocrine care within the transitional process will also be touched upon, with particular reference to children and young people requiring growth hormone therapy, young people with a disorder of sex development, and young people who have undergone cancer treatment as a child. A successful transition process involves the provision of care that is uninterrupted, coordinated, and developmentally appropriate over a period of time before, during, and after a young person transfers to adult services.

Keywords

Transition · Transfer · Adolescent
Coordination · Long-term conditions
Young adult

Abbreviations

CQC	Care quality commission
DSD	Disorder of sex development
NICE	National Institute for Health and Care Excellence
ON TRAC	Taking responsibility for adolescent/adult care
UK	United Kingdom

Key Terms

- **Transition:** A purposeful and planned process of supporting young people and their families/carers to move from child to adult services. 'Transition' refers to the whole process including initial planning and preparation, the actual transfer between services, and continued support after a young person has moved to adult services.
- **Transfer:** Within the transition process 'transfer' occurs. This is the point at which the young person moves to adult services and is discharged from child services.

Key Points

- The transfer of young people from child to adult services is a crucial time in the health of young people who may potentially fall into a poorly managed 'care gap'.
- The young person should be at the centre of transitional care; transition should be developmentally appropriate taking into account the different needs of each young person.
- Transition should be a gradual process which starts in early adolescence and continues until the young person is well established in the adult care setting.
- Parents should be involved in the transition process and gradually prepared to transfer responsibility of health to the young person.

6.1 Introduction

An increasing number of children with long-term health conditions are now surviving into adulthood. Thus, there are a growing number of children with long-term health needs or complex disabilities who will require ongoing specialised care. The provision of health care for this group has been the focus of attention for some time, with numerous reports over the past decade highlighting the need for improvement in order to better meet the needs of young people.

The journey through adolescence to adulthood is a challenging time of psychological, physical, and social change. Young people with a long-term health condition can face even greater challenges as they deal with complex and important changes in the care they need and in the way it is provided. The role of the young person, and also their parents/carers, will evolve with the young person often wanting and indeed being expected to exercise greater independence in the management of their health condition. Health service provision, which fails to meet the needs of young people and families at this time of significant change, may result in deterioration in health or disengagement with services which can have negative long-term consequences. The transition of young people from child to adult services is a crucial period in the health of young people.

Transition services aim to bridge this 'care gap' between child and adult services. 'Transition' can be defined as 'a multi-faceted, active process that attends to the medical, psychosocial and educational/vocational needs of adolescents as they move from the child-focused to the adult-focused health care system' (Blum et al. 1993, p. 573). Within the transition process 'transfer' occurs, which refers the point at which the young person moves to adult health services and is discharged from child health services. On occasion, these two terms, transition and transfer are used interchangeably.

6.2   Issues Within Transitional Care

There are two main challenges to providing transitional care: how care is organised and the impact this has on the continuing delivery of care to young people. Unfortunately, many young people have a very different experience of transition, which does not meet the aspirations of Blum et al.'s (1993) definition. Numerous research studies have reported that some young people experience the transfer to adult care as disjointed and more of a one-off transfer, rather than a process of preparation in which they are involved, that is transition: such experiences seem to be comparable across young people with different diagnoses (for a review see Fegran et al. 2014).

Lack of 'being prepared' was also a finding from the recent report on transition from the Care Quality Commission (CQC) in the United Kingdom (UK) (CQC 2014). Here only 54% of young people described preparation for transition that had enabled them to be involved in the process as much as they wanted to be and 80% of pre-transition case notes reviewed had no transition plans for health (CQC 2014).

Current approaches to transition are often described within three categories (Royal College of Nursing 2013):

1. An abrupt transfer to adult services
2. Staying in the paediatric area longer than is appropriate
3. Leaving medical supervision altogether, voluntarily or by default.

All three are associated with short- and long-term impact on young people with a long-term health condition as receivers of these services. Simple transfer can result in increasing anxiety for young people, this immediate change in a relationship with professionals, often one that is long standing, may leave them feeling isolated from their usual support mechanisms, and they may worry that the adult healthcare team will not be able to meet their needs. A review of qualitative literature on young people's experiences of transition by Fegran et al. (2014) described themes relating to loss of relationships with the child care team combined with insecurity and a feeling of being unprepared for what was ahead. So for some, remaining with a healthcare team they know may be their preferred choice. There is, however, the potential for delayed development into adulthood, and although they may feel safe in an environment and with people they know, some of their needs may not be met if they stay with a child health team too long. Disrupted care, or care that no longer meets their needs, can lead to disengagement from services and may result in deterioration in health.

Within the UK, it has been suggested that this lack of focus on young people as a group with particular healthcare needs in medical training and in the health service underpins the difficulty professionals face in improving transitional care (Gleeson and Turner 2012). The need for transi-

Box 6.1 Differences in Service Provision Between Child and Adult Health Care
- Age range
- Culture of care
- Recognition of growth and development
- Consultation dynamics
- Communication styles
- Role of parents
- Role of family
- Role of peers
- Educational issues
- Vocational issues
- Confidentiality issues
- Tolerance of immaturity
- Spectrum of diseases
- Impact of disease

tion has been created by the structure of healthcare services which focus on either children or adults. Child and adult health care are two very different systems of care, serving different populations with diverse requirements. The differences between these two care systems are summarised below in Box 6.1.

Healthcare professionals are mostly trained with a focus on the care of either adults or children and not young people. Young people are a distinctive group with different needs to children and adults. Core skills training in adolescent health care would help to shift current professional attitudes towards young people and result in professionals being able to offer more rounded support. Healthcare professionals working with young people should receive effective training about the stages of adolescence, how some long-term conditions may affect development, how to care for young people, and how best to communicate with them: core skills needed to provide transitional care.

From focus groups with professionals involved in transitional care, Aldiss et al. (2016) identified a number of factors that were associated with delayed transition. These included factors such as the patients' characteristics (e.g. age, health condition, having complex needs) as well as factors associated with services (such as the availability of equivalent services within adult care and the links between the child and adult team). The

length of a relationship between the young person/family and clinical team was also found to impact on transition; when the team had known the young person since they were very young, transfer to adult services was more likely to be delayed. It is therefore imperative that healthcare professionals consider the population they are working with when planning transitional care and take into account factors which can lead to delayed transition, so that this can be avoided where possible.

6.3 Key Principles of Transition

There is a wealth of discussion in the literature regarding the key principles for transitional care and over the past decade, numerous documents have been produced outlining recommendations for practice (for a review of policy documents, see Hepburn et al. 2015). Within the UK, the latest of these documents is the guidance from the National Institute for Health and Care Excellence (NICE) published in February (2016). Gleeson and Turner (2012) outlined five key principles for transitional care, which are often reflected in other guidelines:

1. The process should consider the holistic nature of transitional care and address both clinical and also psychosocial and educational/vocational issues.
2. The process needs to be flexible and developmentally appropriate to meet the changing needs of young people.
3. The process has also to meet the needs of the parent/carer.
4. The process should span the period from early adolescence to young adulthood: a preparation phase in paediatric care; a transfer phase from paediatric to adult services; and an engagement phase in adult services.
5. Potential interventions to support the process should be considered with a focus on staffing, service delivery, and the young person and their parents/carers.

Transition should be a gradual process which starts in early adolescence (some professionals recommend that preparation for transition starts as early as 10 years old) and ends, not once the young person transfers to adult care, but once the young person is well established within the adult care setting. There is much debate about the best age to transfer young people to adult care and little consensus on when this might be. For many services, the age is arbitrary, fixed at maybe 16 or 18 years old, but a set age of transfer does not consider whether this is developmentally appropriate for that young person. Some young people may be ready to move to adult care sooner than others, having a set age of transfer creates a barrier and can delay the transfer for these young people. Conversely, not having a prescribed age of transfer can mean that services 'hold on' to young people for as long as possible resulting in them remaining in child care for longer than is appropriate (Aldiss et al. 2016). The ideal would be an approach with some flexibility enabling the young person to move to adult health care at a pace that suits them, where they are at the centre of the process.

A key element for successful transition is the relationship between the child and adult care providers. Where there is a good relationship and trust has been established, this usually results in a more positive experience of transition for the young person. This can be easier to achieve if the teams are geographically close to each other and can be more difficult when distance is involved and the child providers transfer young people to multiple care teams: documentation and sharing of information is important to ensure all relevant information about the young person is handed over to the new team.

In Box 6.2, a healthcare professional describes how the above key principles for transition are included in how transition is managed for the young people she works with, including transition being a gradual process, flexibility with the timing of transition, and enabling young people to establish a relationship with adult team prior to transfer.

Box 6.2 Healthcare Professional's Description of a Transition Service (Aldiss et al. 2016)

'In our transition clinic, from the age of fourteen, we discuss transition and we introduce the idea that they are going to be going through a transition process and that is very individual. From mostly sixteen, we see them in a transition clinic, which is jointly held with the adult diabetes team. The adult colleagues come over to our clinic and then from sixteen to eighteen, nineteen, depending on the child and the family, when they want to transition, they will be seen in that transition clinic. It is a very flexible, open clinic in that sense and it is held monthly. They then go to the young adult clinic… and they will see the same team member that they saw here. We have the adult nurse and the adult dietician and the adult diabetologist will come and attend, so we make sure that they have already met them over several years prior and then they go to the young adult diabetes team, which is up to the age of 25. It is a very gentle transition process. We also have several things in place, so we have a diabetes transition passport, which is something that we use with them. It is really to ensure that they understand their condition and it is giving them autonomy. Lots of them are diagnosed as babies or very young children and their parents were very much involved and it is just making sure that they them have much more ownership of their care and their treatment, so that is one thing that we are doing. We are introducing a transition day and graduation day, so it is going to be held twice a year, it is going to be for both the people coming into the transition and also people exiting the transition, so they will be held together. It will be an introduction to what transition is, it will be introducing to them to other various different people, but also taking them over to the adult service, so they can actually see where the adult clinic is, just so they have an idea of where they are going to, sort of, be going in the next couple of years. Also we are going to discuss some of the more adult puberty type of issues, so how to manage diabetes and exams, driving licences, jobs, all that kind of thing, as well as sex and alcohol and that kind of thing we are going to mention as well'.

Good communication between everyone involved, joint planning, and provision of information for young people and parents is essential for a good transition experience. Young people need information about their health condition, the plan for transition, and the adult service they will be transitioned to. This should be provided in an appropriate manner and include different formats where possible (such as verbal, written, and signposting to online resources). The timeline for transition should be shared so that families know what to expect and when transfer is expected to happen. What is expected of young people and parents throughout the transition process should be made clear as well as what they can expect from the professionals involved.

Transition can be a worrying and stressful time for parents. Parents are required to adjust their role, responsibilities, and behaviour to support their child's growing independence in preparation for adulthood. A review of parents' views and experiences of their child's healthcare transition highlighted that transition was characterised by ambiguity and uncertainty, leading to feelings of anxiety and distress (Heath et al. 2017). A strong source of anxiety related to a fear of poor health outcomes from relinquishing control of the health condition to the young person. Thus, it is imperative that transitional care involves parents and takes into account their needs. Parents can be key facilitators of their child's healthcare transition, supporting them to become experts in their own condition and care but in turn parents also need to be supported through this process.

Although what 'should' happen with transitional care is well documented, what is lacking in the literature and documents on transitional care is practical guidance on how professionals might start to make improvements to services in order to meet young people's/families' needs. Working with young people, parents, and professionals, Aldiss et al. (2015) developed benchmarks for transition which consist of eight key statements of best practice for transitional care (Box 6.3) along with associated indicators of best practice. The benchmarks offer a straightforward, practical tool for services to measure themselves against to see how they are doing, identify gaps in the service and provide a platform to share successful practice initiatives. This sharing of best practice is key; services need to learn from each other how to overcome common difficulties and offer each other practical support and encouragement sharing what works and what does not work.

Box 6.3 Best Practice in Transitional Care (from Benchmarks for Transition, Aldiss et al. 2015)

1. Young people are offered advice and information in a clear and concise manner about how to manage their health condition as an adult.
2. The young person as they progress through the transition process is gradually prepared and provided with personally understandable information and support.
3. The young person is supported through a smooth transition by knowledgeable and coordinated child and adult teams.
4. Young people are provided with care and in an environment that recognises and respects that they are a 'young person', not a child or adult.
5. Concise, consistent, and clear written document containing all relevant information about the young person's transition is provided to the teams involved in the transition process.
6. Parents are included in the transition process gradually transferring responsibility for health to the young person.
7. The young person's readiness for transition to adult care is assessed.
8. The young person's General Practitioner (primary care provider) is informed of the plan for transition and is able to liaise with other relevant teams to facilitate services requested/needed by the young person.

6.4 Interventions to Improve Transition

Transition programmes are needed to enhance personal growth, increase control and independence by promoting skills in communication, decision-making, and self-management. There is, however, no 'one-size fits all model of transition'. That approach may in fact be inappropriate, as it may not consider variation in the young people themselves, or their preferred style of engagement (Hislop et al. 2016). Personalised planning for transition seems more appropriate, where young people's preferences, combined with the knowledge healthcare professionals have of their patient population, could lead to more effective and efficient engagement with adult care. Reflecting on a comment made by Allen and Gregory (2009) is helpful when thinking about transitional care: 'rather than asking how best to manage transition, we might ask how best to meet the needs of young people with (a long-term condition) at this stage of their life course'. (p. 162).

The most effective way to achieve a smooth transition has become a topic of considerable debate. There are many examples of services where successful transitional care programmes have been implemented (for a review, see Crowley et al. 2011). What we are short of is evaluation, or empirical evidence from the proposed transitional models of care already in place. A recent Cochrane review on transition found few studies looked at effectiveness of interventions with only four fitting the inclusion criteria for the review (Campbell et al. 2016). The authors concluded that the current evidence is of limited quality and no firm conclusions about the effectiveness of interventions could be drawn: this could be why transitional care programmes are still not fully integrated into clinical services. Transitional care is complex and difficult to evaluate, there are not always clear measurable outcomes (Suris and Akre 2015). One issue surrounds the idea of 'usual care', which is usually used as the control for a comparison study. Usual care in relation to transitional care services is wide-ranging and inconsistent. Additional barriers to the development of robust evaluation studies are the diversity of the health conditions experienced by this patient population and the length of follow-up required to assess the efficacy of interventions over time.

6.5 Models of Transitional Care Interventions

Crowley et al. (2011) described three broad categories of intervention directed at the patient (such as education programmes, skills training), staff (such as a named transition coordinator), and service delivery (such as separate young adult clinics, after-hours phone support, enhanced follow-up). This section provides some examples of such interventions to improve transitional care, drawn from published literature, which could be used in isolation or combined in a multidimensional approach as appropriate for the population. The key features of these interventions are summarised in Table 6.1, with detail of enablers then described.

6.6 Service Delivery-Focused Interventions

6.6.1 Transition Policies and Pathways

In the past, 'transition in healthcare has been a process to get young people to adapt to us and the services we provide rather than us adapting to the needs of young people' (Gleeson and Turner 2012, p. 86). The existence of a transition policy is important to guide services but this needs to be developed in collaboration with young people, parents, and professionals who deliver transition. There needs to be some flexibility with timing of transfer in order to take into account the young person's readiness and what else is happening in their life to

Table 6.1 Key features of transitional care interventions

Intervention	Key features	Example from the literature
Transition policies and pathways	• Written guidance/pathway indicating the process of transitional care • Provides a framework for professionals to use when planning transition • Can help to standardise care for young people ensuring a more equitable access to services	Paone et al. (2006)
Transition clinics and young adult clinics	• Staffed by professionals from the child and adult teams • Enables the young person/family to build a relationship and gain trust in the adult team prior to transfer to adult services • Focuses on preparing the young person for adult services • Opportunity to promote peer interaction/support • Young people may feel less out of place in a young adult clinic than in a general clinic where patients in the waiting room may be older people	Harden et al. (2012)
Enhanced support/follow-up	• Extra support provided for the young person which continues ideally until the young person is well-established within the adult service • Support provided via telephone/text message/email • Contact details for a named person providing the support are given to the young person • Helps the young person to navigate the adult care system	Steinbeck et al. (2014)
Named transition coordinator or key worker	• Named person takes responsibility for a young person's transition • Coordinator has an overarching view of the young person's transition • Ensures effective communication and information sharing between services, professional, and family • Improves continuity of care • Young person/family know who to contact regarding transition	Kelly (2014)
Skills training/education for young people	• Aims to prepare young people for life as an adult with a health condition and help them to develop skills for self-management • Should include education about the young person's health condition, treatment in the past and how the condition will affect them in future • Can be delivered in individual or group sessions • Group sessions enable peer support in addition to education	Mackie et al. (2014)
Assessments of 'Readiness'—transition checklists	• Readiness for transition should be frequently assessed through conversations held during clinic appointments • Checklists can be a useful trigger for engaging young people in conversation to help professionals to speak with young people about readiness • Can help to identify any gaps in a young person's skills, knowledge, or confidence needed to manage their health and transition to adult care • Can be used to track a young person's progress in self-management during the transition process	For a review see Zhang et al. (2014)
Technology-based interventions	• Interventions via internet/mobile apps or text messaging • Allow for remote delivery of an intervention • Uses methods of communication that young people are familiar with and use frequently • Potentially more convenient and easier to access than face-to-face interventions • Can be used to monitor young people, provide self-care advice, reminders or education related to health	Huang et al. (2014)

avoid transferring them at difficult times (e.g. during major exams, during a period of illness crisis/instability). Hospital wide policies and pathways can help to coordinate timing of transition for young people who access more than one service.

The ON TRAC (Taking Responsibility for Adolescent/Adult Care) model of care presents a clinical pathway and framework for transition. This model was originally developed in 1998 at Children's and Women's Health Centre of British Columbia, Canada; it provides a multidisciplinary approach to developmentally appropriate transition planning and skill building (Paone et al. 2006). The model is young people focused and family centred and includes stages of transitional care based on the developmental stages and capabilities of young people. The pathway serves as a healthcare provider's 'tool' to support the planning and preparation of young people with long-term conditions starting at 12 years of age. It outlines the timing, preparation and planning, transfer requirements, roles and tasks that can be embedded into clinical care in the child health, community, and adult settings (a shared care approach) to facilitate preparation for adult services and promote successful transfer. The ultimate goal of transition in the ON TRAC model is for all young people to reach their achievable level of independence, self-confidence, and self-esteem whilst transferring safely and securely into adult healthcare services and adulthood. For further information, see http://www.bcchildrens.ca/health-professionals/clinical-resources/transition-to-adult-care.

6.6.2 Transition Clinics and Young Adult Clinics

If possible, the young person and family should be given the opportunity to build a relationship and establish trust over a period of time with the adult team, prior to be being transferred. This can be achieved through joint clinics being held with members of both the adult and child teams. If these clinics are held in the adult environment, the young person can familiarise themselves with the new environment whilst still under the care of familiar professionals. Joint clinics need to be carefully managed; where there are large teams of professionals it may be overwhelming for the young person to have everyone in the consultation room at one time. Other strategies that can help to ease the way for young people into adult services include: having a 'cross-over' period where the young person has the chance to come back to see the child team following the first appointment within adult services to check all is going well with the transition, being accompanied by a member of the child team on the young person's first visit to the adult clinic and having an accompanied visit to the inpatient area if the young person is likely to require future admissions.

Some adult services offer dedicated young adult clinics, which are separate clinics for young people held within the adult setting. A young person would transition from child health services to the young adult service. This model has the advantage that young people may feel less out of place in the clinic waiting room where they are surrounded by their peers rather than older adults. Usually, these clinics are staffed by professionals from the adult service therefore when the young person moves into the adult clinic; there is some continuity, they can remain with health professionals who are familiar to them.

Harden et al. (2012) describe a model implemented for young people who have undergone a renal transplant which includes joint transition clinics as well as a young adult clinic. Between the ages of 15 and 18 years, patients are seen in a transition clinic staffed by a nephrologist and transplant nurse from the child team and adult team in addition to a youth worker from the adult team. Before transfer to the adult clinic, the young person has the chance to visit and look around the adult unit informally. The young person and family can progressively gain trust in the adult healthcare team before transfer. In addition, the adult team can obtain a thorough de-brief from the child health team, enabling a more effective and comprehensive care plan for the patient. By the age of 18, the young people are transferred to a young adult clinic, held in a student college and sports centre. The aim of holding the clinic in a non-clinical environment is to encourage peer interaction between the patients; this is aided by the youth worker coordinating activities such as having lunch/coffee together and pool competitions in the games room. Timing of transfer to a standard adult clinic varies between the patients and in most cases is determined by them, taking into account their educational, employment, and social development. Harden et al. (2012) compared the rates of transplant loss between two groups of young people: group 1 transitioned to the adult service prior to the implementation of the model above and group 2 experienced the new service. In group 1, 67% of young people lost their transplant, compared to no transplant losses in group 2; Harden et al. (2012) suggest this model improved patient experience with the consequent effect of improving patient adherence to medication and engagement with health professionals.

6.6.3 Enhanced Support/Follow-Up

Enhanced support refers to the extra support provided to a young person as they move into the adult service which continues ideally until they are well established within the new service. The aims of enhanced support are to: improve the experience of transferring to adult services for the young person, help them to navigate the new system, reduce non-attendance, and reduce dropout rates. Such support can be provided to young people moving to adult services in different ways. Steinbeck et al. (2014) describe an intervention which was implemented post-discharge from child health care and sought to promote better use of adult diabetic services. The intervention included a transition coordinator making the first adult diabetes service appointment and provisions of paper and electronic (USB memory stick) copies of information on services and health care for diabetes. This was followed by four standardised telephone calls at week one, three, six and 12 months. These calls aimed to provide support, help the young person to understand the transition process, and discuss the young person's general well-being, life events, transition difficulties, and contact with their adult diabetic services. The intervention described above involved telephone support but it is important that a young person's communication preferences are taken into account when planning such enhanced support, for example, they may prefer

text message or email contact instead of or in addition to telephone support.

6.7 Healthcare Professional-Focused Interventions

6.7.1 Named Transition Coordinator or Key Worker

Good communication between the family and professionals involved in transition is key in the provision of appropriate care and support. It is frustrating and worrying for families when they do not know who to contact regarding transition and are not kept updated on the process. A named person who takes responsibility for a young person's transition can help to resolve some of these issues; a 'key worker' or transition coordinator (see for example Kelly 2014). This is a role usually undertaken by a nurse. The key worker/coordinator has an overarching view throughout the young person's transition process. They play an important role in pulling the different elements of transitional care together, ensuring there is effective communication between services, professionals, and the family. Someone taking on this role is especially vital for young people with complex needs where many services and numerous professionals are involved. In the model for young people with complex health needs described by Kelly (2014), the transition nurse coordinates regular multi-agency transition progress meetings with young people so that information is shared and communicated effectively. The role bridges the gap between child and adult services providing continuity until the young person is established within adult services.

6.8 Young Person-Focused Interventions

6.8.1 Skills Training/Education for Young People

Part of the role of transitional care is to prepare young people for life as an adult with a health condition. The young person needs to understand their health condition; to do this they need information about their treatment when they were younger and how the condition may affect them in the future. Practical information such as how to make appointments, how to get a prescription, and how to contact the healthcare team should be provided along with opportunity to practice these skills before moving to adult care. It is important that the information provided includes 'lifestyle' advice (e.g. about healthy diet, alcohol, smoking, recreational drugs, exercise, sexual health, staying well) as well as information relating to future career/education. Approaches to providing information for young people varies between services, some services run specific education sessions/workshops and others give information routinely in clinic, building up knowledge and skills over time. The advantage of running information/skills training events is that young people can meet others with the same health condition; therefore, peer support is also provided. Such group sessions would also need to be complemented by an individual session(s) for young people where they are able to gain information and ask questions specific to them and their health.

Within children's services, much of the conversation in healthcare consultations is often led by parents. In adult services, the young person will be expected to take the lead. The young person needs to be helped to gain confidence when talking with health professionals without their parent(s) being there. It is important that the young person has the opportunity to practice speaking directly to health professionals whilst they are still seen in children's services with professionals who are more familiar to them. Time without parents present in a consultation also allows the young person to raise any confidential issues they may not wish their parents to know about.

Mackie et al. (2014) describe an intervention delivered by an experienced cardiology nurse that involved a one-to-one teaching session aiming to improve knowledge and self-management skills in preparation for transition to adult care. The elements of this session were tailored to the young person and included: discussion about transition and its importance, issues of confidentiality, issues related to their cardiac condition, review of cardiac anatomy as relevant, discussion of potential future complications, advice about lifestyle issues (smoking, alcohol, and sexual health),

details of adult care team contact names and an introduction to relevant websites. Case studies were used to address health behaviour and written materials were supplied. A 'MyHealth' passport was also created, including the name of the young person's cardiac condition, previous cardiac interventions, and names and purposes of medications. Follow-up emails or text message contact with the nurse were encouraged. An evaluation of this intervention found significant improvement in self-management and cardiac knowledge scores compared to controls not receiving the intervention (Mackie et al. 2014).

6.8.2 Assessments of 'Readiness': Transition Checklists

Readiness for transition should be frequently assessed through conversations held during clinic appointments. A number of checklists/questionnaires are available to assess a young person's readiness to transfer to adult services and provide an indication of the knowledge and skills young people need to acquire to function well in the adult care setting and adult life (Zhang et al. 2014). Figure 6.1 provides an example of a checklist from the Ready Steady Go Transition Programme (www.uhs.nhs.uk/readysteadygo). Such checklists can be a useful trigger for engaging young people in conversation to help professionals to speak with young people about readiness and identify any gaps in skills, knowledge, or confidence needed to manage their health and transition to adult care. They can be used to track a young person's progress in self-management during the transition process. Parents can also be asked for their opinion and feedback about whether or not the young person is ready for transition. It is important to note that checklists rarely assess mastery of knowledge and skills, it is important to check a young person's actual competency (which may be different to their perceived competency).

6.8.3 Technology-Based Interventions

Advances in technology have offered healthcare professionals new opportunities to engage

NHS

The Ready Steady Go transition programme - Go

The medical and nursing team aim to support you as you grow up and help you gradually develop the confidence and skills to take charge of your own healthcare.

Filling in this questionnaire will help the team create a programme to suit you.
Please answer all questions that are relevant to you and ask if you are unsure.

Ready Steady Go programme

Name: Date:

Knowledge and skills	Yes	I would like some extra advice/help with this	Comment
KNOWLEDGE			
I am confident in my knowledge about my condition and its management			
I understand what is likely to happen with my condition when I am an adult			
I look after my own medication			
I order and collect my repeat prescriptions and book my own appointments			
I call the hospital myself if there is a query about my condition and/or therapy			
SELF ADVOCACY (speaking up for yourself)			
I feel confident to be seen on my own in clinic			
I understand my right to confidentiality			
I understand my role in shared decision making with the healthcare team e.g. Ask 3 questions*			
HEALTH AND LIFESTYLE			
I exercise regularly/have an active lifestyle			
I understand the effect of smoking, drugs or alcohol on my condition and general health			
I understand what appropriate eating means for my general health			
I know where and how I can access providers of reliable accurate information about sexual health			
I understand the implications of my condition and drug therapy on pregnancy/parenting (if applicable)			
DAILY LIVING			
I am independent at home – dressing, bathing, showering, preparing meals, etc			
I can or am learning to drive			

*See leaflet or www.advancingqualityalliance.nhs.uk/wp-content/uploads/2013/04/BrochureFinal25.10.12.pdf

Fig. 6.1 Example of a transition checklist—Ready Steady Go Transition programme—'Go' questionnaire 'Ready Steady Go' and 'Hello to adult services' developed by the Transition Steering Group led by Dr. Arvind Nagra, paediatric nephrologist and clinical lead for transitional care at Southampton Children's Hospital, University Hospital Southampton NHS Foundation Trust based on the work of: (1) Whitehouse S, Paone MC. Bridging the gap

The Ready Steady Go transition programme - Go

Knowledge and Skills	Yes	I would like some extra advice/help with this	Comment
DAILY LIVING (CONTINUED)			
I know how to plan ahead for being away from home, overseas, trips e.g. storage of medicines, vaccinations			
I understand my eligibility for benefits (if applicable)			
SCHOOL/CAREER/YOUR FUTURE			
I have had work/ volunteering experience			
I have a Career Plan (please specify)			
I am aware of the potential impact (if any) of my condition on my future career plans			
I know how and what to tell a potential employer about my condition (if applicable)			
I know who to contact for careers advice			
LEISURE			
I can use public transport and access my local community, e.g. shops, leisure centre, cinema			
I see my friends outside school hours			
MANAGING YOUR EMOTIONS			
I know how to deal with unwelcome comments/ bullying			
I know someone I can talk to when I feel sad/fed-up			
I know how to cope with emotions such as anger or anxiety			
I would like more information about where I can get help to deal with my emotions			
I am comfortable with the way I look to others			
I am happy with life			
TRANSFER TO ADULT CARE			
I understand the meaning of 'transition' and transfer of information about me			
I know the plan for my care when I am an adult			
I would like more information about an orientation visit to the adult service I will transfer to for my adult care			

Please list anything else you would like help or advice with:

Thank you

The Ready Steady Go materials were developed by the Transition Steering Group led by Dr Arvind Nagra, paediatric nephrologist and clinical lead for transitional care at Southampton Children's Hospital, University Hospital Southampton NHS Foundation Trust based on the work of: 1. S Whitehouse and MC Paone. Bridging the gap from youth to adulthood. Contemporary Pediatrics; 1998, December. 13-16. 2. Paone MC, Wigle M, Saewyc E. The ON TRAC model for transitional care of adolescents. Prog Transplant 2006;16:291-302 3. Janet E McDonagh et al, J Child Health Care 2006;10(1):22-42. Users are permitted to use 'Ready Steady Go' and 'Hello to adult services' materials in their original format purely for non-commercial purposes. No modifications or changes of any kind are allowed without permission of University Hospital Southampton NHS Foundation Trust.

The following acknowledgement statement must be included in all publications which make reference to the use of these materials: "Ready Steady Go' and 'Hello to adult services' developed by the Transition Steering Group led by Dr Arvind Nagra, paediatric nephrologist and clinical lead for transitional care at Southampton Children's Hospital, University Hospital Southampton NHS Foundation Trust based on the work of: 1. S Whitehouse and MC Paone. Bridging the gap from youth to adulthood. Contemporary Pediatrics; 1998, December. 13-16. 2. Paone MC, Wigle M, Saewyc E. The ON TRAC model for transitional care of adolescents. Prog Transplant 2006;16:291-302 3. Janet E McDonagh et al, J Child Health Care 2006;10(1):22-42." Further information can be found at www.uhs.nhs.uk/readysteadygo   v2.0 2015

Fig. 6.1 (continued) from youth to adulthood. Contemporary Pediatrics. 1998;13–16. (2) Paone MC, Wigle M, Saewyc E. The ON TRAC model for transitional care of adolescents. Prog Transplant. 2006;16:291–302. (3) Janet E, McDonagh et al. J Child Health Care. 2006;10(1):22–42." Further information can be found at www.uhs.nhs.uk/readysteadygo

young people in personal health care and provide support to patients with long-term conditions, which includes the transition period. Mobile phone and tablet mobile technologies featuring software programme apps are already well used by young people for social networking or gaming. They have also been utilised in health care to support personal condition management, using condition-specific and patient-tailored software. In addition to the utilisation of apps, text messaging presents a method of supporting and communicating with young people undergoing transition to adult care. Engaging with young people through technology has many advantages including being easy to access, responsive, convenient, and interactive. Remote delivery as opposed to face-to-face delivery of an intervention potentially reduces cost and increases availability and efficiency. It is essential when developing inter-

ventions involving technology that the end users, in this case young people and healthcare professionals, are involved in the development and testing phases to ensure an intervention that is acceptable and works in practice.

The MD2Me intervention (Huang et al. 2014) is a generic internet and mobile phone delivered disease management intervention which has been evaluated with young people with inflammatory bowel disease, cystic fibrosis, and diabetes. The intervention targets the self-management constructs of monitoring disease symptoms, responding to monitoring with appropriate treatments and actively working with healthcare providers to manage care. Young people log into a secure website weekly to receive theme-based materials about common disease management and communication skills and lifestyle tips (see Fig. 6.2 for a screenshot). Case studies are provided to

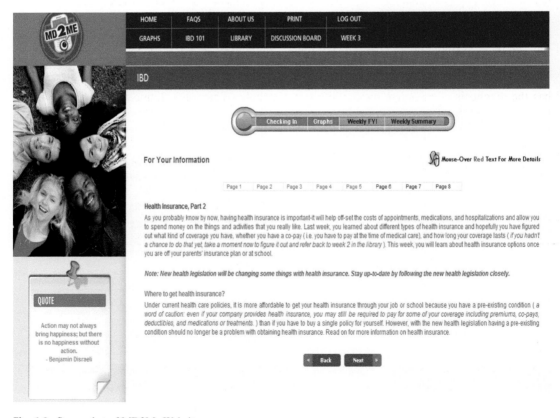

Fig. 6.2 Screenshot of MD2Me Website

increase usability. Tailored text messages and queries are delivered (three to five messages per week) to ensure that participants receive and understand the intervention messages. To encourage more patient-initiated communication, young people can also send text messages to report health concerns to the healthcare team. The intervention was evaluated positively by young people and indicates the potential for generic technology-based interventions which are not disease specific, therefore offering a cost-effective approach to improving transitional care outcomes.

6.9 Transition and Endocrinology

Transitional care is especially important in young people with an endocrine condition. In particular, children who have received growth hormone therapy (see Chap. 2 "GH Therapy in Childhood") need to be re-tested once linear growth is complete, (see Chap. 15) in order to see if growth hormone therapy is still required in adulthood (see Chap. 25 "GH Therapy in Adulthood"), particularly if the young person has the diagnosis of complete hypopituitarism. Paediatric and adult endocrinologists need to work together in order to provide a seamless transition along with the multidisciplinary team, particularly as growth hormone therapy regimes are vastly different in adulthood compared to childhood (Clayton et al. 2005).

The number of cancer survivors is increasing; young people who have undergone treatment for cancer (see Chap. 58) need continued follow-up, sometimes lifelong, and transition guidelines are essential: survivors are at risk of chronic health conditions and require long-term follow-up care (Mulder et al. 2016).

Young people with a disorder of sex development (DSD) (see Chap. 3) present many challenges, particularly concerning disclosure of the condition to the young person, and the requirements for potential genital examinations and potential vaginal treatments (see Chap. 35) Some young people may be diagnosed during

adolescence and spend a short time in paediatric care before transitioning to adult services, particularly patients with gonadal dysgenesis with a Y chromosome where gonadectomy may be advised. It is imperative to include a psychologist within the multidisciplinary team make up, to help underpin the whole transition process, which can take years to complete in a young person with a DSD (Crouch and Creighton 2014).

6.10 Conclusions

Despite professional consensus on the key principles for transitional care, transition programmes are still not fully integrated into health services. There remains much variability in the provision of transitional care for young people. The need for change in order to best meet the needs of young people and parents during transition is very evident in existing literature. A range of approaches to improving the processes and structure of transitional care have been proposed although it is not yet clear how effective these approaches might be in improving health outcomes and the experience of transition for young people. Whatever solution is adopted requires a comprehensive programme that takes into account the young person's psychosocial, lifestyle, and educational/vocational needs in addition to any health needs. Sharing of best practice is key; services need to share successes and failures and learn from each other how to overcome common difficulties in improving transitional care.

6.11 Critical Thinking Points

How and when is the topic of transition introduced to young people and parents in the services you work in? Do you think this is appropriate?

What do you know about the experiences of transition for young people and parents in the service you work in? Is there a mechanism in place for young people and parents to feedback their experiences?

What might the key challenges/barriers be to implementing a seamless transition experience for young people in the service you work in? How might these barriers be overcome?

Are you aware of how transition is implemented in other services within the organisation you work in? How might services improve on sharing best practice and experiences of what works or does not work with regard to transition?

References

Aldiss S, Ellis J, Cass H, Pettigrew T, Rose L, Gibson F. Transition from child to adult care—'it's not a one-off event': development of benchmarks to improve the experience. J Pediatr Nurs. 2015;30:638–47.

Aldiss S, Cass H, Ellis J, Gibson F. "We Sometimes Hold on to Ours"—Professionals' views on factors that both delay and facilitate transition to adult care. Front Pediatr. 2016;4:125. https://doi.org/10.3389/fped.2016.00125.

Allen D, Gregory J. The transition from children's to adult diabetes services: understanding the 'problem'. Diabet Med. 2009;26(2):162–6.

Blum R, Garell D, Hodgman C, Jorissen T, Okinow N, Orr D, Slap G. Transition from child-centred to adult health-care systems for adolescents with chronic conditions: a position paper of the Society for Adolescent Medicine. J Adolesc Health. 1993;14:570–6.

Campbell F, Biggs K, Aldiss S, O'Neill PM, Clowes M, McDonagh J, While A, Gibson F. Interventions to improve transition of care for adolescents from paediatric services to adult services. Cochrane Database Syst Rev. 2016;(4):CD009794. https://doi.org/10.1002/14651858.CD009794.pub2.

Care Quality Commission. From the pond into the sea: children's transition to adult health services. 2014. http://www.cqc.org.uk/content/teenagers-complex-health-needs-lack-support-they-approach-adulthood. Accessed 23 Jan 2017.

Clayton P, Cuneo RC, Juul A, Monson JP, Shalet SM, Tauber M. Consensus statement on the management of the GH treated adolescent in the transition to adult care. Eur J Endocrinol. 2005;152:165–70.

Crouch NS, Creighton SM. Transition of care for adolescents with disorders of sex development. Nat Rev Endocrinol. 2014;10(7):436–2.

Crowley R, Wolfe I, Lock K, McKee M. Improving the transition between child and paediatric healthcare: a systematic review. Arch Dis Child. 2011;96:548–53.

Fegran L, Hall E, Uhrenfeldt L, Aagaard H, Ludvigsen M. Adolescents' and young adults' transition experiences when transferring from paediatric to adult care: a qualitative metasynthesis. Int J Nurs Stud. 2014;51:123–35.

Gleeson H, Turner G. Transition to adult services. Arch Dis Child Educ Pract Ed. 2012;97:86–92.

Harden P, Walsh G, Bandler N, Bradley S, Lonsdale D, Taylor J, Marks S. Bridging the gap: an intergrated paediatric to adult clinical service for young adult with kidney failure. BMJ. 2012;344:e3718.

Heath G, Farre A, Shaw K. Parenting a child with chronic illness as they transition into adulthood. A systematic review and thematic synthesis of parents' experiences. Patient Educ Couns. 2017;100(1):76–92.

Hepburn CM, Cohen E, Bhawra J, Weiser N, Hayeems R, Guttmann A. Health system strategies supporting transition to adult care. Arch Dis Child. 2015;100:559–64.

Hislop J, Mason H, Paar J, Vale L, Colver A. Views of young people with chronic conditions on transition from pediatric to adult health services. J Adolesc Health. 2016;59:345–53.

Huang JS, Terrones L, Tompane T, Dillon L, Pain M, Gottschalk M, Norman G, Bartholomew K. Preparing adolescents with chronic disease for transition to adult care: a technology program. Pediatrics. 2014;133:e1639–46.

Kelly D. Theory to reality: the role of the transition nurse co-ordinator. Br J Nurs. 2014;23:888–94.

Mackie AS, Islam S, Magill-Evans J, Rankin KN, Robert C, Schuh M, Nicholas D, Vonder Muhll I, McCrindle B, Yasui Y, Rempel G. Healthcare transition for youth with heart disease: a clinical trial. Heart. 2014;100:1113–8.

Mulder RL, van der Pal HJH, Levitt GA, Skinner R, Kremer LCM, Brown MC, Bardi E, Windsor R, Michel G, Frey E. Transition guidelines: An important step in the future care for childhood cancer survivors. A comprehensive definition as groundwork. Eur J Cancer. 2016;54:64–8.

National Institute for Health and Care Excellence. Transition from children's to adults' services for young people using health or social care services. 2016. https://www.nice.org.uk/guidance/ng43. Accessed 23 Jan 2017.

Paone MC, Wigle M, Saewyc E. The ON TRAC model for transitional care of adolescents. Prog Transplant. 2006;16(4):291–302.

Royal College of Nursing. Adolescent transition care: RCN guidance for nursing staff. 2013. https://www.rcn.org.uk/library/subject-guides/children-and-young-people-transition-to-adult-services. Accessed 23 Jan 2017.

Steinbeck KS, Shrewsbury VA, Harvey V, Mikler K, Donaghue KC, Craig ME, Woodhead HJ. A pilot randomized controlled trial of a post-discharge program to support emerging adults with type 1 diabetes mellitus transition from pediatric to adult care. Pediatr Diabetes. 2014;16(8):1–6.

Suris J, Akre C. Key elements for and indicators of a successful transition: an international Delphi study. J Adolesc Health. 2015;56:612–8.

Zhang L, Ho J, Kennedy S. A systematic review of the psychometric properties of transition readiness assessment tools in adolescents with chronic disease. BMC Pediatr. 2014;14:4. https://doi.org/10.1186/1471-2431-14-4.

Key Reading

1. Aldiss S, Ellis J, Cass H, Pettigrew T, Rose L, Gibson F. Transition from child to adult care—'it's not a one-off event': development of benchmarks to improve the experience. J Pediatr Nurs. 2015;30:638–47.
2. Campbell F, Biggs K, Aldiss S, O'Neill PM, Clowes M, McDonagh J, While A, Gibson F. Interventions to improve transition of care for adolescents from paediatric services to adult services. Cochrane Database Syst Rev. 2016;(4):CD009794. https://doi.org/10.1002/14651858.CD009794.pub2.
3. Crowley R, Wolfe I, Lock K, McKee M. Improving the transition between child and paediatric healthcare: a systematic review. Arch Dis Child. 2011;96:548–53.
4. Fegran L, Hall E, Uhrenfeldt L, Aagaard H, Ludvigsen M. Adolescents' and young adults' transition experiences when transferring from paediatric to adult care: a qualitative metasynthesis. Int J Nurs Stud. 2014;51:123–35.
5. Heath G, Farre A, Shaw K. Parenting a child with chronic illness as they transition into adulthood. A systematic review and thematic synthesis of parents' experiences. Patient Educ Couns. 2017;100(1):76–92.

Part II

Endocrine Disorders and Genetics in Childhood

Kate Davies and Margaret F. Keil

Genetics and Family History

7

Kelly Mullholand Behm

Contents

K. M. Behm (✉)
Orlando, FL, USA

© Springer Nature Switzerland AG 2019
S. Llahana et al. (eds.), *Advanced Practice in Endocrinology Nursing*,
https://doi.org/10.1007/978-3-319-99817-6_7

Abstract

This chapter describes principles of genetics and family history that are relevant to the practice of clinical endocrinology. It begins with a review of historical eras that provides context for how two seemingly distinct specialties have become intricately interwoven. Genetics concepts are then explained in a progression from basic to complex, each section building on the previous, with clinical examples included to help readers develop a comprehensive understanding without becoming overwhelmed. Topics covered include DNA and RNA structure and function, the genetic code, transcription, translation, exons, introns, gene expression, gene locus, alleles, genotype, phenotype, Mendelian and non-Mendelian patterns of inheritance, epigenetics, gene mutations, chromosomal structural and copy number abnormalities, and cytogenetic and molecular genetic testing methodologies and interpretation.

The Mendelian inheritance section outlines the three laws of Mendelian inheritance and associated inheritance patterns including homozygous and heterozygous, autosomal and pseudoautosomal, dominant and recessive. Non-Mendelian patterns of inheritance described include co-dominance, linkage, sex-linked, multiple alleles, complex polygenic or multifactorial, and mitochondrial.

Gene mutations discussed include point, missense, nonsense, insertion, deletion, duplication, frameshift, substitution, and repeat expansions. Chromosomal abnormalities described include translocations, deletions, duplications, inversions, isochromosomes, dicentric, ring, and aneuploidies resulting from meiotic and mitotic nondisjunction.

The genetic testing section covers karyotyping, fluorescent in situ hybridization, microarrays, gene expression analysis, direct sequencing analysis, and methylation analysis. The section on family history provides information about publicly available tools for collecting genetic and endocrine history data, as well as a detailed description of how to create and use pedigrees to aid in clinical decision-making and communication with patients and their families.

The chapter concludes with a practical discussion of nursing implications, a recommended reading section, and an extensive list of supplemental educational materials and resources. Supplemental materials include a genetics glossary, a list of online resources for information on genetics concepts introduced within the chapter, a list of genetics-based peer-reviewed journals, a list of professional organizations and societies for nurses interested in genetics, and a list of current textbooks on genetics.

The recommended reading section contains a list of online and print publications providing additional in-depth information on genetics in human endocrinology, nursing competencies in genetics, using analogies in patient education, legal and ethical implications of genetics in the clinical setting, issues surrounding disclosure of genetic diagnoses, clinical case studies, interactive pedigree software, epigenetics, molecular genetics testing, gene therapy, additional internet genetics resources, and the future of genetics in endocrinology.

Keywords

Genetics · DNA · Expression · Inheritance · Mutation · Testing · Pedigree

Abbreviations

2n	Diploid
3′	3-prime
3-M	Syndrome causing short stature, unusual facial features, and skeletal abnormalities first identified by researchers named Miller, McKusick, and Malvaux
5′	5-prime
A	Adenine
aCGH	Array comparative genomic hybridization
ACTH	Adrenocorticotropic hormone
AR	Androgen receptor
arr	Array
bp	Base pairs
BWS	Beckwith–Wiedemann syndrome
C	Cytosine
CAG	Cytosine-adenine-guanine nucleotide sequence
CDKN1B	Cyclin dependent kinase inhibitor 1B
cDNA	Complementary DNA
CGH	Comparative genomic hybridization
CH$_3$	Methyl group
CH$_3$CO	Acetyl group
CNV	Copy number variants or copy number variations
CpG	Cytosine-phosphate-guanine (cytosine and guanine separated by a phosphate)
CYP212A	Cytochrome P450 family 21 subfamily A member 2
del or dn	Deletion
der	Derivative chromosome
dp	Duplication
DNA	Deoxyribonucleic acid
FGD	Familial glucocorticoid deficiency
FGFR3	Fibroblast growth factor receptor 3
FISH	Fluorescent in situ hybridization
FMR1	Fragile X mental retardation 1
G	Guanine
GEM	Gene expression microarray
GH	Growth hormone
GNAS	Guanine nucleotide-binding protein alpha subunit or g-protein alpha subunit
HDSNP-array	High-density single nucleotide polymorphism array
i	Isochromosome
ins	Insertion
inv	Inversion
kb	Kilobase pairs
mat	Maternally derived chromosome
Mb	Megabase pairs
MEN1	Multiple endocrine neoplasia type 1 or menin 1
MEN4	Multiple endocrine neoplasia type 4

MIDD	Maternally inherited diabetes and deafness or mitochondrial diabetes and deafness
miRNA	MicroRNAs
MODY5	Maturity-onset diabetes of the young type 5
mRNA	Messenger RNA
mtDNA	Mitochondrial DNA
n	Haploid
NGS	Next-generation sequencing
p	Short arm of a chromosome
PCOS	Polycystic ovarian syndrome
PCR	Polymerase chain reaction
PHEX	Phosphate regulating endopeptidase homolog X-linked
PTPN11	Protein tyrosine phosphatase, non-receptor type 11
q	Long arm of a chromosome
RCAD	Renal cysts and diabetes syndrome
RNA	Ribonucleic acid
rRNA	Ribosomal RNA
SHOX	Short stature homeobox
SNP	Single nucleotide polymorphism
SNP-array	Single nucleotide polymorphism array
SOS1	Son of sevenless homolog 1 or SOS Ras/Rac guanine nucleotide exchange factor 1
SOX3	SRY-box 3 or SRY-related HMG-box 3 (Sex-determining region Y-related high-mobility-group box transcription factor 3)
SRY	Sex-determining region Y
T	Thymine
t	Translocation
tRNA	Transfer RNA
TSH	Thyroid stimulating hormone
U	Uracil
VHL	Von Hippel-Lindau
WES	Whole-exome sequencing
WGS	Whole-genome sequencing
wt	Wild type allele
Xce	X chromosome controlling element
Xic	X-inactivation center
Xist	X inactive specific transcript

Key Terms[1]

- **Autosomal dominant inheritance:** caused by a mutation in a gene located on an autosomal chromosome and occurs when one autosomal allele masks the expression of another allele
- **Autosomal recessive inheritance:** also caused by a mutation in a gene located on an autosome, but in this case, two copies of the recessive gene are needed for the trait to be expressed
- **Chromosomes:** linear end-to-end arrangement of DNA found in tightly coiled packets in the nucleus of every cell
- **Deletion:** a piece of a chromosome breaks off and is lost
- **DNA:** deoxyribonucleic acid; a double chain of linked nucleotides having deoxyribose as their sugars; the fundamental substance of which genes are composed
- **Epigenetics:** heritable changes in gene function that do not involve changes in the DNA sequence
- **Frameshift mutation:** the addition or deletion of a nitrogen base, causing the gene sequence to read out of sequence
- **Functional genomics:** the study of patterns of gene expression and interaction in the genome
- **Gene expression:** the timing, frequency, rate, and efficiency of protein production for a specific gene
- **Genes:** sections of DNA containing coding sequences for making proteins and regulatory sequences for controlling transcription
- **Genome:** the complete set of genes for an organism
- **Genotype:** the pair of alleles a person has at a specific location in the genome
- **Germ mutation:** occur in gametes (reproductive cells)
- **Haplosufficient:** a single copy of a normal gene allele is enough to produce normal function
- **Hemizygous:** there is only one copy of a gene for a specific trait resulting in a recessive phenotype (X-linked genes in human males are hemizygous)

[1] Key terms definitions were derived from National Human Genome Research Institute (2014).

- **Heterozygous:** having differing gene alleles for a trait in an individual, such as Aa
- **Inversion:** a piece of a chromosome breaks off and reattaches itself in reverse order
- **Knockout:** inactivation of one specific gene
- **Locus (gene locus):** the specific place on a chromosome where a gene is located (plural, loci)
- **Mendelian inheritance:** hereditary process which follows Mendel's laws of segregation, independent assortment, and dominance
- **Mitochondrial inheritance:** the passage of mitochondrial DNA from the mother to the offspring through the cytoplasm of the egg
- **Molecular genetics:** the study of the molecular processes underlying gene structure and function
- **Mutant allele:** an allele differing from the allele found in the standard, or wild type
- **Mutations:** less common differences in the sequence of DNA, occurring in less than 1% of the population and having a deleterious effect
- **Nonsense mutation:** a mutation that alters a gene to produce a nonsense codon
- **Null mutation:** a mutation that results in complete absence of function for the gene
- **Phenotype:** the detectable outward manifestations of a specific genotype; the observable effect of an allele, such as eye color or how an individual reacts to a drug
- **Point mutation:** a change in a single nitrogen base in DNA; a mutation that can be mapped to one specific locus
- **Polymorphism:** common variations in the sequence of DNA, occurring in at least 1% of the population; the occurrence in a population of several phenotypic forms associated with alleles of one gene or homologs of one chromosome; useful for genetic linkage analysis
- **Proband:** the family member in which a disease-causing mutation is known to exist; an affected family member coming to medical attention independent of other family members
- **Recessive allele:** an allele whose phenotypic effect is not expressed in a heterozygote

- **RNA:** ribonucleic acid; a single-stranded nucleic acid like DNA but having ribose sugar rather than deoxyribose sugar and uracil rather than thymine as one of the bases
- **SNP (pronounced "snip"):** single nucleotide polymorphism; a type of polymorphism involving variation of a single base pair; the most common type of genetic variation among people
- **Somatic mutation:** occurs in body cells rather than reproductive cells
- **Trait:** the manifestation or phenotype of a specific gene
- **Wild type:** the most common allelic form of a gene; the genotype or phenotype that is found in nature
- **X-linked recessive inheritance:** caused by a gene on the X chromosome rather than on an autosome

Key Points

The content of this chapter will enable the reader to:

- Define at least five genetics concepts not previously known to the reader
- Differentiate between Mendelian and non-Mendelian patterns of inheritance
- Describe the relationship between gene expression and epigenetics
- Give endocrine examples of gene mutations and chromosomal abnormalities
- Explain cytogenetic and molecular genetic test results to patients and families
- Collect a fourth-generation family health history and draw a pedigree depicting genetic relationships

7.1 Introduction

One does not need to be trained as a molecular geneticist to appreciate the intersection of genetics and endocrinology. However, a basic working knowledge of genetics *is* essential in guiding patients to an understanding of the "why?" underlying the disruption to their endocrine physiology. Although not all endocrine disorders with a genetic root cause are inherited, understanding inheritance patterns where they *do* apply is important, as is being able to explain basic principles of non-inherited (acquired) changes resulting from epigenetics, somatic cell line mutations, and errors in mitotic cell division.

Explaining these phenomena to affected patients and their families is not solely the purview of the clinical geneticist. For example, an endocrine health care provider should not deliver the news of a Turner syndrome or non-classical congenital adrenal hyperplasia diagnosis, and then send the overwhelmed and bewildered patient/family off to a consult with the genetics clinic armed *only* with instructions to take the endocrine medications as prescribed and to make a follow-up appointment for a few months down the road. These individuals need to receive basic genetic education from their endocrine provider throughout the entire endocrine workup, beginning with the family history segment of the new patient interview, and continuing through the diagnostic testing process, confirmation of diagnosis, and subsequent follow-up appointments. In addition, maintaining and sharing knowledge of current authenticated patient education resources and support organizations specific to endocrine diagnoses of genetic origin will prevent these individuals from suffering unnecessary fear and anxiety from misinformation that exists on the internet and within their cultural milieu.

The purpose of this chapter is to review principles of genetics and family history that are relevant to the practice of clinical endocrinology. Examples of how these principles might apply to actual patient scenarios are interspersed throughout the chapter to assist in the translation from abstract fact to clinical reality. A list of additional resources and suggestions for further reading and personal education is provided after the main chapter content, as well as a glossary of genetics terminology.

7.2 Historical Eras Linking Genetics and Endocrinology

Putting what we currently know about genetics into historical context brings increased understanding of clinical implications. There are three scientific eras where genetics and endocrinology intersect: the physiologic era, the assay era, and the molecular genetic era (Asa and Mete 2018; Fisher 2004; Marty et al. 2011).

The physiologic era took place pre-Watson and Crick, running from the time of Mendel (mid-1800s) to 1953. In this era, physiologic, biochemical, and cellular anomalies were known, but the specific molecular alteration in a gene as the root cause of the anomaly had not yet been identified. Important scientific milestones of this era included the rediscovery of Mendelian principles of genetic inheritance in the early 1900s, the discovery of insulin in the early 1920s, the discovery of the relationship between genes and proteins in sickle cell anemia, and finally, Watson and Crick's discovery of the three-dimensional double-stranded structure of DNA in 1953, which ushered in the next scientific era (Asa and Mete 2018; Fisher 2004; Marty et al. 2011).

The assay era occurred post-Watson and Crick, from 1953 to 1990, ending just before the Human Genome Project. Scientific discoveries in this era were explosive, focusing on DNA, RNA, mapping, sequencing, and recombination. Important scientific milestones of this era included: discovery of 46 human chromosomes in the mid-1950s, discovery of DNA polymerase I enzyme which led to creation of DNA in a test tube in the late 1950s, development of the plasma insulin immunoassay around 1960, cracking of the genetic code as triplet messenger RNA (mRNA) codons specifying amino acids in the mid-1960s, isolation of the first restriction enzyme, HindII, that could cut DNA molecules within specific recognition sites around 1970, production of the first recombinant DNA (rDNA) molecule in the early 1970s, development of a DNA sequencing method around 1975, production of the first human hormone using rDNA technology in the late 1970s, and finally, the beginning of the Human Genome Project in 1990, which ushered in the current scientific era (Asa and Mete 2018; Fisher 2004; Marty et al. 2011).

The molecular genetic era began with the commencement of the Human Genome Project in 1990 and continues to the present day, and it is the discoveries of this era that have made the genetic diagnosis of many endocrine disorders possible. The genes for insulin and growth hormone were both discovered in the early 1990s, and the final human genome sequence (the complete human DNA sequence) was published in 2003 after the Human Genome Project concluded (Asa and Mete 2018; Fisher 2004; Marty et al. 2011). In terms of significance, this last accomplishment was the equivalent of putting a man on the moon. The discoveries of this era have further defined the fields of genetics and molecular genetics. Genetics is the study of genes and inheritance. Molecular genetics is the study of molecular processes underlying gene structure, function, and behavior; it is analyzing and manipulating individual genes at the DNA level.

7.3 Basic Genetics Review

DNA, genes, chromosomes, genetic code, and genome are terms one may have heard, but not thought to put together in a way that makes practical sense. The analogy of learning to read, i.e., identifying letters in the alphabet, putting those letters together to form words, then linking words to make sentences, sentences to make chapters, and chapters to create a book, can be useful in understanding the connections between basic genetic terminology. This foundation can then be built upon to understand more complex genetic concepts.

7.3.1 DNA (The Genetic Alphabet)

The acronym DNA stands for deoxyribonucleic acid. DNA consists of two parallel linear strands of repeating units called nucleotides. The nucleotides in each parallel strand are joined by weak chemical bonds in a double

helix formation that resembles a twisted ladder. Nucleotides are composed of one deoxyribose sugar-phosphate molecule and one chemical base. The sugar-phosphate portion of each nucleotide forms the outer rails of the ladder, while the base portion faces the center of the ladder. Each center-facing base is joined by a chemical bond to another base connected to the opposite rail of the ladder. The bases are designated by letters: A for adenine, C for cytosine, T for thymine, and G for guanine. During DNA transcription, enzymes forming RNA (a single-stranded ribonucleic acid containing the sugar ribose) substitute the base uracil, designated by the letter U, for the DNA base thymine. When two bases on opposite sides of the ladder are chemically joined together in the center with a weak hydrogen bond to form a rung, they are referred to as base pairs (National Human Genome Research Institute 2015; National Institute of General Medical Sciences 2016; U.S. National Library of Medicine, National Institutes of Health 2017).

This genetic "alphabet" thus contains only five letters representing the five nucleotide bases in DNA and RNA. These bases follow specific rules for pairing with each other to form those "ladder rungs." A and G are purine bases, and T, C, and U are pyrimidine bases. Purines bond to pyrimidines so that A always pairs with T, and C with G in DNA, while A pairs with U in RNA. [One might think of the words "at" and "Catgut" (for A-T and C-G) and the phrase "Hey You!" (for A-U) to remember which bases pair with each other.] Humans have approximately three billion base pairs (six billion bases) contained in the DNA found in most of our cells (National Human Genome Research Institute 2015; National Institute of General Medical Sciences 2016; U.S. National Library of Medicine, National Institutes of Health 2017).

The individual strands within double-stranded DNA are complementary and run in opposite directions due to the rules of base pairing. The direction of the strands is indicated as either 5′ to 3′ or 3′ to 5′. The 5′ and 3′ designations refer to the number of carbon atoms in the sugar-phosphate backbone (National Human Genome Research

Institute 2015; National Institute of General Medical Sciences 2016; U.S. National Library of Medicine, National Institutes of Health 2017). The direction of each strand is important for the processes of transcription and translation, which will be discussed later. Figure 7.1 illustrates the basic structure of DNA described in this section.

7.3.2 Genes (Genetic Sentences)

A gene is a segment of DNA containing a specific sequence of base pairs that provide instructions for making proteins, like sentences and paragraphs made from the nucleotide "alphabet." Humans have approximately 35,000 genes. The smallest genes are about 100 base pairs in length. The largest genes are over one million base pairs long. Base sequence variations occur in only about three million base pairs, 1% of our DNA, yet it is this minute 1% variation that is responsible for the differences that make each individual unique (National Human Genome Research Institute 2015; National Institute of General Medical Sciences 2016; U.S. National Library of Medicine, National Institutes of Health 2017).

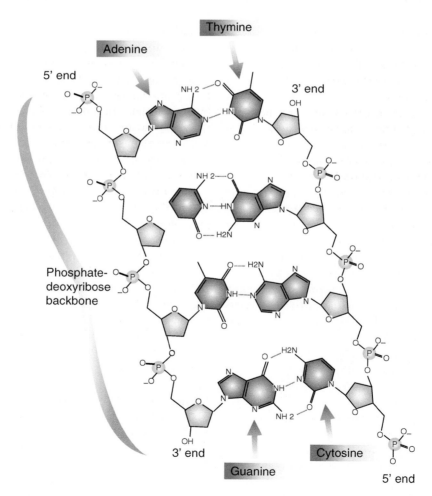

Fig. 7.1 DNA structure (Reproduced from https://www.news-medical.net/image.axd?picture=2016%2F11%2FDNA_structure_-_Zvitaliy_Enlarge_image_.jpg)

7.3.3 Chromosomes and Genomes (Genetic Chapters and Books)

DNA, with its nucleotide base pair "alphabet" sequenced into "sentences" of genes, is contained within tightly coiled packages called chromosomes that are found in the nucleus of every cell. Humans have two types of chromosomes, autosomal chromosomes and sex chromosomes. Autosomal chromosomes are usually referred to as autosomes. There are 22 autosomes (labelled 1 through 22, numbered from the largest to the smallest) and two sex chromosomes (labelled X and Y). The complete set of an organism's DNA (in humans, all the genes within a set of chromosomes) is referred to as a genome (National Human Genome Research Institute 2015; National Institute of General Medical Sciences 2016; U.S. National Library of Medicine, National Institutes of Health 2017). Each chromosome is like a chapter of gene "sentences" in a genome "book."

Each egg or sperm cell contains one "book" or genome in its "library," that is, *one* copy of each of the 22 autosomes and *one* of the two sex chromosomes for a total of 23 chromosomes. This is called the haploid state (one copy). Once an egg is fertilized by a sperm, the resulting zygote has two "books" or genomes in its "library," that is *two* copies of the 22 autosomes, and *two* sex chromosomes, for a total of 46 chromosomes in all its cells. This is called the diploid state (two copies). Eggs and sperm are also referred to as gametes. Cells that develop into gametes are also called germ cells. All other cells are referred to as somatic cells. Germ cells contain one genome, and somatic cells contain two genomes.

If there is a spelling error in a sentence, or if a sentence, paragraph, or chapter is missing, incomplete, or out of order, a book may not make sense to the reader, or it may take on a completely different meaning than its author intended. It is the same with our genome when genetic errors occur. Genetic errors are often referred to as mutations although there are errors that do *not* result from mutation. Mutations that occur in germ cells are called germline mutations, whereas mutations that occur in all other cells are called somatic mutations (National Human Genome Research Institute 2015; National Institute of General Medical Sciences 2016; U.S. National Library of Medicine, National Institutes of Health 2017).

7.4 The Genetic Code

Before one can understand how mutations or other genetic errors occur and what effects they have, one must know what "normal" looks like, just as to recognize that a word has been misspelled, one must already know its correct spelling. We have already established that genes are sections of DNA with a specific sequence of nucleotides whose bases are identified by letters, and that those bases exist in pairs. When a DNA sequence in a gene is transcribed into mRNA, a series of three base pairs forms a codon, which is like a "word" in a gene "sentence." The resulting codons are then translated into amino acids (National Human Genome Research Institute 2015; National Institute of General Medical Sciences 2016; U.S. National Library of Medicine, National Institutes of Health 2017).

The genetic code refers to the list of 64 possible codons (3 base pair combinations) that code for 20 amino acids as well as start and stop sequences. Amino acids are strung together to make proteins. Proteins are molecules that play a critical role in the structure, function, and regulation of the body's cells, tissues, and organs. Proteins are either structural (such as hair and muscle) or functional/regulatory (such as enzymes and transcription factors). Genes thus contain the instructions for making proteins, and act or "express" themselves by dictating the order of amino acids used to make those proteins (National Human Genome Research Institute 2015; National Institute of General Medical Sciences 2016; U.S. National Library of Medicine, National Institutes of Health 2017).

Genetic errors can occur when the order of the base pairs in a codon is disrupted (like a misspelled word), resulting in a premature stop codon (sometimes called a nonsense codon) that causes a shortened protein that doesn't function normally, or a codon for a completely different amino acid resulting in a completely different protein product than what the gene intended to produce (National Human Genome Research Institute 2015; National Institute of General Medical Sciences 2016; U.S. National Library of Medicine, National Institutes of Health 2017). An example of genetic code function is provided in Fig. 7.2.

7.5 Template, Transcription, Translation

Polymerase enzymes are regulatory proteins that synthesize DNA or RNA after the enzyme helicase unwinds the double strands of DNA. Once the strands are separated, the nucleotide sequence in each strand becomes a template for replication or transcription. When DNA duplicates itself, the process is called replication, and DNA polymerase regulates the replication into new double-stranded DNA. When the DNA template is being used to make proteins, the first step in the process is called transcription. Transcription occurs when RNA polymerase copies the DNA template into single-stranded mRNA. Once the DNA template has been transcribed into mRNA, the mRNA copy is referred to as the transcript. It is this transcript that contains the codons for amino acids

that make up proteins. Translation is the process of translational RNA (tRNA) reading the transcript of mRNA and translating it into individual amino acids that are linked together in a chain to form a polypeptide, the main structure of a protein (National Human Genome Research Institute 2015; National Institute of General Medical Sciences 2016; U.S. National Library of Medicine, National Institutes of Health 2017).

7.6 Exons and Introns

DNA in genes contains coding regions for proteins as well as non-coding regions that are transcribed into RNA but not translated into proteins. The coding regions are called exons, and the non-coding regions are called introns. One way to recall the difference is to remember that introns are "in-between" each coding region of a gene. There are additional non-coding regions of DNA that separate the genes from one another. Many non-coding regions of DNA between genes are functional elements that help regulate patterns of gene expression, while the purpose of other non-coding regions is not yet fully understood. Only about 2% of the genome contains genes (DNA sequences encoding proteins) (National Human

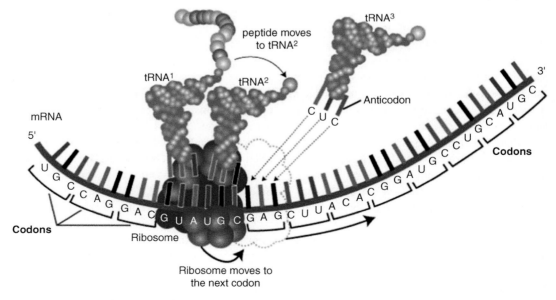

Fig. 7.2 mRNA codons translated into amino acids for protein synthesis (Reproduced from http://cdn.differencebetween.net/wp-content/uploads/2017/12/Difference-Between-Anticodon-and-Codon.jpg)

Genome Research Institute 2015; National Institute of General Medical Sciences 2016; U.S. National Library of Medicine, National Institutes of Health 2017).

The non-coding regions of a gene include a regulatory region at one end that initiates transcription (the 5′ end), and a termination region at the other end that ends transcription (the 3′ end). In between the two ends is the protein encoding sequence (National Human Genome Research Institute 2015; National Institute of General Medical Sciences 2016; U.S. National Library of Medicine, National Institutes of Health 2017). (Remember that the 5′ and 3′ designations merely refer to the number of carbon atoms in the sugar-phosphate backbone.)

When the double strands of DNA are separated, the strand oriented in the 5′ to 3′ direction is known as the sense (coding) strand, while the 3′ to 5′ strand is known as the antisense (anticoding) strand. The 5′ end includes a regulatory region (sometimes referred to as a regulatory box) with a sequence called a promoter. Because this region is located *before* the first exon of a gene begins, it is referred to as "upstream" of the gene. Upstream of the promotor sequence are untranslated enhancer sequences where transcription factors (sequence-specific DNA binding proteins) bind to turn the gene on and control the rate of DNA transcription. The promotor sequences begin as leader sequences called TATA or CCAAT boxes that provide a signal to RNA polymerase telling the enzyme which DNA sequence is ready for transcription. The leader sequences are followed by an initiation codon sequence (ATG on DNA or AUG on RNA) that starts transcription (National Human Genome Research Institute 2015; National Institute of General Medical Sciences 2016; U.S. National Library of Medicine, National Institutes of Health 2017).

The 3′ end includes an untranslated regulatory region with a stop codon sequence (TAG, TAA, TGA on DNA or UAG, UAA, UGA on RNA) that ends transcription. Because this region is located *after* the last exon of a gene ends, it is referred to as "downstream" of the gene. Remember, untranslated doesn't mean untranscribed. Transcribed means DNA is copied into RNA, but that RNA may or may not be translated into an amino acid

depending on whether it has a coding or non-coding sequence. Translation occurs when DNA is copied to RNA with a coding sequence leading to an amino acid (National Human Genome Research Institute 2015; National Institute of General Medical Sciences 2016; U.S. National Library of Medicine, National Institutes of Health 2017).

The initial mRNA transcript (called precursor mRNA) contains the transcribed sequence of both the exons and introns in the sense strand of the DNA template. The introns must be spliced out to produce a mature mRNA transcript before it can exit the nucleus. Introns are identified by specific splice recognition site sequences of two nucleotides (dinucleotides) at each end. Introns begin with the sequence GT (GU on RNA) and end with the sequence AG. Once the introns are spliced out, the mature mRNA transcript contains the sequences of all the exons in the sense strand of DNA and is ready for translation. The stop codon at the 3′ end of the DNA sense strand template mentioned previously is followed by other untranslated sequences that cause capping and tailing of the mature mRNA transcript so that it can exit the nucleus for translation by tRNA mediated by ribosomes in the cytoplasm (National Human Genome Research Institute 2015; National Institute of General Medical Sciences 2016; U.S. National Library of Medicine, National Institutes of Health 2017).

7.7 Gene Expression

Although most of our cells have the same genes, not all genes are active in every cell at the same time.

Genes may be "switched on" (active or expressed) sometimes and "switched off" (inactive or suppressed) at other times. To understand how gene expression occurs, it is important to remember that genes are sequences of DNA that code for proteins; therefore, gene expression refers to the timing, frequency, rate, and efficiency of protein production for that gene (National Human Genome Research Institute 2015; National Institute of General Medical Sciences 2016; U.S. National Library of Medicine, National Institutes of Health 2017).

All DNA exists coiled tightly around histone proteins to form chromatin. Chromatin protects DNA from damage by making it denser and more compact. It also reacts to regulatory proteins, which among other functions, modify its structure to control gene expression and DNA replication. In general, an open chromatin structure is a transcriptionally active state leading to gene activation (expression), while a closed chromatin structure is a transcriptionally inactive state leading to gene inactivation (suppression). Regulatory proteins include transcription factors, activators, repressors, acetyltransferases, deacetylases, methylases, coactivators, corepressors, kinases, and others (National Human Genome Research Institute 2015; National Institute of General Medical Sciences 2016; U.S. National Library of Medicine, National Institutes of Health 2017).

Regulatory proteins regulate the activity of other genes by exerting control of gene expression through four primary mechanisms: (1) attaching to specific DNA binding sites directly (transcription factors, activators, and repressors), (2) modifying chromatin to open its conformation to reveal DNA binding sites for transcription (histone acetyltransferases) or closing its conformation to preventing such access (histone deacetylases and methylases), (3) binding to transcription factors, activators, and repressors to promote or inhibit gene expression (coactivators and corepressors), or (4) chemically altering transcription factors and activators through phosphorylation (kinases) (National Human Genome Research Institute 2015; National Institute of General Medical Sciences 2016; U.S. National Library of Medicine, National Institutes of Health 2017).

Homeobox genes are a family of genes that act during early embryonic development to control the formation of many body structures by coding for regulatory proteins mentioned previously. Homeobox genes exist on every chromosome and usually appear in clusters. Homeobox genes contain a DNA sequence that codes for a 60-amino acid polypeptide chain known as the homeodomain. The homeodomain is the part of the protein that binds directly to sequence-specific binding sites in the regulatory regions of the target genes (National Human Genome Research Institute 2015; National Institute of General Medical Sciences 2016; U.S. National Library of Medicine, National Institutes of Health 2017).

7.8 Gene Locus and Alleles

DNA sequence variations (differences in the order of the nucleotides) occur normally throughout the genome, and the resulting different forms or variants of the same gene are called alleles. Alleles are the cause of normal hereditary variation. The alleles of a gene coding for a functional protein product that are most common or prevalent in a population are called its "wild type," and are usually designated with a plus sign (+) or the abbreviation "wt." Other alleles are considered mutant alleles and are usually designated with a minus sign (−). Only two alleles exist for most genes, but no matter how many alleles exist for a gene, everyone inherits only two of them, one from each parent (National Human Genome Research Institute 2015; National Institute of General Medical Sciences 2016; U.S. National Library of Medicine, National Institutes of Health 2017).

Zygosity refers to similarity between alleles. The inherited alleles for a gene can be identical (homozygous) or different (heterozygous). Locus refers to the location or position of a gene's DNA sequence on a chromosome, and homology refers to similarity in genetic content between chromosomes. Both chromosomes of a homologous pair (a set of matching maternal and paternal chromosomes) have the same loci (gene positions) all the way along their length but may have different alleles at some of the loci. This means that each chromosome in a homologous pair may contain a different variant of a specific gene, but the gene will be in the same position on both chromosomes. Each chromosome of a homologous pair is called a homolog (National Human Genome Research Institute 2015; National Institute of General Medical Sciences 2016; U.S. National Library of Medicine, National Institutes of Health 2017).

All autosomes usually exist in cells as homologous pairs having one homolog from each parent. Sex chromosomes are different. Female sex chromosomes (XX) are homologous, while male sex chromosomes (XY) are not. Since the Y chromosome does not have a homolog, most of the genes on the Y chromosome are unique to that sex chromosome. And although X chromosomes in the cells of females are homologous, most of the genes on one of the X homologs are inactivated to compensate for human males only having one X chromosome. Since X and Y are non-homologous chromosomes, most the genes present on the X chromosome differ from those that exist on the Y chromosome. However, there is an area on the distal end of the short arm of both X and Y called the pseudoautosomal region. Genes in the pseudoautosomal region are present on *both* X and Y chromosomes, and therefore behave like genes on autosomes. Genes in the pseudoautosomal region of the X chromosome also escape inactivation. As a result, both females (who have two X chromosomes) and males (who have one X and one Y chromosome) usually have two functional alleles in each cell for genes from these regions (National Human Genome Research Institute 2015; National Institute of General Medical Sciences 2016; U.S. National Library of Medicine, National Institutes of Health 2017). These concepts are illustrated in Fig. 7.3.

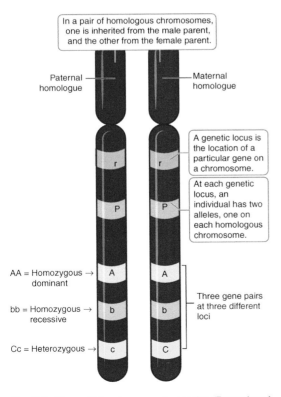

Fig. 7.3 Gene alleles, locus, and zygosity (Reproduced from https://i.stack.imgur.com/16QyG.jpg)

7.9   Genotype and Phenotype

Genotype refers to the pair of alleles an individual has at a specific location (locus) in the genome. Remember that zygosity refers to the degree of similarity between alleles in a genotype. When a pair of alleles for a gene are the same, the genotype is said to be homozygous. When a pair of alleles for a gene are different (heterozygous genotype), one of the alleles can override the other. In this situation, the overriding allele is referred to as the dominant allele, while the other is referred to as recessive. Genotypes can also be homozygous for either the dominant allele or the recessive allele. Genotypes are usually described by labelling the dominant allele with a capital letter and the recessive allele with a lower-case letter. Hemizygous genotypes occur when there is only one allele present for a gene and the other is absent (genes on the X chromosome in cells that contain only one X chromosome in individuals with Turner syndrome), or only one allele exists for that gene (most genes on the Y chromosome in human males) (National Human Genome Research Institute 2015; National Institute of General Medical Sciences 2016; U.S. National Library of Medicine, National Institutes of Health 2017).

Phenotype is the observable effect of the expression of a pair of gene alleles. Phenotype is sometimes referred to as a trait, but this is inaccurate, as there can be more than one phenotype for a given trait. For example, phenotype might mean brown or blue regarding the trait of eye color; or it might mean non-responder regarding the trait of drug response. Phenotypes can represent discontinuous or continuous variation. Discontinuous variation is monogenic, meaning it refers to discrete phenotype alternatives caused by differences in alleles of only one gene. For example, being albino versus pigmented. Continuous variation occurs when a spectrum of differences exist that are not usually traceable to just one gene. This means that the phenotypic differences occur in a continuum rather than as distinct alternatives. Continuous variations are caused by a combination of genes (polygenic) or by the interaction of genes and environment (epigenetic) rather than by just one gene. Examples include height, weight, skin color, or hair color

(National Human Genome Research Institute 2015; National Institute of General Medical Sciences 2016; U.S. National Library of Medicine, National Institutes of Health 2017).

When referring to the number of normal alleles in a genotype required for the gene to produce enough protein product to maintain normal function, the gene involved is described as haplosufficient or haploinsufficient (National Human Genome Research Institute 2015; National Institute of General Medical Sciences 2016; U.S. National Library of Medicine, National Institutes of Health 2017). (This is different from zygosity because zygosity refers to the genotype itself, whereas sufficiency or insufficiency refers to the mechanism through which a genotype produces a phenotype.)

Haplosufficient genes are those in which a single functional allele can compensate for a non-functioning or absent second allele and is thus able to produce sufficient protein product to maintain the gene's normal function. Null alleles of a gene fail to code for a functional protein, and in haplosufficient genes, are usually not expressed if a functional allele is also present. Genes in homologous regions of the X chromosome and most genes on the Y chromosome are examples of haplosufficient genes. One such example is the *SRY* gene located only on the Y chromosome. A single normal *SRY* allele from the Y chromosome is responsible for normal development of male genitalia (National Human Genome Research Institute 2015; National Institute of General Medical Sciences 2016; U.S. National Library of Medicine, National Institutes of Health 2017).

Haploinsufficiency is when a single functional allele of a gene is unable to compensate for a non-functioning or absent second allele and is therefore is insufficient to maintain the gene's normal function. Genes in all autosomes and in the pseudoautosomal regions of the X and Y chromosomes are examples of haploinsufficient genes. One such example is the *SHOX* gene. *SHOX* is the short stature homeobox gene on the X chromosome. Two normal alleles of this gene, one from each sex chromosome, must be present in all cells in both males and females for normal growth and maturation of the skeleton, particu-

larly in the arms and legs. If only one functional allele is present, the amount of *SHOX* protein produced is reduced, and this shortage causes disruption of bone growth beginning in embryonic development. Mutations and deletions in the *SHOX* gene are responsible for the short stature and bone abnormalities observed in Turner syndrome, Léri-Weill dyschondrosteosis, and Langer mesomelic dysplasia (National Human Genome Research Institute 2015; National Institute of General Medical Sciences 2016; U.S. National Library of Medicine, National Institutes of Health 2017).

7.10 Inheritance

Patterns of inheritance can be categorized as Mendelian or non-Mendelian. Mendel described the basic patterns of what is now known as Mendelian inheritance before the existence of genes as the mechanism for inheritance had been discovered. Phenotypic expression of an inherited Mendelian trait depends on the genotype at specific locus. Mendelian traits are inherited in a predictable manner following the laws of segregation, independent assortment, and dominance. Genes on autosomes and the pseudoautosomal regions of the sex chromosomes usually follow Mendelian laws of inheritance (National Human Genome Research Institute 2015; National Institute of General Medical Sciences 2016; U.S. National Library of Medicine, National Institutes of Health 2017).

7.10.1 Mendelian Inheritance

The law of segregation states that the two alleles for one specific trait (one allele on each chromosome of a homologous pair) separate in meiosis during gamete formation (formation of eggs or sperm) so that each gamete has only one allele for that trait. When two gametes randomly fuse at fertilization, the new genotype in the resulting zygote once again contains two alleles for that trait, one from each parent (National Human Genome Research Institute 2015; National

Institute of General Medical Sciences 2016; U.S. National Library of Medicine, National Institutes of Health 2017).

The law of independent assortment states that alleles for two or more *different* traits separate independently from each other during gamete formation, so that an allele for one trait is inherited by offspring independently from the allele for any other trait (National Human Genome Research Institute 2015; National Institute of General Medical Sciences 2016; U.S. National Library of Medicine, National Institutes of Health 2017).

The law of dominance states that there is a dominant allele and recessive allele for each trait. As mentioned previously, dominant alleles are designated by a capital letter and recessive alleles by a lower-case letter. Inherited genotypes are either heterozygous (Aa), homozygous dominant (AA), or homozygous recessive (aa). Heterozygous and homozygous dominant genotypes produce the dominant phenotype for a trait. In the absence of mutation, only homozygous recessive genotypes produce the recessive phenotype for a trait (National Human Genome Research Institute 2015; National Institute of General Medical Sciences 2016; U.S. National Library of Medicine, National Institutes of Health 2017).

Clinical examples of Mendelian inheritance include achondroplasia, multiple endocrine neoplasia, 21-hydroxylase deficiency, Léri-Weill dyschondrosteosis, and Langer mesomelic dysplasia. Achondroplasia can be inherited in an autosomal dominant manner from one affected parent because one mutant allele of the *FGFR3* gene on chromosome 4 is sufficient to cause the phenotype (heterozygous dominant genotype). Inheritance of two mutant alleles from two affected parents is fatal (homozygous dominant genotype) (National Human Genome Research Institute 2015; National Institute of General Medical Sciences 2016; U.S. National Library of Medicine, National Institutes of Health 2017).

Multiple endocrine neoplasia type 1 usually results from autosomal dominant inheritance of mutations in both *MEN1* gene alleles on chromosome 11 (homozygous dominant genotype). All three forms of congenital adrenal hyperplasia resulting from 21-hydroxylase deficiency (classic salt-wasting, classic simple virilizing, and non-classic) are caused by autosomal recessive inheritance of two mutant *CYP21A2* gene alleles on chromosome 6 (homozygous recessive genotype) (National Human Genome Research Institute 2015; National Institute of General Medical Sciences 2016; U.S. National Library of Medicine, National Institutes of Health 2017).

Léri-Weill dyschondrosteosis has a pseudoautosomal dominant pattern of inheritance. The allele for the *SHOX* gene is mutated or missing on the pseudoautosomal region of only one of the two sex chromosomes. Langer mesomelic dysplasia has a pseudoautosomal recessive pattern of inheritance. In this disorder, both alleles for the *SHOX* gene on the pseudoautosomal regions of the sex chromosomes are missing or altered, and the phenotype is more severe (National Human Genome Research Institute 2015; National Institute of General Medical Sciences 2016; U.S. National Library of Medicine, National Institutes of Health 2017).

Lethal genes are those for which one allele is fatal if a genotype with that allele is inherited. Huntington Disease is caused by autosomal dominant inheritance of a lethal mutant *HTT* gene allele on chromosome 4 (National Human Genome Research Institute 2015; National Institute of General Medical Sciences 2016; U.S. National Library of Medicine, National Institutes of Health 2017).

7.10.2 Non-Mendelian Patterns of Inheritance

Non-Mendelian patterns of inheritance include co-dominance, linkage, sex-linked inheritance, multiple alleles, complex inheritance that is polygenic or multifactorial, and mitochondrial inheritance.

Co-dominant inheritance occurs when the effects of both alleles are present in the phenotype so that both traits appear together, and neither is dominant over the other. Human blood type is the most common example. Linkage refers to traits that tend to be inherited together rather separately because the gene alleles for those traits are close enough together on the chromosome to avoid the crossing-over and recombination that occurs during meiosis (National Human Genome Research Institute 2015; National Institute of General Medical Sciences 2016; U.S. National Library of Medicine, National Institutes of Health 2017).

Sex-linked traits are those associated with genes on the non-homologous regions of the X and Y chromosomes. (Remember, genes on non-homologous regions of sex chromosomes contain only one allele in their genotypes, while genes in the pseudoautosomal regions contain two alleles in their genotypes. As noted previously, pseudoautosomal regions of sex chromosomes demonstrate Mendelian inheritance patterns. Sex-linked inheritance can be X-linked or Y-linked (National Human Genome Research Institute 2015; National Institute of General Medical Sciences 2016; U.S. National Library of Medicine, National Institutes of Health 2017).

X-linked inheritance can be X-linked dominant or X-linked recessive. Hereditary hypophosphatemic rickets (X-linked hypophosphatemic rickets) results from a mutation in the *dominant PHEX* gene allele on the X chromosome. It can occur in both males and females but is usually fatal in males. Fragile X syndrome results from a mutation in the *recessive FMR1* gene allele the X chromosome. It also occurs in both males and females, with males being more severely affected. Individuals with complete androgen insensitivity syndrome have both X and Y chromosomes, but they have inherited a *recessive* androgen receptor gene (*AR* gene) allele on their X chromosome and develop external female genitalia but no uterus (National Human Genome Research Institute 2015; National Institute of General Medical Sciences 2016; U.S. National Library of Medicine, National Institutes of Health 2017).

Individuals with *SRY*-related Swyer syndrome (46,XY pure gonadal dysgenesis) also have both X and Y chromosomes in all their cells but have a mutated *SRY* gene allele on their Y chromosome, causing development of both female external genitalia and female reproductive organs, although the gonadal tissue is non-functional.

Most cases develop due to new mutations, but sometimes an individual will inherit the mutation from an unaffected father who is mosaic for the mutation. Mosaicism occurs when the mutation exists in some cells but not in others. Because the mutation is in a gene on the Y chromosome, this is an example of Y-linked inheritance (National Human Genome Research Institute 2015; National Institute of General Medical Sciences 2016; U.S. National Library of Medicine, National Institutes of Health 2017).

The term "multiple alleles" describes a situation in which a gene has *more than* two possible alleles, and the alleles have relative dominance to each other. In Mendelian inheritance, *only* two alleles exist for a gene, and one has absolute dominance over the other (National Human Genome Research Institute 2015; National Institute of General Medical Sciences 2016; U.S. National Library of Medicine, National Institutes of Health 2017).

While monogenic disorders result from mutations in one gene and follow Mendelian patterns of inheritance, complex disorders do not. Complex disorders are often familial but do not have a specific identifiable pattern of inheritance. Complex inheritance is multifactorial, involving the additive effect of many susceptibility genes interacting with each other and with the environment, and is not completely understood. A susceptibility gene is one that confers a risk to develop a disease but is not sufficient by itself to cause the disease. Susceptibility genes can contribute to age of onset and severity of disease or protect against developing the disease. Type 1 diabetes mellitus is an example of a disorder with complex inheritance (National Human Genome Research Institute 2015; National Institute of General Medical Sciences 2016; U.S. National Library of Medicine, National Institutes of Health 2017).

Polygenic inheritance refers to traits in which the phenotype is determined by several different genes. Human stature (height) is an example of this (National Human Genome Research Institute 2015; National Institute of General Medical Sciences 2016; U.S. National Library of Medicine, National Institutes of Health 2017).

Mitochondrial inheritance describes the passing of mitochondrial DNA (mtDNA) from a mother to her offspring through the cytoplasm of her egg cells. All other Mendelian and non-Mendelian inheritance patterns refer to nuclear DNA (DNA that is packaged into chromosomes within the nucleus of cells). Paternal lineage can only be traced through Y-linked DNA in males, while maternal lineage can be traced through mtDNA in both males *and* females. There are 37 genes on mtDNA, 13 of which code for proteins that function as enzymes involved in the energy producing processes within the mitochondria, and the rest provide templates for the synthesis of transfer RNA (tRNA) and ribosomal RNA (rRNA). A clinical example is mitochondrial diabetes and deafness (MIDD), a disorder that results from mutations in at least three mtDNA genes coding for tRNA molecules responsible for synthesis of proteins in the mitochondria of pancreatic beta cells. The mutations impair the ability of the mitochondria to signal insulin release in response to rising glucose levels. The mechanism for the associated deafness is not yet known (National Human Genome Research Institute 2015; National Institute of General Medical Sciences 2016; U.S. National Library of Medicine, National Institutes of Health 2017).

7.11 Epigenetics

Epigenetics is the study of heritable changes that occur *without* a change in DNA sequence. The word "epi" is of Greek origin and means "over" or "above," so epigenetics literally means "above" the genome. The epigenome includes chemical compounds and proteins that mark or tag the genome to provide instructions for turning genes on or off and modifying the way cells produce or use proteins, rather than changing the DNA sequence itself. The epigenome can also change throughout a human's lifespan. Epigenetic changes are passed along as somatic cells divide (National Human Genome Research Institute 2015; National Institute of General Medical Sciences 2016; U.S. National Library of Medicine, National Institutes of Health 2017).

Lifestyle and environmental factors such as diet, medications, smoking, and exposure to pesticides and pollutants can expose a person to chemical tags on the DNA backbone or on histone tails that change the epigenome. Researchers have linked changes in the epigenome to diabetes, autoimmune diseases, and other disorders. Epigenetics explains why although most of all cells in the human body contain the same genes, different cell types behave differently. They behave differently because their epigenetic tags are arranged differently. Epigenetics may also explain differences seen in identical twins (National Human Genome Research Institute 2015; National Institute of General Medical Sciences 2016; U.S. National Library of Medicine, National Institutes of Health 2017).

Epigenetic inheritance involves chemical and structural mechanisms that control gene expression (activation and deactivation of genes), such as chromatin remodelling, X chromosome inactivation, and genetic imprinting. Mechanisms involved in chromatin remodelling via histone modification include methylation and acetylation. During methylation, methyltransferases add methyl groups (CH_3) to histones that close the chromatin structure inducing a transcriptionally inactive state that acts as an off-switch repressing gene expression. During acetylation, acetyltransferases add acetyl groups (CH_3CO) to histones that open the chromatin structure inducing a transcriptionally active state that acts as an on switch activating gene expression. Inappropriate methylation (deactivation) causes a loss of necessary function while inappropriate *de*methylation (removal of a methyl group from the histone causing unintended activation) causes a gain of undesirable function. Similar problems occur when acetylation goes awry (National Human Genome Research Institute 2015; National Institute of General Medical Sciences 2016; U.S. National Library of Medicine, National Institutes of Health 2017).

X chromosome inactivation is an epigenetic form of X chromosome dosage compensation. Dosage refers to the number or "dose" of X chromosomes in a cell. Because cells in human males have one X chromosome while those in human females have two, the species compensates for the extra "dose" females receive by having each cell inactivate (turn off) one of them. This allows males and females to have equal expression of the genes carried on the X chromosome (National Human Genome Research Institute 2015; National Institute of General Medical Sciences 2016; U.S. National Library of Medicine, National Institutes of Health 2017).

The gene that controls which X chromosome remains active is called the X-controlling element (*Xce*), but the mechanism by which it does so is not yet known. The X-chromosomal region that controls the initiation and continuation of X-inactivation is called the X-inactivation center (Xic). The *Xist* gene controls Xic initiation of inactivation (National Human Genome Research Institute 2015; National Institute of General Medical Sciences 2016; U.S. National Library of Medicine, National Institutes of Health 2017).

The exception to this rule is in genes located in the distal region of the short arms of chromosomes X and Y, called the Xp and Yp regions, which demonstrate pseudoautosomal inheritance. In other words, these regions escape X-inactivation and the genes in these regions are inherited in the same manner as genes found on autosomes. This means that two copies of a gene allele are required for expression in these regions instead of the one copy that is required for other genes on the X and Y chromosomes (National Human Genome Research Institute 2015; National Institute of General Medical Sciences 2016; U.S. National Library of Medicine, National Institutes of Health 2017).

Imprinting refers to sex-specific differences in epigenetic methylation patterns. Gene expression is determined by the methylation pattern in the parent of origin (tied to whether it is inherited from mother or father). Unlike histone modification where the methyl groups are attached to the histone tails, during imprinting, the methyl groups are added directly to the DNA without changing the sequence. Cytosine nucleotide bases located next to guanine bases are referred to as CpG dinucleotides. Clusters of CpG repeats are called CpG islands. A different methyltransferase from that used in histone modification adds a methyl group to the cytosine in these islands scattered throughout the genome to inactivate certain genes in only one parent. In some genes, only the copy of the gene from the mother gets turned on, while in others, only the copy from the father. The copy from the opposite parent is turned off. The pattern of methylation is transmitted during replication. Clinical examples include Prader-Willi syndrome and Angelman syndrome which both involve imprinted genes on chromosome 15 (National Human Genome Research Institute 2015; National Institute of General Medical Sciences 2016; U.S. National Library of Medicine, National Institutes of Health 2017).

7.12 Mutations

Genetic alterations in the DNA sequence that occur in *at least* 1% of the population and are common enough to be considered normal variation are referred to as polymorphisms. Polymorphisms are generally considered neutral or not harmful. A single nucleotide polymorphism (SNP) is the smallest possible change in DNA, affecting only one nucleotide. Single nucleotide polymorphisms commonly occur in both coding (exons) and non-coding (introns) regions (National Human Genome Research Institute 2015; National Institute of General Medical Sciences 2016; U.S. National Library of Medicine, National Institutes of Health 2017).

Permanent changes in the DNA sequence that are harmful and rare, occurring in *less than* 1% of the population, are called mutations. Mutations range in size from one nucleotide to large chunks of a chromosome involving many genes. Mutations can be classified as either hereditary (germline) or acquired (somatic). Hereditary mutations are germline mutations because the DNA error occurs in germ cells (egg and sperm, also called gametes). A germline mutation is passed from parent to offspring and remains present in every cell of the offspring's body for the entire lifespan. De novo mutations are defined as new DNA sequence variants that are present in an offspring but absent from both parents. A de novo germline mutation is a new mutation in an egg or sperm cell of a parent or a new mutation that occurs immediately after fertilization before cell division begins. De novo germline mutations can result from DNA errors that occur during meiotic cell division. The mutation is not present in any of the parent's other cells, so the parent is unaffected. The disorder in the offspring caused by the new mutation may be the first appearance of that disorder in the family (there may not be any prior family history of the disorder) (National Human Genome Research Institute 2015; National Institute of General Medical Sciences 2016; U.S. National Library of Medicine, National Institutes of Health 2017).

Acquired mutations are called somatic mutations because they occur in somatic cells (cells that are not egg or sperm cells). All acquired mutations are mutations that cannot be passed on to offspring, are not present in every cell of the body, and can occur at any time from the embryonic period until the end of the individual's lifespan.

DNA errors causing acquired mutations can result from environmental damage to the DNA, errors that occur during DNA replication in mitotic cell division, and problems with DNA repair mechanisms (DNA repair enzymes that find and fix most DNA errors before they can accumulate) (National Human Genome Research Institute 2015; National Institute of General Medical Sciences 2016; U.S. National Library of Medicine, National Institutes of Health 2017). Types of gene mutations with clinical examples are provided in Table 7.1 (Lania et al. 2001; Vassart and Costagliola 2011; Lin et al. 2007; Bashamboo et al. 2016; Birla et al. 2014; Bøe Wolff et al. 2008; Gagliardi et al. 2014; Tonelli et al. 2014; Yamaguchi et al. 2013; Baculescu 2013; Akbas et al. 2012).

Table 7.1 Types of gene mutations with clinical examples (Lania et al. 2001; Vassart and Costagliola 2011; Lin et al. 2007; Bashamboo et al. 2016; Birla et al. 2014; Bøe Wolff et al. 2008; Gagliardi et al. 2014; Tonelli et al. 2014; Yamaguchi et al. 2013; Baculescu 2013)

GENE MUTATION	CLINICAL EXAMPLE
Point—a change in one nucleotide at a single location in a DNA sequence	Loss-of-function germline point mutations in the *GNAS* gene at 20q13.32 can cause pseudohypoparathyroidism type Ia with or without testitoxicosis, while gain-of-function somatic point mutations in the same gene have been linked to McCune-Albright syndrome.
Missense—the change of a single base pair causes the substitution of a different amino acid in the resulting protein	46,XY gonadal dysgenesis with impaired androgen biosynthesis (external female genitalia with palpable bilateral labial testes) was reported in an infant with a heterozygous missense de novo germline mutation.
Nonsense—a change in a single base pair creates a premature stop codon that signals the cell to stop building a protein too soon	A nonsense mutation has been associated with pituitary stalk interruption syndrome resulting in neonatal hypoglycemia, and GH, TSH, and ACTH deficiencies.
Insertion—the addition of genetic material ranging from a single extra DNA base pair to a piece of a chromosome	An insertion mutation was associated with acromegaly and left atrial myxoma in Carney's complex.
Deletion—the removal of genetic material ranging from one DNA base pair within a gene to entire genes	Partial gene deletions contribute to autoimmune polyendocrine syndromes.
Duplication—a piece of DNA is abnormally copied one or more times	A duplication in the aromatase gene results in aromatase deficiency, a rare autosomal recessive disorder that prevents the conversion of androgens to estrogens.
Frameshift—addition or deletion of a nucleotide pair shifts the reading frame of the gene sequence during translation so that all the amino acids after the mutation are altered. Insertions, deletions, and duplications can all be frameshift mutations	A germline heterozygous frameshift mutation of the *CDKN1B* gene has been reported to cause recurrent hyperparathyroidism in the autosomal dominant disorder multiple endocrine neoplasia type 4 (MEN4).
Substitution—one base pair is replaced by a different base pair	A homozygous substitution mutation caused the autosomal recessive disorder familial glucocorticoid deficiency (FGD) in a patient whose parents were heterozygous for the same mutation.
Repeat expansions—a mutation that increases the number of times short nucleotide sequences are repeated in a row	A shorter CAG repeat polymorphism mediates androgen receptor activity contributing to the pathogenesis of polycystic ovarian syndrome (PCOS).

7.13 Chromosomal Abnormalities

Chromosomal abnormalities can be either structural or numerical.

7.13.1 Chromosomal Structural Abnormalities

Abnormal changes in chromosome structure can be inherited or occur randomly during gamete formation or early fetal development (National Human Genome Research Institute 2015; National Institute of General Medical Sciences 2016; U.S. National Library of Medicine, National Institutes of Health 2017). Types of chromosomal structural abnormalities with associated clinical examples and methods for diagnostic testing are provided in Table 7.2 (Akbas et al. 2012; Choi et al. 2013; Stagi et al. 2014; Antonacci et al. 2009; Cetin et al. 2011; Sireteanu et al. 2013; Bellfield et al. 2016).

Table 7.2 Chromosomal structural abnormalities with clinical examples (Akbas et al. 2012; Choi et al. 2013; Stagi et al. 2014; Antonacci et al. 2009; Cetin et al. 2011; Sireteanu et al. 2013; Bellfield et al. 2016)

STRUCTURAL ABNORMALITY	DIAGNOSTIC TESTING	CLINICAL EXAMPLES
Translocations—a broken piece of one chromosome attaches to a non-homologous chromosome	Cytogenetic karyotype analysis	A familial balanced reciprocal translocation 46,XY,t(16;22)(p11;q13) was found in a patient with constitutional short stature. A variety of phenotypes including hypogonadotrophic hypogonadism, precocious puberty, growth hormone deficiency, and idiopathic short stature were identified in patients with 45,XY,t(13;14)(q10;q10) and 45,XX,t(13;14)(q10;q10).
Deletions—a piece of a chromosome breaks off and is lost	Standard karyotype does not detect deletion; requires FISH analysis or other molecular analysis	DiGeorge syndrome results from an autosomal dominant or de novo germline mutation causing deletion of genes on 22q11.2.
Duplications—part of a chromosome is copied too many times resulting in extra copies of genetic material from the duplicated segment	Molecular arrayCGH analysis	Growth hormone deficiency has been associated with *SOX3* gene duplication on chromosome Xq26.3-27.3.
Inversions—a chromosome breaks in two places and the resulting piece reattaches itself into the chromosome in reverse order	Molecular sequence analysis and arrayCGH analysis of inversion breakpoints and FISH analysis of inversions	Renal cysts and diabetes syndrome (RCAD) or maturity-onset diabetes of the young, type 5 (MODY5) is associated with an inversion at chromosome 17q12.
Isochromosome—a chromosome with two identical arms, formed by transverse rather than longitudinal separation of a replicating chromosome, which causes duplication of one arm and loss of the other, with associated gain or loss in copies of the genes on those arms	Cytogenetic karyotype analysis followed by multiple FISH analyses with chromosomes 4, 16, X and centromeric probes	A patient with Turner syndrome was found to have a complex karyotype including both mosaicism of an isochromosome Xq10 and a maternally inherited familial reciprocal translocation between chromosomes 4 and 16 t(4;16)(p15.2;p13.1).
Dicentric chromosomes—a chromosome with two centromeres resulting from the abnormal fusion of two chromosome pieces, each containing a centromere. Some genetic material is usually lost	Cytogenetic karyotype analysis followed by molecular SNP chromosome microarray analysis	A dicentric chromosome 14;18 was found in female with microform holoprosencephaly and Turner-like stigmata.
Ring chromosome—a chromosome that has broken in two places and the ends of the arms fuse to form a circular structure (genetic material at the tip of each arm is usually lost)	Cytogenetic karyotype analysis followed by molecular SNP chromosome microarray analysis	Ring chromosome 18p deletion is associated with anterior pituitary aplasia.

7.13.2 Chromosomal Copy Number Abnormalities

Ploidy refers to the number of sets of chromosomes in the nucleus of a cell. As described earlier in the chapter, diploid somatic cells have two copies of a set of chromosomes (2n), while haploid reproductive cells (germ cells or gametes) have one copy (n). Disorders caused by the presence of an abnormal number of chromosomes are called aneuploidies. Aneuploidies are not mutations, but like de novo germline mutations and acquired somatic mutations, these disorders are not usually inherited. They are present in an offspring but usually absent from both parents (National Human Genome Research Institute 2015; National Institute of General Medical Sciences 2016; U.S. National Library of Medicine, National Institutes of Health 2017).

Disjunction refers to normal homologous chromosome or sister chromatid separation during mitotic or meiotic cell division. Aneuploidies are the result of meiotic or mitotic nondisjunction. Nondisjunction occurs when a pair of chromosomes or chromatids fail to separate during cell division. Endocrine examples include Turner and Klinefelter syndromes (National Human Genome Research Institute 2015; National Institute of General Medical Sciences 2016; U.S. National Library of Medicine, National Institutes of Health 2017).

Meiotic nondisjunction usually occurs randomly during the formation of gametes in a parent resulting in an egg or sperm cell gaining one or more extra chromosome copies (Klinefelter syndrome) or losing a chromosome copy (Turner syndrome). If an abnormal egg or sperm cell is one of the gametes that forms the zygote, the aneuploidy (abnormal chromosome copy number) will be present in every cell of the offspring's body (as is seen in de novo germline mutations). In our example, a 24,XY sperm fertilizes a 23,X egg or a 23,X sperm fertilizes a 24,XX egg resulting in Klinefelter syndrome (47,XXY), or a 23,X sperm fertilizes a 22 egg or a 22 sperm fertilizes a 23,X egg resulting in Turner syndrome (45,X) (National Human Genome Research Institute 2015; National Institute of General Medical

Sciences 2016; U.S. National Library of Medicine, National Institutes of Health 2017).

Mitotic nondisjunction occurs as a random event after conception during cell division early in fetal development and leads to mosaicism. Mosaicism means that the aneuploidy (abnormal chromosome copy number) is present only in some of the cells in the offspring's body, while other cells have the normal chromosome copy number. Following the previous examples, an individual with mosaic Klinefelter syndrome (46,XY/47,XXY) would have one X chromosome and one Y chromosome is some body cells, and an extra copy of the X chromosome in other cells. An individual with mosaic Turner syndrome (46,XX/45X) would have two X chromosomes in some body cells, and only one X chromosome in other cells. Other examples of mosaicism resulting from mitotic nondisjunction in early embryonic development include Down syndrome 46,XY/47,XY,+21, Edward syndrome 46,XX/47,XX,+18, and Patua syndrome 46,XY/47,XY,+13 (National Human Genome Research Institute 2015; National Institute of General Medical Sciences 2016; U.S. National Library of Medicine, National Institutes of Health 2017).

7.14 Interpreting Genetic Test Results

There are two basic types of genetic testing, cytogenetic and molecular. Cytogenetic testing examines chromosomal number and structure using microscopic analysis, whereas molecular genetic testing examines genes and chromosomes at the level of the DNA or RNA molecule using a variety of specialized molecular techniques (National Human Genome Research Institute 2015; National Institute of General Medical Sciences 2016; U.S. National Library of Medicine, National Institutes of Health 2017). The current section will cover basic chromosomal anatomy used to interpret cytogenetic testing, give a detailed explanation of cytogenetic testing methods, and provide an overview of molecular genetic technologies. (Detailed chromosome structural morphology including chromatin, histones, and DNA sequence was covered previously in the chapter section on gene expression and will not be duplicated here.)

The most common cytogenic test result seen in endocrine clinic is the karyotype, while molecular genetic testing results may be from molecular array analyses (SNP-arrays, microarrays, array comparative genomic hybridization), genome-wide or specific gene sequencing, and other molecular methods of mutation detection. Although cytogenetic test interpretation requires knowledge of basic chromosomal anatomy, molecular genetic test interpretation requires additional recollection of concepts such as exons, introns, promoters, and SNPs covered in prior sections of this chapter.

7.14.1 Chromosome Anatomy

Chromosomes can be viewed using a light microscope following treatment with special stains. Stained chromosomes are more easily seen during the phase of mitotic cell division when the chromosomes have replicated and are condensed. Each chromosome has a constriction, called a centromere, which divides the chromosome into short (p) and long (q) arms, and orients the chromosomes during the phases of cell division. The tip of each end is called a telomere (National Human Genome Research Institute 2015; National Institute of General Medical Sciences 2016; U.S. National Library of Medicine, National Institutes of Health 2017).

7.14.2 Cytogenic Testing

7.14.2.1 Karyotyping

A karyotype is a pictorial display of metaphase (standard) or prophase/prometaphase (high resolution) chromosomes from a mitotic cell. Karyotyping can identify abnormalities in chromosome numbers and structure. Standard karyotyping is performed on cells in metaphase when the chromosomes are most condensed, while high resolution karyotyping is performed on cells

in prophase or prometaphase when the chromosomes are slightly more elongated (National Human Genome Research Institute 2015; National Institute of General Medical Sciences 2016; U.S. National Library of Medicine, National Institutes of Health 2017).

The process of obtaining a karyotype involves:

- growing colonies of cells in culture medium until there is sufficient quantity for analysis
- treating the cells with a hypotonic solution to make them swell so that the chromosomes spread out and separate from one another
- arresting mitotic cell division with colchicine in prophase/prometaphase or metaphase
- using special chemicals to digest and remove all chromosomal proteins (such as histones)
- staining the condensed chromosomes with standard dyes (G, C, T, and R banding) or fluorescence (spectral banding)
- and finally, photographing the chromosomes and digitally rearranging them in pairs distinguished by length, size and shape, and unique banding patterns (National Human Genome Research Institute 2015; National Institute of General Medical Sciences 2016; U.S. National Library of Medicine, National Institutes of Health 2017)

Chromosomes are displayed in a karyotype with the autosomes first, arranged by longest (chromosome 1) to shortest (chromosome 22), followed by the sex chromosomes. The unique shape of each chromosome in a karyotype is determined by the location of its centromere. The shape can be described as metacentric (chromosomes 1, 3, 16, 19-20), submetacentric (chromosomes 2, 4-12, 17-18, X), acrocentric (chromosomes 13-15, 21-22, Y), or telocentric (does not exist in humans) (National Human Genome Research Institute 2015; National Institute of General Medical Sciences 2016; U.S. National Library of Medicine, National Institutes of Health 2017).

The lightness or darkness in the banding patterns is determined by the density of the DNA in that region. Darker bands are produced in adenine-thymine-rich areas in G banding, guanine–cytosine-rich areas in R banding, on centromeres in C banding, and on telomeres in T banding. Chromosomes in traditional banding karyotypes appear in black and white. Spectral banding uses multiple fluorescent probes with varying amounts of fluorescent dyes that bind to specific regions of chromosomes resulting in unique spectral characteristics for each chromosome that are detected by computer software that creates a full color digital image of the chromosomes (National Human Genome Research Institute 2015; National Institute of General Medical Sciences 2016; U.S. National Library of Medicine, National Institutes of Health 2017).

Karyotypes can be made at standard or high resolution. Standard metaphase karyotyping can identify 300–600 bands per chromosome, while high resolution prophase/prometaphase karyotyping can identify 700–1200 bands. Just as you were able to see greater detail at higher power magnification when you viewed a slide under a microscope in your high school biology class, higher resolution banding karyotypes can sometimes find chromosomal abnormalities not detected under standard resolution, and spectral karyotypes can sometimes detect translocations not recognizable through standard banding anal-

ysis (National Human Genome Research Institute 2015; National Institute of General Medical Sciences 2016; U.S. National Library of Medicine, National Institutes of Health 2017).

Each arm of the chromosome (p and q) is divided into regions numbered sequentially from the centromere to the telomere. The bands within each region are also numbered sequentially in the same manner, and these bands are further refined by additional levels of sub-band numbering (Fig. 7.4).

A common misperception is that bands represent single genes, but in fact the thinnest bands contain over a million base pairs and potentially hundreds of genes. Gene locations on a chromosome are often shown on a cytogenetic map, which is a diagram displaying the specific banding pattern for that chromosome, with the gene location indicated at a specific distance from the centromere or telomere (National Human Genome Research Institute 2015; National Institute of General Medical Sciences 2016; U.S. National Library of Medicine, National Institutes of Health 2017).

For example, the gene responsible for Kallman syndrome is located at Xp22.3, meaning that it is located within the 3rd sub-band of the 2nd band

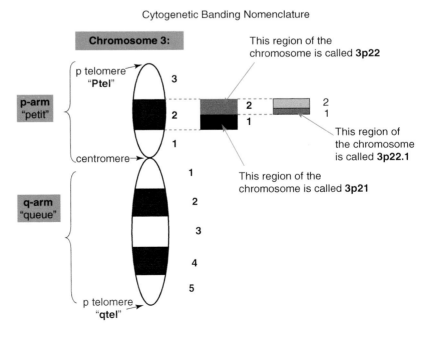

Fig. 7.4 Chromosome anatomy and banding designations (Reproduced from http://cdn.biologydiscussion.com/wp-content/uploads/2015/11/clip_image0222.jpg)

in region 2 of the short arm of the X chromosome. Another example is the area of gene deletion found in patients with Prader-Willi and Angelman syndromes, which is defined as 15q11 to 15q13, meaning that the genetic region is located between the 1st and 3rd bands within the 1st region on the long arm of chromosome 15.

Reading a karyotype report requires an understanding of the terminology used in the description of the analysis. Cells or colonies refer to the number of cells in which the chromosomes were counted, while cultures refer to the number of cell colonies examined to reduce or eliminate the chance of lab error. Cells or metaphases analyzed means the number of cells in which the chromosomes were examined in detail for length, shape, and banding pattern. Images or karyotypes refer to the number of pictures taken, or digital files generated for the report (National Human Genome Research Institute 2015; National Institute of General Medical Sciences 2016; U.S. National Library of Medicine, National Institutes of Health 2017).

Three letter codes are used to describe specific banding techniques. The first letter denotes the type of banding (G, R, C, or T); the second letter indicates the general technique used to remove the chromosomal proteins to permit staining (barium hydroxide, acetic acid, trypsin, BrdU, or heating); and the third letter gives the type of stain used (Giemsa, Wright's). For example, GTG means G banding by trypsin using Giemsa; GTW means G banding by trypsin using Wright's; CBG means C banding by barium hydroxide using Giemsa; RHG means R bands by heating using Giemsa; and RBG means R bands by BrdU using Geimsa (National Human Genome Research Institute 2015; National Institute of General Medical Sciences 2016; U.S. National Library of Medicine, National Institutes of Health 2017).

Karyotype reports use abbreviations to indicate chromosomal abnormalities such as der (derivative chromosome, which is a structurally rearranged chromosome), inv (inversion), ins (insertion), del (deletion), t (translocation), and others (National Human Genome Research Institute 2015; National Institute of General

Medical Sciences 2016; U.S. National Library of Medicine, National Institutes of Health 2017). For example, in a patient with Wittwer syndrome believed to be a variant of Wolf-Hirschhorn syndrome, a karyotype of 46,XY,der(4)t(4;17)(p16.1;q25.3) refers to a derivative chromosome 4 resulting from a translocation between the short arm of chromosome 4 at region 1, band 6, sub-band 1, and the long arm of chromosome 17 at region 2, band 5, sub-band 3 (Wieland et al. 2014). In a patient with Silver-Russell syndrome, a karyotype of 46,XX,der(16)t(11;16)(p15.3;q24.3)mat showed a derivative chromosome 16 resulting from a translocation between the short arm of chromosome 11 at region 1, band 5, sub-band 3, and the long arm of chromosome 16 at region 2, band 4, sub-band 3. The "mat" notation means that further molecular analyses revealed duplications (extra copies) of maternally derived chromosome 11p15 in this patient (Nakashima et al. 2015).

7.14.2.2 Fluorescent In Situ Hybridization

Fluorescent in situ hybridization (FISH) is a cytogenetic technique where a probe is used to locate a specific area of concern on a chromosome. Because FISH targets a specific chromosome region, the test is ordered when clinical findings suggest a specific disorder that isn't confirmed by high resolution karyotyping alone (Anderson 2016). A probe is a manufactured nucleic acid segment (a specific part of a strand of DNA) that seeks out the complementary strand of DNA in the sample and binds to it. The process of binding one complementary strand to another is hybridization. The probe is labelled with fluorescent dye or a radioactive tag for identification when it finds it target. FISH is generally used to detect microdeletions. Laboratory reports for FISH analysis use the abbreviation "ish" followed by the name of the specific probe utilized in the procedure.

7.14.2.3 Cytogenetic Testing Clinical Examples

Table 7.3 contains actual de-identified patient results for cytogenetic testing from an endocrine clinic with author comments added that allow the

Table 7.3 Cytogenetic testing clinical examples

CYTOGENETIC TESTING	
Patient test result	**Author comments**
Case 1 **Cytogenetic Report and Consultation** Quest Diagnostics Age: 7 Sex: Male Specimen Type: Peripheral blood Indication: FISH evaluation for DiGeorge/Velocardiofacial Syndrome [Chromosome analysis (HRO138293) in progress] Summary of Analysis Method: FISH Total Cells: 30 Images: 2 Results ish 22q11.2(TUPLE1x2) Interpretation Negative for DiGeorge/Velocardiofacial syndrome. A fluorescence in situ hybridization (FISH) study, using the probe TUPLE1 (Vysis, Inc.), which hybridizes within band 22q11.2, showed a normal pattern of hybridization. Therefore, the deletion associated with the majority of cases of DiGeorge and Velocardiofacial syndromes is not present in this patient. Deletions contiguous to or smaller than this probe, point mutations and diseases with other genetic etiologies will not be detected by this method.	This patient presented with short stature associated with a heart murmur, low-set ears, and hypotonia. Two tests were subsequently performed for suspicion of DiGeorge/Velocardiofacial syndrome, a FISH evaluation and a chromosome analysis. The result shown here is for the FISH evaluation. DiGeorge/Velocardiofacial syndrome is also referred to as 22q11.2 deletion syndrome. Note the limitations of this type of testing listed in the interpretation section of the results.

Case 2
Cytogenetic Report and Consultation
Quest Diagnostics
 	
Age: 7 y   Sex: Male
Specimen Type: Peripheral blood
Indication: Rule out chromosome abnormality
[FISH for DiGeorge/Velocardiofacial Syndrome (F01 38294)
negative]
 	
Summary of Analysis
Method: GTG
Band Level: 550
Total Cells/Colonies: 20
Cells Analyzed: 5
Images/Karyotypes: 3/2
 	
Results
46,XY, normal male karyotype
 	
Interpretation
The banding level required for high resolution analysis (at least
550 bands per haploid karyotype) was achieved in this study as
requested. The following possibilities, although rare, cannot be
ruled out:
   (a) low level mosaicism,
   (b) very subtle rearrangements, and
   (c) genetic disorders that cannot be detected by cytogenetic
methods.
	This result is for the chromosome analysis
	performed on the same patient as the FISH
	evaluation.
	
	Higher band levels allow greater resolution and
	increase the ability to identify subtler chromosomal
	abnormalities.
	
	Note the limitations of this type of testing listed in
	the interpretation section.
	
	Molecular genetics tests now available for
	diagnosing 22q11.2 abnormalities include:
	  • Deletion/duplication analysis
	  • Sequence analysis of the entire coding region
	  • Targeted variant analysis
	  • Detection of homozygosity.

(continued)

146 K. M. Behm

Table 7.3 (continued)

CYTOGENETIC TESTING	
Patient test result	**Author comments**
Case 3 **Chromosome Analysis** Genzyme Genetics	This patient presented with tall stature and hypothalamic hypogonadism prompting testing for Klinefelter syndrome.
Specimen Type: Peripheral Blood Indications for Study: History of presumed Cornelia de Lange	The test result provides an example of meiotic nondisjunction resulting in aneuploidy. Note the limitations of this type of testing listed in the interpretation section.
Metaphases Counted: 23 Banding Technique: GTW Metaphases Analyzed: 7 Number of Cultures: 2 Metaphases Karyotyped: 3 Banding Resolution: 500	
Results 47,XXY Abnormal karyotype, male	
Interpretation Cytogenetic analysis shows 47,XXY in each metaphase cell examined, consistent with the clinical diagnosis of Klinefelter Syndrome. The clinical manifestations are highly variable, but usually include tall stature, infertility, and a risk for gynecomastia. Mental retardation is unlikely. There is a risk for developmental delays in speech, neuromotor skills, and learning abilities (Robinson, A. et al., Prenatal Diagnosis of Sex Chromosome Abnormalities. In Milunsky, A., ed., Genetic Disorders and the Fetus, 4th edition. Baltimore: The Johns Hopkins University Press, 1998. pp. 249–85). No other chromosome abnormalities are observed. The standard cytogenetic methodology utilized in this analysis does not routinely detect small rearrangements and low-level mosaicism and cannot detect microdeletions. Genetic counseling is recommended for this family.	
Case 4 **Chromosome Analysis Report** Medgenetics Diagnostic Laboratories, Inc.	This patient presented with short stature, dysmorphic facial features, obesity, hypotonia, and mild intellectual disability prompting testing for Prader-Willi syndrome.
Age: 8 y Sex: M Requesting Diagnosis: Dysmorphic features Specimen: Peripheral blood Banding Method: G-banding (GTG) No. Metaphases Analyzed: 20 No. Karyotyped: 2	Follow-up tests that could confirm the diagnosis of Prader-Willi syndrome are listed below.
Cytogenetic Diagnosis 46,XY,del(15)?(q11orq11q12)	Cytogenetics Tests • Fluorescence in situ hybridization (FISH)
Interpretation Deletion of proximal long arm material from one chromosome #15 is apparent in this patient. The question arises as to whether the deletion simply involves part of q11 (generally considered to be benign) or instead encompasses q11 and q12 (associated with the manifestation of Prader-Willi/Angelman syndromes). Materiel on hand is of insufficient quality to discriminate between these two alternatives.	Molecular Genetics Tests • Deletion/duplication analysis • Sequence analysis of the entire coding region • Uniparental disomy study (UPD) • Targeted variant analysis • Methylation analysis • Detection of homozygosity
Recommendations Please repeat for high resolution analysis. Clinical correlation requested.	Prader-Willi and Angelman syndromes involve imprinted genes in sections of chromosome 15. Only the paternal or maternal allele is functional in imprinted genes, while the other allele is inactivated. If both alleles are inherited from one parent instead of one allele from each parent (uniparental disomy), the functional imprinted gene may be missing (the paternal allele in Prader-Willi syndrome and the maternal allele in Angelman syndrome).

(continued)

Table 7.3 (continued)

CYTOGENETIC TESTING	
Patient test result	**Author comments**
Case 5 **Cytogenetic Report and Consultation** Quest Diagnostics Age: 8 Months Sex: Female Indication: FISH evaluation for Prader-Willi-Angelman Syndromes Specimen Type: Peripheral blood Summary of Analysis Method: FISH Total Cells: 20 Images: 2 Results ish 15q12(SNRPNx2) Interpretation Negative for Prader-Willi-Angelman syndromes. A fluorescence in situ hybridization (FISH) study, using the probe SNRPN (Vysis, Inc.), which hybridizes within band 15q12, showed a normal pattern of hybridization, no deletion nor duplication was observed in this patient. Uniparental disomy, mutations affecting imprinting, deletions contiguous to or smaller than this probe, point mutations and diseases with other genetic etiologies will not be detected by this method Genetic counseling is recommended.	This infant presented with failure to thrive, developmental delay, hypotonia, and dysmorphic facial features suspicious for Prader-Willi syndrome. Note the limitations of this type of testing listed in the interpretation section. Recommendations for additional molecular genetic tests noted in previous patient case would also apply to this case. DNA methylation analysis can detect up to 99% of cases and is now the recommended first line test for Prader-Willi syndrome. The FISH test only detects deletions, not methylation defects, imprinting defects, or uniparental disomy.

Case 6
 Cytogenetic Report and Consultation
 Quest Diagnostics
 	
 Age: 11   Sex: Female
 Indication: Rule out Turner's or Mosaic Turner's
 Specimen Type: Peripheral blood
 	
 Summary of Analysis
 Method: GTG
 Total Cells/Colonies: 20
 Band Level: 400–550
 Cells Analyzed: 5
 Images/Karyotypes: 3/2
 	
 Results
 45,X
 	
 Interpretation
 An abnormal female karyotype with a single X chromosome, consistent with the clinical diagnosis of Turner syndrome was noted in all metaphases. Genetic counseling is recommended. The following possibilities, although rare, cannot be ruled out:
     (a) low level mosaicism,
     (b) very subtle rearrangements, and
     (c) genetic disorders that cannot be detected by standard cytogenetic methods.
	This patient presented with severe short stature, hypothyroidism, and features suggestive of Turner syndrome.
	
	 The test result provides an example of meiotic nondisjunction, the failure of homologous chromosomes to separate during the first meiotic cell division, resulting in germline aneuploidy.
	
	 Note the limitations of this type of testing listed in the interpretation section.
	
	 FISH analysis using X and Y probes can identify low-level sex chromosome mosaicism for cryptic Y chromosome material.

(continued)

Table 7.3 (continued)

CYTOGENETIC TESTING	
Patient test result	**Author comments**
Case 7 **Chromosome Analysis** Specimen Type: Peripheral Blood Indication: Pituitary dwarfism Metaphases Counted: 30 Banding Technique: GTW Metaphases Analyzed: 7 Number of Cultures: 2 Metaphases Karyotyped: 3 Banding Resolution: 500 <u>Results</u> 45,X[17]/46,XX[13] Abnormal karyotype, female <u>Interpretation</u> Cytogenetic analysis shows two cell lines: Seventeen (17) of 30 metaphase cells examined show a 45,X Karyotype. A 46,XX karyotype was observed in each of the remaining cells. A 45,X cell line is characteristically associated with Turner syndrome. Patients with 45,X145,XX mosaicism can express a range of clinical features, varying from normal female maturation to full expression of Turner syndrome phenotype (Robinson, A. et al. In Milunsky, A., ed. Genetic Disorders and the Fetus, 4th edition. Baltimore: The Johns Hopkins University Press, 1998. P. 256; and Hsu, L.Y.F. In Milunsky, A., ed. pp. 219–20). No other chromosome abnormalities are observed. The standard cytogenetic methodology utilized in this analysis does not routinely detect small rearrangements and low-level mosaicism and cannot detect microdeletions. Genetic counseling is recommended for this patient/family.	This patient presented with short stature as her chief complaint. The clinic protocol was to test any female presenting with short stature for Turner syndrome. The test result provides an example of mitotic nondisjunction, the failure of sister chromatids to separate during mitosis in early embryonic development, leading to mosaicism of the aneuploidy.

reader to apply concepts covered in this chapter to clinical scenarios. Refer to key terms found at the beginning of this chapter for terminology definitions.

7.14.3 Molecular Genetic Testing

Molecular testing differs from cytogenetic testing in that it looks at changes in DNA sequence or epigenomic modifications to the DNA rather than at chromosomal number and structure within a cell. Three types of molecular genetic testing will be presented here: Microarrays, direct sequencing analysis, and methylation analysis.

7.14.3.1 Microarrays

Microarray technologies fall into two categories: array comparative genomic hybridization (aCGH) and single nucleotide polymorphism array (SNP-array or HDSNP-array). Both aCGH and SNP-array look for copy number variations

(CNV) in the DNA sequence, but aCGH does so by comparing the patient's DNA to reference DNA, while SNP-arrays find CNV directly without the need for reference DNA. Microarrays have a growing number of applications including molecular karyotyping (DNA microarrays) and gene expression studies (RNA microarrays) (Bochud 2012).

Molecular karyotyping via aCGH is able to detect chromosome microdeletions and microduplications not detectable through cytogenetic methods because of its significantly higher resolution (Kirmani 2014). This means that it is able to detect CNV in regions too small to be seen microscopically, and unlike FISH, does not require clinical suspicion of an abnormality in a specific chromosomal location (Anderson 2016). It aCGH is like performing thousands of FISH tests all at one time because it detects missing regions of chromosomes (deletions) or extra segments of chromosomes (duplications) by simultaneously hybridizing the patient's DNA to thousands of reference DNA probes. The probes are unique short DNA segments of every chromosome arranged in a grid attached to a type of glass slide called a gene chip. Because DNA probes are often called oligonucleotides, aCGH is sometimes referred to as oligonucleotide-based array comparative genomic hybridization (oligonucleotide aCGH) (Bochud 2012). The reference DNA is sometimes referred to as the control DNA because it is from individuals with no genetic abnormalities. The genetic regions of the genome represented on the array chip depends on the number of probes in the array (Anderson 2016). The patient's DNA, along with reference DNA, are broken up into fragments and labeled with fluorescent dye (usually green and red) and applied to the chip where the fragments hybridize with matching probes on the array. A microarray scanner machine then analyzes the hybridization patterns. An imbalance in green or red in the analysis indicates duplications or deletions are present (Anderson 2016).

Because there are many different proprietary chip technologies available, aCGH results will look different depending on the specific technology used in the laboratory performing the analysis (Bochud 2012). However, most provide the copy numbers of each chromosome as well as the location and number of deletions (dn) or duplications (dp). Deletions and duplications may be measured in base pairs (bp), kilobase pairs (1000 base pairs per kb), or megabase pairs (one million base pairs per Mb). Here are three examples:

- arr(1-22)x2, (XY)x1 means that the microarray found two copies of chromosomes 1-22 and one copy each of chromosomes X and Y, for a normal male karyotype (Anderson 2016).
- arr(1-22,X)x2 means the array found two copies of chromosomes 1–22 and two copies of chromosome X, for a normal female karyotype (Anderson 2016).
- 46,XY.arr12q24.31(121,332,698-122,486,277) x1dn means that the analysis found the normal number of chromosomes for a male (46,XY), but that on one copy of chromosome 12 at band position 24.31 of the long arm, there was a

deletion (dn) from nucleotide #121,332,698 through nucleotide #122,486,277 (Anderson 2016).

Results may also include a picture of the aCGH analysis and diagrams of the deletions or duplications.

Endocrine examples of disorders detected through microarray technology include Williams syndrome (deletions and duplications) (Henderson et al. 2014), DiGeorge syndrome (deletion) (Henderson et al. 2014), and complex mosaic Turner syndrome (Sdano et al. 2014). Because aCGH technologies are designed to find copy number variations, aCGH analysis does not detect balanced chromosomal abnormalities that do not affect copy number, such as reciprocal translocations, inversions, ring chromosomes, low-level mosaicism, or point mutations (Anderson 2016).

7.14.3.2 Gene Expression Analysis

A detailed description of gene expression analysis or mRNA expression profiling is beyond the scope of this chapter, but an overview as it relates to microarrays is provided here. Gene expression analysis detects the protein product resulting from a gene's activity by analyzing the RNA transcript (message) of DNA rather than a specific DNA sequence. Gene expression analysis is sometimes called functional gene testing because results of gene expression analysis show that a normally functioning gene is making normal protein or that a mutated gene is actively making an abnormal protein or no protein at all. Although there are numerous methods available for measuring mRNA or protein, gene expression microarrays (GEM) using complementary DNA (cDNA) microarray technology make it possible to measure the expression of thousands of genes simultaneously under a variety of conditions (Radha and Rajendiran 2012). Clinical research is now able to predict outcomes by showing gene expression patterns during different developmental and physiological states and in response to experimental interventions (Radha and Rajendiran 2012). The technical process is like aCGH except that RNA is extracted rather than

DNA, and reverse transcription is used to generate cDNA prior to labelling, hybridization, and analysis.

Gene expression analysis research in endocrinology has identified differences in patterns X chromosome gene expression that are associated with the clinical phenotype in Klinefelter syndrome and are responsible for a number of the metabolic abnormalities observed in these patients (Zitzmann et al. 2015).

7.14.3.3 Direct Sequencing

Direct DNA sequencing is the primary molecular method used to detect mutations. Next-generation sequencing (NGS), sometimes referred to as high-throughput sequencing or sequence analysis, determines the order of nucleotide bases in a sample of DNA. NGS technology can be used to sequence a specific gene, whole exomes (all coding regions in the genome), or whole genomes (both coding and non-coding regions of the genome).

NGS is most frequently used to identify a specific mutation at a specific position in a gene when a family member is already affected by a disorder, or when a disorder is suspected for which only a few select mutations are known to be responsible (Kirmani 2014). In these instances, targeted mutation analysis and mutation scanning involves NGS of the exons and introns within one specific gene and can detect mutations scattered throughout the gene (Kirmani 2014).

Whole-exome sequencing (WES) is used when mutations in multiple genes may be involved, whereas whole-genome sequencing (WGS) is used when the genes responsible for the disorder are unknown (Kirmani 2014). Genome sequencing is also used in pharmacogenomic testing to predict an individual's genotype-specific drug responses for commonly used drugs (Harper and Topol 2012).

There are a variety of sequencing technologies available, but the basic process involves preparing a library of DNA, amplifying the DNA segment by polymerase chain reaction (PCR), breaking the amplified DNA into fragments, then sequencing it on a sequencer machine (Buermans and den Dunnen 2014).

Examples of using gene sequencing to diagnose endocrine disorders include *PTPN11* and *SOS1* gene sequencing for Noonan syndrome and *FGFR3* mutational analysis for achondroplasia/hypochondroplasia (Dauber et al. 2013), as well as the identification of numerous gene mutations responsible for idiopathic short stature (Hattori et al. 2017). Clinical investigators have also used whole-exome sequencing to diagnose 3-M syndrome in a patient with a growth disorder previously of unknown origin, as well as finding a new mutation associated with hypergonadotrophic hypogonadism in the same patient (Dauber et al. 2013). For some disorders, a combination of molecular methodologies is required for accurate diagnosis. For example, both deletion/duplication microarray analysis and sequencing of the *VHL* gene is recommended for suspected Von Hippel-Lindau disease (Kirmani 2014).

7.14.3.4 Methylation Analysis

Molecular genetic testing that examines chemical or structural modifications to the DNA affecting gene regulation rather than the DNA sequence itself falls under the umbrella of epigenomic analyses. Much investigation into epigenomic processes such as messenger RNA (mRNA) silencing through microRNAs (miRNAs), chromatin remodelling, and histone modifications is currently confined to research environments (Tapia-Orozco et al. 2017). DNA methylation analysis, however, has moved into the clinical arena in investigations of imprinting disorders, endocrine disrupting chemicals, and cancer screening (Tapia-Orozco et al. 2017; Schenkel et al. 2016). DNA methylation assays require complex DNA pre-treatment steps involving restriction enzymes (REs), bisulfite conversion, and affinity enrichment followed by analysis via microarrays or sequencing (Tapia-Orozco et al. 2017). Of importance are the cytosine-rich areas such as CpG islands where methylation is more likely to occur (see Sect. 7.11 of this chapter).

Researchers have applied methylation analysis to demonstrate the existence of multi-locus methylation defects in imprinted genes in patients with pseudohypoparathyroidism (Rochtus et al. 2016). Others have used a combination of methylation analysis and gene expression analysis to investigate the epigenetic determinants that contribute to the pathogenesis of autoimmune endocrine disorders such as Graves' disease (Cai et al. 2015). An endocrine example of a disorder where methylation analysis has been used as a first-line molecular diagnostic tool is Beckwith–Wiedemann syndrome (BWS) (Lin et al. 2016).

7.14.3.5 Molecular Testing Clinical Examples

Figures 7.5 and 7.6 contain actual de-identified patient results for molecular genetic testing from an endocrine clinic. Author introductory comments precede each figure and allow the reader to apply concepts covered in this chapter to clinical scenarios. Refer to the glossary found at the beginning of this chapter for terminology definitions.

Case 1 The patient result in Figure 7.5 is from a child presenting with severe idiopathic short stature for whom *SHOX* deficiency was part of the differential diagnosis.

The shaded boxes connected by horizontal lines on the report represent the exons in the coding region of the SHOX gene located in the pseudoautosomal region (distal tip) of Xp and Yp.

SHOX is the short stature homeobox gene, a haploinsufficient gene, meaning that normal maternal and paternal alleles must both be present for normal gene expression to occur. Unlike haplosufficient genes, the presence of only one copy of this gene is insufficient for normal gene expression, and deficiency can result in severe short stature and mesomelic bone abnormalities.

Note the limitations of the test listed under the comments section of the report.

A type of molecular test that might address these limitations is called a resequencing array. This is a chip-based sequencing method that looks for point mutations, and small deletions or insertions in the gene. Array-based sequencing may include the entire coding region, gene promoters, and known intronic mutations.

SHO**X**DNA^Dx

Molecular Genetic Assessment for SHOX Deficiency Using Mutation Detection and SNP-Based Detection of Whole Gene Deletions by DHPLC

Genomic DNA is extracted and PCR is used to amplify the SHOX coding exons and selected intragenic markers, SNPs, using custom-designed primers. Heteroduplexes are formed by heating and cooling the PCR-products. These products are then subjected to DHPLC. DHPLC chromatograms from heterozygous mutations, small deletions and small insertions are identified and then confirmed by DNA sequencing (Note that exon 6B is evaluated only by direct DNA sequencing).

Results:

Normal

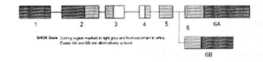

Interpretation:

No SHOX deficiency was detected.

Comments:

SHOX-DNA-Dx detects small mutations and whole gene deletions. SHOX-DNA-Dx does not identify partial SHOX gene deletions or defects in the regulatory elements of the SHOX gene. SHOX-DNA-Dx is also not designed to detect mosaicism of the SHOX gene. If you have any questions concerning SHOX-DNA-Dx or your patient's results, please call the laboratory.

Fig. 7.5 *SHOX* molecular genetic assessment patient result

Molecular Genetic Assessment for MODY3 Using Mutation Detection by DHPLC and Direct Sequencing

Genomic DNA is extracted and PCR is used to amplify the HNF1-a promoter region and coding exons. Heteroduplexes are formed by heating and cooling the PCR products. These products are then subjected to DHPLC. DHPLC chromatograms from heterozygous mutations, small deletions and insertions are identified and then confirmed by DNA sequencing (Note that exons 1, 4 and 7 are evaluated only by direct DNA sequencing).

Results:

| Exon 4: | P291fsinsC = 316X |
| Comprehensive MODY3: | p291fsinsC = 316X |

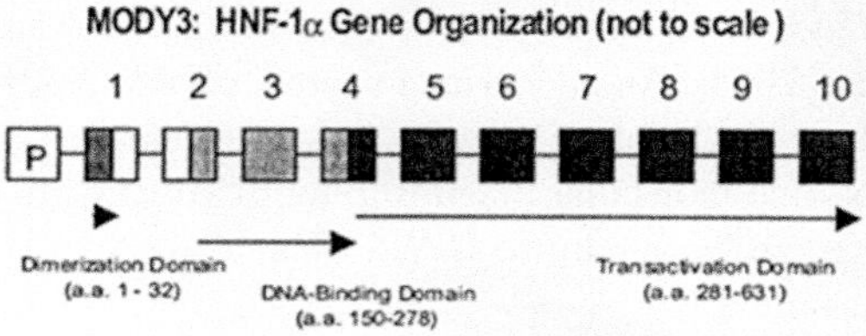

MODY3: HNF-1α Gene Organization (not to scale)

Dimerization Domain (a.a. 1 - 32)
DNA-Binding Domain (a.a. 150-278)
Transactivation Domain (a.a. 281-631)

Interpretation:

Sequencing revealed a nucleotide insertion at position 873. This causes a frameshift which results in a premature stop codon and a truncated protein of 315 amino acids. The patient is heterozygous for the mutation.

Comments:

The mutation (P291fsinsC) has been previously described to co-segregate with the MODY3 phenotype and is likely the cause of your patient's diabetes. (Ellard, S. Hepatocyte Nuclear Factor 1 Alpha (HNF-1a) Mutations in Maturity-Onset Diabetes of the Young. Human Mutation, 16, 377-385). If you have any questions regarding MODY detX or your patient's results, please contact the laboratory.
We strongly recommend genetic counseling as well as testing to identify other affected family members.

Fig. 7.6 MODY3 molecular genetic assessment patient result

Case 2 The patient result in Figure 7.6 is from a an 18 year old presenting with new onset hyperglycemia, polydipsia, polyuria, absence of ketoacidosis, negative antibody testing, and persistently detectable c-peptide.

MODY is maturity-onset diabetes of the young and is inherited through autosomal dominant transmission.

The shaded boxes connected by horizontal lines on the report represent the promotor region and exons of the HNF-1alpha gene on chromosome 12.

7.15 Family History

The family history provides critical data for evaluating an individual's genetic risk for Mendelian or multifactorial disorders. Knowledge of genetic risk promotes frank discussions regarding testing, preventative measures, monitoring, and treatment options if needed (Levy 2013; Owens et al. 2011). Ideally, the family history should include both personal and environmental information for at least 3–4 generations. Personal information refers to gender, current age if living, age and cause of death if deceased, ancestral origin, and all known diagnoses with age at onset. Environmental information refers to the presence or absence of exposure to tobacco, alcohol, recreational drugs, UV or other radiation, toxic chemicals (e.g., lead, asbestos, mercury), or pollutants in the water, air, or soil (e.g., insecticides, radon, smog). Clinicians should encourage patients to discuss their family history with their relatives to increase the accuracy completeness of the data (Levy 2013).

The process of taking a patient's family history is an economically inexpensive diagnostic tool that is often abbreviated in busy clinical settings. There are many templates available to enhance collecting family history data both manually and through an electronic health records (EHR) system. Clinicians with existing EHR systems that do not contain templates or tools for collecting and displaying genetic, personal, and environmental family history data should consult their EHR vendor regarding developing the software changes necessary to provide this resource. The EHR system should be able to organize the family history data into tables and represent it graphically in pedigrees and genograms to enhance patient education (Levy 2013).

An easily accessible publicly available online tool for obtaining a family history is the Surgeon

General's "My Family Health Portrait" (MFHP). Participants in a study evaluating the clinical utility of this tool took an average of 15 min to complete a history, with the longest entry time being 45 min (Owens et al. 2011). Health care providers can use the tool directly within the clinical setting or can instruct patients to complete the tool at home and bring the information with them to clinic. (See Sect. 7.20 at the end of this chapter for the website URL.) Individuals simply go the tool website, click on "create a family history," enter the information, then click "view diagram and chart" (Owens et al. 2011). Once completed, the information can be viewed in a table or as a pedigree.

A pedigree or genogram is like a photographic snapshot of an individual's family health history and genetic relationships expressed graphically through lines and symbols. Using a common set of pedigree lines, symbols, abbreviations, and definitions (a nomenclature) is important so that clinicians can communicate without confusion or inadvertent misinterpretation. The pedigree nomenclature of the National Society of Genetic Counselors is recognized as the international standard for family health histories (Bennett et al. 2008). See Figs. 7.7 and 7.8 for an explanation of pedigree symbols and lines, respectively. An additional set of symbols exist for assisted reproductive technology (Bennett et al. 2008).

Both written family histories and pedigrees can be HIPAA compliant by using initials or first names instead of full names, birth year or age instead of birth date, and year of or age at death instead of date of death (Bennett et al. 2008). Information from family health histories and pedigrees can be used for risk assessment, patient education, treatment planning, health promotion or surveillance, communication between health care professionals, and to enhance communication between patients and their relatives (Bennett et al. 2008). Presymptomatic and susceptibility genetic testing (if indicated by family health history) provide information about increased or decreased disease risk status for the patient, and potential genetic risks for the relatives of that individual (Bennett et al. 2008). Testing options to consider may include expanded genetic panels, full sequencing, or testing for a specific known muta-

tion (Bennett et al. 2008). In addition, genetic testing information and personal/environmental data from family health histories can be entered in evidenced-based algorithms to help guide clinical decisions (Levy 2013).

7.16 Legal/Ethical Issues

Legal and ethical issues related to genetics such as the Genetic Information Non-discrimination Act of 2008 (GINA), patient genetic information stored in electronic medical records, and disclosure of genetic diagnoses are covered elsewhere in this textbook, but additional resources on this topic are listed at the end of this chapter under "Key Reading".

7.17 Nursing Implications

7.17.1 Attitude

Nursing professionals must demonstrate a non-judgmental attitude toward requests for genetic testing. It is critical that nurses at all levels of practice do not inadvertently impose onto families what they might do in similar circumstances. Rather, nurses can impart empathy and compassion by understanding the patient's or parent's point of view.

7.17.2 Disclosure

Genetic testing results should always be given confidentially and in person, never over the telephone or in an impersonal electronic communication. Respect parental wishes regarding disclosure of a genetic diagnosis to a minor child, while encouraging parents to communicate this information to the child at developmentally appropriate levels as the child is growing up. Do not overwhelm families with more information than they can handle at a given time. Provide patient, simple explanations, and never rush, allowing families to digest one concept before moving on to the next. Use analogies to translate complex information and increase comprehension. Educate families to make sure all potential caregivers are present when a diagnosis is discussed so that information isn't passed along 2nd and 3rd hand.

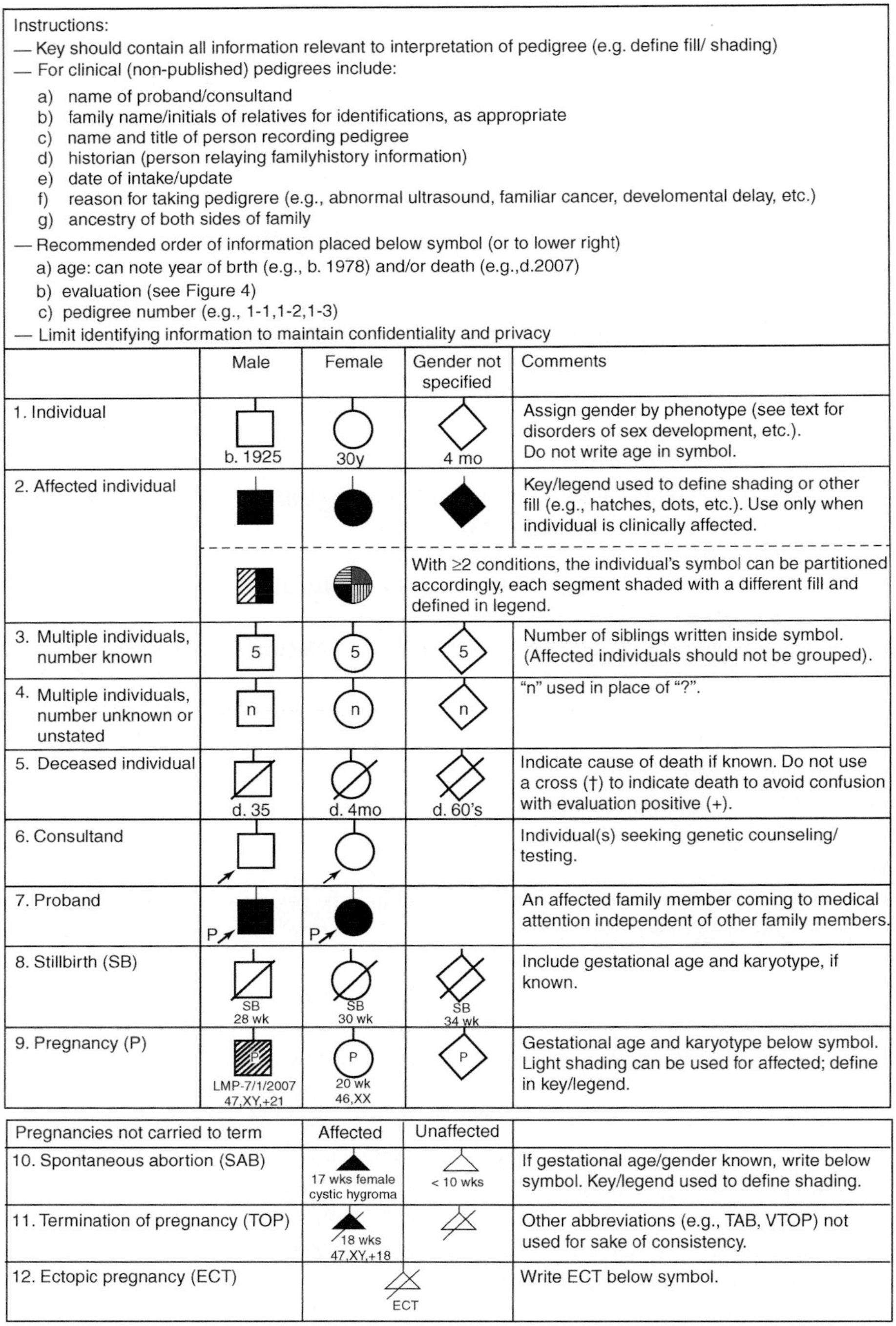

Instructions:
— Key should contain all information relevant to interpretation of pedigree (e.g. define fill/ shading)
— For clinical (non-published) pedigrees include:

   a) name of proband/consultand
   b) family name/initials of relatives for identifications, as appropriate
   c) name and title of person recording pedigree
   d) historian (person relaying familyhistory information)
   e) date of intake/update
   f) reason for taking pedigrere (e.g., abnormal ultrasound, familiar cancer, develomental delay, etc.)
   g) ancestry of both sides of family
— Recommended order of information placed below symbol (or to lower right)
   a) age: can note year of brth (e.g., b. 1978) and/or death (e.g.,d.2007)
   b) evaluation (see Figure 4)
   c) pedigree number (e.g., 1-1,1-2,1-3)
— Limit identifying information to maintain confidentiality and privacy

	Male	Female	Gender not specified	Comments
1. Individual	b. 1925	30y	4 mo	Assign gender by phenotype (see text for disorders of sex development, etc.). Do not write age in symbol.
2. Affected individual				Key/legend used to define shading or other fill (e.g., hatches, dots, etc.). Use only when individual is clinically affected.
				With ≥2 conditions, the individual's symbol can be partitioned accordingly, each segment shaded with a different fill and defined in legend.
3. Multiple individuals, number known	5	5	5	Number of siblings written inside symbol. (Affected individuals should not be grouped).
4. Multiple individuals, number unknown or unstated	n	n	n	"n" used in place of "?".
5. Deceased individual	d. 35	d. 4mo	d. 60's	Indicate cause of death if known. Do not use a cross (†) to indicate death to avoid confusion with evaluation positive (+).
6. Consultand				Individual(s) seeking genetic counseling/ testing.
7. Proband	P	P		An affected family member coming to medical attention independent of other family members.
8. Stillbirth (SB)	SB 28 wk	SB 30 wk	SB 34 wk	Include gestational age and karyotype, if known.
9. Pregnancy (P)	LMP-7/1/2007 47,XY,+21	P 20 wk 46,XX	P	Gestational age and karyotype below symbol. Light shading can be used for affected; define in key/legend.

Pregnancies not carried to term	Affected	Unaffected		
10. Spontaneous abortion (SAB)	17 wks female cystic hygroma	< 10 wks		If gestational age/gender known, write below symbol. Key/legend used to define shading.
11. Termination of pregnancy (TOP)	18 wks 47,XY,+18			Other abbreviations (e.g., TAB, VTOP) not used for sake of consistency.
12. Ectopic pregnancy (ECT)		ECT		Write ECT below symbol.

Fig. 7.7 Pedigree symbols (Reproduced from https://link.springer.com/content/pdf/10.1007%2Fs10897-008-9169-9.pdf)

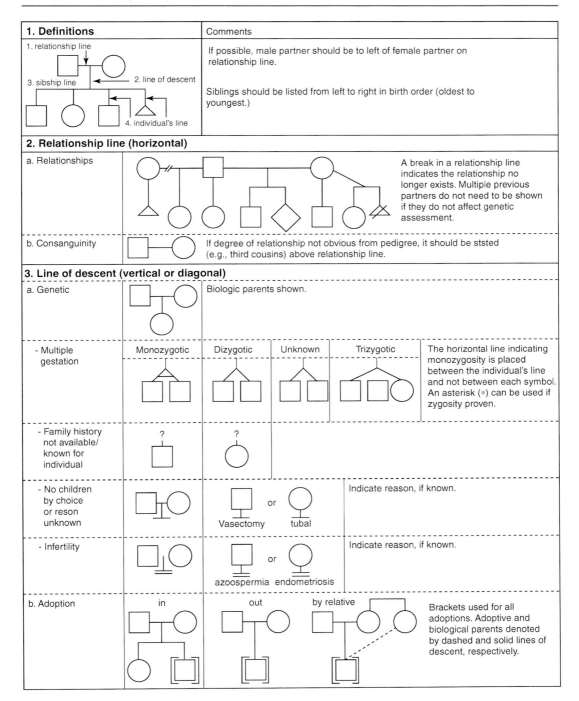

Fig. 7.8 Pedigree line definitions (Reproduced from https://link.springer.com/content/pdf/10.1007%2Fs10897-008-9169-9.pdf)

7.17.3 Care Coordination

Provide anticipatory guidance for comorbidities, and referrals to other specialists as needed, including genetic counselling. Make certain that follow-up appointments are scheduled consistently and kept. Provide information regarding support groups and organizations for families to access as needed. Gently remind families of these resources at successive appointments, realizing that they may not be ready or willing to reach out for help from strangers immediately. Encourage your institution to invest in multidisciplinary clinics that pair endocrinology with other sub-specialists and genetic counsellors. Plan for and initiate pediatric transition to adult care well before it becomes forced at age 18 years. Make sure that transitioning young adults are aware of clinical guidelines for care throughout the lifespan for their disorders, and that they can communicate these to their adult care providers.

7.18 The Future

Evolving issues in genomics affecting endocrinology are not limited to the rapid technological advances in molecular genetics diagnostic testing. Advances in gene therapy research are making the possibility of treating pituitary tumors (Rodriguez et al. 2009) and type I diabetes mellitus (Calne et al. 2010) without surgical or pharmacologic intervention closer to becoming reality. Other endocrine disorders for which gene therapy may become an option include GH deficiency (Racz et al. 2015), hypothalamic diabetes insipidus, and even multifactorial diseases such as type 2 diabetes mellitus and obesity (Yue et al. 2017). Gene therapy is essentially the transfer of genetic material to specific target cells of an individual to prevent or alter a specific disease state. Gene therapy involves the delivery of transgenes through recombinant viral and non-viral vectors. The Key Reading section at the end of the chapter lists additional sources of detailed information regarding viral and non-viral gene therapies.

7.19 Conclusions

While genetics and endocrinology may have begun as unique and separate specialties, they have become intricately interconnected, especially since the turn of the twenty-first century. Advances in molecular genetics laboratory technology have made possible the diagnosis of endocrine disorders resulting from defects in DNA sequence, expression, or regulation. Gene therapy to cure chronic endocrine disorders may become a reality within the next generation. Endocrine nurses at all levels of practice now need to meet competency guidelines in genetics to serve the evolving needs of their patients. Nurses without advanced practice training and qualifications must, at a minimum, be able to provide basic genetics education to patients and their families as related to endocrine diagnoses of genetic origin and their subsequent treatment. Advanced practice nurses must also have enough of an understanding of molecular genetics to order and explain newly available diagnostic testing. Endocrine nurses also need to be aware of ethical and legal issues that may now arise in their practice because of the interconnection of genetics and endocrinology. Such issues include the timing of diagnostic disclosure to minor patients or to individuals outside the immediate family, privacy regulations regarding genetic information contained in electronic health records, and the effects of genetic diagnoses on insurability and employment. Finally, endocrine nurses in the future may become more involved in multidisciplinary clinics where genetics counsellors and clinical geneticists work side by side with endocrine providers to deliver more comprehensive care to endocrine patients.

7.20 Additional Resources

Santos JM, Santos BS, Teixeira L. Interactive clinical pedigree visualization using an open source pedigree drawing engine. In: Kurosu M, editors. Human-computer interaction: eDesign and valuation. HCI 2015, vol. 9169, Lecture notes in computer science. Springer; 2015. https://doi.org/10.1007/978-3-319-20901-2_38. Access can be requested through https://www.

researchgate.net/publication/280446358_Interactive_Clinical_Pedigree_Visualization_Using_an_Open_Source_Pedigree_Drawing_Engine.

7.20.1 Online Software Applications and Tools

1. *List of Medical Analogies*
   www.altoonafp.org/analogies
2. *My Family Health Portrait (MFHP) Tool*
   https://familyhistory.hhs.gov/FHH/html/index.html
3. *American Medical Association Family History Tools*
   https://www.ama-assn.org/delivering-care/collecting-family-history
4. *Cyrillic pedigree drawing software for purchase for professional use*
   http://www.apbenson.com/cyrillic-downloads/
5. *Genealogy and pedigree drawing software for Macintosh*
   http://www.pedigree-draw.com/products.html
6. *CGEN—A clinical GENetics software application*
   http://onlinelibrary.wiley.com/doi/10.1002/humu.21452/full
7. *Create a pedigree*
   http://www.pedigree.varphi.com/cgi-bin/pedigree.cgi
8. *Genogram maker with genogram templates*
   https://www.smartdraw.com/genogram/genogram-maker.htm?id=107977
9. *GenPro Medical Genogram*
   https://www.genopro.com/professions/health-professionals/
10. *f-treeGC*
    A questionnaire-based family tree-creation software for genetic counseling and genome cohort studies
    https://bmcmedgenet.biomedcentral.com/articles/10.1186/s12881-017-0433-4
11. *Progeny Genetics*

Family history, pedigree, risk assessment and EMR clinical tools
http://www.progenygenetics.com/

7.20.2 Online Information on Genetic Concepts

The following online resources are free and publicly available.

1. *GeneEd Genetics, Education, Discovery*
   https://geneed.nlm.nih.gov/topic_sub-topic.php?tid=15&sid=17
   Provides basic education on a variety of topics including DNA, genes, chromosomes, heredity, inheritance patterns, epigenetics, inheritance and the environment, genetic conditions, and more. Provides additional links to animations, videos, articles, games, interactive tutorials, and more.
2. *Genetics Home Reference (GHR)*
   https://ghr.nlm.nih.gov/
   GHR is a guide to understanding genetic conditions, cataloguing more than 1200 health conditions, diseases, and syndrome.
3. *National Human Genome Research Institute (NHGRI)*
   https://www.genome.gov
   The website for the NHGRI, one of the institutes at the National Institutes of Health (NIH), provides current information about news, events, and developments in genomics as well as links to educational information, resources, and research on genetic disorders.
4. *The National Center for Biotechnology Information (NCBI)*
   https://www.ncbi.nlm.nih.gov/
   The NCBI website serves as a gateway to access biomedical and genomic information in scores of databases, including PubMed and all websites in this list with "ncbi" in their URL.
5. *Genes and Disease*
   https://www.ncbi.nlm.nih.gov/books/NBK22183/
   Genes and Disease is an online collection of articles that discuss genes and the diseases

that they cause. These genetic disorders are organized by the parts of the body that they affect. As some diseases affect various body systems, they appear in more than one chapter. With each genetic disorder, the underlying mutation(s) is discussed, along with clinical features and links to key websites.

6. *Genetic Testing Registry (GTR)*

    https://www.ncbi.nlm.nih.gov/gtr/

    The Genetic Testing Registry (GTR®) provides a central location for voluntary submission of genetic test information by commercial test providers. The scope of information provided includes each test's purpose, methodology, validity, evidence of the test's usefulness, and laboratory contacts and credentials.

7. *GeneReviews*

    https://www.ncbi.nlm.nih.gov/books/NBK1116/

    GeneReviews is an online book that serves as an international point-of-care resource for busy clinicians, providing clinically relevant and medically actionable information for inherited conditions in a standardized journal-style format, covering diagnosis, management, and genetic counseling for patients and their families.

8. *MedGen*

    https://www.ncbi.nlm.nih.gov/medgen/

    MedGen is a database on human medical genetics that is searchable by a condition name, the causative gene, a clinical feature, or even an identifier from another database. MedGen also provides links to resources such as genetic tests registered in the NIH Genetic Testing Registry (GTR), information on related genes and disorders with similar clinical features, medical and research literature, practice guidelines, and consumer resources.

9. *NCBI Gene*

    https://www.ncbi.nlm.nih.gov/gene/

    Gene is a database that integrates gene-related information from a wide range of species. A record on a gene may include nomenclature, Reference Sequences (RefSeqs), maps, pathways, variations, phenotypes, and links to genome-, phenotype-, and locus-specific resources worldwide.

10. *Online Mendelian Inheritance in Man (OMIM)*

    www.ncbi.nlm.nih.gov/entrez/query.fcgi?db=OMIM

    OMIM is a comprehensive collection of concise but detailed information on human genes and genetic phenotypes that is updated daily.

7.20.3 Professional Organizations for Nurses Interested in Genetics

1. International Society of Nurses in Genetics (ISONG)

    http://www.isong.org/

2. National Society of Genetic Counselors

    https://www.nsgc.org/

3. Transnational Alliance of Genetic Counselors

    http://igce.med.sc.edu

References

Akbas H, Koksal O, Konca C, Balkan M, Budak T. Familial balanced reciprocal translocation [t(16;22)(p11;q13)mat] in a child with constitutional short stature. J Med Cases. 2012;3(2):149–52. https://doi.org/10.4021/jmc534w.

Anderson S. Chromosome microarray. Am J Matern Child Nurs. 2016;41(5):272–9. https://doi.org/10.1097/NMC.0000000000000260.

Antonacci F, Kidd JM, Marques-Bonet T, Ventura M, Siswara P, Jiang Z, et al. Characterization of six human disease-associated inversion polymorphisms. Hum Mol Genet. 2009;18(14):2555–66. https://doi.org/10.1093/hmg/ddp187.

Asa SL, Mete O. Endocrine pathology: past, present and future. Pathology. 2018;50(1):111–8. https://doi.org/10.1016/j.pathol.2017.09.003.

Baculescu N. The role of androgen receptor activity mediated by the CAG repeat polymorphism in the pathogenesis of PCOS. J Med Life. 2013;6(1):18–25.

Bashamboo A, Bignon-Topalovic J, Rouba H, McElreavey K, Brauner R. A nonsense mutation in the hedgehog receptor CDON associated with pituitary stalk interruption syndrome. J Clin Endocrinol Metab. 2016;101(1):12–5. https://doi.org/10.1210/jc.2015-2995.

Bellfield EJ, Chan J, Durrin S, Lindgren V, Shad Z, Boucher-Berry C. Anterior pituitary aplasia in an infant with ring chromosome 18p deletion. Case Rep Endocrinol. 2016;2016:2853178. https://doi.org/10.1155/2016/2853178.

Bennett RL, French KS, Resta RG, Doyle DL. Standardized human pedigree nomenclature: update and assessment of the recommendations of the National Society of Genetic Counselors. J Genet Couns. 2008;17(5):424–33. https://doi.org/10.1007/s10897-008-9169-9.

Birla S, Aggarwal S, Sharma A, Tandon N. Rare association of acromegaly with left atrial myxoma in Carney's complex due to novel PRKAR1A mutation. Endocrinol Diabetes Metab Case Rep. 2014;2014:140023. https://doi.org/10.1530/EDM-14-0023.

Bochud M. Genetics for clinicians: from candidate genes to whole genome scans (technological advances). Best Pract Res Clin Endocrinol Metab. 2012;26(2):119–32. https://doi.org/10.1016/j.beem.2011.09.001.

Bøe Wolff A, Oftedal B, Johansson S, Bruland O, Løvas K, Meager A, et al. AIRE variations in Addison's disease and autoimmune polyendocrine syndromes (APS): partial gene deletions contribute to APS I. Genes Immun. 2008;9(2):130–6. https://doi.org/10.1038/sj.gene.6364457.

Buermans HP, den Dunnen JT. Next generation sequencing technology: advances and applications. Biochim Biophys Acta. 2014;1842(10):1932–41. https://doi.org/10.1016/j.bbadis.2014.06.015.

Cai TT, Muhali FS, Song RH, Qin Q, Wang X, Shi LF, et al. Genome-wide DNA methylation analysis in Graves' disease. Genomics. 2015;105(4):204–10. https://doi.org/10.1016/j.ygeno.2015.01.001.

Calne RY, Gan SU, Lee KO. Stem cell and gene therapies for diabetes mellitus. Nat Rev Endocrinol. 2010;6(3):173–7. https://doi.org/10.1038/nrendo.2009.276.

Cetin Z, Mendilcioglu I, Yakut S, Berker-Karauzum S, Karaman B, Luleci G. Turner syndrome with iso-chromosome Xq and familial reciprocal transloca-tion t(4;16)(p15.2;p13.1). Balkan J Med Genet. 2011;14(1):57–60. https://doi.org/10.2478/v10034-011-0019-y.

Choi BH, Kim UH, Lee KS, Ko CW. Various endocrine disorders in children with t(13;14)(q10;q10) Robertsonian translocation. Ann Pediatr Endocrinol Metab. 2013;18(3):111–5. https://doi.org/10.6065/apem.2013.18.3.111.

Dauber A, Stoler J, Hechter E, Safer J, Hirschhorn JN. Whole exome sequencing reveals a novel mutation in CUL7 in a patient with an undiagnosed growth disorder. J Pediatr. 2013;162(1):202–204.e1. https://doi.org/10.1016/j.jpeds.2012.07.055.

Fisher DA. A short history of pediatric endocrinology in North America. Pediatr Res. 2004;55(4):716–26. https://doi.org/10.1203/01.PDR.0000113824.18487.9B.

Gagliardi L, Scott HS, Feng J, Torpy DJ. A case of aro-matase deficiency due to a novel CYP19A1 muta-tion. BMC Endocr Disord. 2014;14:16. https://doi.org/10.1186/1472-6823-14-16.

Harper AR, Topol EJ. Pharmacogenomics in clinical practice and drug development. Nat Biotechnol. 2012;30(11):1117–24. https://doi.org/10.1038/nbt.2424.

Hattori A, Katoh-Fukui Y, Nakamura A, Matsubara K, Kamimaki T, Tanaka H, et al. Next generation sequencing-based mutation screening of 86 patients with idiopathic short stature. Endocr J. 2017;64(10):947–54. https://doi.org/10.1507/endocrj.EJ17-0150.

Henderson LB, Applegate CD, Wohler E, Sheridan MB, Hoover-Fong J, Batista DA. The impact of chromosomal microarray on clinical management: a retrospective analysis. Genet Med. 2014;16(9):657–64. https://doi.org/10.1038/gim.2014.18.

Kirmani S. Genetic testing in endocrinology. In: Bandeira F, Gharib H, Golbert A, Griz L, Faria M, editors. Endocrinology and diabetes. New York: Springer; 2014. p. 1–8.

Lania A, Mantovani G, Spada A. G protein mutations in endocrine diseases. Eur J Endocrinol. 2001;145(5):543–59. https://doi.org/10.1530/eje.0.1450543.

Levy HP. Genomic medicine: family history, genetic testing, and the EHR. Intern Med News. 2013;30. https://www.mdedge.com/internalmedicinenews/article/78322/pediatrics/family-history-genetic-testing-and-electronic-health. Accessed 22 Jan 2018.

Lin L, Philibert P, Ferraz-de-Souza B, Kelberman D, Homfray T, Albanese A, Molini V, Sebire NJ, Einaudi S, Conway GS, Hughes IA, Jameson JL, Sultan C, Dattani MT, Achermann JC. Heterozygous missense mutations in steroidogenic factor 1 (SF1/ Ad4BP, NR5A1) are associated with 46,XY disorders of sex development with normal adrenal function. J Clin Endocrinol Metab. 2007;92(3):991–9. https://doi.org/10.1210/jc.2006-1672.

Lin HY, Chuang CK, Tu RY, Fang YY, Su YN, Chen CP, et al. Epigenotype, genotype, and phenotype analysis of patients in Taiwan with Beckwith-Wiedemann syndrome. Mol Genet Metab. 2016;119(1-2):8–13. https://doi.org/10.1016/j.ymgme.2016.07.003.

Marty MS, Carney EW, Rowlands JC. Endocrine disruption: historical perspectives and its impact on the future of toxicology testing. Toxicol Sci. 2011;120(Suppl 1):S93–108. https://doi.org/10.1093/toxsci/kfq329.

Nakashima S, Kato F, Kosho T, Nagasaki K, Kikuchi T, Kagami M, et al. Silver-Russell syndrome without body asymmetry in three patients with duplications of maternally derived chromosome 11p15 involving CDKN1C. J Hum Genet. 2015;60(2):91–5. https://doi.org/10.1038/jhg.2014.100.

National Human Genome Research Institute. Talking glossary of genetic terms. 2014. https://www.genome.gov/glossary/. Accessed Jan 22, 2018.

National Human Genome Research Institute. A brief guide to genomics. 2015. https://www.genome.gov/18016863/a-brief-guide-to-genomics/. Accessed 22 Jan 2018.

National Institute of General Medical Sciences. The new genetics: how genes work. 2016. https://publications.nigms.nih.gov/thenewgenetics/chapter1.html. Accessed 22 Jan 2018.

Owens KM, Marvin ML, Gelehrter TD, Ruffin MT IV, Uhlmann WR. Clinical use of the surgeon general's "My Family Health Portrait" (MFHP) tool: opinions of future health care providers. J Genet Couns. 2011;20(5):510–25. https://doi.org/10.1007/s10897-011-9381-x.

Racz GZ, Zheng C, Goldsmith CM, Baum BJ, Cawley NX. Toward gene therapy for growth hormone deficiency via salivary gland expression of growth hormone. Oral Dis. 2015;21(2):149–55. https://doi.org/10.1111/odi.12217.

Radha R, Rajendiran P. An overview on gene expression analysis. IOSR J Comput Eng. 2012;4(1):31–6. https://doi.org/10.9790/0661-0413136.

Rochtus A, Martin-Trujillo A, Izzi B, Elli F, Garin I, Linglart A, Mantovani G, Perez de Nanclares G, Thiele S, Decallonne B, Van Geet C, Monk D, Freson K. Genome-wide DNA methylation analysis of pseudohypoparathyroidism patients with GNAS imprinting defects. Clin Epigenetics. 2016;8(10). https://doi.org/10.1186/s13148-016-0175-8.

Rodriguez SS, Castro MG, Brown OA, Goya RG, Console GM. Gene therapy for the treatment of pituitary tumors. Expert Rev Endocrinol Metab. 2009;4(4):359–70. https://doi.org/10.1586/eem.09.16.

Schenkel LC, Rodenhiser DI, Ainsworth PJ, Pare G, Sadikovic B. DNA methylation analysis in constitutional disorders: clinical implications of the epigenome. Crit Rev Clin Lab Sci. 2016;53(3):147–65. https://doi.org/10.3109/10408363.2015.1113496.

Sdano MR, Vanzo RJ, Martin MM, Baldwin EE, South ST, Rope AF, Allen WP, Kearney H. Clinical utility of chromosomal microarray analysis of DNA from buccal cells: detection of mosaicism in three patients. J Genet Couns. 2014;23(6):922–7. https://doi.org/10.1007/s10897-014-9751-2.

Sireteanu A, Volosciuc M, Gramescu M, Gorduza E, Vulpoi C, Frunza I, et al. Dicentric chromosome 14;18 plus two additional CNVs in a girl with microform holoprosencephaly and Turner stigmata. Balkan J Med Genet. 2013;16(2):67–72. https://doi.org/10.2478/bjmg-2013-0034.

Stagi S, Lapi E, Pantaleo M, Traficante G, Giglio S, Seminara S, de Martino M. A SOX3 (Xq26.3-27.3) duplication in a boy with growth hormone deficiency, ocular dyspraxia, and intellectual disability: a long-term follow-up and literature review. Hormones (Athens). 2014;13(4):552–60. https://doi.org/10.14310/horm.2002.1523.

Tapia-Orozco N, Santiago-Toledo G, Barron V, Espinosa-Garcia AM, Garcia-Garcia JA, Garcia-Arrazola R. Environmental epigenomics: current approaches to assess epigenetic effects of endocrine disrupting compounds (EDC's) on human health. Environ Toxicol Pharmacol. 2017;51:94–9. https://doi.org/10.1016/j.etap.2017.02.004.

Tonelli F, Giudici F, Giusti F, Marini F, Cianferotti L, Nesi G, Brandi ML. A heterozygous frameshift mutation in exon 1 of CDKN1B gene in a patient affected by MEN4 syndrome. Eur J Endocrinol. 2014;171(2):K7–K17. https://doi.org/10.1530/EJE-14-0080.

U.S. National Library of Medicine, National Institutes of Health. DNA, genes, chromosomes-GeneEd-genetics, education, discovery. 2017. https://geneed.nlm.nih.gov/topic_subtopic.php?tid=15. Accessed 22 Jan 2018.

Vassart G, Costagliola S. G protein-coupled receptors: mutations and endocrine diseases. Nat Rev Endocrinol. 2011;7(6):362–72. https://doi.org/10.1038/nrendo.2011.20.

Wieland I, Schanze D, Schanze I, Volleth M, Muschke P, Zenker M. A cryptic unbalanced translocation der(4) t(4;17)(p16.1;q25.3) identifies Wittwer syndrome as a variant of Wolf-Hirschhorn syndrome. Am J Med Genet Part A. 2014;164A(12):3213–4. https://doi.org/10.1002/ajmg.a.36765.

Yamaguchi R, Kato F, Hasegawa T, Katsumata N, Fukami M, Matsui T, Nagasaki K, Ogata T. A novel homozygous mutation of the nicotinamide nucleotide transhydrogenase gene in a Japanese patient with familial glucocorticoid deficiency. Endocr J. 2013;60(7):855–9. https://doi.org/10.1507/endocrj.EJ13-0024.

Yue J, Gou X, Li Y, Wicksteed B, Wu X. Engineered epidermal progenitor cells can correct diet-induced obesity and diabetes. Cell Stem Cell. 2017;21(2):256–263.e4. https://doi.org/10.1016/j.stem.2017.06.016.

Zitzmann M, Bongers R, Werler S, Bogdanova N, Wistuba J, Kliesch S, Gromoll J, Tüttelmann F. Gene expression patterns in relation to the clinical phenotype in Klinefelter syndrome. J Clin Endocrinol Metab. 2015;100(3):E518–23. https://doi.org/10.1210/jc.2014-2780.

Key Reading

1. Griffiths W, Carroll D. An introduction to genetic analysis. 11th ed. New York: W. H. Freeman; 2015.
2. Kasper CE, Schneidereith TA, Lashley FR. Lashley's essentials of clinical genetics in nursing practice. 2nd ed. New York: Springer; 2016.
3. Strachan T, Read AP. Human molecular genetics. 4th ed. New York: Garland Science; 2010.
4. Goodarzi MO. Genetics of common endocrine disease: the present and the future. J Clin Endocrinol Metab. 2016;101(3):787–94. https://doi.org/10.1210/jc.2015-3640. https://academic.oup.com/jcem/article/101/3/787/2804711.
5. American Nursing Association. Essentials of genetic and genomic nursing: competencies, curricula guidelines, and outcome indicators. 2nd ed; 2009. https://www.genome.gov/pages/careers/healthprofessional-education/geneticscompetency.pdf.
6. Galesic M, Garcia-Retamero R. Using analogies to communicate information about health risks. Appl Cognit Psychol. 2013;27:33–42. https://doi.org/10.1002/acp.2866. https://pdfs.semanticscholar.org/6ad5/41960ed03707c62418bd476b2e901a6b0c1b.pdf.

7. Lough ME, Seidel GD. Legal and clinical issues in genetics and genomics. Clin Nurse Spec. 2015;29(2):68–70. https://doi.org/10.1097/NUR.0000000000000101. https://www.researchgate.net/publication/272079840_Legal_and_Clinical_Issues_in_Genetics_and_Genomics.

8. de Vinck-Baroody O, Weitzman C, Vibbert M, Augustyn M. Disclosure of diagnosis: to tell or not to tell. J Dev Behav Pediatr. 2012;33(5):441–3. https://doi.org/10.1097/DBP.0b013e318258bae6. https://www.researchgate.net/publication/224949987_Disclosure_of_Diagnosis_To_Tell_or_Not_to_Tell.

9. Quigley P. Mapping the human genome: implications for practice. Nursing. 2015;45(9):26–34. https://doi.org/10.1097/01.NURSE.0000470413.71567.fd. https://www.nursingcenter.com/Handlers/articleContent.pdf?key=pdf_00152193-201509000-00008.

10. Zhang X, Ho S-M. Epigenetics meets endocrinology. J Mol Endocrinol. 2011;46(1):R11–32. https://doi.org/10.1677/JME-10-0053. https://www.ncbi.nlm.nih.gov/pmc/articles/PMC4071959/

11. Conley YP, Biesecker LG, Gonsalves S, Merkle CJ, Kirk M, Aouizerat BE. Current and emerging technology approaches in genomics. J Nurs Scholarsh. 2013;45(1):5–14. https://doi.org/10.1111/jnu.12001. http://europepmc.org/articles/PMC3773704.

Congenital Hyperinsulinism (CHI)

8

Claire Gilbert, Kate Morgan, Louise Doodson, and Khalid Hussain

Contents

C. Gilbert (✉) · K. Morgan · L. Doodson
Great Ormond Street Hospital for Children NHS
Trust, London, UK
e-mail: clare.gilbert@gosh.nhs.uk; Kate.morgan@
gosh.nhs.uk; Louise.Doodson@gosh.nhs.uk

K. Hussain
Weill Cornell Medicine-Qatar, Ar-Rayyan, Qatar

Division of Endocrinology, Department of Paediatric
Medicine, Sidra Medicine, OPC, Doha, Qatar
e-mail: khussain@sidra.org

Abstract

The aim of this chapter is to highlight a rare endocrine condition (Congenital Hyperinsulinism, CHI), which can cause low blood glucose levels leading to permanent brain injury. Many Paediatric Nurses are unfamiliar with this condition. CHI is caused by

© Springer Nature Switzerland AG 2019
S. Llahana et al. (eds.), *Advanced Practice in Endocrinology Nursing*,
https://doi.org/10.1007/978-3-319-99817-6_8

unregulated insulin secretion from the pancreas and typically presents in the newborn period, but it can also present later in life. It is imperative for Paediatric Nurses to be knowledgeable on the subject of CHI as they are usually the first to identify the infant's low blood glucose levels, often accompanied by non-specific symptoms such as floppiness, jitteriness, fitting, lethargy, or poor feeding. It is always important to consider CHI if an infant or child presents with unexplained recurrent and persistent hypoglycaemia.

The chapter will focus on understanding how to interpret blood glucose levels, explain the biochemical basis of CHI, provide some background to the genetic causes of CHI, discuss the signs and symptoms of hypoglycaemia and finally, offer guidance for the diagnosis and management of patients with CHI. A case study will be used to illustrate the importance of early identification and prompt treatment.

Keywords
Congenital hyperinsulinism · Brain injury · Insulin · Glucose

Abbreviations

18F-DOPA	Fluorine-18-L-dihydroxyphenylalanine
A&E	Accident and Emergency
ABCC8	ATP Binding Cassette Subfamily C Member 8
ADP	Adenosine diphosphate
ATP	Mitochondrial adenosine triphosphate
b-HOB	Beta-hydroxybutyrate
CHI	Congenital hyperinsulinism
CNS	Clinical Nurse Specialist
CRP	C-reactive protein
EEG	Electroencephalogram
GA	General anaesthetic
GCK	Glu-cokinase
GH	Growth hormone
GLUD1	Glutamate dehydrogenase
G.P	General Practitioner
HADH	Hydroxyacyl-coenzyme A dehydrogenase
HNF1A	Hepatocyte nuclear factor 1A
HNF4A	Hepatocyte nuclear factor 4A
KATP	Mitochondrial adenosine triphosphate-sensitive potassium
KCNJ11	Potassium Voltage-Gated Channel Subfamily J Member 11
Kgs	Kilograms
Kir6.2	Inward rectifying potassium channel
mg/kg/day	Milligram per kilogram per day
mg/kg/min	Milligram per kilogram per minute
mL/kg	Millilitre per kilogram
mLs/kg/day	Millilitres per kilogram per day
mm	Millimetre
mmols/L	Millimoles per Litre
MODY	Maturity onset diabetes of the young
MRI	Magnetic resonance imaging
mTOR	Mechanistic target of rapamycin
mU/L	Milliunits per Litre
NEFA	Non-esterified fatty acids
NHS	National Health Service
nmol/L	Nanomole per litre
PES	Pediatric Endocrine Society
PET	Positron emission tomography
pmol/L	Picomoles per litre
SLC16A1	Solute Carrier Family 16 Member 1
SLE	Systemic lupus erythematosus
SUR 1	Sulfonylurea receptor
μg/L	Micrograms per litre
μmol/L	Micromole per litre

Key Terms
- **Hypoglycaemia screen:** Diagnostic investigation to examine endocrine and metabolic causes of hypoglycaemia.
- **Transient hyperinsulinism:** Usually occurs for a short period post birth. Can occur with or with out associated risk factors.
- **Persistent congenital hyperinsulinism:** Ongoing hypoglycaemia often needing ongo-

ing medical or surgical treatment and can be subdivided into focal or diffuse disease.

- **Focal disease:** A specific area of the pancreas is affected. Focal lesions are usually small, measuring 2–10 mm across.
- **Diffuse disease:** Affects the entire pancreas. It can be inherited in a recessive or dominant manner or can occur sporadically.

Key Points
- If the infant has persistent hypoglycaemia, then the diagnosis of congenital hyperinsulinism (CHI) should be considered.
- Nurses at the bedside should have a low threshold for checking blood glucose level in any infants who are symptomatic of hypoglycaemia.
- Early referral to a specialist CHI centre is important to establish best medical treatment and outcomes.
- A full multidisciplinary team should be in place in order to fully support and guide the family in the treatment needed.

8.1 Introduction

Congenital hyperinsulinism (CHI) is a serious disorder, which, whilst rare, can have lifelong consequences, with severe psychomotor retardation and epilepsy being more common in patients who present in the neonatal period (Menni et al. 2001). The incidence of sporadic forms of CHI is about 1 in 40,000–50,000 with familial forms more common in communities with high consanguinity (Glaser et al. 2000).

CHI is characterized by the presence of insulin in the blood at an inappropriately high level for the concentration of blood glucose (Aynsley-Green et al. 2000). Insulin is a hormone produced by the beta-cells of the pancreas; its purpose is to lower blood glucose levels, facilitating the transport of glucose into the body's cells (Fain 2009). In CHI, the inappropriately

high insulin switches off all alternative fuels for the brain to use (free fatty acids and ketone bodies), hence the risk of brain injury and even death.

There has been much debate over the definition of hypoglycaemia, especially in the neonatal population. This uncertainty has caused confusion in the past as to when to diagnose CHI and how to treat hypoglycaemia. The Pediatric Endocrine Society (PES) considered this gap in evidence-based knowledge and in 2015 convened an expert panel of Paediatric Endocrinologists and Neonatologists. Articles on transitional neonatal hypoglycaemia made recommendations for the diagnosis and management of persistent hypoglycaemia. Stanley et al. (2015) suggests that during the first 24–48 h of life, the normal neonates' blood glucose level is typically lower due to the transitional phase from intrauterine to extra uterine life. This initial period of hypoglycaemia is called transitional neonatal hypoglycaemia and should be managed according to the clinical symptoms and findings at the time. The PES recommends that the focus for the first 24–48 h of life should be on stabilization of glucose levels; however, after this initial transitional period, the physiological and biochemical mechanisms regulate the blood glucose level above 3.5 mmols/L. (Guemes et al. 2016; Thornton et al. 2015) highlights the importance of distinguishing between the normal neonates who may have transitional hypoglycaemia and the infants who have identifiable risk factors for CHI, including those normal neonates whose hypoglycaemia persists beyond 3 days. These neonates need prompt diagnosis and effective treatment to avoid the known serious consequences of hypoglycaemia including seizures and brain injury.

Nurses and midwives by the bedside have the potential to identify these infants with hypoglycaemia and to prevent possible brain injury. If there is any concern that an infant is displaying symptoms such as poor feeding, lethargy, and jitteriness, then a simple blood glucose measurement is essential to identify if the infant is hypoglycaemic. Normal blood glucose values as in Box 8.1.

8.2 Clinical Presentation of CHI

Patients presenting with CHI can have persistent or recurrent hypoglycaemia despite frequent/continuous feeds or intravenous glucose (Kapoor et al. 2009a). Many neonates with CHI typically present at birth though older infants and children can show signs of hypoglycaemia when fasting. As already stated, hypoglycaemic symptoms are often non-specific, but infants are typically lethargic and hypotonic with seizures (Guemes et al. 2016). Parents often describe their infants as "not feeding well, sleepy and jittery". For the nurse by the bedside, a simple blood glucose reading at this time is a powerful tool. Unfortunately, this has been known to be overlooked. Clinical examination may also detect macrosomia, cardiomyopathy, and hepatomegaly, but the absence of these does not exclude CHI.

On taking a clinical history, there are key questions to ask when faced with an infant with CHI, which include the following:

- A thorough neonatal and birth history (looking for risk factors such as prematurity, small size for gestational age, and perinatal stress).
- Length of time for which the infant can fast (is this appropriate for age and weight?).
- Family history of diabetes mellitus (gestational or in any family member).
- Relationship between hypoglycaemic episodes to the timings of feeds or certain foods (e.g. protein or large intakes of glucose).

- In older patients, a potential relationship between hypoglycaemia and exercise. It is important to ask about this.
- Establishing if the infant/child has had any abdominal surgery, e.g. Nissens fundoplication. Again, this may be significant to the diagnosis and the treatment (Bufler et al. 2001).
- Establishing, where appropriate, if hypoglycaemia is only triggered when the infant/child is unwell with an intercurrent illness, as this could be caused by other mechanisms other than CHI.

8.3 Biochemical Basis of CHI

The body maintains blood glucose concentrations within a narrow range, typically 3.5–5.5 mmol/L (Kaufman 2000). In normal physiology, the pancreatic beta-cells are sensitive to the plasma glucose concentration and secrete appropriate amounts of insulin (Hussain 2005). When describing insulin secretion from the pancreatic beta-cell, it is the ATP-sensitive potassium channels (KATP channels) that are thought to play a pivotal role in glucose-stimulated insulin secretion. Figure 8.1 provides an outline of the function of the beta-cell KATP channel.

This channel consists of two proteins, SUR1 and KIR6.2 (encoded by genes *ABCC8* and *KCNJ11*), which are responsible for maintaining the electrical potential of the beta-cell membrane (Inagaki et al. 1995). The KATP channel in the beta-cell is thought to be an "on–off" switch for triggering insulin secretion (Dunne and Petersen 1991). The release of insulin is a result of glucose being metabolized in the beta-cell, and this causes an increase in the intracellular ratio of nucleotides such as ATP/ADP which closes the KATP channel. When the KATP channel is closed, the cell membrane depolarizes, which causes calcium influx via voltage-gated calcium channels, and this is thought to be the stimulus for the release of insulin (insulin exocytosis) into the bloodstream.

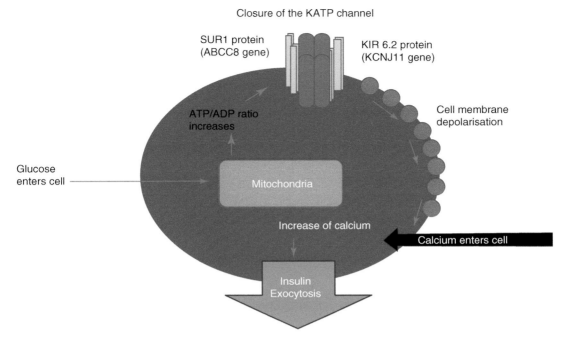

Fig. 8.1 Illustrates the mechanism of insulin secretion when glucose enters the pancreatic beta cell

In CHI, the beta-cells constantly release inappropriate amounts of insulin which is not regulated by the blood glucose level (Aynsley-Green et al. 2000). One of the major causes of this continuous inappropriate insulin production is the "on–off" KATP channel being faulty and permanently in the closed position, resulting in insulin exocytosis. This inappropriate insulin secretion has several effects: it causes glucose to be taken up by insulin-sensitive tissues (such as skeletal muscle, adipose tissue, and the liver); it reduces glucose production in the liver (via glycolysis and gluconeogenesis); and it suppresses fatty acid release and ketone body synthesis (inhibition of lipolysis and ketogenesis) (Kapoor et al. 2009b). This explains the biochemical basis of CHI being hyperinsulinaemic hypoglycaemia, with inappropriately low fatty acids and ketone body formation, hence the increased risk of brain injury (Kapoor et al. 2009b). Simply, this means that the brain is deprived of glucose plus fatty acids and ketone bodies and thus there is a risk of brain injury with this condition.

8.4 Diagnosis of CHI

Persistent hypoglycaemia and an intravenous glucose infusion rate >8 mg/kg/min (normal is 4–6 mg/kg/min) are virtually diagnostic of CHI (Kapoor et al. 2009a). However to confirm the diagnosis, critical blood samples are needed during a controlled hypoglycaemia screen (See Table 8.1) (Steinkrauss et al. 2005). A central venous access device is often the only way to safely administer high concentrations of glucose and to obtain these crucial blood samples. During this hypoglycaemia screen, there are some key factors the nurse must consider.

During the hypoglycaemia screen, the counter-regulatory hormonal response to hypoglycaemia is examined. Glucagon, growth hormone, and cortisol are all endocrine hormones that act against insulin. These hormones all act at various points of glucose metabolism to increase plasma glucose concentration; however, insulin is a glucose lowering hormone. In conclusion, if the hypoglycaemia screen shows that all other causes of hypoglycaemia are ruled out and that the

Table 8.1 Hypoglycaemia Screen

Local practice at a UK tertiary specialist centre when performing a hypoglycaemia screen

1. If the infant has had a general anaesthetic (GA) for a central venous line insertion, then it is important to wait 24 h after the GA to ensure the stress hormones are not raised, thus altering the hypoglycaemia screen results. (This is a practice based on experience in a NHS tertiary hospital.)

2. When weaning the intravenous glucose infusion rate, it is essential to do this slowly to ensure accuracy of the results.

3. All diagnostic bloods (see an example hypoglycaemia screen results) and urine should be taken when the patient is hypoglycaemic <3.0 mmols/L.

4. The laboratory glucose must be a capillary sample. At no time should a true glucose sample be taken from the intravenous line, through which glucose has been administered, as contamination can occur. From clinical experience, capillary samples are always advocated for laboratory glucose samples.

5. Based on clinical practice at an NHS tertiary hospital, the hypoglycaemia screen blood samples are taken when the blood glucose level is <3.0 mmols/L, ensuring the patient is hypoglycaemic for the shortest amount of time possible. Often this means that two nurses are required (one taking the blood samples from the central venous line and the other obtaining the capillary laboratory glucose).

6. Once all the samples are obtained, the hypoglycaemia is corrected by administering. 1 mL/kg 10% glucose bolus and intravenous fluids are recommenced. The blood glucose level is immediately rechecked and checked again after 10 min to ensure the patient is no longer hypoglycaemic.

insulin level is inappropriately raised for the blood glucose level, with corresponding low ketone bodies and fatty acids, then CHI is diagnosed (Aynsley-Green et al. 2000).

8.5 An Example of a Hypoglycaemia Screen

*Plasma glucose 2.0 mmol/L (normal range = 3.5–5.5 mmols/L).
*Insulin 7.5 mU/L (Abnormally raised during hypoglycaemia).
Serum cortisol 450 nmol/L.
Serum glucagon 12 (normal = <50 pmol/L).
Serum GH 1.6 µg/L (normal = 0.9–14.1 µg/L).
Serum ammonia 36 mmol/L (normal = <40 µmol/L).
Plasma lactate 1.3 mmol/L (normal = 0.7–2.1 mmol/L).
*Serum NEFA 0.07 mmol/L (Fatty acids—suppressed).
*Serum b-HOB <0.05 mmol/L (Ketone bodies—suppressed).
Acyl-carnitine profile reported as normal.
Urine organic acids: no abnormality.
*Glucose requirement of 20 mg/kg/min. (Normal = 4–6 mg/kg/min to maintain blood glucose levels above 3.5 mmols/L).
*Indicates results are abnormal.

8.6 Causes of CHI

KAPT channel defects (encoded by genes *ABCC8* and *KCNJ11*) account for the majority of causes of CHI though abnormalities in other genes account for the dysregulation of insulin secretion of approximately 10% of patients with CHI (Nessa et al. 2015). CHI is known to be caused by mutations in certain identified genes (See Table 8.2); however, there is ongoing research to explore other genetic causes.

8.7 Transient CHI

CHI can be subdivided and is distinguished by the length of treatment required and the infant's response to medical management. If CHI is evident for only a short duration and is simply treated with a small dose of diazoxide, then transient CHI is the diagnosis and is usually associated with intrauterine growth retardation, the infants of diabetic mothers, or infants with perinatal asphyxia (Mehta and Hussain 2003). Transient hyperinsulinism can, however, occur in infants with no predisposing factors. Also, some syndromes are also associated with CHI such as Beckwith-Wiedemann syndrome (Munns and Batch 2001).

Table 8.2 Genetics of CHI

Gene	Inheritance
ABCC8/KCNJ11 (Nestorowicz et al. 1996)	*Autosomal recessive* – Diffuse disease, mostly diazoxide unresponsive and often diagnosed within a few days of life *Autosomal dominant* – Often diazoxide unresponsive diffuse disease – Later presentation can be diazoxide responsive plus have family history of type 2 diabetes
GLUD1 (Stanley et al. 1998)	*Autosomal dominant* – Protein (leucine)-sensitive hypoglycaemia which is diazoxide responsive – Asymptomatic hyperammonemia
HADH (Clayton et al. 2001)	*Autosomal recessive* – Diazoxide responsive – In some patients can have abnormal levels of acylcarnitine metabolites present in plasma and urine
GCK (Davis et al. 1999)	*Autosomal dominant* – Can present at any age and variable response to diazoxide
SLC16A1 (Otonkoski et al. 2003)	*Autosomal dominant* – Exercise-induced hyperinsulinaemic hypoglycaemia
HNF4A (Pearson et al. 2007)	*Autosomal dominant* – Patients may go on to develop MODY 1
HNF1A (Stanescu et al. 2012)	*Autosomal dominant* – Diazoxide responsive – May go on to develop MODY 3

8.8 Persistent CHI

Persistent CHI is characterized by ongoing hypoglycaemia, often needing complex medical or surgical treatment. Histological examination of pancreatic tissue from patients who have undergone a pancreatectomy shows that there are two major histological forms of CHI, diffuse, and focal (Rahier et al. 2002). Focal lesions are characterized by beta-cell hyperplasia in a small lesion surrounded by normal pancreatic tissue (See Fig. 8.2).

These small lesions often measure only 2–10 mm and are invisible to the naked eye, though they produce excessive insulin, causing severe hypoglycaemia. Approximately 40–50% of infants with persistent CHI will have the focal form; however, this focal CHI is considered to be sporadic with very low chances of it occurring again in the same family (Ismail et al. 2011). Genetic blood results from the infant and both parents are used to lead the clinician in identifying those patients who need an 18F-DOPA-PET (positron emission tomography) scan to determine if the patient has a focal

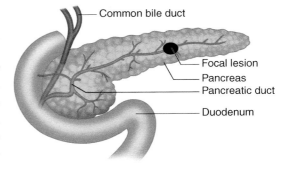

Fig. 8.2 Focal Disease

lesion, and if so, its position in the pancreas (See Fig. 8.3).

Diffuse CHI (See Fig. 8.4) affects the whole of the pancreas and is characterized by beta-cell hypertrophy and hyperplasia of the whole pancreas. Diffuse disease can be familial or sporadic and can result from recessively inherited or dominantly acting mutations (de Lonlay et al. 1997).

If located and completely surgically removed, the focal CHI can be completely cured (Barthlen et al. 2011). However with diffuse CHI, the aim

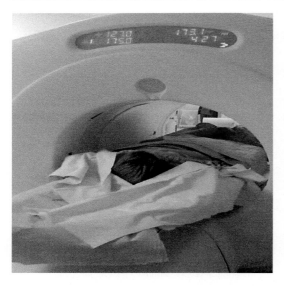

Fig. 8.3 PET scan to localize possible focal lesion

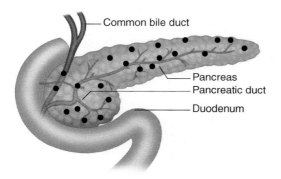

Fig. 8.4 Diffuse disease

of treatment is to medically manage the condition, avoiding surgery if possible, as this could cause the patient to develop diabetes and pancreatic enzyme deficiency in the future. If the patient is unresponsive to all medical therapy, then surgical removal of almost the entire pancreas is occasionally the only option.

8.9 Management of a Patient with CHI

In the acute management phase, high concentrations of intravenous glucose (such as 20% and 30%) are often needed to stabilize the blood glu-

cose levels above 3.5 mmols/L. An intravenous or subcutaneous glucagon infusion is also administered as it releases glycogen stores from the liver (gluconeogenesis and glycogenolysis) (Nessa et al. 2015). A subcutaneous infusion of octreotide (a somatostatin analogue) also inhibits insulin secretion by decreasing insulin gene promoter activity and reducing insulin biosynthesis from pancreatic beta-cells. The aim of this acute treatment is to maintain a safe blood glucose level whilst allowing the infant to establish an oral feeding regimen.

8.10 Medical Therapy

Once the diagnosis of CHI has been established, medical management is trialled. The first-line medication is diazoxide, which needs an intact KATP channel in order for the channels to open and insulin secretion can be inhibited (Aynsley-Green et al. 2000). Diazoxide can cause fluid retention (especially in newborns) and so it must be used with caution, especially in patients who are receiving large volumes of intravenous fluids or oral feeds. There are also a small number of reports that diazoxide can potentially cause pulmonary hypertension and possible cardiopulmonary toxicity (Nebesio et al. 2007). It is recommended that if pulmonary hypertension is identified, then diazoxide should be stopped.

Other medical treatments include subcutaneous octreotide injections four times a day, for patients who show little or no response to oral diazoxide. Long-acting somatostatin analogues such as Lanreotide administered every 28 days are now being used, (see Table 8.3) reducing the intensity of injection therapy of octreotide from four daily subcutaneous injections to one deep subcutaneous injection four weekly.

Lastly, Sirolimus, an immunosuppressant (mTOR inhibitor), has been successfully used in a small number of patients with diffuse CHI who were unresponsive to all previous medical treatments. It is suggested that sirolimus action may affect the number of insulin receptors although the mechanism in treatment of CHI has not been fully delineated (Senniappan et al. 2014). It has been recommended

Table 8.3 Lanreotide

Lanreotide is available in a pre-filled syringe containing 60 mg Lanreotide under the brand name Somatuline® Autogel. It is a white to pale yellow semi-solid gel—a similar texture to petroleum jelly. The starting dose of Lanreotide is often 30 mg but is adjusted according to the child's response to the medicine. The injection is given every 28 days—the aim is that the daily doses of octreotide or diazoxide can be gradually cut down and then stopped.

Before starting Lanreotide injections, a child will need a series of blood tests plus an ultrasound of their liver and gall bladder. During treatment, they will then need to have blood tests along with an ultrasound scan of their gall bladder every 6 months.

Lanreotide is injected into the deep layer of subcutaneous fat under the skin, usually in the upper and outer part of the buttock as there is usually a substantial amount of subcutaneous fat in this area. This also reduces the risk of hitting the sciatic nerve with the injection. One important way to reduce the pain and irritation of injections is to rotate the administration site. Changing injection area also reduces the risk of lipohypertrophy (fatty lump) developing. Whilst this is not dangerous, it will affect how the medicine is absorbed.

It is important that a child is prepared for the injection and distraction therapy can be used whilst the injection is being administered.

Parents and/or Community Children Nurses are trained by the Clinical Nurse Specialists to administer the injection at home, once treatment has been established.

that sirolimus should only be used with caution in CHI specialized centres as adverse events have been reported (Szymanowski et al. 2016). If, after all medical treatment has been trialled, the patient remains unresponsive to medical and dietary interventions, then surgery may be deemed necessary.

8.11 Case Study to Illustrate an Infant's Presentation, Diagnosis, and Treatment for CHI

CT was born at 36 + 4 weeks gestation via a normal vaginal delivery. His birth weight was 2.73 kgs (50th centile). His mother had been treated for the first 12 weeks of pregnancy with oral steroids due to systemic lupus erythematosus (SLE). All her pregnancy scans had been reported as normal and the labour was induced due to her history of SLE. CT's parents were non-consanguineous and were of Filipino origin; he was their first child. At birth, CT was reported to be well and had normal neonatal baby checks. He was discharged after 24 h of birth, but presented in Accident and Emergency (A&E) on day 3 of life with a history of not waking and poor feeding. His mother had been trying to breast feed him but this was not well established and CT received formula top ups from day 2 of life.

On presentation, CT had reportedly had jerky movements over the previous 12–24 h as described by his parents. Seizure activity was witnessed in A&E, which included lip smacking and jerking of all limbs with evident desaturations. A blood glucose level at the time of presentation was 0.4 mmols/L and it was estimated that CT had lost 20% of his body weight since birth. His routine bloods and a blood gas sample were taken and reported as unremarkable. An initial 2 mL/kg bolus of 10% glucose was administered intravenously to correct his hypoglycaemia, which led to a clinical improvement. However, six further seizures were observed and two loading doses of phenobarbitone, one loading dose of phenytoin, and two doses of clonazepam were required to control his seizures. CT was also initially treated for sepsis but his antibiotics were ceased when his CRP was reported as normal as well as microbiologist advice. He was commenced on intravenous fluids containing glucose, though it was noted that whenever his intravenous fluids were interrupted, he would then become hypoglycaemic.

At this time, a referral was made to a tertiary specialist centre and treatment was advised. The initial hypoglycaemia screen showed evidence of CHI as the true glucose was 0.4 mmols/L with corresponding inappropriately raised insulin reported as 86 pmol/L. The protective fuels of fatty acids and ketones were both very low at the time of hypoglycaemia; hence, the diagnosis of CHI was made. All other metabolites were reported as normal. The local hospital reported that CT had abnormal tone but that he had a good suck and was alert on handling. An EEG was reported as normal though an MRI scan showed evidence of cortical necrosis and was sadly grossly abnormal.

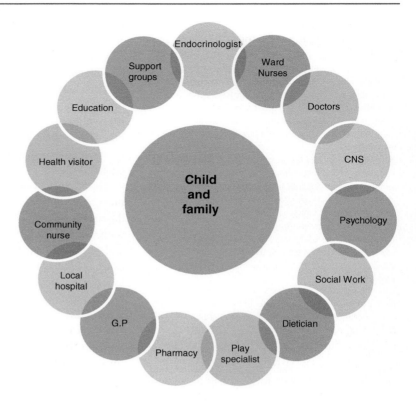

Fig. 8.5 The multidisciplinary team

CT's treatment was to fluid-restrict him to 120 mL/kg/day using a combination of high concentration glucose intravenously via central venous access device and small oral feeds of Aptamil®. On this regime, his blood glucose levels were maintained between 3.6 and 4.8 mmols/L, and his glucose requirement was calculated to be slightly raised at 10 mg/kg/min. On reducing his fluid requirement, this allowed for the safe introduction of diazoxide 5 mg/kg/day with chlorothiazide 7.5 mg/kg/day. Over the next 10 days, CT's intravenous fluids were safely titrated with his oral feeds so that he was eventually on four hourly feeds with no hypoglycaemia, as he was considered to be fully responsive to diazoxide to control his CHI. He was discharged home once his parents were competent in measuring his blood glucose levels pre-feed and in administration of his medications.

After 8 weeks, he was reviewed in the tertiary specialist centre where his dose of diazoxide was calculated to be 2.3 mg/kg/day due to his good weight gain, and there were no hypoglycaemic episodes reported by his parents. It was therefore

decided to admit CT for two nights to reassess his CHI. This was done by safely stopping his medications 3 days prior to admission, then completing a 24 h glucose profile and a 6 h fast off diazoxide and chlorothiazide. The results showed that CT no longer had any hypoglycaemic episodes on his normal feeding regimen and when fasted for 6 h, his blood glucose level no longer dropped and his insulin level remained appropriately low. This means that his CHI had been transient in nature and had successfully resolved after only a short time of treatment with diazoxide. Despite the resolution of the CHI, CT's neurological developmental needed long-term follow-up. A multidisciplinary team approach is essential when caring for children with CHI (See Fig. 8.5).

This case study highlights the importance of early identification and prompt management of CHI, as untreated severe hypoglycaemia can result in severe brain injury and subsequent neurodevelopment handicap. Box 8.2 demonstrates the management pathway from diagnosis to treatment of CHI.

Box 8.2 Management pathway

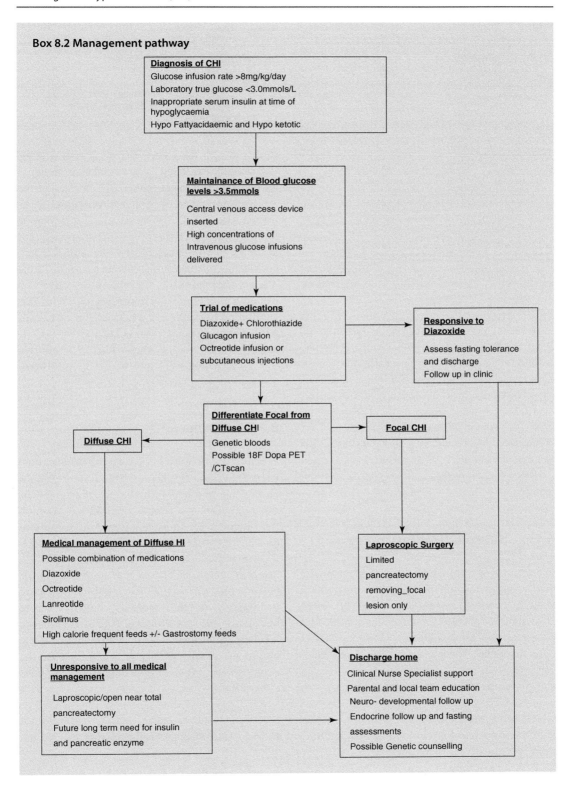

Diagnosis of CHI
Glucose infusion rate >8mg/kg/day
Laboratory true glucose <3.0mmols/L
Inappropriate serum insulin at time of
hypoglycaemia
Hypo Fattyacidaemic and Hypo ketotic

**Maintainance of Blood glucose
levels >3.5mmols**

Central venous access device
inserted
High concentrations of
Intravenous glucose infusions
delivered

Trial of medications
Diazoxide+ Chlorothiazide
Glucagon infusion
Octreotide infusion or
subcutaneous injections

**Responsive to
Diazoxide**

Assess fasting tolerance
and discharge
Follow up in clinic

**Differentiate Focal from
Diffuse CHI**
Genetic bloods
Possible 18F Dopa PET
/CTscan

Focal CHI

Diffuse CHI

Medical management of Diffuse HI
Possible combination of medications
Diazoxide
Octreotide
Lanreotide
Sirolimus
High calorie frequent feeds +/- Gastrostomy feeds

Laproscopic Surgery
Limited
pancreatectomy
removing_focal
lesion only

**Unresponsive to all medical
management**

Laproscopic/open near total
pancreatectomy
Future long term need for insulin
and pancreatic enzyme

Discharge home
Clinical Nurse Specialist support
Parental and local team education
Neuro- developmental follow up
Endocrine follow up and fasting
assessments
Possible Genetic counselling

Table 8.4 Example: hypoglycaemia plan for parents

1. If their blood glucose level is 3.5 mmols or less, re-check after 10 min on an alternative site.
2. If their blood glucose level is still below 3.5 mmols, give one-third of a Glucogel® tube and a small feed.
3. Re-check their blood glucose level 10 min later to ensure their blood glucose level has risen.
4. If they have had a hypo before a feed, give the full feed.
5. If they continue to be hypoglycaemic and do not respond to Glucogel®, please repeat step 2 and call an ambulance to take them to the nearest hospital for management. This may include insertion of an intravenous cannula and intravenous 10% glucose to stabilize their blood glucose levels especially if they are unwell and unable to tolerate feeds.
6. If they present to hospital with a hypoglycaemic episode, they should always be admitted to have their blood glucose levels monitored and corrected with intravenous glucose.

Term infants with no risk factors are often difficult to identify due to non-specific symptoms. Parental education to recognize early symptoms of hypoglycaemia would be recommended, and education plans are drawn up and agreed with families (see Table 8.4) and prompt medical advice should be swiftly sought. Blood glucose levels measurements should be of utmost priority for babies presenting to midwives or A&E nurses with non-specific symptoms such as poor feeding and lethargy.

8.12 Neurological Outcomes

In neonates, the treatment of CHI must be diligently and intensively performed to prevent irreversible brain damage (Hussain et al. 2007). Avatapalle et al. (2013) stated that one-third of patients with CHI developed some form of developmental delay. The degree of brain injury can be variable, with some infants developing seizures and global developmental delay, although some may have very subtle problems with memory, which often manifests itself when the children are of school age. Further studies into the long-term neurological consequence of CHI are needed. The importance of the nursing role in identifying these patients with CHI—leading to a swift diagnosis and implementation of a safe

management plan—cannot be over emphasized. Ultimately, by preventing hypoglycaemia, possible brain injury is also prevented.

8.13 Advances in Treatments for CHI

Research into the causes and treatment of CHI has recently exploded with advances in molecular genetics and medical therapies, including the recent use of Lanreotide and Sirolimus as treatments. The 18F-DOPA-PET imaging technique has revolutionized the diagnostic approach and accuracy of localizing focal CHI, with research continuing to make great advances in this area. The surgical approach to CHI has now advanced to being predominately laparoscopic. With this continuing research and advancement of knowledge, the aim is always to achieve more favourable outcomes for patients with this condition. The far-reaching objective is always to prevent brain injury for this patient group.

8.14 Conclusions

The purpose of this chapter was to briefly illustrate to Paediatric Nurses the importance of monitoring and managing blood glucose levels. Although CHI is a complex endocrine disorder, the outcome for this patient group is continuously improving with evidence-based knowledge and research. The key message is: early detection and treatment is crucial. Nurses at the bedside play a pivotal role in early identification of infants with CHI, and it is vital for them to have a low threshold for checking blood glucose levels in any infant who is symptomatic. If the infant has persistent hypoglycaemia, then the diagnosis of CHI should be considered (Kapoor et al. 2009b).

8.15 Questions to Consider

1. If the bedside blood glucose monitor indicated hypoglycaemia and the hyposcreen results suggested a diagnosis of CHI but the laboratory

glucose was elevated (7.8 mmols), what could this imply?

- Answer—The laboratory glucose is possibly inaccurate as it may have been taken from the intravenous line and contaminated with glucose.
- *Take home message—always take laboratory glucose from a capillary sample, preventing any risk of contamination.*

2. A student nurse has forgotten to inform you that her patient's intravenous glucose infusion is running out and needs changing. What would your actions be?

- Answer—(1) To check blood glucose level, work out how much time you have left before the infusion runs out. (2) Ensure you have an intravenous correction bolus of 1 mL/kg 10% glucose prescribed along with a new bag of fluids. (3) Urgently discuss with medical team appropriate intravenous fluids for the short term as this is an emergency. (4) Do not leave the patient without intravenous glucose and monitor blood glucose levels very closely to prevent hypoglycaemia.

3. What would you do if your central venous access device was to become dislodged and your intravenous glucose infusion was unable to be delivered?

- Check blood glucose levels every 5–10 min.
- Give glucogel in the oral mucosa and assess response.
- Examine the patient and line. If the infant has a central venous device, try to bleed back on this line using Aseptic Non-Touch Technique and flush to check if the line is patent. If the intravenous line is patent, a 1 mL/kg bolus of 10% glucose should be administered. (An emergency prescription of 1 mL/kg 10% glucose should always be written for an infant at risk of hypoglycaemia). A rise in blood glucose level should be seen within 10 min. Always follow the hypo plan in the patient's notes.
- If intravenous access is lost, please have two attempts of peripheral cannulation only. If successful, give 1 mL/kg bolus of 10% glucose to correct hypoglycaemia. Then administer infusion of 10% glucose

maintenance fluids to prevent rebound hypoglycaemia. (Only 10% glucose can be administered safely via a peripheral cannula. For higher concentrations, central access is required).

- In the event cannulation is not promptly obtained, then prescribe and give IM glucagon 1 mg stat dose. This will raise the blood glucose level within 10 min releasing the infants own glycogen stores. However, intravenous access must now be obtained as the infant will become hypoglycaemic once the stores of glycogen are utilized. An anaesthetist should be called to aid in cannulation or for reinsertion of a central line as this is now a clinical emergency.

Acknowledgements *Beki Moult - Health Information & Language Manager*, Great Ormond Street for Children Hospital, Foundation Trust, London, UK. *Dr Maria Guemes—Clinical Fellow—Hyperinsulinism*, Great Ormond Street for Children Hospital, Foundation Trust, London, UK. *Nabilah Begum—Hyperinsulinism Service Coordinator*, Great Ormond Street for Children hospital, Foundation Trust, London UK. *Dr Pratik Shah—Locum Consultant in Paediatric Endocrinology and Honorary Clinical Lecturer*, Great Ormond Street Hospital for Children and UCL Great Ormond Street Institute of Child Health, London. *Dr Ved Bhushan Arya MD PhD—Endocrine Registrar*, Great Ormond Street for Children Hospital, Foundation Trust, London, UK.

References

Avatapalle HB, Banerjee I, Shah S, Pryce M, Nicholson J, Rigby L, Caine L, Didi M, Skae M, Ehtisham S, Patel L, Padidela R, Cosgrove KE, Dunne MJ, Clayton PE. Abnormal neurodevelopmental outcomes are common in children with transient congenital hyperinsulinism. Front Endocrinol. 2013;4(60):1–6.

Aynsley-Green A, Hussain K, Hall J, Saudubray JM, Nihoul-Fekete C, De Lonlay-Debeney P, Brunelle F, Otonkoski T, Thornton P, Lindley KJ. Practical management of hyperinsulinism in infancy. Arch Dis Child Fetal Neonatal Ed. 2000;82:98–107.

Barthlen W, Mohnike W, Mohnike K. Techniques in pediatric surgery: congenital hyperinsulinism. Horm Res Paediatr. 2011;75:304–10.

Bufler P, Ehringhaus C, Koletzko S. Dumping syndrome: a common problem following Nissen fundoplication in young children. Pediatr Surg Int. 2001;7(5):351–5.

Clayton PT, Eaton S, Aynsley-Green A, Edginton M, Hussain K, Krywawych S, Datta V, Malingre HE, Berger R, van den Berg IE. Hyperinsulinism in short-chain L-3-hydroxyacyl-CoA dehydrogenase deficiency reveals the importance of beta-oxidation in insulin secretion. J Clin Invest. 2001;108(3):457–65.

Davis EA, Cuesta-Muñoz A, Raoul M, Buettger C, Sweet I, Moates M, Magnuson MA, Matschinsky FM. Mutants of glucokinase cause hypoglycaemia- and hyperglycaemia syndromes and their analysis illuminates fundamental quantitative concepts of glucose homeostasis. Diabetologia. 1999;42(10):1175–86.

de Lonlay P, Fournet JC, Rahier J, Gross-Morand MS, Poggi-Travert F, Foussier V, Bonnefont JP, Brusset MC, Brunelle F, Robert JJ, Nihoul Fékété C, Saudubray JM, Junien C. Somatic deletion of the imprinted 11p15 region in sporadic persistent hyperinsulinemic hypoglycemia of infancy is specific of focal adenomatous hyperplasia and endorses partial pancreatectomy. J Clin Invest. 1997;100(4):802–7.

Dunne MJ, Petersen OH. Potassium selective ion channels in insulin-secreting cells: physiology, pharmacology and their role in stimulus-secretion coupling. Biochim Biophys Acta. 1991;1071(1):67–82.

Fain JA. Understanding diabetes mellitus and kidney disease. Nephrol Nurs J. 2009;36(5):465–9.

Glaser B, Thornton P, Otonkoski T, Junien C. Genetics of neonatal hyperinsulinism. Arch Dis Child Fetal Neonatal Ed. 2000;82:79–86.

Guemes M, Rahman SA, Hussain K. What is a normal blood glucose? Arch Dis Child. 2016;101(6):569–74.

Hussain K. Congenital hyperinsulinism. Semin Fetal Neonatal Med. 2005;10(4):369–76.

Hussain K, Blankenstein O, de Lonlay P, Christesen HT. Hyperinsulinaemic hypoglycaemia: biochemical basis and the importance of maintaining normoglycaemia during management. Arch Dis Child. 2007;92:568–70.

Inagaki N, Gonoi T, Clement JP, Namba N, Inazawa J, Gonzalez G, Aguilar-Bryan L, Seino S, Bryan J. Reconstitution of IKATP: an inward rectifier subunit plus the sulfonylurea receptor. Science. 1995;270(5239):1166–70.

Ismail D, Smith VV, de Lonlay P, Ribeiro MJ, Rahier J, Blankenstein O, Flanagan SE, Bellanne-Chantelot C, Verkarre V, Aigrain Y, Pierro A, Ellard S, Hussain K. Familial focal congenital hyperinsulinism. J Clin Endocrinol Metab. 2011;96(1):24–8.

Kapoor R, James C, Hussain K. Advances in the diagnosis and management of hyperinsulinemic hypoglycaemia. Nat Clin Pract Endocrinol Metab. 2009a;5(2):101–12.

Kapoor R, Flanagan SE, James C, Shield J, Ellard S, Hussain K. Hyperinsulinaemic hypoglycaemia. Arch Dis Child. 2009b;94:450–7.

Kaufman FR. Role of the continuous glucose monitoring system in pediatric patients. Diabetes Technol Ther. 2000;2(Suppl 1):49–52.

Mehta A, Hussain K. Transient hyperinsulinism associated with macrosomia, hypertrophic obstructive cardiomyopathy, hepatomegaly and nephromegaly. Arch Dis Child. 2003;88(9):822–4.

Menni F, de Lonlay P, Sevin C, Touati G, Peigne C, Barbier V. Neurologic outcomes of 90 neonates and infants with persistent hyperinsulinemic hypoglycaemia. Pediatrics. 2001;107:476–9.

Munns C, Batch J. Hyperinsulinism and Beckwith-Wiedemann syndrome. Arch Dis Child Fetal Neonatal Ed. 2001;84(1):67–9.

Nebesio TD, Hoover WC, Caldwell RL, Nitu ME, Eugster EA. Development of pulmonary hypertension in an infant treated with diazoxide. J Pediatr Endocrinol Metab. 2007;20(8):939–44.

Nessa A, Asim Rahman S, Hussain K. Molecular mechanisms of congenital hyperinsulinism and prospective therapeutic targets. Expert Opin Orphan Drugs. 2015;3(8):1–11.

Nestorowicz A, Wilson BA, Schoor KP, Inoue H, Glaser B, Landau H, Stanley CA, Thornton PS, Clement JP IV, Bryan J, Aguilar-Bryan L, Permutt MA. Mutations in the sulonylurea receptor gene are associated with familial hyperinsulinism in Ashkenazi Jews. Hum Mol Genet. 1996;5(11):1813–22.

Otonkoski T, Kaminen N, Ustinov J, Lapatto R, Meissner T, Mayatepek E, Kere J, Sipilä I. Physical exercise-induced hyperinsulinemic hypoglycemia is an autosomal-dominant trait characterized by abnormal pyruvate-induced insulin release. Diabetes. 2003;52(1):199–204.

Pearson ER, Boj SF, Steele AM, Barrett T, Stals K, Shield JP, Ellard S, Ferrer J, Hattersley AT. Macrosomia and hyperinsulinaemic hypoglycaemia in patients with heterozygous mutations in the HNF4A gene. PLoS Med. 2007;4(4):0760–9.

Rahier J, Guiot Y, Sempoux C. Persistent hyperinsulinaemic hypoglycaemia of infancy: a heterogeneous syndrome unrelated to nesidioblastosis. Arch Dis Child Fetal Neonatal Ed. 2002;82(2):F108–12.

Senniappan S, Alexandrescu S, Tatevian N, Shah P, Arya V, Flanagan S, Ellard S, Rampling D, Ashworth M, Brown RE, Hussain K. Sirolimus therapy in infants with severe hyperinsulinemic hypoglycaemia. N Engl J Med. 2014;370(12):1131–7.

Stanescu DE, Hughes N, Kaplan B, De León DD. Novel presentations of congenital hyperinsulinism due to mutations in the MODY genes: HNF1A and HNF4A. J Clin Endocrinol Metab. 2012;97(10):E2026–30.

Stanley CA, Lieu YK, Hsu BY, Burlina AB, Greenberg CR, Hopwood NJ, Perlman K, Rich BH, Zammarchi E, Poncz M. Hyperinsulinism and hyperammonemia in infants with regulatory mutations of the glutamate dehydrogenase gene. N Engl J Med. 1998;338(19):1352–7.

Stanley CA, Rozance PJ, Thornton PS, De Leon DD, Harris D, Haymond MW, Hussain K, Levitsky LL, Murad MH, Simmons RA, Sperling MA, Weinstein DA, White NH, Wolfsdorf JI. Re-evaluating "transitional neonatal hypoglycemia": mechanism and implications for management. J Pediatr. 2015;166(6):1520–5.

Steinkrauss L, Lipman TH, Hendell CD, Gerdes M, Thornton PS, Stanley CA. Effects of hypoglycemia on developmental outcome in children with congenital hyperinsulinism. J Pediatr Nurs. 2005;20(2):109–18.

Szymanowski M, Estebanez MS, Padidela R, Han B, Mosinska K, Stevens A, Damaj L, Pihan-Le Bars F, Lascouts E, Reynaud R, Ferreira C, Bansept C, de Lonlay P, Saint-Martin C, Dunne MJ, Banerjee I, Arnoux JB. mTOR inhibitors for the treatment of severe congenital hyperinsulinism: perspectives on limited therapeutic success. J Clin Endocrinol Metab. 2016;101(12):4719–29.

Thornton P, Stanley CA, De Leon DD, Harris D, Haymond MW, Hussain K, Levitsky LL, Murad MH, Rozance PJ, Simmons RA, Sperling MA, Weinstein DA, White NH, Wolfsdorf JI. Recommendations from the Pediatric Endocrine Society for evaluation and management of persistent hypoglycemia in neonates, infants, and children. J Pediatr. 2015;167(2):238–45.

Genetic Syndromes Presenting in Childhood Affecting Hypothalamic Function

9

Kathryn Clark

Contents

Abstract

This chapter will focus on two genetic syndromes affecting hypothalamic function that typically present in childhood, Prader-Willi syndrome, and congenital optic nerve hypoplasia.

Prader-Willi syndrome (PWS) is a complex and challenging rare disorder resulting from the absence of gene expression on the paternal chromosome 15q11.2–q13. First described in 1956 as a medical syndrome, the chromosome 15 deletion was discovered in 1981. PWS is a spectrum disorder with a complex phenotype. The universal hallmark is hypotonia with decreased foetal activity noted during pregnancy. Most neonates are born with a lack of suck and respiratory irregularities. They are sleepy and seldom cry. Hypotonia and failure to thrive in infancy evolve into rapid weight gain in early childhood often with insatiable appetite and food seeking; this will lead to profound life-threatening obesity if not well managed at home and in school. Hypothalamic impairments complicate day-to-day life—high pain tolerance, temperature dysregulation, sleepiness, and

K. Clark (✉)
Prader-Willi Syndrome Association (USA),
Sarasota, FL, USA

University of Michigan Hospital,
Ann Arbor, MI, USA
e-mail: kclarkscio@comcast.net

© Springer Nature Switzerland AG 2019
S. Llahana et al. (eds.), *Advanced Practice in Endocrinology Nursing*,
https://doi.org/10.1007/978-3-319-99817-6_9

constant drive to eat. Pituitary deficiencies of growth hormone and GnRH require skilled endocrine care throughout the lifespan. Children with PWS are at risk for respiratory crises from central apnoea and hypotonia with poor ventilatory effort in infancy and aspiration from impaired swallowing motility. Intellectual abilities span a wide spectrum although many children are successful in mainstream classrooms. Unique behavioural patterns including perseveration, skin picking, anxiety, and difficulty with task switching are common. With early diagnosis and intervention, developmental progress, health, and family stress can be significantly improved. Families need diagnosis-specific interventions with specialized medical care throughout the lifespan. Researchers are expanding understanding of PWS. Children born in the past two decades enjoy improved quality of life over previous generations. Treatment remains symptom driven, with no cure for the gene deletion.

Congenital optic nerve hypoplasia is correlated with pituitary dysfunction and developmental brain abnormalities. Nystagmus in infancy should be promptly assessed in the endocrine setting as pituitary deficiencies can include life-threatening hypoglycaemia and shock. Newborn screening programmes designed for congenital hypothyroidism seldom detect thyroid stimulating hormone (TSH) deficiency leaving these babies at high risk of hypothyroidism at the most critical time. Visual impairment ranges from unilateral visual field defects to bilateral complete blindness; pituitary deficiencies can be complete deficiencies of all hormones with prenatal onset, or development of insufficiencies over time. Brain abnormalities noted on magnetic resonance imaging (MRI) have relevance in predicting developmental and intellectual challenges, which occur in a wide spectrum. Endocrine nurses have a critical role in supporting and educating these families, and in helping them understand the unique impact of visual impairment on the child's development and behaviour.

Keywords

Growth hormone · Hypothalamic dysfunction · Hypotonia · Obesity · Optic nerve hypoplasia · Prader-Willi syndrome · Septo optic dysplasia

Abbreviations

ACTH	Adrenocorticotropic hormone
ADH	Antidiuretic hormone
APGAR	Appearance-Pulse-Grimace-Activity-Respiration
BMI	Body mass index
cm	Centimetre
DNA	Deoxyribonucleic acid
FDA	Food and Drug Administration
FISH	Florence in situ hybridization
FPWR	Foundation for Prader-Willi Research
GH	Growth hormone
GnRH	Gonadotropin releasing hormone
hCG	Human chorionic gonadotropin
IGF-1	Insulin like growth factor 1
IPWSO	International Prader-Willi Syndrome Organization
kg	Kilogram
mg	Milligram
MRI	Magnetic resonance imaging
NIH	National Institutes of Health
ONH	Optic nerve hypoplasia
OT	Occupational therapy
PC1	Prohormone convertase
PT	Physical therapy
SOD	Septo optic dysplasia
TSH	Thyroid stimulating hormone
USA	United States of America

Key Terms

- **Uniparental disomy:** This occurs when a person receives two copies of a chromosome from one parent but no copy from the other parent.
- **Genomic imprinting:** Epigenetic phenomenon that causes genes to be expressed in a

parent-of-origin specific way; it is a process of silencing genes through DNA methylation.

- **Food security:** Condition that relates to the availability of a food supply that allows a person to meet their dietary needs in a safe and healthy way. No hope of independent access to food.
- **Oral aversion:** Refers to the avoidance, reluctance or fear/anxiety of eating, drinking, or allowing sensation in or around the mouth.

Key Points

- PWS is a genetic imprinting mutation resulting in a spectrum of diverse medical problems, cognitive effects, and behavioural challenges. Early diagnosis improves outcomes.
- Families require hope, support, and education in raising a medically fragile and complex child with unique medical problems and unusual behaviour patterns. Families with rare conditions can feel isolated and need significant support.
- Food security (no hope of independent access to food) is essential to control troublesome behaviours and preventing life-threatening obesity.
- Children with PWS are at risk in the health care setting because of high pain tolerance and unusual responses to medications including anaesthesia. Providers are often unaware of these unusual morbidities and parents must learn to advocate for their child within the health care system. Printed medical alert booklets are available from international advocacy groups which outline these findings.
- This chapter will describe the physical findings in children born with optic nerve hypoplasia and the pathophysiology associated with the syndrome known as septo optic dysplasia. The spectrum of physical and developmental

challenges will be explained. Visual impairment beginning at birth results in unique learning needs which will be described. Nurses in the endocrine setting should acquire the experience and wisdom needed to help these families.

- The endocrine needs of an individual with this disorder are the same as other types of pituitary and hypothalamic insufficiencies and the reader is encouraged to review those chapters.

9.1 Introduction

This chapter will provide an overview of two genetic syndromes affecting hypothalamic function that typically present in childhood, Prader-Willi syndrome, and congenital optic nerve hypoplasia.

9.2 Prader-Willi Syndrome

9.2.1 Pathophysiology

Chromosome 15 includes a 5–6 Mb gene region in which the maternal gene is silenced and only the paternal region is expressed, one of the few patterns of imprinting in the human genome. In PWS, region 15q11.2–q13 is not active due to random loss (paternal deletion), or maternal disomy with paternal loss (uniparental disomy). An extremely rare inherited imprinting defect has also been identified (Butler et al. 2016b). There are a variety of identified genes in this region, none of which completely explains the complex phenotype. This rare disorder affects males and females equally; estimated incidence is 1:10,000–30,000 live births. Specific testing is required with all subtypes of PWS detected by deoxyribonucleic acid (DNA)-based methylation testing or chromosomal microarray. Inadequate genetic testing (e.g. fluorescence in situ hybridization (FISH)) will not detect all the subtypes and is not the recommended initial test. Further testing for IC micro deletions are also recommended (Butler et al. 2016b). There are consensus guidelines to make this diagnosis using specific weighted clinical criteria when genetic testing is unavailable, but genetic testing is the standard of care.

The mechanisms of hunger in PWS do not follow typical hunger hormonal patterns such as blood sugar and insulin, ghrelin, and leptin. Bariatric surgery does not interrupt the hunger and satiety cycle, and it is not recommended by PWS experts. Bariatric surgery creates significant risks with anaesthesia metabolism, gut motility impairment, impaired pain sensation, and high risk of picking the surgical sites. Of greatest concern is that the individual with PWS will return to the same environment that allowed profound weight gain to occur in the first place—no food security.

9.2.2 Clinical Characteristics

At birth, profound hypotonia generally alerts the medical team to the possible diagnosis. APGAR (Appearance-Pulse-Grimace-Activity-Respiration) scores will be low. Suck and cry may be absent. The baby may not be easily stimulated to fully awaken. Few of these children would survive without a stay in the neonatal intensive care unit (NICU). Early failure to thrive is common and support is needed to ensure weight gain in a sleepy child with poor suck and no sense of hunger. Nasogastric feedings of formula or breast milk may be required to supply adequate nutrition; enrichment may be needed. Most babies progress over a few weeks to an adequate suck, with feeding specialist expertise in selecting a nipple. In some cases, hypotonia, sleepiness, or swallowing abnormalities are so profound that gastric tube feedings are needed to send the baby safely home. Swallowing is often abnormal and presents an aspiration risk.

Babies need hip examinations to look for the common dysplasia seen in PWS, related to hypotonia. Early scoliosis often responds well to bracing or serial casting. A standard back examination for scoliosis screening is inadequate in

this population, due to hypotonia masking curves; a scoliosis series is recommended at age one year, and examination and X rays throughout childhood. Curves progress very quickly in this population and surgery can lead to many unique risks and challenges for those with PWS.

Strabismus is common. Eyeglasses, patching, or surgery are commonly required.

Persons with PWS also have low muscle mass, which reduces metabolic rate, even if hypotonia improves. Facial features are affected by hypotonia; babies may have a longer face, almond-shaped eyes, and a downturned mouth (Butler et al. 2016b; Irizarry et al. 2016). Hypopigmentation is typical but not universal. It is a subtle and appealing phenotype.

Gastric and intestinal motility are erratic, and constipation is very common. Infants have poor suck and swallow, and children have delayed milestones in eating skill attainment. Impairments in swallowing may not improve over time and could explain higher rates of respiratory infections (Gross et al. 2017; Tan and Urquhart 2017). Saliva tends to be thick and sticky, a challenge for swallowing and chewing and impairing dental health.

Hypothalamic impairment contributes to poor temperature control, reduced sensation of pain, reduced respiratory drive, and pituitary dysfunction. GnRH deficiency and gonadal dysfunction are common (Butler et al. 2016b; Irizarry et al. 2016). Most boys with PWS are born with undescended testes and often micro phallus. This indicates prenatal GnRH deficiency. PWS experts recommend 6–10 weeks of human chorionic gonadotropin (hCG) treatment to attempt to stimulate testicular growth and spontaneous descent prior to consider surgery. These testes are often very high in the abdomen and difficult to locate without this stimulatory boost. HCG also prompts a small boost in natural testosterone levels and can improve phallic size and muscular strength. Micro phallus may require testosterone treatment, and while this is not urgent, valuable improved muscle strength is a side benefit of testosterone injections (Angulo et al. 2015; Bakker et al. 2015; Irizarry et al. 2016). There have been no reports of fertility in men with PWS; three births have occurred in women with the syndrome. Female puberty is often incomplete due to GnRH deficiency.

9.2.3 Clinical Management

Prompt treatment with growth hormone (GH) is highly recommended by PWS experts (Butler et al. 2016b; Deal et al. 2013a; Emerick and Vogt 2013; Irizarry et al. 2016). There are myriad studies of the impact of GH beyond physical growth—breathing strength, suck ability, social engagement, learning, and improved milestone attainment. Different protocols are used for deciding when to treat, with some babies treated while still in the NICU. Sleep and breathing issues must be explored, either prior to or shortly after beginning GH. Weight gain must be established for adequate response to GH. Sleep apnoea and tube feedings are not contraindications to beginning GH therapy. GH deficiency is common, but the use of GH is more global, with significant benefits not seen in other GH-deficient populations. Long-term treatment has a lasting impact on body mass index (BMI), strength, cognitive improvements, and energy, in addition to growth (Bakker et al. 2013; Butler et al. 2016b; Deal et al. 2013a; Dykens et al. 2017; Emerick and Vogt 2013; Irizarry et al. 2016). Optimal dosing is not well understood, but many children respond well to lower doses than typical in the GH-deficient population, often with robust IGF-1 responses (Bakker et al. 2013).

Somewhere between ages 1 and 3 years, most children with PWS will begin to become more interested in food. Weight gain increases even without an increase in caloric intake. Meals need to be well regulated, nutrient balanced with a multivitamin, and snacks should be provided on a schedule. Caloric needs are between 60 and 80% of typical children; there is a movement toward lower carbohydrate diets (Emerick and Vogt 2013). Parents need to establish food rules early—adults control the food, which is never provided upon request. This approach builds a solid framework for the future and is known to decrease anxiety in children with PWS, as well as control weight. Spontaneous treats or unexpected changes in dinnertime or what food is being served can lead to emotional breakdowns in these children. For many families, locking cupboards and the refrigerator is the best solution to food security and also diminishes anxiety about available food for the person with PWS.

Hydration can become a problem, as many persons with PWS do not like to drink water. This may be related to swallowing coordination issues (Gross et al. 2017). Constipation may occur, and daily bulking agents are often indicated. Poor sensation of the need to defecate is common.

Children with PWS have a wide variety of educational needs, with some requiring special education throughout the day and others thriving in typical classrooms. One central need is complete food security—no candy from teachers, no surprise cupcake treats for birthdays, no donut sales in the school hallway. Any food events must be well planned to avoid tantrums and behaviour problems. Many children need the assistance of an aide to ensure a smooth day, with routines that cannot always be controlled, but can be managed. During the school day, therapies such as speech, occupational or physical therapy (OT, PT) can be provided. Children with PWS benefit from daily exercise as a part of their education plan, in addition to recess or classroom gym time. As children get older and playtime is eliminated, many children with PWS should continue with a daily exercise plan to benefit both weight and behaviour.

Developmental patterns may be delayed, sometimes through poor muscle tone and the lack of experiences due to sleepiness and decreased activity. Speech may be delayed, and apraxia is not uncommon. Speech therapists are essential team members, not just for communication skills but also to assist with the transition to pureed and table foods.

A small insect bite can become a sore that does not heal for years because people with PWS have an unusual habit of picking at sores, surgical scars, and sometimes the rectum. Open wounds must be kept covered, insect bites avoided, and attention redirected.

The personality style of persons with PWS is often described as charming and loving, with an affectionate nature and desire to please others. The need for routines and a love of repetitive behaviours is common (Whittington and Holland 2010). Tantrums of epic proportion often accompany thwarted expectations or unexpected changes in routines. Since pleasing others and appearing "good" is highly valued by persons with PWS, telling the truth is often difficult. The drive for food is variable, but most individuals will take any opportunity to rapidly eat food, which is suddenly unguarded. Choking, often during a furtive food binge, is a significant cause of early death. Stubbornness is common.

The phenotype of PWS has changed significantly over the past decades due to the action of GH on muscle development and parental empowerment to limit food and optimize development through a variety of therapies. Older individuals with PWS, without exposure to GH in childhood, have short stature, with small hands and feet, and poor muscle development. Excessive fat is often deposited on hips and thighs, even with normal BMI. If the individual has not been prevented from overeating, profound obesity will result with the expected dire medical outcomes including early death.

9.2.4   Clinical Investigations

No single gene has been shown to contain all impaired functions seen in PWS, but identifying the gene for each cluster of problems has been rapidly advancing (Angulo et al. 2015). Prohormone convertase (PC1) deficiency, linked to a critical region in the deleted gene has been identified as the likely source of the major neuroendocrine features of PWS (Burnett et al. 2017). Scientific research and treatment options for any of the many problems in PWS would have potential impact on much larger populations, especially those affecting hunger and obesity.

Given the known hypothalamic dysregulation, oxytocin replacement has promising potential, with decreased oxytocin neurons noted in adults. Preliminary trials in infants (Tauber et al. 2017) demonstrated improved sucking and swallowing and maternal-infant gaze (bonding) after a short course of intranasal oxytocin. Miller et al. (2017) found less robust effect in a 2017 study of older children.

Orexin a (hypocretin 1) is a hypothalamic neuropeptide which is an important regulator of appetite and feeding behaviour, as well wakefulness, gut motility, and pleasure seeking and may be dysfunctional in PWS (Manzardo et al. 2016).

Anxiety can become a more challenging problem than hunger. Typical psychotropic medications may be prescribed but often do not always manage the symptoms. The basis of anxiety in PWS is multifactorial, with hypothalamic factors and gene deletions known to have an impact on anxiety. Other behavioural patterns, such as psychosis risk, skin picking, and repetitive behaviours are targets for research.

Once profound obesity has occurred, survival may be in jeopardy. Caloric needs are extremely low after infancy, and normal diets and lack of food security will lead to profound obesity. Medications are in clinical trials to both decrease hunger and appetite and cause weight loss. The broad utility of these medications would benefit more people than just those with PWS. One promising trial was withdrawn by the manufacturer after two deaths occurred due to thrombotic events. Thrombotic events may be a significant cause of mortality in PWS, rather than a response to a study medication, and data is being collected to better understand this risk.

Behaviours seen in autism overlap much of the behavioural phenotype of PWS. These include repetitive behaviours, repeated questioning, and an insistence on sameness and routines. Language delays such as apraxia may mimic the communication issues seen in autism spectrum disorders (ASD). One study of 146 children found that while many children with PWS have ASD behaviours, only 12% meet diagnostic criteria for ASD. This number is much greater than the current average of 1–2% of the population (Dykens et al. 2017), but it is certainly not universal and did not follow the typical ASD gender as the PWS group were equally female and male. PWS is of interest to autism researchers because of a shared gene mutation, which has been found in some children with autism.

9.2.5 Nursing Assessment

Assess family systems and coping. Post-partum issues such as physical separation of mother and baby or maternal health challenged are immediate priorities.

Expert Quote: Greet the new family with congratulations on the birth of their beautiful child. Admire and praise the baby—this is not just a child with a rare genetic disorder, but an anticipated and beloved new family member. Provide the family with hope before providing education or a treatment plan.

Physical assessment will always focus on growth patterns, weight and length/height, BMI. There are PWS-specific growth charts for children with PWS who are on GH (Butler et al. 2016a). Rate of weight gain is important, with failure to thrive dominating in infancy and rapid fat gain beginning between age 1 and 3 years. Diet should be discussed at each encounter. Obtain specific information about supplements.

Document the genetic subtype and the results of all genetic tests. There are different health risks associated with the two most common subtypes, paternal deletion and mUPD.

Developmental assessment at each visit should include asking parents for positive changes and progression. Assess language skills, receptive and expressive.

Assess whether parents have PWS-specific emergency medical information to share with providers who are unfamiliar with the syndrome. These are available from the PWS advocacy organizations and are available online.

9.2.6 Nursing Care and Management

Children with PWS require a team of specialists for optimal care. Endocrinology, genetics, sleep, orthopaedic surgery, dietician, behaviour/developmental, ophthalmology, and gastroenterology will all be consulted in the first years of life. This is in addition to the therapists—feeding expert, physical therapist, occupational therapist, and speech therapist. Coordination of these visits

relieves a travel and communication burden for families and promotes interdisciplinary care and understanding of this rare disorder.

Advocacy and education are primary roles of the nurse (Vitale 2016). Assist parents by providing the resources, which are available through national and international support groups. If the child is in the NICU, help parents obtain the booklet available at this website: www.pwsausa. org. National and international organizations maintain up-to-date educational materials for professionals and parents. Support groups can offer trained parent mentors and group meetings. Some parents may need repeated encouragement to connect with this invaluable resource.

Early therapies such as OT, feeding specialists, and PT are essential. With poor upper body strength, babies will need help with tummy time and safe positioning in car seats and carriers. Sleepy babies miss opportunities to learn, and parents need help in making choices that optimize brain development. Parents should be encouraged to stimulate development during wakeful times and not let these windows of energy be missed.

Parents must wake the baby for scheduled feedings, as hunger is generally absent for the first year of life. Careful tracking of weight gain is important. Diet management will require a dietician to stay up to date on the unique and emerging dietary approaches to PWS. In the neonatal period, weight gain is essential for brain growth. The transition to oral feedings is often slow and many infants require nasogastric feedings for 3–6 months. Oral feedings should be limited to 20 min to avoid exhausting the baby. Feedings may need to be thickened. Breast milk may require fortification to meet caloric needs.

As children transition to oral feedings, parents may fear obesity and underfeed the child. There will be a wide range of needs, as some children will have significant delays in motor skills and thus require fewer calories than a typical toddler. After age 1 year, 10 kilocalorie/cm/day is a good starting point for most children. There is emerging evidence that a very low carbohydrate diet (45%) can decrease hunger. Many children with PWS require 60% of typical calories in order to manage weight gain. Multivitamins are needed due to the low volume of foods. There is evidence that high quantities of raw foods, such as salads, which was a common approach in the past, may lead to more digestive motility problems. Softer cooked vegetables or soups may help avoid bowel obstructions. Be aware that over the counter supplements are very popular with young parents. These include coenzyme Q10, carnitine, coconut oil, and MCT oil.

Endocrine nurses will already be familiar with GH treatment. These children are most rewarding to treat with significant changes in body composition and muscle tone along with improved growth. Parents see this therapy as life changing and issues of access to care or changes in doses or brands of GH can be significantly more stressful for them than for other patient populations. Nurses should be proactive in prescription renewals and authorizations to avoid stress on the family.

Constipation is almost universal, likely from multiple factors, including poor muscle tone, delayed motor milestones, and intestinal dysmotility. Polyethylene glycol is generally well tolerated and may be needed daily. High-fibre diets or increased raw foods are not recommended due to known risks of bowel obstruction.

When interacting with children who have PWS, thoughtful communication is key. As concrete thinkers, persons with PWS will respond poorly to teasing or figurative speech. Auditory processing is slow; so allow time to answer questions without rushing them. Avoid "thinking out loud"—they will count on the nurse to be consistent and not change the plans. Children with PWS are eager to please; give them a chance to shine. Asking questions about negative behaviours will often be met with anxiety and outright lies. For example, there is no point in asking if someone is following the correct diet if the nurse has determined that weight gain has been excessive. Speak privately with parents when complex issues need discussion.

Genetic diagnoses come with guilt, shame, and blame. Parents and grandparents will need repeated explanations over the years. While the geneticist and genetic counsellor are the experts in explaining the genetic details, families will continue to seek answers from other providers. The genetics visit may have been a time of shock, grief, and exhaustion, so prepare for further questions. Invite extended family members to clinic visits to directly educate them and to help parents by addressing difficult topics with family members.

Expert Quote: Specifically, state that PWS is not caused anything that the parents did or were exposed to, that it does not "run in families" (check first to determine whether the child has the very rare familial imprinting disorder instead of the more common paternal deletion or mUPD). Paternal deletion may be misunderstood to mean that it is the father's "fault"—specifically state that many fathers or mothers interpret the genetic terminology to mean that PWS was because of something defective on their part, but that this is not the case.

To advance the understanding of rare disorders, the National Institutes of Health (NIH) in the USA has developed sophisticated data base platforms for data collection voluntarily provided by parents through an online portal. This international registry is cross-cultural and includes historic data; it will allow researchers to seek participants for clinical trials. Encourage parents to enrol their child in the Global Registry at www.pwsregistry.org.

Connections to the local, national, and international parent support and advocacy groups are a lifeline for parents struggling with a rare diagnosis that includes a potentially frightening future. In 1975, an American parent and professional group was formed (Prader-Willi Syndrome Association (USA)) for the purpose of family support, education, and the advancement of research. The organization continues to provide new parents with peer mentors, local chapters, advocacy, and educational materials for parents and professionals. Professionals interested in the syndrome have benefitted from this and other organizations which supply funding for research. Many countries (UK, Australia) have their own independent organizations with similar websites, with extensive materials for families and professionals. Foundation for Prader-Willi Research

(FPWR) was formed with the goal of finding a cure. Their website provides information for families interesting in joining in clinical trials and reading about breakthroughs in research. International Prader-Willi Syndrome Organization (IPWSO) can help families locate PWS clinicians and parent groups around the world and includes links to the most vital written materials, translated into many languages. This organization also offers free genetic testing for PWS to those families unable to access this in their own country. Nurses should encourage connection to these groups. Internet information can also exhaust a parent who cannot filter out fears and negative thoughts, so also ask whether these groups are helpful or draining, and give permission to parents to take time off from their groups, if needed. IPWSO.org, pwsausa.org, and fpwr. org are excellent resources. These resources are also the most up-to-date source for providers and the nurse should access these as a primary source of information.

Skin picking often starts with an insect bite. Recommend skin protection when outdoors, and covering any small lesion. Distraction and redirection can be helpful; chastising them or punishment can increase the picking through anxiety and stubbornness.

Recognize the patterns of behaviour change, such as repetitive play, repeated questioning, and tantrums. Children who have these challenges benefit from behaviour plans that include understanding of the syndrome. While some families will naturally provide structure and routine, this may be very challenging for other families. Sleepiness and low energy should be addressed as these interfere with learning and social time.

Health supervision guidelines and anticipatory guidance for children with PWS are outlined in the American Academy of Paediatrics 2010 Clinical Report—Health Supervision for Children with PWS (McCandless 2011).

The following resource has specific guidelines for the endocrine specialist (Table 9.1).

Case Study: Prader-Willi Syndrome

With a primiparous mother, reports about poor foetal activity were minimized. Samuel was born at 34-week gestation with Apgar score of 2 and 4. He was admitted to the NICU for poor respiratory effort and failure to suck. He had profound hypotonia with atypical neonate positioning, arms and legs fully extended. He was on a ventilator for 3 weeks and was fed by nasogastric tube with no attempt to suck. On physical examination, he had very low muscle tone, was difficult to arouse; he was blond and pale, different from his dark-haired parents. He had bilaterally undescended testes with the right palpable in the inguinal canal. Phallic size was abnormal at 2.0 cm. Scrotum was small. NICU physicians immediately suspected PWS and sent DNA methylation studies, which confirmed the diagnosis of PWS.

When he was born, the Food and Drug Administration (FDA) in the United States of America (USA) had not yet approved GH for PWS. After contacting the national PWS organization, his parents took him to another academic institution where a pioneer in the care of PWS children assessed him and urged GH therapy. He returned to his home setting and was tested for growth hormone deficiency using standard testing. IGF-1 was low and GH peaks were less than 5 ng/dL. At age 3 months, GH was started at a very low dose, 0.1 mg daily. He was still on oxygen at night and using a nasogastric tube to complete his feedings, beginning to suck and swallow. He did not smile, but made good eye contact and was a cuddly baby, although he slept for about 16 h daily and needed to be woken for therapies and feedings. Parents pursued all early intervention therapies and he was involved in occupational therapy, speech/feeding, and physical therapy. They maintained contact with the local and national support groups for up-to-date information and shared this with his providers.

At age 5 months, he returned to the paediatric endocrine clinic. He was smiling and kicked his legs to show happiness. He had poor head control. The nasogastric tube was gone; he was feeding by mouth, and was awake for at least 10 h per day. Weight gain was excellent and he was growing well. He was no longer on oxygen.

He was given hCG 500 units intramuscular injection twice weekly for 6 weeks with resulting

Table 9.1 Endocrine management of patients with Prader-Willi syndrome (Emerick 2013)

Age	Area to address	Testing/treatment
Birth to 3 months or at diagnosis	Diagnosis	• DNA methylation analysis as initial test
		• Subsequent determination of genetic subtype
	Hypothyroidism	• TSH, FT4
		• Start treatment if hypothyroxinemic
	Growth hormone	• Initiate discussion of hGH therapy
3 months through childhood	Hyperphagia	• Provide education on: nutritional phases, need for food security, strict dietary control and routine, regular physical
		• Nutrition referral
	Cryptorchidism	• Urology referral
		• Consider trial of hCG
	Hypothyroidism	• Annual TSH and FT4 starting at age 1
	Growth hormone	• Consider starting therapy in the first few months of life, or prior to onset of obesity
		• No pre-treatment testing required
		• Starting dose: 0.5 mg/m^2/day with progressive increase to 1 mg/m^2/day
		• Aim to keep IGF-1 levels between +1 and + 2 SDS
	Growth hormone monitoring	Prior to starting therapy:
		1. Otolaryngology referral if there is a history of sleep disordered breathing, snoring, or enlarged tonsils or adenoids are present, with consideration of tonsillectomy and adenoidectomy
		2. Referral to a pulmonologist or sleep clinic
		3. Sleep oximetry in all patients, preferably polysomnographic evaluation
		4. Spine film with orthopaedic referral if significant scoliosis present
		5. Bone age film if at appropriate chronologic age
		6. Consider body composition evaluation (e.g. DXA)
		Contraindications to therapy:
		1. Untreated severe OSA
		2. Uncontrolled diabetes
		3. Severe obesity
		4. Active malignancy
		5. Active psychosis
		While on therapy:
		1. IGF-1 every 6–12 months
		2. Repeat polysomnography within the first 3–6 months of initiating hGH therapy
		3. Spine film and/or orthopaedic assessment if concerns for scoliosis progression
	Adrenal insufficiency	• Consider obtaining cortisol and ACTH levels during acute illness or other stressful situation to clarify diagnosis
		• Consider stress dose steroids for all patients with PWS during stress to include mild upper respiratory infections and the perioperative period

Table 9.1 (continued)

Age	Area to address	Testing/treatment
Puberty through adulthood	Hypogonadism	• Sex steroid therapy as needed to promote normal timing and progression of puberty in males and females • Adult females: sex steroid replacement if oligo/amenorrhoea or low BMD in the setting of a low oestradiol level • Adult males: testosterone replacement as for hypogonadal males. May be behavioural benefits from topical androgen formulations
	Growth hormone	• Adults: evaluate the GH/IGF-1 axis prior to initiating hGH • Adult staring dose: 0.1–0.2 mg/day • Aim to keep IGF-1 0 to +1 SDS
	Diabetes	• Screen prior to initiation of and annually during growth hormone therapy in patients ≥ 12 years of age • Screen in obese individuals as is recommended for the general population
	Obesity	Periodic monitoring of/for: 1. Lipid profiles 2. Hepatic steatosis

complete descent of the right testis. Phallic size increased to normal for 6 months. Strength was improved by parental report. Urology assessed him and scheduled surgery for left orchiopexy, which he tolerated well. Special attention was given to anaesthesia risks and he stayed overnight for this typically outpatient procedure.

Sam continued on growth hormone with normal growth and height throughout childhood. He always had a normal BMI and appeared slender; at times, his parents were urged to increase his calories to improve weight gain. He did not seek food or binge eat. Sam enjoyed obeying the rules and being a "good" boy; he also had a family who kept a very solid routine for Sam and his younger brother, with excellent food security at home.

Kindergarten was delayed due to speech delays and poor motor skills, but when he entered kindergarten, it was in a mainstream classroom, with OT, PT, and speech therapies at the school. He was an excellent reader but required academic support throughout his schooling. Sam developed into a charming happy child, eager to please others, energetic, and very positive—a joy to be around. By high school, he had achieved a black belt in Tae Kwon Do and he finished his Eagle Scout aware by graduation. Scoliosis developed rapidly and he had surgery for rod placement at age 15 years; he recovered easily from this, determined to be as healthy as possible. This surgery

improved his height by 3 in. and his adult height is 173 cm with a weight of 60 kg.

During early adolescence, Sam became aware of his limitations and developed anxiety, which was treated with medications. This anxiety increased in high school, as he considered what his future would hold. He is now attending community college and living with his parents, considering moving to a PWS community in the future.

9.3 Optic Nerve Hypoplasia

When a child is noted to have unusual eye movements, a prompt ophthalmologic evaluation is essential. If small optic discs, consistent with optic nerve hypoplasia (ONH) are noted, an endocrine evaluation and brain magnetic resonance imaging (MRI) are required, regardless of the lack of other symptoms. These children must be promptly evaluated to rule out hypoglycaemia, thyroid deficiency, and adrenocorticotropic hormone (ACTH) or cortisol deficiency, all critically important in the neonatal period. MRI imaging is needed for assessment of the entire brain as well as special attention to the pituitary/hypothalamic/optic chiasm.

Septo optic dysplasia (SOD) is diagnosed when there are two abnormalities in this triad: pituitary/hypothalamic disorders; visual deficits or blindness; and/or abnormalities of brain structures. For example, a child with optic nerve hypoplasia and pituitary deficiencies has SOD, as does the child who has a hypoplastic corpus callosum and optic nerve hypoplasia (ONH), without pituitary deficiencies. The impairments and life challenges in SOD are primarily related to the degree of brain abnormalities rather than the degree of pituitary hypofunction or visual loss.

Visual impairment at birth results in a unique developmental pattern. A multidisciplinary team is needed for optimal development of these children, as well as for support of the parents and family. SOD babies are often first-born children of young mothers, and experience in parenting is often limited. Endocrine care and support is not different in this population from that of other patients who have pituitary deficiencies. However, expert-nursing involvement is essential for parental confidence and competency and for best outcomes for the child with this challenging diagnosis.

9.3.1 Pathophysiology

The connection between underdevelopment of the optic nerves and pituitary function was first made in 1970 (Borchert 2012). For many years, this heterogeneous developmental condition was referred to as "De Morsier's Syndrome" and septo optic dysplasia (SOD), despite the negligible role of the septum pellucidum. SOD now is used to describe the condition when there are at least two of three abnormalities: optic nerve hypoplasia, abnormalities of midline brain structures, and hypothalamic/pituitary dysfunction. Thus, some individuals diagnosed with SOD will not have endocrine disorders, and most do not have abnormalities of the septum pellucidum.

A genetic cause of ONH is found in only a small minority of patients tested (McCabe and Dattani 2014), and it is very rare for families to have more than one child with this disorder (Borchert 2012). Genes responsible for the development of pituitary and optic nerve (Deal et al. 2013b). *HESX1* effects are variable but have been associated with pituitary dysfunction and ONH

(McCabe and Dattani 2014). *Sox 2*, *Sox 3* and *Sox 3* are required for anterior pituitary development. PROP1 stimulates pituitary cell differentiation; TBX19 is involved in ACTH deficiency (McCabe and Dattani 2014).

Risk factors for SOD include young maternal age, primiparous state (Borchert 2012; Garcia-Filion and Borchert 2013), "unhealthy behaviour, and poor pre-conception health" (Garcia-Filion and Borchert 2013). However, there is a dearth of findings of risky behaviours in mothers (Garcia-Filion and Borchert 2013) and no data found on the fathers. First trimester vaginal bleeding has been noted to be more common (Ryabets-Lienhard et al. 2016).

Optic nerve hypoplasia is the second leading cause of blindness in neonates (Borchert 2012; Garcia-Filion and Borchert 2013) and the leading cause of permanent blindness in children in the western world (Ryabets-Lienhard et al. 2016). Incidence around the world has been increasing since the 1980s (Ryabets-Lienhard et al. 2016) with Sweden reporting 17.3 per 100,000 in 2014 and the United Kingdom (UK) reporting 10.9 per 100,000 (Garcia-Filion and Borchert 2013; Ryabets-Lienhard et al. 2016). Lack of central registries and schools for the blind in the USA may be explanations for the somewhat lower incidence of 9.7 per 100,000 (Ryabets-Lienhard et al. 2016).

9.3.1.1 Clinical Characteristics

Optic nerve hypoplasia is expressed with a broad range of visual function, from minor unilateral visual field impairment, to complete bilateral blindness. Actual visual ability is uncertain in infancy, and initial exams cannot predict eventual visual ability. Improvement in vision has been noted in the first years of life in some children (Ryabets-Lienhard et al. 2016).

Nearly 80% of children with bilateral optic nerve hypoplasia will have pituitary dysfunction (Garcia-Filion and Borchert 2013) and developmental delays. Those with unilateral ONS have less risk of developmental delay and pituitary problems (70%) (Borchert 2012; Garcia-Filion and Borchert 2013). Hypothalamic impairment is not uncommon in SOD and is more likely than primary pituitary dysgenesis (Borchert 2012). Hypothalamic impairment can cause temperature dysregulation, abnormal thirst, abnormal hunger, and sleep disturbances.

Brain abnormalities may include absent or hypoplastic corpus callosum, white matter hypoplasia, schizencephaly, and arachnoid cysts. These findings carry a higher probability of impaired cognitive function.

Isolated absence of the corpus callosum is related to significant risk of developmental delay. When seen in combination with pituitary dysfunction and/or optic nerve hypoplasia (SOD), children with abnormalities of the corpus callosum generally face significant developmental challenges. Cortical (brain) abnormalities are prognostic of the greatest challenges, including seizures, motor development delay, and global cognitive impairment (Signorini et al. 2012).

Endocrine abnormalities may not all present at the time of diagnosis, so surveillance is needed during childhood. The most common abnormality in SOD is growth hormone deficiency, seen in 70%. Thyroid secreting hormone (TSH) deficiency is diagnosed in 43%, ACTH deficiency in 27%, and ADH deficiency, diabetes insipidus, 5% (Ryabets-Lienhard et al. 2016; Cemeroglu et al. 2015). Abnormalities of gonadotropin releasing hormone (GnRH) function can also occur, with micro phallus noted at birth and GnRH deficiency, and paradoxically, precocious puberty (Borchert 2012).

The initial endocrine evaluation includes the entire array of pituitary hormones, insulin like growth factor 1 (IGF-1) as proxy for growth hormone (GH), cortisol, free thyroxine and TSH, prolactin, and electrolytes. If the child presents in infancy, gonadotropins and the sex appropriate gonadal hormone (oestradiol or testosterone) should be measured, as these early levels are predictive of gonadotropin releasing hormone (GnRh) deficiency in adolescence (Borchert 2012). In infancy, the danger of hypoglycaemia from cortisol deficiency cannot be overstated. Growth hormone also plays a significant role in homeostasis although the role of GH in linear growth is not significant until the child is 6–9 months old. Treatment guidelines are the same as for any individual with multiple hormone deficiencies; for example, cortisol must be replaced before starting thyroid replacement. Treatment of micro phallus in infancy, once the child is stable, can make toilet training easier, which is not an insignificant challenge.

Sleep issues are significant in the blind population. These children often lack normal sleep patterns, and parents require significant support to handle the challenges of poor or absent sleep. Melatonin may help some children with sleep initiation, but other children and adults may not acquire a true diurnal rhythm; the assistance of a sleep specialist may be essential.

9.3.1.2 Nursing Care and Management

Early intervention for developmental delays is essential. Children with visual impairment will not proceed through the typical patterns of other children (Garcia-Filion and Borchert 2013). They may be fearful of moving, and delay creeping and walking. Motor delays are common (75% of children with SOD) (Borchert 2012). Some are very quiet and watchful babies, as they take in auditory information; they may be overwhelmed by stimulation, responding by crying or by tuning out the world. Well-meaning adults may provide too many musical toys, for example. Close work with occupational (OT) and physical therapy (PT) and vision consultants can help the parents understand their child's unique needs. These babies are especially prone to plagiocephaly, as they resist "tummy time", lacking the visual motivation to lie prone.

Blind children often develop routinized behaviours, called "blindisms", which are self-stimulatory behaviours, such as rocking, head bobbing, hand flapping, and eye tapping. A diagnosis of autism spectrum is found in 33% of children with SOD (Jutley-Neilson et al. 2013). It is more common (57%) in children with near total visual loss, and in 12.5% of those with mild to moderate visual impairment (Garcia-Filion and Borchert 2013). This is a higher rate of autism than in the general blind population (Borchert 2012).

Oral aversion is a common problem in the visually impaired child. They lack the anticipation of a bottle coming near, and do not see others eating at the table; spoon-feeding is a mystery to them, and they may respond with distress. In addition, many of these children lack oral coordination, which can lead to unnecessary upper gastrointestinal evaluations. Instead, intensive OT and speech therapy can assist with the slower progression many of these children need on the path to competent eating. For many children with oral aversion, chronic constipation is also an issue and should be considered part of this cluster of developmental challenges.

Case Study: Optic Nerve Hypoplasia

Maria was born at 41-week gestation at 2720 g 48 cm to a gravida 1- para-1, 17-year-old woman. Prenatal care did not begin until 15-week gestation, but the pregnancy was uneventful. Maria's father was not involved or aware of the pregnancy. Maria's mother was planning to finish high school and had good support from her mother.

The baby demonstrated poor sucking and lethargy in the newborn nursery. Blood glucose level was 45 mg/dL, but she was sent home without concerns. Newborn screening for thyroid levels (TSH) was not abnormal. During the first 2 weeks of her life, mother fed her every 3 h using formula and a premature nipple. Maria was a good sleeper and had to be woken for feedings. At age 2 weeks, she had not gained any weight. She was noted to be slightly jaundiced, but no other abnormalities were noted. Mother expressed concern that Maria did not make eye contact, and that her eyes "looked funny" but this was not observed by her paediatrician.

At her 1-month visit, her yellowish skin colour had not resolved. She had periods of shakiness, and mother continued to worry about her "shaking" eyes. Weight gain and growth had been poor (3000 g, 49 cm); the paediatrician noted nystagmus and referred her to a paediatric ophthalmologist. Mother was encouraged to wake the baby more often and continue 3-h feedings around the clock.

The ophthalmologist diagnosed optic nerve hypoplasia and referred her urgently to a paediatric endocrinologist. An MRI was ordered but was delayed until the hormone evaluation was com-

pleted. At her endocrine visit, cortisol was undetectable, TSH was 0.3 miu/L, free T4 was 0.5 ng/dL, and IGF-1 less than 10 ng/mL. Non-fasting glucose was 55 mg/dL. Liver enzymes were slightly elevated, but all other labs were within normal limitations for her age. Clinical exam was consistent with panhypopituitarism, including small labial folds. Maria's mother had done a remarkable job of keeping her fed and well hydrated.

Maria was diagnosed at age 2 months with ACTH, TSH, and probable GH deficiency. Cortisol replacement began first, followed by thyroid replacement. When she was stable, an MRI of the brain revealed bilateral optic nerve hypoplasia and a thin corpus callosum. Initiation of the hormone replacement resulting in immediate improvement in her wakefulness and eating behaviour. She began to gain weight well and to grow. Glucose level normalized immediately.

The nurse provided education on the complex medications. She assured the mother and grandmother that this disorder has no known cause, and that while feelings of guilt are normal, there is not a known cause or any way to prevent this condition. The nurse followed up with frequent phone contact and made referrals for social services and early intervention services. At each visit, the nurse assessed the baby's developmental progress and pointed out progress typical of a child with a visual impairment.

9.4   Conclusions

PWS is a complex rare genetic disorder. The current generation of children has a different and more hopeful health and behavioural profile than in the past. Researchers are rapidly identifying specific gene actions, which are responsible for the phenotype and medical complications. While targeted treatments are still under investigation, the mainstay of health care for children with PWS is avoidance of obesity, proactive approaches to behaviour problems, and detection and treatment of known medical risks. Intensive early therapies, especially growth hormone treatment, have been instrumental in the development of a very different outcome for the youngest generations with this rare disorder. Parents must learn to become advocates and to educate the providers. They will need ongoing education as new therapies and treatments emerge. Nurses caring for children with this rare disorder need to stay up to date as research is rapidly changing the focus of care and recommended practices.

In addition to the challenges of managing multiple pituitary deficiencies in childhood, children with SOD may have the additional burdens of visual impairment and brain abnormalities. There are challenges in childhood, including motor development, feeding, risk of autism and seizure disorders, sleep disturbances, and uncertainty of cognitive potential. Parents are often young and require guidance and support.

Acknowledgements With special thanks to Kathy Clark, Medical Coordinator for Prader-Willi Syndrome Association (USA), for including information about the Patient Advocacy Groups: Prader-Willi Syndrome Association (USA) (https://www.pwsausa.org), Foundation for Prader-Willi Research (FPWR) (https://www.fpwr.org), and the International Prader-Willi Syndrome Organization (IPWSO) (https://www.ipwso.org).

Web Resources for Families

http://www.onesmallvoicefoundation.org/
http://www.onhconsulting.com/
https://www.familyconnect.org/parentsitehome.aspx
https://www.magicfoundation.org
https://www.chla.org/the-vision-center-ophthalmology
(United States Resource).

References

Angulo MA, Butler MG, Cataletto ME. Prader-Willi syndrome: a review of clinical, genetic, and endocrine findings. J Endocrinol Investig. 2015;38(12):1249–63.

Bakker NE, Kuppens RJ, Siemensma EP, Tummers-de Lind van Wijngaarden RF, Festen DA, Bindels-de Heus GC, Bocca G, Haring DA, Hoorweg-Nijman JJ, Houdijk EC, Jira PE, Lunshof L, Odink RJ, Oostdijk W, Rotteveel J, Schroor EJ, Van Alfen AA, Van Leeuwen M, Van Pinxteren-Nagler E, Van Wieringen H, Vreuls RC, Zwaveling-Soonawala N, de Ridder MA, Hokken-Koelega AC. Eight years of growth

hormone treatment in children with Prader-Willi syndrome: maintaining the positive effects. J Clin Endocrinol Metab. 2013;98(10):4013–22.

Bakker NE, Wolffenbuttel KP, Looijenga LH, Hokken-Koelega AC. Testes in infants with Prader-Willi syndrome: human chorionic gonadotropin treatment, surgery and histology. J Urol. 2015;193(1):291–8.

Borchert M. Reappraisal of the optic nerve hypoplasia syndrome. J Neuroophthalmol. 2012;32(1):58–67. https://doi.org/10.1097/WNO.0b013e31824442b8.

Burnett LC, LeDuc CA, Sulsona CR, Paull D, Rausch R, Eddiry S, Carli JF, Morabito MV, Skowronski AA, Hubner G, Zimmer M, Wang L, Day R, Levy B, Fennoy I, Dubern B, Poitou C, Clement K, Butler MG, Rosenbaum M, Salles JP, Tauber M, Driscoll DJ, Egli D, Leibel RL. Deficiency in prohormone convertase PC1 impairs prohormone processing in Prader-Willi syndrome. J Clin Invest. 2017;127(1):293–305.

Butler MG, Lee J, Cox DM, Manzardo AM, Gold JA, Miller JL, Roof E, Dykens E, Kimonis V, Driscoll DJ. Growth charts for Prader-Willi syndrome during growth hormone treatment. Clin Pediatr (Phila). 2016a;55(10):957–74.

Butler MG, Manzardo AM, Forster JL. Prader-Willi syndrome: clinical genetics and diagnostic aspects with treatment approaches. Curr Pediatr Rev. 2016b;12(2):136–66.

Cemeroglu AP, Coulas T, Kleis L. Spectrum of clinical presentations andendocrinological findings of patients with septo-optic dysplasia: a retrospective study. J Pediatr Endocrinol Metab. 2015;28(9–10):1057–63.

Deal CL, Tony M, Höybye C, Allen DB, Tauber M, Christiansen JS. 2011 Growth Hormone in Prader-Willi Syndrome Clinical Care Guidelines Workshop Participants. Growth Hormone Research Society workshop summary: consensus guidelines for recombinant human growth hormone therapy in Prader-Willi syndrome. J Clin Endocrinol Metab. 2013a;98(6):E1072–87.

Deal C, Hasselmann C, Pfäffle RW, Zimmermann AG, Quigley CA, Child CJ, Shavrikova EP, Cutler GB Jr, Blum WF. Associations between pituitary imaging abnormalities and clinical and biochemical phenotypes in children with congenital growthhormone deficiency: data from an International Observational Study. Horm Res Paediatr. 2013b;79(5):283–92.

Dykens EM, Roof E, Hunt-Hawkins H. Cognitive and adaptive advantages of growth hormone treatment in children with Prader-Willi syndrome. J Child Psychol Psychiatry. 2017;58(1):64–74.

Emerick JE, Vogt KS. Endocrine manifestations and management of Prader-Willi syndrome. Int J Pediatr Endocrinol. 2013;2013(1):14.

Garcia-Filion P, Borchert M. Optic nerve hypoplasia syndrome: a review of theepidemiology and clinical associations. Curr Treat Options Neurol. 2013;15(1):78–89.

Gross RD, Gisser R, Cherpes G, Hartman K, Maheshwary R. Subclinical dysphagia in persons with Prader-Willi syndrome. Am J Med Genet A. 2017;173(2):384–94.

Irizarry KA, Miller M, Freemark M, Haqq AM. Prader Willi syndrome: genetics, metabolomics, hormonal function, and new approaches to therapy. Adv Pediatr Infect Dis. 2016;63(1):47–77.

Jutley-Neilson J, Harris G, Kirk J. The identification and measurement of autistic features in children with septo-optic dysplasia, optic nerve hypoplasia and isolated hypopituitarism. Res Dev Disabil. 2013;34(12):4310–8.

Manzardo AM, Johnson L, Miller JL, Driscoll DJ, Butler MG. Higher plasma orexin a levels in children with Prader-Willi syndrome compared with healthy unrelated sibling controls. Am J Med Genet A. 2016;170(9):2328–33.

McCabe MJ, Dattani MT. Genetic aspects of hypothalamic and pituitary gland development. Handb Clin Neurol. 2014;124:3–15.

McCandless SE. Committee on Genetics. Clinical report—health supervision for children with Prader-Willi syndrome. Pediatrics. 2011;127(1):195–204.

Miller JL, Tamura R, Butler MG, Kimonis V, Sulsona C, Gold JA, Driscoll DJ. Oxytocin treatment in children with Prader-Willi syndrome: a double-blind, placebo-controlled, crossover study. Am J Med Genet A. 2017;173(5):1243–50.

Ryabets-Lienhard A, Stewart C, Borchert M, Geffner ME. The optic nerve hypoplasia spectrum: review of the literature and clinical guidelines. Adv Pediatr Infect Dis. 2016;63(1):127–46.

Signorini SG, Decio A, Fedeli C, Luparia A, Antonini M, Bertone C, Misefari W, Ruberto G, Bianchi PE, Balottin U. Septo-optic dysplasia in childhood: the neurological, cognitive and neuro-ophthalmological perspective. Dev Med Child Neurol. 2012;54(11):1018–24.

Tan HL, Urquhart DS. Respiratory complications in children with Prader-Willi syndrome. Paediatr Respir Rev. 2017;22:52–9.

Tauber M, Boulanouar K, Diene G, Çabal-Berthoumieu S, Ehlinger V, Fichaux-Bourin P, Molinas C, Faye S, Valette M, Pourrinet J, Cessans C, Viaux-Sauvelon S, Bascoul C, Guedeney A, Delhanty P, Geenen V, Martens H, Muscatelli F, Cohen D, Consoli A, Payoux P, Arnaud C, Salles JP. The use of oxytocin to improve feeding and social skills in infants with Prader-Willi syndrome. Pediatrics. 2017;139(2).

Vitale SA. Parent recommendations for family functioning with Prader-Willi syndrome: a rare genetic cause of childhood obesity. J Pediatr Nurs. 2016;31(1):47–54.

Whittington J, Holland A. Neurobehavioral phenotype in Prader-Willi syndrome. Am J Med Genet C Semin Med Genet. 2010;154C(4):438–47.

Key Reading

1. Irizarry KA, Miller M, Freemark M, Haqq AM. Prader-Willi syndrome: genetics, metabolomics, hormonal function, and new approaches to therapy. Adv Pediatr. 2016;63(1):47–77.
2. Emerick JE, Vogt KS. Endocrine manifestations and management of Prader-Willi syndrome. Int J Pediatr Endocrinol. 2013;2013(1):14.
3. McCandless SE. Committee on Genetics. Clinical report—health supervision for children with Prader-Willi syndrome. Pediatrics. 2011;127(1):195–204.
4. Borchert M. Reappraisal of the optic nerve hypoplasia syndrome. J Neuroophthalmol. 2012;32(1):58–67.
5. Garcia-Filion P, Borchert M. Optic nerve hypoplasia syndrome: a review of the epidemiology and clinical associations. Curr Treat Options Neurol. 2013;15(1):78–89.
6. Ryabets-Lienhard A, Stewart C, Borchert M, Geffner ME. The optic nerve hypoplasia spectrum: review of the literature and clinical guidelines. Adv Pediatr. 2016;63(1):127–46.

Genetic Syndromes Presenting in Childhood Affecting Gonadotropin Function

Sharron Close, Ana Claudia Latronico, and Marina Cunha-Silva

Contents

S. Close (✉)
Emory School of Medicine, Emory University School of Nursing, The eXtraordinarY Clinic at Emory, Atlanta, GA, USA
e-mail: sharron.m.close@emory.edu

A. C. Latronico · M. Cunha-Silva
Unidade de Endocrinologia do Desenvolvimento de Hormônios e Genética Molecular LIM42, Disciplina de Endocrinologia e Metabologia do Hospital das Clínicas da Faculdade de Medicina da Universidade de São Paulo, Brazil, São Paulo, Brazil

Abstract

This chapter will focus on two genetic syndromes affecting gonadotropin function that typically present in childhood, Klinefelter syndrome, and testotoxicosis.

Klinefelter syndrome (47,XXY) is the most common sex chromosome aneuploidy with a prevalence of 1 in 450–500 male births. Unless detected by prenatal screening or prenatal diagnosis, this chromosome variation diagnosis is frequently missed in children. Physical, neurocognitive, and psychosocial phenotypes of boys with 47,XXY

© Springer Nature Switzerland AG 2019
S. Llahana et al. (eds.), *Advanced Practice in Endocrinology Nursing*,
https://doi.org/10.1007/978-3-319-99817-6_10

are extremely variable, making a typical case difficult to characterize. Health care needs of boys born with 47,XXY are complex including the need for monitoring growth, pubertal development, optimization of reproductive capacity, bone health, and acknowledgement of physical symptoms such as fatigue, hypotonic muscle strength, tremors, tics, and pain. Physical health risks associated with 47,XXY include: metabolic syndrome, Type II diabetes, cardiovascular disease, immunological issues, bone loss, and certain types of malignancies. Boys with 47,XXY frequently show executive function issues, language-based learning difficulties, problems with communication, and struggles with behavior that contribute to stressors for the boys as well as for their families. Psychosocial manifestations of these stressors include low self-esteem, increased risk for depression, difficulties maintaining personal relationships, and adverse quality of life. There is a general lack of awareness in the health care community about the complexities of care required for families who have sons with 47,XXY. Since puberty is a sentinel time for diagnosing and monitoring hypogonadism, families often depend on professionals in the specialty of endocrinology to address their many concerns. Families seeking anticipatory guidance about how 47,XXY will influence the growth and development of their sons often look to the specialty of endocrinology to help them navigate a health care environment that is confusing to them. This chapter will describe the physical, neurocognitive, and psychosocial phenotype of 47,XXY in childhood and provide suggestions for endocrine-related health surveillance for advanced practice nurses (APRN). APRNs in endocrinology practice are perfectly positioned to assess, coordinate, and provide family-centered navigation for health surveillance according to child's level of development.

Testotoxicosis or familial male-limited precocious puberty is a rare dominant form of gonadotropin-independent precocious puberty caused by constitutively activating mutations of the luteinizing hormone receptor. Affected males present premature and progressive virilization associated with accelerated growth and advanced bone age between 2 and 4 years of age. Hormonal profile is characterized by elevated testosterone levels, despite prepubertal levels of luteinizing hormone. Treatment typically consists of reducing hyperandrogenism with ketoconazole or a combination of antiandrogens and aromatase inhibitors.

Keywords

Klinefelter syndrome · 47,XXY
Sex chromosome aneuploidy · Phenotype
Androgen deficiency · Puberty · Receptor
Mutations · Virilization

Abbreviations

APN	Advanced Practice Nurse
BA	Bone age
c-AMP	cyclic adenosine monophosphate
cm	Centimeter
FSH	Follicle stimulating hormone
GnRH	Gonadotropin releasing hormone
G-protein	Guanine-protein
hCG	Human chorionic gonadotropin
IU/L	International unit/Liter
kg	Kilogram
KS	Klinefelter syndrome
LH	Luteinizing hormone
LHCGR	Luteinizing hormone receptor gene
mg	Milligram
ng/dL	Nanogram/deciliter
SD	Standard deviation

Key Terms

- **Sex chromosome aneuploidy:** Chromosomal disorder characterized by the loss or gain of one or more of the sex chromosomes.
- **Hypergonadotropic hypogonadism:** Also known as primary hypogonadism, which involves an impaired response of the gonads to gonadotropins (FSH, LH) and results in

lack of sex steroid production and delayed sexual development.

- **Activating mutations:** Also known as gain-of-function mutation, which changes the gene product and results in enhanced activation and abnormal function.
- **Virilization:** Development of male secondary sex characteristics in prepubertal males and females (i.e. facial and body hair, male pattern hair growth, enlarged clitoris, enlarged penis, masculinization of urogenital tract) associated with androgen excess.

Key Points
- Boys born with an extra X chromosome have complex health care and social needs that are not easily recognized or addressed by health care providers.
- While boys with 47,XXY are known to demonstrate hypergonadotropic hypogonadism beginning in puberty, androgen deficiency alone does not account for many characteristics and symptoms associated with 47,XXY.
- Testotoxicosis is a rare cause of peripheral precocious puberty that affects boys exclusively. The pattern of inheritance is autosomal dominant in the familial form of testotoxicosis.
- The hormonal profile of testotoxicosis is characterized by elevated serum levels of testosterone, contrasting with prepubertal basal and GnRH-stimulated LH levels. Rapid and progressive virilization, growth acceleration, and skeletal maturation are typical manifestations.
- Constitutively activating mutations of the luteinizing hormone receptor gene represent the genetic basis of testotoxicosis.
- APRNs in endocrinology practice are perfectly positioned to assess, coordinate, and provide family-centered navigation for health surveillance according to child's level of development.

10.1 Introduction

This chapter will provide an overview of two genetic syndromes affecting gonadotropin function that typically present in childhood, Klinefelter Syndrome, and testotoxicosis familial male-limited precocious puberty.

10.2 Klinefelter Syndrome

Knowledge of genetics and the ability to develop an index of suspicion for the genetic basis of endocrine-based problems are important aspects of practice for APRNs (refer to Chap. 7). Sex chromosome variations are among the many genetic conditions that require endocrine management in coordination with other treatment or therapy. Several variations of sex chromosomes exist involving additional Xs or Ys that are associated with a number of physical, psychological, and medical issues that require coordinated multidisciplinary care (Tartaglia et al. 2015). The most common of these variations is the karyotype 47,XXY, also known as Klinefelter Syndrome (KS). The prevalence of KS is estimated to be about 1 in 450–600 male births (Bojesen et al. 2003; Herlihy et al. 2011). While the prevalence of KS is not rare, it is not commonly diagnosed and is often discovered incidentally when mothers undergo prenatal screening for other genetic conditions. Even with the advent prenatal screening, only 10% of affected individuals are diagnosed during childhood and almost 75% are unaware that they carry an extra X (Abramsky and Chapple 1997). Diagnosis of KS is done by chromosomal analysis, a study of the structure, and number of chromosomes that is also known as a karyotype. This section will discuss the background of KS, genetic mechanism underlying the karyotype, the physical, neurocognitive, and psychosocial phenotype, the endocrine basis for symptoms, treatment, associated health risks and issues regarding the complexities of care for patients.

10.2.1 Background of KS

The syndrome known as 47,XXY was originally described in 1942 by Dr. Harry S. Klinefelter and colleagues in a case series of 9 patients with similar physical characteristics (Klinefelter et al. 1942). These characteristics included tall stature, light or absent facial hair, small testes, low testosterone levels, and azoospermia. In 1959, using radiographic imaging of chromosomal structures, Patricia Jacobs and colleagues discovered that men with KS characteristics also had an extra X resulting in the karyotype 47,XXY (Jacobs and Strong 1959). Since the original report of physical characteristics, clinicians and scientists have expanded the physical phenotype to include descriptions of neurocognitive and psychosocial characteristics as well (Close et al. 2015; van Rijn et al. 2014a; Nieschlag 2013; Tartaglia et al. 2010; Boada et al. 2009).

10.2.2 Genetic Mechanism for KS

Klinefelter syndrome is not an inherited condition. It is not passed down from one generation to the next by autosomal dominant or autosomal recessive pattern. Rather, the genetic mechanism is the result of non-disjunction of sex chromosomes during development of gametes (sperm or eggs) or during Meiosis I or II in the embryological phase of development. During formation of gametes, cells divide to distribute one sex chromosome (and X or a Y) to each gamete. On occasion, sex chromosomes fail to divide properly thereby distributing more than one X or Y. If one gamete has more than one sex chromosome present, it combines with the other parental gamete to develop an embryo with multiple sex chromosomes. Extra Xs may come from paternal or maternal origin. Parental contribution occurs 50% of the time from the father and 50% of the time from the mother (Jacobs et al. 1988). The extra X in the XXY karyotype may have variable effects due to the processes of activation, inactivation, or partial activation of one or both X chromosomes (Zitzmann et al. 2004). Gene "dosage" is highly variable and thought to contribute the variable phenotypes observed in KS.

Non-disjunction may also occur after fertilization and this can lead to mosaicism when the developing embryo has a cell line of 46 XY as well as 47,XXY. Individuals with 46 XY/47,XXY mosaicism are reported to have milder physical and neurocognitive characteristics (Paduch et al. 2008).

10.2.3 Diagnosis of KS

Prenatal testing is usually performed as a screening measure to detect trisomies such as 13, 18, and 21 in women of advanced maternal age. Until recently, this testing was done via amniocentesis or chorionic villi sampling. Due to the advent of non-invasive prenatal screening (NiPS), risk for these chromosomal trisomies along with sex chromosome aneuploidies, such as 47,XXY, are being detected early and is becoming standard practice for many prenatal clinics across the country (Bianchi et al. 2012). When parents first learn of risk or receive confirmatory results of 47,XXY, consultation with a specialist in endocrinology becomes a priority concern. Diagnosis, however, is not always made prior to birth. A frequent scenario with 47,XXY occurs when a young man attains adulthood and encounters difficulties in achieving pregnancy with his partner. After consultation with a urologist, the patient may learn that his testes are small and firm, with evidence of low sperm count or azoospermia. These clinical observations usually initate a plan that includes ordering a karyotype to turl our 47,XXY. For undiagnosed boys, many important signs, symptoms, and clinical observations often do not trigger a health care provider to consider inquiry into a genetic diagnosis. Signs that are frequently missed in children include speech and language delay, learning issues, and behavioral struggles.

10.2.4 Case Presentation of KS

JT is a 16-year-old male with a history of learning difficulties and early speech and language delay. He reports that he is unable to keep up with other kids his own age in sports and other physical activities. Parent reports that during JT's early childhood, he was bullied by other children and frequently not chosen by his peers for group activities. Patient reports that now that he is self-conscious about his body because he is much taller than his peers (>99%), that he is not developing facial hair and that his breast area is becoming protuberant. Parent reports that teachers have described him as lazy and disorganized. JT has expressed to his parents recently that he is too tired to care anymore and that he wishes he could just disappear. At first glance, this case description may sound like a typical disenfranchised teenage boy. On closer examination, however, there are important observations to be made that require further clinical inquiry. On physical examination, this young man was found to have a number of physical features such as tall stature, eunuchoid body proportion, gynecomastia, diminished upper body muscle bulk and strength, Tanner stage V pubertal development, and testicular volume of 8 mL.

Laboratory findings demonstrated elevated luteinizing hormone (LH), and follicle stimulating hormone (FSH) with serum testosterone at 320 mg/dL that suggested hypergonadotropic hypogonadism. Based upon clinical observations, a chromosomal analysis was ordered revealing that this child had 47 chromosomes in the pattern of 47,XXY, also known as Klinefelter Syndrome (KS).

10.2.5 KS Physical Health and Other Health Characteristics

One of the earliest features of KS in child development is a rapid rise in linear growth during the school years with stature greater than the 99th percentile. Tall stature, however, is not always observed. Long legs relative to torso and very long arms may give the child a "eunuchoid" proportion. The onset of puberty and its progression during the Tanner stages of sexual development may demonstrate more emerging features such as low upper body muscle bulk and strength, light facial hair, development of gynecomastia, and small testes. Testicular development in a child should roughly follow Tanner staging. In later

Tanner stages IV-V, if testicular volume remains small, this is a sign that genetic testing for 47,XXY should be ordered.

A problem exists, sometimes, in pediatric primary care, when health care providers defer genital examinations in boys to save them from embarrassment. Failure to observe small testes is another reason why the diagnosis of 47,XXY frequently missed during the course of normal care. Physical, neurocognitive, and psychosocial health characteristics associated with 47,XXY vary widely from person to person. Due to the wide range of variability, "textbook" examples are rarely seen. There are, however, several characteristics that, in combination, may elicit a suspicion of 47,XXY in an undiagnosed child. Boys with 47,XXY may also express a variable psychosocial phenotype that is shaped by inherent personality characteristics, yet-to-be-understood mechanisms involved with the supernumerary X, factors of nurture within the family and their social environment. Many boys with 47,XXY show social cognitive deficits that may contribute to social dysfunction (van Rijn et al. 2014b). Social dysfunction has been described as autistic-like without necessarily meeting the full diagnostic requirement for the designation of autism spectrum disorder. Some of these features include deficits in social communication, reciprocal social interaction and restricted, repetitive patterns of behavior (Tartaglia et al. 2017). Neurocognitive features of boys with 47,XXY include normal to low-normal intelligence with specific language-based learning difficulties. Speech and language delays may exist in early childhood along with slow auditory processing, problems with memory, visual-motor difficulties, and fine motor control issues. These variable features may manifest as learning issues that require special attention at school either in the form of individualized education plans, or 504 accommodations for disability. The diagnosis of 47,XXY is not considered a physical or neurocognitive disability per se although many boys and men with 47,XXY demonstrate specific disabilities in learning that impair school and work performance.

10.2.6 Endocrine Basis for Symptoms and Treatment in KS

The feature of hypogonadism and androgen deficiency is due to progressive hyalinization of testicular tissue and the seminiferous tubules. As boys enter puberty, the pituitary gland systematically pulses LH and FSH to signal the testes to begin manufacture and secretion of testosterone. Depending on how fibrotic the testicular tissue has become, the testes become increasingly unable to produce levels of testosterone enough to suppress LH and FSH. As a result, LH and FSH remain high while serum testosterone begins to wane as the child progresses through puberty. Androgen deficiency in adults is associated with fatigue, lack of maintaining upper body muscle bulk, decreased facial hair, lack of libido, azoospermia, osteoporosis irritability, and depression (Styne and Puberty 2015). While boys with 47,XXY are expected to eventually show androgen deficiency in early childhood through adolescence, their serum levels of testosterone remain roughly in the normal to low-normal range. Evidence-based clinical guidelines and clinical consensus documents from professionals in endocrinology currently do not currently exist for how and when to treat children.

Since androgen treatment clinical guidelines and consensus documents do not currently exist for pediatric populations, health care providers are reluctant to treat young boys with testosterone in the absence of identifiable deficiency. Some youth with 47,XXY report bothersome symptoms such as fatigue, lack of motivation, irritability, lack of upper body strength, low self-esteem, and depression. It is unclear, and so far, unsupported by scientific evidence that exogenous testosterone treatment will improve these symptoms in children.

There currently exists conflicting and provocative scientific work with infants with regard to early treatment (Ross et al. 2005; Lahlou et al. 2011), but no body of evidence has yet emerged to support its use unless urogenital anomalies such as microphallus exist. A study completed in 2005 with 29 boys between the ages of 1 month

and 23 months suggested that testicular volume and phallic length were diminished, indicating early androgen deficiency (Ross et al. 2005). In 2011, however, researchers found in 72 boys who were less than 2 years of age, that the majority had normal external genitalia (Lahlou et al. 2011). While testosterone replacement therapy is often employed to mitigate physical symptoms, a body of literature is emerging concerning its affect in cognition and behavior in children. In a 2015 study of boys between the ages of 36 and 72 months results suggested that boys with microphallus during infancy who were treated with testosterone had improved scores for social communication, social cognition, and total (T) score on the Child Behavior Checklist along with improvements in the Behavior Rating Inventory of Executive Function compared to untreated controls (Samango-Sprouse et al. 2015). In a 2017 randomized control study with 84 boys between the ages of 4 and 12 years comparing a low-dose oral testosterone treatment group with a no-treatment group. Results from this study showed improvement in only 1 out of 5 endpoints (visual-motor function) (Ross et al. 2017). A secondary analysis of the data in this study showed positive effects of psychosocial function including anxiety, depression, and social problems. No significant effects were observed on cognitive function or behaviors such as hyperactivity or aggression. While evidence continues to be generated, results thus far do not provide strength of evidence to direct the use of testosterone as a clinical treatment for behavior and cognition.

For adolescents aged 18 years and older who demonstrate androgen deficiency with serum levels consistently below normal range for age, there are a variety of testosterone products available as seen in Table 10.1. The Endocrine Society has established clinical guidelines for treating men, age 18 years and older with androgen deficiency syndromes (Bhasin et al. 2010). For adolescents with 47,XXY entering puberty (and/or age of 13 years), it is recommended to begin initial therapy with testosterone enanthate 50 mg intramuscularly every month for about 9 months (Styne and Puberty 2015).

Table 10.1 Testosterone replacement therapy for boys 18 years of age and older

Formulation	Route	Dose and schedule
Testosterone enanthate or cypionate	IM	150–200 mg IM every week OR 75–100 mg IM every 2 weeks
Long-acting testosterone undecanoate in oil	IM	European regimen: 1000 mg IM followed by 1000 mg at 6 weeks, and 1000 mg every 10–14 weeks
1% testosterone gel	Transdermal	5–10 g of testosterone gel containing 50–100 mg testosterone every day
Testosterone patch	Transdermal	1–2 patches designed to deliver 5–10 mg testosterone over 24 h applied every day to non-pressure areas
Testosterone-in-adhesive matrix patch	Transdermal	2 × 60 cm² patches delivering approximately 4.8 mg of testosterone per day
Buccal bioadhesive testosterone tablets	Trans-oral mucosa	30 mg controlled release bioadhesive tablets twice daily
Oral testosterone undecanoate[a]	Oral	40–80 mg twice daily or three times daily with meals
Testosterone pellets	Subcutaneous	3–6 pellets implanted subcutaneously; dose and regimen vary with formulation

Adapted from Endocrine Society Clinical Practice Guidelines for men with androgen deficiency syndromes (Bhasin et al. 2010)

[a]Not approved for clinical use in the United States, but available in many other countries

Regular assessment of adolescents' adherence to therapy and monitoring of symptoms is a key part of patient care for the Advanced Practice Nurse (APRN). While monitoring serum testosterone levels when an adolescent is on treatment provides biological feedback in terms of serum levels, it is important to monitor changes in symptoms as well. Some adolescents may report improvements for specific symptoms such as facial hair growth and muscle bulk while other symptoms such as irritability, mood, and tremors may be exacerbated.

10.2.7 Health Surveillance of KS

A number of health risks exist for patients born with 47,XXY that need to be surveilled throughout the lifespan. A recommended health surveillance schedule according to age is shown in Table 10.2. Many physical health risks are endocrine in nature such as: hyperinsulinism, metabolic syndrome, Type II diabetes, thyroid disease, and osteopenia or osteoporosis. Other physical health risks include: hyperlipidemia, hypertension, cardiovascular disease, vascular leg ulcerations, arthritis, breast cancer, tremors, and tics. Psychological health risks include anxiety, depression, suicide, and risk of substance abuse. Recommended best practice for the APRN who monitors boys and adolescents with 47,XXY is to annually conduct a thorough physical exam that includes all systems, screening for depression, anxiety, and substance use.

10.3   Testotoxicosis

Testotoxicosis or familial male-limited precocious puberty is a rare cause of peripheral precocious puberty that affects exclusively boys (Schedewie et al. 1981). It is caused by constitutively activating mutations of the luteinizing hormone receptor gene (*LHCGR*). The pattern of inheritance is autosomal dominant in familial cases, but sporadic cases can occur (Kremer et al. 1999; Laue et al. 1995).

Affected boys typically develop rapid and progressive virilization characterized by penile growth, pubic hair development, minimal testicular enlargement, growth acceleration, and skeletal maturation before the age of 4 (Table 10.3) (Schedewie et al. 1981; Kremer et al. 1999; Laue et al. 1995; Reiter and Norjavaara 2005; Egli et al. 1985). The hormonal profile is characterized by elevated serum levels of testosterone, despite prepubertal basal and GnRH-stimulated LH levels. Normal adrenal precursors and undetectable serum β-hCG should exclude adrenal abnormalities and hCG-producing germ-cell tumors, respectively, in these boys. Testosterone levels can widely range and very high testosterone levels have been reported (>1000 ng/dL)

Table 10.2 Schedule of Recommended Health Surveillance for KS

Areas of specialty or evaluation	Birth–4 years11 months	5 years–9 years 11 months	10–18 years	>18 years
Chromosome testing	Confirm prenatal	Post-natal diagnosis		
Parent/family counseling	Annual	Annual	Annual	Annual
Developmental exam	Annual	Annual	Annual	as needed
Neuropsychology		Initial to biannual	Initial to biannual	Initial to biannual
Endocrinology	Infancy and/or genital anomalies	Annual Beginning at 8 years Peri-pubertal consult	Annual Pubertal progression HRT and bone Sexuality	Semiannual to annual HRT and bone Sexuality
Educational and behavioral psychology and social cognition assessment	as needed	as needed	as needed	as needed
Psychiatry		as needed	as needed	as needed
Urology/fertility	as needed or for urogenital anomalies	as needed or for urogenital anomalies	as needed	as needed
Speech and language	Initial and annual	as needed	as needed	
Occupational therapy	Initial and annual	as needed	as needed	as needed
Physical therapy	as needed	as needed	as needed	as needed
Social work	as needed	as needed	as needed	as needed
Immunology	as needed	as needed	as needed	as needed
Pulmonology	as needed	as needed	as needed	as needed
Neurology	as needed	as needed	as needed	as needed
Sleep apnea			as needed	as needed
Cardiovascular			as needed	as needed

HRT hormone replacement therapy
Reprinted with permission from Pediatric Endocrinology Review (Close et al. 2017)

(Egli et al. 1985). Interestingly, family members with the same mutation may present with phenotypes of variable severity (Laue et al. 1995).

Notably, activating mutations in the LHCG receptor do not cause hyperandrogenism, polycystic ovary syndrome, or reproductive abnormality in women. The lack of clinical manifestations in female carriers suggests that ovarian function is dependent of the activation of both LH and FSH receptors (Eunice et al. 2009).

The LH receptor (LHCGR) is a G protein-coupled receptor with a large amino-terminal extracellular domain, seven-membrane traversing α-helices, and carboxyl-terminal intracellular domain (Themmen and Huhtaniemi 2000; Macedo et al. 2016). The *LHCGR* gene, located on chromosome 2p21, contains 11 exons. Although the reported mutations in familial and sporadic cases had a genetic heterogeneity, they were usually sited in exon 11 of the *LHCGR* gene (Themmen

and Huhtaniemi 2000). The p.Asp578Gly mutation in the sixth transmembrane domain has been the most frequent LH receptor alteration. All mutations identified in boys with testotoxicosis were in the heterozygous status, except one (p.Ala568Val), which was caused by maternal isodisomy (Laue et al. 1995; Macedo et al. 2016). However, the clinical and hormonal features of the affected boy with this homozygous mutation were similar with those previously reported. Activating mutations in *LHCGR* have been characterized by a constitutive activity, leading to increased production of c-AMP due to activation of adenylate cyclase (Themmen and Huhtaniemi 2000). Interestingly, a somatic activating mutation (p.Asp578His) of the *LHCGR* has been identified in boys displaying Leydig cell tumors. Concomitant activation of phospholipase C and adenylate cyclase has been proposed as a mechanism determining tumorigenicity in Leydig cell (Liu et al. 1999).

Table 10.3 Clinical, hormonal, and genetic criteria for testotoxicosis

Clinical criterion	
Pubertal development	Progressive and rapid virilization before 4 years of age. Possible family history of precocious puberty
Testicular size	Symmetric and minimally increased (> 2.5 cm or 4 mL)
Growth velocity	Accelerated (> 6 cm per year)
Bone age	Advanced (at least 1 year)
Hormonal criterion	
Testosterone (ng/dL)	Elevated (widely range)
Basal LH (UI/L)	Prepubertal range
LH peak after GnRH or GnRH agonist (UI/L)	Suppressed or blunted
Serum β-hCG (UI/L)	Undetectable
Adrenal androgen precursors	Normal
Genetic criterion	
Gene analysis	Activating mutation of LH receptor gene

10.3.1 Treatment of Testotoxicosis

Treatment typically consists of reducing hyperandrogenism in boys with testotoxicosis with ketoconazole or a combination of anti-androgens and aromatase inhibitors. Long-term treatment with both therapies resulted in similar outcomes and limited efficacy in attaining normal adult height (Almeida et al. 2008). Central precocious puberty typically follows over time, requiring the addition of a GnRH analog (Macedo et al. 2016). After the maturation of hypothalamic-pituitary-testicular axis, normal adult function appears to range from normal paternity to reduced testicular volume or oligospermia (Egli et al. 1985). Untreated boys can present behavioral disturbance and short adult height due to premature closure of the epiphyses (Almeida et al. 2008).

Case Study

A 2.6-year-old boy had penile enlargement, frequent erections, accelerated growth velocity, deepening voice, and aggressive behavior. His height was 115 cm (6 standard deviation (SD)) and

weight was 24.3 kg. Penile length was 10.3 cm, testicular size was 2.0 × 1.0 cm² at right and 2.0 × 1.0 cm² at left, and pubic hair was Tanner stage 4. Bone age (BA) was advanced, 6.0 years. His basal testosterone levels ranged from 1.5 to 40 nmol/L (prepubertal range: <1.0 nmol/L). Basal serum LH and FSH levels were both undetectable. Additionally, a GnRH stimulation test (gonadorelin 0.1 mg, intravenous) indicated suppressed LH and FSH levels (LH < 0.6 IU/L and FSH < 1.0 IU/L) at all-time points. He was treated with cyproterone acetate and aromatase inhibitor (anastrozol 1 mg/day). At the end of treatment, his chronological age was 9.3 years, BA was 16 years, and his height was 158 cm (4 SD).

10.4 Nursing Role

10.4.1 Complexity of Care for Patients Diagnosed with Klinefelter Syndrome or Testotoxicosis

Care for infants, boys, and adolescents diagnosed with 47,XXY or testotoxicosis is best accomplished by building and working with an interprofessional team that may include advanced practice nursing, developmental pediatrics, neuropsychology, endocrinology, urology, psychiatry, psychology, speech and language (47,XXY), occupational therapy, and physical therapy (47,XXY) (Tartaglia et al. 2015). Whether under the auspices of one institution, or by referral to local or regional specialists, the integration and coordination of care is best accomplished by the APRN. As nurses, we see the child and his health care needs within the context of himself, his diagnosis, his family, school, community, and the greater world. To provide patient- and family-centered care, we must be mindful of needs, desires, preferences, and resources available to provide the best care according to the child's developmental status and his developmental trajectory. Patients and families often seek a roadmap to anticipate physical, neurocognitive, and psychosocial needs as children grow. The APRN is called upon to help them navigate this path.

Table 10.4 Web Resources for Information About Klinefelter Syndrome

Resource	Contact information
Association of X and Y variations (AXYS)	www.genetic.org
Genetic Alliance	www.geneticalliance.org
eXtraordinarY Kids Clinic University of Colorado Denver Children's Hospital Denver, CO	www.childrenscolorado.org/conditions/behavior/xychromosome.aspx
eXtraordinarY Kids Clinic Nemours/Alfred DuPont Hospital Wilmington, DE	http://www.nemours.org/about/mediaroom/press/dv/introduces-extraordinary-kids-clinic.html
eXtraordinarY Clinic Emory Health Care Division of Pediatric Genetics Atlanta, GA	https://genetics.emory.edu/patient-care/index.html
Johns Hopkins Klinefelter Syndrome Center Johns Hopkins Medical Center Baltimore, MD	http://klinefelter.jhu.edu
NORD National Association for Rare Disorders	www.rarediseases.org
National Institutes of Health Genetics Home Reference Klinefelter Syndrome	https://ghr.nlm.nih.gov/condition/klinefelter-syndrome

Since endocrinology is a central point of care for boys with 47,XXY or testotoxicosis, the endocrinology APRN is perfectly positioned to assess, monitor, and provide consistent customized treatment plans and support for patients and families. When patients and families first receive the diagnosis of 47,XXY or testotoxicosis they are often stunned, confused, and left to their own devices to probe and learn as much as they can. Much information probing is conducted from Internet-based resources and on social media. The APRN may be most effective during a clinical visit by first assessing major concerns of the patient and family and addressing them systematically with complexity of care in mind. While the Internet is rich with good and poor information, the APRN can be instrumental in guiding patients and families toward information that is up-to-date and reliable. (For 47,XXY several helpful resources can be found in Table 10.4). The National Advocacy Association for X & Y Chromosome Variations known as "AXYS" has formed a Clinical and Research Consortium composed of medical centers interested in developing regional multidisciplinary care for patients

and families. The website for this organization and current regional clinics may also be found in Table 10.4. Patient- and family-centered care is the hallmark of practice for APRNs. Our knowledge, accessibility, and willingness to navigate complex patterns of care contributes greatly to achieving best clinical outcomes for patients and families affected by 47,XXY.

10.5 Conclusions

KS and testotoxicosis (familial male precocious puberty) are complex genetic conditions that require careful assessment and follow-up across the lifespan. Beginning in childhood, patient and family-centered care requires navigation by a multidisciplinary team that includes APRNs. Since alterations in hormone levels alone does not account for many characteristics associated with KS or testotoxicosis, the role of APRNs is to help patients and families navigate the process of securing physical, neurocognitive, and psychosocial assessments that will meet targeted needs for each patient. APRNs in endocrinology practice are perfectly positioned to assess, coordinate, and provide family-centered navigation for health surveillance according to each child's level of development.

References

Abramsky L, Chapple J. 47,XXY (Klinefelter syndrome) and 47,XYY: estimated rates of and indication for postnatal diagnosis with implications for prenatal counselling. Prenat Diagn. 1997;17(4):363–8.

Almeida MQ, Brito VN, Lins TS, Guerra-Junior G, de Castro M. Antonini SR, et al. ong-term treatment of familial male-limited precocious puberty (testotoxicosis) with cyproterone acetate or ketoconazole. Clin Endocrinol. 2008;69(1):93–8.

Bhasin S, Cunningham GR, Hayes FJ, Matsumoto AM, Snyder PJ, Swerdloff RS, et al. Testosterone therapy in men with androgen deficiency syndromes: an Endocrine Society clinical practice guideline. J Clin Endocrinol Metab. 2010;95(6):2536–59.

Bianchi DW, Platt LD, Goldberg JD, Abuhamad AZ, Sehnert AJ, Rava RP, et al. Genome-wide fetal aneuploidy detection by maternal plasma DNA sequencing. Obstet Gynecol. 2012;119(5):890–901.

Boada R, Janusz J, Hutaff-Lee C, Tartaglia N. The cognitive phenotype in Klinefelter syndrome: a review of the literature including genetic and hormonal factors. Dev Disabil Res Rev. 2009;15(4):284–94.

Bojesen A, Juul S, Gravholt CH. Prenatal and postnatal prevalence of Klinefelter syndrome: a national registry study. J Clin Endocrinol Metab. 2003;88(2):622–6.

Close S, Fennoy I, Smaldone A, Reame N. Phenotype and adverse quality of life in boys with Klinefelter syndrome. J Pediatr. 2015;167(3):650–7.

Close S, Talboy A, Fennoy I. Complexities of care in Klinefelter syndrome: an APRN perspective. Pediatr Endocrinol Rev. 2017;14(Suppl 2):462–71.

Egli CA, Rosenthal SM, Grumbach MM, Montalvo JM, Gondos B. Pituitary gonadotropin-independent male-limited autosomal dominant sexual precocity in nine generations: familial testotoxicosis. J Pediatr. 1985;106(1):33–40.

Eunice M, Philibert P, Kulshreshtha B, Audran F, Paris F, Sultan C, et al. Mother-to-son transmission of a luteinizing hormone receptor activating mutation in a prepubertal child with testotoxicosis. J Pediatr Endocrinol Metab. 2009;22(3):275–9.

Herlihy AS, Halliday JL, Cock ML, McLachlan RI. The prevalence and diagnosis rates of Klinefelter syndrome: an Australian comparison. Med J Aust. 2011;194(1):24–8.

Jacobs P, Strong J. A case of human intersexuality having a possible XXY sex-determining mechanism. Nature. 1959;183:302–3.

Jacobs PA, Hassold TJ, Whittington E, Butler G, Collyer S, Keston M, et al. Klinefelter's syndrome: an anal-ysis of the origin of the additional sex chromosome using molecular probes. Ann Hum Genet. 1988;52(Pt 2):93–109.

Klinefelter HF, Reifensten EC, Albright F. Syndrome characterized by gynecomastia, asermatogenesis without a-leydigism and increased secretion of follicle-stimulating hormone. J Endocrinol Metab. 1942;2:615–22.

Kremer H, Martens JW, van Reen M, Verhoef-Post M, Wit JM, Otten BJ, et al. A limited repertoire of mutations of the luteinizing hormone (LH) receptor gene in familial and sporadic patients with male LH-independent precocious puberty. J Clin Endocrinol Metab. 1999;84(3):1136–40.

Lahlou N, Fennoy I, Ross JL, Bouvattier C, Roger M. Clinical and hormonal status of infants with non-mosaic XXY karyotype. Acta Paediatr. 2011;100(6):824–9.

Laue L, Chan WY, Hsueh AJ, Kudo M, Hsu SY, Wu SM, et al. Genetic heterogeneity of constitutively activating mutations of the human luteinizing hormone receptor in familial male-limited precocious puberty. Proc Natl Acad Sci U S A. 1995;92(6):1906–10.

Liu G, Duranteau L, Carel JC, Monroe J, Doyle DA, Shenker A. Leydig-cell tumors caused by an activating mutation of the gene encoding the luteinizing hormone receptor. N Engl J Med. 1999;341(23):1731–6.

Macedo DB, Silveira LF, Bessa DS, Brito VN, Latronico AC. Sexual precocity-genetic bases of central precocious puberty and autonomous gonadal activation. Endocr Dev. 2016;29:50–71.

Nieschlag E. Klinefelter syndrome: the commonest form of hypogonadism, but often overlooked or untreated. Dtsch Arztebl Int. 2013;110(20):347–53.

Paduch DA, Fine RG, Bolyakov A, Kiper J. New concepts in Klinefelter syndrome. Curr Opin Urol. 2008;18(6):621–7.

Reiter WO, Norjavaara E. Testotoxicosis: current viewpoint. Pediatr Endocrinol Rev. 2005;3(2):77–86.

Ross JL, Samango-Sprouse C, Lahlou N, Kowal K, Elder FF, Zinn A. Early androgen deficiency in infants and young boys with 47,XXY Klinefelter syndrome. Horm Res. 2005;64(1):39–45.

Ross JL, Kushner H, Kowal K, Bardsley M, Davis S, Reiss AL, et al. Androgen treatment effects on motor function, cognition, and behavior in boys with Klinefelter syndrome. J Pediatr. 2017;185:193–199.e4.

Samango-Sprouse C, Stapleton EJ, Lawson P, Mitchell F, Sadeghin T, Powell S, et al. Positive effects of early androgen therapy on the behavioral phenotype of boys with 47,XXY. Am J Med Genet C Semin Med Genet. 2015;169(2):150–7.

Schedewie HK, Reiter EO, Beitins IZ, Seyed S, Wooten VD, Jiminez JF, et al. Testicular leydig cell hyperplasia as a cause of familial sexual precocity. J Clin Endocrinol Metab. 1981;52(2):271–8.

Styne D, Puberty GM. Ontogeny, neuroendocrinology, physiology and disorders. In: Kronenberg H, Melmed A, Polonsky K, Larsen P, editors. Williams textbook of endocrinology. Philadelphia, PA: Saunders; 2015. p. 13.

Tartaglia N, Cordeiro L, Howell S, Wilson R, Janusz J. The spectrum of the behavioral phenotype in boys and adolescents 47,XXY (Klinefelter syndrome). Pediatr Endocrinol Rev. 2010;8(Suppl 1):151–9.

Tartaglia N, Howell S, Wilson R, Janusz J, Boada R, Martin S, et al. The eXtraordinarY Kids Clinic: an interdisciplinary model of care for children and adolescents with sex chromosome aneuploidy. J Multidiscip Healthc. 2015;8:323–34.

Tartaglia NR, Wilson R, Miller JS, Rafalko J, Cordeiro L, Davis S, et al. Autism spectrum disorder in males with sex chromosome aneuploidy: XXY/Klinefelter syndrome, XYY, and XXYY. J Dev Behav Pediatr. 2017;38(3):197–207.

Themmen APN, Huhtaniemi IT. Mutations of gonadotropins and gonadotropin receptors: elucidating the physiology and pathophysiology of pituitary-gonadal function. Endocr Rev. 2000;21(5):551–83.

van Rijn S, Stockmann L, Borghgraef M, Bruining H, van Ravenswaaij-Arts C, Govaerts L, et al. The social behavioral phenotype in boys and girls with an extra X chromosome (Klinefelter syndrome and Trisomy X): a comparison with autism spectrum disorder. J Autism Dev Disord. 2014a;44(2):310–20.

van Rijn S, Stockmann L, van Buggenhout G, van Ravenswaaij-Arts C, Swaab H. Social cognition and underlying cognitive mechanisms in children with an extra X chromosome: a comparison with autism spectrum disorder. Genes Brain Behav. 2014b;13(5):459–67.

Zitzmann M, Depenbusch M, Gromoll J, Nieschlag E. X-chromosome inactivation patterns and androgen receptor functionality influence phenotype and social characteristics as well as pharmacogenetics of testosterone therapy in Klinefelter patients. J Clin Endocrinol Metab. 2004;89(12):6208–17.

McCune–Albright Syndrome

11

Beth Brillante and Lori Guthrie

Contents

B. Brillante (✉) · L. Guthrie
National Institutes of Health, National Institute of
Dental and Craniofacial Research, Skeletal Disorders
and Mineral Homeostasis Section,
Bethesda, MD, USA
e-mail: bbrillante@mail.nih.gov;
guthriel@mail.nih.gov

© Springer Nature Switzerland AG 2019
S. Llahana et al. (eds.), *Advanced Practice in Endocrinology Nursing*,
https://doi.org/10.1007/978-3-319-99817-6_11

Abstract

McCune–Albright syndrome (MAS) is a rare, non-hereditable genetic disorder classically defined by a clinical presentation of bone (fibrous dysplasia), skin (café-au-lait macules), and/or endocrine abnormalities. Sporadic occurrence of an activating mutation in the *GNAS* gene creates a mosaic tissue environment marked with normal and mutated cells. Mutation effect is variable with ability to cause significant disruption to various organs. Bone abnormalities include deformities and fractures, which may lead to pain, disability, and immobility. Visible irregularly shaped skin markings may be large and pronounced. Hyperfunctioning endocrinopathies pose challenges to normal growth, development, and function. Individual presentation is unique in extent and severity with a range from mild, barely recognizable symptoms to severe, disfiguring disease. MAS commonly presents in childhood with a fracture or endocrine abnormality, which leads to a diagnosis. Individual variation drives the need for medical and nursing care that is centered on an accurate diagnosis. Management and treatment of bone and endocrine disease enhances and promotes patient well-being and optimal physical functioning. Despite the complexity and challenges, the majority of individuals affected appear to be psychologically well adjusted and live productive lives (Kelly et al., Bone 37(3):388–394; 2005).

Keywords

McCune–Albright syndrome · Gsα mutation
Fibrous dysplasia · Endocrinopathy (ies)
Café-au-lait macules

Abbreviations

CF	Craniofacial
FD	Fibrous dysplasia
GHX	Growth hormone excess
GNAS	Guanine nucleotide binding protein alpha stimulating activity polypeptide
MAS	McCune–Albright syndrome
NTX	N-telopeptide
OTC	Over-the-Counter
PP	Precocious puberty

Key Terms

- *GNAS* **activating mutation:** Genetic mutation resulting in abnormal version of the G protein, which causes the Gsα pathway to be constantly turned on, leading to overproduction of hormones or increased cell proliferation that results in abnormal cell differentiation and malfunction.

- **Fibrous dysplasia:** Skeletal disorder where normal bone and bone marrow is replaced with fibrous or connective tissue that may result in pain, misshapen bone, functional impairment, and fractures.

- **Café-au-lait macules:** light hyperpigmented (light or dark brown) skin lesions.

Key Points

- McCune–Albright syndrome (MAS) is a rare, complex, non-hereditary genetic disorder.
- MAS is characterized by the presence of two or more abnormalities of the bone (fibrous dysplasia), skin (café-au-lait), endocrine (endocrinopathies), and/or more rarely, other systems.
- Individual variation drives the need for medical and nursing intervention that is centered on an accurate diagnosis and appreciation of the spectrum of the disease.
- Optimal individual well-being and physical functioning is achievable through individualized management and treatment plans focused on bone, endocrine, and other abnormalities.
- Most individuals with MAS adjust psychologically well to their disease and lead productive lives.

11.1   Introduction

McCune–Albright syndrome is a rare non-hereditary genetic disorder affecting approximately 1/100,000 to 1/1,000,000 individuals worldwide (Dumitrescu and Collins 2008). Diagnosis most often occurs in childhood and is classically defined by a clinical presentation of simultaneously occurring bone, skin, and/or endocrine features (Weinstein et al. 1991). Due to the random nature and sporadic rise of a *GNAS* (guanine nucleotide binding protein alpha stimulating activity polypeptide) mutation, clinical manifestations are dependent on the specific tissues affected and the extent of tissue involvement (Collins et al. 2013). Individual presentation is

unique. Prognosis and clinical management is based on location and severity of disease.

The syndrome was first described in the medical literature by Donovan McCune (1936) and Fuller Albright et al. (1937). Both reported an unusual syndrome in females characterized by three distinguishing features: irregular pigmentations of the skin; symptoms of precocious puberty (PP); and bone abnormalities with bowing, fractures, and deformities. Since these initial reports a broader scope of the syndrome has emerged. In contrast to what was originally postulated, MAS affects males equally as much as females and features associated with the syndrome are more extensive than previously reported (Collins et al. 2013; Collins 2006; Collins and Shenker 1999). Due to the unique clinical presentation, a thorough clinical assessment coupled with a comprehensive evaluation and individualized approach to treatment/management is required.

11.2   McCune–Albright Syndrome: Mutation Effect on Embryonic Development

MAS is the result of a postzygotic somatic mutation (Dumitrescu and Collins 2008). There is no identified cause for this non-heritable mutation which occurs randomly in the general population (Riminucci et al. 2007). Genetic changes are caused by an activating mutation of the gene *GNAS* (Weinstein et al. 1991). Specifically, the Gsα, which is responsible for cellular development/function, is affected. Gsα serves as the "on/off" switch for cell activity and proliferation for tissues including the bone, skin, pituitary, thyroid, and gonadal organs. In MAS, the Gsα pathway is constantly turned on leading to overproduction of hormones, or increased cell proliferation and resulting in abnormal cell differentiation and malfunction. Tissue effect is sporadic, dependent upon when the mutation occurs during embryogenesis.

In normal human embryogenesis, growth and development originate as a single stem cell. This single cell proceeds through an orderly process of differentiation to form three germ layers known as the ectoderm (outer), endoderm (inner), and mesoderm (middle). The ectoderm and endoderm form first followed by the mesoderm. Each layer has a predetermined role in the development of specific tissues that emerge into mature organs. Examples of tissue development for each layer are provided in Table 11.1.

A generally accepted model of pathogenesis proposes that once a mutation occurs within a stem cell the mutated cell is carried through the normal process of differentiation creating various alterations in cellular development along the way. Figure 11.1 illustrates this effect in MAS.

MAS mutations may cause abnormalities in any or all tissues under the influence of Gsα (Weinstein et al. 1991; Weinstein and Shenker 1993; Shenker et al. 1993). Commonly affected include bone, skin, pituitary, thyroid, and gonadal organs. Mutations occurring early in development have the potential for significant disruption to all three layers, therefore affecting multiple tissues (widespread disease). Mutations emerging later in development establish limited disease. Germline *GNAS* mutations are believed to result in neonatal lethality (Happle 1986).

Table 11.1 Germ layer tissue development

Germ layer	Examples of tissue development
Ectoderm	Epidermis, pituitary gland, adrenal medulla, jaw
Mesoderm	Bone, reproductive organs, adrenal cortex
Endoderm	Thymus, thyroid, parathyroid glands, digestive tract, liver, pancreas, epithelial lining of respiratory, excretory and reproductive organs

Adapted from Tortora and Derrickson (2017)

11.3 MAS: Diagnostic Criteria, Differential Diagnosis, and Clinical Characteristics

Diagnosis is clinical, based on the presence of any combination of *two or more* of the following: skeletal (fibrous dysplasia), skin (café-au-lait macules), and endocrine abnormalities (Collins and Shenker 1999). Diagnostic imaging

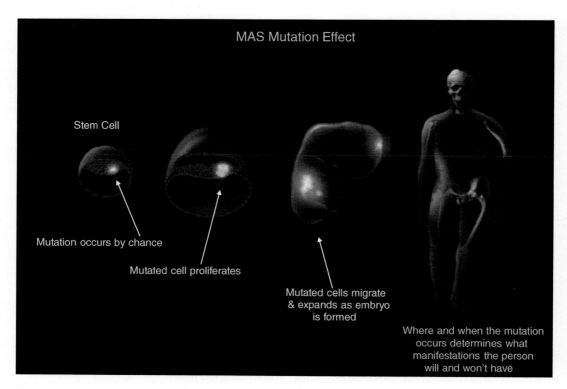

Fig. 11.1 MAS mutation effect (Dumitrescu and Collins 2008)

can also be used to diagnose and/or confirm FD or endocrine findings. Histological (i.e., biopsy) testing of *GNAS* may confirm a diagnosis but is not required. Genetic tests for mutation detection exist but are not routinely available; reliability of these tests depends on the degree of tissue mosaicism and sensitivity of technique (Agopiantz et al. 2016). Genetic testing is not required to establish a diagnosis, but may be useful when there is clinical uncertainty.

11.3.1 Differential Diagnosis

Differential diagnosis includes:

- Neurofibromatosis type I
- Osteofibrous dysplasia
- Non-ossifying fibromas
- Idiopathic central precocious puberty
- Osteogenesis imperfecta
- Ovarian neoplasm
- Cherubism

11.3.2 Clinical Characteristics: Bone, Skin, and Endocrine Abnormalities

Individuals usually present with at least two out of the three characteristics of bone, skin, and/or endocrine abnormalities. Bone lesions are the most common finding followed by café-au-lait macules, and endocrinopathies (Collins et al. 2012). Less common other manifestations include renal, liver, and pancreatic abnormalities but are not part of the diagnostic criteria (Agopiantz et al. 2016). Manifestations of the syndrome are usually evident by 5 years of age, but occasionally the diagnosis is made later in life. Understanding the clinical characteristics of MAS is important for diagnosis, management, and treatment.

11.3.2.1 Skeletal System: Fibrous Dysplasia

11.3.2.1.1 Characteristics and Features
Fibrous dysplasia (FD) is characterized by benign, scar-like (fibrotic) lesions in the bone.

Excess activation of Gsα generates an increased production and clustering of immature bone cells which limit hematopoietic cell action within the bone marrow (Riminucci et al. 2007). This process forms a weak abnormal fibrotic lesion that replaces normal bone. Due to poor infrastructure, these lesions are unable to provide optimal bone support or function which leads to weakness, deformities, and breaks. Clinical morbidities include fractures, disabilities, limps, and pain.

FD lesions do not usually present clinically or radiographically at birth (Boyce and Collins 2015). Diagnosis of FD in infancy is rare except in severely affected individuals with deformities or fractures. Within the first few years of life, FD lesions become more apparent due to bone expansion during linear growth in childhood. Lesion expansion is progressive through adolescence with a typical slowing into adulthood (Boyce and Collins 2015). The extent of FD disease can usually be determined by the age of 10 years, with no new clinically significant lesions emerging after the age of 15 years (Leet and Collins 2007). The one skeletal exception may be rib involvement (Kelly et al. 2008).

The timing of the mutation during embryogenesis dictates which bones are affected, the number of bones affected, and the extent of disease in affected bones. FD lesions may form in any one or all the bones of the human skeleton (Robinson et al. 2016). Lesions may occur in one bone (monostotic), multiple bones (polyostotic), or nearly every bone in the body (panostotic).

Clinical (physical exam) and radiologic evaluations are the most common methods of diagnosis of FD (Boyce and Collins 2015). Skeletal X-ray images best capture clinically evident lesions, whereas bone scans (99TcMDP or Sodium Fluoride (NaF)) best capture lesions that are not clinically obvious. In individuals age 6 and above, an initial bone scan is recommended to determine the extent of bone disease (Stanton et al. 2012). In children under age 6, radiographs may be used to determine extent of bone disease. A bone biopsy of a lesion may be done in cases where a diagnosis cannot be determined; however, it is not required for an FD diagnosis (Stanton et al. 2012). Figure 11.2 illustrates examples of FD bone disease on radiographic imaging (a, b, c, d) and bone

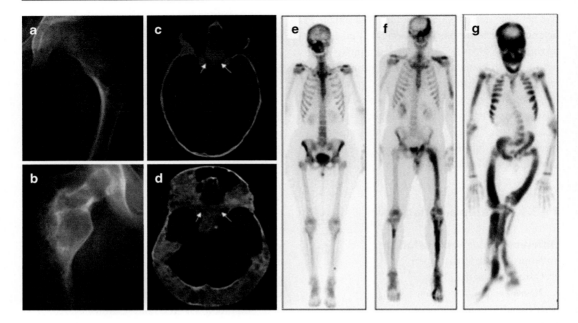

Fig. 11.2 FD bone disease on radiographic and nuclear medicine imaging, (Dumitrescu and Collins 2008)

scan images of three individuals with varying degrees of FD ((e) mild, (f) moderate, (g) severe), FD lesions appear as dark areas in the bones.

Identification of the specific bone(s) to which FD lesion(s) are present is important to establish and predict functional and mechanical effects. The most commonly affected are the skull and facial bones (~85%), pelvic (~57%), and femur (~56%) (Kelly et al. 2008). Skeletal bones are often classified together regionally as appendicular, axial, or craniofacial. Individuals may have lesions in one, two, or three of these areas. Important differences in FD features and characteristics exist for these regions.

11.3.2.2 Appendicular Fibrous Dysplasia

Appendicular lesions are found in the shoulder, pelvic, and long bones (i.e., arms, legs) of the skeleton. On physical exam, these bones may appear normal, especially in infants and young children. However, as the child grows, the bones may become more distorted with changes in contour and width size. On radiographs, appendicular lesions appear in the bone shaft as lytic or ground glass circumscribed lesions surrounded by a very thin bone cortex (Boyce and Collins

2015). Appendicular lesions expand within the bone cortex but do not cross out of the bone into other tissues (Hart et al. 2007). Expansion within the bone cortex may become quite large. Progressively through the age spectrum these lesions change in appearance becoming more sclerotic possibly due to slowing of bone activity (Boyce and Collins 2015; Leet and Collins 2007; Hart et al. 2007). Complications that arise from these lesions result in leg length discrepancies, deformities, and fractures (Leet et al. 2004).

11.3.2.3 Axial Fibrous Dysplasia

Axial lesions are located in the sternum, spine, and ribs. On radiographs they appear as cystic lesions within the bone cortex; they do not expand out of the bone (Collins et al. 2013). Lesions in the spine are a common finding (~63%) with scoliosis being the most significant clinical complication (Leet et al. 2004). Rib fractures with pain are common in adulthood (Kelly et al. 2008).

11.3.2.4 Craniofacial Fibrous Dysplasia

Craniofacial (CF) lesions are located in the skull, face, and/or jawbones. They are dense and hard fibrous tissue (Collins 2006). Initially these lesions present as small lumps or bumps on the head, cheekbone, or jaw bone. In infants, CF FD lesions may not be detected on exam; however, with growth they may become more evident. CF lesions are best characterized on computed tomography (CT) appearing as homogeneous ground glass tissue with expansile features (Lee et al. 2012). On radiographs they appear as sclerotic lesions (Akintoye et al. 2003). These lesions have the potential to expand and compress vital structures, most critically the cranial nerves (Lee et al. 2002; Cutler et al. 2006). Most complications that occur with CF FD are related to bone expansion. Fortunately, in the majority of individuals with optic nerve encasement, CF FD disease appears to remain stable without progressive optic neuropathy (Cutler et al. 2006). Unlike appendicular lesions, CF lesions may continue to progress through adulthood (Collins 2006).

11.3.3 Clinical Outcomes Associated with FD

11.3.3.1 Bone Pain
Bone pain is a common feature reported in up to 67% of the FD population (Kelly et al. 2008). Pain related to FD is hard to predict, is not well understood and does not directly correlate with the number of bone lesions or extent of disease (Kelly et al. 2008). The etiology of pain may be due to the lesion itself, fracture, phosphate wasting, or hypophosphatemia (Boyce and Collins 2015). Pain perception is individualized. Some individuals do not report bone pain and in those that do report pain, intensity varies from mild to severe. Children with FD report bone pain less frequently (49%) than adults (81%) (Kelly et al. 2008; Chapurlat et al. 2012). In children, FD does not typically present with pain unless associated with a fracture. Pain appears to become a more significant consequence starting in late adolescence. In adults FD bone pain is more likely, with lower extremity, rib, and spinal pain as the most common sites (Kelly et al. 2008). Headaches associated with CF FD appear to emerge in late adolescence and early adulthood, especially in patients with growth hormone excess (GHX) (Kelly et al. 2005).

11.3.3.2 Fractures
Pathologic fractures are a common feature of FD. Appendicular bones are the most common sites of fracture, with femoral fractures occurring most frequently in childhood. Long bone fractures most often occur between the ages of 6 and 10 years of age with a slowing into adulthood (Leet et al. 2004). Rib fractures occur frequently in adults but rarely occur in children (Hart et al. 2007). Individuals with hypophosphatemia are at higher risk for fractures (Leet et al. 2004). Fractures of the skull are rare.

11.3.3.3 Clinical Morbidities Associated with Fibrous Dysplasia
Alteration in normal bone growth causes clinical morbidities. In the appendicular bones, leg length discrepancy may become obvious during growth and is usually a sign of bone disease progression (Stanton et al. 2012). FD lesions located in the proximal femur frequently cause weakness, bowing, and changes to the femoral neck shaft angle, which results in two commonly known deformities: (1) Shepherd Crook deformity occurs when the femoral head of the bone bows outward as shown in Fig. 11.3a. (2) Windswept deformity occurs when the femur head bows inward, as shown in Fig. 11.3b.

FD lesions in the spine may lead to scoliosis with varying degrees of deformity. The prevalence rate of scoliosis is estimated at 40–52% (Leet et al. 2004). Respiratory compromise due to collapse of spine may occur which has led to death in few cases (Mancini et al. 2009). CF lesions initially appear as facial asymmetry with a small population progressing to disfigurement (Collins et al. 2013; Boyce and Collins 2015; Kelly et al. 2008; Lee et al. 2012). CF FD may also cause narrowing of the auditory canal, deformities of the jaw and cranial area, dentition changes, and facial deformities (Lee et al. 2012). A very small subset of individuals is at risk for partial or complete blindness or hearing loss due to compression of the cranial nerves (Lee et al. 2002; Boyce et al. 2013a). These risks are particularly significant in the setting of untreated GHX.

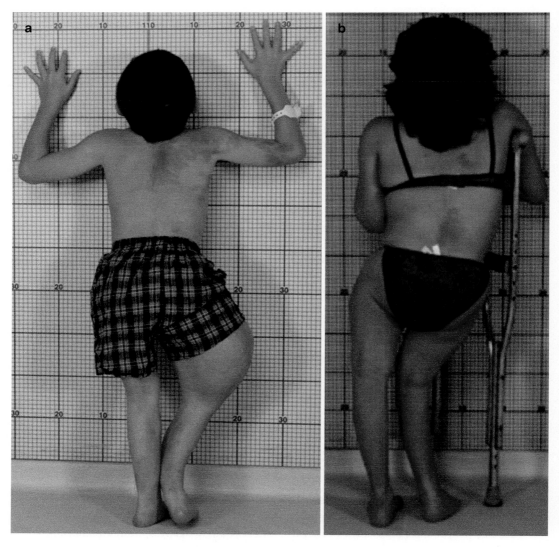

Fig. 11.3 (**a**) Shepherd Crook. (**b**) Windswept deformity. Copyright permission received from ENDOTEXT

11.3.3.4 Aneurysmal Bone Cysts

On occasion a rapidly expanding fluid-filled cyst known as an aneurysmal bone cyst forms in FD bone, often in the skull or long bones. Symptoms are acute with rapid onset of pain, increased size and deformity of bone. Aneurysmal bone cysts carry the potential for severe morbidity related to expansion into neighboring tissues. Although rare, there have been reports of sudden blindness due to a rapidly expanding skull cyst compressing the optic nerve (Lee et al. 2002, 2012). Aneurysmal bone cysts are considered emergent

and should be followed with immediate MRI and evaluation by a surgeon (Lee et al. 2012).

11.3.3.5 Psychosocial Impact on Quality of Life

FD is a complex bone disorder with the potential to affect physical as well as social aspects of life. Social and emotional functioning were studied and correlated to individual skeletal disease in a large FD population by Kelly et al. (2005). The data show that adult and children with FD report high levels of self-esteem and social function despite impaired physical function. Quality of life (QOL) parameters were equivalent to the normal (United States) population despite low physical scores, suggesting that individuals adapt well to their disease. Social data from the study indicates that affected individuals succeed at all levels of education and employment and perceive themselves as leading meaningful, productive lives (Kelly et al. 2005).

11.4   Integumentary System: Cafe-Au-Lait Macules

The Gsα mutation effect on the integumentary system results in the formation of light brown skin spots referred to as café-au-lait macules. These spots can also be identified by their irregularly shaped jagged borders, which bear resemblance to topographical areas of the United States

(i.e., "the coast of Maine"). Café-au-lait macules are not unique to MAS and are a very common finding among the general population.

Café-au-lait macules are present at birth and may be the first symptom in the diagnosis of MAS. However, some macules may be small, faint, or not easily visible, and can be missed on early assessment. These macules are uniquely individual with a wide variation in color, size, shape, and anatomical location. Macules frequently appear to start or end at a midpoint on the body. Some spots expand unilaterally down the body while others wrap entirely around the torso. Figure 11.4 illustrates the wide range in presentation of MAS-associated café-au-lait macules. Even though café-au-lait lesions are commonly located on the same side as bone involvement, skin and bone involvement do not necessarily correlate (Collins et al. 2012; Boyce and Collins 2015).

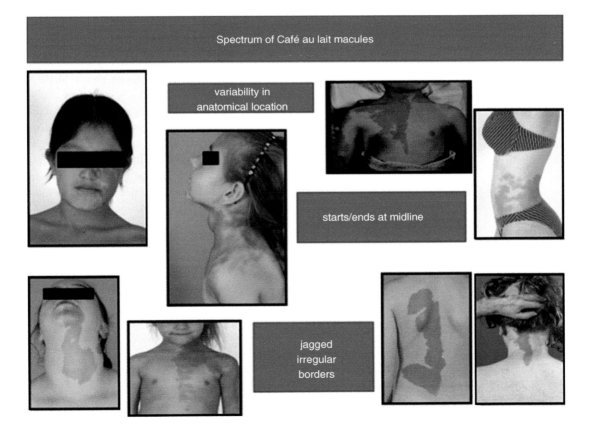

Fig. 11.4 Spectrum of Café-au-lait Macules (Leet and Collins 2007; Dumitrescu and Collins 2008; Collins et al. 2012)

11.5 Endocrine System: Endocrinopathies

Dysfunction of endocrine tissue is the result of altered signal transduction pathways responsible for regulating endocrine cell functions and bodily hormones. Overproduction of hormones alters the intrinsic pathways causing deleterious effects to organs. Any or all endocrine organs may be affected. Individuals may present with one or multiple endocrinopathies.

11.5.1 Gonadal Abnormalities

Gonadal abnormalities are common. Gonadotropin-independent precocious puberty arises from early activation of the gonads in both males and females. PP occurs in ~ 85% of the girls and ~10–15% of the boys with MAS (Boyce and Collins 2015). Manifestations of PP occur before age 8 in girls and before age 9 in boys.

In girls, intermittent autonomous activation of ovarian tissue produces high serum estradiol levels resulting in early vaginal bleeding, breast development and/or (recurrent) ovarian cysts (Boyce and Collins 2015; Foster et al. 1986). PP is often the first clinical symptom of MAS in infants and young girls. Symptoms such as vaginal bleeding, rapid breast development, and abdominal pain (ovarian pain) are usually concerning to the child and parents and often get the attention of a clinician.

In boys, autonomous testosterone production results in increased growth of testicles and/or penis, early sexual behavior/aggression, and/or growth of pubic and axillary hair. PP in boys sometimes goes undetected. Untreated PP in both males and females results in increased growth velocity and bone age advancement leading to a reduced final adult height. Occasionally a child with peripheral PP (with or without adequate treatment) will later develop central PP due to the early activation of the pituitary gland.

Gonadal involvement occurs at an approximate equal rate in both males and females (Boyce et al. 2012; Akintoye et al. 2013). Adult women may experience menstrual irregularities with or with-

out recurrent ovarian cysts (Foster et al. 1986). Ultrasounds of the ovaries often show benign ovarian cysts. Erratic functioning of ovaries may cause a delay in fertility for some women (Boyce and Collins 2015). Most women with MAS can become pregnant, maintain a viable pregnancy, and produce healthy offspring.

In adult males, testicular lesions interspersed with hyperplasia of the Leydig/sertoli cells (gonadal tissue) are commonly observed on ultrasound (Boyce et al. 2012). These lesions are not normally visible or palpable on exam and do not cause symptoms. Lesions may be associated with gonadotropin-independent PP and should be clinically correlated. Testicular lesions are usually benign; however, there have been rare cases that have emerged as malignant (Boyce et al. 2012).

11.5.2 Thyroid Abnormalities

Thyroid abnormalities include clinical hyperthyroidism (with and without goiter) and abnormal thyroid tissue with cysts and nodules. Hyperthyroidism occurs in approximately one-third of the population (Boyce and Collins 2015). The mutation causes sustained hypersecretion of thyroid hormones with cellular proliferation (Feuillan et al. 1990). Diagnosis of hyperthyroidism prior to the age of 5 is rare and primarily subclinical. Hyperthyroidism becomes more evident after the age of 5 but may remain undetected until laboratory tests or ultrasounds are performed to confirm disease (Boyce and Collins 2015). Young children rarely exhibit signs of hyperthyroidism. In older children and adults, common symptoms of hyperthyroidism include goiter, weight loss, sweating, nervousness, anxiety, and fatigue. Persistent hyperthyroidism is common and many individuals will eventually require a thyroidectomy (Boyce and Collins 2015).

Thyroid cysts and/or nodules observed on ultrasound (with or without hyperthyroidism) occur in approximately 54% of the MAS population (Boyce and Collins 2015). Measurement of serum thyroid levels should be performed to correlate thyroid function with ultrasound findings. Lesions appearing in the absence of hyperthyroidism are rarely symptomatic. There is slight risk of thyroid cancer in the MAS population therefore periodic follow-up with examination, laboratory tests, and ultrasound should be performed in the setting of abnormal ultrasound findings (Collins et al. 2003).

11.5.3 Pituitary Gland Abnormalities

Growth hormone excess occurs less frequently (~10–15%) than other endocrinopathies (Boyce and Collins 2015). Mutation effect results in unregulated production of excess growth hormone by the pituitary gland (Akintoye et al. 2002). Presentation is subtle, typically with subclinical findings until the age 7. The main symptoms include accelerated bone growth exhibited by increased height; significant increase in bone growth of the hands, feet, and head; and/or excessive sweating. Radiographic images may reveal "tufting" of fingers or toes. In the absence of clinical symptoms, diagnosis is based on laboratory and overnight serum growth hormone testing.

Untreated GHX in children may result in gigantism due to accelerated growth of the long bones before closure of growth plate. Individuals with GHX are at higher risk for certain morbidities due to the rapidly expanding and thickening bone. CF bone is most susceptible to GHX often causing asymmetry of the face with widened facial bones of the forehead, nose, and jaw. Thickened jaw bones may cause loosening of teeth and changes to dentition (Lee et al. 2012). In rare cases, rapid expansion in bone growth may cause impingement of cranial nerves, causing blindness and/or diminished hearing (Lee et al. 2012; Akintoye et al. 2002). Individuals with MAS and GHX are also at risk for hypertension and high cardiac output due the higher bone burden, which taxes the cardiovascular system (Collins et al. 2012). Rarely a benign pituitary tumor may be detected. In these cases, surgery is recommended which is typically curative (Boyce and Collins 2015).

11.5.4 Adrenal Abnormalities

Cushing's syndrome (neonatal hypercortisolism) is a rare complication of MAS and occurs almost exclusively during the first year of life. It is the result of bilateral autonomous neonatal adrenal hyperfunction caused by the Gsα mutation (Brown et al. 2010). Adrenal tissue manifests with diffuse nodular hyperplasia and cortical atrophy (Carney et al. 2011). Symptoms may be subtle to include moon or rounded face, low birth weight, and abnormal weight gain, especially in the face and trunk. Diabetes and hyperlipidemia may be present. Infants with Cushing's syndrome can become severely ill with the risk of death. Approximately half of MAS related cushing's syndrome cases have spontaneously resolved on their own (Boyce and Collins 2015).

11.6 Other Manifestations

11.6.1 Renal Effect

Phosphate wasting by the kidneys is a prevalent finding in up to 50% of the population, especially those with significant bone disease (Collins et al. 2001, 2012; Riminucci et al. 2003). The MAS mutation causes overproduction of fibroblast growth factor-23 (FGF23), a hormone responsible for regulating phosphorus in the kidneys (Riminucci et al. 2003). Increased levels of FGF23 trigger the kidney(s) to release extra phosphorus into the urine. This effect signals the bones to release additional phosphorus to the kidney. Constant recurrence of this cycle leads to osteomalacia/rickets of the bone (Robinson et al. 2016). Phosphate wasting may or may not lead to hypophosphatemia. Symptoms of phosphate wasting include bone pain, muscle weakness, and increased fractures (Boyce et al. 2013b).

11.6.2 Less Common Manifestations

Less common manifestations have been reported in the literature. These include various abnormal-

Table 11.2 Less common manifestations

Organ system	Manifestations
Liver	Hepatitis (infancy) and hepatic adenomas (Parvanescu et al. 2014)
Gastrointestinal	Gastroesophageal tract abnormalities (Wood et al. 2017) Gastrointestinal polyps (Zacharin et al. 2011)
Pancreas	Pancreatitis, intraductal papillary mucinous neoplasms (Gaujoux et al. 2014; Parvanescu et al. 2014; Wood et al. 2017)
Muscle	Intramuscular myxomas (Biazzo et al. 2017)

Adapted from Boyce and Collins (2015)

ities of the liver, gastrointestinal tract, pancreas, and musculature. Table 11.2 summarizes these findings.

Although rare, malignancies have been reported in association with MAS to include bone (Ruggieri et al. 1995), thyroid (Collins et al. 2003), testicle (Boyce et al. 2012), and breast (Majoor et al. 2018).

11.7　Age of Diagnosis

Diagnosis may occur anytime throughout the lifespan and is based on manifestations of the disease.

11.7.1　Infancy Presentation

Diagnosis shortly after birth is possible based on the presence of café-au-lait macules, Cushing's syndrome, and/or early vaginal bleeding. In females, early vaginal bleeding may be the first and only presenting symptom.

Case Scenario 1
A 12-month female presents with bloody discharge in her diaper. Physical exam findings include increased growth velocity of 14–15 cm per year (>95%), Tanner stage 2 breasts, and a large, light brown irregular bordered macule on posterior neck and chest. Bone age is advanced 2 years from chronological age.

Nursing Assessment: What MAS manifestations does this infant have? Would you anticipate further workup? If so, what other manifestations would you be looking for? What type of education would you provide to the family?

11.7.2　Childhood Presentation

Childhood is the most common time for diagnosis. Rapid growth coupled with high levels of physical activity contributes to identification of symptoms. Incidental findings of FD are commonly found on X-rays and/or other images. Bone features leading to diagnosis include abnormal gait with limp, signs of leg length discrepancy, and scoliosis. Pain is a rare first finding in children, however if present, imaging should be done to rule out fractures and/or any other bone abnormalities. Other findings include those related to endocrinopathies. PP with bleeding and/or breast development is often the first signs in girls. Attention should be made in children with accelerated growth which may indicate GHX, PP, or hyperthyroidism.

Case Scenario 2
A 7-year-old boy presents with a left femur mid-shaft fracture obtained while playing soccer. Radiographs show the fracture at the site of a bony lesion is described as "ground glass." Physical exam reveals two light brown jagged edged birthmarks near the crease of his buttocks that respect the midline and an increased testicular volume. Endocrine testing reveals high testosterone levels. Bone scan and X-rays show numerous, bilateral bone lesions in extremities and the skull; bone age is advanced by 3 years.

Nursing Assessment: What MAS manifestations does this child have? What germ layers would you predict were affected in embryogenesis? Which manifestations require follow-up?

Case Scenario 3
A 10-year-old girl presents to the emergency department with complaints of sudden decreased

vision in one eye. The ER physician notes some mild facial asymmetry. An MRI shows an extensive bony lesion surrounding the right orbit and a fluid-filled cyst compressing the right optic nerve. An ophthalmology exam reveals a pale optic disk. Uncorrected vision shows 20/500 vision on the right with normal vision on the left. Further evaluation reveals a small brown skin macule and tall stature. Routine bloodwork is normal.

Nursing Asssessment: Does this child meet the criteria for diagnosis of MAS? Why? If so, what manifestations does she exhibit? What manifestation would be the most critical to manage and how? What other endocrinopathy/ies should be ruled out?

11.7.3 Adulthood Presentation

Diagnosis of MAS in adulthood occurs mostly as the result of symptoms related to FD including fractures, pain, or an incidental finding on imaging. Initial findings of endocrine abnormalities are rare, but possible (e.g., thyroid).

11.8   MAS: Diagnostic Methods

A comprehensive initial evaluation should be done to establish a diagnosis and to determine the facets of disease. This should include a physical exam with medical history, blood and urine laboratory tests, and diagnostic imaging. Additional evaluations are required based on specific clinical findings.

11.8.1 Physical Exam and Medical History

A detailed clinical history coupled with a thorough physical exam are critical diagnostic tools in the establishment of a MAS diagnosis. In children, Tanner staging should be performed in addition to height, weight, and bone age on X-ray (captured on a growth chart). Common findings are indicated below.

Box 11.1 Physical Exam/Medical History

Manifestation	Common findings
BONE	• Limp or abnormal patterns of walking • Asymmetric overgrowth or deformity of bone(s) • Decreased vision or hearing • Decreased activities of daily living (ability) • Pain (note location and severity) • Growth chart—accelerated growth with bone age advancement
SKIN ENDOCRINE	• Variable size lesions, brown in color with jagged, irregular borders
Precocious puberty	• Advanced growth velocity • Advanced bone age • Short or tall stature • Reduced predicted final adult height • Advanced Tanner staging • **(Girls)** presence (or history) of vaginal bleeding, breast development, pubic hair • **(Boys)** pubic and axillary hair, increased testicular/penis size for age, early sexual behavior/aggression
Growth hormone excess	• Tall stature for age • Rapid increase in height • Enlarged hands and feet • Widened or expanded cranial/facial bones • Bone age advancement • Sweating
Hyperthyroidism	• Palpable nodules • Goiter • Accelerated growth on growth chart • Bone age advancement • Symptoms of hyperthyroidism
Cushing's syndrome	• Moon/round face • Low birth weight
OTHER	• Abnormal weight gain
Liver	• Symptoms of hepatitis (jaundice, etc.)
Gastrointestinal	• Complaints of gastroesophageal reflux • Pain
Pancreatitis	• Symptoms of pancreatitis
Myxomas	• Palpable mass in muscle

11.8.2 Laboratory Tests

Perform to assess general health, bone and endocrine abnormalities.

Box 11.2 Laboratory Tests

Test	Common results/rationale
Blood tests	
Routine (CBC, PT/PTT, chemistries)	• Hematological values within normal range • High alkaline phosphatase due to bone effect • Low phosphorus, calcium, and/or vitamin D if phosphate wasting is present • Abnormal chemistry values consistent with endocrine/bone organ effect (repeat testing or additional testing and/or imaging required) *Note: Not all abnormal laboratory values are indicative of MAS. Values should be correlated with clinical workup*
Endocrine	• Abnormal thyroid results support hyperthyroid diagnosis • Elevated cortisol (with hyperlipidemia) indicates Cushing's syndrome (neonates/early toddlerhood) • Elevated prolactin suggests pituitary tumor • Elevated luteinizing hormone, follicle stimulating hormone, testosterone, estrogen—perform further clinical workup for GHX and PP *Note: a single elevated GH with elevated IGF-1 requires further testing to determine source of GHX; a single GH value is not conclusive in the diagnosis of GHX*
Overnight serial serum test for hormonal axes (if GHX suspected)	• Non-suppressible GH levels indicate GHX
Bone and mineral blood tests (assess bone turnover, formation, resorption)	• Low ionized calcium with high PTH may indicate secondary hyperparathyroidism due to vitamin D deficiency • High alkaline phosphatase, bone specific alkaline phosphatase (BSAP) and osteocalcin (due to bone disease) *Note: BSAP is specific to bone disease; high BSAP levels indicate extensive bone disease; low BSAP indicate low bone disease*

Test	Common results/rationale
Urine tests	
Random urine and/or 24-h sample for: • Mineral metabolism (calcium, magnesium, phosphorous) • Cortisol • Bone turnover markers—N-telopeptide (NTX), pyridinoline, and deoxypyridinoline (24 h)	• High-normal levels of phosphate (urine) with low TMP-GFR indicate phosphate wasting • High cortisol levels in 24-h specimen indicate Cushing's syndrome • High bone turnover markers indicative of bone disease

11.8.3 Radiographic Imaging and Nuclear Medicine Bone Scans

Perform to assess bone and endocrine effect.

Box 11.3 Imaging

Test	Rationale	Common findings
Skeletal radiographs (limited or whole body)	Easy, quick, minimal risk	• Appendicular and axial lesions appear ground glass in bone shaft with thin cortex; fractures • Craniofacial lesions appear sclerotic
Bone age (children ≤18 years of age)	Provides bone growth information. Provides guidance in the treatment of bone growth and endocrinopathies	• Advanced bone age > 2 years could indicate PP, GHX, hyperthyroidism, pituitary tumor—further workup indicated
99TcMDP or NaF bone scan (≥ 5 years of age)	Determine extent of bone disease	• Increased tracer uptake in bones indicative of FD lesions or other bone abnormalities (fractures)

11.8.4 Additional Diagnostic Workup Based on Clinical Findings

Additional diagnostic workup should be done to characterize the extent of disease. Guidance for specific findings is provided below.

Box 11.4 Additional Diagnostic Workup

Clinical findings	Additional diagnostic/medical testing	Common findings
Craniofacial FD	• Computed tomography (skull)	CF FD lesions appear ground glass Aneurysmal bone cysts Pituitary gland adenomas Cranial nerve compression
	• Ophthalmology, audiology, otolaryngology examination and testing	Cranial nerve compression Narrowing of auditory canal Sinus narrowing/obliterations
	• Dental examination	Dentition and jaw abnormalities
	• Craniofacial surgical exam (if needed)	
Appendicular FD	• Rehabilitation medicine • Physical therapy • Occupational therapy (as needed) • Pain consultation (as needed) • Orthopedic consultation (as needed)	Abnormalities in function and mobility (range-of-motion, activities of daily living, gait)
Scoliosis	• Scoliosis radiographs • Pulmonary function test to assess lung volume/parameters • Rehabilitation medicine evaluation • Orthopedic consultation (as needed)	Lesions in the spine, varying degrees of curve angle Diminished lung volume Abnormalities in gait, posture, function
Rib fractures/rib abnormalities	• Chest radiographs • Bone scan • Rehabilitation medicine evaluation • Pain consultation (as needed)	Rib fractures/abnormal growth Abnormalities in gait, posture, function Rib pain
Growth hormone excess	• Serial blood testing (growth hormone suppression test, growth hormone stimulation test) • MRI pituitary, to identify pituitary adenoma • Echocardiogram to evaluate cardiac output	Increased height and bone age advancement Hands/feet show tufting on imaging GH does not suppress Pituitary adenoma Note: IGF-1 blood test should be used to monitor treatment effect in GHX Abnormal cardiac results
Thyroid disease	• Thyroid ultrasound, if abnormal lab tests/ultrasound	Tissue appears swiss cheese like with cystic and solid lesions embedded in normal tissue
Precocious puberty/ gonadal abnormalities (female)	• Ovarian (bilateral) pelvic ultrasound	Ovarian cysts (recurrent) Large or mature uterus for girls Thickened endometrial tissue *Note: Ultrasound abnormalities may or may not correlate to clinical symptoms*
Precocious puberty/ gonadal abnormalities (male)	• Testicular (bilateral) ultrasound	Hyperechoic and hypoechoic lesions interspersed with hyperplastic testicular tissue *Note: Ultrasound abnormalities may or may not correlate to clinical symptoms*

(continued)

Box 11.4   (continued)

Clinical findings	Additional diagnostic/medical testing	Common findings

Cushing's syndrome	• 24-h urine collection for free cortisol
	• Low-dose dexamethasone suppression test (measures AM serum level)
	• Diurnal serum or salivary cortisol test
	• Additional tests to determine the source of tumor (pituitary or adrenal):
	  – ACTH blood test
	  – MRI (pituitary)
	  – CT (adrenals)
		High cortisol levels

Pancreatic abnormalities	Laboratory tests	Elevated amylase + lipase
	MRI abdomen/MRCP with contrast	Pancreatic pathology
Gastrointestinal abnormalities	Endoscopy/colonoscopy	Gastroesophageal reflux Polyps

11.9   MAS: Management and Treatment

MAS is a complex disorder with many manifestations. There is no treatment or cure for MAS. Clinical intervention requires a multidisciplinary team experienced in endocrine, orthopedics, pain management, and rehabilitation. After the initial evaluation, clinical evaluations should occur at regular intervals to assess, manage, and treat manifestations.

In children, a comprehensive yearly evaluation with repeat testing related to diagnosed or suspected bone and/or endocrine disease is recommended (Boyce and Collins 2015; Stanton et al. 2012). Attention to CF FD, GHX, and/or scoliosis should be made due to the high risk for morbidities; frequent interval consultations with appropriate specialists are prudent. Into adolescence and adulthood, gonadal and thyroid abnormalities warrant frequent (1–2 year) imaging for progression of disease and possibility of malignancy, which is rare (Boyce and Collins 2015). Those with GHX should be monitored frequently for changes in vision, hearing, and/or cardiovascular issues. Successful management of symptoms may be achieved through established therapies, treatments, and/or surgeries which enhance overall well-being, improve physical function, and ameliorate clinical symptoms.

Management and treatment is based on presenting manifestations.

11.9.1   Café-Au-Lait Macules: Management

There is no cure or treatment for café-au-lait macules. Methods to diminish lesion color and size have not been effective (Collins et al. 2012). Cosmetic makeup may help to temporarily diminish lesion color.

11.9.2   Fibrous Dysplasia: Management and Treatment

There are no proven medical treatments and/or therapies that eradicate or alter FD lesions. Management efforts are focused on optimizing physical function while minimizing morbidities. In the absence of pain, fracture, or deformity, frequent clinical observation with interval radiograph imaging is sufficient for the management of FD bone disease over time (Stanton et al. 2012). Bone scans ($\geq$ age 6) may be repeated in 3–5 year intervals to monitor bone disease throughout childhood (Stanton et al. 2012). Into adulthood repeat bone scan images may not be needed if disease is stable. Throughout the life spectrum, CF and axial FD lesion progression are best followed by radiographs and conservative use of CT imaging.

11.9.3 FD: Preventative and Therapeutic Measures

Early identification of bone involvement is the key to understanding the effect of the disease on bone. With knowledge of bone location and extent of disease, functional impact is better anticipated and predicted to identify preventative measures aimed at lowering overall morbidity.

Prophylactic non-weight bearing activities is *not recommended* in the absence of pain, fractures, or deformities (Stanton et al. 2012). Active, natural, low risk movement based on individual ability should be encouraged and optimized by all. Routine muscle conditioning and strengthening is also important for bone support (Paul et al. 2014). Individuals should be encouraged to participate in activities with low risk of injury to bones such as swimming or stationary biking to avoid fractures and other injuries (Paul et al. 2014). Those with moderate or severe appendicular and/or axial FD should be instructed to minimize or eliminate contact sports and other high-risk activities (e.g., horseback riding, skiing).

Individuals with appendicular and axial FD should be evaluated by rehabilitation medicine as early as possible to assess overall function and mobility. Those with appendicular FD are at risk for limb length discrepancies, deformities, and fracture. Those with spinal FD are at risk for progression of scoliosis. Routine physical therapy can minimize pain and enhance mobility (Paul et al. 2014). Physical therapists should develop individualized plans to include exercises for proper movement and form as well as those to increase muscle strength. Dependent on the involved bone(s), equipment such as canes, walkers, and wheelchairs may be recommended as preventative or therapeutic measures for individuals with lower extremity disease (Paul et al. 2014). Physical supports such as customized orthotics or shoe lifts can easily correct leg length differences or assist with hip/pelvis malalignment (Paul et al. 2014). In addition to physical therapy, individuals may benefit from a consultation with an occupational therapist if FD disease interferes with their ability to carry out functions of daily living and/or performance in a job or school. Nurses can encourage and assist individuals in finding accessory aids and developing functional plans to meet their specific needs to achieve optimal function.

11.9.4 FD: Surgical Management

11.9.4.1 Appendicular FD

In the setting of fractures and/or deformities, surgical intervention is required (Stanton et al. 2012). Surgical intervention is challenging and should be performed by a surgeon experienced working with FD bone. Traditional orthopedic techniques such as bone grafting and curettage of FD lesions have proven ineffective due to regeneration and regrowth of dysplastic bone lesion (Boyce and Collins 2015). Similarly, standard screws and plates have been found ineffective due to the soft consistency of the FD bone (Leet and Collins 2007; Stanton et al. 2012). External fixation devices and bracing have also proven ineffective (Boyce and Collins 2015). Closed management systems such as casting and conventional surgical procedures have proven suitable for limited situations of FD including non-weight bearing upper limb lesions as well as monostotic lesions located in other bones (Stanton et al. 2012). Treatment with these modalities warrants careful clinical monitoring to ensure proper alignment of the newly formed dysplastic bone.

Internal fixation devices, specifically intramedullary (IM) devices, have been shown to be the most effective as corrective surgical treatment particularly for weight bearing bones, as these devices provide additional support to strengthen the weakened bone (Stanton et al. 2012). In individuals with upper limb weight bearing ability (i.e., crutches), internal fixation is useful. Despite surgical corrective measures, recurrent fractures and deformities of the surgically corrected bones may still occur requiring individuals to have multiple surgeries.

11.9.4.2 Axial FD

Progression of scoliosis can be stopped by surgical fusion in effort to prevent morbid outcomes (Stanton and Diamond 2007).

11.9.4.3 CF FD

Surgical management of CF FD is often difficult due to lesion location and expansile features. In the setting of CF FD, a craniofacial surgeon with expertise in FD should be consulted prior to surgery. In most instances, FD lesions cannot be fully excised, there is a 68% probability of regrowth of partially resected lesions (Boyce et al. 2016). In individuals with GHX, regrowth incidence increases to 88% (Boyce et al. 2016). The most common indication for surgery is debulking of bone. Other indications include the removal of aneurysmal bone cysts and correction of jaw malformations. Optic canal encasement, a common feature, should be conservatively managed as the risk of blindness from surgery is high (Cutler et al. 2006; Lee et al. 2002). The benefits of CF surgery should be carefully measured against the potential outcomes of surgery.

11.9.5 FD: Pain Management

There is no medical treatment or therapy that permanently eradicates FD bone pain. Several treatments are effective in managing pain including non-pharmaceutical and pharmaceutical options. Non-pharmaceutical therapies include the use of heat, gentle massage, acupuncture, and biofeedback. Pharmaceutical treatments include the use of over-the-counter (OTC) pain relievers, bisphosphonates, and narcotic medications. OTC pain relievers such as acetaminophen, ibuprofen, and naproxen are the most commonly used and the most effective treatment for mild to moderate FD bone pain (Kelly et al. 2008). OTC pain relievers may also be combined with non-pharmaceutical therapies to enhance pain relief.

For severe pain, intravenous (IV) bisphosphonates such as pamidronate or zoledronate can be used for pain relief in the appendicular and axial skeleton. The pharmacological action of bisphosphonates is aimed at reducing bone turnover and has been proven effective in reducing bone pain (Boyce et al. 2014). One dose of IV bisphosphonate provides a longer duration of pain relief than OTCs with effects usually lasting several months. Bisphosphonate intervals should be scheduled based on pain (Boyce 2000). There are a few significant side effects of IV bisphosphonate treatment. A common first administration reaction may occur resulting in a "flu-like" reaction with chills, fever, and general ill-feeling. To avoid this reaction, individuals should be pre-medicated with a non-steroidal anti-inflammatory drug (NSAID) treatment before the first administration. Most individuals tolerate repeat IV bisphosphonate therapy without reaction. A long-term serious side effect of this drug class is osteonecrosis of the jaw. The incidence of development of osteonecrosis of the jaw in the FD population is unknown but appears infrequent (Boyce and Collins 2015). Individuals should have a thorough dental hygiene exam to address any dental abnormalities (i.e., cavities, extractions, root canal) before starting treatment and should be monitored routinely while receiving therapy. If OTC pain relievers and bisphosphonates are not effective, narcotic medications may be considered as a last option. A pain consultant should be sought in these cases.

11.9.6 Endocrinopathies: Management and Treatment

The goal of treatment is to control hormone overproduction and minimize target organ effects. Treatment for endocrinopathies should be individualized based on organ involvement. Standard medical treatment can ameliorate and/or manage endocrinopathies associated with MAS.

11.9.7 Phosphate Wasting: Management and Treatment

The goal of treatment is to control phosphorus retention by the kidney. Treatment includes the use of oral phosphate supplement and active vitamin D (Boyce et al. 2013b).

11.10 Psychosocial Considerations of FD/MAS: Management and Treatment

11.10.1 Parental Considerations

A significant finding among parents with children diagnosed with FD/MAS is that they suffer more emotionally than the child himself, and more emotionally than parents without a chronic illness (Kelly et al. 2005). These parental reactions are like those observed in parents with children that have similar other chronic illnesses (i.e., asthma or rheumatoid arthritis). Parental reactions may be of concern, fear, worry, and/or a sense of being overwhelmed. Nurses should make every effort to reassure parents that despite physical impairments children and adults with MAS appear to adjust and cope well with their medical condition. Individuals with MAS have been shown to be fully capable of succeeding in education and employment (Kelly et al. 2005). Factual information should be provided to child and family. Discussions related to bone and endocrine disease should emphasize a realistic prognosis highlighting appropriate supports, medical management plans, and treatment. Parents should be empowered to become advocates for their child. Families should be encouraged to connect with local, regional, and international FD and MAS support groups.

11.10.2 Genetic Education

Parents should be educated and reassured that MAS is non-heritable; there are no instances of vertical transmission of MAS (Happle 1986; Boyce and Collins 2015; Boyce 2000). Emphasis should be made that neither parent passed the mutation onto the child. Parents should be informed that siblings have the same probability of acquiring MAS as the general public (Boyce and Collins 2015; Boyce 2000). Individuals with MAS should be reassured that the mutation cannot be passed on to the offspring of an affected individual.

11.10.3 Adjustment/Management of MAS

MAS is a complex disorder. Understanding the various facets and management of disease may be a challenge for parents as well as individuals. Clinicians should provide clear instructions as well as rationale for diagnoses, tests, evaluations, and therapies/treatments. Written information for both the parent and child (age appropriate) should be provided. Parents and children (age appropriate) should be involved in the decision-making and should be encouraged to keep copies of their medical records at home.

For individuals with moderate-severe FD, a change in physical activity may be warranted. Clinical recommendation may include having a child change his current activity from high impact (i.e., soccer) to low impact (i.e., swimming). In some individuals, preventative measures may require assistive equipment including wheelchair, crutch, or cane use. In both situations, parents may have difficulty psychologically adjusting to this change, even more so than the child (Kelly et al. 2005). Despite the psychological difficulty, parents should be supported and strongly encouraged to move toward these changes to avoid future physical complications for their child. Nurses can play an active role in providing recommendations for activities based on the child's and parent's interest. Physical activity, even with supports, should be encouraged within the individual's ability.

11.11 Conclusions

MAS is a complicated disease that may present a complex clinical picture to those not familiar with the syndrome. Due to the multiple facets of the disease, individual presentation is unique; no two individuals present with the same clinical features. Individual prognosis is contingent upon an early accurate diagnosis followed by long-term management. Diagnosis is dependent upon identification of the clinical signs and symptoms related to fibrous dysplasia, café-au-lait macules, and endocrinopathies, particularly in infancy and childhood. A comprehensive initial evaluation should include detailed assessments, evaluations, laboratory tests, and radiologic imaging to define the manifestations of the disease. Long-term management involves routine interval follow-up for identified endocrine or bone abnormalities. Clinical interventions are aimed at minimizing potential adverse outcomes related to bone and endocrine disease. Management of fibrous dysplasia includes therapies for pain control coupled with surgical and rehabilitation interventions. Management of endocrinopathies is accomplished with standard medical therapies and surgical interventions. Even though adults and children with MAS appear well adjusted and live productive lives, parents of children with MAS are emotionally affected by the disease and may need additional support. Successful management of the disease is possible with medical and nursing care which is individually tailored.

References

Agopiantz M, Journeau P, Lebon-Labich B, Sorlin A, Cuny T, Weryha G, et al. McCune-Albright syndrome, natural history and multidisciplinary management in a series of 14 pediatric cases. Ann Endocrinol. 2016;77(1):7–13.

Akintoye SO, Chebli C, Booher S, Feuillan P, Kushner H, Leroith D, et al. Characterization of gsp-mediated growth hormone excess in the context of McCune-Albright syndrome. J Clin Endocrinol Metab. 2002;87(11):5104–12.

Akintoye SO, Lee JS, Feimster T, Booher S, Brahim J, Kingman A, et al. Dental characteristics of fibrous dysplasia and McCune-Albright syndrome. Oral Surg Oral Med Oral Pathol Oral Radiol Endod. 2003;96(3):275–82.

Akintoye SO, Boyce AM, Collins MT. Dental perspectives in fibrous dysplasia and McCune–Albright syndrome. Oral Surg Oral Med Oral Pathol Oral Radiol. 2013;116(3):149–55.

Albright FBA, Hampton AO, Smith P. Syndrome characterized by osteitis fibrosa disseminata, areas of pigmentation, and endocrine dysfunction with precocious puberty in females: report of 5 cases. N Engl J Med. 1937;216:727–46.

Biazzo A, Di Bernardo A, Parafioriti A, Confalonieri N. Mazabraud syndrome associated with McCune-Albright syndrome: a case report and review of the literature. Acta Biomed. 2017;88(2):198–200.

Boyce AM. Fibrous dysplasia. In: De Groot LJ, Chrousos G, Dungan K, Feingold KR, Grossman A, Hershman JM, et al., editors. Endotext. South Dartmouth, MA: MDText.com; 2000.

Boyce AM, Collins MT. Fibrous dysplasia/McCune HYP Albright syndrome. In: Pagon RA, Adam MP, Ardinger HH, Wallace SE, Amemiya A, Bean LJH, et al., editors. GeneReview. Seattle, WA: University of Washington; 2015.

Boyce AM, Chong WH, Shawker TH, Pinto PA, Linehan WM, Bhattacharryya N, et al. Characterization and management of testicular pathology in McCune-Albright syndrome. J Clin Endocrinol Metab. 2012;97(9):E1782–90.

Boyce AM, Glover M, Kelly MH, Brillante BA, Butman JA, Fitzgibbon EJ, et al. Optic neuropathy in McCune-Albright syndrome: effects of early diagnosis and treatment of growth hormone excess. J Clin Endocrinol Metab. 2013a;98(1):E126–34.

Boyce AM, Bhattacharyya N, Collins MT. Fibrous dysplasia and fibroblast growth factor-23 regulation. Curr Osteoporos Rep. 2013b;11(2):65–71.

Boyce AM, Kelly MH, Brillante BA, Kushner H, Wientroub S, Riminucci M, et al. A randomized, double blind, placebo-controlled trial of alendronate treatment for fibrous dysplasia of bone. J Clin Endocrinol Metab. 2014;99(11):4133–40.

Boyce AM, Burke A, Cutler Peck C, DuFresne CR, Lee JS, Collins MT. Surgical management of polyostotic craniofacial fibrous dysplasia: long-term outcomes and predictors for postoperative regrowth. Plast Reconstr Surg. 2016;137(6):1833–9.

Brown RJ, Kelly MH, Collins MT. Cushing syndrome in the McCune-Albright syndrome. J Clin Endocrinol Metab. 2010;95(4):1508–15.

Carney JA, Young WF, Stratakis CA. Primary bimorphic adrenocortical disease: cause of hypercortisolism in McCune-Albright syndrome. Am J Surg Pathol. 2011;35(9):1311–26.

Chapurlat R, Gensburger D, Jimenez-Andrade J, Ghilardi J, Kelly MH, Mantyh P. Pathophysiology and medical treatment of pain in fibrous dysplasia of bone. Orphanet J Rare Dis. 2012;7:S3.

Collins MT. Spectrum and natural history of fibrous dysplasia of bone. J Bone Miner Res. 2006;21(Suppl 2):99–104.

Collins MT, Shenker A. McCune HYP Albright syndrome: new insights. Curr Opin Endocrinol Diabetes. 1999;6:119–25.

Collins MT, Chebli C, Jones J, Kushner H, Consugar M, Rinaldo P, et al. Renal phosphate wasting in fibrous dysplasia of bone is part of a generalized renal tubular dysfunction similar to that seen in tumor-induced osteomalacia. J Bone Miner Res. 2001;16(5):806–13.

Collins MT, Sarlis NJ, Merino MJ, Monroe J, Crawford SE, Krakoff JA, et al. Thyroid carcinoma in the McCune-Albright syndrome: contributory role of activating Gs alpha mutations. J Clin Endocrinol Metab. 2003;88(9):4413–7.

Collins MT, Singer FR, Eugster E. McCune-Albright syndrome and the extraskeletal manifestations of fibrous dysplasia. Orphanet J Rare Dis. 2012;7(Suppl 1):S4.

Collins MT, Riminucci M, Bianco P. Fibrous dysplasia. In: Rosen CJ, editor. Primer on the metabolic bone diseases and disorders of mineral metabolism. 8th ed. Ames, IA: Wiley-Blackwell; 2013. p. 786–91.

Cutler CM, Lee JS, Butman JA, FitzGibbon EJ, Kelly MH, Brillante B, et al. Long-term outcome of optic nerve encasement and optic nerve decompression in patients with fibrous dysplasia: risk factors for blindness and safety of observation. Neurosurgery. 2006;59(5):1011–7.

Dumitrescu CE, Collins MT. McCune-Albright syndrome. Orphanet J Rare Dis. 2008;3:12.

Feuillan P, Shawker T, Rose S, Jones J, Jeevanram RK, Nisula BC. Thyroid abnormalities in the McCune-Albright syndrome: ultrasonography and hormonal studies. J Clin Endocrinol Metab. 1990;71(6):1596–601.

Foster CM, Feuillan P, Padmanabhan V, Pescovitz OH, Beitins IZ, Comite F, et al. Ovarian function in girls with McCune-Albright syndrome. Pediatr Res. 1986;20(9):859–63.

Gaujoux S, Salenave S, Ronot M, Rangheard AS, Cros J, Belghiti J, et al. Hepatobiliary and pancreatic neoplasms in patients with McCune-Albright syndrome. J Clin Endocrinol Metab. 2014;99(1):E97–101.

Happle R. The McCune HYP Albright syndrome: a lethal gene suviving by mosaicism. Clin Genet. 1986;29(4):321–4.

Hart ES, Kelly MH, Brillante B, Chen CC, Ziran N, Lee JS, et al. Onset, progression, and plateau of skeletal lesions in fibrous dysplasia and the relationship to functional outcome. J Bone Miner Res. 2007;22(9):1468–74.

Kelly MH, Brillante B, Kushner H, Gehron Robey P, Collins MT. Physical function is impaired but quality of life preserved in patients with fibrous dysplasia of bone. Bone. 2005;37(3):388–94.

Kelly MH, Brillante B, Collins MT. Pain in fibrous dysplasia of bone: age-related changes and the anatomical distribution of skeletal lesions. Osteoporos Int. 2008;19(1):57–63.

Lee JS, FitzGibbon E, Butman JA, Dufresne CR, Kushner H, Wientroub S, et al. Normal vision despite narrowing of the optic canal in fibrous dysplasia. N Engl J Med. 2002;347(21):1670–6.

Lee JS, FitzGibbon EJ, Chen YR, Kim HJ, Lustig LR, Akintoye SO, et al. Clinical guidelines for the management of craniofacial fibrous dysplasia. Orphanet J Rare Dis. 2012;7(Suppl 1):S2.

Leet AI, Collins MT. Current approach to fibrous dysplasia of bone and McCune-Albright syndrome. J Child Orthop. 2007;1(1):3–17.

Leet AI, Chebli C, Kushner H, Chen CC, Kelly MH, Brillante BA, et al. Fracture incidence in polyostotic fibrous dysplasia and the McCune-Albright syndrome. J Bone Miner Res. 2004;19(4):571–7.

Majoor BC, Boyce AM, Bovee JV, Smit VT, Collins MT, Cleton-Jansen AM, et al. Increased risk of breast cancer at a young age in women with fibrous dysplasia. J Bone Miner Res. 2018;33(1):84–90.

Mancini F, Corsi A, De Maio F, Riminucci M, Ippolito E. Scoliosis and spine involvement in fibrous dysplasia of bone. Eur Spine J. 2009;18(2):196–202.

McCune DJ. Osteitis fibrosa cystica: the case of a nine year old girl who also exhibits precocious puberty, multiple pigmentation of the skin and hyperthyroidism. Am J Dis Child. 1936;52:743–4.

Parvanescu A, Cros J, Ronot M, Hentic O, Grybek V, Couvelard A, et al. Lessons from McCune-Albright syndrome-associated intraductal papillary mucinous neoplasms: GNAS-activating mutations in pancreatic carcinogenesis. JAMA Surg. 2014;149(8):858–62.

Paul SM, Gabor LR, Rudzinski S, Giovanni D, Boyce AM, Kelly MR, et al. Disease severity and functional factors associated with walking performance in polyostotic fibrous dysplasia. Bone. 2014;60:41–7.

Riminucci M, Collins MT, Fedarko NS, Cherman N, Corsi A, White KE, et al. FGF-23 in fibrous dysplasia of bone and its relationship to renal phosphate wasting. J Clin Invest. 2003;112(5):683–92.

Riminucci M, Robey PG, Bianco P. The pathology of fibrous dysplasia and the McCune-Albright syndrome. Pediatr Endocinol Rev. 2007;4(Supplement 4):401–11.

Robinson C, Collins MT, Boyce AM. Fibrous dysplasia/McCune-Albright syndrome: clinical and translational perspectives. Curr Osteoporos Rep. 2016;14(5):178–86.

Ruggieri P, Sim FH, Bond JR, Unni KK. Osteosarcoma in a patient with polyostotic fibrous dysplasia and Albright's syndrome. Orthopedics. 1995;18(1):71–5.

Shenker A, Weinstein LS, Moran A, Pescovitz OH, Charest NJ, Boney CM, et al. Severe endocrine and nonendocrine manifestations of the McCune-Albright syndrome associated with activating mutations of stimulatory G protein GS. J Pediatr. 1993;123(4):509–18.

Stanton RP, Diamond L. Surgical management of fibrous dysplasia in McCune-Albright syndrome. Pediatr Endocinol Rev. 2007;4(Supplement 4):446–52.

Stanton RP, Ippolito E, Springfield D, Lindaman L, Wientroub S, Leet A. The surgical management of fibrous dysplasia of bone. Orphanet J Rare Dis. 2012;7(Suppl 1):S1.

Tortora GJ, Derrickson BH. Principles of anatomy & physiology. 15th ed. New York: Wiley; 2017. p. 658–60. 1107–1126.

Weinstein LS, Shenker A. G protein mutations in human disease. Clin Biochem. 1993;26(5):333–8.

Weinstein LS, Shenker A, Gejman PV, Merino MJ, Friedman E, Spiegel AM. Activating mutations of the stimulatory G protein in the McCune-Albright syndrome. N Engl J Med. 1991;325:1688–95.

Wood LD, Noe M, Hackeng W, Brosens LA, Bhaijee F, Debeljak M, et al. Patients with McCune-Albright syndrome have a broad spectrum of abnormalities in the gastrointestinal tract and pancreas. Virchows Arch. 2017;470(4):391–400.

Zacharin M, Bajpai A, Chow CW, Catto-Smith A, Stratakis C, Wong MW, et al. Gastrointestinal polyps in McCune Albright syndrome. J Med Genet. 2011;48(7):458–61.

Key Reading

1. Boyce AM, Collins MT. Fibrous dysplasia/McCune HYP Albright syndrome. In: Pagon RA, Adam MP, Ardinger HH, Wallace SE, Amemiya A, Bean LJH, et al., editors. GeneReview. Seattle, WA: University of Washington; 2015.

2. Collins MT, Singer FR, Eugster E. McCune-Albright syndrome and the extraskeletal manifestations of fibrous dysplasia. Orphanet J Rare Dis. 2012;7(Suppl 1):S4.

3. Chapurlat R, Gensburger D, Jimenez-Andrade J, Ghilardi J, Kelly MH, Mantyh P. Pathophysiology and medical treatment of pain in fibrous dysplasia of bone. Orphanet J Rare Dis. 2012;7:S3.

4. Kelly MH, Brillante B, Kushner H, Gehron Robey P, Collins MT. Physical function is impaired but quality of life preserved in patients with fibrous dysplasia of bone. Bone. 2005;37(3):388–94.

5. Robinson C, Collins MT, Boyce AM. Fibrous dysplasia/McCune-Albright syndrome: clinical and translational perspectives. Curr Osteoporos Rep. 2016;14(5):178.

Part III

Hypothalamus and Pituitary

Christine Yedinak and Judith P. van Eck

Anatomy and Physiology of the Hypothalamic-Piuitary Axis

12

Kathryn Evans Kreider

Contents

Abstract

The pituitary gland is a small gland located in the sella turcica, a cavity in the base of the brain. The pituitary gland measures less than 1 cm and weighs less than 1 g but is responsible for maintaining critical homeostatic functions that sustain life. Almost all of the functions of the pituitary are regulated by input from the hypothalamus, and the two glands are connected through the hypophyseal

(pituitary) stalk. The pituitary has 3 lobes—anterior (adenophyophysis), posterior (neurohypophysis), and intermediate (pars intermedia) lobe. The anterior, intermediate, and posterior sections of the pituitary act synergistically and are independently functional, each section producing different hormones and regulatory processes. The anterior pituitary produces six hormones in peptide form, including thyroid stimulating hormone (TSH), corticotropin or adrenocorticotrophic hormone (ACTH), follicle stimulating hormone (FSH), lutenizing hormone (LH), growth hormone (GH), and prolactin (PRL). All of the anterior pituitary hormones except PRL act by

K. E. Kreider (✉)
Duke University School of Nursing and Duke University Medical Center, Durham, NC, USA
e-mail: kathryn.evans@duke.edu

© Springer Nature Switzerland AG 2019
S. Llahana et al. (eds.), *Advanced Practice in Endocrinology Nursing*,
https://doi.org/10.1007/978-3-319-99817-6_12

stimulating other glands to release additional hormones. The release and production of these hormones is controlled through a classic feedback loop. The posterior lobe of the pituitary, also known as the neurohypophysis, secretes oxytocin and anti-diuretic hormone (ADH), also known as vasopressin. Release of the posterior pituitary hormones is regulated by neuronal activity.

Disruption to the pituitary gland may cause dysregulation to hormone production or secretion. The etiology of dysregulation is varied but the majority of dysfunction is related to the presence of a pituitary tumor or adenoma. However, hypopituitarism may be congenital, caused by an unrelated illness, injury and in some cases is the result of treatment for other diseases. Patients may present with a wide range of pathophysiologic symptoms, including bone growth disruption, infertility, galactorrhea, muscle wasting, headaches, fatigue, poor blood pressure homeostasis, or disruption to normal fluid balance. Patients with pituitary diseases often require lifelong treatment and require intense education regarding their disease and treatment, management of comorbidities and psychological support.

Advances in medicine now allow replacement of all pituitary deficiencies so that patients, even with panhypopituitarism, have the potential to lead a full and productive life. Early detection and appropriate medical therapies for all pituitary dysfunctions are critical.

Keywords

Anterior pituitary · Posterior pituitary Infundibulum · Neurohypophysis · Pituitary hormones

Abbreviations

ACTH	Adrenocorticotropic hormone
ADH	Anti-diuretic hormone
AP	Anterior pituitary
FSH	Follicle stimulating hormone
GH	Growth hormone
GIH	Growth hormone inhibiting hormone/somatostatin
GRH	Growth hormone releasing hormone
LH	Luteinizing hormone
POMC	Pro-opiomelanocortin
PP	Posterior pituitary
PRL	Prolactin
TRH	Thyroid releasing hormone
TSH	Thyroid stimulating hormone

Key Terms

- **Hypophyseal-portal circulation**: The circulatory system connecting the hypothalamus and pituitary gland.
- **Anterior pituitary**: The front lobes of the pituitary gland, responsible for secreting TSH, LH, FSH, PRL, GH, and ACTH.
- **Posterior pituitary:** The rear lobes of the pituitary, responsible for producing ADH and oxytocin.
- **Thyroid stimulating hormone**: The hormone responsible for the secretion of free T3 and Free T4, primary regulators of metabolism, cardiovascular function, and growth/development.
- **Adrenocorticotropic hormone:** The hormone responsible for stimulating cortisol production from the adrenal glands.
- **Follicle** stimulating hormone: The hormone responsible for female ovulation and menstruation, as well as male testosterone production.
- **Luteinizing hormone:** A hormone important in regulating ovulation and menstruation in females and spermatogenesis in males.
- **Growth hormone:** A hormone critical for human growth and development, including bone development and remodeling, metabolism, and muscle strength.
- **Prolactin:** A hormone responsible for milk production in pregnant women.
- **Pro-opiomelanocortin**: A precursor glycoprotein that assists in the production of other hormones.
- **Thyroid stimulating hormone:** A hormone regulating the synthesis of T4 and T3 in the thyroid.

- **Thyroid releasing hormone:** The hormone originating in the hypothalamus, triggering the pituitary to release TSH.
- **Vasopressin/Anti-diuretic hormone (ADH):** This hormone is responsible for maintaining fluid homeostasis in the body.
- **Oxytocin:** A hormone that facilitates uterine contractions and delivery.

Key Points
- The pituitary gland measures less than 1 cm and weighs less than 1 g, but is responsible for secreting hormones that maintain critical homeostatic functions to sustain life. As a result, it is commonly referred to as the "master gland."
- Almost all functions of the pituitary are regulated by input from the hypothalamus, and the two glands are connected through the hypophyseal (pituitary) stalk.
- The anterior pituitary (AP), also known as the adenohypophysis, comprises the largest territory of the gland. The anterior pituitary produces six hormones in peptide form, including thyroid stimulating hormone, corticotropin/adrenocorticotrophic hormone, follicle stimulating hormone, lutenizing hormone, growth hormone, and prolactin.
- The posterior lobe of the pituitary, also known as the neurohypophysis, secretes oxytocin and anti-diuretic hormone, also known as vasopressin.
- Disruption of these hormone cascades can cause a variety of pathophysiologic processes including (but not limited to) disorders of growth and development, gonadal and reproductive dysfunction, dysregulation of metabolism, emotional disturbances, fluid imbalance, cardiovascular disorders, and possibly death.

12.1 Introduction

12.1.1 Pituitary Gland Introduction and Gross Anatomy

The pituitary gland is a small gland located in the sella turcica, a cavity in the base of the brain (Fig. 12.1). The pituitary gland measures less than 1 cm (0.4 in.) and weighs less than 1 g (0.03 oz), but is responsible for maintaining critical homeostatic functions that sustain life (Amar and Weiss 2003). Almost all of the functions of the pituitary are regulated by input from the hypothalamus, and the two glands are connected through the infundibulum or the hypophyseal (pituitary) stalk. There are several connections from the hypothalamus to the pituitary, including one from the median eminence, the primary functional link between the two glands. It contains connecting axons and releasing factors which are responsible for hormone production and/or release. Hormone releasing factors are rapidly distributed from the hypothalamus to the pituitary via the hypophyseal-portal circulation, which is derived from the internal carotid arteries and provides blood circulation to the pituitary (Melmed 2017) (Fig. 12.2). The anterior pituitary is the most richly vascularized of all mammalian tissues, receiving approximately 0.8 mL/g/min of blood from the portal system (Amar and Weiss 2003).

The hypothalamic-pituitary axis facilitates signaling between the brain and hormone-secreting target glands through positive and negative feedback responses (Fig. 12.3). These signals sustain end-organ function and the cycle of hormone production and inhibition to support the bodies cycle of hormonal needs. The pituitary gland is controlled by positive feedback from the hypothalamus and negative feedback from end-organ hormone production. The negative feedback system works through self-regulation, whereby, when a released hormone achieves a preset level, either the hormone itself or products of the hormone release will trigger the system to stop releasing the stimulating hormone and/or trigger the release of inhibiting hormones to avoid oversecretion (Amar and Weiss 2003). In contrast, a

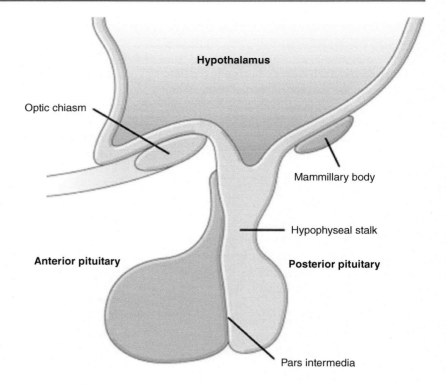

Fig. 12.1 Anatomy of the pituitary gland. Reprinted from Hall J. Pituitary hormones and their control by the hypothalamus. Guyton and Hall textbook of medical physiology. 13th ed. pp. 939–950. Copyright (2016), with permission from Elsevier

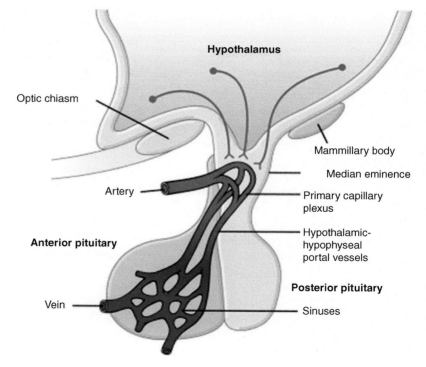

Fig. 12.2 Hypophyseal portal vessels. Reprinted from Hall J. Pituitary hormones and their control by the hypothalamus. Guyton and Hall textbook of medical physiology. 13th ed. pp. 939–950. Copyright (2016), with permission from Elsevier

Fig. 12.3 Negative feedback system (thyroid hormone). Hall J. Pituitary hormones and their control by the hypothalamus. Textbook of medical physiology. 13th ed. pp. 939–950. Copyright (2016), with permission from Elsevier

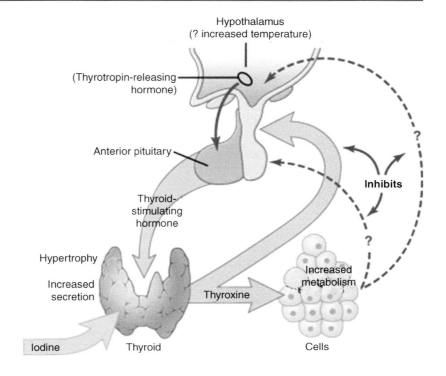

positive feedback loop stimulates the production of a specific releasing hormone from the hypothalamus and pituitary when levels at the end organ decline below a set threshold. For example, during the female menstrual cycle, low estrogen and progesterone levels from the ovaries and uterus provide a negative feedback signal to the hypothalamus to produce GnRH and provide positive feedback to the pituitary to manufacture luteinizing hormone (LH) and follicle stimulating hormone (FSH). These subsequently rise, triggering ovulation. If the egg is not fertilized, there is a sharp drop in estrogen and progesterone levels (negative feedback), stimulating menses and resetting the cycle when threshold low levels of estrogen and progesterone are reached. Therefore, the release of a hormone serves to control its own production (Hall 2016). Other factors are involved in maintaining the delicate balance of hormones release and inhibition, including cytokines, growth factors, nutrients, and neurotransmitters (Melmed 2017).

The pituitary has 3 lobes—anterior (adenophyophysis), posterior (neurohypophysis), and intermediate (pars intermedia). The anterior,

intermediate, and posterior sections of the pituitary act synergistically and independently, each section producing different hormones and regulatory processes or functioning as a specific hormonal axis.

The endocrine hormones are carried by the circulatory system to cells throughout the body where they bind to cell receptors and initate cell reactions, usually resulting in an end-organ function completing the axis (Fig. 12.4). Proper functioning of the hypothalamus, pituitary, and end organ is required for completion of the axis. Some endocrine hormones produce effects throughout the body (example: growth hormone) while others act directly on target tissues (such as adrenocorticotropic hormone) (Hall 2016).

Most of the hormones of the pituitary gland are released in a cyclical manner. These cycles may vary based on a clock mechanism, such as a 24-h circadian rhythm, by season, development and age, diurnal patterns, or association with the sleep-wake cycle (Hall 2016). Other patterns of hormone release also exist, such as pulsatile or with acute brain stimulation (Melmed 2017). Most hormones also have a continuous or tonic

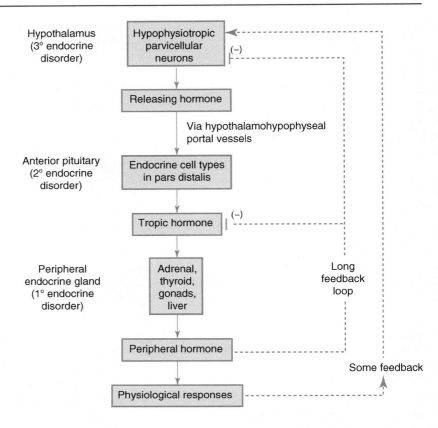

Fig. 12.4 Endocrine axis. Reprinted from White BA, Porterfield SP. Endocrine and reproductive physiology. 2013. Figure 5.10

production so levels never fall to zero (White and Porterfield 2013).

12.2 Anterior Pituitary

The anterior pituitary (AP), also known as the adenohypophysis, comprises the largest territory of the gland. The anterior pituitary produces six hormones in peptide form including thyroid stimulating hormone (TSH), corticotropin or adrenocorticotrophic hormone (ACTH), follicle stimulating hormone (FSH), lutenizing hormone (LH), growth hormone (GH), and prolactin (PRL) (Amar and Weiss 2003). All of the hormones except PRL act by stimulating other glands to release additional hormones (Fig. 12.5). PRL acts on breast tissue directly to stimulate milk production (Hall 2016).

Secretion of anterior pituitary hormones occurs episodically, stimulated by the hypothalamus. Hypothalamic releasing hormones and hypothalamic inhibiting hormones are sent to the anterior pituitary through the hypothalamic-hypophyseal portal vessels. These hormones act on the specific cells to control release or inhibition of their respective hormones (positive feedback). Each secretion may last a few minutes, with a longer duration of action (90–140 min), depending on physiologic stimulation (Amar and Weiss 2003).

There are six currently recognized cell types in the anterior pituitary. The first and most common are somatotropes which secrete GH. The somatotropes make up 40–50% of the cells in the AP and are located primarily in the lateral section of the AP. Mammotrophs (also known as lactotrophs) secrete PRL and make up 10–25% of the cells in the AP. Mammotrophs are located throughout the AP. Corticotrophs, which manufacture corticotrophin (ACTH) and POMC, comprise an additional 15–20% of cells. Corticotrophs are generally located in the anteriomedial part of the AP. Gonadotrophs secrete FSH and LH, make

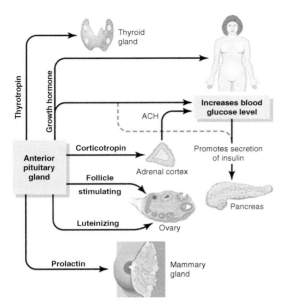

Fig. 12.5 Metabolic functions of the anterior pituitary gland. Reprinted from Hall J. Pituitary hormones and their control by the hypothalamus. Guyton and Hall textbook of medical physiology. 13th ed. pp. 939–950. Copyright (2016), with permission from Elsevier

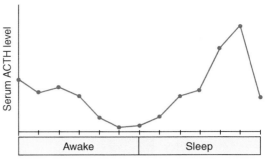

Fig. 12.6 Diurnal pattern for serum adrenocorticotropic hormone (ACTH). Reprinted from White BA, Porterfield SP. Endocrine and reproductive physiology. 2013. Figure 5.14

up 10–15% of cells, and are located throughout the gland. Thyrotrophs secrete TSH, only accounting for 3–5% of AP cells (Hall 2016).

12.2.1 Corticotropin/Adrenocorticotrophic Hormone (ACTH)

Corticotrophic cells in the anterior lobe produce pro-opiomelanocortin (POMC), a precursor glycoprotein that cleaves to produce hormones such as ACTH. In addition, POMC produces melanocyte stimulating hormones in the pars intermedia and is responsible for the production of opioid peptides (endorphins) in the brain. POMC is also produced in the hypothalamus, placenta, lungs, and gastrointestinal tract (Amar and Weiss 2003). Corticotroph cells are responsive to stimulation from corticotrophin-releasing hormone (CRH) from the hypothalamus, and are inhibited by the production of the glucocorticoid cortisol from the zona fasciculata of the adrenal glands.

Corticotropin (adrenocorticotrophic hormone) is essential to life. The primary action of this hormone is to stimulate the adrenal glands to produce glucocorticoids, aldosterone, and androgens. The half-life of corticotropin is approximately 10 min, allowing for rapid adjustments in levels based on physiologic needs. Corticotropin is released on a 24-h circadian recurring pattern. The lowest levels usually occur around normal bedtime or 11 pm to midnight and the highest levels in the morning hours, typically 2–4 h before awakening (Fig. 12.6). Secretion of corticotropin is regulated by corticotropin-releasing hormone (CRH), produced in the hypothalamus in medial paraventricular nuclei and in response to low circulating levels of cortisol. Additionally, CRH, and thus corticotropin, is released in response to physiologic stressors such as physical injury, pain or emotional fear, stress and strain, and is a central mechanism in the "flight or fight" phenomena (Fig. 12.7). The physiology of ACTH in the body is broad and includes maintaining blood pressure, heart rate, and blood sugar levels for cell metabolism to maintain environmental adaptation and create conditions that favor survival in times of acute threat or stress (Melmed 2017). In addition, ACTH, supported by the hypothalamic, pituitary, adrenal axis (HPA axis), responds to stressors by reducing blood flow or constricting blood vessels particularly of the GI tract, increasing heart rate blood pressure, blood sugar, increasing cellular metabolism, and focusing attention and cognition. The production of CRH and corticotropin are

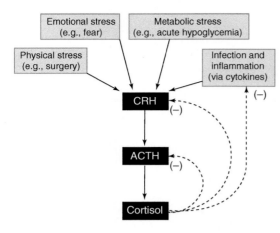

Fig. 12.7 Factors regulating secretion of CRH and ACTH. Reprinted from White BA, Porterfield SP. Endocrine and reproductive physiology. 2013. Figure 5.15

inhibited when glucocorticoids (cortisol) ciculating in the blood stream are sufficient to maintain homeostasis and/or the threat has resolved (Amar and Weiss 2003).

12.2.2 Thyroid Stimulating Hormone

The TSH molecule is a glycoprotein that has a half-life of 60 min. The primary action of TSH is to promote the synthesis and secretion of thyroxine (T4) and triiodothyronine (T3) in the thyroid. Thyroid hormone secretion is dependent on the feedback loop between TSH and thyrotropin releasing hormone (TRH). Secretion of TSH is stimulated by TRH, while somatostatin (produced in the hypothalamus) inhibits the release (Amar and Weiss 2003). Cold temperatures can increase the production of TRH, stimulating more TSH production. TSH binds to the receptors on thyroid cells, which causes production of thyroxine (T4) and triiodothyronine (T3). T3 and T4 are recognized by the hypothalamus and pituitary, which block the secretion of TSH when appropriate or supraphysiologic levels are achieved. Thyroid hormone acts on almost all cells and tissues in the body. Thyroid hormone is essential for supporting oxygenation of cardiovascular tissue by increasing cardiac output (White and Porterfield 2013). In addition, thyroid hormone is responsible for maintaining basal metabolic rate, respiratory effort and oyxgen supply, function and growth of bone and muscle, regulation of the reproductive system, and fetal brain development (White and Porterfield 2013).

12.2.3 Follicle Stimulating Hormone and Luteinizing Hormone

Follicle stimulating hormone (FSH) and luteinizing hormone (LH) are responsible for the gonadal development in both men and women, gametogenesis (germ cell production), the production of androgens and estrogens, and regulating ovulation in women (Amar and Weiss 2003). In women, FSH and LH both increase prior to ovulation, with FSH being the primary driver for follicular development each month. LH stimulation occurs in concert with FSH, creating a more rapid increase in follicular secretion. LH is primarily responsible for the final stages of follicular growth leading to ovulation (Fig. 12.8).

In men, LH is the primary stimulator of testosterone production in the testes and FSH stimulates spermatogenesis (Hall 2016). LH has a half-life of around 60 min while the half-life of FSH is around 170 min. Stimulation of FSH and LH is regulated by gonadotropin-releasing hormone (GnRH), a peptide produced in the hypothalamus. Secretion of FSH and LH occurs in a pulsatile manner. Inhibition of FSH occurs with the hormone inhibin, a polypeptide produced in the gonads of both sexes (Hall 2016).

12.2.4 Growth Hormone

Growth hormone (GH) is the most abundant of the hormones produced in the anterior pituitary gland. GH leads to the production of polypeptide growth factors secreted by the liver, cartilage, and other tissues. The effects of GH are seen throughout the body in protein synthesis and promoting the growth of cells and tissues (Fig. 12.9). Actions include growth of long bones, increase in lean body mass and decrease in body fat, increasing hepatic glucose output and acting as an anti-insulin effect in muscles (Amar and Weiss 2003). GH also stimulates general metabolic rate. The half-life of GH is between 10 and 20 min (Faria et al. 1989). Secretion of GH is stimulated by growth hormone releasing hormone (GRH) and growth hormone inhibiting hormone (GIH, also known as somatostatin), both produced in the hypothalamus. GH release is pulsatile and there are very low basal levels in between bursts (Melmed 2017) (Fig. 12.10). GH release is stimulated by hypoglycemia, sleep, exercise, and stressors. Chronic malnutrition or fasting causes dramatically elevated GH levels. GH is inhibited by glucose and cortisol. IGF-1 also inhibits secretion of GH from the pituitary (Hall 2016). Growth hormone is essential for human development, but continues to be a critical hormone throughout adulthood. In adulthood, GH is essential for bone metabolism and remodeling; metabolism of carbohydrates, protein, and lipids; and muscle strength and exercise. There is some data to suggest that GH is essential for cognitive development and function (Wass and Reddy 2010) as well as maintaining quality of life (McKenna et al. 1999). Insulin-like growth factors (IGF-1 and IGF-2) regulate many of the actions of GH. IGF-1

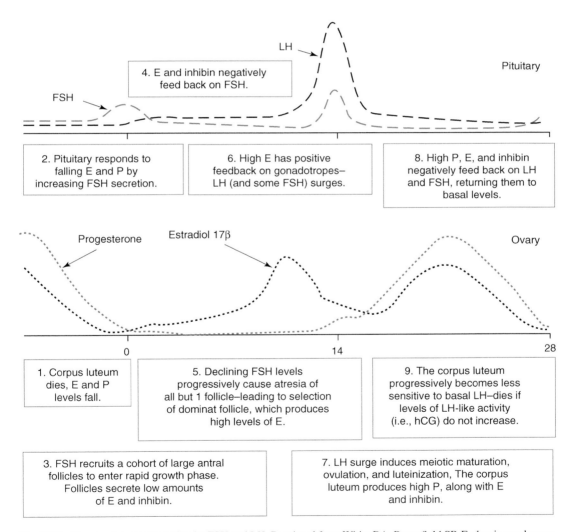

Fig. 12.8 Menstrual cycle regulation by FSH and LH. Reprinted from White BA, Porterfield SP. Endocrine and reproductive physiology. 2013. Figure 10.14

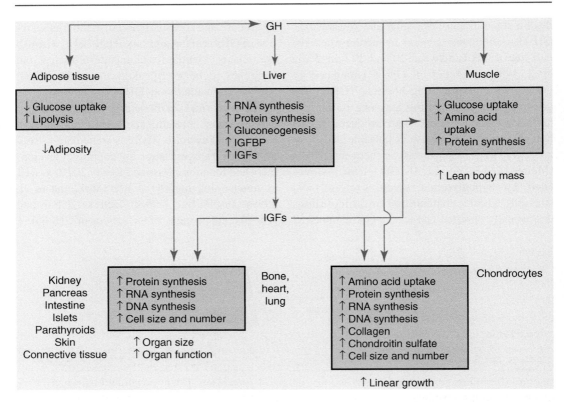

Fig. 12.9 Biologic actions of growth hormone. Reprinted from White BA, Porterfield SP. Endocrine and reproductive physiology. 2013. Figure 5.21

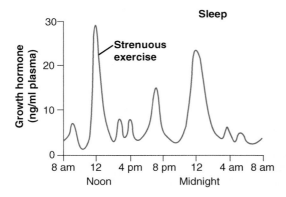

Fig. 12.10 Pulsatile release of growth hormone. Reprinted from Hall J. Pituitary hormones and their control by the hypothalamus. Guyton and Hall textbook of medical physiology. 13th ed. pp. 939–950. Copyright (2016), with permission from Elsevier

peaks in puberty and declines with advancing age. IGF-2 plays a large role in the development of the fetus before birth. IGF-1 is monitored more commonly than GH in laboratory testing because it does not fluctuate significantly during the day in the same manner that GH does, allowing for more consistent testing results.

12.2.5 Prolactin

Prolactin (PRL) works with progesterone and estrogen to assist in the development of the female breast and promote milk secretion from the breast. It also works to inhibit the actions of gonadotropins on the ovary. The role of prolactin in men is unclear, but high levels can lead to impotence and infertility. High levels of prolactin can also lead to female infertility and should be assessed during an infertility evaluation. Hyperprolactinemia may contribute to an increased risk of osteoporosis due to the secondary lowering of estrogen and testosterone. Women with hyperprolactinemia are 2–4.5 times more likely to develop an osteoporotic fracture, compared to age and BMI-matched controls

(Hui et al. 1988). The risk of osteoporosis related to elevated prolactin levels dissipates with normalization of the prolactin levels. TRH stimulates PRL and prolactin-inhibiting factor (PIF, or dopamine) inhibits-proalctin production. Exercise, stress, sleep, pregnancy, and nipple stimulation can all increase PRL release (Amar and Weiss 2003).

12.2.6 Physiology of the Posterior Lobe

The posterior lobe of the pituitary, also known as the neurohypophysis, secretes oxytocin and antidiuretic hormone (ADH), also known as vasopressin. Both of these peptides are produced in the hypothalamus, pass through nerve fibers in the hypothalamo-hypophyseal tract, and are released from the pars nervosa (posterior lobe) in response to stimuli (Amar and Weiss 2003). Release of these hormones is regulated by calcium-dependent exocytosis in response to action potentials arriving at the nerve ending. Exocytosis occurs into the extracellular fluid,

gaining access to the peripheral circulation. The posterior lobe is primarily made up of axon endings that originate in the hypothalamus. The axon terminals are in close proximity to blood vessels, which allows the hormones to be secreted into the bloodsteam (Hall 2016) (Fig. 12.11).

12.2.7 Oxytocin

Oxytocin acts on the breast and uterus. In breast tissue, oxytocin causes the flow of milk from the alveoli to the nipples. Oxytocin release is caused by nipple stimulation, which communicates with neurons in the hypothalamus that discharge action potentials and cause the release of oxytocin from the posterior pituitary gland (Amar and Weiss 2003). Oxytocin also assists in labor, causing contractions of the uterine muscles. Some research supports the idea that oxytocin may stimulate the passage of sperm to the fallopian tubes in nonpregnant women. In men, oxytocin also increases around ejaculation, which may assist with contraction of smooth muscle tissue that propels sperm to the urethra (Ganong 2001).

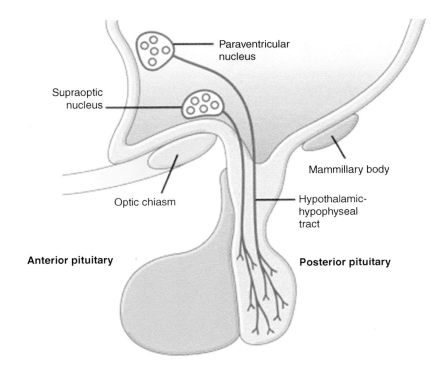

Fig. 12.11 Posterior pituitary relationship to hypothalamus. Reprinted from Hall J. Pituitary hormones and their control by the hypothalamus. Guyton and Hall textbook of medical physiology. 13th ed. pp. 939–950. Copyright (2016), with permission from Elsevier

Paraventricular nucleus

Supraoptic nucleus

Optic chiasm

Anterior pituitary

Mammillary body

Hypothalamic-hypophyseal tract

Posterior pituitary

12.2.8 Vasopressin

Vasopressin, also known as anti-diuretic hormone or ADH, has its primary action in the renal system, where it acts to concentrate urine. Its primary objective is to balance concentration by regulating circulating volume. In the collecting ducts of the kidney, vasopressin causes aquaporins (water channels) to translocate from the endosomal to the luminal membranes. This action causes increased permeability of the collecting duct which allows water to enter the hypertonic interstitium. This causes urine volume to decrease and the urine concentration to increase. Subsequently, specific gravity increases and triggers a decrease in plasma osmolality (the concentration of solutes in the solution), increasing circulating blood volume and subsequently decreasing serum sodium.

Vasopressin is secreted in a variety of situations such as decreased circulating volume in hemorrhage, pain, exercise, and nausea and vomiting. In addition to the renal actions, vasopressin also acts to constrict vascular muscle tissue, which can assist in blood pressure regulation (Amar and Weiss 2003). Alcohol is an inhibitor of ADH release, which subsequently decreases circulating volume and increases serum sodium or promotes dehydration.

12.3 Nursing Process

An understanding of normal pituitary anatomy and physiology establishes a basis for helping the patient navigate personalized treatment goals. Patient-centered care and adherence to the principles as described by the Picker Institute are purposed to engage and empower patients to achieve self-efficacy with respect to these goals (Picker Institute 2017).

Pituitary dysfunction can lead to significant morbidity and mortality. Recognition of the normal physiology and impact of hormone secretion is often revealing for both nurse and patient. In the context of the nursing process assessment of patient reported signs and symptoms, vital signs,

growth and development (auxology), vision, reproductive functions, metabolic indices, bone density, sleep parameters, mental status, stress response, and fluid balance all involve an understanding of normal pituitary function. Each hormonal axis requires assessment for dysfunction, which will be further described in subsequent chapters.

A nursing action plan for patients with pituitary dysfunction is dynamic and goal directed and includes an appropriate education program that aims to empower participation in self-care and collaborative decision making regarding their treatment (Marks et al. 2005a, b; Bennett et al. 2010). Promotion of treatment adherence improves outcomes and quality of life. The dynamics inherent in this concept require the nurse to participate in ongoing evaluation, reviewing the literature for new knowlege with respect to pituitary function and for changes in the individual's function over time and the life cycle.

Assessing symptoms based on pituitary hormone function may include the determination of alterations to the HPA axis function during an acute phase of illness, when the patient is undergoing a surgical procedure or with the diagnosis of a pituitary tumor. Monitoring for signs and symptoms of other hormonal dysfunction enables early diagnosis and prompt treatment.

Patient education and understanding of normal gland function and alterations in function in all with pituitary disease, as in those with other diseases, lays the foundation for self-care and treatment adherence for best outcomes (Adams 2010). Patients must be counseled on actual or potential symptoms that can result from their disease process. Advances in medicine now allow patients with every type of pituitary deficiency, including panhypopituitarism, to lead a full life, although quality of life can vary. However, the best outcomes can be achieved with early detection and prompt and appropriate medical therapies. Additionally, patients identified with pituitary dysfunction should be immediately referred to a specialty provider in endocrinology for a prompt evaluation.

12.4 Conclusions

The pituitary gland is a small but crucial master gland in the body that is closely associated with the hypothalamus and is responsible for regulating many essential physiologic and end-organ processses. The anterior pituitary gland has six types of cells that assist in a variety of hormone production and regulation including corticotropin, thyroid stimulating hormone, follicle stimulating hormone, luteinizing hormone, growth hormone, and prolactin. The posterior pituitary produces two additional types of hormones: vasopressin and oxytocin. Each of these pituitary hormones plays a key role in a variety of physical functions and sustaining life. Any disruption of these hormone cascades can cause a variety of pathophysiologic processes. Apoplexy or bleeding into the pituitary gland can lead to death if not immediately identified and treated with glucocorticoids (cortisol replacement). Nurses in all environments, particularly advanced practice nurses, should understand the key features of the pituitary gland as a primary foundation for the study of endocrinology.

References

Adams RJ. Improving health outcomes with better patient understanding and education. Risk Manag Healthc Policy. 2010;3:61–72. https://doi.org/10.2147/RMHP.S7500

Amar AP, Weiss MH. Pituitary anatomy and physiology. Neurosurg Clin N Am. 2003;14(1):11–23.

Bennett HD, Coleman EA, Parry C, Bodenheimer T, Chen EH. Health coaching for patients with chronic illness. Fam Pract Manag. 2010;17(5):24–9.

Faria AC, Veldhuis JD, Thorner MO, Vance ML. Half-time of endogenous growth hormone (GH) disappearance in normal man after stimulation of GH secretion by GH-releasing hormone and suppression with somatostatin. J Clin Endocrinol Metab. 1989;68(3):535–41.

Ganong WF. Central regulation of visceral function. In: Review of medical physiology. 20th ed. New York: McGraw Hill; 2001. p. 224–47.

Hall JE. Guyton and hall textbook of medical physiology. 13th ed. Philadelphia: Elsevier; 2016. p. 925–50.

Hui SL, Slemenda CW, Johnston CC. Age and bone mass as predictors of fracture in a prospective study. J Clin Invest. 1988;81:1804–9.

Marks R, Allegrante JP, Lorig K. A review and synthesis of research evidence for self efficacy-enhancing interventions for reducing chronic disability: implications for health education practice (part I). Health Promot Pract. 2005a;6(1):37–43.

Marks R, Allegrante JP, Lorig K. A review and synthesis of research evidence for self-efficacy-enhancing interventions for reducing chronic disability: implications for health education practice (part II). Health Promot Pract. 2005b;6(2):148–56.

McKenna SP, Doward LC, Alonso J, Kohlmann T, Niero M, Prieto L, Wíren L. The QoL-AGHDA: an instrument for the assessment of quality of life in adults with growth hormone deficiency. Qual Life Res. 1999;8(4):373–83.

Melmed S. The pituitary. 4th ed. San Diego: Elsevier Academic Press; 2017.

Picker Institute. Picker Institute's eight principles of patient-centered care. 2017. http://cgp.pickerinstitute.org/?page_id=1319. Accessed 23 Oct 2017.

Wass JA, Reddy R. Growth hormone and memory. J Endocrinol. 2010;207(2):125–6.

White BA, Porterfield SP. Endocrine and reproductive physiology. 4th ed. Philadelphia: Elsevier; 2013. p. 99–128.

Key Reading

1. Amar AP, Weiss MH. Pituitary anatomy and physiology. Neurosurg Clin N Am. 2003;14(1):11–23.
2. Ben-Shomo A, Melmed S. In: Melmed S, editor. Hypothalamic regulation of the anterior or pituitary function in pituitary. 4th ed. San Diego: Elsevier Academic Press; 2017.
3. Marks R, Allegrante JP, Lorig K. A review and synthesis of research evidence for self efficacy-enhancing interventions for reducing chronic disability: implications for health education practice (part I). Health Promot Pract. 2005a;6(1):37–43.
4. Marks R, Allegrante JP, Lorig K. A review and synthesis of research evidence for self-efficacy-enhancing interventions for reducing chronic disability: implications for health education practice (part II). Health Promot Pract. 2005b;6(2):148–56.

Metabolic Effects of Hypothalamic Dysfunction

13

Cecilia Follin

Contents

Abstract

The hypothalamus is a very small, key regulator of endocrine, metabolic, and behavioral functions. The hypothalamus controls the release of 8 major hormones by the pituitary and is involved in temperature regulation, control of food and water intake, sexual behavior and reproduction. Hypothalamus neuronal bodies that produce factors controlling the pituitary are clustered in different nuclei which have specific functions. The clinical syndrome will depend on the location and extent of the underlying lesion. The lesion may be very small and only affect specific hypothalamic nuclei. The lateral hypothalamus contains the thirst center and controls thirst. Neurons from the supraoptic and PVN of the hypothalamus terminate in the posterior pituitary and control the release of ADH (antidiuretic hormone) which then acts on the kidneys to prevent loss of water. Osmotic sensors in the hypothalamus work with ADH to maintain water metabolism.

Destruction of the VMN in hypothalamus induces hyperphagia, hyperinsulinemia, and weight gain. The same neurons in the hypothalamus express high levels of leptin and ghrelin receptors. Hypothalamic damage can result in "leptin resistance," which means a decreased sensitivity to leptin and resulting in an inability to detect satiety despite high energy stores. Ghrelin is known as the "hunger hormone" and is mainly produced by the stomach. Circulating

C. Follin (✉)
Department of Oncology, Skane University Hospital, Lund, Sweden
e-mail: cecilia.follin@med.lu.se

© Springer Nature Switzerland AG 2019
S. Llahana et al. (eds.), *Advanced Practice in Endocrinology Nursing*,
https://doi.org/10.1007/978-3-319-99817-6_13

ghrelin is increased under fasting and reduced after refeeding. When the hypothalamus is damaged and disturbances in energy expenditure and appetite-regulation occur, a syndrome of severe weight gain ensues, termed "hypothalamic obesity." Hypothalamic obesity can occur as a consequence of acquired anatomic hypothalamic damage including various types of hypothalamic tumors, inflammatory diseases, head injury, cranial radiotherapy, and cerebral aneurysm.

Childhood onset craniopharyngioma (CP) is a rare intracranial tumor that frequently affects hypothalamic/pituitary regions. CP patients suffer from increased morbidity, primarily due to hypothalamic damage. Understanding the central role of the hypothalamus in the regulation of feeding and energy metabolism is important in the care of the patients with hypothalamic disorders. The care should be conducted by experienced multidisciplinary teams, with the nurse as a key team member.

Keywords
Hypothalamus · Hypothalamic obesity
Energy homeostasis · Appetite control
Temperature regulation · Thirst center
Neuronal bodies

Abbreviations

ALL	Acute lymphoblastic leukemia
ACTH	Adrenocorticotropin hormone
ADH	Antidiuretic hormone
ARC	Arcuate nucleus
AGRP	Agouti-related peptide
CO	Childhood onset
CRH	Corticotropin-releasing hormone
CRT	Cranial radiotherapy
CP	Craniopharyngioma
DMN	Dorsomedial nucleus
GnRH	Gonadotropin-releasing hormone
GH	Growth hormone
GHRH	Growth hormone releasing hormone
HT	Hypothalamus
INF	Infundibular nucleus
NPY	Neuropeptide Y

PVN	Paraventricular nucleus
PWS	Prader–Willi syndrome
TRH	Thyrotropin-releasing hormone
VMN	Ventromedial nucleus

Key Terms
- **Energy homeostasis:** A biological process that involves the coordinated homeostatic regulation of food intake and energy expenditure.
- **Afferent neurons:** Sense stimuli and send information to the brain.
- **Hyperphagia:** Abnormally increased appetite.
- **Leptin:** The "satiety hormone," is a hormone made by adipose cells that helps to regulate energy balance by inhibiting hunger.
- **Ghrelin:** The "hunger hormone," is a hormone produced by ghrelinergic cells in the gastrointestinal tract regulating appetite.
- **Hypothalamic obesity:** A syndrome of severe weight gain due to damage to the hypothalamus when disturbances in energy expenditure and appetite-regulation occur.

Key Points
- Hypothalamus is important in coordinating signals between nervous system and the endocrine system and it influences hormonal and behavioral system, as well as, the control of body temperature, hunger and thirst.
- Damage to the hypothalamus will lead to significant clinical morbidity and can result in metabolic complications, such as disturbed energy balance, hypothalamic obesity, insulin and leptin resistance.
- Hypothalamus releases ADH (antidiuretic hormone) which acts on the kidneys to prevent loss of water through the urine. Diabetes insipidus is a rare water metabolism disorder which is caused by ADH deficiency.
- The pathogenic mechanism underlying hypothalamic obesity is complex and multifactorial. Weight gain results from

damage to hypothalamus, which leads to hyperphagia, low-resting metabolic rate, and hormone deficiency. The weight gain is unlike that of normal obesity. The patients gain weight even if caloric restriction and lifestyle modification are provided.

- As no non-surgical therapeutic option is currently available for hypothalamic obesity, prevention of hypothalamic injury should be the preferred strategy. The care should be conducted by experienced multidisciplinary teams, including nurses providing comprehensive coordinated care and promoting healthy lifestyle behavior.

13.1   Introduction

The hypothalamus is a very small, but important area of the brain and a key regulator of endocrine, metabolic, and behavioral functions. The hypothalamus controls the release of 8 major hormones by the pituitary (Fig. 13.1) and is involved in temperature regulation, control of food and water intake, sexual behavior and reproduction, control of behavior, and mediation of emotional responses. It may be very difficult to differentiate between hypothalamic and pituitary disease as the endocrine abnormalities are often similar. As the hypothalamus regulates both endocrine and autonomic function, there is usually a combination of endocrine and neurological disturbance in hypothalamic damage.

The hypothalamus is a small cone shaped structure, weights about 4 g, below the thalamus and on both sides of the third cerebral ventricle. The hypothalamus is connected to the pituitary through the pituitary stalk. The portal system is a unique arrangement of capillaries and veins located in the stalk, allowing the hypothalamic hormones to pass directly to the anterior pituitary. Hypothalamus neuronal bodies that produce factors controlling the pituitary are clustered in different nuclei which have specific functions (Schneeberger et al. 2014). The clinical syn-

drome will depend on the location and extent of the underlying lesion. The lesion may be very small and only affect specific hypothalamic nuclei (Schneeberger et al. 2014).

Disturbed energy balance with intractable weight gain, termed hypothalamic obesity, is one of the most agonizing late complications after hypothalamic damage (Lustig 2002). The pathogenesis of hypothalamic obesity involves the inability to transduce afferent hormonal signals of adiposity. However, efferent sympathetic activity persists resulting in reduced energy expenditure and increased vagal activity results in increased insulin secretion and adipogenesis.

The hypothalamus is thought to contain the "biological clock" that regulates certain body functions that vary at different times of the day (e.g., body temperature, hormone secretion, hunger) or those that vary over a period of many days (e.g., menstrual cycle). Lesions of the hypothalamus often disrupt the state of the sleep-waking cycle (Schneeberger et al. 2014).

13.2   Hypothalamus

13.2.1   Thirst Control/Fluid Balance

The lateral hypothalamus contains the thirst control center. When blood that is too concentrated or dehydrated reaches the hypothalamus, the patient becomes thirsty. In response, the PVN and supraoptic nuclei of the hypothalamic are activated producing antidiuretic hormone (ADH) which is released as a chemical signal at the terminus of their respective neurons in the posterior pituitary and subsequently secreted into the blood stream. ADH, in turn, acts on the kidneys to prevent loss of water through the urine. ADH constantly regulates and balances the amount of water in the blood. Higher water concentration increases the volume and pressure of the blood and osmotic sensors in the hypothalamus work with ADH to maintain water metabolism. The effect on the body is to conserve water by returning it to the blood and stop it from being lost by excretion. Decreased levels of ADH in the blood can also be caused by compulsive water drinking or low serum osmolality in the blood, e.g., concentration of particles in the blood.

Fig. 13.1 The hypothalamus controls the release of 8 major hormones by the pituitary and is involved in temperature regulation, control of food and water intake, sexual behavior and reproduction, control of behavior, and mediation of emotional responses. (Used with permission from Jameson, J. L. (ed.) *Harrison's Endocrinology, 4th Edition.* New York: McGraw Hill Education)

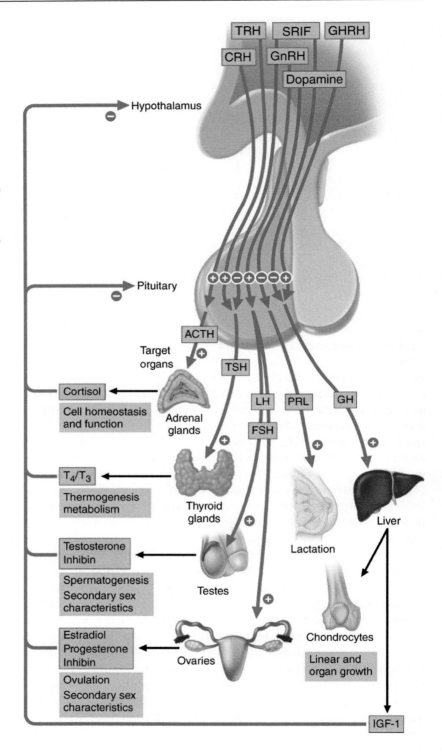

Central diabetes insipidus is a rare water metabolism disorder which is caused by ADH deficiency. The symptoms include excessive urination (polyuria) followed by extreme thirst (polydipsia). The patients are often extremely tired because their sleep is frequently interrupted by the need to urinate. In severe cases urination may occur more frequently than every 30 min. The urine is clear and has an abnormally low concentration of particles. Specific gravity is low. Diabetes insipidus can lead to severe dehydration with high serum levels of sodium if it is left untreated (Higham et al. 2016).

13.2.2 Appetite Control

Energy homeostasis is a biological process that adjusts food intake over time to promote stability in the amount of body fuel stored as fat. The regulation of appetite and body weight involves the human brain and in particular the hypothalamus. Information regarding nutrient status and energy stores is communicated to the brain through diverse afferent neuronal signals. The hypothalamus consists of groups of nerve cells bodies forming distinct nuclei including the arcuate nucleus (ARC), (also known as infundibular nucleus (INF)), the paraventricular nucleus (PVN), the dorsomedial nucleus (DMN), and the ventromedial nucleus (VMN). Destruction of these nuclei induces hyperphagia, hyperinsulinemia, and weight gain (Schneeberger et al. 2014). Animal studies have shown the ventromedial nucleus as the satiety center which inhibits feeding when stimulated and leads to hyperphagia when destroyed. The ARC is a very important area in the control of energy homeostasis. It is located on both sides of the third ventricle (Fig. 13.2). In the ARC there are two populations of neurons controlling appetite and energy expenditure. Neuropeptide Y (NPY) and agouti-related peptide (AGRP) control energy expenditure and anorexigenic neuropeptides, cocaine-and amphetamine-regulated transcript (CART), and α-melanocyte-stimulating hormone (α-MSH). This neuronal circuit is crucial for sensing and integrating a number of peripheral signals allowing for a precise control of food intake and energy expenditure. The neurons in the ARC

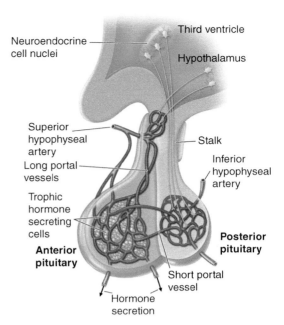

Fig. 13.2 The hypothalamus is a small cone shaped structure, weights about 4 g, below the thalamus and on both sides of the third cerebral ventricle. The hypothalamus is connected to the pituitary through the pituitary stalk. The portal system is a unique arrangement of capillaries and veins located in the stalk, allowing the hypothalamic hormones to pass directly to the anterior pituitary. (Used with permission from Jameson, J. L. (ed.) *Harrison's Endocrinology, 4th Edition.* New York: McGraw Hill Education)

express high levels of leptin and ghrelin receptors (Kamegal et al. 2000; Horvath et al. 2001). Leptin is derived from adipose cells and interacts with leptin receptors to regulate energy balance by inhibiting hunger. Hypothalamic damage can result in "leptin resistance," which means a decreased sensitivity to leptin and resulting in an inability to detect satiety despite high energy stores. Ghrelin is known as the "hunger hormone" and is mainly produced by the stomach. Circulating ghrelin is increased under fasting and reduced after refeeding (Tschöp et al. 2000). Central and peripheral administration of ghrelin in rodents has been shown to robustly promote food intake causing adiposity and weight gain (Tschöp et al. 2000). Ghrelin also enhances appetite in humans, but ghrelin levels have been shown to decrease in obese humans (Wren et al. 2001) (Figs. 13.3 and 13.4).

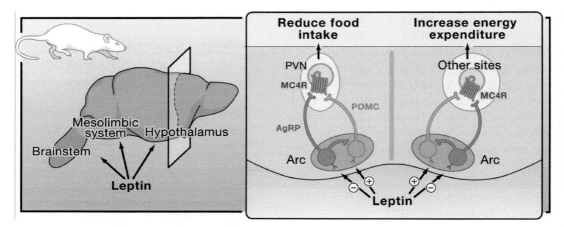

Fig. 13.3 Control of food intake by the hypothalamic leptin-melanocortin pathway. The hypothalamus receives and integrates neural, metabolic, and hormonal signals to regulate energy homeostasis. In particular, the adipocyte-derived hormone leptin and the melanocortin pathway have a critical role in the control of food intake. *AgRP* Agouti-related protein; *Arc* arcuate nucleus; *MC4R* melanocortin 4 receptor; *POMC* pro-opiomelanocortin; *PVN* paraventricular nucleus. Reprinted by Creative Commons License: Coll AP, Farooqi IS, O'Rahilly S. Hormonal control of food intake. Cell. 2007;129(2):251–262

13.2.2.1 Childhood Onset Craniopharyngioma

Childhood onset craniopharyngioma (CP) is a rare intracranial embryonal malformation of the sellar region. These tumors frequently affect hypothalamic/pituitary regions. CP patients suffer from increased morbidity, primarily due to hypothalamic (HT) damage (Holmer et al. 2010; Müller et al. 2000). Contributing factors to a high BMI among CP patients do not include higher energy intake but rather low basal metabolic rate and low levels of physical activity (Holmer et al. 2010). Another important factor is autonomic imbalance, including vagally mediated hyperinsulinemia (Lustig et al. 2003; Bray and Gallagher 1975). Further, CP patients are leptin resistant and ghrelin levels decrease in parallel with the HT involvement by the tumor (Holmer et al. 2010).

13.2.2.2 Cranial Radiotherapy and Hypothalamic Dysfunction in Children

Childhood brain tumor survivors treated with cranial radiotherapy (CRT) with hypothalamic damage are at increased risk for obesity (Holmer et al. 2010; Müller et al. 2000). It is established that the largest childhood cancer group, the acute lymphoblastic leukemia (ALL) survivors, treated

with CRT suffer from obesity and lipid abnormalities (Link et al. 2004). Further, the metabolic hormones insulin and leptin have shown resistance (Follin et al. 2016; Sklar et al. 2000) among ALL survivors (Brennan et al. 1999), suggesting a radiation-induced hypothalamic dysfunction.

Prader–Willi syndrome (PWS) is a genetic neurodevelopmental disorder due to loss of genes within a critical chromosomal region. These genes are widely expressed in the brain, including the hypothalamus. This results in a number of neuroendocrine abnormalities, including hyperphagia and morbid obesity, hypogonadism and GH deficiency. In contrast, ghrelin levels are increased in populations with a possible hypothalamic dysfunction e.g., PWS (Delparigi et al. 2002), and in childhood leukemia survivors treated with cranial radiotherapy (Link et al. 2004).

13.2.3 Temperature Regulation

The functions of the hypothalamus are of a homeostatic nature, such as temperature regulation. If the internal temperature drops or rises outside the normal range, the hypothalamus will take steps to adjust it to avoid potentially dangerous

Fig. 13.4 Hormones from the gut and endocrine organs affect food intake. Reprinted by Creative Commons License: Coll AP, Farooqi IS, O'Rahilly S. Hormonal control of food intake. Cell. 2007;129(2):251–262

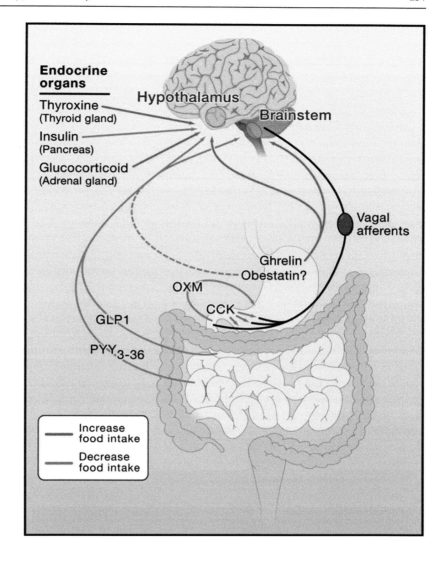

conditions by sending signals to muscles, organs, glands, and nervous system. When body temperature increases, neurons in the anterior part of the hypothalamus turn on mechanisms for heat dissipation that include sweating and dilation of blood vessels in the skin. When body temperature decreases, neurons in the posterior part of the hypothalamus are responsible for heat production through shivering, vasoconstriction in the skin, and blockage of perspiration. Lesions in the anterior part can result in hyperthermia and lesions in the caudal part can result in hypothermia when the environmental temperature is low (Morrison and Nakamura 2011).

13.2.4 Hypothalamic Obesity

When the hypothalamus is damaged and disturbances in energy expenditure and appetite-regulation occur, a syndrome of severe weight gain ensues. This syndrome is termed "hypothalamic obesity" and its weight gain is unlike that of normal obesity. The patient gains weight even if caloric restriction and lifestyle modification are implemented. Hypothalamic obesity can occur as a consequence of acquired anatomic hypothalamic damage and includes various types of hypothalamic tumors, inflammatory diseases, head injury, cranial radiotherapy, and cerebral aneurysm. Complications related to obesity are the major causes of morbidity, such as diabetes type 2 and cardiovascular disease (Kim et al. 2016). Obesity alone is also associated with increased mortality (Adams et al. 2006).

Studies of childhood acute lymphoblastic leukemia (ALL) and brain tumor populations report an abnormal increase in weight long after cancer therapy has been discontinued. Many of these studies demonstrate that cranial radiotherapy is an important risk factor (Lustig et al. 2003). The finding of increased levels of leptin/kg fat mass or fat mass associated with a reduced HT volume among the ALL survivors indicates a hypothalamic involvement after CRT treatment (Follin et al. 2016).

In childhood onset CP, an extremely high frequency of hypothalamic obesity of 30–77% has been reported after treatment. Tumor location, e.g., HT involvement, has been suggested to be the most important risk factor for obesity (Müller et al. 2000). Elevated serum leptin levels have been found in CP patients with suprasellar tumor component (Roth et al. 2015), suggesting that normal inhibition fails to occur due to disruption of the negative feedback loop in which leptin binds to hypothalamic receptors. Studies also report that CP patients continue to have a lower than normal level of physical activity (Harz et al. 2003). Attempts to control hypothalamic obesity with diet, exercise, and pharmacological treatments have not been successful in patients with a history of CP.

In patients with PWS, hypothalamic dysfunction manifests as temperature dysregulation, central sleep apnea and obesity with insatiable hunger and reduced muscle mass. Caloric needs of persons with PWS are significantly lower than norms for age or weight (Cataletto et al. 2011). Endocrine issues include GH deficiency, hypogonadotropic hypogonadism and less often, central hypothyroidism and central adrenal insufficiency.

13.2.5 Hypothalamic Hormones and Actions

Neurons from the nuclei in the supraoptic region of the hypothalamus stimulate the secretion of vasopressin (ADH, antidiuretic hormone), oxytocin from the posterior pituitary, and CRH (corticotropin-releasing hormone) from the hypo-

thalamus. ADH and oxytocin are transported down the axons from cells in the supraoptic and paraventricular nuclei through the stalk to the posterior pituitary, where they are stored and released as needed into the blood stream (Fig. 13.1). Damage to the anterior hypothalamus blocks the production of ADH, resulting in central diabetes insipidus, which is characterized by rapid water loss from the kidneys. Hypothalamic neurons that produce growth hormone releasing hormone (GHRH), corticotropin-releasing hormone (CRH), thyrotropin-releasing hormone (TRH), and gonadotropin-releasing hormone (GnRH) send their axons through the median eminence to terminate and release their hormones into the hypophyseal-portal circulation. This network of blood vessels penetrates into the anterior lobe of the pituitary. The hypothalamic neurohormones stimulate responsive anterior pituitary cells to secrete growth hormone (GH), adrenocorticotropin hormone (ACTH), thyroxin-stimulating hormone (TSH), lutenizing hormone (LH), and follicular-stimulating hormone (FSH). Dopaminergic neurons are responsible for tonic inhibition of prolactin secretion from the anterior pituitary, while somatostatin released from somatostatinergic neurons inhibits GH and TRH release (Higham et al. 2016).

Exposure to cranial radiotherapy impacts the hypothalamus more than the anterior pituitary and GH deficiency is often the first endocrine sequelae post therapy (Littley et al. 1988; Chrousos et al. 1982). It has been shown that patients treated with cranial radiotherapy, e.g., ALL survivors, have a blunted GH response to insulin tolerance test (ITT) and a low GH peak during GHRH-arginine testing (Björk et al. 2005). Damage of the lateral hypothalamus by cranial radiotherapy is a possible explanation for this phenomenon, because this area contains neurons responsible for promoting GH secretion after stimulation by hypoglycemia (Maghnie et al. 2002).

13.3 Nursing Process

Evaluate the patient's health status. Take a detailed medical and family history. Identify the patient's behavior regarding food intake, physical activity, and lifestyle. Identify deficits in fluid balance and temperature regulation. Recognize abnormal findings, including psychological effects such as depression. Provide a detailed explanation to the patient and family of the function of the hypothalamus, how damage occurs and affects behaviors. Identify the patient/family knowledge gaps regarding healthy lifestyle behaviors and plan together a personalized education program. Offer follow-up with continuity and support. Facilitate referrals and contact with the endocrinologist, dietician, physiotherapist, and psychologist.

13.4   Conclusions

The hypothalamus is a key regulator of body clock functions, pituitary functions, weight and water homeostasis. Information regarding nutrient status and energy stores is communicated to the brain through diverse afferent neuronal signals. The hypothalamus consists of groups of nerve cells bodies forming distinct nuclei including the arcuate nucleus, (also known as infundibular nucleus), the paraventricular nucleus, the dorsomedial nucleus, and the ventromedial nucleus. Destruction of these nuclei induces hyperphagia, hyperinsulinemia, and weight gain. Hypothalamic injury can result in "leptin resistance," which means a decreased sensitivity to leptin and results in an inability to detect satiety despite high energy stores. Further, ghrelin levels have been shown to decrease in obese humans. In craniopharyngioma patients, a rare intracranial embryonal malformation of the sellar region, frequently affects the hypothalamic/pituitary regions with ghrelin levels decreasing in parallel with tumor involvement on the HT. The weight gain of hypothalamic obesity is unlike that of normal obesity. The patients gain weight even if caloric restriction and lifestyle modification are provided.

Understanding the central role of the hypothalamus in the regulation of food and energy metabolism is important in the care of the patients with hypothalamic disorders. As no medical/non-surgical therapeutic option is currently available to treat hypothalamic obesity, prevention of hypothalamic injury should be the preferred strategy. Care should be provided by experienced

multidisciplinary teams that include nurses. The nurse should provide psychological support and a personalized plan of care that includes facilitating communication with the multidisciplinary team and educating the patients in healthy lifestyle choices and behaviors.

References

Adams KF, Schatzkin A, Harris TB, Kipnis V, Mouw T, Ballard-Barbash R, Hollenbeck A, Leitzmann MF. Overweight, obesity, and mortality in a large prospective cohort of persons 50 to 71 years old. N Engl J Med. 2006;355(8):763–78.

Björk J, Link K, Erfurth EM. The utility of the growth hormone (GH) releasing hormone-arginine test for diagnosing GH deficiency in adults with childhood acute lymphoblastic leukemia treated with cranial irradiation. J Clin Endocrinol Metab. 2005;90(11):6048–54.

Bray GA, Gallagher TF. Manifestations of hypothalamic obesity in man: a comprehensive investigation of eight patients and a review of the literature. Medicine. 1975;54(4):301–30.

Brennan B, Rahim A, Blum W Adams JA, Eden OB, Shalet SM. Hyperleptinemia in young adults following cranial irradiation in childhood cancer survivors: growth hormone deficiency or leptin insensitivity? Clin Endocrinol (Oxf). 1999;61:683–91.

Cataletto M, Angulo M, Herz G, Whitman B. Prader-Willi syndrome: a primer for clinicians. Int J Pediatr Endocrinol. 2011;2011(1):12.

Chrousos GP, Poplack D, Brown T, O'Neill D, Schwade J, Bercu BB. Effects of cranial radiation on hypothalamic-adenohypophyseal function: abnormal growth hormone secretory dynamics. J Clin Endocrinol Metab. 1982;54:1135–9.

Delparigi A, Tschöp M, Heiman M, Salbe AD, Vozarova B, Sell SM, et al. High circulating ghrelin: a potential cause for hyperphagia and obesity in Prader-Willi syndrome. J Clin Endocrinol Metab. 2002;87: 5461–4.

Follin C, Gabery S, Petersén Å, Sundgren P, Björkman-Burtcher I, Lätt J, Mannfolk P, Erfurth EM. Metabolic risk is associated with reduced hypothalamic volume in individuals treated with cranial radiotherapy for childhood leukemia. PLoS One. 2016;29:7–12.

Harz KJ, Müller HL, Waldeck E, Pudel V, Roth C. Obesity in patients with craniopharyngioma: assessment of food intake and movement counts indicating physical activity. J Clin Endocrinol Metab. 2003;88(11):5227–31.

Higham CE, Johannsson G, Shalet SM. Hypopituitarism. Lancet. 2016;388(10058):2403–15.

Holmer H, Pozarek G, Wirfält E, Popovic V, Ekman B, Björk J, et al. Reduced energy expenditure and impaired feeding-related signals but not high energy intake reinforces hypothalamic obesity in adults with childhood onset craniopharyngioma. J Clin Endocrinol Metab. 2010;95:5395–402.

Horvath T, Diano S, Sotonyi P, Heiman TM. Minireview: ghrelin and the regulation of energy balance—a hypothalamic perspective. Endocrinology. 2001;142:4163–9.

Kamegal J, Tamura H, Shimizu T, Ishi S, Hitochi S, Wakabayashi I. Central effect of ghrelin, an endogenous growth hormone secretagogue, on hypothalamic peptide gene expression. Endocrinology. 2000;114:4797–9.

Kim SH, Despres JP, Koh KK. Obesity and cardiovascular disease: friend or foe? Eur Heart J. 2016;37(48):3560–8.

Link K, Moell C, Garwicz S, Cavallin-Ståhl E, Björk J, Thilén U, Erfurth EM. Growth hormone deficiency predicts cardiovascular risk in young adults treated for acute lymphoblastic leukemia in childhood. J Clin Endocrinol Metab. 2004;89:5003–12.

Littley MD, Shalet SM, Beardwell CG, Ahmed SR, Applegate G, Sutton ML. Hypopituitarism following external radiotherapy for pituitary tumors in adults. Q J Med. 1988;262:145–60.

Lustig RH. Hypothalamic obesity: the sixth cranial endocrinopathy. Endocrinologist. 2002;12:210–2174.

Lustig R, Post S, Srivannaboon K, Rose SR, Danish RK, Burghen GA. Risk factors for the development of obesity in children surviving brain tumours. J Clin Endocrinol Metab. 2003;88:611–6.

Maghnie M, Cavigioli F, Tinelli C, Autelli M, Arico M, Aimarett G, Ghigo E. GHRH plus arginine in the diagnosis of acquired GH deficiency of childhood-onset. J Clin Endocrinol Metab. 2002;87:2740–4.

Morrison SF, Nakamura K. Central neural pathways for thermoregulation. Front Biosci. 2011;16(1):74–104.

Müller HL, Gebhardt U, Teske C, Faldum A, Zwiener I, Warmuth-Metz M, Pietsch T, Pohl F, Sörensen N, Calaminus G, Study Committee of KRANIOPHARYNGEOM. Post-operative hypothalamic lesions and obesity in childhood craniopharyngioma: results of the multinational prospective trial KRANIOPHARYNGEOM 2000 after 3-year follow-up. Eur J Endocrinol. 2000;165(1):17–24.

Roth CL, Eslamy H, Werny D, Elfers C, Shaffer ML, Pihoker C, Ojemann J, Dobyns WB. Semiquantitative analysis of hypothalamic damage on MRI predicts risk for hypothalamic obesity. Obesity. 2015;23(6):1226–33.

Schneeberger M, Gomis R, Claret M. Hypothalamic and brainstem neuronal circuits controlling energy balance. J Endocrinol. 2014;220:T25–46.

Sklar CA, Mertens AC, Walter A, Mitchell D, Nesbit ME, O'Leary M. Changes in body mass index and prevalence of overweight in survivors of childhood acute lymphoblastic leukemia: role of cranial irradiation. Med Pediatr Oncol. 2000;35:91–5.

Tschöp M, Weyer C, Tataranni A, Devanarayan V, Ravussin E, Heiman M. Circulating ghrelin levels are decreased in human obesity. Diabetes. 2000;50:707–9.

Wren AM, Seal LJ, Cohen MA, Brynes AE, Frost GS, Murphy KG, Dhillo WS, Ghatel MA, Bloom SR. Ghrelin enhances appetite and increases food intake in humans. J Clin Endocrinol Metab. 2001;86:5992.

Sella and Suprasellar Brain Tumours and Infiltrarive Disorders Affecting the HPA-Axis

14

Christine Yedinak

Contents

C. Yedinak (✉)
Northwest Pituitary Center, Oregon Health and
Sciences University, Portland, OR, USA
e-mail: yedinakc@ohsu.edu

© Springer Nature Switzerland AG 2019
S. Llahana et al. (eds.), *Advanced Practice in Endocrinology Nursing*,
https://doi.org/10.1007/978-3-319-99817-6_14

Abstract

The pituitary is a unique organ that is key to maintaining end organ function. However, it is particularly susceptible to some tumors, cysts, and infiltrates. Disruption of pituitary function may help target symptom etiology, but can lead to significant morbidity and mortality if not treated effectively.

Patients can present with similar symptom of mass effect, headaches, and pituitary deficiencies despite disparate types of lesions. In some cases, the patient is asymptomatic, and the lesion is found incidentally on Computerized Tomography (CT)/Magnetic resonance imaging (MRI) imaging. Treatment may depend on the type of lesion found on MRI or after surgical pathology when a definitive diagnosis is acquired.

Disorders such as empty sella syndrome may be primary or secondary to other disorders such as intracranial hypertension or occur after tumor resection. Infiltrative and infective disorders may be primary or localized to the pituitary, or may result secondarily from other system diseases. Cysts or tumors beginning in embryonic development can become symptomatic, with growth impacting the optic apparatus resulting in mass effect symptoms such as headaches and/or visual changes. Other tumors may originate in the hypothalamus, grow downward and impact the optic apparatus and the pituitary gland.

Assessment includes a detailed history and physical, MRI and biochemical and dynamic testing for pituitary dysfunction. MRI may have characteristics suggestive of a diagnosis but surgical pathology is often required for a definitive diagnosis. Treatment is often dictated by tumor or lesion histology.

Nursing assessment includes patient emotional, social and executive functions, resources, family history including parental and personal exposures. Together these form the basis of patient education, preparation for further testing and treatment planning decisions. The patient's family can be important historians of patient symptoms particularly in the event of cognitive and memory dysfunction.

Keywords

Pituitary infiltrative disorders · Hypothalamic tumors · Intracranial hypertension · Pituitary dysfunction · Parasellar cysts

Abbreviations

ACTH	Adrenocorticotrophic hormone
AIP	Aryl hydrocarbon–interacting protein gene
CP	Craniopharyngioma
CSF	Cerebrospinal fluid
CT	Computerized tomography
DI	Diabetes insipidus
ES	Empty sella
FSH	Follicle stimulating hormone
GSU	Glycoprotein hormone subunits
HPA	Hypothalamic-pituitary-adrenal (axis)
ICP	Intracranial pressure
IIH	Idiopathic intracranial hypertension
LAR	Long acting release
LCH	Langerhans Cell Histiocytosis
LDL	Low density lipoprotein
LH	Luteinizing hormone

LHH   Lymphocytic hypophysitis
LINH   Lymphocytic infundibuloneurohy
         pophysitis
MEN-1   Multiple endocrine neoplasia-type 1
MRI   Magnetic resonance imaging
PC   Pituitary carcinoma
PES   Primary empty sella
PH   Pituitary hypophysitis
QoL   Quality of life
RCC   Rathke's cleft cysts
SES   Secondary empty sella
SSA   Somatostatin analogues (ligands)
SSTR   Somatostatin receptor
TSH   Thyroid stimulating hormone
WHO   World Health Organization

Key Terms
- **Sella turcica:** the saddle like bony compartment in which the pituitary sits.
- **Suprasellar:** above the sella turcica.
- **Parasellar:** the region next to the pituitary.
- **Histopathology:** microscopic examination of tissue obtained during surgery.
- **Dynamic testing:** involves the stimulation or suppression of one or more pituitary hormones after the administration of a specific agent.
- **Hypopituitarism:** insufficient hormone production from one or more pituitary hormonal axes.
- **Panhypopituitarism:** inadequate hormonal production of all pituitary hormones.
- **Optic apparatus:** includes the optic nerves and optic chiasm.
- **Optic chiasm:** the point above the pituitary gland where the optic nerves from the eye cross over each other and enter the opposite side of the brain.

Key Points
- Pituitary function can be disrupted by benign cysts and tumors, locally aggressive and cancerous lesions or infiltrative disorders from remote system disease.
- Tumors may be asymptomatic until they exert mass effect or pressure on surrounding structures within the Sella such as the pituitary stalk or optic nerves.

- Patient symptoms may be similar at presentation despite different etiologies and often center symptoms of mass effect. Surgical pathology may be needed to guide treatment.
- A detailed patient intake history, including exposure risks, recent illnesses, family history, current symptoms of systems dysfunction and functional limitations for all patients is recommended to aid diagnosis. Family input is valuable.
- Pituitary dysfunction may be evident at presentation and require immediate evaluation and treatment, particularly if HPA axis dysfunction is present.
- Children are afflicted with some tumors with greater frequency than adults. Consideration may need to be given to growth hormone deficiency and replacement therapy after tumor control.

14.1   Introduction

The pituitary gland is aptly lauded as the body's *master gland*. However, the function of the gland is influenced by numerous genetic and genomic, anatomic, vascular, biochemical and metabolic and environmental factors. These factors can interact at all levels in relation to the gland modifying its actions and downstream impact on end organs.

The pituitary largely lies outside the protection of the blood–brain barrier, and thus is not protected from invasion of some pathologic species. Systemic inflammatory diseases, infectious, metastatic and immune disorders can infiltrate the pituitary, inflicting transient or devastating consequences on pituitary function. Biochemical changes from chemotherapeutic agents can result in partial or panhypopituitarism. Genetic and genomic changes secondary to metabolic and environmental exposures have been shown to negatively impact the pituitary hormonal functions.

Sella, parasellar, and suprasellar tumors can significantly change the pituitary structure, its functions, and patient symptomatology. Tumors can arise from multiple cell types, mostly from local cells within the sella and suprasellar region, but can also result from distant metastasis or infection, albeit less frequently. Germ cell tumors, and epidermoid cysts and Rathke's cleft cysts (RCCs) are tumors that arise from developmental cells. Meningiomas are tumors derived from the protective meninges covering of the brain, including the pia mater, the arachnoid and the dura mater. Gliomas are tumors that arise from the supporting cells in the brain. Metastatic tumors originate in another part of the body and spread to the brain, but are extremely rare. Diseases such as tuberculosis, fungal infections, and inflammatory disorders usually originate in other body systems and may migrate to the pituitary.

The treatment goal in all cases is to minimize pituitary hormonal dysfunction, restore function and vision, and prevent secondary end organ dysfunction. This may involve the removal of a tumor or cyst and/or pituitary hormone replacement. Patient and family education and support is a vital component in treatment adherence to aid preservation of functional capacity and to improve quality of life.

14.2 Empty Sella Syndrome: Primary Empty Sella (PES) and Secondary Empty Sella (SES)

14.2.1 Definition

Empty sella (ES) occurs when there is a weakness or failure of the diaphragma sella and the subarachnoid space that allows cerebral spinal fluid (CSF) to herniate into the sella turcica resulting in compression or flattening of the pituitary gland (Tyrrell et al. 1994; Auer et al. 2018). This may produce a partial or a complete empty sella (>50% of sella fluid filled) (Carmichael 2017). As a result, the sella itself may become enlarged (Carmichael 2017). ES can be primary (PES) such as in the case of a congenital weakness (or absence) of the diaphragma sella or of an unknown etiology. Secondary empty sella (SES)

may occur after a surgical tumor removal, radiation, trauma, increased intracranial pressure or pituitary infarction or necrosis, such as in postpartum Sheehan's syndrome (Tyrrell et al. 1994; Carmichael 2017). Other contributory conditions include hydrocephalus, intracranial hypertension (pseudotumor cerebri), thrombus, brain tumor, and Chiari malformation, all of which promote ES by increasing intracranial pressure (ICP). Other factors that have been associated with PES include obesity, hypertension, and sleep apnea, but the mechanisms are unclear (Fig. 14.1).

14.2.2 Epidemiology

Empty sella is relatively common, with a prevalence ranging from 5 to 35% of the general population as drawn from cases found on autopsy and from clinical practice imaging reports (Tyrrell et al. 1994). However, this may be an overestimate (Auer et al. 2018). Females are affected 5 times more than males particularly if they have a history of pregnancy (Tyrrell et al. 1994). Peak age at diagnosis is 30–40 years, perhaps earlier in females than in males. However, PES can also be found associated with genetic disorders or perinatal complications in children (Tyrrell et al. 1994). An estimated 8–15% of patients presenting with ES subsequently develop intracranial hypertension (IIH).

14.2.3 Presenting Symptoms

PES may be asymptomatic and an incidental finding on imaging obtained for other reasons. However, when symptoms occur, they include headaches, fatigue, and/or symptoms of anterior pituitary dysfunction. Women may present with menstrual irregularities, galactorrhea (often with normal prolactin), infertility, and hirsutism. Male presentation is often sexual dysfunction and gynecomastia (Tyrrell et al. 1994). On rare occasions, the pulsatile nature of CSF fluid in the sella may erode the bony sella floor, resulting in CSF rhinorrhea (a "CSF" leak) (Tyrrell et al. 1994). In the presence of a CSF leak, patients report a

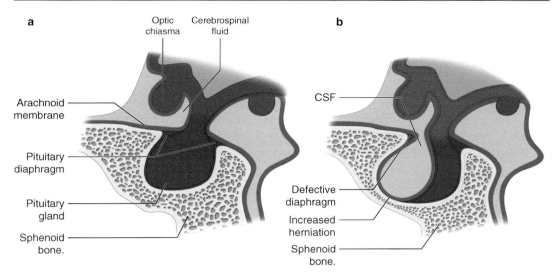

Fig. 14.1 Empty Sella Syndrome. (**a**) Normal pituitary and sella (color hatching green). (**b**) Partial Empty Sella with arachnoid membrane herniation and flattening of normal pituitary

severe, positional headache on standing and experience clear, salty fluid draining from the nares (usually unilaterally) with bending forward (Schlosser and Bolger 2003). Visual field deficits are an uncommon presentation. More severe forms of PES are associated with debilitating headache, increased intracranial pressure, possibly projectile vomiting, papilledema on fundal exam, and rarely seizures. ES can be confirmed by MRI or CT of the sella and suprasellar region (Tyrrell et al. 1994).

14.2.4 Assessment and Testing

The presence of hypopituitarism is controversial, but some studies indicate one or more pituitary axis dysfunctions may be present in up to 53% of cases (Auer et al. 2018; Li et al. 2017). Panhypopituitarism may be present in around 4% of cases (Tyrrell et al. 1994; Carmichael 2017). Pituitary functions testing is warranted even in asymptomatic patients (Auer et al. 2018). Ophthalmology evaluation is indicated to assess for any visual field deficits.

MRI is recommended for diagnosis and CT if MRI is otherwise contraindicated. Characteristic findings of ES on imaging include a fluid density

filling the sella indicative of CSF, thinning of the pituitary stalk, and semilunar flattening of the pituitary against the sella floor. The stalk may be distorted to one side if unilateral ES is present (Chiloiro et al. 2017).

14.2.5 Treatment

Treatment is based on the etiology of ES. Replacement of pituitary hormonal deficiencies is warranted, particularly glucocorticoids, in the event of hypothalamic pituitary adrenal (HPA) axis dysfunction and adrenal insufficiency. Hydrocortisone is recommended as first replacement if needed followed by thyroxine. Sex hormones can be introduced when the patient is stable. However, growth hormone (GH) is not recommended in patients with intracranial hypertension (Tyrrell et al. 1994).

14.2.6 Summary

Overall, obese females 30–40 years with a history of pregnancy, headaches, hypertension, and sleep apnea may be at increased risk for PES. Assessment of these risk factors may be helpful in guiding clinical decisions. Despite an asymptomatic presentation, pituitary function testing is recommended. Diagnostic MRI is recommended along with ophthalmology review for any involvement of the optic apparatus or visual field changes.

14.2.6.1 Intracranial Hypertension (Pseudotumor Cerebri)

14.2.6.1.1 Definition

Idiopathic intracranial hypertension or pseudotumor cerebri (IIH) is a disorder usually presenting with high CSF pressure when brain parenchyma is normal. This is not associated with a cerebral tumor, enlarged ventricles, or malignancy (Friedman et al. 2013). The mechanism of increased intracranial pressure in intracranial hypertension is unknown. Risk factors are as described above for PES. Although the course is mostly benign, there is a risk of vision loss in one or both eyes in 8–10% of cases and vision compromise in an estimated 50% of cases (Ball et al. 2011). Both steroid withdrawal and hyperparathyroidism have been linked to the development of IIH (Wall 2010).

14.2.6.1.2 Epidemiology

The incidence worldwide is reported as 0.5–2/100,000 people per year in the general population (Chatziralli et al. 2018). However, the prevalence increases to 3.5–19/100,000 in young overweight women (usually >20% overweight) (Wall 2010; Chatziralli et al. 2018). In pediatric populations, although there is no gender difference in prevalence, there is a trend toward a higher prevalence with age. There is also a higher prevalence in boys at a younger age than girls and in young adolescents with a higher in body mass index (BMI) (Sheldon et al. 2016). From 53.2 to 77.7% of pediatric cases are thought to be secondary to other known systemic changes, such as endocrine disorders, drugs, infections and/or trauma and, as such, may occur in children with average BMI (Per et al. 2013). The disorder is rare in children younger than 3 years and adults more than 60 years of age (Friedman et al. 2013).

14.2.6.1.3 Presenting Symptoms

Patients will usually present with bilateral headache behind the eyes that may be pulsatile and/or associated with tinnitus (pulse-synchronous tinnitus) (Wall 2010; Chatziralli et al. 2018). They may also report photophobia, nausea and dizziness, plus transient visual blurring of 30 seconds or less (Wall 2010). Headaches may be daily and pulsatile and become worse with coughing, straining, lying down, bending over or with other Valsalva maneuvers (Wall 2010; Chatziralli et al. 2018). Some features may be transient, but headaches most often last more than 1 h. Patients may report intermittent diplopia, that may be worse when looking toward the affected side and is associated with cranial nerve V1 involvement (Chatziralli et al. 2018). If cranial nerve V11 is involved, a slower blink reflex, difficulty in tightly closing the eye on the affected side, and/or sensory changes around and behind the ear may be found (González-Andrades et al. 2016). Children (females <7 years, males <8.5) may be asymptomatic (Sheldon et al. 2016).

14.2.6.1.4 Assessment and Testing

Papilledema is usually found on fundal exam in most patients and is an indication for further evaluation. Referral to neuro-ophthalmology and MRI are warranted. Emerging technologies now recommended include: Ophthalmic echography (ultrasound) and Optical Coherence Tomography (OCT); infrared reflectance imaging; computerized visual field exam; and visual evoked potential exams. These can be used as both diagnostic and follow-up testing to evaluate IIH. They evaluate the morphology of the optic nerve to determine the presence of vascular or CSF flow anomalies or neoplasms (Tyrrell et al. 1994; Chatziralli et al. 2018).

Although neurologic exam is invariably normal, other testing is recommended. Brain imaging with MRI/CT is essential to rule out other lesions. There are usually no cerebral ventricular abnormalities, but empty sella is found in up to 94% of patients with IIH (Tyrrell et al. 1994; Friedman et al. 2013). MRI is often followed by a lumbar puncture (spinal tap), to measure opening pressure of CSF, which has been a diagnostic standard. However, this is currently controversial as CSF pressure changes during the day. Therefore, repeat testing is discouraged in favor of new optical diagnostics. The diagnosis criteria that have been used in adults and children were derived from the Dandy criteria with some modifications over the years (Friedman et al. 2013; Wall 2010; Rangwala and Liu 2007) (Table 14.1). The CSF opening pressure on spinal tap is largely considered diagnostic of IIH when pressures are >250 mm H_2O in obese adults and > 200 mm H_2O in non-obese adults (Friedman et al. 2013; Wall 2010). In children, particularly over 8 years of age, the opening pressure may be normal up to 250–280 mm H_2O, with lower pressures for younger children (Friedman et al. 2013; Rangwala and Liu 2007). A CSF sample is often collected for analysis to look for potential causes of IIH. Lumbar puncture may also cause a temporary reduction in CSF pressure and symptoms (Wall 2010; Idiopathic Intracranial Hypertension 2014).

Table 14.1 Recommended diagnostic criteria for pediatric IIH

1. Patient is pre-pubertal
2. If symptoms or signs present, they may only reflect those of generalized intracranial hypertension of papilledema. Normal mental status
3. Documented elevated intracranial pressure (age appropriate) measured in the lateral decubitus position *Neonates: >76 mm H_2O *Age less than 8 with papilledema: >180 mm H_2O *Age 8 or above or less than 8 without papilledema: >250 mm H_2O
4. Normal CSF composition except in neonates who may have up to 32 WBC/mm³ and protein as high as 150 mg/dL
5. No evidence of hydrocephalus, mass, structural, or vascular lesion on MRI, with and without contrast, and MR venography. Narrowing of the transverse sinuses is allowed
6. Cranial nerve palsies allowed if they are of no other identifiable etiology and improve with reduction in cerebrospinal fluid pressure or resolution of other signs and symptoms of intracranial hypertension
7. No other identified cause of intracranial hypertension

Reference and permission: Rangwala and Liu (2007)

Accurate weight measurement is important. The risk and prevalence of IIH rises concomitantly with BMI in children and in adults (Friedman et al. 2013; Sheldon et al. 2016; Rangwala and Liu 2007). In children, the risk is higher with adolescent weight gain and obesity by early adolescence (Sheldon et al. 2016; Rangwala and Liu 2007). This was also positively correlated with the onset of puberty as defined by tanner criteria and not by age (Sheldon et al. 2016). Girls with IIH may also be taller than boys using standardized anthropometrics. In a random controlled study, the risk of developing IIH in adults was also shown to be progressively higher with higher classes of obesity (Daniels et al. 2007).

Pituitary dysfunction in IIH is usually associated with a high prevalence of ES syndrome and should be evaluated in this context. Elevated prolactin and/or deficiencies in one or more axes functions or panhypopituitarism can occur (Table 14.1) (Chiloiro et al. 2017).

14.2.6.1.5 Treatment and Long-Term Management

There are no guidelines for the management of IIH. The main goals are to reduce ICP, preserve vision, and reduce disability (Chatziralli et al. 2018). Weight loss remains a principle goal in treatment and bariatric surgery may be indicated. A weight loss of 5–10 lbs (2–4.5 kg) has been shown to significantly reduce ICP and papilledema (Tyrrell et al. 1994; Chatziralli et al. 2018).

Medical therapies with diuretics (Acetazolamide and Furosemide) and the antiepileptic, topiramate have been shown to improve symptoms over placebo treatments in clinical trials (Chatziralli et al. 2018). Surgical intervention with CSF diversion (ventriculoperitoneal shunt) may be required to control ICP for intractable headaches if medical therapy fails. Although effective in some cases, up to 50% of patients may subsequently need a shunt revision (Wall 2010). Optic nerve fenestration or cutting window or slits in the fibrous strands that form the optic sheath behind the globe of the eye has been reported as improving or relieving headaches in 50% or more of patients so treated (Wall 2010).

Recurrence may occur many years after initial diagnosis and treatment. This is apparent after weight gain, particularly in children, and reported from long-term medical follow-up well into adulthood (Friedman et al. 2013). Corticosteroids may be useful, but a slow taper is recommended to avoid recurrent papilledema (Wall 2010).

14.2.6.1.6 Quality of Life (QoL)

Although few studies have focused on QoL, changes in both visual and general QoL have been reported (Ball and Clarke 2006). In one report, no difference was found in patients with IIH with respect to anxiety and depression on QoL short form SF-36 and the hospital anxiety and depression scale (HADS) questionnaires versus a standardized population (Ball and Clarke 2006). Measures for pain and change in health status were higher than in the general population. In another study comparing women with and without IIH with age and weight matched women and normal weight subjects, the patient group was found to have significantly increased anxiety, depression, and hardship related to health issues than other women (Kleinschmidt et al. 2000). Assessment of visual QoL using a standardized instrument at diagnosis of IIH revealed an association between visual acuity in the worst eye, visual symptoms, and pain symptoms (headache, neck pain) with decreased QoL. Obesity was not found to be associated (Digre et al. 2015). More QoL studies are needed, particularly regarding pre- and post-treatment effects.

14.2.6.1.7 Nursing Care

Assess the patients in the context of the impact of their symptoms on current functioning and lifestyle to develop a patient-centered management plan. Evaluate the lifestyle factors that may precipitate symptoms and discuss alternate strategies to avoid increased ICP. These should include: monitor fluid intake and balance intake of electrolyte containing solutions and water; monitor and avoid activities that may precipitate a Valsalva maneuver that increases intrathoracic pressure and subsequently ICP (i.e., breath holding, heavy lifting, straining with defecation, and coughing) (Perry et al. 2014). Encourage the patient to keep a headache diary for long-term assessment of features and pain level throughout treatment.

Weight loss and medication adherence are major foci of treatment. Discuss and implement weight loss strategies, particularly if the patient's BMI is >30 and offer nutritional counseling. If appropriate, refer the patient for consultation with a bariatric surgeon. Stress the need for medication adherence, particularly taking regular doses of antihypertensives and diuretics. If the patient is treated with glucocorticoids, establish a taper schedule in writing for the patient to follow. Review when and how the patient typically takes each medication and discuss alternate strategies and medication reminders as needed.

Regular and long-term monitoring of visual changes is essential to avoid vision loss. Referral for a formal neuro-ophthalmology review and regular follow-up for monitoring to assess papilledema is essential. Provide patient education regarding monitoring symptoms, emphasizing the importance of self-care. Outline an ongoing monitor plan to include symptom review, weight management review, ophthalmology, and MRI as needed.

14.3 Infiltrative Disorders

14.3.1 Definition

Infiltrative disorders occur with the deposition of cells or substances not normally found in the pituitary that originate from distal disease (McDermott 1997). These disorders are often classified as inflammatory, infectious, neoplastic or from other etiologies such as hemochromatosis or cancer immunotherapy (McDermott 1997; Iwama et al. 2014) (Table 14.2).

The impact on the anterior or posterior pituitary may vary by disorder, and some authors report this is influenced by differential vascular supply. The hypothalamus and the anterior pituitary are supplied by the hypophyseal portal circulation from the superior hypophyseal artery, and the posterior pituitary is supplied largely by arterial blood from the inferior hypophyseal artery. This may explain the higher prevalence of some disorders in the anterior versus the posterior pituitary (McDermott 1997).

Table 14.2 Classifications of infiltrative disorders

Inflammatory
Sarcoidosis
Histiocytosis
Hypophysitis
Lymphocytic
Granulomatous
Necrotizing infundibulohypophysitis
Wegener's granulomatosis
Infectious
Tuberculosis
Syphilis
Fungi
Parasites
Viruses
Neoplastic
Metastatic carcinomas
Lymphoma
Leukemia
Other
Hemochromatosis
Cancer immunotherapy

Adapted from McDermott (1997)

These disorders may be asymptomatic and found incidentally on brain imaging for unrelated injuries or for symptoms such as headaches, visual changes, or other pituitary deficiencies.

14.3.2 Hypophysitis

Pituitary hypophysitis (PH) is the result of infiltration into the pituitary of lymphocytes, macrophages, and plasma cells that can lead to temporary or permanent pituitary dysfunction in one or more axes (Glezer and Bronstein 2012). PH is considered a rare disease, with an estimated incidence of one case in nine million individuals per year or approximately 1% of all pituitary adenomas on postoperative histology. PH may be primary or only affecting the pituitary or secondary to other systemic diseases (Glezer and Bronstein 2012). Several types of primary hypophysitis have been identified, including: Lymphocytic (LYH), granulomatous, xanthomatous, mixed forms (lymphogranulomatous, xanthogranulomatous), necrotizing and Immunoglobulin-G4 (IgG4) plasmacytic types or related to immunotherapy or cancer chemotherapy with ipilimumab (Glezer

and Bronstein 2012; Shi et al. 2009; Mittal et al. 2012; Faje 2016). Although anti-pituitary or autoantibodies can be measured, the literature reports variable results (Crock 1998; Gellner et al. 2008). Secondary PH is associated with other autoimmune diseases such as thyroiditis, diabetes, hypoparathyroidism, Graves' disease, Addison's disease, multiple autoimmune endocrinopathies, or other organ-specific immune diseases (Mittal et al. 2012). Definitive diagnosis and determination of Infiltrative cell types is only found on histopathology.

14.3.2.1 Lymphocytic Hypophysitis (LYH)

LYH can be classified by location within the pituitary, such as lymphocytic adenohypophysitis (focal lesion), lymphocytic infundibuloneurohypophysitis ((LINH) involving the pituitary stalk and posterior pituitary function), and lymphocytic panhypophysitis (generalized) (Glezer and Bronstein 2012).

14.3.2.2 Epidemiology

In LYH, females are more likely to be affected than males 6:1 with an average age of 34.5 and 44.7 respectively years. The highest risk period for the development of PH is during pregnancy or immediately postpartum (usually within 2 months), when approximately 57% of cases are found (Melmed and Kleinberg 2016). Pediatric cases of LYH are extremely rare, but there is a similar preponderance of females, as in adult cases (Gellner et al. 2008). However, in immunotherapy CTLA-4 mediated hypophysitis, males are affected more commonly than females (Faje 2016).

14.3.2.3 Course and Symptoms of LYH

The course of PH in both adults and children may be short and spontaneously resolved but may also be progressive and result in pituitary cell destruction, atrophy and subsequent ES or fibrosis (Gellner et al. 2008; Melmed and Kleinberg 2016). In the Lymphocytic Infundibuloneurohypophysitis (LINH) subtype that affects the pituitary stalk (or if the posterior pituitary is involved), the patient usually presents with symptoms of diabetes insipidus and elevated prolactin (Mittal et al. 2012; Melmed and Kleinberg 2016). Presenting symptoms are similar in adults and children, and include headache, symptoms of diabetes insipidus (DI) with polyuria and polydipsia DI or compressive symptoms with VF loss (Gellner et al. 2008). Symptoms of pituitary dysfunction may manifest immediately or be delayed as pituitary cells are progressively destroyed as inflammation is replaced by fibrosis (Gellner et al. 2008; Melmed and Kleinberg 2016). Prolactin may be elevated due to stalk involvement or compression, and hypogonadism is estimated to occur in 56% of patients. Hypothyroidism may be a late appearing deficiency. Growth hormone deficiency is also reported in LYH, but is not as common as in other types of PH (Melmed and Kleinberg 2016).

14.3.2.4 Patient Assessment
Assessment of the HPA axis with dynamic testing, along with serum analysis for gonadal functions (Follicle Stimulating Hormone (FSH), Luteinizing hormone (LH), and testosterone), prolactin, Thyroid stimulating hormone (TSH), Thyroxine (FT4), and Insulin-like growth factor 1 (IGF-1) is recommended. In early studies, serum autoantibodies to 49-kDa cytosolic protein were found in 70% of patients with histology-confirmed PH (Crock 1998). Assessment of anti-pituitary antibodies may be helpful in some cases (Glezer and Bronstein 2012; Gellner et al. 2008).

MRI is recommended for diagnosis and management. Characteristic changes found on MRI include: homogenous enlargement of the pituitary, a lesion that is indistinguishable from an adenoma, widening of the pituitary stalk, and loss of the pituitary bright spot in the posterior pituitary. The pituitary gland may appear pear shaped on coronal (frontal) images (Mittal et al. 2012; Melmed and Kleinberg 2016; Laws et al. 2006). As PH resolves, these changes normalize. Although MRI is useful in diagnosis, a definitive diagnosis requires histopathology after a biopsy or removal of the lesion or pituitary tissue.

14.3.2.5 Treatment
Supportive treatment is usually recommended, including the management of pituitary deficiencies (Fleseriu 2017). The need for pituitary hormonal replacement therapy may be prolonged. Glucocorticoids may be needed if adrenal hypofunction is evident. The risk of thyroid dysfunction in cytotoxic T-lymphocyte antigen 4 (CTLA4) mediated hypophysitis is higher and occurs earlier than in lymphocytic hypophysitis, so replacement may be indicated early in the course of the disorder (Dillard et al. 2010).

High dose steroids have been used to treat inflammation and avoid pituitary cell destruction. This remains controversial as results of studies has been equivocal (Faje 2016; Laws et al. 2006). However, high dose glucocorticoids of approximately 1 mg/kg prednisone (or equivalent such as methylprednisolone) with a slow taper may be used. In cases of ipilimumab therapy related PH, steroids the and cessation of the drug may be considered (Faje 2016). Vasopressin replacement with desmopressin may be used to treat symptoms of DI. All pituitary functions should be tested (including testing the HPA axis function) and monitored at regular intervals.

Surgery is usually not indicated if the diagnosis can be made clinically. With clear clinical and biochemical evidence of PH, the patient can be monitored by yearly MRIs for a minimum of 5 years or until stable (Laws et al. 2006). However, surgery is recommended when there is progressive vision loss or there is a need for histology with suspicion or risk of metastatic disease (Faje 2016; Melmed and Kleinberg 2016).

14.3.2.6 Histopathology
Histopathology does provide a definitive diagnosis, and is useful in differentiating the specific infiltrative cells to classify the type of PH (Table 14.3).

14.3.2.7 Immunotherapy-Related Autoimmune Hypophysitis
Hypophysitis associated with the treatment of metastatic cancers with immunotherapies such as Ipilimumab has become more frequent (Dillard et al. 2010). Ipilimumab is a monoclonal antibody that downregulates the immune response by

Table 14.3 Classifications of pituitary hypophysitis

Hypophysitis type	Characteristics
Lymphocytic	Anterior pituitary with diffuse T and B lymphocyte infiltrates (Melmed and Kleinberg 2016)
Granulomatous	Granulomatous areas, multinucleated giant cells (Elgamal et al. 2017)
Xanthomatous	Cholesterol clefts
IgG4	A high ratio of IgG4/IgG-positive cells (>40%) (Bernreuther et al. 2017)
Necrotic	Necrotic tissue, mononuclear cell, and CD8-positive cytotoxic T cells (Gutenberg et al. 2012)

blocking the CTLA4 receptors expressed on pituitary cells, thereby allowing T cell infiltration and triggering an autoimmune response (Faje 2016; Dillard et al. 2010). This may occur preferentially in PRL, TSH, and adrenocorticotropic hormone (ACTH) producing cells (Iwama et al. 2014; Fleseriu 2017). Recent studies indicate that 8–15% of patients treated with ipilimumab may develop PH, men more frequently than women (Faje 2016; Melmed and Kleinberg 2016). Recognition of clinical symptoms is key. Symptoms may appear after 1–2 months of treatment and include headaches, easy fatigability, weakness, anorexia, and nausea. Hyponatremia may develop in some cases. Visual symptoms and DI appear to be rare (Iwama et al. 2014; Faje 2016). Symptoms may be vague and non-specific or severe, particularly when adrenal insufficiency is the presenting symptom. Evidence of pituitary enlargement on MRI may present before other symptoms of pituitary dysfunction (Faje 2016). PH appears to be rare when other immunotherapies are used (Faje 2016).

14.3.2.8 Nursing Care

Patient assessment is centered on symptomatology and long-term management. If treatment with high dose glucocorticoids is initiated, family and patient education regarding side effects and management strategies for mood changes, and increased appetite may be useful to support treatment adherence. A written schedule of taper for patient self-care guidance is helpful. Patients

should be aware of the risks of tapering too quickly and the nurse alert for worsening symptoms that may be indicative of recurrent hypophysitis, IIH, or adrenal insufficiency. Dynamic testing of the HPA axis may be indicated before and after glucocorticoid taper. Patient and family members require education regarding the signs and symptoms of adrenal insufficiency. Both symptom evaluation and regular MRIs are used as a means of monitoring treatment efficacy. MRIs may be indicated every 6–12 months until stable or hypophysitis is resolved.

Management of fluids may vary with the patient's climatic environment and is paramount in cases with DI. Provide the patient with the resources to assess under and over treatment of DI as a component of education. Fluid status, hypo- and hypernatremia require close monitoring.

Long-term management of pituitary deficiencies may be required. These needs may change across the lifespan or with changes in accessibility to treatment. The need for replacement may be lifelong and also require a transition plan in the case of patients re-locating or transferring care, particularly to local primary care or general practice services.

14.3.3 Sarcoidosis

Sarcoidosis is an immune disease in which inflammatory cells form abnormal lumps or granulomas. The disease most often begins in the lungs, skin, or lymph system, but may affect any tissue. The hypothalamus and pituitary gland are affected in an estimated 5–10% of cases. Formed of macrophages and T cells during the inflammatory phase, over time, the affected tissue becomes fibrotic (McDermott 1997; Moshkin et al. 2011). Patients present with symptoms of anterior and posterior pituitary insufficiency including DI and adrenal insufficiency. Surgical pathology is needed for definitive diagnosis. Treatment with corticosteroids is the primary therapy (Moshkin et al. 2011). The nursing response is similar to that described for other infiltrative disorders (See above).

14.3.4 Histiocytosis

14.3.4.1 Definition
Langerhans cells are dendritic cells of the immune system that reside in the basal epidermal layers. They process and present antigens to T cells and trigger activation of other lymphocytes to fight disease (Néel et al. 2015). Histiocytes are immature cells. Langerhans cell histiocytosis (LCH) is a rare form of cancer where Langerhans cells proliferate into numerous immature cells in one or in multiple body organs or tissues, forming granulomas (Néel et al. 2015). Mutations of the BRAF, MAP 2 K1, RAS, and ARAF genes have been found to be associated with LCH (PDQ® Pediatric Treatment Editorial Board 2018). Risk factors include: parental exposures to metal, granite, or wood dust in the workplace, parental history of cancer (including LCH) or thyroid disease, Hispanic descent, smoking, newborn infection or lack of inoculations in childhood (PDQ® Pediatric Treatment Editorial Board 2018).

14.3.4.2 Epidemiology
The pituitary is a susceptible site for LCH, but the prevalence is low and estimated at less than one-third of all cases (Néel et al. 2015; PDQ® Pediatric Treatment Editorial Board 2018). Although both adult and childhood cases occur, LCH is more common in children, with a prevalence of 1:200,000 children, with the highest incidence in newborns (Néel et al. 2015; Tillotson and Bhimji 2018). However, some studies indicate that 58% of patients are adults (Néel et al. 2015). Mortality is low if the disease is limited to a single area such as in the pituitary.

14.3.4.3 Symptoms of LCH
Pituitary LCH is often associated with DI as the presenting symptom. In 50% of children, LCH is accompanied by growth hormone deficiency plus DI. When the hypothalamus is involved, children may present with significant weight gain. With anterior pituitary involvement puberty may be early or delayed (Melmed and Kleinberg 2016; PDQ® Pediatric Treatment Editorial Board 2018). Adult onset pituitary LCH also presents with DI and one or more pituitary deficiencies.

Hypogonadism is most frequently reported (Catford et al. 2016). The disease may be self-limiting or, in an estimated 6% of cases, progress to panhypopituitarism in both adults and children (Catford et al. 2016).

14.3.4.4 Patient Assessment
Evaluation in all cases includes MRI and assessment of all pituitary functions. Dynamic testing for the evaluation of HPA axis function is critical. Assessment for multisystem disease may be indicated based on the patients' history and physical exam (Catford et al. 2016). A water deprivation test may be needed for diagnosis of DI. Genetic testing is recommended, particularly in cases with a family history of LCH (PDQ® Pediatric Treatment Editorial Board 2018). A history of parental exposures is needed, particularly in pediatric cases. MRI may show enlargement of the pituitary, stalk thickening, and loss of the posterior pituitary bright spot (Melmed and Kleinberg 2016).

14.3.4.5 Treatment
Treatment recommendations vary. Some authors recommend a trial of high dose glucocorticoids prior to surgical biopsy, which may ultimately be necessary for definitive diagnosis (Néel et al. 2015; Catford et al. 2016). High dose glucocorticoids plus cancer chemotherapy are indicated in some cases, particularly in childhood LCH (Melmed and Kleinberg 2016; Carroll et al. 2018). This requires collaboration with pediatric or adult oncology for clinical management. Pituitary replacement therapy with vasopressin for DI control, growth hormone replacement in children, and replacement of gonadal hormones in adults are commonly required. However, all pituitary hormones may require replacement in severe cases (Catford et al. 2016). Chemotherapy and radiation treatments have also been used, but there are no randomized controlled studies that have established the most effective treatment (Carroll et al. 2018).

14.3.4.6 Outcome and Nursing Care
Long-term outcomes depend upon the patient's age and disease severity. Ongoing monitoring

is required with MRI for normalization of the pituitary stalk and gland size, anterior pituitary hormonal functions and electrolytes for control of DI. In children, monitoring growth and diet and for evidence of secondary cancers may be indicated, particularly after early chemotherapy or radiation treatment (Néel et al. 2015). An individual approach to treatment is essential, as some children may suffer neurological deficit and need multidisciplinary approach to care, whereas adults may suffer from issues such as infertility. Childhood survivors may suffer from quality of life issues that need evaluation and intervention appropriate to their life stage needs (PDQ® Pediatric Treatment Editorial Board 2018).

LCH patient and provider support and information available online includes: The Histiocytosis Study Group (GEH) Website http://www.histiocytose.org/geh/ which is described as "An association of health professionals whose purpose is to improve the medical management of patients with histiocytosis as well as the development of medical and scientific research on these pathologies," and the Histiocytosis association https://www.histio.org.

14.3.5 Fungal Infection

Fungal infections of the pituitary associated primarily with sphenoid aspergillus have been reported, but are rare (Sajko et al. 2015). These pituitary lesions show characteristic changes, such as high and low intensity regions on CT or MRI associated with aspergillus proliferation (Sajko et al. 2015). The incidence is reported to be increasing secondary to immunocompromise associated with diabetes mellitus and treatment with immunosuppressive therapies. CNS fungal infections are associated with a mortality of 50–100% and require aggressive treatment with antifungal medications (Iplikcioglu et al. 2004; Dubey et al. 2005).

Patients largely present with headache, vomiting, proptosis, sinus congestion, weakness, and altered sensorium. Although Aspergillus was found in the majority of reported cases, infection with Cryptococcus and Candida has also been found on histopathology (Dubey et al. 2005).

14.3.6 Pituitary Abscess

An abscess in the pituitary is extremely rare, with very few reported cases. These usually present as a pituitary adenoma and the patient reports headaches and visual changes with larger lesions. Pathologic etiology may be fungal, such as in aspergillus abscess, bacterial or sterile (Iplikcioglu et al. 2004). Radiographic findings on MRI or CT are not useful in the diagnosis, and transsphenoidal surgery with biopsy or resection of the lesion is needed for diagnosis and to provide definitive treatment. Antifungal or antibiotic therapy is recommended (Iplikcioglu et al. 2004).

14.3.7 Infectious Disorders

Tuberculosis, syphilis, acquired immune deficiency syndrome (AIDS), hemorrhagic fever, and other viral syndromes may present as pituitary lesions or can result in pituitary dysfunction (Fleseriu 2017). A tuberculin lesion in the pituitary may be indistinguishable on MRI from other pituitary lesion and may present as syndrome of inappropriate antidiuretic hormone (SIADH with hyponatremia), mass effect or may be asymptomatic. These infections may rarely result in a pituitary abscess or fungal infection. ACTH deficiency may be present, in association with AIDS infection or hypogonadism and/or sick thyroid syndrome requiring glucocorticoid replacement. Pituitary atrophy and empty sella syndrome can occur as a result of hemorrhagic fever (Fleseriu 2017). Pituitary deficiencies up to panhypopituitarism may be the end result of infection.

14.3.8 Primary Pituitary and Metastatic Carcinomas

Pituitary carcinomas (PC) are rare but carry a high mortality rate. At 5 years after diagnosis the estimated mortality is over 66 and 80% of patients by 8 years after diagnosis. However, the estimated prevalence is low, occurring in only 0.1–0.2% of all pituitary tumors (Yoo et al. 2018). Two distinct groups of patients have been described with PC: those with pituitary adenomas having slow progression and recurrence over a number of years from a pituitary adenoma and those with rapid oncogenesis and death. Most PC fall into the former category (Yoo et al. 2018).

Elevation of the histologic proliferative marker Ki67 may be an indicator of tumor aggression but the cutoff percentage of cells required for this to be a sensitive predictor of recurrence or oncogenesis is unclear and not defined by WHO (Yoo et al. 2018). Likewise, the use of tumor suppressor p53 immunopositivity as a malignant marker is also debated. The European Endocrine Society Guidelines recommend the measurement of p53 and a mitotic count if Ki67 is >3% (Raverot et al. 2018).

Once diagnosed with a pituitary tumor, many patients express fears of brain cancer. Based on these statistics, they can be quickly reassured that cancer is most unlikely.

14.3.9 Hemochromatosis

Iron overload associated with high ferritin and total iron binding capacity in hemochromatosis is a hereditary autosomal recessive disorder. The disorder is related to excess absorption of iron from dietary sources (Carmichael 2017). The uptake of iron in the pituitary, preferentially by gonadotroph cells, leads to hypogonadism. Other anterior pituitary hormones may also be affected to a lesser degree (Carmichael 2017). Genetic testing and pituitary function testing are indicated in the presence of hemochromatosis.

14.4 Development and Hypothalamic Tumors

14.4.1 Germ Cell Tumors

Germinomas or germ cell tumors are rare, with reports of prevalence varying by age and country. In children, CNS cases represent 0.5–2.1% of all intracranial tumors reported in western countries but are reported in up to 16% of intracranial tumors in Japan (Moshkin et al. 2011; Guedes et al. 2018). It is very rare that the tumor is focused in the pituitary (Moshkin et al. 2011).

The etiology of germ cell tumors is presumed to be from residual or displaced embryonic cells with tumors most commonly found in the midline suprasellar and pineal regions. Tumors are classified according to stage of embryonic development that the tumor cells most closely resemble such as germinoma, teratoma, choriocarcinoma, or mixed types. The peak incidence occurs in the second decade of life with males more commonly presenting with pineal tumors and females with suprasellar tumors (Moshkin et al. 2011; Guedes et al. 2018). An association with syndromes such as Downs, Klinefelter's, and Cornelia de Lange has also been reported (Moshkin et al. 2011).

Patients with suprasellar lesions usually present with mass effect or compression of the optic chiasm with visual changes, precocious puberty, hypothalamic or pituitary dysfunction (including hypothyroidism, delayed growth hormone deficiency, and/or diabetes insipidus) (Moshkin et al. 2011; Guedes et al. 2018). A biopsy and surgical debulking of the tumor may be needed for diagnosis and for treatment in the event of mass effect. Teratomas may be removed by surgical resection, but germinomas are known to be sensitive to radiation, with an excellent prognosis. However, late effects of radiation therapy need to be considered, including the development of hypopituitarism as the individual ages (Guedes et al. 2018). Some types of germ cell tumors may need the addition of chemotherapies.

14.4.2 Rathke's Cleft Cyst (RCC)

14.4.2.1 Definition

RCCs are thought to form from the remnants of the Rathke's pouch during embryogenesis (Moshkin et al. 2011). They are differentiated from other cysts by their mucoid colloid content (Huo et al. 2018). RCCs are usually small (<5 mm) and asymptomatic, but may grow large enough to cause compression of the optic apparatus and mass effect symptoms or may be incidentally found on imaging for other purposes. The majority of RCCs are between 10 and 20 mm, but cases up to 50 mm have been reported (Larkin et al. 2014).

14.4.2.2 Epidemiology
Females are affected over males 2:1 with a peak age of 30–40 years (Moshkin et al. 2011). This ratio may be higher in pediatric populations with reports of up to 3.7: 1 female to male case (Larkin et al. 2014).

14.4.2.3 Symptoms
Typical symptoms are headaches that may occur even with small tumors and are a presenting feature in approximately 40% of cases (Larkin et al. 2014; Fleseriu et al. 2009). Visual deficits may begin with increasing mass effect with growth of the cyst. Symptoms of pituitary deficiencies are reported in up to 81% of patients (Larkin et al. 2014). Hypogonadism, menstrual abnormalities, and prolactinemia are most common. Rupture of the cyst can occur resulting in inflammation, headache, and symptoms of aseptic meningitis. Sphenoid sinusitis, syncope, and seizures can also occur (Larkin et al. 2014).

14.4.2.4 Treatment
Treatment varies with the patient's symptoms and size of cyst. Up to one-third of patients may have spontaneous resolution of the cyst but 5.3–31% grow slowly during a watch period and required surgery (Larkin et al. 2014). Transsphenoidal surgical removal of the cyst is the treatment of choice after replacement of glucocorticoids in cases of hypoadrenalism. The use of intraoperative ethanol infusion to remove any residual cell wall has been described, but studies have not shown significant benefit in recurrence rates (Larkin et al. 2014). The need for radiation therapy is rare. Headaches are significantly improved or resolved after cyst removal, and pituitary deficiencies may be resolved (Larkin et al. 2014; Fleseriu et al. 2009). Recurrence usually occurs within the first 5 years postoperatively and can occur in up to 48% of cases. Multiple relapses may occur, but remain rare (Larkin et al. 2014).

14.4.3 Epidermoid and Dermoid Cysts

These are cysts that are formed in early development, either in or around the sella, and are lined with keratinized squamous epithelium. Dermoid cysts contain sebaceous or apocrine glands and/or hair follicles (Moshkin et al. 2011; Huo et al. 2018). Less the 1% of intracranial lesions are epidermoid or dermoid cysts. Similar to other cystic sella and parasellar lesions, the patient usually presents with symptoms of mass effect such as headache and visual disturbances. Males are affected more frequently than females 1.7:1 and with dermoid cysts presenting in early adulthood and epidermoid cyst in mid-40s. Pituitary deficits may also be present and should be evaluated but are not common (Huo et al. 2018).

Surgical resection remains the treatment of choice. However, chemical meningitis may occur if the cyst ruptures and keratinous material is spilled (Moshkin et al. 2011). It is important that the capsule also be removed to avoid recurrence (Huo et al. 2018). Cases of squamous cell carcinoma in the cyst have also been reported (Moshkin et al. 2011).

14.4.3.1 Arachnoid Cyst
Arachnoid cysts are suprasellar cysts that are developmental defects in the arachnoid membrane. Fluid accumulates in the defect and may eventually grow large enough to apply mass effect on the optic apparatus. The patient may present with visual deficits and visual field deficiency, but usually the pituitary is spared and there is no impact to pituitary function (Shin et al. 1999; Gustina et al. 2017). In congenital cases, obstructive hydrocephalus may be found with symptoms of increased intracranial pressure. These patients will often present before the age of 5 years and concomitant ACTH, GH deficiency and/or precocious puberty may be evident (Gustina et al. 2017). In adulthood, arachnoid cysts may be asymptomatic or an incidental finding on a head CT or MRI for other reasons. However, these may grow slowly and present with symptoms of mass effect over time. Pituitary deficiencies are rare in adulthood (Shin et al. 1999). Treatment to remove or fenestrate the cyst

usually resolves the symptoms with very rare recurrence (Shin et al. 1999).

14.5 Meningioma

14.5.1 Definition

An estimated one-fifth of all meningiomas occur in the sella and parasellar regions (Melmed and Kleinberg 2016; Dolecek et al. 2012). These are tumors that arise from the arachnoid and Meningothelial cells. They may invade the pituitary but rarely originate in the pituitary. They normally migrate downwards into the sella and may affect both the optic nerve causing mass effect. Impact on the pituitary stalk can result in elevated prolactin levels.

14.5.2 Epidemiology

Meningiomas represent approximately 30% of all intracerebral tumors (Melmed and Kleinberg 2016; Dolecek et al. 2012). More females are affected than males (2.8:1 in adulthood). However, no gender difference is found for the rare meningiomas found in children and adolescents. The prevalence does increase with age, and most patients present in middle age (40–55 years) (Gustina et al. 2017). Estrogen receptors in meningiomas make these tumors susceptible to growth during pregnancy, during the menstrual cycle, or during the use of estrogen containing birth control or with hormone replacement therapy.

14.5.3 Symptoms

Patient symptoms are dependent on the area affected. In suprasellar tumors, the patient often reports slow vision loss, usually in one eye associated with mass effect (Gustina et al. 2017). Headaches, deterioration in hearing and cognition, short-term memory loss, and confusion are reported in approximately 20% of patients. Up to 40% of patients are obese at the time of presenta-

tion (Gustina et al. 2017). Pituitary dysfunction varies but hypogonadism and menstrual disorders are most common (Gustina et al. 2017). On MRI, meningiomas have a characteristic encapsulated appearance and create their own cavity within the brain parenchyma (Gustina et al. 2017).

14.5.4 Treatment

Tumor resection may be achieved in some cases using a transsphenoidal approach. However, meningiomas are very vascular lesions, and may hemorrhage with tumor resection (Melmed and Kleinberg 2016). Craniotomy may to needed and also tumor embolization for safety. Evaluation and monitoring of both visual acuity and visual fields is indicated. Monitoring of pituitary function status pre- and postoperatively is recommended.

14.5.5 Outcome and Recurrence

Short-term outcomes show restoration or improvement of visual deficits in 60% or more of patients. However, recurrence rates are high. Numerous histological variants have been described, and tumors are graded using the World Health Organization (WHO) classification: grade I (benign, 90%), grade II (atypical, 8%), and grade III (anaplastic/malign, 2%) (Shivapathasundram et al. 2018). The higher the grade, the higher the risk of tumor recurrence, with up to 80% recurrence if grade III. However, even WHO grade I meningiomas reoccur in about 20% of patients, particularly when histology indicates a Ki67 index of 3% or higher (Shivapathasundram et al. 2018). Men are more likely to have tumor recurrence than women. Redo surgery and radiation therapy may be necessary for tumor control. Several researchers have found the presence of cancer stem cells in meningiomas that may present a treatment target for the future (Shivapathasundram et al. 2018). Patients require close follow-up and monitoring with MRI every 6–12 months until stable and at least yearly over the first 5 years. Once stable the patient may be able to transition to MRI every 5 years.

14.6 Harmatoma

These are rare benign pedunculated tumors found on the hypothalamus and the floor of the third ventricle that are composed of ganglion cells (Moshkin et al. 2011). Most patients present before the age of 4 years with precocious puberty (90%), "laughing" seizures, behavioral issues, and developmental delay (Gustina et al. 2017). Patients may become obese over time. Harmatomas may also be associated with other inherited autosomal dominant disorders such as Pallister–Hall syndrome (Gustina et al. 2017).

The treatment of precocious puberty is the downregulation of GnRH receptors with long acting GnRH analogues. Surgical options are not usually indicated secondary to increased risk to local structures, but radiation therapy may have a role (Gustina et al. 2017).

14.7 Craniopharyngioma

14.7.1 Definition and Epidemiology

Craniopharyngiomas (CP) are benign, slow growing tumors that account for approximately 3–4.6% of all intracranial tumors (Fahlbusch and Buchfelder 2017; Algahtani et al. 2018). About 9% of all childhood intracranial tumors are CPs, with a peak incidence between 15 and 20 years of age. In adulthood, the peak incidence is between 50 and 74 years (Shin et al. 1999; Gustina et al. 2017). There is no significant difference in prevalence by gender (Fahlbusch and Buchfelder 2017).

14.7.2 Etiology

Pituitary CPs originate from epithelial cells on the surface of the pituitary gland and are thought to arise from the remnants of Rathke's pouch. These often develop along the infundibulohypophysial axis in the region between the sella and hypothalamus, and present treatment challenges associated with tumor growth, associated morbidities and recurrence (Algahtani et al. 2018; Bi et al. 2018). CPs grow to fill the sella and parasellar regions and extend either in front of or behind the optic chiasm, in approximately 4–5.9% of cases (Algahtani et al. 2018).

Two histological subtypes of CP have been identified: adamantinomatous and papillary. Adamantinomatous or cystic CPs are found in most pediatric cases and representing about 60% of all CPs; papillary CPs mostly found in adults in whom 81–95% of which have been found to harbor a *BRAFV600E* mitogenic mutation (Bi et al. 2018). In childhood and adolescent CP, 70% of the adamantinomatous type of CPs bear a mutation of the β-catenin gene (Müller 2016). These may represent a future treatment target (Bi et al. 2018). Tumors are often large and locally aggressive. The majority of children (91%) present with tumors >3 cm.

14.7.3 Symptoms

Patients often present with diabetes insipidus and impaired gonadal function. Hypopituitarism is present in 95% of cases (Shin et al. 1999). The majority of patients present with ophthalmologic complaints, neurological deficits and up to one-third have psychiatric manifestations (Shin et al. 1999). Children often present with intermittent and early morning headache, vomiting (possibly projectile), and changes in visual acuity. Short stature is reported in approximately 43% of children, and sleep disturbances are common (Gustina et al. 2017). Visual changes in acuity and asymmetric visual field deficits are more common in adults (Gustina et al. 2017). Seizures may be a presenting symptom if there is temporal lobe involvement. Ataxia can occur with midbrain involvement (Gustina et al. 2017).

14.7.4 Assessment

On MRI, CPs present with characteristic cystic and solid components or areas of calcification and hemorrhage (Maya and Pressman 2017). Prechiasmic lesions may have symptoms of optic atrophy, and, if the tumor is retrochiasmatic, papilledema may be present on formal ophthalmologic exam. If there is extension of the tumor into the cavernous sinuses, visual exam may show signs of cranial nerve III, IV, and V1 damage with symptoms of diplopia and disconjugate gaze even on a visual confrontational exam (Gustina et al. 2017). Assessment of anterior and posterior pituitary functions and full neurologic examination are recommended.

14.7.5 Treatment

First-line treatment is surgical excision of the tumor and confirmation of histopathology. CPs are described as technically difficult to remove due to adherence of the tumor to local structures. Removal of the tumor can cause further damage to structures such as the optic apparatus, hypothalamus, carotid and basilar arteries, and third ventricle which accounts for some of the associated post-surgical morbidity (Bal et al. 2016; Prieto et al. 2018). Microscopic and endoscopic surgical techniques have improved both mortality and morbidity, but recurrence rates remain at 21–25% (Gustina et al. 2017). Even in the hands of experienced surgeons, historical surgical approaches have resulted in 53–80% of patients requiring postoperative pituitary replacement and management of DI long term (Algahtani et al. 2018). Some surgeons report this can be significantly improved in adults and children using an endonasal endoscopic transsphenoidal surgical approach (Bal et al. 2016). However, higher rates of CSF leak have been reported (Bal et al. 2016; Patel et al. 2017). Radiation may be still indicated for tumor regrowth or large residual lesions.

Postoperative evaluation for persistent or new onset anterior and pituitary deficits is needed. Diabetes insipidus is anticipated postoperatively, given that most tumors are proximate or adherent to the pituitary stalk (Patel et al. 2017). However, this may be transient and resolve postoperatively. Visual acuity and visual field testing postoperatively reveals improved vision in the majority of patients (>60%) (Müller 2016; Patel et al. 2017). Hypothalamic dysfunction and obesity is also apparent in the majority of patients (55–85%) and results in significant morbidity, mortality, and poor quality of life (Müller 2016). Other associated changes include daytime sleepiness, disturbed circadian rhythm, behavioral changes, and imbalances in regulation of thirst, body temperature, heart rate, and/or blood pressure.

14.7.6 Nursing and Long-Term Care

Treatment recommendations include encouraging activity, dietary counseling, and management of hunger, although hypothalamic obesity is usually not responsive to conventional lifestyle modifications. There are few long-term studies to confirm best practice. However, a planned home care environment with respect to diet and exercise has been shown to be somewhat effective (Müller 2016). Antiglycemic medications have been found to be effective for weight reduction in some patients as has lap band bariatric surgery. However, long-term outcomes demonstrated weight gain. Replacement of melatonin to improve sleep, and/or assessment and treatment of sleep apnea and narcolepsy is recommended (Müller 2016). Patients may require long-term replacement of pituitary hormones and associated education and support.

14.8 Conclusions

For all tumors that impact the pituitary, hormonal function, and vision may be compromised. Assessment of all pituitary functions and formal ophthalmology review, both acutely at patient presentation, and with long-term monitoring, is indicated. A comprehensive history and physical including environmental exposures, historical and current medications, symptom review, and a thorough clinical examination are critical in the diagnosis and to guide treatment. MRI may be diagnostic even when clinical findings are negatives.

Surgical treatment may be indicated when vision is threatened or to enable a definitive diagnosis. The need for replacement of pituitary deficiencies and particularly growth hormone in children is common. Likewise, treatment for adrenal insufficiency is indicated in some children and adults and may be required lifelong. When hypothalamic damage is apparent, home management of weight gain is currently the most effective treatment. In the treatment of hypophysitis, the use of high dose glucocorticoids is controversial, but may be useful in some cases.

Nursing care includes attention to a broad spectrum of patient functions. This extends from the time of patient diagnosis through long-term treatment. Patient needs may change across the lifespan necessitating an adaptive treatment plan. Patient and family teaching are tailored to each diagnosis.

References

Algahtani AY, Algahtani HA, Jamjoom AB, Samkari AM, Marzuk YI. De novo craniopharyngioma of the fourth ventricle: case report and review of literature. Asian J Neurosurg. 2018;13(1):62–5. https://doi.org/10.4103/1793-5482.185063.

Auer MK, Stieg MR, Crispin A, Sievers C, Stalla GK, Kopczak A. Primary empty Sella syndrome and the prevalence of hormonal dysregulation—a systematic review. Dtsch Arztebl Int. 2018;115:99–105. https://doi.org/10.3238/arztebl.2018.0099.

Bal E, Öge K, Berker M. Endoscopic endonasal transsphenoidal surgery, a reliable method for treating primary and recurrent/residual craniopharyngiomas: nine years of experience. World Neurosurg. 2016;94:375–85.

Ball AK, Clarke CE. Idiopathic intracranial hypertension. Lancet Neurol. 2006;5:433–42.

Ball AK, Howman A, Wheatley K, Burdon MA, Matthews T, Jacks AS, Lawden M, Sivaguru A, Furmston A, Howell S, Sharrack S, Davies MB, Sinclair AJ, Clarke CE. A randomised controlled trial of treatment for idiopathic intracranial hypertension. J Neurol. 2011;258:874–81. https://doi.org/10.1007/s00415-010-5861-4.

Bernreuther C, Illies C, Flitsch J, Buchfelder M, Buslei R, Glatzel M, Saeger W. IgG4-related hypophysitis is highly prevalent among cases of histologically confirmed hypophysitis. Brain Pathol. 2017;27(6):839–45. https://doi.org/10.1111/bpa.12459. Epub 2017 Jan 11.

Bi WL, Larsen AG, Dunn IF. Genomic alterations in sporadic pituitary tumors. Curr Neurol Neurosci Rep. 2018;18:4. https://doi.org/10.1007/s11910-018-0811-0.

Carmichael JD. Anterior pituitary failure. In: Melmed S, editor. Pituitary. 4th ed. London: Elsevier; 2017. p. 329–63.

Carroll KT, Lochte BC, Chen JY, Snyder VS, Carter BS, Chen CC. Intraoperative magnetic resonance imaging-guided biopsy in the diagnosis of suprasellar langerhans cell histiocytosis. World Neurosurg. 2018;112:6–13. https://doi.org/10.1016/j.wneu.2017.12.184. Epub 2018 Jan 6.

Catford S, Wang YY, Wong R. Pituitary stalk lesions: systematic review and clinical guidance. Clin Endocrinol. 2016;85:507–21.

Chatziralli I, Theodossiadis P, Theodossiadis G, Asproudis I. Perspectives on diagnosis and management of adult idiopathic intracranial hypertension. Graefes Arch Clin Exp Ophthalmol. 2018;256(7):1217–24. https://doi.org/10.1007/s00417-018-3970-4. Accessed 26 Mar 2018.

Chiloiro S, Giampietro A, Bianchi A, Tartaglione T, Capobianco A, Anile C, De Marinis L. Diagnosis of endocrine disease: primary empty Sella: a comprehensive review. Eur J Endocrinol. 2017;177(6):R275–85.

Crock PA. Cytosolic autoantigens in lymphocytic hypophysitis. J Clin Endocrinol Metab. 1998;83:609–18.

Daniels AB, Liu GT, Volpe NJ, et al. Profiles of obesity, weight gain and quality of life in idiopathic intracranial hypertension (pseudotumor cerebri). Am J Opthalmol. 2007;143:635–41.

Digre KB, Bruce BB, McDermott MP, Galetta KM, Balcer LJ, Wall M. Quality of life in idiopathic intracranial hypertension at diagnosis: IIH treatment trial results. Neurology. 2015;84(24):2449–56. https://doi.org/10.1212/WNL.0000000000001687.

Dillard T, Yedinak CG, Alumkal J, Fleseriu M. Anti-CTLA-4 antibody therapy associated autoimmune hypophysitis: serious immune related adverse events across a spectrum of cancer subtypes. Pituitary. 2010;13:29–38.

Dolecek TA, Propp JM, Stroup NE, Kruchko C. CBTRUS statistical report: primary brain and central nervous system Tumors diagnosed in the United States in 2005–2009. Neuro-Oncology. 2012;14(Suppl 5):v1–v49. https://doi.org/10.1093/neuonc/nos218.

Dubey A, Patwardhan RV, Sampth S, Santosh V, Kolluri S, Nanda A. Intracranial fungal granuloma: analysis of 40 patients and review of the literature. Surg Neurol. 2005;63:254–60.

Elgamal ME, Mohamed RMH, Fiad T, Elgamal EA. Granulomatous hypophysitis: rare disease with challenging diagnosis. Clin Case Rep. 2017;5(7):1147–51. https://doi.org/10.1002/ccr3.1007.

Fahlbusch R, Buchfelder M. Pituitary surgery. In: Melmed S, editor. The pituitary. 4th ed. London: Elsevier; 2017. p. 671–87.

Faje A. Immunotherapy and hypophysitis: clinical presentation, treatment, and biologic insights. Pituitary. 2016;19:82–92. https://doi.org/10.1007/s11102-015-0671-4.

Fleseriu M. Pituitary dysfunction in systemic disorders. In: Melmed S, editor. The pituitary. 4th ed. London: Elsevier; 2017. p. 365–38.

Fleseriu M, Yedinak C, Campbell C, Delashaw JB. Significant headache improvement after transsphenoidal surgery in patients with small sellar lesions.

J Neurosurg. 2009;110(2):354–8. https://doi.org/10.31 71/2008.8.JNS08805.

Friedman DI, Liu GT, Digre KB. Revised diagnostic criteria for the pseudotumor cerebri syndrome in adults and children. Neurology. 2013;81(13):1159–65. https://doi.org/10.1212/WNL.0b013e3182a55f1.

Gellner V, Kurschel S, Scarpatetti M, Mokry M. Lymphocytic hypophysitis in the pediatric population. Childs Nerv Syst. 2008;24(7):785–92. https://doi.org/10.1007/s00381-007-0577-1. Epub 2008 Feb 26.

Glezer A, Bronstein MD. Pituitary autoimmune disease: nuances in clinical presentation. Endocrine. 2012;42:74–9. https://doi.org/10.1007/s12020-012-9654-7.

González-Andrades M, García-Serrano JL, Gallardo MCG, Mcalinden C. Multiple cranial nerve involvement with idiopathic intracranial hypertension. QJM. 2016;109(4):265–6. https://doi.org/10.1093/qjmed/hcv217.

Guedes BF, Souza MNP, Barbosa BJAP, et al. Intracranial germinoma causing cerebral haemiatrophy and hypopituitarism. Pract Neurol. 2018;18(4):306–10. https://doi.org/10.1136/practneurol-2017-001771.

Gustina A, Frara S, Spina A, Mortini P. The hypothalamus. In: Melmed S, editor. The pituitary. 4th ed. London: Elsevier; 2017. p. 291–327.

Gutenberg A, Caturegli P, Metz I, et al. Necrotizing infundibulo-hypophysitis: an entity too rare to be true? Pituitary. 2012;15(2):202–8. https://doi.org/10.1007/s11102-011-0307-2.

Huo CW, Caputo C, Wang YY. Suprasellar keratinous cyst: a case report and review on its radiological features and treatment outcome. Surg Neurol Int. 2018;9:15. https://doi.org/10.4103/sni.sni_269_17.

Idiopathic Intracranial Hypertension. National Eye Institute. Last reviewed April 2014. https://nei.nih.gov/health/iih/intracranial.

Iplikcioglu AC, Bek S, Bikmaz K, Ceylan D, Gokduman CA. Aspergillus pituitary abscess. Acta Neurochir. 2004;146:521–4. https://doi.org/10.1007/s00701-004-0256-x.

Iwama S, De Remigis A, Callahan MK, Slovin SF, Wolchok JD, Caturegli P. Pituitary expression of CTLA-4 mediates hypophysitis secondary to administration of CTLA-4 blocking antibody. Sci Transl Med. 2014;6:230ra45.

Kleinschmidt JJ, Digre KB, Hanover R. Idiopathic intracranial hypertension: relationship to depression, anxiety and quality of life. Neurology. 2000;54:319–24.

Larkin S, Karavitaki N, Ansorg O. Chapter 17: Rathke's cleft cyst. In: Fliers E, Korbonits M, Romijn JA, editors. Handbook of clinical neurology (3rd series), vol. 124. Amsterdam: Elsevier B.V; 2014.

Laws ER, Vance ML, Jane JA Jr. Hypophysitis. Pituitary. 2006;9:331–3.

Li J, Jia HW, Wang CL, Zhang R, Qu MY, Li W, Yuan MH, Cui J, He Q, Wei HY, Zhu TH, Ma ZS, Liu W, Dong ZL, Gao ZG. Primary empty Sella of 123 cases of clinical analysis. Chin J Intern Med.

2017;56(4):268–72. https://doi.org/10.3760/cma.j.issn.0578-1426.2017.04.006.

Maya MM, Pressman BK. Piutitary imaging. In: Melmed S, editor. The pituitary. 4th ed. London: Elsevier; 2017. p. 645–70.

McDermott MT. Infiltrative diseases of the pituitary gland. In: Wierman ME, editor. Diseases of the pituitary. Contemporary endocrinology, vol. 3. New York: Humana Press; 1997. p. 395–6.

Melmed S, Kleinberg D. Chapter 9—pituitary masses and tumors. In: Melmed S, Kenneth S, Polonsky P, Larsen R, Kronenberg HM, editors. Williams textbook of endocrinology. 13th ed. Philadelphia, PA: Elsevier; 2016. p. 232–99.

Mittal R, Kalra P, Dharmalingam M, Verma RG, Kulkarni S, Shetty P. Lymphocytic hypophysitis masquerading as pituitary adenoma. 1. Lymphocytic hypophysitis masquerading as pituitary adenoma. Indian J Endocrinol Metab. 2012;16(8):304–6.

Moshkin O, Albrecht S, Bilboa JM, Kovacs K. Nonpituitary tumors of the sellar region. In: Melmed S, editor. The pituitary. 3rd ed. London: Elsevier; 2011. p. 119–66. https://doi.org/10.1016/B978-0-12-380926-1.10015-X.

Müller HL. Craniopharyngioma and hypothalamic injury: latest insights into consequent eating disorders and obesity. Curr Opin Endocrinol Diabetes Obes. 2016;23(1):81–9. https://doi.org/10.1097/MED.0000000000000214.

Néel A, Artifoni M, Donadieu J, Lorillon G, Hamidou M, Tazi A. Langerhans cell histiocytosis in adults. Rev Med Interne. 2015;36(10):658–67.

Patel VS, Thamboo A, Quon J, Nayak JV, Hwang PH, Edwards M, Patel ZM. Outcomes after endoscopic endonasal resection of craniopharyngiomas in the pediatric population. World Neurosurg. 2017;108:6–14. https://doi.org/10.1016/j.wneu.2017.08.058.

PDQ® Pediatric Treatment Editorial Board. PDQ Langerhans Cell Histiocytosis Treatment. Bethesda, MD: National Cancer Institute. 2018. https://www.cancer.gov/types/langerhans/patient/langerhans-treatment-pdq. Accessed 28 Apr 2018.

Per H, Canpolat M, Gümüş H, Poyrazoğlu HG, Yıkılmaz A, Karaküçük S, Doğan H, Kumandaş S. Clinical spectrum of the pseudotumor cerebri in children: etiological, clinical features, treatment and prognosis. Brain and Development. 2013;35(6):561–8. https://doi.org/10.1016/j.braindev.2012.08.008. Epub 2012 Sep 13.

Perry BG, Cotter JD, Mejuto G, Mündel T, Lucas SJE. Cerebral hemodynamics during graded Valsalva maneuvers. Front Physiol. 2014;5:349. https://doi.org/10.3389/fphys.2014.00349.

Prieto R, Pascual JM, Rosdolsky M, Barrios L. Preoperative assessment of craniopharyngioma adherence: magnetic resonance imaging findings correlated with the severity of tumor attachment to the hypothalamus. World Neurosurg. 2018;110:e404–26. https://doi.org/10.1016/j.wneu.2017.11.012. Epub 2017 Nov 11.

Rangwala LM, Liu GT. Pediatric idiopathic intracranial hypertension. Surv Ophthalmol. 2007;52(6):597–617.

Raverot G, Burman P, McCormack A, Heaney A, Petersenn S, Popovic V, Trouillas J, Dekkers OM. The European Society of Endocrinology European Society of endocrinology clinical practice guidelines for the management of aggressive pituitary tumours and carcinomas. Eur J Endocrinol. 2018;178:G1–G24. https://doi.org/10.1530/EJE-17-0796.

Sajko T, Gnjidić Ž, Sesar N, Malenica M. Sphenoid sinus aspergilloma in trans-sphenoidal surgery for pituitary adenomas. Acta Neurochir. 2015;157(8):1345–51 discussion 1351. https://doi.org/10.1007/s00701-015-2485-6.

Schlosser RJ, Bolger WE. Spontaneous nasal cerebrospinal fluid leaks and empty Sella syndrome: a clinical association. Am J Rhinol. 2003;17(2):91–6.

Sheldon CA, Paley GL, Xiao R, Kesler A, Eyal O, Ko MW, Boisvert CJ, Avery RA, Salpietro V, Phillips PH, Heidary G, McCormack SE, Liu GT. Pediatric idiopathic intracranial hypertension: age, gender, and anthropometric features at diagnosis in a large, retrospective multisite cohort. Ophthalmology. 2016;123(11):2424–31. https://doi.org/10.1016/j.ophtha.2016.08.004. Epub 2016 Sep 28.

Shi J, Zhang J, Wu Q, Chen G, Zhang H, Bo W. Granulomatous hypophysitis: two case reports and literature review. J Zhejiang Univ Sci B. 2009;10(7):552–8. https://doi.org/10.1631/jzus.B0820355.

Shin JL, Asa SL, Woodhouse LJ, Smyth HS, Ezzat S. Cystic lesions of the pituitary: clinicopathological features distinguishing craniopharyngioma, Rathke's cleft cyst, and arachnoid cyst. J Clin Endocrinol Metab. 1999;84(11):3972–82.

Shivapathasundram G, Wickremesekera AC, Tan ST, et al. Tumour stem cells in meningioma: a review. J Clin Neurosci. 2018;47:66–71.

Tillotson CV, Bhimji SS. Histiocytosis, Langerhans cell. In: StatPearls [internet]. Treasure Island, FL: StatPearls; 2018. https://www-ncbi-nlm-nih-gov.liboff.ohsu.edu/books/NBK430885.

Tyrrell JB, Finding W, Aron DC. Hypothalamus and pituitary: chapter 2. In: Greenspan FS, Baxter JD, editors. Basic & clinical endorinology. 4th ed. Norwalk, CT: Appelton & Lange; 1994. p. 91.

Wall M. Idiopathic intracranial hypertension. Neurol Clin. 2010;28(3):593–617. https://doi.org/10.1016/j.ncl.2010.03.003.

Yoo F, Kuan EC, Heaney AP, et al. Corticotrophic pituitary carcinoma with cervical metastases: case series and literature review. Pituitary. 2018;21:290. https://doi.org/10.1007/s11102-018-0872-8.

Dynamic Investigations and Diagnostic Testing

15

Christine Yedinak and Kate Davies

Contents

C. Yedinak (✉)
Northwest Pituitary Center, Oregon Health and
Sciences University, Portland, OR, USA
e-mail: yedinakc@ohsu.edu

K. Davies
Department of Advanced and Integrated Practice,
London South Bank University, London, UK
e-mail: kate.davies@lsbu.ac.uk

© Springer Nature Switzerland AG 2019
S. Llahana et al. (eds.), *Advanced Practice in Endocrinology Nursing*,
https://doi.org/10.1007/978-3-319-99817-6_15

Abstract

The evaluation of pituitary function is complex and critical. Pituitary dysfunction causes a wide range of physical, emotional, social, and potentially spiritual changes, all of which compound the process of evaluation. Patient and family anxieties are heightened given either symptoms of unknown etiology or a new discovery of a "brain tumor," which can influence testing outcomes and requires nursing expertise in management.

Infants and children are affected by pituitary dysfunction that can present with life-threatening symptoms and parents in need of significant support. Both issues pose a challenge to the endocrine nurse involved in the child's evaluation. Most testing is not emergent and appropriate patient and parent preparation with attention to factors that can invalidate testing is vital. Explanations and/or literature provided to the patient and family must be age and language appropriate.

There is a broad range of diagnostic techniques that may be employed in diagnosis and ongoing patient management for patients with pituitary diseases. Knowledge of the testing purpose, procedure, and result interpretation is essential for the endocrine nurse performing testing and advance practice nursing for long-term patient management.

Keywords

Provocative testing · Dynamic testing · Pituitary dysfunction · Patient preparation · Anterior pituitary · Posterior pituitary

Abbreviations

17KG	17-ketogenic steroid
17OHCS	17-hydroxycorticosteroid
17OHP	17-hydroxyprogesterone
ACTH	Adrenocorticotropic hormone
ADA	American Diabetic Association
ADH	Anti-diuretic hormone
AI	Adrenal insufficiency
AVP	Arginine vasopressin
CAH	Congenital adrenal hyperplasia
Cm	Centimeter
CRH	Corticotropin releasing hormone
CSF	Cerebral spinal fluid
CT	Computed tomography
DDAVP	Synthetic desmopressin
DI	Diabetes insipidus
dL	Deciliter
EMR	Electronic Medical Record
FSH	Follicle stimulating hormone
G	Gram
GH	Growth hormone
GHD	Growth hormone deficiency
GHRH	Growth hormone releasing hormone
GnRH	Gonadotropin releasing hormone
GST	Glucagon stimulation test
HCG	Human chorionic gonadotropin
HPA	Hypothalamic pituitary adrenal
HPG	Hypothalamic pituitary gonadal
HPT	Hypothalamic–pituitary thyroid
IGF-1	Insulin-like growth factor 1
IPSS	Inferior petrosal sinus sampling
ITT	Insulin tolerance test
IV	Intravenous
IVP	Intravenous push
Kg	Kilogram
LH	Luteinizing hormone
LNSC	Late night salivary cortisol
m²	Meter squared
mL	Milliliter
mOsm	Milli-osmolarity
MRI	Magnetic resonance imaging
Na	Sodium
Ng	Nanogram
nmol/L	Nanamole/liter
PCOS	Polycystic ovarian syndrome
PET-CT	Positron emission tomography with computerized tomography
rhGH	Recombinant growth hormone
SAI	Secondary adrenal insufficiency
SHBG	Sex hormone binding globulin
SRS	Somatostatin receptor scintigraphy
T3	Triiodothyronine
T4	Thyroxine
TRH	Thyrotropin releasing hormone
TSH	Thyroid stimulating hormone
WDT	Water deprivation test
μg	Microgram

Key Terms

- **Provocative/dynamic/stimulation testing:** is the exposure of the patient to a substance or drug to evaluate their bodies' response. This response is compared to average responses from unaffected individuals.
- **Testing protocol:** describes the standardized method or procedure used to perform a test.
- **Cut-off values:** differentiate normal responses from abnormal or dysfunctional responses.
- **Informed consent:** is a process of explanation to a patient and family, in an understandable language and age-appropriate manner, the proposed procedure, risks and benefits, and anticipated outcome(s) of testing. The patient must be given ample opportunity to ask questions and consider the information provided. This must be provided for all procedures with written consent for any invasive or experimental procedures.

Key Points

- Many pediatric dynamic/provocative function tests are based on adult protocols, with weight-related dosages of medication.
- All patients require age-appropriate preparation for provocative testing. Parents of pediatric patients also require preparation with respect to the developmental medical needs of their child.
- Provocative testing is often time intensive for staff and time consuming for the

patient. Some tests are carried out over a number of days.

- Medical testing is anxiety provoking and some invasive tests may require the patient to be pretreated with anxiolytics or receive sedation, particularly in children. Thoughtful preparation can reduce anxiety and the need for other medications.
- In order to fully prepare a patient for testing, the nurse must have detailed knowledge of why and how the test is performed, and the meaning of the results.

15.1 Introduction

Both random and provocative or dynamic blood tests are the cornerstone of diagnosis in pituitary diseases and dysfunction. However, there is substantial variability in testing protocols between countries and between individual testing sites. Standardization is inhibited in some cases by lack of consensus regarding the timing of blood collections and drug dosages that will reliably arrive at a consistent diagnosis. There is variability in assays used between studies that make results difficult to compare. Likewise, cut-off point variability is apparent between different protocols adding further complexity.

Given these challenges, the information in this chapter attempts to provide some standardized recommendations for patient preparation and testing procedures and highlights some of the significant differences in process and/or interpretation of results. This chapter is meant as a guide and must be interpreted in the context of the reader's clinical site.

15.2 Basal Testing and Random Serum Analysis

15.2.1 Corticotropin Assessment

Corticotropin levels are assessed to determine adequacy of adrenal function or the presence of cortisol excess. Low cortisol levels may be associated with primary or secondary adrenal insufficiency. Likewise, cortisol excess may be associated with pituitary-derived adrenocorticotropic hormone (ACTH) excess or adrenal hypersecretion. Both clinical assessment and biochemical testing are used in diagnosis (Nieman 2003). When cortisol levels are high, it is important that further testing distinguish between Cushing's and pseudo-Cushing's syndrome (Nieman 2018). Prior to a blood draw the patient must be screened for all forms of cortisol suppressive or corticosteroid containing agents both prescribed and over the counter (creams, lotions, sprays, supplements, herbal preparations, tonics, and skin bleaching agents, joint injections, etc.) as well as estrogen use (effects cortisol binding globulin) (Nieman 2018).

Random cortisol levels must be interpreted in the context of the time of day the sample was drawn, as these levels display a variable circadian or 24 h pattern of production (see Anatomy & Physiology). The highest cortisol levels are found in the early morning and lowest at midnight. Random cortisol levels are therefore not diagnostic and further dynamic testing modalities are usually required.

In primary adrenal failure or dysfunction, a morning cortisol of less than 140 nmol/L (5 g/dL) with a concomitant ACTH level that is twofold the upper limit of the reference range is diagnostic for primary adrenal insufficiency. However, a dynamic corticotropin stimulation test to confirm the diagnosis is recommended (Bornstein et al. 2016).

In secondary adrenal insufficiency (SAI), impaired corticotropin releasing hormone (CRH) and/or ACTH secretion lead to low adrenal cortisol production. A baseline cortisol measurement of <3 μg/dL (83 nmol/) is indicative of SAI. Conversely, a cortisol >18 μg/dL (500 nmol/L) excludes a diagnosis of adrenal insufficiency. The cortisol level should be evaluated in the context of factors such as the time of day, specific assay cut-off, the presence of liver dysfunction, and the use of estrogen in women. However, many cases of SAI may not be quite so overt. Therefore, dynamic corticotropin testing is recommended (Nieman 2003; Bornstein et al. 2016).

In addition, the mineralocorticoid axis remains intact in untreated SAI, resulting in a subsequent increase in arginine vasopressin (AVP)/antidiuretic hormone (ADH) level, water retention, and hypervolemic hyponatremia (Wallace et al. 2009).

In cases of cortisol excess, random elevated ACTH and/or cortisol requires further evaluation, as described below.

15.2.2 Somatotrophs: Growth Hormone Assessment

Growth hormone (GH) levels may be measured using a random GH level plus an insulin growth hormone-1 (IGF-1) measurement from a single draw blood sample. The diagnostic use of random GH measurement is limited by its short half-life, which is estimated at a mean of 13.6 min (range 11.9–19.4) (Mullis et al. 1992). A mean of 5 time point draws at 30 min intervals has shown to be effective in measuring GH excess in patient with active or treated acromegaly (Roelfsema et al. 2016). Growth hormone measurement in children explores implications for growth (see Chap. 2), and stimulation testing is necessary.

GH excreted from the pituitary attaches to receptor sites on liver cells. This stimulates the liver to produce IGF-1 which can be measured at any time of day (Schilbach et al. 2017). IGF-1 levels are adjusted for gender and age. Both low and elevated levels require further evaluation for GH deficiency and excess (Roelfsema et al. 2016).

15.2.3 Gonadotroph Assessment

The measurement of follicle stimulating hormone (FSH) and luteinizing hormone (LH), testosterone and estrogen levels assess pituitary production along with ovarian and testicular function. In women, the estrogen level rises to inhibit the production of FSH. LH then rises with the inhibition of FSH, matures the ovum, and results in ovulation. The empty ovum produces progesterone to support a pregnancy but falls again if pregnancy does not occur. The levels of FSH and LH will vary according to the woman's age and the timing of the blood draw with respect to the menstrual cycle (Ben-Schomo and Melmed 2011). Reference ranges are usually provided by the laboratory according to the woman's age and time of cycle. Testosterone levels may also be measured in woman suspected of having polycystic ovarian syndrome (PCOS). The performing laboratory publishes reference levels.

In males, FSH and LH stimulate the production of testosterone from the Leydig cells in the testes. When the secretions of FSH and LH from the pituitary are impaired, there is resultant hypogonadotropic hypogonadism (Kaiser 2016). Testosterone production is diurnal with the highest surges in the morning, particularly in young men. Measurement, therefore, is best attempted in the morning. For a full evaluation of gonadal function, total testosterone and a testosterone profile can be ordered which includes a total and free testosterone plus a sex hormone binding globulin (SHBG) (Kaiser 2016).

15.2.4 Thyrotroph Assessment

Hypothalamic thyrotropin stimulating hormone (TRH) stimulates the production of pituitary thyroid stimulating hormone (TSH). In turn, TSH binds to receptors on the cell surface in the thyroid gland and results in the production and release of thyroid hormones triiodothyronine (T3) and thyroxine (T4). TSH is often measured as an indicator of thyroid function and is usually a reliable facsimile, except in the context of pituitary dysfunction. Measurement of free T4 is recommended as the most sensitive indicator of central hypothyroidism in the context of pituitary disease (Carmichael 2016).

15.2.5 Lactotrophs Assessment

Prolactin level is measured in non-pregnant females or with concomitant pregnancy testing in sexually active females. Avoidance of breast stimulation or stressful venipuncture is recommended prior to measurement of prolactin. A number of medications may elevate the prolactin level and need to be discontinued, when possible, prior to level assessment. Levels above normal range when patients demonstrate symptoms, need further evaluation for the presence of a prolactinoma (see Chap. 19) (Melmed et al. 2011).

15.2.6 Posterior Pituitary Assessment

The neurohypophysis releases AVP, which influences the anterior pituitary ACTH secretion, as well as responding to osmotic changes, hemorrhage, or the concentration of sodium (Na) in cerebrospinal fluid (CSF). AVP release is increased to reabsorb water from the kidneys when Na levels are high and decreases in order to allow diuresis when Na levels are low (Bichet 2016). Serum sodium levels, urine and serum osmolality, and AVP levels are useful in the management of dysfunction. Full evaluation of the posterior pituitary function requires a water deprivation test.

15.2.6.1 Water Deprivation Test (WDT)

A WDT needs to be undertaken when diagnosis of diabetes insipidus (DI) is suspected. DI occurs when insufficient anti-diuretic hormone (ADH) is produced by the posterior pituitary gland or when the target organs (kidneys), do not respond by adequately concentrating urine. The former is known as central diabetes insipidus and the latter nephrogenic DI (Davies and Collin 2015). Patients with both diagnoses will present with polydipsia and polyuria.

Initial investigations would include a full screening of blood and urine tests. Plasma sodium, potassium, bicarbonate, chloride, urea, creatinine, phosphate, calcium, glucose, liver function tests, and full blood count are usually performed. Both a serum and urine will also be investigated for osmolality. Plasma copeptin (a stable peptide stoichiometrically co-secreted with AVP) is a promising new marker for the diagnosis of AVP-dependent fluid disorders (Timper et al. 2015).

If indicated, a WDT is performed. The goal of this test is to determine if the patient's posterior pituitary is able to excrete adequate amounts of AVP/ADH and/or if the renal tubules in the kidneys are able to concentrate urine (Davies and Collin 2015).

15.2.6.1.1 Patient Preparation
Adults are asked to take all regular medications and eat the morning of testing, avoid alcohol for 48-h, and caffeine for 12–24 h prior to testing. Smoking is also discouraged. Many centers allow fluids and normal diet until the time of admission. All fluids are restricted at the time of admission and throughout the test. The test must be done under medical supervision as it can potentially cause dehydration with elevated sodium.

Children may be admitted, in some centers, for a 24 h fluid balance assessment, to confirm polyuria and polydipsia and also to rule out psychogenic or habitual, excessive drinking (Cheetham and Baylis 2002; Raine et al. 2011). Usually during this time, children should be restricted to solids and water only, omitting flavored or sugary drinks. If flavored drinks are withheld and the child refuses water, if the posterior pituitary and renal function is normal, the polyuria will cease. However, if the symptoms continue, the investigation should progress to the water deprivation test. Children are usually permitted to eat and drink until they arrive at the testing center (Cheetham and Baylis 2002).

Clear, age-appropriate, explanation of the testing purpose and procedure is essential, particularly as water intake during testing will invalidate the test.

15.2.6.1.2 Procedure
The WDT is a standardized 6–7 h test in adults and children, during which the patient is able to eat foods such as toast, biscuits but no water. The patient is closely observed during testing to avoid inadvertent fluid intake. Children may need to be accompanied to the lavatory.

(a) Baseline measurement of weight is done on admission to the testing unit and 97% of this weight is calculated and recorded.

(b) Baseline vital signs (blood pressure and heart rate) are taken and recorded on admission.

(c) The patient voids and discards first void.

(d) An intravenous catheter (cannula) is placed in the patients arm.

(e) A sample of blood for serum sodium and osmolality is collected at the beginning of the study (usually around 9 a.m.) and sent to the laboratory for STAT analysis.

(f) Urine samples are collected and measured hourly (volume, specific gravity, osmolality).

(g) Blood samples are collected hourly for STAT analysis.

(h) Vital signs are assessed hourly.

(i) The patients are weighed hourly and weight is compared to baseline. (See Table 15.1) (Cheetham and Baylis 2002; Raine et al. 2011).

The test is discontinued if:

– The first urine osmolality is >600 mOsmol/kg and subsequent sample is >750 mOsmol/kg the test can be aborted as results are normal.

– The child or adult has more than a 3% loss in body weight indicating moderate dehydration.

– Plasma osmolality >295 mOsm/kg (where normal values are 285–295) and sodium (Na) >145 mmol/L–confirms central (cranial) DI.

– Urine osmolality >800 mOsm/kg*—this would exclude DI, and the urine will be concentrated (normal values are 500–800: lower values would indicate dilute urine) or if the

thirst is intolerable (Wong and Man 2012). * In some reports urine osmolality >700 mOsm/kg.

– The urine output has not decreased, and the urine: plasma ratio is less than two, but plasma osmolality remains below 295, continue the test (Wong and Man 2012).

– Urine osmolarity is greater than 800 mOsmol/ kg after fluid deprivation, and greater than 800 mOsmol/kg after desmopressin suggests primary polydipsia.

15.2.6.1.3 Additional Procedure/Step 2

If 3–5% of body weight is lost, the patient has continued to have urine output which is not decreasing, urine has not concentrated and plasma osmolality has risen to >300 mOsmol/kg, desmopressin is administered by subcutaneous or intramuscular injection.

Patients with central/cranial DI (vasopressin deficiency or insufficiency) will respond to desmopressin administration by concentrating urine output. The urine osmolality will rise to >700 mOsm/kg. In patients with nephrogenic DI who have renal resistance to vasopressin, the urine continues to have a low osmolality of less than 700 mOsm/kg (Moore et al. 2003; Dashe et al. 1963).

DDAVP (desmopressin) can be administered, usually 0.4 µg (under 2 years of age) to 1 µg (over 2 years of age), to assess the renal desmopressin response (Cheetham and Baylis 2002; Raine et al. 2011). Samples for plasma and urine osmolality, and plasma sodium need to be measured for a further 4 h, and the child or adult can eat and

Table 15.1 Water Deprivation Test sampling (adapted from Butler and Kirk 2011)

	Time	Weight (kg)[a]	HR (bpm)	BP (mmHg)	Urine volume (mL)	Specific gravity	Samples
$T = 0$	0830						*, **
$T = 1$ h	0930						**
$T = 2$ h	1030						*, **
$T = 3$ h	1130						**
$T = 4$ h	1230						*, **
$T = 5$ h	1330						*, **
$T = 6$ h	1430						**
$T = 7$ h	1530						*, **

*Blood and **urine specimens to be sent for Na + and osmolality
Plasma osmolality: 0830, 1030, 1230, 1330, 1530 h
Urine osmolality: 0830, 0930, 1030, 1130, 1230, 1330, 1430, 1530, 1630, 1730 h
[a]Notify Doctor if body weight drops by 5% or more of the weight at the start of the test

drink normally. This part of the test can sometimes be performed at a later date if need be.

15.3 Hypopituitarism

15.3.1 Combined Pituitary Function Test (ITT/TRH/GnRH)

Pituitary reserve is completely assessed by using a combined pituitary function test. Some studies have combined an insulin tolerance test (ITT), TRH and GnRH tests, CRH, GRH, TRH, LH-RH, and lysine vasopressin. However, reports of efficacy vary (Burke 1992; Hashimoto et al. 1990). In practice, the TRH and GnRH tests are criticized for providing little clinically useful data beyond the basal hormone measurements: TFTs and prolactin; gonadal steroids; and gonadotropins. There have been reports that TRH and GnRH may be associated with a risk of pituitary apoplexy (Burke 1992). Additionally, others suggest that random basal samples should be drawn prior to doing provocative or dynamic testing in order to avoid unnecessary testing (Howlett 1997).

15.4 Corticotroph Function Testing

15.4.1 Diurnal Curves (Cortisol Day Curve/24 h Cortisol Profile/ Hydrocortisone Day Curve)

1. *A cortisol day curve* is used to determine the individual's endogenous cortisol production over a defined period during the day or for up to 24 h. This allows closer examination of adrenal response to endogenous ACTH production. The patient may be monitored as frequently as hourly with serum cortisol/ACTH levels (after the placement of an intravenous access), or at 3 or more time points during the day using salivary cortisol sampling (Selmaoui and Touitou 2003; Charles et al. 2016).
2. *The hydrocortisone day curve* is a means of assessing the adequacy of hydrocortisone replacement therapy over an average 24-h

period. The goal is to determine appropriate dosing and dose intervals based on cortisol levels drawn in the morning, mid-day, and in the evening prior to bedtime. The patient is administered their usual replacement doses of hydrocortisone during testing (Howlett 1997). Similarly, salivary cortisol levels collected have also been shown to be an effective means of assessment (Ross et al. 2013).

3. *A single morning plasma cortisol level* of <3 μg/dL (83 nmol/L) is considered indicative of AI and a plasma cortisol level > 19 μg/dL (524 nmol/L) excludes adrenal insufficiency (Nieman 2003). Dynamic testing is recommended for values in between.

15.4.2 Hypocortisolism

15.4.2.1 Insulin Tolerance Test (ITT)

The insulin tolerance test (ITT) is the "gold standard" for cortisol stimulation testing. Testing with ITT is used in the assessment of ACTH and cortisol reserve, growth hormone deficiency in adults and children, and to differentiate Cushing's syndrome from depression or pseudo-Cushing's (Nieman 2003; Carmichael 2016).

The ITT involves precipitating hypoglycemia with subcutaneous insulin injection, inducing a rise in cortisol and GH in normal individuals. However, it is contraindicated in patients with ischemic heart disease, epilepsy, type 2 diabetes mellitus, untreated hypothyroidism, patients over the age of 60 and should be used with caution for patients over the age of 55 years. ITT is not recommended when a random morning cortisol is <100 nmol/L (3 μg/dL) (Carmichael 2016).

Alternatives are the glucagon stimulation test, which is a central test of GH and cortisol reserve, and thus comparable to the ITT, or the short Synacthen test. The latter is disadvantaged by of only testing adrenal reserve and may give a false-positive result if performed soon after pituitary surgery/damage (Burke 1992).

ITT can be performed in children over the age of 10 years when the diagnosis of panhypopituitarism is suspected, such as after radiotherapy of a brain tumor (see Sect. 10 Chaps. 58–60). It cannot be performed following an HCG stimulation test, or after priming with sex steroids (Butler and Kirk 2011). ITT is recognized as the gold standard test for growth hormone deficiency diagnosis in children by the BSPED (British Society of Paediatric Endocrinology and Diabetes). Some centers in the UK advocate varying the procedure protocol by excluding the 120-min sample and also administering IV 10% dextrose after the 20-min sample has been taken. There is no proven benefit to these practices (Lone et al. 2011).

ITT should only be administered by trained/experienced, licensed medical professionals due to the risks associated to hypoglycemia. Hypoglycemic rescue must be available at the bedside in case of a severe hypoglycemic crisis.

Patient Preparation: Patients are asked to fast for 8–10 h prior to testing and should hold their morning medications prior to arrival but bring these medications with them to the testing center. All usual medications can be taken following the end of testing. Continued intake of water is recommended to allow better venous access. To allow IV placement, comfortable attire should allow access to both the right and left arm. In some centers, patients may be asked to bring a sandwich or a meal to be consumed at the completion of testing. Patients should not drive for 2 h after testing. It is recommended that patients receive written instructions at the time of appointment scheduling.

Children: Sex steroid priming remains controversial in the literature but guidelines by the Drug and Therapeutics Committee and Ethics Committee of the Pediatric Endocrine Society do recommend sex steroid priming prior to provocative GH testing in prepubertal boys older than 11 and in prepubertal girls older than 10 years. This is proposed as a means of addressing age-related deficiencies to allow comparison with established norms. Estrogen is administered to girls 2 days prior to testing and testosterone to boys 1 week prior to testing.

Girls: 2 mg (1 mg for body weight <20 kg) of β-estradiol (not ethinyl estradiol) orally for 2 evenings prior to testing.

Boys: Intramuscular testosterone 50–100 mg of a depot formulation administered 1 week before the test.

Procedure: On admission to the testing unit, patients will be weighed to allow calculation of the appropriate insulin dosage. Vital signs will also be taken and recorded at this time. If the unit is using electronic medical records, the data is entered directly. However, templates of testing records are often practical to use at the bedside to record data such as glucose measurements, signs and symptoms, or other notes during testing.

Regular insulin is used in testing. The dose is weight based and is administered to the patient via intravenous push (IVP) to induce hypoglycemia. The dose required ranges from 0.05 to 0.15 IU/kg. There is some variability between centers. The dose of 0.1 IU/kg (maximum 0.015 IU/kg) is standard in children, particularly if panhypopituitarism is suspected or the patient has low morning cortisol (Butler and Kirk 2011).

Baseline and fasting labs will be drawn prior to the insulin administration. Venous samples for glucose and GH are collected at 0, +15, +30, +60, +90, and +120. Bedside monitoring of blood glucose with a glucometer is advised, particularly in response to patient symptoms. Vital signs and patient symptoms are also measured and all information is recorded at each time point.

To be a valid test, the patient's glucose must drop to either 40 mg/dL or below OR 50% of their baseline fasting glucose (Carmichael 2016). If the post-dosing glucoses do not meet this criterion, another dose of insulin can be administered under the supervision of the licensed medical professional's discretion. If glucoses still do not drop to either of these levels, the test should be terminated and rescheduled for another time.

Upon completion of the test, the patient should have a meal prior to discharge and their glucose should be back to baseline. In children, parents are advised to observe their children at home for signs of rebound hypoglycemia, treat with orange juice and protein snack, and contact the testing unit as needed. All contact phone numbers should be given to the parents at patient discharge.

Hypoglycemic Symptoms: Patients need to be closely monitored throughout the testing with venous sampling and/or bedside blood glucose finger stick monitoring to prevent serious hypoglycemia. Symptoms of hypoglycemia include sweating, heart palpitations, clammy skin, fatigue, headache, thirst, confusion, pallor, and dizziness. If not monitored closely, severe hypoglycemia can lead to seizures, coma, or, in extreme cases, death. Therefore, patients must be able to communicate during this test and must be kept awake (Butler and Kirk 2011). Pediatric nurses should fully understand hypoglycemic symptoms, as children may not be able to verbalize their symptoms.

Hypoglycemic Rescue: If blood glucose is <40 mg/dL (≤2.2 mmol/L) with symptoms a glucose drink of at least 30 mL is given orally. If blood glucose does not rise within 15–30 min, decreases further or if oral glucose is not tolerated then IV glucose is administered. Dextrose-50 (or 10% glucose in the UK) must be at the bedside in case of a severe hypoglycemic emergency. For management of hypoglycemia in children, a rescue dose of 200 mg/kg of 10% dextrose (2 mL/kg) administered IVP slowly over about 3 min if the blood glucose falls below <40 mg/dL (2.2 mmol) although some authors recommend treatment at <4 mmol/L. (Butler and Kirk 2011) Overzealous management of hypoglycemia has been proven to be complex and sometimes fatal (Shah et al. 1992). This underscores the importance of experienced medical management of ITT in children. In children, if hypopituitarism is suspected, 100 mg hydrocortisone should also be prepared for IV administration.

Test Interpretation: There continues to be debate regarding lower cut-off levels indicative of GHD, particularly as levels are currently not BMI adjusted. Peak levels of <3.1 μg/L or <5.0 μg/L indicate pituitary dysfunction and the presence of growth hormone deficiency syndrome in adults and children, respectively (Grimberg et al. 2016).

15.4.2.2 ACTH Stimulation Testing

ACTH stimulation test is performed to measure the adrenal stress response to ACTH. These tests are used to diagnose or exclude primary and secondary adrenal insufficiency, Addison's disease, and other related conditions. The tests are also used distinguish whether the cause is from the adrenal glands (low cortisol and aldosterone pro-

duction) or the pituitary gland (low ACTH production). Significant variability has been reported in a UK regarding patient preparation, laboratory reported normal ranges, and procedure protocols (Chatha et al. 2010).

There continues to be debate regarding the optimal testing to determine adrenal hypofunction or insufficiency. No current test is safe, economic, convenient, and has a high sensitivity and specificity (Nieman 2003). Some centers use a low dose or a 1 μg dose of Synacthen while others only use 250 μg testing (Nieman 2003). In the evaluation of primary adrenal insufficiency, the Endocrine Society guidelines recommend the 1 μg test as a screening test but favor the 250 μg (standard dose) test when available (Bornstein et al. 2016).

15.4.2.2.1 Short ACTH (Synacthen/ Cosyntropin)/Low Dose (1 μg)

Although advocated, as a sensitive test there is some debate about false-positive results (Nieman 2003; Dickstein and Saiegh 2008; Fleseriu et al. 2010). Additionally, there is no commercially available 1 μg preparation necessitating dilution of 250 μg doses introducing a risk of dilutional error. This test is used to identify secondary adrenal insufficiency or to test the HPA axis function following prolonged steroid treatment (Carmichael 2016; Butler and Kirk 2011; Moloney et al. 2015; Broersen et al. 2015). In children, the short Synacthen test is also used for the investigation and diagnosis of congenital adrenal hyperplasia (Trapp et al. 2011). (See Chap. 35).

Patient Preparation: This is minimal, with instructions to hold all glucocorticoid medications and treatments (including steroid creams and sprays) the morning of testing. In some countries, children may be admitted the evening before the test for safety. Anesthetic cream can be applied to both arms in the antecubital space and the back of both hands an hour prior to arrival in the testing unit.

Procedure: An intravenous cannula (IV) is placed in a vein, typically in the inside of the elbow or in the back of the hand on admission to the testing unit. If there is concern regarding the viability of an IV for subsequent blood draws, a second cannula may be placed, particularly in children where the access may not be maintained after several draws. This also allows blood draws to be obtained without the potential for drug contamination. As this procedure is stressful, particularly in children, and ACTH and cortisol may rise, the patient is allowed to rest for 30–60 min prior to initiating testing. Blood is drawn for baseline measurement of blood cortisol and ACTH levels. Beginning the procedure by 9 a.m. is recommended in children (Butler and Kirk 2011).

Drug Preparation and Administration: A dose of 1 µg of ACTH (Synacthen/Cosyntropin/Synacthen = **SYN**thetic **ACTH**) is prepared by:

(a) Inject a 250 µg of drug into a solution of 249 mL of normal saline and mix well. The solution is prepared and 1 mL (1 µg) is withdrawn for administration immediately prior to testing to avoid adherence of the medication to the syringe walls or tubing.

(b) Dilute 250 µg of drug in 50 mL of normal saline giving a solution of 250 µg in 50 mL. Take 1 mL of this solution and dilute with 9 mL of saline giving 5 µg in 10 mL. Withdraw 2 mL (1 µg) for administration.

 – This test requires accuracy in dilution and administration technique for best results.

 – *Adult and Pediatric dose:* One µg of drug (milliliters as per dilution) is withdrawn and administered to the patient via IVP (Carmichael 2016).

 – The IV catheter is flushed with 3–4 mL of normal saline after drug administration. After 2–4 mL of saline is withdrawn and from the catheter and discarded, a second cortisol level is drawn at 30 min after drug administration. This test is usually well tolerated and without side effects (Chitale et al. 2013).

 – *Interpretation:* Peak serum levels above 18 µg/dL (500 nmol/L) indicated and adequate adrenal response in adults or 19 µg/dL > 550 nmol/L in children (Nieman 2003; Bornstein et al. 2016; Carmichael 2016; Butler and Kirk 2011).

15.4.2.2.2 Standard Dose ACTH Test/High Dose (25 mg/250 µg)

A supraphysiologic dose of 250 µg ACTH (1000 times higher than normal peak production) is effective in identify primary adrenal insufficiency (AI), but although used to identify secondary AI may have limited ability to detect secondary adrenal hypofunction unless the adrenal glands have atrophied over time from lack of pituitary ACTH stimulation (Nieman 2003; Bornstein et al. 2016; Carmichael 2016). In pediatrics a newborn baby with ambiguous genitalia will need immediate testing (see Chaps. 3 and 35) or when the child's levels of 17-hydroxyprogesterone (17OHP) are elevated above 30 nmol/L and is indicative of CAH (Butler and Kirk 2011).

Patient Preparation: The test can be performed at any time of the day (Carmichael 2016). However, the patient is instructed to hold any glucocorticoid replacement the day of testing which may risk symptomatic adrenal insufficiency, such as after long-term glucocorticoid use. Performance of the test early in the day may avoid this. This is especially pertinent in children. Patients should be instructed to bring their normal dose of glucocorticoid to clinic for administration at the completion of the test. In children, anesthetic cream can be applied to both antecubital spaces and the backs of both hands about an hour prior to arrival at the testing unit. This test is usually well tolerated.

Procedure: An angio-catheter (IV) is usually placed in a vein, typically in the inside of the elbow or in the back of the hand. In children two sites may need to be cannulated. Blood is drawn for baseline measurement of blood cortisol and ACTH levels.

Adult Dose: A solution of 250 µg/2 mL of sterile saline is prepared and administered IVP. Note: Synachten may be supplied in a 250 µg lyophilized vial or as 1 mL solution. The drug must be prepared according to package instructions.

Dose for Children: The dose of Synachten should be 500 ng(0.5 µg)/1.73 m^2 body surface area/(BSA). (To calculate BSA, = [height(cm) × weight (kg)/3600]m^2). Therefore, it is imperative that the child's weight

AND height is recorded upon admission. This may be administered IV or IM (Butler and Kirk 2011).

Usual doses:

0–6 months	62.5 µg
6 months–2 years	125 µg
>2 years	250 µg

Dilution: The dose and dilution of Synacthen may be different in each country or testing center. Most preparations require dilution. Check the package insert for dilution instructions. The dosage must be calculated according to the dilution. The solution also needs to be well mixed prior to drawing up the required dosage.

Recommended start time for testing in children is 9 a.m. At this time, baseline samples for cortisol and ACTH and 17OHP are drawn. A second baseline cortisol level is drawn 1 h later at some facilities. Synacthen is then administered, and sampling for cortisol continues at 30 and 60 min (Carmichael 2016; Butler and Kirk 2011). The test is well tolerated with very rare hypersensitivity reaction.

Interpretation: Peak serum levels above 18 µg/dL (500 nmol/L) indicated and adequate adrenal response (Nieman 2003; Bornstein et al. 2016; Carmichael 2016).

15.4.3 Metyrapone (Metopirone) Dynamic Testing

Metyrapone stimulation test is used to assess pituitary function. The drug blocks the conversion of 11-deoxycortisol to biologically active cortisol. In normal subjects, this stimulates the production of CRH and ACTH by negative feedback. Therefore, this test is useful to evaluate adrenal hypo- or hyperfunction. A failure to increase ACTH indicates either ACTH deficiency or primary adrenal disease and excludes a diagnosis of Cushing's disease (Newell-Price JDC 2016).

This drug can be used in two different ways, including an overnight single-dose test (OMT) or a multiple-dose test (STD). These tests are contraindicated in patients who are hypersensitive to metyrapone or its components. Common to both

tests, the procedure is performed under medical supervision (Fiad et al. 1994; Berneis et al. 2002).

Common side effects for either test can include hypotension, nausea, vomiting, abdominal discomfort, headache, dizziness, and allergic rash. As with all clinical testing, check with the patient's health insurance to ensure testing is covered (Fiad et al. 1994; Berneis et al. 2002).

OMT Procedure: Metyrapone is a 250 mg oral capsule taken with milk. Adults are dosed at 30 mg/kg at midnight with a maximum of 3 g given. A single blood sample is taken between 0730 and 0800 for 11-deoxycortisol (11-DOC) and/or adrenocorticotropic hormone (ACTH) levels.

Interpretation: A normal response is indicated in a rise of plasma ACTH levels of 44 pmol/L or 200 ng/L or an increase in 11-DOC to over 0.2 µmol/L or µg/L. (Fiad et al. 1994; Berneis et al. 2002)

STD Procedure: Patients are hospitalized for 24 h and administered six divided doses of 750 mg every 4 h over 24 h for a cumulative dose of 4.5 g. Patients collect a total of three 24 h urine specimens (the day prior to dosing, the day of dosing, and the day after dosing). Samples are measured for 17-hydroxycorticosteroids (17-OHCS) and/or 17 ketogenic steroids (17-KGS) levels.

Interpretation: A doubling of 17-KGS or a two- or fourfold increase in 17-OHCS indicates a normal response. Abnormal responses are indicative of partial or full panhypopituitarism, Cushing's syndrome, and/or adrenal hyperplasia.

These tests are limited by the availability of metyrapone and clinical laboratories able to perform the analysis (Newell-Price JDC 2016; Fiad et al. 1994; Berneis et al. 2002).

15.5 Hypercortisolism

The protocol for investigating Cushing's syndrome in children is the same in adults. Cushing's syndrome, especially Cushing's disease, is very rare in children. Close contact between adult and pediatric endocrine teams during pediatric investigations is vital (Savage et al. 2008).

15.5.1 Urinary Free Cortisol: 24 h (UFC)

Urinary cortisol excretion over a 24 h period has been considered the gold standard of adrenocortical activity for the diagnosis of Cushing's syndrome. There is currently some debate about this status and the cut-off values used for the upper limit of normal, based on new assay methods (Raff et al. 2015). Regardless, it remains a highly sensitive marker of cortisol production and useful in the diagnosis of both low and excess cortisol (Newell-Price JDC 2016; Nieman et al. 2008). However, cortisol only appears in the urine when it exceeds the binding capacity in plasma (Raff et al. 2015).

The purpose of this test is to assess how much free (unbound) cortisol is in urine. This level is correlated with blood levels of free cortisol over the previous 24 h period (Newell-Price JDC 2016). Two collections are recommended (Nieman et al. 2008).

Patient preparation: includes avoidance of medications including all steroid creams, oral or injected glucocorticoids (including intraarticular injections), ketoconazole, estrogens, carbamazepine, fenofibrate, and mitotane that interfere with the assay and provide false cortisol levels (Nieman et al. 2008). When the glomerular filtration rate less than 30 mL/min or if the patient is drinking more than 3–5 L of fluid daily, the testing results may be inaccurate (Nieman 2018).

Procedure: The patient is instructed to void on awakening and discard the first morning urine. However, the time of this void is recorded and initiates the 24 h of the collection. All urine is collected in jugs provided by the laboratory or large clean containers for exactly 24 h from the start time. This includes the first morning void on the following day. All urine collected must be kept refrigerated or on ice during the collection and until deposited at the laboratory (Nieman 2018). Check with the laboratory that will perform the assay regarding what type of urine preservative may be required.

Interpretation: The results are interpreted in the context of the urine volume and creatinine and in children, corrected for body surface area.

Cut-off values are published by the lab performing the test based on the specific assay used.

15.5.2 Late Night Salivary Cortisol (LNSC)

In people with normal cortisol production, cortisol nadir or the lowest level, is immediately before sleep with a circadian rise in the early morning. The loss of this circadian pattern is the hallmark of Cushing's syndrome (Yaneva et al. 2004). However, in shift workers with a variable schedule, LNSC may not be reliable (Nieman 2018).

Patient Preparation: Patient should not be taking glucocorticoids and women are instructed to discontinue estrogen about 2 weeks prior to testing. The patient must not take anything by mouth for an hour prior to collecting the salivary sample. This includes glucocorticoid medications or creams, food, fluids, gum, toothpaste, and cigarettes. Gentle teeth cleaning is recommended in order to avoid blood contamination of saliva.

Appropriate selection of saliva collection device for use in children takes into account the age and cooperation level of the child (e.g. whole saliva sampling, passive drool or spitting in tube, braided cotton dental rope, polymer rolls, mucous extractors, or modified eye sponges) (Keil 2011). Typically for children, an assistant using disposable gloves can place the pledget under the tongue and assist to replace the pledget inside the collection tube. There are a number of styles of collection devices and new devices and apps are available for some smartphones (Fig. 15.1).

Patients should receive clear written instructions regarding sample collection (Hodgson and Granger 2013): Emphasis should be placed on labeling all tubes with collection times, name, birthdate, and date of collection. The pledget or swab should not be touched but tipped directly into saliva pooled on the floor of the mouth. This should be saturated before it is returned to the storage tube. The specimen does not require refrigeration and can be delivered to laboratory at room temperature (Hodgson and Granger 2013). Check with the laboratory performing the assay if refrigeration is required for other types of spec-

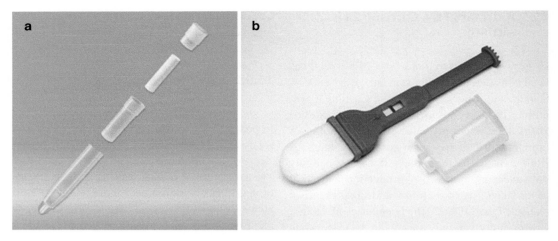

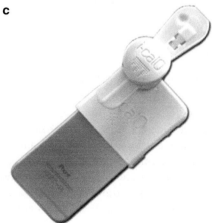

Fig. 15.1 Salivary cortisol testing devices (**a**, **b**) cotton pledgets (**c**) Smart phone based cortisol measuring systems. From: Choi S, et al. Real-time measurement of human salivary cortisol for the assessment of psychological stress using a smartphone. Sens BioSens Res. 2014;2:8–11

imens. Any required health insurance/authorization forms to accompany the samples should be fully completed.

Result interpretation: An LNSC level > than 145 ng/dL (4 nmol/L) is indicative of Cushing's syndrome (Nieman et al. 2008; Papanicolaou et al. 1998). Two specimens are recommended for diagnosis (Nieman et al. 2008).

15.5.3 Low Dose Dexamethasone Suppression Test (DST)

This test is used to assess hypercortisolism, differentiating between those patients with, and

without, Cushing's syndrome (Newell-Price JDC 2016). In normal subjects, a dose of 0.5 mg of dexamethasone every 6 h for 8 doses has been shown to suppress urinary 17 hydroxycorticosteroid excretion by the second day of administration in patients without Cushing's disease. This suppression is not evident in patients with Cushing's syndrome (Newell-Price JDC 2016; Liddle 1960).

Patient Preparation and Procedure: The patient is given a clear written schedule to time dose administration every 6 h for 8 doses. Usually recommended beginning at 9:00 a.m. day 1. Following this schedule, patients are instructed to present to a laboratory at 9 a.m. day 3, 6 h after the last dose of dexamethasone. A cortisol level is drawn on presentation. A salivary cortisol collection at precisely 2 h after the last dose of dexamethasone may also be used (Newell-Price JDC 2016).

Dose adjustment in children: 2 mg/day per 1.73 m^2. Body surface area in children less than 40 kg or 30 μg/kg/day in divided doses. The dose required in adults or in pediatric patients is the same when the patient's weight is over 40 kg (88.2 lb) (Butler and Kirk 2011; Newell-Price JDC 2016).

Interpretation: A morning serum cortisol level is normal if less than 1.8 μg/dL (50 nmol/L) ruling out Cushing's syndrome (Nieman et al. 2008).

15.5.4 Overnight Dexamethasone Suppression Test (O/N DST)

As for DST, the overnight test is based on the suppression of urinary 17 hydroxycorticosteroid excretion. It is advocated as a practical alternative screening test for Cushing's syndrome, but does not differentiate the sources of cortisol. The patient is administered 1 mg of dexamethasone between 11:00 and 12:00 p.m. and serum cortisol is measured by venipuncture the next morning between 8:00 and 9:00 a.m. (Newell-Price JDC 2016)

Interpretation: Cut-off for normal levels remains less than 1.8 μg/dL (50 nmol/L) although there is some ongoing debate. The specificity of ON/DST is low (Newell-Price JDC 2016; Nieman et al. 2008).

15.5.5 High Dose Dexamethasone Suppression Test/2 Day DST

A high dose of dexamethasone is used to differentiate pituitary-dependent Cushing's for adrenal sources of hypercortisolism. It is also useful but not conclusive in excluding ectopic Cushing's. This test is useful only after Cushing's syndrome has been diagnosed (Newell-Price JDC 2016).

Procedure: A baseline 24 h urine free cortisol (UFC) or morning serum cortisol level is drawn. A morning serum cortisol is recommended as more accurate and convenient (Nieman et al.

2008). Dexamethasone 2 mg is administered orally every 6 h for 2 days (for a total of 8 mg). A second 24 h UFC is collected or a serum cortisol level is after the last dose of dexamethasone. Two protocols have been described; initiation of dexamethasone at 9 a.m. with cortisol level drawn at 9 a.m. or 6 h after the last dose; or the first dose of dexamethasone at 12 noon with the cortisol level drawn at 8 a.m., exactly 2 h after the last dose (Hashimoto et al. 1990; Yanovski et al. 1998).

Interpretation: If the level of cortisol suppresses to less than 50% of the baseline levels in either test, or if cortisol level is >1.8 μg/dL (50 nmol/L) pituitary-dependent Cushing's disease is confirmed (Newell-Price JDC 2016; Nieman et al. 2008).

15.5.6 Corticotropin Releasing Hormone (CRH) Test

CRH is the releasing factor for pituitary ACTH. CRH testing is used to confirm ACTH-dependent source of excess ACTH, establishing a diagnosis of Cushing's disease. Pituitary ACTH producing tumors, but not ectopic ACTH tumors respond to CRH stimulation. It can also be used to diagnose and to differentiate the source of adrenal insufficiency as primary or suprapituitary to diagnose hypercortisolism or to evaluate adrenal function post-pituitary surgery. In patients with ACTH deficiency causing adrenal insufficiency, ACTH does not rise in response to CRH. In Cushing's disease, there is a significant rise in ACTH (Trainer et al. 1995).

Although both ovine and human forms of CRH are available, only ovine CRH such as Corticorelin Ovine Triflutate/Acthrel is FDA approved for use in the USA. Ovine CRH is about five times more potent, mainly because it has a longer effect on ACTH and subsequent cortisol secretion (Trainer et al. 1995).

Patient Preparation: Patients should not be taking glucocorticoids or estrogen as in all testing for hypercortisolism. Anticipated side effects of drug administration including facial, neck, and upper body flushing and an increase in heart rate are described to the patient prior to testing. Patients also report sensing the need to take a deep breath immediately after drug administration. Side effects are minimized by slow bolus over 30 s or more. The procedure is the same for adults and children.

Procedure:

- Schedule a start time preferably at 8–9 a.m.
- Encourage children to void prior to the start of the procedure.
- Establish IV access and secure cannula, particularly in young children.
- Draw baseline ACTH and cortisol level at −15 min. Place ACTH specimen on ice.
- Administer Ovine* (or human) CRH. 1.0 µg/kg body weight is injected intravenously as a bolus over 30 s for adults and children. Maximum dose is 100 µg or one vial reconstituted with 2 m of sterile saline for 50 µg/mL dilution.
- Saline flush IV cannula with 5–10 mL.
- Serum ACTH and cortisol are measured at 5 time points: baseline, 15, 30, 45, and 60 min after drug administration.

Result interpretation: A 35% rise in ACTH and a 20% rise in cortisol compared to baseline at 15–30 min after administration is diagnostic of Cushing's disease and excludes pseudo-Cushing's syndrome (Chitale et al. 2013; Batista et al. 2007).

The response is increased in persons with hypothyroidism, ethanol withdrawal, and some acute and chronic illnesses. Pregnancy and renal failure may decrease the response.

There is no apparent difference in ACTH response between children and adults (Newell-Price JDC 2016; Batista et al. 2007).

15.5.7 Dexamethasone Suppression and CRH Stimulation Test (DST/CRH)

A combination of dexamethasone and CRH testing has been advocated to improve diagnostic accuracy for Cushing's syndrome and exclude pseudo-Cushing's. Reason for testing is as described previously. This test may also be use-

ful in discriminating mild or cyclical cases of Cushing's disease (Erickson et al. 2007; Moro et al. 2000).

Patient Preparation: Evidence indicates improved test accuracy when medication use, particularly antidepressant medications and some cardioactive drugs are used at the time of testing (Valassi et al. 2009). When possible, estrogen and antidepressant medications should be held during testing. The patient is given written instructions with the dexamethasone prescription with medication start time and subsequent dose times.

Procedure: Eight doses of oral dexamethasone 0.5 mg every 6 h for 48 h. The patient presents to the testing unit and has an IV cannula placed within 1.5 h of the last dose of dexamethasone. An IV infusion of 100 mg of CRH is administered as per CRH protocol described previously.

Interpretation: A serum cortisol threshold of 1.4 µg/dL (38 nmol/L) 15 min after CRH is diagnostic for Cushing's syndrome. Simultaneous baseline measurement of dexamethasone, cortisol, and ACTH is recommended to assess dexamethasone metabolism and improve the diagnostic accuracy of testing. Dexamethasone level must be adequate to suppress ACTH/cortisol prior to CRH administration (Raff et al. 2015). An adequate dexamethasone level is considered to be >5.6 nmol/L (160 ng/dL) (Nieman et al. 2008).

15.5.8 Insulin Tolerance Test (ITT)

This test is used to assess cortisol respone for both hypo and hypercortisol states. (See Sect. 15.4.2.1) for a detailed description.

15.5.9 Central Venous Sampling: Inferior Petrosal and Cavernous Sinus Sampling

Central venous sampling is used to determine a pituitary ACTH-dependent source of hypercortisolism or Cushing's syndrome. In some patients, it may also help to determine the lateralization or the location (right or left) of the hypersecreting tumor in the pituitary. There are two methods of venous sampling: Inferior petrosal sinus sampling and cavernous sinus sampling.

15.5.9.1 Inferior Petrosal Sinus Sampling (IPSS)

Bilateral inferior petrosal sinus sampling (IPSS) is considered the single most accurate test for the differentiation of ACTH-dependent Cushing's syndrome in adults and children. IPSS is recommended in cases where less invasive biochemical testing has confirmed hypercortisolism or has been equivocal and when the MRI of the pituitary is normal or contains a small mass less than 6 mm. This procedure is best performed by an experienced neuroradiologist (Newell-Price JDC 2016).

This is an invasive procedure involving the direct catheterization of both right and left petrosal sinuses to measure ACTH in the blood draining from vessels each side of the pituitary. Central ACTH levels are compared with ACTH levels from peripheral vein samples, which are drawn simultaneously (Sharma and Nieman 2011; Lindsay and Nieman 2005). This helps to determine the side with the highest production of ACTH.

Patient Preparation: This includes an explanation of risks and benefits and requires the patients' written informed consent. The procedure is usually well tolerated with mild discomfort with bilateral catheter placement. Rare serious side effects have been reported and include vascular damage and venous thromboembolism, sixth nerve palsy, venous subarachnoid hemorrhage, brain stem infarction, and acute renal insufficiency due to contrast dye (Newell-Price JDC 2016; Lindsay and Nieman 2005; Miller and Doppman 1991). Preparation with an age-appropriate explanation of the procedure is particularly important for children and the procedure is typically performed with sedation for safety.

Procedure: A peripheral IV catheter is placed on admission to the interventional radiation center and conscious sedation is usually administered prior to and during the procedure. The use of local anesthetic creams applied to the antecubital spaces bilaterally and the back of both hands about an hour prior to admission to the procedure center is recommended for children.

The patient is placed in supine position and under fluoroscopy; catheters are placed in the femoral veins bilaterally at the groin and advanced to the right and left petrosal sinus. ACTH sample are drawn from the peripheral IV cannula along with simultaneous samples drawn from both the right and left petrosal sinuses catheters. Blood samples are drawn for baseline measurement at −3 min and 0 time points. CRH is administered peripherally and serial samples are taken at 3–5 min intervals for 2–3 measures. Desmopressin can also be used to stimulate the release of ACTH during IPSS (Machado et al. 2007; Oldfield et al. 1985).

Interpretation: For the diagnosis of Cushing's disease, a basal central to peripheral ACTH gradient (comparison of ACTH from petrosal vein to peripheral source) of more than 2:1 or more than 3:1 after administration of CRH is required. The absence of a gradient indicates an ectopic source of Cushing's syndrome outside of the pituitary gland (Sharma and Nieman 2011). When performed by a skilled and experienced radiologist; accuracy can be as high as 99%. However, false negatives and false positives can occur due to unsuccessful catheterization, inappropriate catheter placement, performance during normocortisolemic periods, and in the case of CRH secreting tumors. In order to increase accuracy, concurrent sampling of prolactin can be used to normalize ACTH ratios. While still highly accurate as a differential diagnostic tool, the use of IPSS to lateralize a tumor within the pituitary gland is still a matter of controversy, with its accuracy somewhere between 50 and 100%.

Post-procedure, pressure is applied to both venous access sites, typically the groin, to prevent bleeding (Miller and Doppman 1991). The most common complication of IPSS is a groin hematoma, seen in 3–4% of patients (Fig. 15.2).

15.5.9.2 Cavernous Sinus Sampling (CSS)

Cavernous sinus sampling (CSS) is recommended as an alternative to IPSS as the cavernous sinuses are closer to the pituitary gland and may provide a higher central to peripheral gradient without the use of CRH. However, no studies have concluded

Fig. 15.2 Catheter placement for bilateral simultaneous blood sampling of the inferior petrosal sinuses

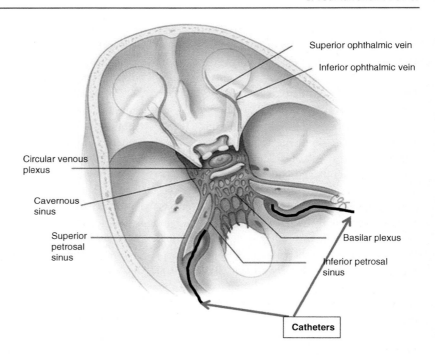

Superior ophthalmic vein

Inferior ophthalmic vein

Circular venous plexus

Cavernous sinus

Superior petrosal sinus

Basilar plexus

Inferior petrosal sinus

Catheters

that it offers any additional advantages. There is additional risk of complications from entering the cavernous sinus as compared to the petrosal sinuses, as well as increased cost (Lindsay and Nieman 2005).

Other alternative methods of venous sampling may be used due to the risk of complications and technical difficulty of performing IPSS. Some centers have suggested the use of jugular venous sampling (JVS) with the administration as it is safer and requires less expertise. However, accuracy is lower than that of IPSS (Ilias et al. 2004).

15.6 Growth Hormone Testing

Dynamic/provocative testing is used to evaluate both growth hormone deficiency (stimulation testing) and growth hormone excess (suppression testing).

15.6.1 Growth Hormone Stimulation Testing

Although initially associated with children with idiopathic short stature, growth hormone deficiency (GHD) is now recognized in both adults

and children (Gupta 2011). More recently GHD has been associated with a history of traumatic brain injury (TBI). Stimulation testing determines the presence of GHD. Several tests may be used for this evaluation including IGF-1 generation test or stimulation with: glucagon, arginine, GHRH (semorelin acetate), ITT, L-Dopa, or clonidine. Two tests may be required to demonstrate GHD.

Children with a bone age of >10 years who are not yet in puberty may not show an optimal response to GH stimulation. Hence, they may be "primed" with sex steroids, such as estrogen, testosterone, or stilbestrol (Butler and Kirk 2011). Priming has been used to increase the GH peak response in testing in prepubertal children to levels equivalent of children already in puberty and remains controversial (Strich et al. 2009). Accurate pubertal staging is required prior to this test. Some advocates of priming before GH testing indicate that the timing of "priming" is important with respect to puberty. They observe that this method should be used only within 5 years before normal pubertal onset (Rosenbloom 2011). Others believe priming is unnecessary and simply reduces the number of "non-responders" by artificially raising the GH peak level (Soliman et al. 2014; Lazar and Phillip 2010).

Nevertheless, priming protocols include:

- Ethinyl estradiol 10 µg orally once a day for 5 days prior to the test for girls
- Testosterone esters 100 mg IM 1 week before the test for boys
- Oral stilbestrol 1 mg daily for 3 days before the test, or twice daily for 2 days before the test
- If priming is taking place, steps should be taken to ensure test continuity with GH testing at the appropriate testing center. Either ITT, glucagon, or GHRH testing is used after "priming."

15.6.1.1 Insulin Tolerance Testing (ITT)

This has been previously described in (See Sect. 15.4.2.1).

15.6.1.2 IGF-1 Generation Test

Dysfunction in the GH-IGF-1 axis is apparent in children with idiopathic short stature related to growth hormone insensitivity. This test measures circulating IGF1 levels generated in response to subcutaneous injections of recombinant human GH (rhGH) administration. Growth hormone insensitivity (GHIS) is apparent when growth hormone levels are high, but baseline IGF-1 remains low (Cotterill et al. 1998). Some authors suggest that the IGF-1 generation test is less sensitive for diagnosing mild GHIS, yet it is still widely used to confirm a diagnosis of GHD (Coutant et al. 2012).

Procedure. There are a number of protocols described for this test. The most common is performed over 5 days and requires four rhGH injections (33 mg/kg per day; total dose of 132 mg/kg) (Coutant et al. 2012). The patient presents on day 1 for a serum IGF-1 level. After returning home, the child can eat and drink as normal. On the following 4 days, a dose of GH is administered to the child, usually by a visiting nurse. Twelve hours after the administration of the last dose of GH, the child returns to the testing clinic for another serum IGF-1 level to be drawn.

Interpretation: Failure to increase IGF-1 levels on growth hormone administration and/or IGF-1 increment of <15 ng/mL is indicative of GHIS

and is discussed in more detail in the Chap. 2. In the case of GHD, the IGF-1 is increased (Blair et al. 2004). Although used frequently as a diagnostic tool in Europe, this test has been criticized for its inability to identify mild and some more severe cases of GHD in children (Coutant et al. 2012).

15.6.1.3 Glucagon Stimulation Test (GST)

The glucagon test is commonly used in adults and in children under the age of 12 years of age, whereas the insulin tolerance test is commonly used for children over this age. The GST is used as an alternative in adult patients where ITT is contraindicated. The GST is a very effective and safe way to measure pituitary function with fewer side effects than ITT, as hyperglycemia and not hypoglycemia is induced (Yuen et al. 2013).

Patient preparation: This is a 3–4 h test. Adults and children are fasted for at least 12–24 h and present to the testing site early morning (8 a.m.). Intake of water is encouraged. Patients are asked to hold morning medications but can take medications at the completion of testing. Common side effects can include headache, sweating, nausea, and vomiting. Children are particularly susceptible to vomiting. Rebound hypoglycemia may occur later in the day if the child does not eat or drink after testing. Most centers keep the children long enough to ensure tolerance of a normal diet has resumed (Butler and Kirk 2011).

Procedure: An IV cannula is inserted and sampling commences with samples of glucose and growth hormone at 0, 60, 90, 120, 150, and 180 min in children (25, 2011). In some centers, more frequent samples are obtained at time 0, +15, +30, +45, +60, +90, + 120, +180, +210, and + 240 min. However, standard draws in adults are every 20 min for 4 h (Bonert 2016). Cortisol levels may also be measured.

A dose of glucagon is administered via an intramuscular (IM) injection, usually in the buttock after baseline (0) serum samples are drawn. This drug is contraindicated in the presence of pheochromocytoma or insulinoma. There are two ways of determining the dose of glucagon needed: the fixed dose and the weight-based dose.

Patients are dosed with 1 mg (10 µg) of glucagon IM for weights under 90 kg and 1.5 mg (15 µg) of glucagon for weights above 90 kg in a fixed dose GST. For the weight-based dosing GST, patients are dosed at 0.03 mg/kg of glucagon. This dose is used in children to a maximum of 1 mg and can be administered subcutaneously (Carmichael 2016).

Interpretation: Patients whose response peaks >3 ng/mL have a normal test and their pituitary is functioning appropriately. Results under 3 ng/mL (3 µg/L) demonstrate pituitary dysfunction and pharmacologic treatment could be required. In children, 3–6 µg/L is considered partial growth hormone deficiency. Consider a cut-off of 1 ng/mL for obese patients (Yuen et al. 2013; Bonert 2016; Hamrahian et al. 2016).

15.6.1.4 Arginine Stimulation Testing

Arginine is seldom used as a single agent for the diagnosis of growth hormone deficiency secondarily to efficacy; it is often used in combination testing. In some countries, the availability of arginine also limits its use. Arginine is also not as commonly used in children. Most frequent combination use is with either L-DOPA or GHRH. Arginine is an intravenous stimulant to the pituitary for the release of HGH in patients where the measurement of pituitary reserve for HGH can be diagnostic for GHD.

Patient Preparation: The patient is usually fasted overnight or for 8–10 h. Infants may eat up to 4 h prior to the procedure. Consumption of water is encouraged. Morning medications are usually held. The most common side effects are nausea, headache, and complaints of a metallic taste in the mouth or polyuria. Children are encouraged to bring a favorite activity, DVD, or comfort toy. Application of anesthetic cream to antecubital areas or forearms for IV placement can be done by parents prior to arrival at the testing site. Arginine may exacerbate acidosis in patients with renal failure and may be hazardous in patients with liver disease; other stimulatory agents should be used in persons with these disorders (R-Gene 2016). This drug is also contraindicated in persons having highly allergic tendencies.

Procedure: After arrival in clinic, an IV cannula is placed and baseline levels of IGF-1 and GH are drawn. An arginine dose of 0.5 g/kg (maximum 30 g) is infused via IV infusion over 30 min (Carmichael 2016). Dose must be double checked, as arginine overdose in children can be fatal. Excessive rates of infusion may result in local irritation and in flushing, nausea, or vomiting. Inadequate dosing may diminish the stimulus to the pituitary and nullify the test (R-Gene 2016).

If this is to be a combined test with glucagon, the lyophilized glucagon must be reconstituted and a dose of 30 µg/kg (maximum 1 mg) of body weight is administered IM (thigh or buttocks). GH, glucose (and cortisol levels if needed) blood samples are drawn every 30 min for 2 h (Glucagon 2017).

Similar to the arginine/L-DOPA test, the arginine/GHRH test also takes place over 120 min. Baseline labs, including GH, are drawn prior to the GHRH 1 µg/kg via IVP for patients weighing over 60 kg (consult the package insert for patients weighing less than 60 kg). Arginine dosing of 30 g is then infused over 30 min with GH blood draws thereafter every 30 min for 2 h (GNRH Ferring 2012).

Interpretation: A peak value under 3 ng/mL is considered abnormal and could warrant a second confirmation test. Some authors define levels <3 ng/mL as severe GHD and < 5 ng/mL as GHD (Hamrahian et al. 2016).

- A normal response is a peak >5 ng/mL or increase of 5 ng/mL over basal level.
- A blunted response occurs in hypothalamic-pituitary dwarfism.
- Lack of response also is found in persons with hypothyroidism.
- Response is inversely proportional to basal GH; no response may be seen if basal level is >5 ng/mL.
- GH levels may be decreased in hyperglycemia, obesity, and during treatment with cimetidine. GH levels may increase if the patient is treated with diethylstilbestrol, propranolol, indomethacin, glucocorticoids.

15.6.1.5 Growth Hormone Releasing Hormone Stimulation Testing (GHRH)

Growth hormone releasing hormone is often combined with other tests such as arginine stimulation to evaluate GHD. The purpose is to confirm new or persistent GHD in adulthood or adolescence, particularly after final height is achieved, or to diagnose GHD when ITT is contraindicated (GNRH Ferring 2012; Molitch et al. 2011).

Preparation: The patient is instructed to fast overnight or for 8–12 h. Continued intake of water is encouraged. GH treatment should be held for 1 month prior to testing. Side effects may include Facial flushing, rare paresthesia, nausea, and abnormal taste sensation after GHRH administration.

Procedure:

- An IV cannula is placed on admission and the patient allowed to rest for 45 min.
- Baseline GH and IGF-1 measurement are drawn (−15 mins), and GH at 0 min.
- GHRH (Somatorelin, Ferring, Geref) 1 µg/kg (maximum dose 100 µg) is injected through IV as a bolus injection (GNRH Ferring 2012).
- If a combined test, infuse 0.5 g/kg L-arginine monohydrochloride (maximum dose 30 g) as a 10% solution (30 g/300 mL) in normal saline over 30 min.
- Blood samples for further GH estimation are drawn at 30, (45), 60, 90, 120, and 150 min after the start of the arginine infusion.
- Patient is able to eat lunch at +150 min or after the last blood test.
- Pulse and BP are monitored and recorded during the procedure.

Interpretation: Cut-offs for diagnosis of GH deficiency remain unclear, but may depend on peak GH, age, and BMI and waist circumference (Colao et al. 2009). Using GHRH-arginine test is most sensitivity and specific to GHD, at a GH cut-off of <4.1 µg/L and has been shown to be comparable to ITT (Molitch et al. 2011). Higher cut-off of ≤8.0 µg/L have been recommended for patients with BMI ≥25 and <30 (Carmichael 2016).

15.6.1.6 L-DOPA Stimulation Test

Similar to the test listed above, the L-DOPA stimulation test can be used as an independent test of GHD but results are inferior to ITT or combination testing. It is administered over 2 h with fasting GH levels taken at baseline and every 30 min thereafter via an IV line. After baseline samples are obtained, patients are dosed with 125 mg of oral L-DOPA if weighing <10 kg, 250 mg if 10–30 kg and 500 mg orally if >30 kg. The most common side effect is nausea. L-DOPA is contraindicated in patients with a history of cardiac arrhythmia. The maximum GH secretion occurs after 60–90 min (Bonert 2016).

15.6.1.7 Clonidine Test

Clonidine was found to stimulate a profound rise in GH levels in oral, and subsequently intravenous doses (Gil-Ad et al. 1979). This is used more frequently in children (Coutant et al. 2012).

Procedure: The child is placed in the supine position for venous cannulation. After rest, a sample of whole blood is collected for baseline GH. After obtaining the baseline sample, a dose of 0.10–0.15 mg/m². Clonidine is administered orally and subsequent blood samples for GH are collected after 30, 60, 90, and 120 min (Gil-Ad et al. 1979). Side effects are reported as mild including fatigue and somnolence and mild postural hypotension (Bonert 2016).

Interpretation: A cut-off level of >3.0 ng/mL is reported as indicating normal GH levels (De Fátima Borges et al. 2016).

15.6.2 Growth Hormone Excess

Growth hormone (GH) is secreted in bursts with higher amplitude burst during sleep. The half-life of GH is short, around 11–19 min, making a random single sample unreliable to diagnose acromegaly (Faria et al. 1989). Two tests are typically used for this diagnosis: A growth hormone profile and an oral glucose tolerance test (OGTT) which will suppress normal but not excess GH secretions and thereby confirm growth hormone excess or acromegaly.

15.6.2.1 Growth Hormone Profile

This test is typically done after an 8–12 h fast. A growth hormone 5-point profile is an average of serum GH levels collected at intervals of 30 min, usually over a 2 h time period. Baseline IGF-1 and GH levels are collected. A mean GH >2.5 µg/L (6.9 nmol/L) is indicative of acromegaly.

15.6.2.1.1 Oral Glucose Tolerance Test (OGTT) for Growth Hormone Suppression

This test is rarely done in children, as growth hormone excess is rare in children. However, the protocol is the same as that for adults.

Patient preparation: The patient is fasted for 8–12 h, usually from midnight prior to the test. On admission to the testing area, an IV cannula is placed for peripheral access, and baseline serum glucose and growth hormone levels are drawn. Side effects are usually mild and include nausea, vomiting, abdominal bloating, and/or headache.

Procedure: Baseline levels of serum glucose, growth hormone, and IGF-1 are drawn prior to glucose administration and at 30, 60, 90, and 120 min following ingestion of glucose. The patient is given 75 g of glucose to drink. In children, the oral glucose solution is calculated at 1.75 g/kg, up to the maximum 75 g (Butler and Kirk 2011). This is usually flavored orange, fruit punch or lemon lime, and most contain corn-derived dextrose, citric acid, flavoring, sodium benzoate, yellow #6, and purified water.

Interpretation: A lack of suppression to <1 µg/L occurs in pituitary tumors secreting GH or in ectopic GHRH production (Melmed 2016). Lack of suppression also is common in patients with Cushing's syndrome, affective disorders, and anorexia nervosa. In acute illness, acromegaly, or chronic renal failure, a paradoxic rise in GH may occur.

15.6.2.1.2 Glucose Tolerance Test (GTT) for Insulin Resistance

Insulin resistance and type 2 diabetes is common in the general population but is often a hallmark of pituitary disease. This test also performed frequently in children, with the rise in pediatric obesity and type 2 diabetes (Conwell and Batch 2004). The testing protocol is the same as for adults.

Patient preparation and procedure as per OGTT for GH suppression.

Patients are encouraged to withhold drugs that will increase or decrease glucose levels.

Oral contraceptives, estrogens, glucocorticoids, thiazides, phenytoin, lithium, ranitidine, propranolol, and tetrahydrocannabinol can increase glucose levels and guanethidine, clofibrate, and salicylates can decrease glucose levels.

Interpretation as per American Diabetic Association (ADA) criteria (American Diabetes Association 2015):

Diabetes: Peak glucose level over 2 h > 200 mg/dL.

Impaired glucose tolerance: Peak glucose level over 2 h > 140–200 mg/dL

15.7 Gonadotroph Assessment

15.7.1 Clomiphene Stimulation Test/ Clomiphene Citrate Challenge Test (CCCT)

The purpose of the CCCT is to predict ovarian reserve and the prognosis for future pregnancy. Clomiphene has an antiestrogenic effect, stimulating GnRH and LH and FSH production from the pituitary (Kaiser 2016).

Procedure: Baseline FSH and LH and estrogen are measured on cycle day 3. Patients are administered 100 mg Clomiphene orally daily for 1–4 weeks or two pills per day cycle days 5–9. FSH and LH are drawn on day 10.

Interpretation: A doubling of LH and a 20–50% rise in FSH indicates normal pituitary response. Failure to increase may indicate decreased ovarian reserve or fewer remaining quality eggs (Carmichael 2016).

15.7.2 Human Chorionic Gonadotropin (HCG) Stimulation Test

In adult males, the HCG stimulation test is used to assess Leydig cell function and their capacity to produce testosterone. This is particularly pertinent in the evaluation of infertility (Kaiser 2016; Carmichael 2016).

Procedure: A baseline total testosterone level is drawn, followed by an injection of 5000 IU hCG (Pregnyl) in the gluteal muscle. A follow-up blood sample is taken 72 h later.

Interpretation: A rise of >7.5 nmol/L indicates normal Leydig cell function (Bang et al. 2017).

In pediatrics: The HCG stimulation test is widely considered the gold standard for investigating children with ambiguous genitalia (Grant et al. 1976). The 4-day test is discussed in more detail in the Chap. 3. A prolonged HCG stimulation test is performed when primary hypogonadism is suspected, or when exploring the causes for delayed puberty (Butler and Kirk 2011). This test takes over 3 weeks and requires frequent IM injections of HCG. Liaison with the local general or primary care practitioner or community nursing team will decrease the family's burden of travel for injections.

Procedure: Baseline plasma total testosterone, LH and FSH are drawn on day 1 prior to administration of 2000 IU HCG IM twice weekly for 3 weeks. Testosterone levels are drawn 24 h after the last injection (Butler and Kirk 2011). The dose may vary from 1000 to 5000 IU administered every day for 3–5 days. Testosterone levels may be sampled at 0, 48, and 72 h.

Interpretation: A flat response to HCG indicates testicular agenesis or hypogonadotropic hypogonadism. A rise in the testosterone levels >5 nmol/L (or 8 nmol/L in some studies) indicates adequate Leydig cell function or constitutional delay in puberty in adolescents (Butler and Kirk 2011; Carmichael 2016).

15.7.3 Gonadotropin Releasing Hormone Test (GnRH Test)

The GnRH test assesses the child for precocious puberty (see Chap. 4) and is a simple and most accurate way to assess the hypothalamic pituitary gonadal axis (Davies and Collin 2015). This test confirms a diagnosis of central gonadotropin-dependent precocious puberty (Eckert et al. 1996). It is not useful in determining pubertal signs such as premature thelarche (Bizzarri et al. 2014).

Procedure: The test takes 1 h to perform. Samples for LH, FSH, and estrogen or testosterone are drawn at 0, 20, and 60 min. GnRH is administered intravenously after the 0 sample is

Table 15.2 Responses to GnRH stimulation

Diagnosis	Response
Normal child	FSH and LH both rise at 20, decreases at 60 min
Central precocious puberty	Pubertal response
Gonadotropin-independent precocious puberty	LH and FSH levels are suppressed
Gonadal failure	Basal LH and FSH values are increased, and the response to the GnRH is vastly increased
Delayed puberty	Response is either poor or absent
Hypogonadotropic hypogonadism	Response is either poor or absent

Adapted from Davies and Collin (2015)

drawn. A dose of 2.5 μg/kg, with a maximum dose of 100 μg, is administered (Butler and Kirk 2011). The test can be performed at any time of the day and does not require fasting.

Interpretation: Central precocious puberty is diagnosed if the LH level rises and gives a "pubertal response" in response to GnRH. The differences in the LH and FSH responses indicate the cause, as seen in the Table 15.2 (Davies and Collin 2015).

15.8 Thyrotroph Assessment

15.8.1 Thyroid Releasing Hormone (TRH) Test

The TRH test is rarely used in adults or children, given the availability of sensitive TSH assays. TRH testing was used to assess hyperthyroidism and suppression of TSH, TSH resistance, or a TSH secreting tumor (Butler and Kirk 2011). The test involves measuring baseline TSH levels via an IV cannula, administration of TRH, and subsequent draws for serum TSH after 15 and 30 min. In children, measurement at 60 and 120 min is also required. There is some associated discomfort including nausea, vomiting, bitter taste in the mouth, flushing and an urge to urinate, which is especially difficult for children (Table 15.3) (Mehta et al. 2003).

Table 15.3 Interpretation of TRH testing

Dysfunction	TSH after TRH administration
Primary hyperthyroidism	No change in TSH levels
Low TSH: end organ failure	Immediate increase in TSH
Secondary hypothyroidism (pituitary disease)	No increase in TSH
Tertiary hypothyroidism (hyperthalamic disease)	Delayed response (60–120 min)

Moncayo et al. (2007)

15.9 Conclusions

Testing for hypothalamic and pituitary dysfunction is complex and often requires multiple modalities to confirm a diagnosis. Random blood testing is not always diagnostic and dynamic or provocative testing may be required for a definitive diagnosis. Some provocative tests require complex patient preparation and are anxiety provoking. It is recommended that detailed written instructions be provided to the patient in order for testing to provide accurate, useful information in diagnosis.

In pediatric patient, preparation for testing is directed at both the child and the parent, and should be age-appropriate. Topical, light, or conscious sedation may be used for some testing modalities.

To instill confidence in patients during the critical, and emotion laden, diagnostic period the nurse must be knowledgeable in all facets of testing preparation, performance, and interpretation according to their role.

References

American Diabetes Association. Classifications and diagnosis of diabetes. Diabetes Care. 2015;38(Supplement 1):S8–S16. https://doi.org/10.2337/dc15-S005. Accessed 20 Jun 2018.

Bang AK, Nordkap L, Almstrup K, Priskorn L, Petersen JH, Rajpert-De Meyts E, Andersson AM, Juul A, Jørgensen N. Dynamic GnRH and hCG testing: establishment of new diagnostic reference levels. Eur J Endocrinol. 2017;176(4):379–91. https://doi.org/10.1530/EJE-16-0912.

Batista DL, Riar JR, Keil M, Stratakis CA. Diagnostic tests for children who are referred for the investigation of Cushing syndrome. Pediatrics. 2007;120(3):575–86.

Ben-Schomo A, Melmed S. Hypothalamic regulation of anterior pituitary function. In: Melmed S, editor. The pituitary. 3rd ed. London: Elsevier; 2011. p. 261–99. https://doi.org/10.1016/B978-0-12-380926-1.10015-X.

Berneis K, Staub JJ, Gessler A, Meier C, Girard J, Müller B. Combined stimulation of adrenocorticotropin and compound-S by single dose Metyrapone test as an outpatient procedure to assess hypothalamic-pituitary-adrenal function. J Clin Endocrinol Metab. 2002;87(12):5470–5. https://doi.org/10.1210/jc.2001-011959.

Bichet DG. The posterior pituitary. In: Melmed S, editor. The pituitary. 3rd ed. London: Elsevier; 2016. p. 251–88.

Bizzarri C, Spadoni GL, Bottaro G, Montanari G, Giannone G, Cappa M, Cianfarani S. The response to gonadotropin releasing hormone (GnRH) stimulation test does not predict the progression to true precocious puberty in girls with onset of premature thelarche in the first three years of life. J Clin Endocrinol Metab. 2014;99(2):433–9.

Blair JC, Camacho-Hubner C, Miraki-Moud F, Rosberg S, Burren CP, Lim S, Clayton PE, Bjarnason R, Albertsson-Wikland K, Savage MO. Standard and low-dose IGF-I generation tests and spontaneous growth hormone secretion in children with idiopathic short stature. Clin Endocrinol. 2004;60:163–8.

Bonert VS, Melmed S. Growth hormone. In Melmed S Pituitary 4th. London. Elsevier 2016:85–127.

Bornstein SR, Allolio B, Arlt W, Barthel A, Don-Wauchope A, Hammer GD, Husebye ES, Merke DP, Murad MH, Stratakis CA, Torpy DJ. Diagnosis and treatment of primary adrenal insufficiency: an Endocrine Society clinical practice guideline. J Clin Endocrinol Metabol. 2016;101(2):364–89. https://doi.org/10.1210/jc.2015-1710.

Broersen LH, Pereira AM, Jorgensen JO, Dekkers OM. Adrenal insufficiency in corticosteroids use: systematic review and meta-analysis. J Clin Endocrinol Metab. 2015;100(6):2171–80.

Burke CW. The pituitary megatest: outdated? Clin Endocrinol. 1992;36:133–4.

Butler G, Kirk J. Paediatric endocrinology and diabetes. Oxford: OUP Press; 2011.

Carmichael J. Anterior pituitary failure pituitary. In: Melmed S, editor. Pituitary. 4th ed. London: Elsevier; 2016. p. 329–64.

Charles LE, Fekedulegn D, Burchfiel CM, et al. Shiftwork and diurnal salivary cortisol patterns among police officers. J Occup Environ Med. 2016;58(6):542–9. https://doi.org/10.1097/JOM.0000000000000729.

Chatha KK, Middle JG, Kilpatrick ES. National UK audit of the short synacthen test. Ann Clin Biochem. 2010;47(Pt 2):158–64. https://doi.org/10.1258/acb.2009.009209.

Cheetham T, Baylis PH. Diabetes insipidus in children. Pediatr Drugs. 2002;4(12):785–96.

Chitale A, Musonda P, McGregor AM, Dhatariya KK. Determining the utility of the 60 min cortisol measurement in the short synacthen test. Clin Endocrinol. 2013;79(1):14–9.

Colao A, Di Somma C, Savastano S, Rota F, Savanelli MC, Aimaretti G, Lombardi G. A reappraisal of diagnosing GH deficiency in adults: role of gender, age, waist circumference, and body mass index. J Clin Endocrinol Metab. 2009;94:4414–22.

Conwell LS, Batch JA. Oral glucose tolerance test in children and adolescents: Postives and pitfalls. J Paediatr Child Health. 2004;40:620–6.

Cotterill A, Camacho-Hubner C, Savage MO. Changes in serum IGF-1 and IGFBP3 concentrations during the IGF-1 generation test performed prospectively in children with short stature. Clin Endocrinol. 1998;48:719–24.

Coutant R, Dorr HG, Gleeson H, Argente J. Diagnosis of endocrine disease: limitations of the IGF1 generation test in children with short stature. Eur J Endocrinol. 2012;166(3):351–7.

Dashe AM, Cramm RE, Crist CA, Habener JF, Solomon DH. A water deprivation test for the differential diagnosis of polyuria. JAMA. 1963;185:699–703.

Davies K, Collin J. Understanding clinical investigations in children's endocrinology. Nursing children and young people. 2015;27(8):26–36.

De Fátima Borges M, Teixeira FCC, Feltrin AK, et al. Clonidine-stimulated growth hormone concentrations (cut-off values) measured by immunochemiluminescent assay (ICMA) in children and adolescents with short stature. Clinics. 2016;71(4):226–31. https://doi.org/10.6061/clinics/2016(04)09.

Dickstein G, Saiegh L. Low-dose and high-dose adrenocorticotropinvtesting: indications and shortcomings. Curr Opin Endocrinol Diabetes Obes. 2008;15:244–9.

Eckert KL, Wilson DM, Bachrach LK, Anhalt H, Habiby RL, Olney RC, Hintz RL, Neely EK. A single sample, subcutaneous gonadotropin releasing hormone test for central precocious puberty. Pediatrics. 1996;97(4):517–9.

Erickson D, Natt N, Nippoldt T, Young WF Jr, Carpenter PC, Petterson T, Christianson T. Dexamethasone-suppressed corticotropin-releasing hormone stimulation test for diagnosis of mild hypercortisolism. J Clin Endocrinol Metab. 2007;92(8):2972–6. Epub 2007 May 8.

Faria AC, Veldhuis JD, Thorner MO, Vance ML. Half-time of endogenous growth hormone (GH) disappearance in normal man after stimulation of GH secretion by GH-releasing hormone and suppression with somatostatin. J Clin Endocrinol Metab. 1989;68(3):535–41.

Fiad TM, Kirby JM, Cunningham SK, McKenna TJ. The overnight single-dose metyrapone test is a simple and reliable index of the hypothalamic-pituitary-adrenal axis. Clin Endocrinol. 1994;40:603–9. https://doi.org/10.1111/j.1365-2265.1994.tb03011.x.

Fleseriu M, Gassner M, Yedinak C, Chicea L, Delashaw JB Jr, Loriaux DL. Normal hypothalamic-pituitary-adrenal axis by high-dose cosyntropin testing in patients with abnormal response to low-dose cosyntropin stimulation:

a retrospective review. Endocr Pract. 2010;16(1):64–70. https://doi.org/10.4158/EP09153.OR.

Gil-Ad I, Topper E, Laron Z. Oral clonidine as a growth hormone stimulation test. Lancet. 1979;2(8137):278–9.

Glucagon. Glucagon [package insert]. New York: Eli Lilly and Company; 2017.

GNRH Ferring. GNRH Ferring (Somatorelin) [package insert]. Saint Prex: Ferring Pharmaceuticals; 2012.

Grant DB, Laurance BM, Atherden SM, Ryness J. HCG stimulation test in children with abnormal sexual development. Arch Dis Child. 1976;51:596–601.

Grimberg A, DiVall SA, Polychronakos C, Allen DB, Cohen LE, Quintos JB, Rossi WC, Feudtner C, Murad MH. Guidelines for growth hormone and insulin-like growth factor-I treatment in children and adolescents: growth hormone deficiency, idiopathic short stature, and primary insulin-like growth factor-I deficiency. Horm Res Paediatr. 2016;86:361–97.

Gupta V. Adult growth hormone deficiency. Indian J Endocrinol Metab. 2011;15(Suppl 3):197. https://doi.org/10.4103/2230-8210.84865.

Hamrahian AH, et al. Revised GH and cortisol cut-points for the glucagon stimulation test in the evaluation of GH and hypothalamic-pituitary-adrenal axes in adults: results from a prospective randomized multicenter study. Pituitary. 2016;19:332–41.

Hashimoto K, Makino S, Hirasawa R, Takao T, Kageyama J, Ogasa T, Ota Z. Combined anterior pituitary function test using CRH, GRH, LH-RH, TRH and vasopressin in patients with non-functioning pituitary tumors. Acta Med Okayama. 1990;44(3):141–7.

Hodgson NA, Granger DA. Collecting saliva and measuring salivary cortisol and alpha-amylase in frail community residing older adults via family caregivers. J Vis Exp. 2013;82:50815. https://doi.org/10.3791/50815.

Howlett TA. An assessment of optimal hydrocortisone replacement therapy. Clin Endocrinol. 1997;46(3):263–8.

Ilias I, Chang RE, Pacak K, et al. Jugular venous sampling: an alternative to petrosal sinus sampling for the diagnostic evaluation of adrenocorticotropic hormone-dependent Cushing's syndrome. J Clin Endocrinol Metab. 2004;89:3795.

Kaiser S. Conadotropin hormones. In: Melmed S, editor. Pituitary. 4th ed. London: Elsevier; 2016. p. 205–50.

Keil MF. Salivary cortisol: a tool for biobehavioural research in children. J Ped Nurs. 2011;27(3):287–9.

Lazar L, Phillip M. Is sex hormone priming in peripubertal children prior to growth hormone stimulation tests still appropriate? Horm Res Paediatr. 2010;73(4):299–302.

Liddle GW. Tests of pituitary-adrenal supressibility in the diagnosis of Cushing's syndrome. J Clin Endocrinol Metab. 1960;20:1539–60.

Lindsay JR, Nieman LK. Differential diagnosis and imaging in Cushing's syndrome. Endocrinol Metab Clin North Am. 2005;34(2):403–21.

Lone SW, Khan YN, Qamar F, Atta I, Ibrahim MN, Raza J. Safety of insulin tolerance test for the assessment of growth of growth hormone deficiency in children. J Pak Med Assoc. 2011;61(2):153–7.

Machado MC, de Sa SV, Domenice S, et al. The role of desmopressin in bilateral and simultaneous inferior petrosal sinus sampling for differential diagnosis of ACTH-dependent Cushing's syndrome. Clin Endocrinol. 2007;66:136–42.

Mehta A, Hindmarsh PC, Stanhope R, Brain CE, Preece M, Dattani MT. Is the thyrotropin releasing hormone test necessary in the diagnosis of central hypothyroidism in children. J Clin Endocrinol Metab. 2003;88(12):5696–703.

Melmed S. Acromegaly. In: Melmed S, editor. Pituitary. 4th ed. London: Elsevier; 2016. p. 423–66.

Melmed S, Casanueva FF, Hoffman AR, Kleinberg DL, Montori VM, Schlechte JA, Wass JAH. Diagnosis and treatment of hyperprolactinemia: an Endocrine Society clinical practice guideline. J Clin Endocrinol Metab. 2011;96(2):273–88. https://doi.org/10.1210/jc.2010-1692.

Miller D, Doppman J. Petrosal sinus sampling: technique and rationale. Radiology. 1991;178:37–47.

Molitch ME, Clemmons DR, Malozowski S, Merriam GR, Mary Lee Vance M. Evaluation and treatment of adult growth hormone deficiency: an Endocrine Society clinical practice guideline. J Clin Endocrinol Metab. 2011;96(6):1587–609. https://doi.org/10.1210/jc.2011-0179.

Moloney S, Murphy N, Collin J. An overview of the nursing issues involved in caring for a child with adrenal insufficiency. Nurs Child Young People. 2015;27(7):28–36.

Moncayo H, Dapunt O, Moncayo R. Diagnostic accuracy of basal TSH determinations based on the intravenous TRH stimulation test: an evaluation of 2570 tests and comparison with the literature. BMC Endocr Disord. 2007;7:5. https://doi.org/10.1186/1472-6823-7-5.

Moore K, Thompson CJ, Trainer P. Disorders of water balance. Clin Med. 2003;3:28–33.

Moro M, Putignano P, Losa M, Invitti C, Maraschini C, Francesco Cavagnini F. The desmopressin test in the differential diagnosis between Cushing's disease and Pseudo-Cushing states. J Clin Endocrinol Metab. 2000;85(10):3569–74. https://doi.org/10.1210/jcem.85.10.6862.

Mullis PE, Pal BR, Matthews DR, Hindmarsh PC, Phillips PE, Dunger DB. Half-life of exogenous growth hormone following suppression of endogenous growth hormone secretion with somatostatin in type I (insulin-dependent) diabetes mellitus. Clin Endocrinol. 1992;36(3):255–63.

Newell-Price JDC. Cushing's disease. In: Melmed S, editor. Pituitary. 4th ed. London: Elsevier; 2016. p. 515–71.

Nieman LK. Dynamic evaluation of adrenal hypofunction. J Endocrinol Investig. 2003;26(7 Suppl):74–82.

Nieman LK. Diagnosis of Cushing's syndrome in the modern era. Endocrinol Metab Clin N Am. 2018;47(2):259–73. Review. PMID: 29754631. https://doi.org/10.1016/j.ecl.2018.02.001.

Nieman LK, Biller BMK, Findling JW, et al. The diagnosis of Cushing's syndrome: an Endocrine Society clinical practice guideline. J Clin Endocrinol Metab. 2008;93(5):1526–40. https://doi.org/10.1210/jc.2008-0125.

Oldfield E, Chrousos G, Schulte H, et al. Preoperative lateralization of ACTH-secreting microadenomas by bilateral and simultaneous inferior petrosal venous sinus sampling. N Engl J Med. 1985;312:100–3.

Papanicolaou DA, Yanovski JA, Cutler GB, Chrousos GB, Nieman LK. A single sleeping midnight serum cortisol measurement distinguishes Cushing's syndrome from pseudo-Cushing's states. J Clin Endocrinol Metab. 1998;83:1163–7.

Raff H, Auchus RJ, Findling JW, Nieman LK. Urine free cortisol in the diagnosis of Cushing's syndrome: is it worth doing and, if so, how? J Clin Endocrinol Metab. 2015;100(2):395–7. https://doi.org/10.1210/jc.2014-3766.

Raine JE, Donaldson MDC, Gregory JW, van Vliet G, editors. Practical endocrinology and diabetes in children. Chichester: Wiley-Blackwell; 2011.

R-Gene. R-Gene (Arginine) [package insert]. New York: Pharmacia & Upjohn; 2016.

Roelfsema F, Biermasz NR, Pereira AM, Veldhuis JD. Optimizing blood sampling protocols in patients with acromegaly for the estimation of growth hormone secretion. J Clin Endocrinol Metab. 2016;101(7):2675–82. https://doi.org/10.1210/jc.2016-1142.

Rosenbloom AL. Sex hormone priming for growth hormone stimulation testing in pre- and early adolescent children is evidence based. Horm Res Paediatr. 2011;75(1):78–80.

Ross IL, Levitt NS, Van der Walt JS, Schatz DA, Johannsson G, Haarburger DH, Pillay TS. Salivary cortisol day curves in Addison's disease in patients on hydrocortisone replacement. Horm Metab Res. 2013;45(1):62–8. https://doi.org/10.1055/s-0032-1321855. Epub 2012 Aug 14.

Savage MO, Chan LF, Afshar F, Plowman PN, Grossman AB, Storr HL. Advances in the management of paediatric Cushing's disease. Horm Res. 2008;69:327–33.

Schilbach K, Strasburger CJ, Bidlingmaier M. Biochemical investigations in diagnosis and follow up of acromegaly. Pituitary. 2017;20(1):33–45. Review. PMID: 28168377. https://doi.org/10.1007/s11102-017-0792-z.

Selmaoui B, Touitou Y. Reproducibility of the circadian rhythms of serum cortisol and melatonin in healthy subjects: a study of three different 24-h cycles over six weeks. Life Sci. 2003;73:3339–49.

Shah A, Stanhope R, Matthew D. Hazards of pharmacological tests of growth hormone secretion in childhood. Br Med J. 1992;304:173–4.

Sharma ST, Nieman LK. Cushing's syndrome: all variants, detection, and treatment. Endocrinol Metab Clin N Am. 2011;40(2):379–91.

Soliman A, Adel A, Sabt A, Elbukhari E, Ahmed H, De Sanctis V. Does priming with sex steroids improve the diagnosis of normal growth hormone secretion in short children? Indian J Endocrinol Metab. 2014;18(Suppl 1):S80–3.

Strich D, Terespolsky N, Gillis D. Glucagon stimulation test for childhood growth hormone deficiency: timing of the peak is important. J Pediatr. 2009;154:415–9.

Timper T, Fenske W, Kuhn F, Frech N, Arici B, Rutishauser J, Kopp P, Allolio B, Stettler C, Muller B, Katan M, Christ-Crain M. J Clin Endocrinol Metab. 2015;100(6):2268–74.

Trainer PJ, Faria M, Newell-Price J, Browne P, Kopelman P, Coy DH, Besser GM, Grossman AB. A comparison of the effects of human and ovine corticotropin-releasing hormone on the pituitary-adrenal axis. J Clin Endocrinol Metab. 1995;80(2):412–7.

Trapp CM, Speiser PW, Oberfield SE. Congenital adrenal hyperplasia: an update in children. Curr Opin Endocrinol Diabetes Obes. 2011;18(3):166–70.

Valassi E, Swearingen B, Lee H, et al. Concomitant medication use can confound interpretation of the combined dexamethasone-corticotropin releasing hormone test in Cushing's syndrome. J Clin Endocrinol Metab. 2009;94(12):4851–9. https://doi.org/10.1210/jc.2009-1500.

Wallace I, Cunningham S, Lindsay J. The diagnosis and investigation of adrenal insufficiency in adults. Ann Clin Biochem. 2009;46(5):351–67. https://doi.org/10.1258/acb.2009.009101.

Wong LM, Man SS. Water deprivation test in children with polyuria. J Pediatr Endocrinol Metab. 2012;25(9–10):869–74.

Yaneva M, Mosnier-Pudar H, Dugue M-A, Grabar S, Fulla Y, Bertagna X. Midnight salivary cortisol for the initial diagnosis of Cushing's syndrome of various causes. J Clin Endocrinol Metab. 2004;89(7):3345–51.

Yanovski JA, Cutler GB Jr, Chrousos GP, Nieman LK. The dexamethasone-suppressed corticotropin-releasing hormone stimulation test differentiates mild Cushing's disease from normal physiology. J Clin Endocrinol Metab. 1998;83(2):348–52.

Yuen KC, et al. Clinical characteristics, timing of peak responses and safety aspects of two dosing regimens of the glucagon stimulation test in evaluating growth hormone and cortisol secretion in adults. Pituitary. 2013;16:220–30.

Key Reading

1. Dashe AM, Cramm RE, Crist CA, Habener JF, Soloman DH. A water deprivation test for the differential diagnosis of polyuria. JAMA. 1963;185(9):699–703.

2. Lienhardt A, Grossman AB, Dacie JE, Evanson J, Huebner A, Afshar F, Plowman PN, Besser GM, Savage MO. Relative contributions of inferior petrosal sinus sampling and pituitary imaging in the investigation of children and adolescents with ACTH dependent Cushing's syndrome. J Clin Endocrinol Metab. 2001;86(12):5711–4.

3. Pavord SR, Girach A, Price DE, Absalom SR, Falconer-Smith J, Hewlett TA. A retrospective audit of the combined pituitary function test, using the insulin stress test, TRH and GnRH in a district laboratory. Clin Endocrinol (Oxf). 1992;36(2):135–9.

4. Jenkins RC, Ross RJM. Protocols for common endocrine tests. In: Grossman A, editor. Clinical endocrinology. 2nd ed. Oxford: Blackwell Science; 1998. p. 1117–34.

5. Nieman LK. Dynamic evaluation of adrenal hypofunction. J Endocrinol Invest. 2003;26(7 Suppl):74–82.

6. Nieman LK. Diagnosis of Cushing's syndrome in the modern era. Endocrinol Metab Clin North Am. 2018;47(2):259–73. https://doi.org/10.1016/j.ecl.2018.02.001. Review. PMID: 29754631

7. Carmichael J. Anterior pituitary failure pituitary. In: Melmed S, editor. Pituitary. 4th ed. London: Elsevier; 2016. p. 329–64.

8. Miller D, Doppman J. Petrosal sinus sampling: technique and rationale. Radiology. 1991;178:37–47.

9. Molitch ME, Clemmons DR, Malozowski S, Merriam GR, Mary Lee Vance M. Evaluation and treatment of adult growth hormone deficiency: an Endocrine Society clinical practice guideline. J Clin Endocrinol Metabol. 2011;96(6):1587–609. https://doi.org/10.1210/jc.2011-0179.

10. Wong LM, Man SS. Water deprivation test in children with polyuria. J Pediatr Endocrinol Metab. 2012;25(9–10):869–74.

Diagnostic Imaging

16

Christine Yedinak

Contents

C. Yedinak (✉)
Northwest Pituitary Center, Oregon Health and
Sciences University, Portland, OR, USA
e-mail: yedinakc@ohsu.edu

Keywords

Pituitary · Imaging · Suprasella · Sella
Tumours · Ectopic hormone secretion

Abbreviations

CSF	Cerebrospinal fluid
CT	Computed tomography
DWI	Diffusion weighted images
FLAIR	Fluid attenuated inversion recovery
Gy	Grey
MRI	Magnetic resonance imaging
T	Tesla
T1	Longitudinal (parallel to the magnetic field)
T2	Transverse (perpendicular to the magfield)
TE	Echo time
TR	Repetition time (TR)

Key Terms

- **Dynamic sequencing:** a rapid sequences of imaging obtained after contrast administration
- **Imaging planes:** planes that divide up the body directionally. By convention the divided body is facing the observer.
- **Paramagnetic contrast:** a contrast agent used to enhance delineation of tumors on imaging.
- **Ectopic tumors:** the production of peptides by neuroendocrine tumors outside the pituitary.

© Springer Nature Switzerland AG 2019
S. Llahana et al. (eds.), *Advanced Practice in Endocrinology Nursing*,
https://doi.org/10.1007/978-3-319-99817-6_16

- **Ionizing radiation:** X-rays, or gamma rays with sufficient energy to cause ionization in the medium through which it passes.
- **Non-iodizing radiation:** does not have sufficient energy to remove atoms but can create heat.
- **Diffusion weighted images:** detect the movement of water particles in tissue and help to identify ischemic characteristics of tumors.

Key Points
- Although CT and MRI are both used to image the sella and suprasella region, MRI is the preferred modality to delineate a pituitary tumour.
- Anyone entering an MRI suite, or preparing patients for MRI, must be trained and adhere to MRI safety precautions.
- Paramagnetic contrast agents and dynamic sequenced imaging are used to highlight small tumours and other structures.
- Current concerns regarding the use of gadolinium as a contrast media have resulted in the development and use of alternate solutions.
- Localizing ectopic tumours may require the administration of sophisticated nuclear tagged agents and scintigraphy techniques. These require special patient education and preparation.

16.1 Introduction

Both Computed tomography (CT) and Magnetic resonance imaging (MRI) are used in the diagnosis of hypothalamic/pituitary tumours and have replaced plain radiography and pneumoencephalograms for imaging of the sella region. Angiography continues to be useful, and is often combined with MRI for visualization of the sella and masses and for vessel anatomy and pathology. The advent of tomography allowed for multidirectional thin anatomic section analysis and,

along with the development of computer assisted tomography (CAT scans) and magnetic resonance imaging (MRI), (particularly when combined with angiography), allows significant resolution of pathology in the pituitary region. MRI is now the imaging of choice when evaluating space occupying lesions in the hypothalamic and pituitary sella regions (Maya and Pressman 2011; Basics, neuroradiology 2018).

Imaging is captured in several planes: (Fig. 16.1)

- Axial plane: Transverse images represent 'slices' of the body perpendicular to the spine that divides the body into superior and inferior sections.
- Sagittal plane: Images taken perpendicular to the axial plane which separate the left and right sides (lateral view).

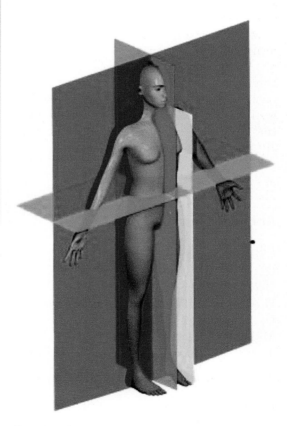

Fig. 16.1 Anatomical imaging planes. Blue: Coronal plane. Red: Sagittal (medial). Green: Axial or transverse plane. Yellow: Sagittal (lateral) plane

- Coronal plane: Images taken perpendicular to the sagittal plane, which separate the front from the back (frontal view).

16.2 CT Scan vs MRI

Both CT and MRI are used in imaging the hypothalamus and sella region. However, there are differences in these imaging modalities. Generally, contrast enhanced MRI is considered a superior modality for the assessment and monitoring of sella and suprasellar tumours (Basics, neuroradiology 2018; Weidman et al. 2015).

CT images are only acquired in the axial plane. This data is then used to reconstruct images in other planes. When reading CT images, air is displayed as black (such as in the sinuses), and brain parenchyma is Grey (Gy), while bone of the skull is seen as bright white (Basics, neuroradiology 2018).

MRI can be acquired in any plane. Each MR image is captured as a sequence. The primary MR sequences include: T2, T1, T1 with contrast, Diffusion and FLAIR. Because of the number of sequences, each being separately acquired, an MRI takes much longer to complete than a CT (Basics, neuroradiology 2018; Weidman et al. 2015; Radue et al. 2016).

The colour of the same structure in MRI may be light or dark according to the type of sequence. Fluid, such as CSF and blood, appears bright on T2 and dark on T1. White structures are subcutaneous fat (Basics, neuroradiology 2018; Weidman et al. 2015; Radue et al. 2016).

No ionizing radiation is used in MRI. A powerful magnet creates a magnetic field around the patient. Magnet strengths range from 0.3 to 3 T (1.5 and 3 T most common) which re-align the protons in cell nuclei of water molecules in the body (Basics, neuroradiology 2018; Weidman et al. 2015; Yousem and Grossman 2010). Pulsed radio waves (radiofrequency) are then directed at the patient. These are absorbed by, and disturb, the proton alignment. Subsequently, the magnet 'relaxes' and the protons return to their original state emitting the radiofrequency energy (echo signal). This *relaxation time* is the time it takes for the protons to regain their original equilibrium state. After repeated pulses to the same slice, the energy is converted to a digital image, based on the intensity of the echo signal, the relaxation time, and the density of the proton. Two types of relaxation time differentiate the direction of the images displayed: T1—Longitudinal (parallel to the magnetic field) and T2—transverse (perpendicular to the magfield) (Weidman et al. 2015; Yousem and Grossman 2010).

The contrast in the image is referred to as '*weighting*' and is determined by:

1. Repetition Time (TR)—the time between successive RF pulses
2. Echo Time (TE)—time between the arrival of the RF pulse that excites and the arrival of the return signal at the detector.

Therefore, T1 weighted images show CSF as dark versus T2 images in which CSF appears bright (Basics, neuroradiology 2018; Yousem and Grossman 2010).

Fluid Attenuated Inversion Recovery (FLAIR) refers to images with a long TR and TE time. This accentuates pathology with abnormalities remaining bright in FLAIR images (Basics, neuroradiology 2018) (Fig. 16.2).

Diffusion weighted images (DWI) on the other hand are a sensitive means of detecting stroke and random movement of water protons. Water in the brain moves freely in the extracellular spaces, but is restricted within intracellular spaces. During ischemia, the sodium-potassium pump fails and sodium accumulates prompting water to move into the cell due to the osmotic gradient. This is seen as on DWI as an extremely bright signal (area) (Radue et al. 2016; Yousem and Grossman 2010).

16.3 MRI

Identification of specific types of lesions or masses of the sella and suprasellar region on MRI is made based on key features. Masses are described by the location and extension of the mass (such as above the sella or to one or both

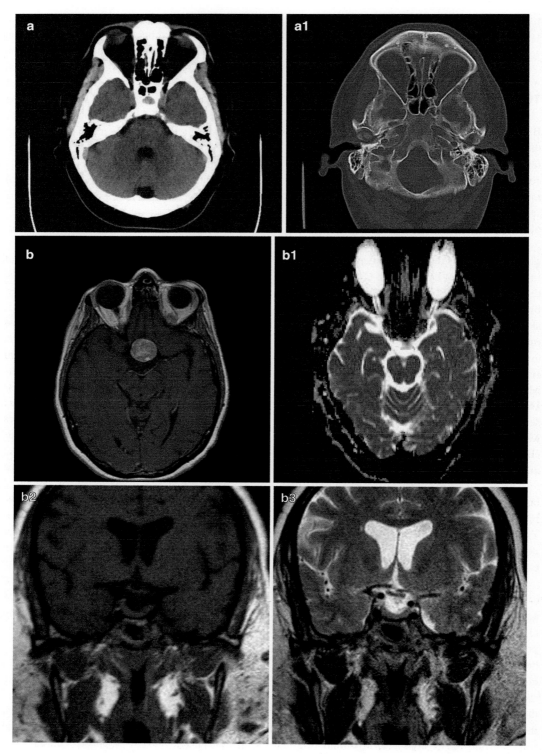

Fig. 16.2 (**a** and **a1**). CT and (**b**) MRI Images. (**b**) Axial Flair post contrast. (**b1**) DWI. (**b2**) Coronal T1 pre contrast (fluid/dark, tissue/white, brain parenchyma/grey). (**b3**) Coronal T2 pre contrast (fluid/white, air/dark, tissue/light, brain parenchyma/grey). (**b4**) Coronal T1 post contrast (fluid/dark, enchanced pituitary and tissue white)

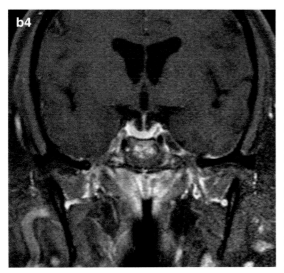

Fig. 16.2 (continued)

cavernous sinuses beside the pituitary gland), the uniformity of the image (the pattern of contrast enhancement described as the intrinsic signal), and other distinguishing features such as cystic areas and calcifications (See burg et al. 2017).

Procedure: The use of MRI may be limited when the patient has implanted metals and other magnetizable materials. Therefore, all patients must be assessed prior to MRI. MRI *incompatible* implants include non-titanium joint replacements, orthodontic braces, surgical aneurysm clips, cochlear implants, some artificial heart valves, implanted cardiac pacemakers, cerebral shunts, etc. Some cobalt-chromium and stainless steel implantable products *are* MR compatible (Koch et al. 2010). Concern for intraocular metals or the potential for metal shrapnel may need to be assessed prior to MRI with x-ray images in patients with an occupational exposure risk. Metals can cause local distortion and degrade the MRI image. The magnet can also cause motion in magnetizable materials with potential for tissue damage and burns (Koch et al. 2010). Implantable devices can also be damaged. Some reprogrammable CSF shunts will require resetting after MRI. Patients are advised to remove medication patches to avoid burns and are usually asked to disrobe and dress in a hospital gown to avoid skin contact with snaps, zippers or other metal in clothing (Weidman et al. 2015). The use of handheld ferrous detectors has also been recommended, particularly for use with children (See burg et al. 2017).

An intravenous paramagnetic contrast enhancement agent is used to help improve the quality of images and enhance visualization of pathology such as microadenomas. Likewise, it improves the visibility of inflammation, blood supply and vessels in the sella and suprasella region. Gadolinium contrast is used to assess brain lesions due to its ability to cross the blood brain barrier. However, iodinated IV contrast can also be used to assess the pituitary gland, which is outside the blood brain barrier (Maya and Pressman 2011). It contains a gadolinium molecule bonded to a chelating agent to prevent toxicity. However, there remains some concern regarding accumulation of gadolinium in the brain and in 2017, the European Medicines Agency (EMA) restricted it use (EMA's final opinion confirms restrictions on use of linear gadolinium agents in body scans 2017). The use of Dotarem (gadoteric acid/gadoterate meglumine) has been maintained. To date, the FDA in the USA has not followed suit but studies are ongoing. Many US imaging centres have adopted Dotarem as an alternative to gadolinium. Although gadolinium is usually reported as well tolerated it is contraindicated in pregnancy, in cases of sensitivity to the drug and in renal impairment. A creatinine is usually drawn prior to contrast administration to ensure administration is safe (Yousem and Grossman 2010).

Side effects are rare and most patients feel no effects. Some patients report a sensation of cold in the arm during injection, which takes about 30 s. Up to 4/100 patients report mild nausea or headache and vomiting occurs for less than 1/100 patients after injection. Mild itching occurs in 1/1000 patients (Ramalho et al. 2016). Some patients will also require treatment with an oral anxiolytic agent prior to MRI to avoid a sense of panic associated with being confined within the MRI unit (claustrophobia). In severe cases, or in paediatrics, IV conscious sedation or anaesthesia may be required (See burg et al. 2017).

Additionally, motion artefact degrades the quality of MR images. In some cases, the use of an 'open' MRI may be useful.

Special Considerations: Although MRI can be performed during pregnancy, it is only performed with an urgent indication. Gadolinium is known to cross the placenta and may be retained in amniotic fluid during pregnancy. Given the unknown impact on the foetus, administration of contrast is not recommended during pregnancy (Bulas and Egloff 2013). Gadolinium is water soluble and very little is reported to cross into breast milk during 24 h after MRI. Guidelines from the American College of Obstetricians and Gynaecologists recommend continuing breastfeeding after MRI (Copel et al. 2017).

An imaging study is usually composed of coronal and sagittal images and in some centres dynamic scanning techniques are used to enhance or differentiate small pituitary masses from normal tissue. Dynamic sequencing involves the rapid acquisition of images immediately after the administration of contrast (Maya and Pressman 2011). Standard MR imaging of the sella and perisellar region are captured in thin slices of 2–3 mm.

Paediatric patients may require sedation. However, for infants, sleeping images may be obtained by feeding and swaddling the infant prior to imaging. Videos and stories delivered via earphones may also be useful. A clear description of the reason and process of imaging that is appropriate to the child's age is recommended (Raschle et al. 2012).

The choice of wording is important in early childhood. MRI may be described as a 'brain camera' that takes pictures of the brain and scanner noise as 'camera clicks' (Raschle et al. 2012). In preparation, showing the child 'photographs' depicting MRI images and allowing them to walk around the imaging room and scanner to familiarize them with the equipment may help to allay anxiety and promote cooperation. Incorporating verbal games into the process such as counting 'clicks' and 'de-medicalizing' the event is useful (Raschle et al. 2012). The parent must also be prepared in advance and can be directed to vetted web-sites to understand why and how the images are obtained.

16.3.1 Sella Imaging

16.3.1.1 Normal Imaging

High resolution 1.5 or 3 T imaging is preferred for imaging the sella to improve the diagnostic capacity. Coronal and sagittal views are usually obtained with contrast enhancement and dynamic sequences.

The normal anterior pituitary tissue usually enhances homogeneously or in a uniform colour (signal). The intensity of the colour should be approximately the same as that of the brain tissue (i.e. it is isointense). After contrast administration, the signal in the anterior pituitary is much lighter (hyperintense). The colour of the cavernous sinuses lateral to the pituitary is darker relative to the rest of the brain (hypointense). The carotid arteries (flow or signal voids) are seen clearly as dark areas and can be tracked through each image slice. The optic chiasm and the optic nerves can be seen clearly on T1 weighted images, and do not enhance with contrast administration because of their blood brain barrier. The pituitary stalk (infundibulum) does enhance similarly to the anterior pituitary (Maya and Pressman 2011; Weidman et al. 2015; Yousem and Grossman 2010). The normal pituitary size reaches about 7–8 mm (less than 9 mm) in an adult male and the infundibulum measures 2 mm at the point of insertion into the gland. The gland in children and women of childbearing years may be more superiorly convex (Maya and Pressman 2011; Yousem and Grossman 2010; Buchfelder and Schlaffer 2014). This size increases in pregnant females and returns to normal size around 6 months post-partum (Buchfelder and Schlaffer 2014). All pituitary dimensions may decrease in the elderly (Maya and Pressman 2011).

The posterior pituitary is usually hyperintense on T1 weighted images and is often described as the pituitary bright spot. After contrast administration, this distinction between the anterior and posterior pituitary is not as apparent (Maya and Pressman 2011) (Fig. 16.3).

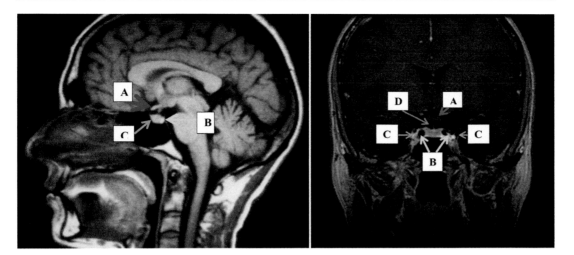

Fig. 16.3 Normal pituitary: sagittal view. A: Optic apparatus/nerves. B: Posterior 'bright spot'. C: Anterior pituitary. T1 normal pituitary gland: coronal view. A: Optic chiasm. B: Flow voids, internal carotid arteries. C: Cavernous sinuses. D: Pituitary stalk (infundibulum)

16.3.1.2 Non-functioning Microadenoma

Microadenomas have been reported as a common finding in the general population with an incidence up to 27% (Maya and Pressman 2011). They are often an incidental finding on imaging for other purposes, such as after a head injury, and are frequently asymptomatic.

A paramagnetic contrasted MRI with multiple views through the pituitary may be needed to identify a small microadenoma. Microadenomas, by definition, are <10 mm in any dimension. It is usually easier to identify those >4 mm so smaller lesions may go undetected (Buchfelder and Schlaffer 2014). They are usually round ovoid or flattened and are *hypo*intense in T1 images compared to the surrounding pituitary tissue. They usually have minimal effect on the infundibulum (pituitary stalk) but when this is no longer midline and is deviated to one side, then closer examination is indicated for a lesion on the opposite side to the deviation (Maya and Pressman 2011). The lesion itself is often uniform in intensity and may cause bulging in the affected side of the pituitary. Dynamic images may be especially useful in locating small tumours not visible on other images (Buchfelder and Schlaffer 2014). Other imaging techniques may also be applied to identify small tumours such as in Cushing's disease.

When a convex gland is seen on MRI in females of childbearing age, without areas of hypoenhancement, checking for pregnancy is recommended. When no tumour is found and the patient's biochemical testing indicates Cushing's syndrome, the presence of ectopic sources of ACTH production may need to be evaluated (Maya and Pressman 2011) (Fig. 16.4).

16.3.1.3 Non-functioning Macroadenoma

By definition, a macroadenoma is mass that is greater than 10 mm (1 cm). Non-contrasted MRI usually demonstrates the enlargement of the sella turcica in the presence of a large mass but contrasted views further differentiate the tumour from surrounding structures. There may be some changes to the sella floor with erosion into the bone. The infundibulum may be significantly deviated or not distinguishable from the tumour. The gland itself may be convex and also not distinguishable from the mass. This may impinge on, compress or elevate the optic chiasm (apparatus). This may be seen best in coronal views, and is a most important assessment (Maya and Pressman 2011; Buchfelder and Schlaffer 2014). There may be invasion of the cavernous sinuses either on one side or both sides of the pituitary, which becomes most obvious when the internal

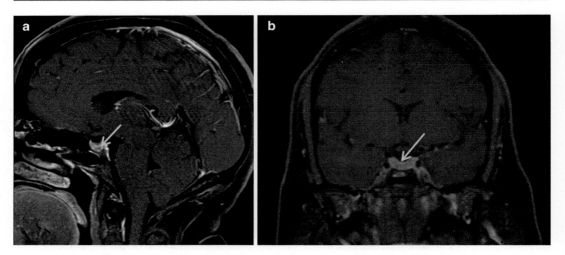

Fig. 16.4 Non-functioning microadenoma. T1 images (**a**) sagittal, (**b**) coronal view

carotid artery (arteries) are completely surrounded. The tumour mass may also extend inferiorly down into the sphenoid sinus (Maya and Pressman 2011; Buchfelder and Schlaffer 2014).

Benign adenomas are differentiated from carcinoma by associated bony changes and irregular shaped infiltrative features of the latter (Maya and Pressman 2011). They may also have some darker areas contained within the boundaries of the tumour that may represent cysts, necrosis or areas of haemorrhage. Macroadenomas usually appear uniformly solid or homogenously enhance with contrast. If they extend to the suprasella region they give a characteristic 'snowman' appearance (Gupta et al. 2018) (Fig. 16.5).

16.3.1.4 Empty Sella
In empty sella syndrome, the pituitary appears as a half-moon with thin enhancing tissue. This appears squashed against the floor of the sella (Ranganathan et al. 2013). The sella fills with CSF fluid, appearing dark on imaging. Empty sella can be partial or complete, and pituitary function testing is indicated (Fig. 16.6).

16.3.1.5 Prolactin Producing Adenoma
Prolactinomas represent about 41% of all microadenomas. A lesion or mass found on MR imaging is confirmed as prolactin secreting based on

elevated serum prolactin. Lactotrophs are usually located in the lateral areas of the anterior pituitary; therefore, prolactinomas are often seen in the posterolateral aspects of the gland (Maya and Pressman 2011) (Fig. 16.7).

16.3.1.6 ACTH Producing Adenoma
Typically, ACTH tumours are microadenomas and may be difficult to distinguish from the normal gland. MR images are usually captured in 2–3 mm slices, particularly through the anterior pituitary, where most ACTH secreting tumours are found (Sahdev et al. 2007). Some clinicians feel dynamic images are more sensitive in identifying small ACTH producing tumours (Friedman et al. 2007). An estimated 40–50% of these tumours are not found on imaging (Fig. 16.8).

16.3.1.7 Growth Hormone (GH) Producing Adenoma
Often GH producing tumours are found as macroadenomas. Assessment of the extent of tumour invasion into the cavernous sinuses and supra sella is helpful in determining post-surgical prognosis for disease remission and clinical management. In several studies, a characteristic tumour hypointensity in T2 images is seen in patients with high insulin-like growth factor 1 (IGF-1), and has been found in up to 50% of patients with GH secreting adenomas (Hagiwara et al. 2003; Potorac et al. 2015) (Fig. 16.9).

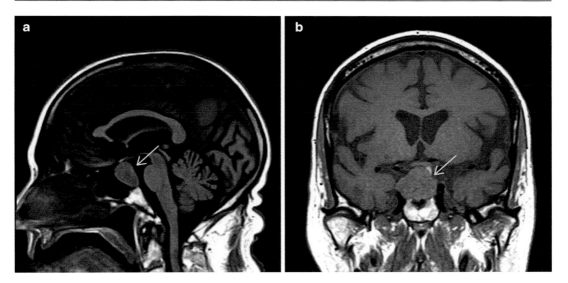

Fig. 16.5 Non-functional macroadenoma. (**a**) FLAIR sagittal image. (**b**) T1 coronal image

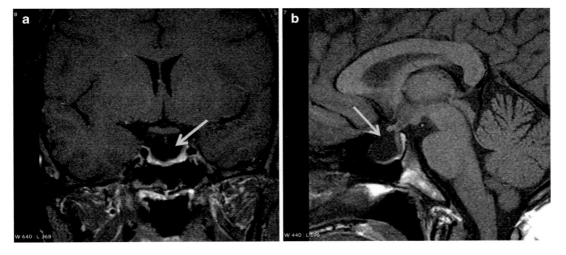

Fig. 16.6 Empty sella syndrome (arrow indicates CSF fluid). (**a**) T1 coronal view. (**b**) T1 sagittal view. Case courtesy of Dr. Sandeep Bhuta, Radiopaedia.org, rID: 5484

16.3.1.8 Rathke's Cleft Cyst

Rathke's cleft or pouch is formed from the invagination of the roof of the mouth during embryonic development. This eventually forms the anterior and the intermediate lobes of the pituitary gland. Cysts forming in this region are referred to as pars intermedia cysts or Rathke's cleft cysts. Lined with epithelial cells, they contain mucoid and serous material (Maya and Pressman 2011).

Bounded by a cyst wall, they are clearly defined and typically in front of the infundibulum (pituitary stalk) (Maya and Pressman 2011). They usually appear uniform in intensity, but this may vary from hypointense to hyperintense depending on the fluid content. Characteristic features on imaging include intracystic nodules with low to iso signal intensity (Byun et al. 2000).

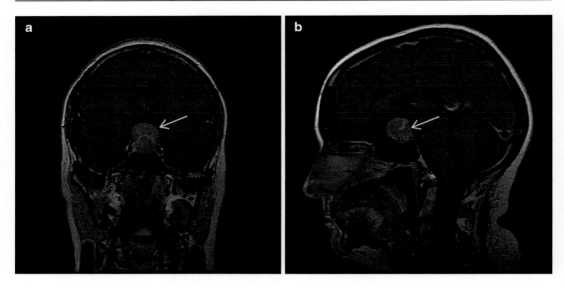

Fig. 16.7 Prolactinoma. (**a**) T1 coronal image. (**b**) T1 sagittal image

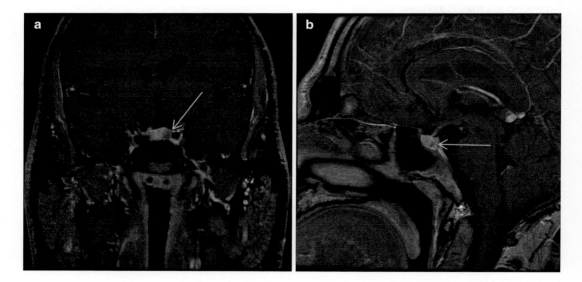

Fig. 16.8 ACTH producing adenoma (arrow indicates tumour). (**a**) T1 coronal view. (**b**) T1 sagittal view

Pars media (pituitary intermediate or middle lobe) cysts are a frequent finding and are usually seen best on sagittal T1 views (Fig. 16.10).

16.3.1.9 Hypophysitis

Hypophysitis is frequently misdiagnosed as a macroadenoma. With clear identification of features on diagnostic imaging, the patient may be treated medically and avoid the need for surgi-cal intervention (Gutenberg et al. 2009). Two clear distinguishing features found on imaging are symmetric enlargement of the pituitary gland and a thickened non-tapering pituitary stalk. Comparatively, macroadenomas are usu-ally irregular in shape and the pituitary stalk is deviated. In addition, a homogeneous appear-ance, both on pre- and post-gadolinium images, and an intense gadolinium enhancement were

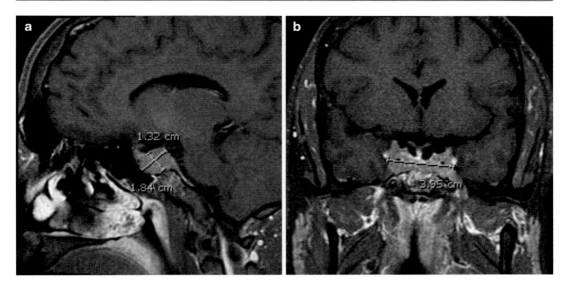

Fig. 16.9 Growth hormone producing adenoma. (**a**) T1 sagittal view. (**b**) T1 coronal view

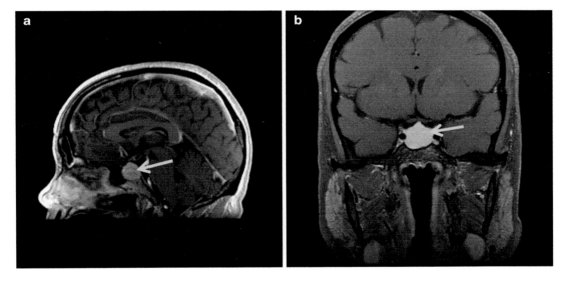

Fig. 16.10 Rathke's cleft cyst (arrow indicates cyst). (**a**) T1 sagittal view. (**b**) T1 coronal view

found to be characteristic of hypophysitis (Gutenberg et al. 2009). The pituitary bright spot may be absent. Dynamic images may be helpful in differentiating hypophysitis from other infective aetiologies (Fig. 16.11).

16.3.1.10   Craniopharyngioma

These tumours also arise from remnants of Rathke's pouch, but may originate anywhere along the infundibulum and midline up to the floor of the third ventricle (Maya and Pressman 2011; Buchfelder and Schlaffer 2014). They are differentiated from Rathke's cleft cysts by the incorporation of solid and cystic regions. Areas of calcifications and haemorrhage are more commonly found on MR images in paediatric populations than in adults (Maya and Pressman 2011) (Fig. 16.12).

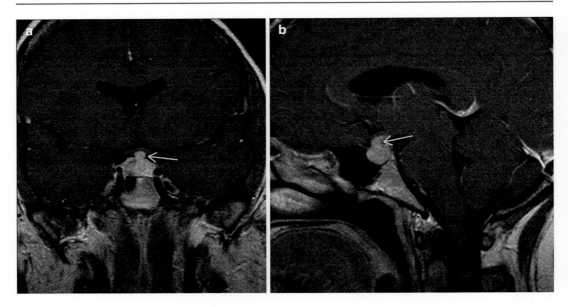

Fig. 16.11 Hypophysitis. (**a**) T1 coronal view. (**b**) T1 sagittal view

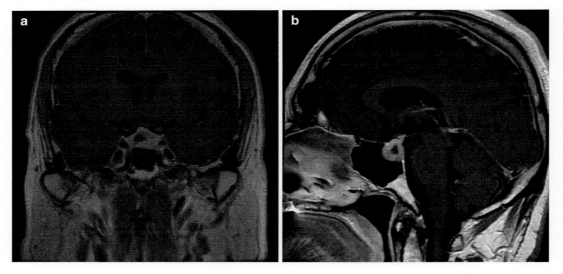

Fig. 16.12 Craniopharyngioma. (**a**) T1 coronal image. (**b**) T1 sagittal view

16.3.1.11 Meningioma

Arising from above the pituitary (suprasella), meningiomas are more likely to invade the pituitary. On imaging, both T1 and T2 images are isointense with the brain parenchyma (Maya and Pressman 2011). Post contrast administration, meningiomas enhance evenly (homogeneously) and intensely. A tail of enhancing tissues may be seen projecting from the tumour. The pituitary itself can usually be identified as separate from the tumour (Fig. 16.13).

16.4 Octreotide Scan

In ACTH-dependent Cushing's syndrome, there is an ectopic source of ACTH in 10–20% of cases (Ilias et al. 2005). An octreotide scan is a nuclear

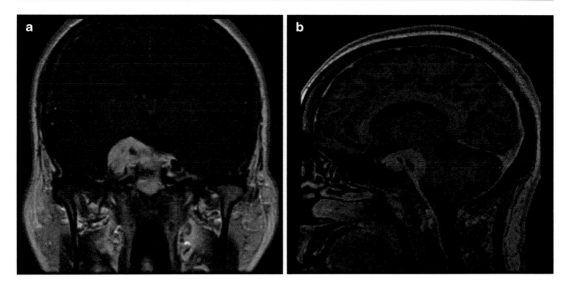

Fig. 16.13 Meningioma. (**a**) T1 coronal view. (**b**) T1 sagittal view

medicine test used to isolate a neuroendocrine tumour. Somatostatin receptor scintigraphy (SRS) using radiolabeled ^{111}In-DTPA octreotide is the conventional imaging methodology for identifying neuroendocrine tumours, ectopic ACTH and GH tumours, particularly when other modalities have failed to do so. Some report a chelating agent, DOTA (1,4,7,10-tetraazacyclodo decane-N,N=,N,N tetraacetic acid), has been added to the octreotide for increased attraction to tumour cells. Octreotide has an affinity for somatostatin receptors SSR-2 and -5 which are over-expressed on neuroendocrine tumour cell membranes, tagging or identifying tumour on scintigraphy or with combined CT or PET scanning (Rufini et al. 2006).

Procedure: No fasting is required, but patients must be withdrawn from somatostatin therapy prior to scan. An IV cannula is placed and the patient is injected with In-DTPA octreotide. Single-photon emission computed tomography (SPECT) scans are obtained 4, 24 and 48 h later (Rufini et al. 2006). The patient is advised to drink water to help flush the radiolabeled tracer out through urine and stool. This will be excreted in 1–2 days and is not harmful to others.

16.5   DOTA-Peptide PET-CT Scanning

When ectopic sources of ACTH or growth hormone (GH) have not been identified by usual imaging, the somatostatin analogues DOTA-peptides may be utilized and have been proposed as superior in efficacy to octreotide (Deppen et al. 2016). This is a radioactive tracer that, once administered, will adhere to or 'tag' somatostatin receptors (SSR) expressed on both ACTH and GH tumours. Several DOTA-peptides such as [68]DOTATOC and [68]DOTATATE that have an affinity for SSR-2 and -5 are used in conjunction with Positron Emission Tomography with Computerized Tomography (PET-CT) scanning, and have been efficacious in identifying ectopic tumour anywhere in the body (Gilardi et al. 2014; Venkitaraman et al. 2014).

Procedure: The patient must avoid any treatment with somatostatin drugs (SSAs) the month prior to testing. No fasting is required, and normal medications (exclusive of SSAs) can be taken the morning of testing. The drug is prepared once the patient has arrived to the testing centre because of its short half-life. An IV cannula is placed, and the drug administered. After a 60-min wait, the patient is asked to void prior to scanning. Once scanning begins, the process will take approximately 30–45 min, and requires the patient to be as still as possible. After scanning, the images will be reviewed for quality prior to the patient's discharge. Fluid consumption and frequent voiding to eliminate the tracer is important after scanning. The procedure is usually tolerated well without side effects (The Christie Patient Information Service 2016).

As for all nuclear testing, breastfeeding should be discontinued for 24–48 h after administration of the agent. It is recommended that women with young children avoid contact with them for at least 24 h after testing (Venkitaraman et al. 2014).

16.6   Conclusions

Radiographic, tomographic and nuclear studies may be indicated for the diagnosis of pituitary or ectopic hypersecretory disorders. These are often time consuming and some patients may require an anxiolytic medication in order to complete imaging.

MRI is usually preferred over CT for the identification of sella and suprasella tumours. Safety is paramount when preparing a patient for MRI. This includes screening for magnet incompatible items, renal disorders, and prior reactions to contrast media. Paramagnetic contrast agents are administered intravenously to enhance the recognition of abnormalities.

Education and preparation is needed for all imaging and is particularly pertinent for patients undergoing nuclear medicine scans. Throughout testing, clear information, answered questions and psychological support are essential to achieve effective diagnosis and treatment outcomes.

References

Basics, neuroradiology. University of Wisconsin Updated Jan 4, 2018, 9:10 AM.

Buchfelder M, Schlaffer S. Imaging if the pituitary. In: Fliers E, Korbonits M, Romijn JA, editors. Handbook of clinical neurology. Vol. 124. 3rd series, Clinical neuroendocrinology. Elsevier B.V.; 2014.

Bulas D, Egloff A. Benefits and risks of MRI in pregnancy. Semin Perinatol. 2013;37(5):301–4.

Byun WM, et al. MR imaging findings of Rathke's cysts: significance if intracystic nodules. AJNR Am J Neuroradiol. 2000;21:485–8.

Copel J, El-Sayed Y, Heine RP, Wharton KR. Committee Opinion No. 723: guidelines for diagnostic imaging during pregnancy and lactation. Obstet Gynecol. 2017;130(4):e210–6. https://doi.org/10.1097/AOG.0000000000002355.

Deppen SA, Blume J, Bobbey AJ, Shah C, Graham MM, Lee P, Delbeke D, Walker RC. 68Ga-DOTATATE compared with 111In-DTPA-octreotide and conventional imaging for pulmonary and gastroenteropancreatic neuroendocrine tumors: a systematic review and meta-analysis. J Nucl Med. 2016;57(6):872–8. https://doi.org/10.2967/jnumed.115.165803. Epub 2016 Jan 14.

EMA's final opinion confirms restrictions on use of linear gadolinium agents in body scans. 23/11/2017. EMA/625317/2017 http://ema.europa.eu. Accessed 6.13.18.

Friedman TC, Zuckerbraun E, Lee ML, Kabil MS, Shahinian H. Dynamic pituitary MRI has high sensitivity and specificity for the diagnosis of mild Cushing's syndrome and should be part of the initial workup. Horm Metab Res. 2007;39(6):451–6.

Gilardi L, Colandrea M, Fracassi SL, Sansovini M, Paganelli G. 68Ga-DOTA0-Tyr3octreotide (DOTATOC) positron emission tomography (PET)/CT in five cases of ectopic adrenocorticotropin-secreting tumours. Clin Endocrinol. 2014;81:152–3.

Gupta K, Sahni S, Saggar K, Vashisht G. Evaluation of clinical and magnetic resonance imaging profile of pituitary macroadenoma: a prospective study. J Nat Sci Biol Med. 2018;9(1):34–8. https://doi.org/10.4103/jnsbm.JNSBM_111_17.h.

Gutenberg A, Larsen J, Lupi I, Rohde V, Caturegli P. A radiologic score to distinguish autoimmune hypophysitis from nonsecreting pituitary adenoma preoperatively. Am J Neuroradiol. 2009;30(9):1766–72. https://doi.org/10.3174/ajnr.A1714.

Hagiwara A, Inoue Y, Wakasa K, Haba T, Tashiro T, Miyamoto T. Comparison of growth hormone-producing and non-growth hormone-producing pituitary adenomas: imaging characteristics and pathologic correlation. Radiology. 2003;228(2):533–8. Epub 2003 Jun 20.

Ilias I, Torpy DJ, Pacak K, Mullen N, Wesley RA, Nieman LK. Cushing's syndrome due to ectopic corticotropin secretion: twenty years' experience at the National Institutes of Health. J Clin Endocrinol Metab. 2005;90(8):4955–62.

Koch KM, Hargreaves BA, Butts K, Chen PW, Gold GE, King KF. Magnetic resonance imaging near metal implants. J Magn Reson Imaging. 2010;32(4):773–87.

Maya MM, Pressman BD. Pituitary imaging. In: Melmed S, editor. The pituitary. 4th ed. London: Elsevier; 2011. p. 645–69.

Potorac I, Petrossians P, Daly AF, Schillo F, Ben Slama C, Nagi S, Sahnoun M, Brue T, Girard N, Chanson P, Nasser G, Caron P, Bonneville F, Raverot G, Lapras V, Cotton F, Delemer B, Higel B, Boulin A, Gaillard S, Luca F, Goichot B, Dietemann JL, Beckers A, Bonneville JF. Pituitary MRI characteristics in 297 acromegaly patients based on T2-weighted sequences. Endocr Relat Cancer. 2015;22(2):169–77. https://doi.org/10.1530/ERC-14-0305. Epub 2015 Jan 2.

Radue E-W, Weigel M, Wiest R, Urbach H. Introduction to magnetic resonance imaging for neurologists. Continuum: Lifelong Learning in Neurology. 2016;22(5, Neuroimaging):1379–98.

Ramalho J, Ramalho M, Jay M, Burke LM, Semelka RC. Gadolinium toxicity and treatment. Magn Reson Imaging. 2016;34(10):1394–8. https://doi.org/10.1016/j.mri.2016.09.005. ISSN: 0730-725X, 1873-5894.

Ranganathan S, Lee SH, Checkver A, et al. Magnetic resonance imaging finding of empty sella in obesity related idiopathic intracranial hypertension is associated with enlarged sella turcica. Neuroradiology. 2013;55(8):955–61. https://doi.org/10.1007/s00234-013-1207-0.

Raschle N, Zuk J, Ortiz-Mantilla S, et al. Pediatric neuroimaging in early childhood and infancy: challenges and practical guidelines. Ann N Y Acad Sci. 2012;1252:43–50. https://doi.org/10.1111/j.1749-6632.2012.06457.x.

Rufini V, Calcagni ML, Baum RP. Imaging of neuroendocrine tumors. Semin Nucl Med. 2006;36(3):228–47.

Sahdev A, Reznek RH, Evanson J, Grossman AB. Imaging in Cushing's syndrome. Arq Bras Endocrinol Metabol. 2007;51(8):1319–28.

Seeburg DP, Dremmen MHG, Huisman TAGM. Imaging of the sella and parasellar region in the pediatric population. Neuroimaging Clin N Am. 2017;27:99–121. https://doi.org/10.1016/j.nic.2016.08.004.

The Christie Patient Information Service June 2016 CHR/NM/1157/24.05.16 Version 1 Review June 2019 www.christie.nhs.uk.

Venkitaraman B, Karunanithi S, Kumar A, Bal C, Ammini AC, Kumar R. ^{68}Ga-DOTATOC PET-CT in the localization of source of ectopic ACTH in patients with ectopic ACTH-dependent Cushing's syndrome. Clin Imaging. 2014;38(2):208–11. https://doi.org/10.1016/j.clinimag.2013.10.007. Epub 2013 Nov 7.

Weidman EK, Dean KE, Rivera W, Loftus ML, Stokes TW, Min RJ. MRI safety: a report of current practice and advancements in patient preparation and screening. Clin Imaging. 2015;39(6):935–7. https://doi.org/10.1016/j.clinimag.2015.09.002. Epub 2015 Sep 4.

Yousem DM, Grossman RI. Chapter 11: The sella and central. Skull base neuroradiology, The requisites. Mosby; 2010. p. 356–83. ISBN: 0323045219.

Key Reading

1. Radue E-W, Weigel M, Wiest R, Urbach H. Introduction to magnetic resonance imaging for neurologists. Continuum: Lifelong Learning in Neurology. 2016;22(5, Neuroimaging):1379–98.
2. Seeburg DP, Dremmen MHG, Huisman TAGM. Imaging of the sella and parasellar region in the pediatric population. Neuroimaging Clin N Am. 2017;27:99–121. https://doi.org/10.1016/j.nic.2016.08.004.
3. Weidman EK, Dean KE, Rivera W, Loftus ML, Stokes TW, Min RJ. MRI safety: a report of current practice and advancements in patient preparation and screening. Clin Imaging. 2015;39(6):935–7. https://doi.org/10.1016/j.clinimag.2015.09.002. Epub 2015 Sep 4.

Non-functioning Pituitary Adenomas

17

Judith P. van Eck
and Sebastian J. C. M. M. Neggers

Contents

J. P. van Eck (✉) · S. J. C. M. M. Neggers
Department of Medicine, Section Endocrinology,
Erasmus Medical Centre,
Rotterdam, The Netherlands
e-mail: j.vaneck@erasmusmc.nl;
s.neggers@erasmusmc.nl

Abstract

Non-functioning pituitary adenomas (NFPAs) occur in a substantial proportion of the population. Non-functioning pituitary adenomas occur sporadically and seldom arise as components of familial tumour syndromes. Treatment of non-functioning pituitary adenomas depends on the clinical signs and symptoms, comorbidities and patient preferences. It is a process of shared decision making between the patient and a multidisciplinary team. Surgery is indicated when the pituitary adenoma abuts or compresses the optic chiasm and causes visual field loss or vision loss. The goal of pituitary surgery for NFPA is to prevent patients from incurring bitemporal hemianopsia or restore visual field deficits and/or double vision. In most cases, patients diagnosed with a NFPA need long-term follow-up in order to monitor for tumour growth, alterations in visual field examination, biochemical assessment of the anterior pituitary functions and hormone replacement therapy if needed. Endocrine nurses play a key role in educating patients about the aetiology of NFPA, surgical treatments and hormone replacement therapy.

Keywords

Non-functioning pituitary adenoma
Microadenoma · Macroadenoma
Incidentaloma · FSH · LH

Abbreviations

ACTH	Adreno corticotroph hormone
AIP	Aryl hydrocarbon receptor-interacting protein
BTH	Bitemporal hemianopsia
CT	Computed tomography
E2	Estradiol
FIPA	Familial isolated pituitary adenomas
FSH	Follicle stimulating hormone
FT4	Free thyroxine-4 hormone
HFA	Humphrey field analyser
IGF-1	Insulin-like growth factor-1
LH	Luteinizing hormone
MEN-1	Multiple endocrine neoplasia type 1 syndrome
MRI	Magnetic resonance imaging
NFPA	Non-functioning pituitary adenoma
PRL	Prolactin
T	Testosterone
TSH	Thyroid stimulating hormone

Key Terms

- **Non-functioning pituitary adenoma:** Non-functioning pituitary adenomas are slowly growing adenomas that originate in the pituitary gland. Non-functioning pituitary adenomas do not produce hormones that lead to classical endocrine syndromes.

- **Compression of the optic chiasm:** The optic chiasm is the area of the brain where the optic nerves partially cross over. Pituitary adenomas are the most common cause of compression of the optic chiasm. This may lead to bitemporal hemianopsia.

- **Bitemporal hemianopsia:** Bitemporal hemianopsia is a type of blindness or visual field deficit in which all the vision in the peripheral temporal field segments of both eyes is lost, leaving only the central, nasal fields to be perceived.

- **Hypopituitarism:** The loss of one or more anterior pituitary hormones leading to deficient hormone production in the corresponding target gland.

- **Panhypopituitarism:** The loss of all pituitary hormonal production.

- **Transsphenoidal pituitary surgery:** Transsphenoidal pituitary surgery can be done by an endoscope or a microscope. Surgical instruments are inserted into part of the brain by going through the nose and the sphenoid bone into the sphenoidal sinus cavity. Transsphenoidal surgery is used to remove tumours of the pituitary gland.

Key Points

- The prevalence of non-functioning pituitary adenomas based on population studies is 14–46 per 100,000. Of all pituitary adenomas 25% is clinically non-functioning. The clinical importance of a NFPA depends on the size and compression on surrounding structures.
- NFPA are classified by size, based on radiological imaging. A microadenoma is smaller than 1 cm, macroadenomas are larger than 1 cm. Incidentalomas are found by coincidence on imaging and can be a micro- and macroadenoma.
- When a NFPA is found, biochemical hormonal assessment is needed to exclude hypopituitarism. Visual field examination is needed when the NFPA abuts or compresses the optic chiasm.
- Pituitary surgery is indicated when compression of the optic chiasm leads to visual fields deficits and/or loss of visual acuity. Radiotherapy can be used after pituitary surgery for (re-growth of) the remnant.
- Endocrine nurses play a key role in educating patients about the treatment of pituitary adenomas, alarming symptoms, hypopituitarism hormone replacement therapy and long-term follow-up.

17.1 Introduction

Non-functioning pituitary adenomas and prolactinomas represent the largest group of all pituitary adenomas. Non-functioning pituitary adenomas are mostly slow growing benign tumours that are often detected incidentally. Patients may remain asymptomatic and a tumour may be found during imaging procedures for unrelated causes such as after a closed head injury or accident. In symptomatic patients, complaints secondary to mass effect on surrounding structures such as visual changes or headaches may prompt imaging and reveal a pituitary lesion. Incidentalomas can be a micro- or a macroade-

noma. Symptomatic patients most often are found to have a macroadenoma. These complaints include: visual field deficits, loss of visual acuity, headaches and hypopituitarism and critically, apoplexy.

17.2 Aetiology and Prevalence

17.2.1 Aetiology

The aetiology of NFPAs to date remains uncertain. Pituitary adenomas represent a heterogeneous group of tumours. Pituitary adenomas are mostly benign monoclonal neoplasms that arise from any of the five hormone secreting cell types of the anterior lobe of the pituitary gland (Alexander et al. 1990). Most non-functioning pituitary tumours are sporadic mutations (95%), with only 5% arising as components of familial tumour syndromes such as multiple endocrine neoplasia type 1 (MEN-1) (Marques and Korbonits 2017). A number of different molecular mechanisms that lead to pituitary adenomas have been identified, although in the majority of the sporadic cases, the exact molecular pathogenesis remains unknown (Caimari and Korbonits 2016). Factors hypothesized to contribute to develop non-functioning pituitary adenomas include altered hypothalamic hormones, growth hormones, growth factors, proliferation factors, proteins and (proto) onco-genes (Herder et al. 2011). Also, research has demonstrated that growth hormone producing pituitary adenomas are more prevalent in highly polluted areas. The high prevalence was not explainable on the basis of a familial susceptibility or on a known genetic predisposition. More research is needed to study the prevalence of non-functioning pituitary adenomas and the role of environmental and industrial pollution in the formation of these tumours (Cannavò et al. 2010).

17.2.2 Prevalence

The majority of data on the prevalence of pituitary adenomas are extracted from morphological studies or from old clinical surveys, which are based either on tertiary referral hospital census or on nation-wide cancer registries and likely under-represent prevalence (Fernandez et al. 2010). Anatomical studies with results extracted either from serial autopsies or from magnetic resonance imaging have suggested the presence of a pituitary tumour in the general population is approximately 16.7% of cases (Ezzat et al. 2004). It is only within the last decade that more intensive population-based studies have been performed. Population-based studies give more reliable information about the clinical relevant non-functioning pituitary adenomas. The estimated prevalence of non-functioning pituitary adenomas based on population studies currently is 14–46 per 100,000 (Fernandez et al. 2010; Daly et al. 2006; Agustsson et al. 2015; Gruppetta et al. 2013). Non-functioning pituitary adenomas account for 25–30% of all pituitary adenomas (Alexander et al. 1990).

17.3 Genetic Causes of Non-functioning Pituitary Adenomas

Five percent of all pituitary adenomas (PAs) occur in a family setting, because of a genetic defect that predisposes family members to pituitary adenoma development, either in isolation or as part of a syndrome. Despite their relative rarity, hereditary PAs are important entities because they often present in younger patients, have a more aggressive course, and are more refractory to therapy (Gadelha et al. 2013). Non-functioning pituitary adenomas occur in families with FIPA (Familial Isolated Pituitary adenomas) and MEN-1 (Multiple Endocrine Neoplasia type 1).

17.3.1 Familial Isolated Pituitary Adenomas (FIPA)

FIPA is characterized by the occurrence of two or more cases of pituitary adenomas in a family in the absence of other associated tumours (Beckers et al. 2013). In FIPA families, individuals may

have the same PA subtype among affected subjects (homogeneous FIPA), or a mixture of different types of PAs may occur in the same kindred (heterogeneous FIPA) (Daly and Beckers 2015). In 25% of individuals in FIPA families, a germline mutation of the aryl hydrocarbon receptor-interacting protein (AIP) gene can be identified. AIP mutation was also found in >10% of patients with a macroadenoma prior to age 30 and in 20% of children with macroadenomas (Vasilev et al. 2012).

17.3.2 Multiple Endocrine Neoplasia Type 1 Syndrome (MEN-1)

MEN-1 is a rare hereditary cancer syndrome characterized by the occurrence of endocrine and non-endocrine tumours. The three main components of MEN-1 are primary hyperparathyroidism, duodenopancreatic neuroendocrine tumours and pituitary adenomas (Chandrasekharappa et al. 1997). MEN-1 pituitary disease is dominated by prolactinomas, but systematic screening of MEN-1 patients shows a large number of non-symptomatic small non-functioning pituitary adenomas (De Laat et al. 2015). The diagnosis of MEN-1 is established in one of these scenarios: a patient with 2 or more MEN-1-associated tumours; a patient with one MEN-1-associated tumour and a first-degree relative with MEN-1; a mutant gene carrier, that is, an individual with a MEN1 mutation but no clinical, biochemical or structural evidence of MEN-1 (Thakker et al. 2012). Genetic counselling and testing is recommended for family members diagnosed with MEN-1.

17.4 Clinical Manifestations of Non-functioning Pituitary Adenomas

Non-functioning pituitary adenomas account for 25–30% of all pituitary adenomas (Alexander et al. 1990). Non-functioning pituitary adenomas (NFPAs) produce small quantities of hormones (e.g. gonadotrophins

(LH, FSH), TSH or fragments of hormones (e.g. alpha subunits). The production of small quantities of these hormones does not lead to classic clinical syndromes like acromegaly and Cushing's disease (see Chaps. 8 and 9). Also, alpha subunits are not biologically active when beta-subunits are not produced (Edmonds et al. 1975). These adenomas are therefore considered as 'non-functioning'. Individuals harbouring a NFPA usually present with one or a combination of symptoms secondary to mass effect on surrounding tissues and include: visual field defects, double vision, loss of visual acuity, headache and hypopituitarism (Ferrante et al. 2006; Greenman and Stern 2015).

Visual field deficits are caused by suprasellar extension of the adenoma leading displacement of the optic pathways (Fig. 17.1). It results often in a unique bitemporal hemianopsia which is typical for large pituitary adenomas, or other visual field defects (Lee et al. 2015). Bitemporal hemianopsia is a visual field deficit in which all the vision in the peripheral temporal fields of both eyes is lost, leaving only the nasal or central visual fields to be perceived (Lee et al. 2015). Incomplete bitemporal visual field defects are much more common than true hemianopsia (Lee et al. 2015). The visual acuity may also be decreased (Ogra et al. 2014). 40–70% of the patients with NFPA present with visual field defects (Ferrante et al. 2006; Lee et al. 2015; Ogra et al. 2014). When bitemporal hemianopsia and/or decreased visual acuity has/have been demonstrated, there is a need for neurosurgical intervention in order to restore visual functions. When compression of the optic chiasm is left untreated complete blindness can ensue (Müslüman et al. 2011).

Headache is a common presenting symptom and occurs in approximately 40–60% of patients harbouring a non-functioning pituitary adenoma (Ferrante et al. 2006; Ebersold et al. 1986; Comtois et al. 1991). The aetiology is not very clear, but studies have demonstrated an association between the presence of headache and tumour size, optic chiasm compression, sellar destruction and cavernous sinus invasion (Gondim et al. 2009; Cottier et al. 2000). Also,

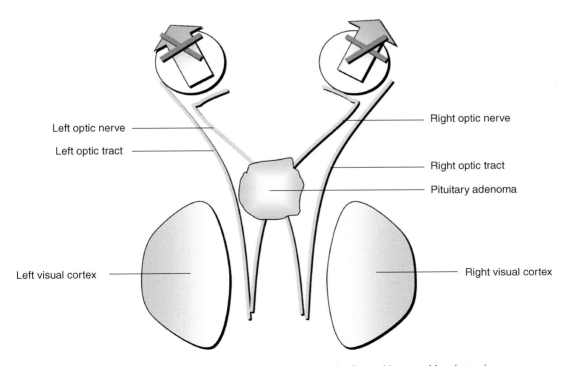

Left optic nerve

Left optic tract

Right optic nerve

Right optic tract

Pituitary adenoma

Left visual cortex

Right visual cortex

Fig. 17.1 Compression of the optic chiasm by the pituitary adenoma leading to bitemporal hemianopsia

a family history for headaches is a risk factor for patients harbouring a pituitary adenoma (Yu et al. 2017). There are studies that show that neurosurgical resection of the pituitary adenoma may relieve the patients of some chronic headaches (Ebersold et al. 1986; Comtois et al. 1991; Wolf et al. 2016). Another recent study demonstrated no significant improvement in headaches after pituitary surgery (Siegel et al. 2017). For this reason headache alone may not be a valid indication for transsphenoidal pituitary surgery.

Hypopituitarism. Hypopituitarism is the lack of production of one or more anterior pituitary hormones. It may result in growth hormone deficiency, hypogonadotropic hypogonadism, secondary hypothyroidism and secondary adrenal insufficiency. Hypopituitarism occurs in variable degrees and when assessed, found in the majority of patients with non-functional pituitary adenomas (Ferrante et al. 2006; Jaffe 2006; Nomikos et al. 2004). Hypopituitarism is caused by the mass effect of the pituitary adenoma on normal pituitary tissue or as a result of compression of the hypophyseal portal circulation by the tumour mass. Recovery from hypopituitarism after decompression surgery has been described (Berg et al. 2010; Fatemi et al. 2008; Jayasena et al. 2009; Yedinak et al. 2015), but is unlikely if hypothalamic or pituitary tissue has been destroyed (e.g. by radiation therapy, haemorrhage or surgery) (Vance 1994).

Pituitary apoplexy is a rare endocrine emergency caused by an acute bleeding in a pituitary macroadenoma, resulting in a rapid increase in tumour size, that may lead to acute severe headache, visual field deficits, loss of vision and hypopituitarism (Rolih and Ober 1993; Brougham et al. 1950). Diagnosis is confirmed by Magnetic Resonance Imaging (MRI) and visual field examination. MRI is the radiologic investigation of choice and much more sensitive than a CT scan (Rajasekaran et al. 2011). Emergency pituitary surgery is indicated in case of severe visual field deficits, loss of visual acuity or severe headaches. Stress dose glucocorticoid replacement may be lifesaving in apoplexy.

17.5 Micro- Versus Macroadenomas

Pituitary adenomas are being classified by size, confirmed by radiology assessment. Microadenomas have a tumour size smaller than 10 mm on radiology imaging. Tumours that exceed the size of 10 mm are classified as macroadenomas. In macroadenomas, the sella turcica is enlarged. Macroadenomas are often symptomatic due to the mass effect of the tumour.

Microadenomas are located within the normal borders of the sella turcica. Symptomatology in non-functional microadenomas is often absent, due to normal secretion patterns of pituitary hormones and the fact that microadenomas also rarely give compression to surrounding structures. Small intrasellar non-functioning pituitary lesions occur in 10–20% of the population or more in some reports. They may require monitoring for growth but if non-functioning are not usually of clinical importance (Agustsson et al. 2015). They may need to be further evaluated in the presence of symptoms of hypopituitarism.

17.5.1 Pituitary Incidentalomas

Pituitary incidentalomas are lesions that are detected on examination of a patient for other reasons. Patients are most often asymptomatic with respect to the tumour. Incidentalomas may be found during imaging procedures for symptoms such as headaches, after head trauma or symptoms involving the neck or central nerve system (Paschou et al. 2016). Pituitary incidentalomas can be microadenomas or macroadenomas. They can be functional and non-functional. When a pituitary incidentaloma is detected on imaging, hypopituitarism and hypersecretion need to be excluded (Molitch and Russell 1990). Non-functioning macro-incidentalomas should either be surgically removed or, if completely asymptomatic, followed closely with repeat scans (Molitch and Russell 1990). Recommendations vary regarding the interval of scanning. The interval decision is often based on symptoms, tumour growth, proximity to the optic chiasm and can be recommended from every 6 months up to every 5 years.

17.6   Assessment and Therapeutic Options

17.6.1 Radiology Assessment

17.6.1.1   Magnetic Resonance Imaging (MRI)

An MRI scan is considered the imaging modality of choice for the diagnosis of pituitary disorders because of its multiplanar capability and its good soft tissue contrast (Ezzat et al. 2004). The use of MRI has preferred over the use of CT because MRI allows better recognition of normal structures and has a higher resolution in defining tumours. Imaging of the pituitary has been performed in coronal and sagittal planes at 1.5–2 mm interval. Using this procedure, microadenomas of 3–5 mm can be detected. Gadolinium is a non-iodinated and most often the contrast agent of choice during this procedure and gives the opportunity to detect the smallest pituitary lesions distinguishing between pituitary tissue and the pituitary lesion (Gao et al. 2001). It also clarifies the position of the adenoma in relation to surrounding structures, e.g. the optic chiasm, and arteria carotis interna (the internal carotid arteries). It is important to note that patients with high creatinine or renal disease are not candidates for gadolinium contrast. Patients should be screened closely for metal implants or occupational risk of retained metal fragments and may need x-rays prior to MR scanning.

17.6.1.2   Computed Tomography (CT)

In known pituitary lesions, computed tomography is used to evaluate bone changes of the sella and calcifications in suspected craniopharyngiomas. CT is a second choice procedure for imaging pituitary lesions in patients when there is a contra-indication for MRI because of metal items in situ, e.g. a pacemaker or arterial/peripheral stents and claustrophobia (Pressman 2017).

17.6.2 Hormonal Assessment

In patients harbouring non-functioning pituitary adenomas, biochemical hormonal assessment is essential in diagnosing and treatment of hypopituitarism. Hypopituitarism in patients with pituitary adenomas is caused by interruption of the hypothalamic-pituitary-portal circulation by the tumour mass or by a direct destruction of hormone-producing tissue of the anterior pituitary. Both contribute to possible necrosis of normal pituitary gland which results in irreversible hypopituitarism and possibly panhypopituitarism (loss of all anterior pituitary functions) (Arafah 1986).

In cases with pituitary insufficiency, deficiency of the target organ hormones is found, without the expected compensatory rise in pituitary hormone levels. Therefore, measuring pituitary hormones alone is of limited or no value in diagnosing hypopituitarism.

In addition to measuring pituitary hormones, blood levels of target gland hormones are measured by immunoassays under standardized circumstances or conditions in order to interpret the results correctly (Table 17.1).

The anterior part of the pituitary produces stimulating hormones for the production of

1. *The adrenal hormone cortisol*
   The hypothalamus-pituitary-adrenal axis (HPA) has a diurnal day rhythm. The adrenal hormone cortisol reaches a peak level between 8.00 and 9.00 A.M. To evaluate the HPA-axis integrity morning cortisol is measured (Fig. 17.2). Further dynamic testing may also be needed (See Chap. 5).

Table 17.1 Anterior pituitary functions and end-organ hormones

Pituitary hormone	Pituitary end organ and hormones
Thyroid Stimulating Hormone—TSH	Thyroid—FT4
Adreno corticotroph releasing hormone—ACTH	Adrenals—cortisol
Gonadotrophic hormones: LH/FSH	Ovaries—estrogens (F)/ testis—testosterone (M)
Growth hormone—GH	Liver—IGF-1
Prolactin	

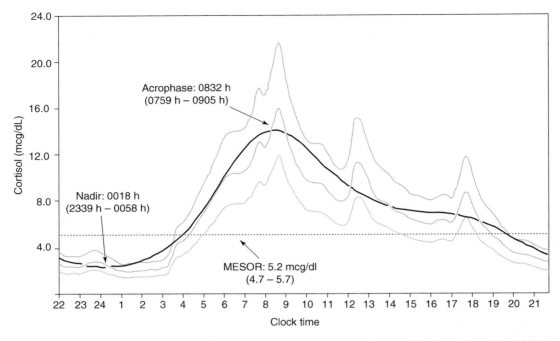

Fig. 17.2 Circadian rhythm of cortisol. Adapted from: Debono, M., et al. (2009). 'Modified-release hydrocortisone to provide circadian cortisol profiles'. The Journal of Clinical Endocrinology & Metabolism **94**(5): 1548–1554

Fig. 17.3 Circadian rhythm of testosterone in men. Adapted from: Bremner, W. J., et al. (1983). 'Loss of circadian rhythmicity in blood testosterone levels with ageing in normal men'. The Journal of Clinical Endocrinology & Metabolism **56**(6): 1278–1281

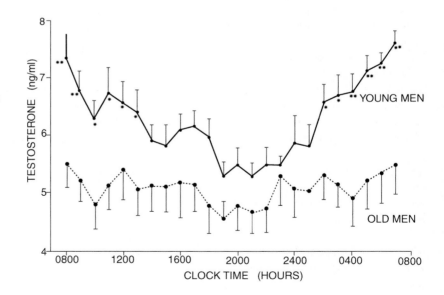

2. *Thyroid hormone*

   To evaluate the hypothalamus-pituitary-thyroid axis, FT4 is measured. TSH levels in pituitary patients are normal to low-normal and with pituitary damage and surgery TSH is no longer a reliable contribution in the evaluation of the hypothalamus-pituitary-thyroid axis.

3. *Gonadal hormone*

   Gonadal hormones are stimulated by LH and FSH and produced in the ovaria and testes (Fig. 17.3). LH, FSH and testosterone are measured in men. Testosterone reaches a peak level between 08:00 and 10:00 A.M. and therefore it is best measured in the morning.

In women, LH, FSH and oestradiol are measured for evaluation of the hypothalamus-pituitary-gonadal axis and results are time of the menstrual cycle and menopausal status dependent.

4. *Growth hormone (GH)*
   To evaluate the hypothalamus-pituitary-growth hormone axis, insulin-like growth factor-1 (IGF-1) is measured. It is produced by the liver after stimulation from growth hormone produced in the pituitary. Growth hormone is secreted in a pulsatile fashion by the anterior pituitary and therefore a random sample is of little value in the evaluation of growth hormone deficiency or excess. The GH axis function requires further evaluation by dynamic tests (See Chap. 5).

5. *Prolactin*
   Prolactin is inhibited by the production of dopamine in the hypothalamus, but can be slightly elevated in patients with a large non-functioning pituitary adenoma due compression of the pituitary stalk that can disrupt the dopamine inhibition of prolactin production in the anterior pituitary (Chahal and Schlechte 2008).

   For more information about pituitary function and dynamic pituitary testing, see Chaps. 1 and 5.

17.7 Visual Field Examination

Visual field analyses reflect the degree of the compression to the optic nerve that results the structural damage of the nerve. Visual fields can be evaluated by Goldmann and Humphrey perimetry. The Goldmann perimeter is a hollow white spherical bowl positioned at set distance in front of the patient (Fig. 17.4). An examiner presents a test light of variable size and intensity in a variety of visual fields. The Humphrey perimetry is an automated test. The patient is required to fixate at a central point with each eye while a light of variable intensity is flashed in the peripheral field of vision. The patient is required to acknowledge the flashing light by pressing a button.

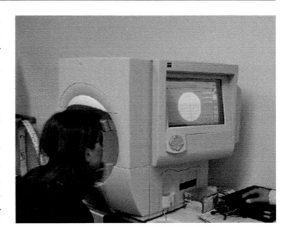

Fig. 17.4 Humphrey's visual field examination

Informal visual field exams by confrontation can also be accomplished in clinic with the practitioner seated 3–4 ft from the patient. With both practitioner and patient facing each other, each cover one eye as the practitioner holds up fingers equidistant between them. Each visual quadrant is tested when the patient correctly perceives the number of digits displayed in each visual field quadrant. Formal testing is indicated with any deficiencies when compared with the examiner's field of vision.

Formal evaluation of visual fields pre- and postoperatively or during long-term follow-up provides a standard quantitative method in assessing the progression of visual field loss (Anik et al. 2011). Other causes of visual field deficits should be ruled out by the ophthalmologist, such as glaucoma and cataract.

17.8 Therapeutic Options

Treatment of non-functioning pituitary adenomas depends on the clinical signs and symptoms, comorbidities and personal circumstances. It is a process of shared decision making of the multidisciplinary team, together with the patient.

17.8.1 Pituitary Surgery

In patients harbouring a non-functional pituitary adenoma, pituitary surgery is indicated when the pituitary adenoma abuts or compresses the optic chiasm. The goal of pituitary surgery is to prevent patients from incurring bitemporal hemianopsia or to restore visual field deficits and visual field acuity loss. Pituitary surgery can be performed by transsphenoidal approach with a microscope or endoscope. In giant adenomas, a transcranial surgery is usually indicated (See Pituitary Surgery Chap. 12).

17.8.2 Radiotherapy

In NFPA radiotherapy is commonly used for postoperative adenoma remnants with invasive character that are not accessible surgically. The timing of radiation for NFPA is a current subject of controversy. Some radiotherapists recommend radiotherapy after initial surgery. Others use radiotherapy only if further growth of the residual adenoma is observed. Read more about radiotherapy in Chap. 12.

17.8.3 Expectative Approach

In patients harbouring a non-symptomatic non-functioning pituitary adenoma with no compression to the optic chiasm, one can 'wait and scan' or 'wait and watch'. This approach is to closely monitor the evolution of the adenoma. When, or if, growth of the adenoma occurs and/or visual field deficits are demonstrated, the indication for pituitary surgery needs to be reconsidered.

17.8.4 Medical Treatment

In NFPA, the goal of treatment is tumour reduction or stabilization of tumour size in order to reduce signs and symptoms caused by compression of the tumour on surrounding structures (e.g. optic chiasm). Currently, no treatment medical treatment modality has been found that has demonstrated reliable reduction in tumour size of NFPA (Greenman 2007).

There were attempts to use dopamine agonists to address tumour growth after surgical resection of a NFPA macroadenomas. In two small nonrandomized studies it was found that with D2 tumour expression some benefit may be achieved with respect to stabilization of any residual tumour in 61–70% (Greenman et al. 2005; Pivonello et al. 2004). There may also be some potential benefit in rare cases in whom radiotherapy and a second surgical intervention are less attractive (Neggers and Lelij van der 2014). However, overall there seems to be a limited role for dopamine agonists in NFPA.

17.8.5 Headaches Assessment and Management

Assessment of pain should be integrated in the diagnostic workup and follow-up of patients with a non-functioning pituitary adenoma. Headaches assessment can be performed by using structured questionnaires, or in a less structured way, as long as pain is not neglected. In a proportion of patients, a referral to a neurologist may be useful. Different treatment strategies are often necessary (optimization of endocrinological treatment, pharmaceutical pain management, physiotherapy, behavioural psychotherapy when appropriate, etc.) (Dimopoulou et al. 2014).

17.9 Long-Term Management

Patients with a non-functioning pituitary adenoma, especially when patients have undergone pituitary surgery, in most cases need lifelong follow-up of the adenoma. Radiologic assessment by MRI is needed to follow the size of the pituitary adenoma or any residual tumour. When the optic chiasm is involved, repeated perimetry to follow the visual fields and visual acuity is also needed. Usually this can be discontinued or performed less frequently during long-term follow-up after pituitary surgery. Regular biochemical assessment is essential to follow up the anterior pituitary functions. Long-term hypopituitarism after surgery is possible and may be more frequent if the patient received additional radiotherapy. However, hormonal assessment is essential to optimize hormone replacement therapy. Treatment of hypopituitarism with hormone replacement therapy is needed to improve symptomatology associated with hypopituitarism, to avoid potentially life-threatening situations in the case of adrenal insufficiency and to protect patients from the long-term sequela of untreated hypopituitarism such as osteoporosis and cardio-vascular disease.

17.10 Nursing Interventions

At the point of diagnosis, patients often fear this tumour is cancerous and will spread to other parts of the body. Patient education may start with reassurance and a description of the characteristics of adenomas versus cancerous tumours (See Imaging Chap. 5). The prevalence of pituitary carcinomas is less than 0.1% and if surgery is needed, the diagnosis will be confirmed by pathology (Heaney 2011). Explain that if metastasis occurs it is usually related to cancer from other locations such as lung or breast to the pituitary and not from the pituitary to other organs. Patients meeting criteria for MEN-1, however, will need further evaluation and psychological support as described above.

Patients often require multiple tests (as described above) and if better informed can more actively participate in and adhere to a plan of assessment and care. Patient preparation enhances trust, decreases anxiety and achieves a more seamless transition between disciplines such as neuro-ophthalmologists, neurosurgeons, neuro-radiologists, ear-nose and throat (ENT) specialists, dynamic or invasive testing units or genetic testing and counsellors.

Involving the patients' family or support person(s) in disease-related education efforts using multiple educational modalities such as print, audio-visual methods, demonstration and verbal instruction is important for understanding and retention of information. It is important to take into account learning styles, literacy and culture (Marcus 2014). Referral to and/or the use of websites with endorsed patient educational material such as provided by the European Society of Endocrinology, the Endocrine Society (USA)

Hormone Health Network and patient support organizations such as the World Alliance of Pituitary Organizations (WAPO) can provide both education and direct patient access to appropriate support.

How the information regarding the patient's tumour is delivered sets the stage for patient trust and subsequent learning, particularly at an initial visit after tumour discovery. Using approaches such as a modification of the SPIKE protocol for giving 'bad' news may be useful (Baile et al. 2000). This involves setting up the encounter in a private consultation, making a connection with the patient, preparing for the discussion and avoiding highly emotive wording such as 'brain tumour' or technical jargon. Check the understanding of the patient and family members to critical information given and invite them to ask questions regarding the information they require. Provide information as requested by both the patient and family and use references, written materials, etc. that can read in a more relaxed manner at home. Lastly address the patient and families emotions and immediate concerns such as preparation for surgery, work-related issues, expectations postoperatively such as steroids, monitoring of blood levels of some hormones for events while inpatient or after discharge such as diabetes insipidus, syndrome of inappropriate antidiuretic hormone and adrenal insufficiency (See Chap. 12).

Patient need to be aware that they will have regular, often lifelong, follow-up, although the follow-up interval may vary according to the patient's clinical needs, treatment location and patient access to care. It is important for the patient to be aware of unexpected signs and symptoms occurring in the meantime. Symptoms such as severe, sudden onset headache (often described as the 'worst headache of my life'), progressive headache, particularly associated with nausea and vomiting, and any new visual changes should be evaluated by the pituitary team immediately (See Endocrine Emergencies). Given the long-term relationship these patients form with their pituitary team, endocrine nurses play a key role in educating patients about signs and symptoms of changes in pituitary function and normal and abnormal symptoms across the life cycle. Nurses support the patient maximizing their functional capacity and quality of life in the context of pituitary diseases.

References

Agustsson TT, Baldvinsdottir T, Jonasson JG, Olafsdottir E, Steinthorsdottir V, Sigurdsson G, et al. The epidemiology of pituitary adenomas in Iceland, 1955–2012: a nationwide population-based study. Eur J Endocrinol. 2015;173(5):655–64.

Alexander JM, Biller BM, Bikkal H, Zervas NT, Arnold A, Klibanski A. Clinically nonfunctioning pituitary tumors are monoclonal in origin. J Clin Investig. 1990;86(1):336.

Anik I, Anik Y, Koc K, Ceylan S, Genc H, Altintas O, et al. Evaluation of early visual recovery in pituitary macroadenomas after endoscopic endonasal transphenoidal surgery: quantitative assessment with diffusion tensor imaging (DTI). Acta Neurochir. 2011;153(4):831–42.

Arafah BM. Reversible hypopituitarism in patients with large nonfunctioning pituitary adenomas. J Clin Endocrinol Metab. 1986;62(6):1173–9.

Baile WF, Buckman R, Lenzi R, Glober G, Beale EA, Kudelka AP. SPIKES—a six-step protocol for delivering bad news: application to the patient with cancer. Oncologist. 2000;5(4):302–11.

Beckers A, Aaltonen LA, Daly AF, Karhu A. Familial isolated pituitary adenomas (FIPA) and the pituitary adenoma predisposition due to mutations in the aryl hydrocarbon receptor interacting protein (AIP) gene. Endocr Rev. 2013;34(2):239–77.

Berg C, Meinel T, Lahner H, Mann K, Petersenn S. Recovery of pituitary function in the late-postoperative phase after pituitary surgery: results of dynamic testing in patients with pituitary disease by insulin tolerance test 3 and 12 months after surgery. Eur J Endocrinol. 2010;162(5):853–9.

Brougham M, Heusner AP, Adams RD. Acute degenerative changes in adenomas of the pituitary body—with special reference to pituitary apoplexy. J Neurosurg. 1950;7(5):421–39.

Caimari F, Korbonits M. Novel genetic causes of pituitary adenomas. Clin Cancer Res. 2016;22(20):5030–42.

Cannavò S, Ferraù F, Ragonese M, Curtò L, Torre ML, Magistri M, et al. Increased prevalence of acromegaly in a highly polluted area. Eur J Endocrinol. 2010;163(4):509–13.

Chahal J, Schlechte J. Hyperprolactinemia. Pituitary. 2008;11(2):141.

Chandrasekharappa SC, Guru SC, Manickam P, Olufemi S-E, Collins FS, Emmert-Buck MR, et al. Positional cloning of the gene for multiple endocrine neoplasia type 1. Science. 1997;276(5311):404–7.

Comtois R, Beauregard H, Somma M, Serri O, Aris-Jilwan N, Hardy J. The clinical and endocrine outcome to trans-sphenoidal microsurgery of nonsecreting pituitary adenomas. Cancer. 1991;68(4):860–6.

Cottier JP, Destrieux C, Brunereau L, Bertrand P, Moreau L, Jan M, et al. Cavernous sinus invasion by pituitary adenoma: MR imaging. Radiology. 2000;215(2):463–9.

Daly AF, Beckers A. Familial isolated pituitary adenomas (FIPA) and mutations in the aryl hydrocarbon receptor interacting protein (AIP) gene. Endocrinol Metab Clin N Am. 2015;44(1):19–25.

Daly AF, Rixhon M, Adam C, Dempegioti A, Tichomirowa MA, Beckers A. High prevalence of pituitary adenomas: a cross-sectional study in the province of Liege, Belgium. J Clin Endocrinol Metabol. 2006;91(12):4769–75.

De Laat JM, Dekkers OM, Pieterman CRC, Kluijfhout WP, Hermus AR, Pereira AM, et al. Long-term natural course of pituitary tumors in patients with MEN1: results from the DutchMEN1 study group (DMSG). J Clin Endocrinol Metabol. 2015;100(9):3288–96.

Dimopoulou C, Athanasoulia AP, Hanisch E, Held S, Sprenger T, Toelle TR, et al. Clinical characteristics of pain in patients with pituitary adenomas. Eur J Endocrinol. 2014;171(5):581–91.

Ebersold MJ, Quast LM, Laws ER Jr, Scheithauer B, Randall RV. Long-term results in transsphenoidal removal of nonfunctioning pituitary adenomas. J Neurosurg. 1986;64(5):713–9.

Edmonds M, Molitch M, Pierce JG, Odell WD. Secretion of alpha subunits of luteinizing hormone (LH) by the anterior pituitary. J Clin Endocrinol Metabol. 1975;41(3):551–5.

Ezzat S, Asa SL, Couldwell WT, Barr CE, Dodge WE, Vance ML, et al. The prevalence of pituitary adenomas. Cancer. 2004;101(3):613–9.

Fatemi N, Dusick JR, Mattozo C, McArthur DL, Cohan P, Boscardin J, et al. Pituitary hormonal loss and recovery after transsphenoidal adenoma removal. Neurosurgery. 2008;63(4):709–18.

Fernandez A, Karavitaki N, Wass JAH. Prevalence of pituitary adenomas: a community-based, cross-sectional study in Banbury (Oxfordshire, UK). Clin Endocrinol. 2010;72(3):377–82.

Ferrante E, Ferraroni M, Castrignano T, Menicatti L, Anagni M, Reimondo G, et al. Non-functioning pituitary adenoma database: a useful resource to improve the clinical management of pituitary tumors. Eur J Endocrinol. 2006;155(6):823–9.

Gadelha MR, Trivellin G, Ramírez LCH, Korbonits M. Genetics of pituitary adenomas. Endocrine tumor syndromes and their genetics. Front Horm Res. 2013;41:111–40. Karger Publishers.

Gao R, Isoda H, Tanaka T, Inagawa S, Takeda H, Takehara Y, et al. Dynamic gadolinium-enhanced MR imaging of pituitary adenomas: usefulness of sequential sagittal and coronal plane images. Eur J Radiol. 2001;39(3):139–46.

Gondim JA, de Almeida JP, de Albuquerque LA, Schops M, Gomes E, Ferraz T. Headache associated with pituitary tumors. J Headache Pain. 2009;10(1):15–20.

Greenman Y. Dopaminergic treatment of nonfunctioning pituitary adenomas. Nat Rev Endocrinol. 2007;3(8):554.

Greenman Y, Stern N. Optimal management of nonfunctioning pituitary adenomas. Endocrine. 2015;50(1):51–5.

Greenman Y, Tordjman K, Osher E, Veshchev I, Shenkerman G, Reider-Groswasser II, et al. Postoperative treatment of clinically nonfunctioning pituitary adenomas with dopamine agonists decreases tumour remnant growth. Clin Endocrinol. 2005;63(1):39–44.

Gruppetta M, Mercieca C, Vassallo J. Prevalence and incidence of pituitary adenomas: a population based study in Malta. Pituitary. 2013;16(4):545–53.

Heaney AP. Clinical review: pituitary carcinoma: difficult diagnosis and treatment. J Clin Endocrinol Metab. 2011;96(12):3649–60.

Herder dWW, Feelders RA, Van der Lelij AJ. Clinically non-functioning tumors and gonadotropinomas. In: Wass JAH, editor. Oxford textbook of endocrinology and diabetes. Oxford; 2011. p. 209–18.

Jaffe CA. Clinically non-functioning pituitary adenoma. Pituitary. 2006;9(4):317–21.

Jayasena CN, Gadhvi KA, Gohel B, Martin NM, Mendoza N, Meeran K, et al. A single early morning serum cortisol in the early post operative period following transphenoidal surgery for pituitary tumours accurately predicts hypothalamo-pituitary-adrenal function. Endocr Abstr. 2009;19((Jayasena C.N.; Gadhvi K.A.; Gohel B.; Martin N.M.; Meeran K.; Dhillo W.S.) Department of Investigative Medicine, Imperial College London, Hammersmith Hospital, London, United Kingdom):P272.

Lee IH, Miller NR, Zan E, Tavares F, Blitz AM, Sung H, et al. Visual defects in patients with pituitary adenomas: the myth of bitemporal hemianopsia. AJR Am J Roentgenol. 2015;205(5):W512–8.

Marcus C. Strategies for improving the quality of verbal patient and family education: a review of the literature and creation of the EDUCATE model. Health Psychol Behav Med. 2014;2(1):482–95.

Marques P, Korbonits M. Genetic aspects of pituitary adenomas. Endocrinol Metab Clin. 2017;46(2):335–74.

Molitch ME, Russell EJ. The pituitary "incidentaloma". Ann Intern Med. 1990;112(12):925–31.

Müslüman AM, Cansever T, Yılmaz A, Kanat A, Oba E, Çavuşoğlu H, et al. Surgical results of large and giant pituitary adenomas with special consideration of ophthalmologic outcomes. World Neurosurg. 2011;76(1):141–8.

Neggers S, Lelij van der A-J. Medical approach to pituitary tumors. In: Clinical neuroendocrinology. Elsevier; 2014.

Nomikos P, Ladar C, Fahlbusch R, Buchfelder M. Impact of primary surgery on pituitary function in patients with non-functioning pituitary adenomas—a study on 721 patients. Acta Neurochir. 2004;146(1):27–35.

Ogra S, Nichols AD, Stylli S, Kaye AH, Savino PJ, Danesh-Meyer HV. Visual acuity and pattern of visual field loss at presentation in pituitary adenoma. J Clin Neurosci. 2014;21(5):735–40.

Paschou SA, Vryonidou A, Goulis DG. Pituitary incidentalomas: a guide to assessment, treatment and follow-up. Maturitas. 2016;92:143–9.

Pivonello R, Matrone C, Filippella M, Cavallo LM, Di Somma C, Cappabianca P, et al. Dopamine receptor expression and function in clinically nonfunctioning pituitary tumors: comparison with the effectiveness of cabergoline treatment. J Clin Endocrinol Metab. 2004;89(4):1674–83.

Pressman BD. Pituitary imaging. Endocrinol Metab Clin N Am. 2017;46(3):713–40.

Rajasekaran S, Vanderpump M, Baldeweg S, Drake W, Reddy N, Lanyon M, et al. UK guidelines for the management of pituitary apoplexy. Clin Endocrinol. 2011;74(1):9–20.

Rolih CA, Ober KP. Pituitary apoplexy. Endocrinol Metab Clin N Am. 1993;22(2):291–302.

Siegel S, Carneiro RW, Buchfelder M, Kleist B, Grzywotz A, Buslei R, et al. Presence of headache and headache types in patients with tumors of the sellar region—can surgery solve the problem? Results of a prospective single center study. Endocrine. 2017;56(2):325–35.

Thakker RV, Newey PJ, Walls GV, Bilezikian J, Dralle H, Ebeling PR, et al. Clinical practice guidelines for multiple endocrine neoplasia type 1 (MEN1). J Clin Endocrinol Metab. 2012;97(9):2990–3011.

Vance ML. Hypopituitarism. N Engl J Med. 1994;330(23):1651–62.

Vasilev V, Daly A, Naves L, Zacharieva S, Beckers A. Clinical and genetic aspects of familial isolated pituitary adenomas. Clinics. 2012;67:37–41.

Wolf A, Goncalves S, Salehi F, Bird J, Cooper P, Van Uum S, et al. Quantitative evaluation of headache severity before and after endoscopic transsphenoidal surgery for pituitary adenoma. J Neurosurg. 2016;124(6):1627–33.

Yedinak C, Hameed N, Gassner M, Brzana J, McCartney S, Fleseriu M. Recovery rate of adrenal function after surgery in patients with acromegaly is higher than in those with non-functioning pituitary tumors: a large single center study. Pituitary. 2015;18(5):701–9.

Yu B, Ji N, Ma Y, Yang B, Kang P, Luo F. Clinical characteristics and risk factors for headache associated with non-functioning pituitary adenomas. Cephalalgia. 2017;37(4):348–55.

Key Reading

1. Agustsson TT, Baldvinsdottir T, Jonasson JG, Olafsdottir E, Steinthorsdottir V, Sigurdsson G, et al. The epidemiology of pituitary adenomas in Iceland, 1955–2012: a nationwide population-based study. Eur J Endocrinol. 2015;173(5):655–64.
2. Marques P, Korbonits M. Genetic aspects of pituitary adenomas. Endocrinol Metab Clin North Am. 2017;46(2):335–74.
3. Dimopoulou C, Athanasoulia AP, Hanisch E, Held S, Sprenger T, Toelle TR, et al. Clinical characteristics of pain in patients with pituitary adenomas. Eur J Endocrinol. 2014;171(5):581–91.
4. De Laat JM, Dekkers OM, Pieterman CRC, Kluijfhout WP, Hermus AR, Pereira AM, et al. Long-term natural course of pituitary tumors in patients with MEN1: results from the DutchMEN1 study group (DMSG). J Clin Endocrinol Metabol. 2015;100(9):3288–96.

Thyroid Stimulating Hormone Secreting Adenoma (TSHoma)

18

Christine Yedinak

Contents

Abstract

Pituitary thyroid stimulating hormone (TSH) hypersecreting adenomas are rarer than any other hypersecretory pituitary adenoma. The etiology of these tumors is not known. TSHomas cause central hyperthyroidism, with elevation of the thyroid hormones without suppression of TSH. Although reported to occur at most ages, there is a higher prevalence with increasing age.

Most patients present with macroadenomas (>1 cm), headaches, and visual changes associated with tumor enlargement and optic nerve pathway compression. Others present with symptoms of thyrotoxicosis. Early diagnosis and treatment is recognized as the best means of avoiding complications such as vision loss, cardiac arrhythmias, or bone loss. New imaging modalities have improved diagnosis and made early treatment possible.

Treatment has two goals: normalization of TSH hypersecretion and tumor control. Primary therapy is aimed at tumor removal in order to normalize TSH, but medical therapy may be indicated if hypersecretory tumor remnants remain or

C. Yedinak (✉)
Northwest Pituitary Center, Oregon Health and Sciences University, Portland, OR, USA
e-mail: Yedinakc@ohsu.edu

© Springer Nature Switzerland AG 2019
S. Llahana et al. (eds.), *Advanced Practice in Endocrinology Nursing*,
https://doi.org/10.1007/978-3-319-99817-6_18

there is tumor regrowth. There is little data regarding long-term outcomes, late effects, or quality of life. This is likely related to the rarity of the disease.

Thyroid stimulating hormone · TSHoma · Pituitary adenoma · Central hyperthyroidism · Thyrotoxicosis

Abbreviations

ACTH	Adrenocorticotrophic hormone
AIP	Aryl hydrocarbon receptor-Interacting Protein gene
CT	Computerized tomography
FSH	Follicle stimulating hormone
FT4	Free thyroxine
GSU	Glycoprotein hormone subunits
HPA	Hypothalamic–pituitary–adrenal (axis)
HPT	Hypothalamic–pituitary–thyroid axis
LAR	Long acting release
LH	Luteinizing hormone
MEN-1	Multiple endocrine neoplasia type 1
MRI	Magnetic resonance imaging
PET	Positron emission tomography
SSA	Somatostatin analogues (ligands)
SSTR	Somatostatin receptor
TRH	Thyroid releasing hormone
TSH	Thyroid stimulating hormone
TSHoma	Thyroid stimulating hormone producing pituitary adenoma

Key Terms

- **Central hyperthyroidism:** over production of thyroid stimulating hormone from the pituitary leading to enlargement of the thyroid and thyrotoxicosis.
- **Thyroid ablation:** the destruction of the thyroid gland using radioactive iodine.
- **TSH β subunit**: the portion of TSH that determines the THS receptor activity in thyroid follicular cells.
- **Thyroid feedback loop:** the production and release of thyroid hormones T3 and T4 act on the hypothalamus and the pituitary to regulate their own production.

Key Points
- TSHomas are rare pituitary adenomas, frequently misdiagnosed as hyperthyroidism.
- Thyroid levels are regulated by the Hypothalamic–Pituitary–Thyroid (HPT) axis feedback loop.
- A detectable TSH level when FT4 levels are high is suggestive of a pituitary source of hyperthyroidism or TSHoma.
- Exogenous administration of T3 suppresses TSH β transcription and production.
- There has been a significant increase in the diagnosis of TSHomas, likely related to better imaging and diagnostic testing.
- Treatment options are similar to other pituitary adenomas with surgery as first-line and medical therapy as second-line therapies. Radiation therapy remains an option in unresponsive tumors.
- Research data is limited, particularly with respect to long-term impact on the patient and their quality of life.

18.1 Introduction

The diagnosis of TSHoma has increased fivefold in some countries, attributed to better and more frequent imaging (Tjörnstrand and Nyström 2017) and likely more awareness of the disorder. The mean age at presentation is in the fourth decade in both genders with age impacting the size of the tumor. Younger patients tend to present with smaller tumors that are more amenable to surgical removal and enjoy a higher frequency of remission (Tjörnstrand and Nyström 2017).

Early treatment requires the recognition that symptoms and biochemistry are associated with central and not primary hyperthyroidism. Historically misdiagnosed, this disorder has been associated with inappropriate thyroid ablation and thyroidectomies (Tjörnstrand and Nyström 2017; Greenman 2017). Improved biochemical test accuracy, ultrasound, and newer imaging techniques such as PET/CT scans with 68Ga-DOTATOC promise even more accurate tumor location and more specific treatment. Improved histopathology allows the determination of tumor cell receptors that may help predict response to medical therapies and potential indicators of tumors more likely to recur (Greenman 2017).

Delay in diagnosis continues to be 6–12 years, depending on prior treatment and data regarding long-term outcomes is scarce (Greenman 2017). However, increased incidence has generated more interest in research for future impact.

18.2 Definition

Central hyperthyroidism is the result of autonomous secretion of Thyroid Stimulating Hormone (TSH) and may present with symptoms of thyrotoxicosis. First recognized in the 1960s, central hyperthyroidism is caused by a pituitary TSH secreting adenoma that causes excess production of active thyroxine from the thyroid gland, which subsequently fails to suppress the production of TSH (Tjörnstrand and Nyström 2017). TSH cells only represent about 5% of all pituitary cells which may help to explain the lower prevalence of TSHomas.

18.3 Epidemiology

Among pituitary adenomas, TSHomas are the most rare and represent about 0.4–3% of all pituitary adenomas based on postsurgical and postmortem reports (Tjörnstrand and Nyström 2017; Beck-Peccoz et al. 2015). However, there has been a significant increase in the incidence, which is likely related to a combination of better and more frequent use of imaging and greater recognition of the disease (Tjörnstrand and Nyström 2017). Prevalence of TSHomas is similar in both genders, with a mean age at presentation of 45 years. However, the reported ages at diagnosis range from 8 to 84 years (Beck-Peccoz et al. 2013). Familial cases have been reported in MEN-1 in association with AIP mutations (Beck-Peccoz et al. 2013).

18.4 Hypothalamic–Pituitary–Thyroid (HPT) Axis

TSH is produced by thyrotropes in the pituitary gland and comprises both α (alpha) and β (beta) subunits (Sarapura and Samuels 2017). These are genetically coded by two different genes on two different chromosomes. The genes are transcribed in the thyrotropes and combined to produce TSH. The β-subunit determines the downstream activity of TSH. The TSH α-subunit is a gene promotor important in the regulation of thyroid releasing hormone (TRH). TSH production is regulated by thyroid releasing hormone (TRH) from the hypothalamus which in turn is inhibited after thyroid hormones T4 (thyroxine) and T3 (triiodothyronine) are produced from the thyroid (Sarapura and Samuels 2017) (Fig. 18.1).

TRH is transported from the hypothalamus to the pituitary via the hypophyseal portal system (the blood vessels connecting the hypothalamus and the pituitary) where it binds to the surface of thyrotrope cells (Sarapura and Samuels 2017). This starts a cascade of events within the cell to produce TSH. TSH enters the portal circulation and attaches to the cell surface of the thyroid follicular cells to stimulate iodinated thyroglobulin to release T4 and T3. Although T4 has some independent activity peripherally, it is essentially a prohormone for the more metabolically active T3 in peripheral cells. Some T4 is de-iodinated and converted to T3 in the thyroid itself, but the majority is converted in the liver (Nomura et al. 1975). T3 promotes metabolic activity and numerous life sustaining activities in almost all body cells including myocardial contractility, rate and relaxation, fetal neurologic development, and more (Cooper and Ladenson 2011). T3 production is the main regulator of TSH β transcription (Sarapura and Samuels 2017). Therefore, this activity is inhibited by administration of exogenous forms of T3 (triiodothyronine). The serum measurement of free T4 and T3 (T4 and T3 that are not bound to protein) is a more accurate measurement of the levels of both that are available to exert cellular effects (Sarapura and Samuels 2017) (for more details, see Sect. 4 Chap. 26).

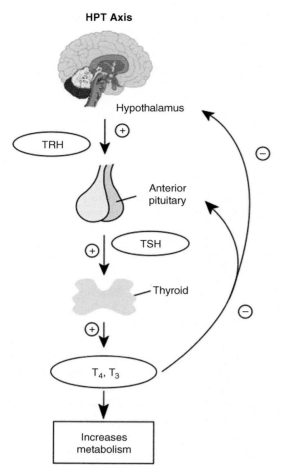

Fig. 18.1 Thyroid feedback loop. The hormones that make up the HPT axis control the metabolic processes of all cells in the body. The secretion of TRH from the hypothalamus activates the pituitary to release of TSH, which in turn promotes the production and release of T4 and T3 by the thyroid gland. Negative feedback effects of T4 and T3 on both the hypothalamus and the pituitary regulate the HPT axis function. Permission: https://embryology.med.unsw.edu.au/embryology/index.php?curid=10638; http://tedct.org.uk

18.5 Pathology

Although the cause of these tumors is unknown, multiple factors such as genetic mutations, over-activation of cell proliferation, and lack of TSH suppression are suspected (Sarapura and Samuels 2017). Defective negative feedback with decreased levels of T3, defective enzy-

matic deiodination, or increased conversion of T4 to inactive reverse T3 (rT3) may also be pathologic mechanisms. Reverse T3 levels have been found to be significantly elevated in the sera of patients with TSHomas (Greenman 2017). There may also be a relationship between defective TRH suppression and significant elevations in serum levels of free α-subunits (Sarapura and Samuels 2017).

Dopamine and somatostatin both inhibit TSH. TSH tumor cells are also known to express somatostatin receptor subtypes 1, 2, 3, and 5 which present a target for medical therapy (Greenman 2017). Detailed postoperative histopathology reports including this information can help direct medical therapies if needed.

During pituitary cell embryonic development, TSH, Growth Hormone (GH), and prolactin (PRL) are generated from the Prop-1/Pit 1 lineage. Most TSHomas secrete only excess TSH, but up to 1/3rd may co-secrete growth hormone (GH), prolactin (PRL) or have pluri-hormonal secretion (Greenman 2017; McDermott and Ridgway 1998). Despite co-secretion, few patients appear to present with symptoms associated with co-secreted hormones. Co-secretion may be found clinically and confirmed on microscopic histopathology of tumor samples taken intraoperatively (Tjörnstrand and Nyström 2017).

The majority of TSHomas are macroadenomas (80–90%) that are often found to be invasive. Increased mitotic activity has also been reported based on positive staining on pathology of >3% of cells for p53 and Ki67, although reports vary in this regard (Tjörnstrand and Nyström 2017; Greenman 2017). Prior to the development of sensitive TSH immunoassays, many patients were misdiagnosed and underwent thyroid ablation, which may have contributed to late diagnosis and increased incidence of large and more invasive tumors (Greenman 2017; McDermott and Ridgway 1998).

The patient may present with mild, inappropriately mild (given biochemistry), or severe symptoms of thyrotoxicosis, such as weight loss, nervousness, irritability, easy fatigability, muscle spasms, intolerance to hot weather, excessive sweating, shakiness and fine motor tremors, palpitations, increased bowel movements, and muscle weakness with loss of muscle mass and bone density. Reports of headaches, changes in vision, and visual field deficits secondary to mass effect as the tumor expands are not uncommon (Greenman 2017) (Fig. 18.2). Symptoms of hyperthyroidism may also be masked by those of co-secreted hormones such as growth hormone or prolactin and include: amenorrhea, galactorrhea, hypogonadism, decreased libido, infertility, breast discomfort or discharge or growth of hand or shoe size, sweating, widening gaps between teeth (Tjörnstrand and Nyström 2017). On physical examination, ophthalmopathy and pretibial myxedema are usually absent or if present orbitopathy may be unilateral (Fig. 18.3). A large goiter is usually present (even after partial thyroidectomy) and skin may be hot, moist, and velvety. Tachycardia and/or atrial fibrillation may be present or symptoms of cardiac failure (Beck-Peccoz et al. 2013, 2015 Brucker-Davis et al. 1999).

18.6 Assessment

Assessment includes biochemical assessment, thyroid ultrasound, and MRI. Both a random serum free T4 (FT4) and TSH should be measured. Serum TSH may be normal or elevated, but free T4 and T3 are significantly elevated and are considered the most sensitive indicator of the presence of a TSHoma (Greenman 2017; Beck-Peccoz et al. 2015). Measurement of glycoprotein hormone subunits (GSU) may reveal an imbalance of α-subunit and β-subunit (GSU) with an elevated α-GSU. This may only be useful in the presence of a macroadenoma (Greenman 2017). An elevated α-subunit/TSH ratio has also been reported as a sensitive indicator of TSHoma in a patient with an intact thyroid (Carmichael 2017). Elevated FT4 and FT3, in the presence of a detectable TSH, rules out Grave's disease and argues for TSHoma (Beck-Peccoz et al. 2015).

In the presence of elevated or detectable TSH with elevated FT4 and FT3 and/or compressive symptoms (headache and visual deficits), a head CT or MRI should be performed to confirm a pituitary tumor. Rare ectopic TSH secretion (usu-

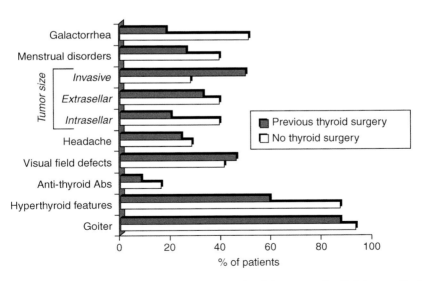

Fig. 18.2 Clinical manifestations in patients with TSH-secreting adenomas. The presence of goiter is indicative of TSHoma, even in patients after partial thyroidectomy. Hyperthyroid features may be overshadowed by those of associated hypersecretion/deficiency of other pituitary hormones. Invasive tumors are seen in about half of the patients with previous thyroidectomy and in 1/4 of untreated patients (permission Beck-Peccoz 2015)

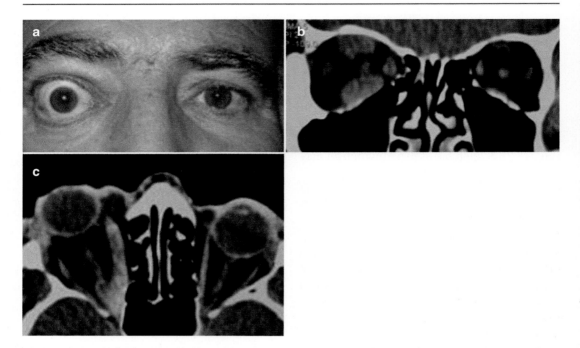

Fig. 18.3 (**a**) right unilateral orbitopathy. (**b**) bilateral orbitopathy (**c**) left orbitopathy. From: Kashkouli MB, et al. Indian J Ophthalmol. 2011 Sep-Oct; 59(5): 363–366. doi: https://doi. org/10.4103/0301-4738.83612. This is an open-access article distributed under the terms of the Creative Commons Attribution-Noncommercial-Share Alike 3.0 Unported

ally pharyngeal) has been described (Beck-Peccoz et al. 2013). If the lesion on CT/MRI is a microadenoma, resistance to thyroid hormone needs to be considered and an incidentaloma ruled out (Beck-Peccoz et al. 2015). Thyroid ultrasound and fine needle biopsy are recommended for nodular goiter, in consideration of a higher risk of thyroid cancer in TSHomas (4.8% of cases) (Beck-Peccoz et al. 2015). Guidelines suggest that other biomarkers such as cholesterol, LDL, triglycerides, ferritin, erythrocyte microcytosis, resting energy expenditure, and cardiac function parameters are of limited diagnostic value (Beck-Peccoz et al. 2013).

Dynamic testing may be indicated if no defined pituitary or ectopic mass is found or when there is concern for resistance to thyroid hormone. A TRH test and/or T3 suppression test are first-line tests and an octreotide infusion to suppress TSH may be useful. TRH dynamic testing measures the increase in TSH after adminis-

tration of exogenous TRH, with doubling of baseline levels considered a positive test (Tjörnstrand and Nyström 2017). This test is done infrequently and TRH is no longer available in some countries including the USA (Salvatori et al. 2010). Scintigraphy radiolabeled octreotide scans and PET/CT scans with 68Ga-DOTATOC may be useful in locating a rare ectopic source of TSH (Tjörnstrand and Nyström 2017).

18.7 Treatment

First-line treatment is tumor removal in appropriate cases and suppressive therapy if the patient is not a candidate for surgical options. Surgical tumor resection can achieve a remission rate of 60% in patients with macroadenomas in the hands of an experienced surgeon (Beck-Peccoz et al. 2013, 2015). Although controversial, antithyroid drugs such as methimazole or propylthiouracil and/or medical suppressive therapies with cabergoline or somatostatin therapy are recommended by some clinicians prior to surgical tumor removal to decrease TSH (Beck-Peccoz et al. 2015).

If TSH remains elevated after tumor removal, medical suppressive therapy is indicated. Although TSHomas express several somatostatin receptors (SSTR 1, 2, 3, and 5), SSTR2 is most frequently expressed in subtypes 2A and 2B (Tjörnstrand and Nyström 2017). First-generation somatostatin ligands/analogues (SSAs) such as octreotide LAR®, lanreotide SR®, or lanreotide Autogel® are recommended for suppressive therapy based on their affinity to act on SSTR2 and SSTR5 receptors (Tjörnstrand and Nyström 2017; Beck-Peccoz et al. 2013). All preparations may not be available in some countries. There is evidence that euthyroidism is restored in up to 90% of cases with goiter and tumor shrinkage achieved in 30 and 40% of cases respectively after medical therapy (Beck-Peccoz et al. 2013). Patients report side effects of treatment including diarrhea and should be monitored for symptoms of cholelithiasis.

Ongoing follow-up is recommended, but data regarding appropriate intervals is scarce (Beck-Peccoz et al. 2013). Likewise there are few reports of recurrence rates and even fewer regarding quality of life in patients after treatment of a TSHoma.

18.8 Nursing Care

Assessment of patient history with emphasis on their past medical history and family history of pituitary, thyroid, or parathyroid tumors is important. Evaluate the patient's and families understanding of the process of medical evaluation and the path to the anticipated diagnosis. This process may be complex if multiple imaging modalities, fine needle biopsy, cardiac and bone evaluations are required. Preparation for some procedures is essential and must be reviewed with the patient in advance. Determine if the patient/family has adequate resources at their disposal and if further support is required in any functional domain.

Patient education may be a staged process, as each test is resulted and the diagnosis is confirmed. Disease-related education along with information and coordination of care for any concomitant diseases revealed in the process of assessment may be indicated. Preparation for surgery and pretreatment with an antithyroid medication involves coordination between the patient and the operative team.

Further assessment postoperatively may reveal persistent TSH secretion, indicating the need for medical therapy. A detailed explanation of the purpose for treatment and treatment options that demonstrate clear value to the patient both with respect to short-term symptoms and long-term outcomes will enhance adherence. SSA therapies are currently injectable, some of which have been shown to be safe and effectively administered at home by the patient or family (Salvatori et al. 2010). Assessment of the patient/family's capacity and willingness to deliver this treatment as prescribed in the home is required in some countries. Drug administration may also involve coordinating home nursing support and/or in office teaching. The treatment plan should evolve as an interaction between patient, family, and all health care providers.

Long-term follow-up will be required. At each visit, assessment of the patient's understanding of the disease and treatment in the context of their changing symptoms and understanding is advised to facilitate self-care. Regular biochemical testing, including liver function testing, TSH and FT4 are recommended. This may need to be done as frequently at least 2–3 times in the first year postoperatively or until the patient is stable (Beck-Peccoz et al. 2013). Ophthalmologic and visual field examinations are recommended as a baseline pre- and postoperatively for patients with a history of large macroadenomas. These may be best obtained in between MRIs that are recommended every 1–2 years at least for the first 5 years postoperatively (Beck-Peccoz et al. 2013). Coordination of follow-up at a location that is convenient for the patient is more likely to result in long-term adherence (Yedinak et al. 2018; Craig et al. 2014).

18.9 Conclusions

Historically, many patients with elevated TSH and symptoms of hyperthyroidism were inappropriately treated with thyroid ablation or thyroidectomy. This may have inadvertently promoted TSHoma growth. With improved ultrasonic techniques and TSH sensitivities and the availability of sophisticated CT/MRI techniques, the incidence and prevalence of the disease has significantly increased but diagnostic accuracy has substantially improved. This has also spurred a substantial increase in research. Despite diagnostic advances, treatment delays are estimated to be over 6 years from the onset of symptoms and over 12 years for patients post thyroid ablation or thyroidectomy. TSHomas are still most often found as macroadenomas and present with symptoms of mass effect and/or thyrotoxicosis.

Treatments include surgical and medical approaches, with surgical removal of the TSHoma as the first choice in therapy. Somatostatin ligands remain the next most effective treatment in cases of residual or recurrent disease. There is limited data about the long-term outcomes and quality of life for these patients, but best outcomes are achieved with early diagnosis and treatment of microadenomas. The minimum follow-up recommendations are for monitoring of MRI and serum biochemistries yearly for the first 5 years postoperatively. However, lifelong intermittent follow-up may be indicated.

References

Beck-Peccoz P, Lania A, Beckers A, Chatterjee K, Wemeau JL. 2013 European thyroid association guidelines for the diagnosis and treatment of thyrotropin-secreting pituitary tumors. Eur Thyroid J. 2013;2:76–82. https://doi.org/10.1159/000351007.

Beck-Peccoz P, Lania A, Persani L. Chapter 24: TSH-producing adenomas. In: Jameson JL, DeGroot LJ, editors. Endocrinology. 7th ed. Philadelphia: W.B. Saunders Pub.; 2015. p. 266–74.

Brucker-Davis F, Oldfield EH, Skarulis MC, Doppman JL, Weintraub BD. Thyrotropin-secreting pituitary tumors: diagnostic criteria, thyroid hormone sensitivity, and treatment outcome in 25 patients followed at the National Institutes of Health. J Clin Endocrinol Metab. 1999;84:476–86.

Carmichael JD. Anterior pituitary failure. In: Melmed S, editor. The pituitary. 4th ed. London: Elsevier; 2017. p. p329–63.

Cooper DS, Ladenson PW. The thyroid gland. In: Gardner DG, Shoback DM, editors. Greenspan's basic and clinical endocrinology. 9th ed. The McGraw-Hill Companies, Inc.; 2011. p. 170–89.

Craig BM, Reeve BB, Brown PM, et al. US valuation of health outcomes measured using the PROMIS-29. Value Health. 2014;17(8):846–53. https://doi.org/10.4172/clinical-practice.1000386. Review.

Greenman Y. Thyrotropin-secreting pituitary tumors. In: Melmed S, editor. The pituitary. 4th ed. London: Elsevier; 2017. p. 573–88.

McDermott MT, Ridgway C. Central hyperthyroidism. Endocrinol Metab Clin N Am. 1998;27(10):187–203.

Nomura S, Pittman CS, Chambers JB, Buck MW, Shimizu T. Reduced peripheral conversion of thyroxine to triiodothyronine in patients with hepatic cirrhosis. J Clin Invest. 1975;56(3):643–52.

Salvatori R, Nachtigall LB, Cook DM, Bonert V, Molitch ME, Blethen S, Chang S, SALSA Study Group. Effectiveness of self- or partner-administration of an extended-release aqueous-gel formulation of lanreotide in lanreotide-naïve patients with acromegaly. Pituitary. 2010;13(2):115–22.

Sarapura VD, Samuels MH. Thyroid-stimulating hormone. In: Melmed S, editor. The pituitary. 4th ed. London: Elsevier; 2017. p. 163–201.

Tjörnstrand A, Nyström HF. Diagnosis of Endocrine Disease: diagnostic approach to TSH-producing pituitary adenoma. Eur J Endocrinol. 2017;177(4):R183–97.

Yedinak C, Pulaski-Liebert K, Adelman DT, Williams J. Acromegaly: current therapies benefits and burdens. Clin Pract. 2018;15(2):499–511.

Key Reading

1. Greenman Y. Thyrotropin-secreting pituitary tumors. In: Melmed S, editor. The pituitary. 4th ed. London: Elsevier; 2017. p. 573–88.
2. Beck-Peccoz P, Lania A, Persani L. Chapter 24: TSH-producing adenomas. In: Jameson JL, DeGroot LJ, editors. Endocrinology. 7th ed. Philadelphia: W.B. Saunders Pub.; 2015. p. 266–74.

Prolactin Producing Adenomas: Prolactinomas and Hyperprolactinemia

19

Christine Yedinak

Contents

Abstract

Prolactinomas (PPAs) are the most common type of secretory pituitary adenomas. The majority of prolactinomas are found in women on evaluation of amenorrhea, infertility, and new onset or persistent lactation after discontinuation of breastfeeding. Although galactorrhea may also be a sentinel symptom in males, this is not as common, and is often preceded by sexual dysfunction. Diagnosis may not occur, particularly in males or postmenopausal women, until midlife when tumor growth impacts the optic chiasm and/or visual deficits are found, prompting ophthalmology review and subsequent imaging. Likewise, pituitary adenomas may be an incidental finding on a head CT or MRI obtained during a workup for headaches, after a head trauma, or other symptoms.

C. Yedinak (✉)
Northwest Pituitary Center, Oregon Health and Sciences University, Portland, OR, USA
e-mail: yedinakc@ohsu.edu

© Springer Nature Switzerland AG 2019
S. Llahana et al. (eds.), *Advanced Practice in Endocrinology Nursing*,
https://doi.org/10.1007/978-3-319-99817-6_19

343

In addition to a brain MRI to determine tumor size, location, and characteristics, all pituitary hormonal expressions are usually evaluated. Both macroadenomas (MA) and microadenomas (mA) may cause anterior pituitary hormone deficits, and further dynamic testing may be needed. Posterior pituitary hormone deficits are quite rare and would only occur with very large tumors. Prolactin (PRL) assays may vary, so obtaining a diluted PRL level is necessary when levels are high in patients with large tumors (usually >3 cm diameter) to avoid misinterpretation of results secondary to the assay "hook effect." Evaluation of macroprolactin (biologically inactive PRL) may also be needed in patients without symptoms in order to avoid unnecessary treatment.

Treatment may depend on presenting symptoms and deficiencies. However, prolactinomas are most frequently responsive to dopamine agonist (DA) medications that both normalize prolactin levels and can shrink tumors. Normalization of PRL most often restores fertility, resolves galactorrhea, and significantly improves headaches. Likewise, visual deficits will often resolve or significantly improve with tumor shrinkage. Intolerance or resistance to dopamine agonists, tumor growth while on dopamine agonists, co-secretion with another hormone or a need for a biopsy for histopathology are criteria for transsphenoidal tumor resection. Best postoperative results are achieved by an experienced neurosurgeon. However, treatment with medical therapies (DA), other hormone replacements, or radiation therapy may still be needed postoperatively to control prolactin levels or residual tumor growth.

Keywords

Prolactin · Prolactinoma · Hyperprolactinemia Hypogonadism · Infertility · Galactorrhea

Abbreviations

AP   Anterior pituitary
DA   Dopamine agonist
FSH   Follicle stimulating hormone
GH   Growth hormone
GnRH   Gonadotropin releasing hormone
ICD   Impulse control disorder
LH   Luteinizing hormone
MA   Macroadenomas/adenomas >1 cm
mA   Microadenomas/adenomas <1 cm
MRI   Magnetic resonance imaging
PA   Pituitary adenoma
PPA   Prolactin producing adenoma/ prolactinoma
PRF   Prolactin releasing factors
PRL   Prolactin
QoL   Quality of life

Key Terms

- **Prolactin receptor:** is a cell surface molecule to which prolactin binds, causing attachment to a second receptor that changes the configuration of the cell membrane and allows the movement of prolactin into the cell.
- **Prolactin transcription:** is the first step in encoding the RNA within the cell with the functional instructions from the prolactin DNA molecule.
- **Dopamine inhibition:** occurs when dopamine, manufactured in the hypothalamus, travels down neuronal projections into the pituitary gland. It is released and attaches to dopamine-2 (D2) receptors on lactotrophs in the pituitary inhibiting the production of dopamine.
- **Dopamine agonists:** act on the D2 receptors on lactotrophs to inhibit the production of prolactin from the pituitary.
- **Hyperprolactinemia:** occurs when the blood levels of prolactin are above the normal range. The normal range is gender specific.
- **Hypogonadism:** occurs when GnRH and subsequent LH/FSH release from the pituitary is suppressed resulting in ovarian or testicular dysfunction.

Key Points

- Prolactin is a hormone with a primary role in lactation but a broad range of biologic activity.
- Hyperprolactinemia has a range of physiologic, pharmacologic and pathologic etiologies.
- Prolactinomas occur in children and adults of all ages.
- Dopamine agonists are effective and are recommended as first line medical treatment for prolactinomas.
- Macroprolactinomas are more common in adolescent boys, women after menopause and older men and have a high lifetime rate of recurrence.
- Surgery and radiation therapy are only required to treat prolactinomas when first line treatment fails.

19.1 Introduction

Understanding of the role of PRL in lactation began emerging in the late 1920s, and by 1950s it was demonstrated that PRL secretion was inhibited by dopamine from the hypothalamus. However, isolation of the hormone PRL in humans did not occur until around 1971 (Grattan 2015).

Normal lactotrophs or prolactin producing cells make up an estimated 15–50% of all the anterior pituitary cells in males and females (Gillam and Molitch 2011a). Inhibition of prolactin production largely stems from dopamine release by the hypothalamus that travels down the portal venous system and attaches to the D2 receptors in the pituitary (Melmed et al. 2011). There are PRL releasing factors as well.

The major function of PRL is to promote lactation in humans, but it is also involved in numerous other adaptive functions in various systems in animals (Grattan 2015). During pregnancy, hyperplasia of the lactotrophs occurs which substantially increases the PRL level, promoting proliferation of the mammary glands and lactation. This level is sustained through breastfeeding, and will slowly return to normal after delivery and cessation of breastfeeding (Klibanski 2010).

Hyperprolactinemia can occur related to disruption of the pituitary stalk (such as in the case of a large macroadenoma) due to decreased dopamine reaching the lactotrophs, from over production from a PRL adenoma cell overproduction (prolactinoma) in the pituitary, poor clearance of prolactin (particularly macroprolactin), and/or other drug effects (Romijn 2014). Some herbal preparations such as Milk Thistle (not Blessed Thistle) and Fennel have been shown to increase PRL in clinical studies. Signs and symptoms associated with elevated prolactin are similar, despite the etiology of the elevation. Hypogonadism and infertility commonly result from elevated PRL levels in both sexes.

Prolactinomas comprise approximately 50–66% of all pituitary adenomas, are frequently microadenomas and more common in woman between 20 and 50 years (Molitch 2017). Diagnostic criteria for a prolactinoma are elevated blood levels of prolactin and the presence of a pituitary tumor on MRI (Melmed et al. 2011). Although prolactinomas are also found in children, they are rare, being more common in females during adolescence (Salenave et al. 2015; Hoffmann et al. 2018).

High PRL levels can be accompanied by symptoms such as headaches, menstrual abnormalities and galactorrhea (lactation) or visual deficits (Gillam and Molitch 2011a; Romijn 2014; Molitch 2017). Restoration of fertility, relief of symptoms, and tumor shrinkage can usually be achieved with dopamine agonist therapies (DA) which is most often first line therapy. Transsphenoidal surgery may be necessary in cases resistant to DA, when CSF leak develops and/or in cases with a large aggressive tumor not responding to the DA. There remains ongoing debate regarding the need for lifelong treatment, the cost-effectiveness of DA therapies versus surgical resection, and the risks and benefits of both surgery and long-term treatment (Gillam and Molitch 2011a; Romijn 2014; Molitch 2017; Ikeda et al. 2013; Jethwa et al. 2016; Zygourakis et al. 2017).

19.2 Prolactin Physiology

Prolactin is produced in lactotroph cells of the pituitary gland. Primarily associated with lactation, recent studies are revealing that prolactin is also produced in numerous extra pituitary tissues, such as the endothelial cells, mammary cells, the decidua, immune cells, skin and hair follicles, adipose tissue, the cochlea, the brain, the thymus, and more (Marano and Ben-Jonathan 2014). In fact, PRL may be produced in most tissues and either independently or cooperatively have a wide range of regulatory and biologic functions, although these other functions in humans are of uncertain physiologic significance (Marano and Ben-Jonathan 2014). PRL exerts its effects in an autocrine, paracrine, and/or endocrine fashion by attaching to a diversity of prolactin receptors expressed in various tissues including in the pituitary gland itself (Ignacak et al. 2012).

19.2.1 Embryonic Cell Differentiation and Lactotrophs Proliferation

During embryonic development, there is continual interaction between the hypothalamus and the pituitary during which transcription factors are produced that determine the differentiation of cell lines in the pituitary (Gillam and Molitch 2011a). Prophet of Pit-1 (Prop1) gene/transcription factor controls the development of all non-corticotroph cells including PRL, whereas POU1F1 (Pit-1) transcription factor is necessary for the development and proliferation of thyrotrophs and somato-mammotrophs. The differentiation of somatomammotrophs to somatotrophs and lactotrophs and proliferation of lactotrophs occurs under the influence of estrogen (Gillam and Molitch 2011a). Transcription factor Pit-1 and other factors also regulate the cellular level synthesis of PRL. Pit-1 interacts with other regulatory proteins, specific DNA elements, and target promotors of the gene altering the structure of the signal that either allows or inhibits transcription and thereby influencing PRL production (Gillam and Molitch 2011a) (Fig. 19.1). The structure of PRL is similar to that of GH with many lactotrophs arising for GH cells and approximately 25% of GH adenomas co-secreting prolactin (Bernard et al. 2015; Grossman and Besser 1985). Lactotrophs comprise 10–50% of all adenohypophyseal cells, are reported to be similar in number for both genders, and remain relatively stable with age in women but may decrease in men (Gillam and Molitch 2011a; Romijn 2014).

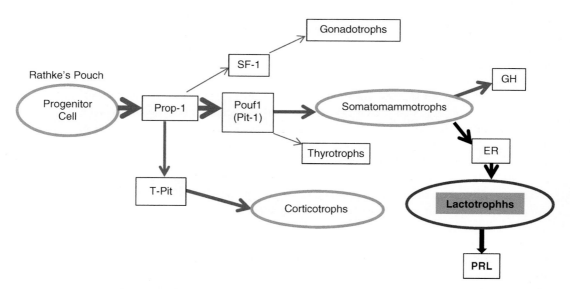

Fig. 19.1 Cell differentiation: Mammotrophs Prop-s and Pouf1 (Pit-1) are transcription factors that differentiate cell lineage. Estrogen stimulates the final differentiation of somatomammotrophs to lactotrophs (mammotrophs)

19.2.2 Prolactin Production

19.2.2.1 Dopamine Inhibition

The hypothalamus controls the secretion of PRL from the pituitary lactotrophs by using an inhibitory mechanism that is different than the control mechanisms of other anterior hormone production, which is predominantly stimulatory. Tonic basal PRL control is achieved through neuronal dopaminergic inhibition, which is considered the chief prolactin inhibiting factor, although other factors such as GABA may be contributory (Grattan 2015; Gillam and Molitch 2011a; Grossman and Besser 1985). Dopamine is manufactured in cell bodies in the arcuate nucleus of the hypothalamus, and delivered to the median eminence where it is released into the proximal portal vessel plexus and then transported down the portal vessels of the infundibulum (pituitary stalk) to the lactotrophs where it inhibits prolactin production (Fig. 19.2) (Grattan 2015). Prolactin itself may also provide some negative feedback to limit its

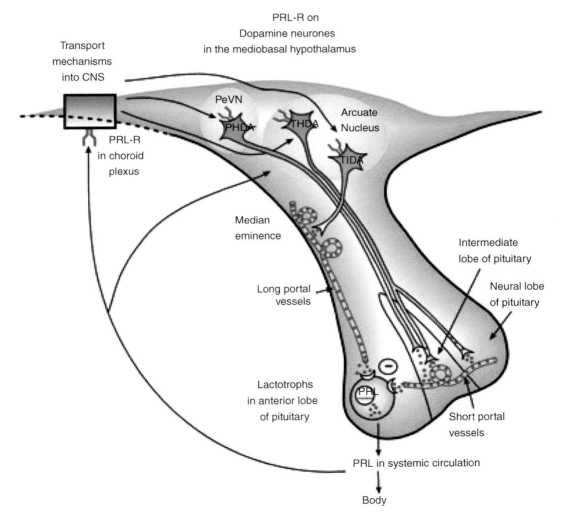

Fig. 19.2 In most conditions, the secretion of prolactin (PRL) from the anterior pituitary gland is predominantly under inhibitory control from the hypothalamus. Dopamine released from the Arcuate Nucleus in the median eminence of the hypothalamus travels down the pituitary stalk to attach to D2 receptors on lactotroph cells in the anterior pituitary inhibiting PRL production. From: Andrews ZB. Neuroendocrine Regulation of Prolactin Secretion During Late Pregnancy: Easing the Transition into Lactation. Journal of Neuroendocrinology, 2005, Vol. 17, 466–473. Figure 1. P 467. Copyright Permission: John Wiley and Sons

own production by attaching to prolactin receptors on dopamine neurons to control its own production in a tonic or basal fashion, although this has only been shown in animals (Grattan 2015).

19.2.2.2 Prolactin Releasing Factors (PRFs)

Prolactin Releasing Factors (PRFs) mediate rapid and slow prolactin release under demand conditions such as pregnancy, lactation, and/or physiologic stress (Low 2016). This mechanism maintains tight homeostatic control of blood levels of PRL1. Thyrotropin releasing Hormone (TRH) causes rapid release of PRL in human studies. The neuropeptide Vasoactive Intestinal Peptide (VIP) when released from the median eminence of the hypothalamus, has an additive effect to TRH to stimulate pituitary PRL secretion (Gillam and Molitch 2011a). Other PRFs include serotonin, opioids, and possibly other neuroactive peptides and neurotransmitters still under investigation in humans. PRL levels also rise as a result of the blockade or suppression of dopamine inhibition by neuroleptic and other drugs that block the dopamine receptor (Low 2016).

Pulsatile secretion of PRL occurs in a sleep dependent circadian pattern with highest levels being produced during non-REM sleep independent of breast stimulation (Gillam and Molitch 2011a; Dk et al. 1985). Lower pulse amplitude secretions occur during awake hours.

19.2.3 Prolactin Variants

Pituitary PRL is an anterior pituitary polypeptide hormone composed of 199 amino acids and produced by pituitary lactotroph cells (Gillam and Molitch 2011a). PRL is encoded by a single gene. However, a number of prolactin variants are known (Bernard et al. 2015). Many variants result from posttranslational changes associated with processes such as phosphorylation, glycosylation, sulfation, and deamidation causing structural changes to the PRL protein, impacting its end function or biological activity (Bernard et al. 2015). The majority of circulating pituitary prolactin is in the form of small or monomeric prolactin (molecular weight of 23 kDa) but both "big"(a covalently

bound dimer of prolactin with a molecular weight 48–56 kDa), and "big big" (molecular weights >100 kDa) forms of prolactin have been found in plasma and in the pituitary gland (Romijn 2014; Bernard et al. 2015; Freeman et al. 2000). These heteromers and PRL complexed with immunoglobulins may cause an accumulation of large prolactin moieties termed "macroprolactin." These are less biologically active forms of prolactin.

Other PRL variants such as 14 kDa, 16 kDa, and 22 kDa are the result of cleavage of the "small" 23 kDa protein which is thought to happen outside the cell. These variants subsequently act at PRL receptor sites to independently or synergistically regulate target tissue activities such as in the retina, myocardium, chondrocytes, and mammary gland in animal studies (Bernard et al. 2015). Some studies have shown that 16 kDa PRL isoform has potent antiangiogenic and antitumoral effects and several researchers have connected 16 kDa PRL with peripartum cardiomyopathy and impaired cardiac capillary function (Bernard et al. 2015; Horseman and Gregerson 2014; Hilfiker-Kleiner et al. 2006, 2012; Dalzell et al. 2011).

19.2.4 Prolactin Receptor Activity

The PRL molecule attaches to receptor sites not only in the mammary glands but in diverse tissues. This attachment recruits and binds to a second receptor which changes the membrane conformation and PRL is transported into the cell. Although some forms of PRL use different cell signaling pathways, monomeric 23 kDa PRL transmits instructions to the cell nucleus for gene transcription, (cell proliferation or inhibition) via what is known as Janis Kinase 2-Signal Transduction and Activator of Transcription 5 (JAK2-STAT5) signaling pathway (Fig. 19.3) (Ignacak et al. 2012; Gorvin 2015). Instructions for both cell and receptor site proliferation are required for mammary gland development and lactation. This requires the cooperative activities of estrogen, progesterone, and other growth factors (Romijn 2014; Gorvin 2015). In the same way, PRL also affects fertility by inhibiting gonadotropin secretion and downstream testosterone production in men and egg development,

Fig. 19.3 Signal transduction pathways of the prolactin receptor activation. Prolactin effects target tissue changes by attaching to cell membrane receptors which activates a JAK-2/ STAT cascade. This is transcribed in the cell nucleus to regulate gene expression. Ignacak A, Kasztelnik M, Sliwa T, Korbut RA, Rajda K, Guzik TJ. Prolactin - not only lactotrophin a "new" view of the "old" hormone. J Physiol Pharmacol. 2012 Oct;63(5):435–43. Fig. 2. p437. Reprinted with permission

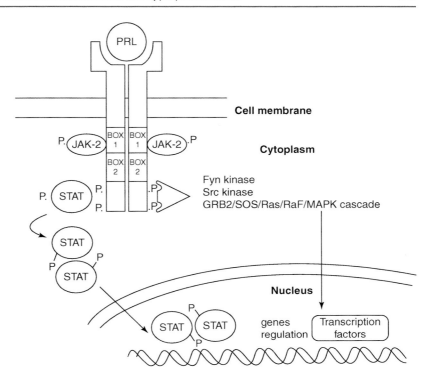

ovulation, and blastocyst implantation in women (Gorvin 2015). PRL receptor site isoforms or mutations in different tissues could potentially affect the downstream signaling and ultimately alter the function(s) of PRL (Ignacak et al. 2012). Increased expression of PRL receptors and/or alterations in the JAK2-STAT5 signaling pathway have been implicated in tumorigenesis or tumor progression and have generated particular research interest with respect to the development of breast cancer (Bernard et al. 2015; Gorvin 2015). There is also much interest in the association of tumor invasiveness with the interaction between PRL and estrogen receptors.

19.2.4.1 Prolactin Receptors Expression

PRL receptors have been found to be expressed in most tissues. In mouse models they are highly expressed in the pancreatic B cell, impacting glucose-mediated insulin secretion, particularly during pregnancy. It is hypothesized that this mechanism may be associated with gestational diabetes in humans, but current evidence is not convincing (Gorvin 2015). Increased adipose tissues and changes in fat storage distribution,

leptin and adiponectin levels have also been demonstrated in mice when PRL levels are increased during pregnancy (Gorvin 2015). Likewise, weight gain and insulin resistance have also been demonstrated in hyperprolactinemia in humans (Gillam and Molitch 2011a). PRL receptors expressed on leukocytes in the spleen and thymus suggest a role in the immune system function by enhancing T-cell activation and proliferation (Gorvin 2015). In humans, elevated prolactin levels have been found in patients with immune diseases such as lupus, rheumatoid arthritis, psoriasis, Sjogren's syndrome, uveitis, and multiple sclerosis, diseases that have been improved with therapy to lower PRL levels (Gillam and Molitch 2011a). Bone mass was also found to be decreased in hyperprolactinemic women that normalized with treatment to lower PRL levels but appears to be mediated primarily by the restoration of normal estrogen levels (Klibanski 2010). In mammals, prolactin has also been shown to reduce Na + and K+ renal excretion and adenosine triphosphatase activity, thereby affecting osmoregulation and, in particular, affecting human amniotic fluid transport (Ignacak et al. 2012).

19.3 Causes of Elevated Prolactin

Elevated prolactin (hyperprolactinemia) can be related to physiologic, pharmacologic, or pathologic causes including poor renal prolactin clearance. Hyperprolactinemia is idiopathic in up to 40% of cases (Romijn 2014; Ignacak et al. 2012; Majumdar and Mangal 2013). Normal physiologic causes are adaptive such as pregnancy and lactation (milk production). Other causes, particularly pathologic etiologies, effect biologic change and dysfunction (Grattan 2015) (Table 19.1).

19.3.1 Physiologic

Physiologic hyperprolactinemia is a response to pregnancy, nipple stimulation, exercise, and stress (Romijn 2014). The dominant physiologic role of prolactin in women is the development of the mammary glands in pregnancy and lactogenesis (milk production). Estrogen, progesterone, placental lactogen, insulin growth hormone, and cortisol also play a synergistic role (Gillam and Molitch

2011b). Recent studies have shown that the PRL level doubles from pre-pregnancy levels in the first trimester, during which time the size of the pituitary gland itself enlarges. PRL levels continue to climb to over 30 times above baseline with highest levels 24–48 h after delivery (vaginal or cesarean section) (Hu et al. 2017). Levels decrease again to normal in the first week postpartum in the absence of breastfeeding or are maintained throughout breastfeeding (Klibanski 2010; Cocks Eschler et al. 2018). An early study demonstrated that PRL levels in breastfeeding mothers during the first 6 weeks postpartum peak to 8.5 times baseline with suckling. After this time, and at least through to 28 week period of the study, prolactin levels normalized but increased to an average of 6 times baseline with suckling (Noel et al. 1974). Mothers who used a breast pump experienced similar elevated PRL levels after pumping.

Current evidence, from animal models, suggests that low maternal PRL levels at the end of pregnancy and high prolactin levels in the early postpartum period may negatively affect maternal nurturing behavior and may also be a factor in

Table 19.1 Etiology of hyperprolactinemia

Physiological	Pituitary	Other
Coitus	Acromegaly	Surgery
Exercise	Idiopathic	Trauma
Lactation	Lymphocytic hypophysitis or parasellar mass	Systemic disorders
Pregnancy	Macroadenoma (compressive)	Chest—neurogenic chest wall trauma, surgery, herpes
Sleep	Macroprolactinemia	Zoster
Stress	Plurihormonal adenoma	Chronic renal failure
Menses		
Pathological	Prolactinoma	Cirrhosis
Hypothalamic-pituitary stalk damage	Pituitary	Cranial radiation
Granulomas	Acromegaly	Epileptic seizures
Infiltrations	Idiopathic	Polycystic ovarian disease
Irradiation	Lymphocytic hypophysitis or parasellar mass	Surgery
Rathke's cyst	Macroadenoma (compressive)	Trauma
Trauma: pituitary stalk section, suprasellar surgery	Macroprolactinemia	Systemic disorders
Tumors: craniopharyngioma, germinoma, hypothalamic	Plurihormonal adenoma	Chest—neurogenic chest wall trauma, surgery, herpes
Metastases, meningioma	Suprasellar pituitary mass extension	Zoster
		Chronic renal failure

Ref: Melmed S, Kleinberg D 2008 Anterior pituitary. In: Kronenberg HM, Melmed S, Polonsky KS, Larsen PR eds. Williams textbook of endocrinology 11th ed. Philadelphia: Saunders Elsevier; 185–261

poor transgenerational nurturing behaviors in offspring (Sairenjia et al. 2017; Mitani et al. 2018). Higher levels during pregnancy not only support lactation but play a significant role in inhibiting pregnancy during breastfeeding by suppressing gonadotropin release and thereby, ovulation (Majumdar and Mangal 2013).

Vigorous exercise induced elevations of PRL have been reported to briefly increase prolactin levels, especially under the influence of serotonin in depressed subjects (E et al. 2004; Noel et al. 1972). Other studies reported increased core body temperature and not exercise per se significantly increases PRL levels (Chang et al. 1986).

Major stress such as surgery and severe illness has been shown to transiently increase prolactin levels up to an average of 2–5 times baseline. Smaller increases were found after minor procedures, such as during colonoscopy and venipuncture (Melmed et al. 2011; Gillam and Molitch 2011b; Noel et al. 1972). With prolonged stress, levels decrease.

19.3.2 Pharmacologic

Pharmacologic causes are numerous and must be considered, particularly when the patient presents with no classical clinical symptoms associated with hyperprolactinemia and other causes (pregnancy, renal failure, hypothyroidism, and macroprolactin) have been excluded. Close scrutiny of the patient's history and concomitant medications is recommended (Table 19.2). To confirm a pharmacologic etiology, if possible, the offending medication should be withdrawn for 3–4 days and PRL rechecked (Molitch 2005). Withdrawal of antipsychotic and anti-depressive therapies requires consultation with the patient's psychiatric provider. Treatment options include discontinuing or switching from the offending agent to another therapeutic option.

19.3.3 Pathologic

Pituitary adenomas producing excess prolactin are the main cause of pathologic hyperprolactinemia. This may be the result of PRL receptor and/or transcription mutations and alterations in

Table 19.2 Drugs that interfere with dopaminergic function

Class	Drug
Major Tranquillizers	Thiazides
	Butyrophenones
Antipsychotics	Phenothiazines
	Haloperidol
	Amisulpride
	Atypical
	Risperidone
	Molindone
Antidepressants	*Serotonin Reuptake Inhibitors* (SSRIs) (minimal)
	Tricyclics
	Amitriptyline
	Desipramine
	Clomipramine
	Monoamine oxidase inhibitors
	Pargyline
	Clorgyline
Antihypertensives	Verapamil
	Methyldopa
Dopamine receptor blockers	Reserpine
	Alcohol
	Cocaine
	Heroin
Prokinetics (GI motility)	Metoclopramide (Reglan)
	Domperidone
	Diabeticorum
Serotonin 5-HT3 receptor antagonists	*Proton Pump Inhibitors (PPIs)*
	Omeprazole
Estrogens	Oral contraceptives
Opiates	Morphine

Ref: Molitch, Molitch (2005); and Chahal and Schlechte (2008)

prolactin stimulating factors that inhibit dopamine tone (Glezer and Bronstein 2015). Systemic diseases such as liver failure, ACTH dependent Cushing's disease, and hypothyroidism can be contributory. Large sellar masses and inflammatory disorders that impinge on the pituitary stalk can interrupt dopaminergic inhibition of prolactin production causing serum PRL levels to rise (Klibanski 2010; Romijn 2014; Chahal and Schlechte 2008).

Poor renal clearance of prolactin causes elevated serum prolactin, particularly in chronic renal failure or related to the presence of large molecular weight prolactin. "Big" prolactin (a covalently bound dimer of prolactin with a molecular weight 48–56 kDa) and "big big" (molecular weights >100 kDa) forms of prolactin have been found both in plasma and in the pituitary gland (Romijn 2014; Bernard et al. 2015; Freeman et al. 2000). These macroprolactins are aggregate forms of prolactin or complexes of PRL and IgG that are less biologically active and usually do not cause clinical symptoms. However, they can confound clinical diagnosis (Klibanski 2010; Bernard et al. 2015; Freeman et al. 2000; Gillam and Molitch 2011b). Women with macroprolactinemia may present with menstrual irregularities. Therefore, measurement of the bioactive monomeric prolactin is recommended using subfractionation (polyethylene glycol (PEG) precipitation) to avoid unnecessary treatment (Romijn 2014; Bernard et al. 2015; Gillam and Molitch 2011b; Olukoga and Kane 1999). Approximately 10–20% of patients presenting with hyperprolactinemia are found to have macroprolactinemia (Chahal and Schlechte 2008; Olukoga and Kane 1999; Smith et al. 2007).

19.3.3.1 Prolactinoma
Prolactinomas are benign pituitary tumors producing excess prolactin, resulting in hyperprolactinemia. They represent up to 66% of all pituitary adenomas (Grossman and Besser 1985; Cocks Eschler et al. 2018). Prevalence is estimated at 400–500 cases per million, with higher prevalence in females of childbearing age between 20 and 50 years than in men 10:1 (Ciccarelli et al. 2008; Chanson and Maiter 2017). Postmenopausal prevalence is similar for females and males but males tend to have larger and more aggressive tumors (Cocks Eschler et al. 2018).

Prolactinomas are classified by size with microadenomas (mA) being <10 mm and Macroadenomas (MA) >10 mm. In women with prolactinoma, 60% are found to have mA (Glezer and Bronstein 2015). MA have an estimated prevalence of 100 per million but a ratio of 1:8–9 females to males (Chanson and Maiter 2017). Prolactin levels correlate with tumor size with higher levels associated with larger tumors. Cancerous or malignant PPAs are extremely rare and estimated to represent one-third of the 0.1–0.2% occurrence of all malignant pituitary

adenomas (Glezer and Bronstein 2015; Chanson and Maiter 2017).

The pathogenesis of prolactinomas is not fully understood, however, as in most pituitary adenomas, PPAs are monoclonal. It is hypothesized that PPAs develop as the result of a cascade of events that include genetic translational mutations, microRNA alterations, and/or epigenetic changes (Chanson and Maiter 2017). Aggressive PPAs may result from disinhibition of proliferation, lack of sensitivity to inhibitory signals, or lack of cell apoptosis (cell death) (Chanson and Maiter 2017).

Giant prolactinomas are defined as PPAs with the greatest diameter 40 mm or greater, with suprasellar extension and a baseline PRL level of more than 100 ng/L (Chanson and Maiter 2017). These tumors are more prevalent in adolescent boys and middle aged males.

19.3.3.1.1 Signs and Symptoms of Prolactinoma
Most commonly, patients present with symptoms of hypogonadism secondary to the suppression of pulsatile GnRH and subsequent low expression of pituitary gonadotrophs (LH/FSH), testosterone and decreased ovulation (Majumdar and Mangal 2013). Therefore, women present more frequently with oligomenorrhea, amenorrhea, and infertility. Males often present with erectile dysfunction. Both genders present with poor libido, although elevated prolactin may go undiagnosed in males much longer than females. After the age of 50, hypogonadism is often attributed to age and therefore this may further delay the correct diagnosis (Klibanski 2010; Chanson and Maiter 2017). Galactorrhea is more common in women, is not independently diagnostic of a prolactinoma and may not even be present, as estrogen and progesterone are required to prime lactation (Glezer and Bronstein 2015). Conversely, isolated galactorrhea may occur in the context of normal PRL if increased breast sensitivity to lactotrophic stimulation is present, increasing the clinical challenge in diagnosis (Chanson and Maiter 2017). As a result of prolonged hyperprolactinemia resulting in amenorrhea and chronic estrogen suppression, osteopenia and osteoporosis may develop

(Klibanski 2010). Decreased bone mass and anemia also occur in males secondary to low testosterone (Klibanski 2010). Headache is a common presenting symptom regardless of the size of tumor but is more common in men with larger tumors, as are visual changes and visual field deficits (Klibanski 2010).

Approximately 10–15% of patients with macroadenomas present with quadratic visual field deficits due to compression of the optic chiasm. Ophthalmoplegia (eye muscle paralysis) with the involvement of cranial nerves III, IV, and VI is present in approximately 10% of MA with cavernous sinus invasion (Chanson and Maiter 2017). Headaches, in clusters, are common in these patients, particularly when the tumor extends into the cavernous sinuses (Chanson and Maiter 2017).

19.3.3.1.2 Diagnosis

In the presence of symptoms, a serum prolactin level greater than 100 μg/L is suggestive of prolactinoma, and levels >250 μg/L and in particular >500 μg/L are indicative of a MA (Melmed et al. 2011; Gillam and Molitch 2011b). Levels <40 μg/L may be elevated by medications, chest stimulation, or stress. However, medication associated elevations can be as high as 200 μg/L. Impact of a tumor or disruption to the pituitary stalk can likewise present with high PRL, but usually <100 μg/L (Melmed et al. 2011). This is known as stalk effect.

Hyperprolactinemia in the context of associated symptoms warrants a gadolinium enhanced brain magnetic resonance imaging (MRI) to evaluate the presence, size, and location of a pituitary tumor, and to provide confirmation of a diagnosis of prolactinoma. If the tumor on MRI is shown to be compressing the optic chiasm, then formal visual field testing should be done. Surgical pathology is rarely needed (Cocks Eschler et al. 2018).

19.3.3.1.3 Measurement of Prolactin: Laboratory Assay

A venous blood sample is drawn to assess prolactin levels. Although dynamic tests have been employed in the past using provocative agents such as thyrotropin releasing hormone (TRH), chlorpromazine, levodopa domperidone and insulin induced hypoglycemia, these tests are now largely abandoned due to lack of specificity, expense, and effort (Chahal and Schlechte 2008). However, a repeat level is indicated to confirm PRL results in the event of a minimal increase (Gillam and Molitch 2011b).

Serum PRL has been shown to rise rapidly, although minimally in some subjects after breast stimulation or manipulation. Avoidance of these activities prior to drawing a PRL level is recommended. Vigorous exercise, high stress prior to a blood draw and/or the stress of venipuncture may also minimally increase levels (Melmed et al. 2011). Evaluation of renal and thyroid function and the possibility of pregnancy in sexually active females of child bearing age may need to be concurrently evaluated (Klibanski 2010).

Timing of blood draws may have an impact on PRL levels. Serum PRL level varies during the day, with highest pulsatile production occurring during sleep (Dk et al. 1985). Nadir levels occur around midday or 3–4 h after waking (Spiegel et al. 1994). To avoid medication effects, withdraw known confounding medications at least 3–4 days or more prior to the blood draw. Fasting is not required. However, there is some data that indicates higher PRL levels immediately after eating and with increased body temperature after vigorous exercise (Christensen et al. 1985). An early study found that normal levels for females were significantly higher than for males 1–25 ng/ml vs 1–20 ng/ml, respectively (Kleinberg et al. 1977).

Assay methodologies, reference ranges, and reporting units vary between laboratories and may impact comparison or trending of results (Farzami and Aliasgharpour 2017). A sandwich type 2 site immunoradiometric (IRMA) or chemiluminometric assay is preferred in clinical laboratories secondary to higher sensitivity. It is referenced to the fourth IS (2016 International Standard) 83/573 set by WHO (Medicines and Healthcare Regulatory Agency 2016). In this test, the PRL molecules become sandwiched between antibody layers, unbound PRL is washed off, and the level read. However, in some patients with very high PRL levels due to very large tumors

(>3 cm), the PRL (antigen) binding to the anti-body is overwhelmed and only the remaining unbound prolactin is measured, resulting in a falsely low PRL measurement (Gillam and Molitch 2011b; Comtois et al. 1993). This is known as the "Hook Effect." A diluted prolactin assay is recommended to avoid false negative results associated with the effect reported using international standardization (IS) units-μg/L (Jeffcoate et al. 1986).

To test for macroprolactin, a polyethylene gly-col precipitation method (PEG) or the gold stan-dard method of gel filtration chromatography is used (Farzami and Aliasgharpour 2017).The lat-ter is reportedly slow, costly, and labor intensive. Using PEG precipitation, monomeric 23 kDa PRL is separated from immunoglobulins that form "big" and "big big" forms of PRL to allow accurate evaluation of prolactin levels for clinical interpretation.

19.3.3.1.4 Treatment

Treatment is indicated for hyperprolactinemia in the presence of symptoms, and when MRI indi-cates a pituitary MA or an enlarging tumor (Klibanski 2010) (Table 19.3).

The Endocrine Society guidelines (2011) recommend that patients with Ma, no symp-toms, and minimal PRL elevations be monitored with 1–2 yearly interval PRL levels and MRI,

Table 19.3 Indications for medical/surgical treatment

Surgical therapy	Medical therapy
Mass effects	*Effects of hyperprolactinemia*
Hypopituitarism	Hypogonadism
Visual field defects due to pressure on the optic chiasm	Amenorrhea or oligomenorrhea
Cranial nerve deficits	Infertility
Headaches	Impotence
Other	Osteoporosis or osteopenia
Tumor growth	*Relative indications*:
Resistance to treatment	Bothersome galactorrhea
Risk of cardiac valvulopathy	Bothersome hirsutism
Expense of lifelong treatment	Headaches

Ref: Gillam and Molitch (2011b); and Klibanski (2010)

given current evidence of low risk of tumor growth (Melmed et al. 2011; Klibanski 2010). The optimal monitoring interval is unknown. However, treatment of amenorrhea with birth control (oral contraceptives) is recommended. Spontaneous resolution of hyperprolactinemia may occur in postmenopausal women and has been reported in up to 30% of women after DA induced pregnancy (Klibanski 2010; Crosignani et al. 1981).

In medication induced hyperprolactinemia, particularly when asymptomatic, no treatment is recommended (Melmed et al. 2011). Withdrawal of the offending medication is preferred but an alternate medication may be appropriate. However, treatment for hypogonadal symptoms or low bone mass with estrogen or testosterone therapy may be indicated (Melmed et al. 2011). Likewise, no treatment is indicated in the case of patients with PRL elevations determined to be related to macroprolactins.

Treatment is indicated in the presence of symptoms when other causes have been excluded. The goals of treatment are: normalization of PRL, tumor shrinkage and the relief of symptoms such as headache, visual disturbances, restoration of fertility and hypopituitarism (Romijn 2014; Glezer and Bronstein 2015).

Dopamine agonists are the first line of treat-ment for prolactinomas. By binding to (Gillam and Molitch 2011a) dopamine receptors sites, DA inhibits the production of PRL from both normal lactotrophs and tumor cells (Romijn 2014). A number of DAs are available including bromocrip-tine (Parlodel®), lisuride (Dopergine®), quina-golide (Norprolac®), cabergoline (Dostinex®), and pergolide (Permex®) (Chanson et al. 2007a). These are both ergot and non-ergot preparations with ergot drugs being more vasoactive. Pergolide (an ergot) is now considered a second line drug because of its particularly high tendency towards valvular heart disease and quinagolide (a non-ergot) is not available in the USA but is available in Europe (Gillam and Molitch 2011b).

Overall DAs have demonstrated efficacy in meeting all treatment goals. In long-term, largely uncontrolled observational studies, a mean of 68% (20–100%) of patients receiving DA (bromocriptine, cabergoline or quinagolide) normalized PRL and tumor size reduction was achieved in a mean of 62% (20–100%) of cases (Melmed et al. 2011). The majority of patients treated with medical therapy had significant improvement or resolution in: visual field deficiencies 67% (33–100%), amenorrhea 78% (40–100%), infertility 53% (10–100%), sexual dysfunction 67% (6–100%), galactorrhea 86% (33–100%) (Melmed et al. 2011). Interestingly, if PRL remains somewhat elevated after significant improvement, resolution of symptoms, and tumor shrinkage, there is currently no evidence of harm (Klibanski 2010).

DAs differ in their respective dosing profiles, efficacy, and side effects. Bromocriptine has a short elimination half-life of 3.3 h and duration of action of 12–14 h requiring more frequent dosing from 1 to 3 times a day (2.5–15 mg daily) (Romijn 2014). Cabergoline has a longer half-life up to 65 h and duration of action of 7–14 days, allowing a longer dosing interval of 1–2 times weekly, whereas quinagolide with a 22 h half-life and duration of action of 24 h is dosed daily (Barlier and Jaquet 2006). The conventional dose of cabergoline is up to 2 mg/week (Molitch 2017). Drug resistance and intolerance occurs in 10–35% of cases and with higher frequency for those taking bromocriptine (Romijn 2014; Kars et al. 2009). Likewise, cabergoline, which is a more specific D2 receptor agonist, effectively shrinks up to 90% of tumors, compared with 50% in those treated with bromocriptine (Melmed et al. 2011; Romijn 2014; Glezer and Bronstein 2015).

Although side effects of DA are similar for all medications, there are some striking differences. Most common side effects are nausea, vomiting, postural hypotension and dizziness with rare nasal congestion, cramps, psychiatric disorders, and cerebrospinal fluid leaks (Glezer and Bronstein 2015). Cabergoline and quinagolide have been shown to have fewer side effects than bromocriptine (Klibanski 2010; Barlier and Jaquet 2006). Cabergoline and pergolide have been associated with a possible risk of cardiac valvulopathy associated with high doses and long duration of therapy. As ergot alkaloids, these DA may stimulate the serotonin $5HT_{2B}$ receptor activity in cardiac valves, resulting in fibromyoblast proliferation and valvular thickening (Klibanski 2010). Only one study, to date, has shown increased, dose dependent risk of tricuspid regurgitation while several studies have shown no association (Klibanski 2010; Glezer and Bronstein 2015). However, regular monitoring of echocardiogram in patients requiring higher doses of cabergoline is recommended (Molitch 2017).

DA have also been associated with impulse control disorder (ICD) associated with a high affinity for D3 receptors. A dose dependent, anti-anhedonic potency leads to disinhibition of impulse control (Noronha et al. 2016). This includes repetitive and compulsive activities such as shopping, gambling, eating and hypersexuality. A warning to this effect is advised to both patients and families when starting treatment with DA.

Surgical treatment is usually reserved for patients presenting with macroadenomas that continue to grow while on DA and those with, resistance and intolerance to DA (see Chap. 12). Some authors recommend considering surgical intervention to treat severe, unremitting symptoms, when there is a need to "debulk" tumors to improve response to DA, in order to avoid long-term or lifetime treatment with DA or when there is a high risk of cardiac valvular damage or other severe side effects. Radiotherapy is required in <5% of cases for tumor control (Molitch 2017) (see Chap. 13). A single site cost analysis in the USA revealed a significant age based cost and quality-adjusted life years (QALYs) advantage for surgical treatment over long-term medical therapy, but further confirmation of life quality is warranted (Zygourakis et al. 2017).

The duration of therapy continues to be a matter of debate. The current Endocrine Society guidelines (2011) recommend a slow withdrawal of medication while monitoring PRL levels. The most appropriate candidates should have a 2 year history of normal PRL levels and no visible tumor on MRI prior to withdrawal (Melmed et al. 2011). Current studies indicate that approximately 21% of patients have sustained normal PRL after treatment withdrawal (Klibanski 2010).

19.3.3.1.5 Prolactinoma and Pregnancy

Elevated prolactin levels inhibit GnRH release which decreases pituitary LH pulsatility amplitude and subsequently decreases estradiol levels necessary for ovulation resulting in menstrual irregularities and infertility (Cocks Eschler et al. 2018).

Treatment with dopamine agonist (DA) not only aims to reverse hyperprolactinemia and hypogonadism but to restore fertility. Although both cabergoline and bromocriptine can be used when fertility is desired, bromocriptine is the DA of choice. Neither either have been shown to affect fetal development or spontaneous abortions (Melmed et al. 2011; Molitch 2017; Colao et al. 2008). However, quinagolide has been associated with fetal risk and is not recommended in women desiring pregnancy. Regardless, it is recommended that DA be withdrawn as soon as pregnancy is confirmed (Melmed et al. 2011; Molitch 2017; Chanson and Maiter 2017). Successful pregnancy is reported in 75–90% of women treated with DA (Cocks Eschler et al. 2018).

The increased estrogen levels stimulate lactotrophs proliferation and increasing PRL levels during pregnancy and, along with cessation of the DA, there is a risk of tumor growth. In pregnancy there is a physiologic increase in the size of the pituitary gland of up to 136%, reaching maximum size immediately after delivery (Bronstein 2005). In patients with mA, tumor growth is usually minimal (and estimated at 2–3% of cases) and reports up to, and above, 21% for patients with MA (Molitch 2017; Cocks Eschler et al. 2018; Bronstein 2005). Taken together, there is an increased risk to the optic apparatus with a higher risk in patients with MA.

Monitoring during pregnancy is paramount. In the presence of a MA, formal visual field monitoring every 1–3 months is indicated (Klibanski 2010; Bronstein 2005). Measurement of PRL level during pregnancy is not recommended (Melmed et al. 2011). Both imaging and treatment with DA can be resumed during pregnancy only in the presence of signs and symptoms of tumor growth and/or if optic apparatus compression becomes apparent (Glezer and Bronstein 2015; Bronstein 2005). Bromocriptine is frequently recommended over cabergoline during pregnancy, as

there is recorded use in over 6000 pregnancies vs 900 women using cabergoline, but both are considered safe (Melmed et al. 2011; Cocks Eschler et al. 2018). Emergent transsphenoidal surgery may be indicated during pregnancy in the case of apoplexy, failed DA therapy or significant visual loss and delivery may be considered if the pregnancy is sufficiently advanced (Glezer and Bronstein 2015; Bronstein 2005).

Re-evaluation for changes in tumor volume and prolactin level is undertaken as soon as is practical postpartum. Although tumor volume may increase during pregnancy, both tumor volume decrease and remission of hyperprolactinemia have been reported in over 10% of patients who normalized PRL level, menses, and ovulation after pregnancy (Cocks Eschler et al. 2018; Glezer and Bronstein 2015). For women with Ma, the basal PRL secretion is reported to be reduced following pregnancy and lactation which may contribute to the resolution of hyperprolactinemia for these women (Bridges 2018).

PRL is high immediately after delivery and slowly returns to normal the week after delivery in non-breastfeeding mothers. Basal levels decrease by about 4–6 weeks postpartum but will sharply increase for short periods with suckling during breastfeeding (Gillam and Molitch 2011b; Bronstein 2005). Intense and frequent suckling inhibits ovulation and menses and has been used as a means of birth control in some settings (Gillam and Molitch 2011b). In the presence of a prolactinoma, levels may remain elevated but there is no evidence of tumor growth during breastfeeding in mothers with either a mA or MA (Bronstein 2005).

Mood shifts postpartum have been associated with changes in PRL levels. High PRL levels have been associated with increased anxiety during gestation and may also be related to postpartum mood changes and depressive-like behaviors (Bridges 2018). Higher PRL has also been implicated in the development of maternal nurturing behaviors (Grattan 2015).

19.3.3.1.6 Prolactin in Males

The actions of prolactin in males remain unclear. Males with prolactinomas usually present after a number of years of impotence and decreased libido but may also have normal testosterone levels (Ciccarelli et al. 2008). However, infertility is common, as in females, secondary to the suppression of GnRH secretion and decreased pituitary LH/FSH pulsatile secretion and subsequent testosterone production. Gynecomastia and galactorrhea are not common in men (10–20%) and it has been suggested that after long-term hypogonadism, aromatization of testosterone to estrogen and associated mammary gland hyperplasia is no longer apparent (Chanson and Maiter 2017). Additionally, breast stimulation in males does not result in lactation (Grattan 2015). Osteoporosis/osteopenia, anxiety, and depression may be present (Ignacak et al. 2012). Some studies have also reported an association between an increase in PRL level and parental behaviors in men but this remains controversial (Grattan 2015). An association between prostate hypertrophy and hyperprolactinemia has also been found that normalizes after treatment with DA (Ciccarelli et al. 2008).

Headaches and visual changes may be presenting symptoms in men with MA (Ignacak et al. 2012) Males with prolactinomas are on average 10 years older than females. It is unclear if delayed diagnosis accounts for the higher prevalence of MA in men or whether they have, for unknown reasons, more aggressive forms of tumors (giant invasive and malignant). In tumor histopathology, higher cell proliferative indexes (Ki-67, Proliferating Cell Nuclear Antigen) have been found in men (Ciccarelli et al. 2008; Chanson and Maiter 2017). However, some studies have found no gender or difference with respect to response to DA in mA or MA or in dose required for PRL normalization or tumor shrinkage (Ciccarelli et al. 2008; Colao et al. 2003).

Treatment with DA remains first line treatment for males with prolactinomas. Surgery is usually reserved for indications of tumor growth while on DA, DA resistance, apoplexy, acute visual field changes, or when there is a need for histopathology. Although transsphenoidal approach is most common, craniotomy is performed when the lesion is not accessible using the former approach (Chanson and Maiter 2017).

Hypogonadism will usually resolve with the normalization of PRL level (Melmed et al. 2011). Due to PRL action on male germ cells, sperm counts and motility may be low for up to 2 years after PRL normalizes. In up to 20% of patients, sperm counts remain low (Chanson and Maiter 2017). Additionally, in a large UK based retrospective open-cohort study, men with prolactinomas were found to have significantly increased cardiovascular risk compared to a non-affected population, whereas there was no increased risk found for age similar females (Toulis et al. 2018).

19.3.3.1.7 Prolactinoma in Childhood

Prolactinomas are rare in childhood and more likely to occur in adolescence at the beginning of puberty (Hoffmann et al. 2018). Prolactinomas represent about 50% of all pediatric pituitary adenomas but only about 2% of all pediatric intracranial tumors (Hoffmann et al. 2018). Some studies report the prevalence of macroadenomas in children is almost twice that of adults (37.5 vs 19.4%) (Cocks Eschler et al. 2018). Apoplexy in adolescents (14–23 years) with macroprolactinomas may be occur with a similar frequency in adults (approximately 17% vs 20%) (Jankowski et al. 2015; Sarwar et al. 2013).

The clinical presentation and symptoms in children may vary with age, tumor size, and prolactin level (Cocks Eschler et al. 2018). The majority of pediatric prolactinomas (75%) occur in girls who typically present with primary amenorrhea or menstrual disorders (up to 96%), galactorrhea, and headaches associated with mA (Hoffmann et al. 2018; Cocks Eschler et al. 2018; Chanson and Maiter 2017; Catli et al. 2012). Pubertal development may otherwise remain normal in girls, likely related to the higher prevalence of microadenomas (Cocks Eschler et al. 2018). Boys present at an earlier age with headaches, visual changes, delayed pubertal development (50%), and growth retardation (20–25%) with more invasive and aggressive macroadenomas (Hoffmann et al. 2018; Chanson and Maiter 2017; Catli et al. 2013). Other than hypogonadism, panhypopituitarism, thyroid or corticotroph deficiency remains rare in children (Salenave et al. 2015). However, two studies reported that one-third to one half of patients were obese at diagnosis (Salenave et al. 2015; Catli et al. 2012). In newborns of mothers with high prolactin, the infants PRL will often be markedly elevated until about 3 months of age when it normalizes (Chahal and Schlechte 2008).

Few patients are diagnosed before puberty with several recent studies reporting a mean age at presentation of 14–16.5 years (Salenave et al. 2015; Catli et al. 2012). Basal prolactin levels were significantly higher in boys than girls, likely related to larger tumor size in boys (Salenave et al. 2015; Hoffmann et al. 2018; Catli et al. 2012).

Most prolactinomas in children are thought to result from sporadic genetic mutations. AIP gene mutations are reportedly more frequent in children than adults with prolactinomas, particularly with GH-PRL secreting macroadenomas (Salenave et al. 2015). The possibility of MEN-1 also needs to be evaluated in apparently sporadic pituitary adenomas in children. Salvenave et al. (in a large pediatric cohort, found that patients with DA-resistant tumours were younger, had higher baseline PRL and were more likely to have MEN-1 mutations (Salenave et al. 2015). From the Dutch MEN-1 study of 325 patients >16 years, tumor control was achieved in those with prolactinomas (n = 52) using dopamine agonists (de Laat et al. 2015).

Testing and treatment options are the same for pediatric as in adult patients. Medical therapy with dopamine agonist therapy will normalize PRL levels in approximately 75% of cases (Salenave et al. 2015; Hoffmann et al. 2018; Catli et al. 2012). Few patients require surgical transsphenoidal tumor debulking, usually secondary to visual disorders or loss, DA intolerance or nonadherence. Surgical intervention in order to avoid long-term or lifelong treatment with DAs remains in debate (Chanson and Maiter 2017; Chanson et al. 2007b). However, this may be a cost-effective option given the anticipated length of treatment but the immediate potential operative complications must always be considered (Zygourakis et al. 2017). There are few longitudinal prospective studies regarding the risk of cardiac valvulopathies after long-term treatment with cabergoline from childhood. Avoidance of this risk may be another consideration for surgical intervention in patients requiring large doses of cabergoline. Radiation therapy remains an option in recurrent and aggressive tumors that are unremitted by other therapies, but is limited by concern for hypopituitarism, possibly neurological damage and infertility (Cocks Eschler et al. 2018).

19.4   Tumor Recurrence

Postoperative tumor recurrence in early reports was higher in patients with macroadenoma but some author question the source as new versus "old" or residual tumor (Rodman et al. 1984). Chanson and Maiter highlight the subjective nature of reported data that skews recurrence rates (Spiegel et al. 1994). Some data supports estimates that approximately 75–80% of patients with a history of macroadenoma will require resumption of therapy (Klibanski 2010). Kim et al. (2017) reported a higher frequency of recurrence in males in a median of 8.9±6.6 year follow-up and others have found a higher recurrence with a baseline PRL >200 ng/L (Chanson and Maiter 2017; Kim et al. 2017). Recurrence rates for patients with microadenomas ranges from 10 to 15% postoperatively (Chanson and Maiter 2017). Few patients require radiation treatment for tumor control after failing to respond to DA.

19.5   Quality of Life (QoL)

Few studies of QoL in patients with hyperprolactinemia or prolactinomas were found in a review of the literature. Children treated with DA were found to have no difference in survival or functional capacity compared with long-term survivors of different sellar masses (Hoffmann et al. 2018). Premenopausal women with DA-treated macroprolactinomas had lower physical functioning, physical role and pain scores compared to age matched controls using SF-36 questionnaire (Kim et al. 2017). In other small studies, social functioning and mental health, vitality, role emotion, and mental summary scores were found to be lower in patients with prolactinoma even after normalization of PRL levels when compared to unaffected controls (Kim et al. 2017; Johnson et al. 2003). Patient scores were not differentiated by tumor size in these studies. There remains no substantial evidence that QoL is changed or improved by treatment or normalization of PRL.

19.6   Nursing Care Summary

19.6.1   Assessment

Assessment at presentation requires the collection of detailed and often sensitive information. Data collected in referral information and patient completed questionnaires requires verification. Patients require assurance of privacy before being comfortable divulging personal information, particularly regarding hypogonadism and sexual activity. The comfort level of the interviewer will often frame the patient's response. In many countries, personal medical information is protected by law unless it is medically necessary to be shared with other medical professionals.

Full disclosure regarding psychiatric history, all medications (including those purchased "over the counter"), other drug use including illicit drugs used by the patient is vital. Direct inquiry may be necessary by the health care provider regarding more sensitive drug use such as alcohol volumes, marihuana, cocaine, and morphine that may decrease or increase PRL levels (Ranganthan et al. 2009; Torre and Falorni 2007). Again, reassurance of confidentiality and information security is needed in order to obtain accurate information for the provision of appropriate care.

Anecdotally, by the time the patient consults in endocrinology, they have many unanswered questions. Initial assessment includes the patients understanding of the reason for the referral and their expectations regarding ongoing evaluation and treatment. Many have little knowledge of the pituitary and its function and may have been told they have a "brain tumor." Connotations of malignancy serve to increase the anxiety of patient and family. Information regarding the benign nature of prolactinomas in 99.8–99.9% of cases is helpful.

Health and illness beliefs and practices vary according to cultures and may need to be made explicit in order for the patient to fully understand the etiology of any pathology and their role in self-care. Identify the key symptoms that the patient wishes to address and clarify these based on known data to support and frame realistic expectations. As with headaches, complete resolution may not be achievable but jointly establish symptom remission goals that would be acceptable and improve his/her quality of life. Coordination and consultation with other services is often necessary.

19.6.2   Diagnosis

Diagnostic testing may be limited to a simple blood draw or may be more extensive and is based on the patient's symptoms. In asymptomatic patients, a macroprolactin level may need to be assessed to determine bioactive PRL levels. If the patient has symptoms and prior PRL levels have been normal, ensuring that a diluted assay has been done may change the course of further evaluation and treatment.

Patient instructions for blood draws should ensure that all medications and drugs that may affect the PRL level have been withdrawn for at least 3–4 days. The patient may need to hold estrogen-based birth control and use other forms of birth control during evaluation. Avoidance of breast stimulation and vigorous exercise before the draw is recommended (Chang et al. 1986). Although midday is usually nadir PRL level, there is no clear recommendations for a specific time of day for samples to be obtained. Nadir levels may vary for shift workers. Repeat samples may be needed prior to a final diagnosis. A pregnancy test may need to be performed simultaneously in woman of child bearing age in order to ensure that an elevated level is not related to an unanticipated pregnancy.

MRI is recommended in symptomatic patients with elevated diluted PRL levels. If the patient is anxious regarding this procedure, pre-treatment with an anxiolytic may be indicated. In the USA, a prior authorization from the patients insurance is usually required prior to the procedure. Interpretation by an experienced neuroradiologist may be needed to evaluate small mA. Patients with MA that impact the optic apparatus require further evaluation with a formal ophthalmologic exam to identify visual changes and deficits. Both the MRI and ophthalmologic exam will serve as baseline evaluations for comparison after treatment.

Further evaluation of pituitary functions may be needed such as evaluation of cortisol, ACTH levels, thyroid function (TSH/FT4), LH, FSH, testosterone (males) and in addition, renal function. Bone density scanning is recommended to evaluate bone density in patients with prolonged hypogonadism. Males may need further assessment for CVD.

19.6.3 Implementation

With a diagnosis of prolactinoma a detailed patient education is warranted. The goal of patient education is to promote self-care and improve treatment adherence. Visual aids such as the patient's own MRI images are powerful messages and can frame the patient's understanding of the disease. The use of media such as vetted online and YouTube videos and resources such as www.pituitarysociety.org /patient education, the European Society of Endocrinology https://www.ese-hormones.org/for-patients/ and Hormone Health https://www.hormone.org/ that can be readily accessed on mobile devices are valuable educational tools. These resources can be used in an office setting and continue to provide a reference for patients after an introductory discussion. It is important to remember that, under stress, information retention is limited and repetition of material with subsequent visits is essential.

Treatment planning requires patient involvement in decision making. A clear understanding of the risk, benefits, and side effects of each option includes a discussion of the implications for each individual patient. Patient treatment tolerance and adherence may begin with a discussion of coping strategies and practices to minimize the effects of the most common side effects. High risk side effects such as DA behav-

ioral changes and impulse control disorders must be clearly described to the patient and relatives along with a discussion of an effective management plan should these occur. For treatment planning and management of patient pre and post-surgery, see Chap. 23.

Emergency guidelines should be provided in written form and reinforced with each visit. Communicate key events that represent a need for immediate medical intervention and a plan to seek emergency care. These events should include: sudden severe onset of headache, peripheral vision loss, clear nasal drainage usually along with severe headache (cerebrospinal fluid (CSF) leak), and acute psychotic behaviour changes and severe depression with suicidal ideation.

Pregnancy may or may not be a desired outcome but is a risk in sexually active child bearing age women once treatment with DA is initiated and PRL is normalized. If pregnancy is not desired, then a form of birth control should be started concomitantly with DA, particularly when using cabergoline, which can normalize PRL levels quickly. At the confirmation of pregnancy, the DA is withdrawn and the patient is monitored every trimester for compressive symptoms and visual field exams are recommended for patients with MA.

19.6.4 Evaluation

Follow-up may occur in various settings from a general practitioner office to specialty endocrine or pituitary centers or with endocrine consultants and advance practice providers. This may depend on accessibility and convenience for the patient, the complexity of the patient's care needs, and/or the comfort level of the provider. However, the key components of follow-up evaluations include: side effects review, particularly the identification of critical side effects; medication review including usage, dosing interval and timing, consistency and continuity of use; desire for or restoration of fertility; symptom changes or improvement; biochemical assessment; and interval review of MRI (every 6–12 months until stable then every 2 years) (Klibanski 2010). All reviews may require adjustment to a management plan.

Acknowledgement The author acknowledges Mark Molitch MD who is the Professor of Medicine (Endocrinology), Feinberg School of Medicine, Northwestern Memorial Hospital, Chicago, IL USA.

References

Barlier A, Jaquet P. Quinagolide – a valuable treatment option for hyperprolactinaemia. Eur J Endocrinol. 2006;154:187–95.

Bernard V, Young J, Chanson P, Binart N. New insights in prolactin: pathological implications. Nat Rev Endocrinol. 2015;11(5):265–75. https://doi.org/10.1038/nrendo.2015.36. Epub 2015 Mar 17. Review. PMID:25781857

Bridges, RS. Prolactin: Regulation and actions. Neuroscience 2018. Online Jan 2018. https://doi.org/10.1093/acrefore/9780190264086.013.61.

Bronstein MD. Prolactinomas and pregnancy. Pituitary. 2005;8:31–8. https://doi.org/10.1007/s11102-005-5083-4.

Catli G, Abaci A, Altincik A, Demir K, Can S, Buyukgebiz A, Bober E. Hyperprolactinemia in children: clinical features and long-term results. J Pediatr Endocrinol Metab. 2012;25(11–12):1123–8.

Catli G, Abaci A, Bober E, Büyükgebiz A. Clinical and diagnostic characteristics of hyperprolactinemia in childhood and adolescence. J Pediatr Endocrinol Metab. 2013;26(1–2):1–11. https://doi.org/10.1515/jpem-2012-0327.

Chahal J, Schlechte J. Hyperprolactinemia. Pituitary. 2008;11:141. https://doi.org/10.1007/s11102-008-0107-5.

Chang FE, Dodds WG, Sullivan M, Kim MH, Malarkey WB. The acute effects of exercise on prolactin and growth hormone secretion: comparison between sedentary women and women runners with normal and abnormal menstrual cycles. J Clin Endocrinol Metab. 1986 Mar;62(3):551–6.

Chanson P, Maiter D. Prolactinoma. In: Melmed S, editor. The pituitary. 4th ed. London: Elsevier; 2017. p. 467–514.

Chanson P, Borson-Chazot F, Chabre O, Estour B. Drug treatment of hyperprolactinemia. Ann Endocrinol (Paris). 2007;68(2–3):113–7. Epub 2007 May 29. Review

Chanson P, Borson-Chazot F, Chabre O, Estour B. Drug treatment of hyperprolactinemia. Ann Endocrinol. 2007;68(2–3):e30–4.

Christensen SE, Jørgensen O, Møller J, Møller N, Orskov H. Body temperature elevation, exercise and serum prolactin concentrations. Acta Endocrinol. 1985;109(4):458–62.

Ciccarelli A, Guerra E, De Rosa M, Milone F, Zarrilli S, Lombardi G. PRL secreting adenomas in male patients. Pituitary. 2008;8:29–32.

Cocks Eschler D, Javanmard P, Cox K, Geer EB. Prolactinoma through the female life cycle. Endocrine. 2018;59:16.

Colao A, Di Sarno A, Cappabianca P, et al. Gender differences in the prevalence, clinical features and response to cabergoline in hyperprolactinemia. Eur J Endocrinol. 2003;148(3):325–31.

Colao A, Abs R, Bárcena DG, Chanson P, Paulus W, Kleinberg DL. Pregnancy outcomes following cabergoline treatment: extended results from a 12-year observational study. Clin Endocrinol. 2008;68:66–71.

Comtois R, Robert F, Hardy J. Immunoradiometric assays may miss high prolactin levels. Ann Intern Med. 1993;119:173.

Crosignani PG, Ferrari C, Scarduelli MC, Picciotti R, Malinverni AC. Spontaneous and induced pregnancies in hyperprolactinemic women. Obstet Gynecol. 1981;58(6):708–13.

Dalzell JR, Jackson E, Gardner RS. An update on peripartum cardiomyopathy. Exp Rev Cariovasc Ther. 2011;9:1155–60. https://doi.org/10.1586/erc.11.121.

de Laat JM, Dekkers OM, Pieterman CR, Kluijfhout WP, Hermus AR, Pereira AM, van der Horst-Schrivers AN, Drent ML, Bisschop PH, Havekes B, de Herder WW, Valk GD. Long-term natural course of pituitary tumors in patients with MEN1: results from the DutchMEN1 Study Group (DMSG). J Clin Endocrinol Metab. 2015;100(9):3288–96. https://doi.org/10.1210/JC.2015-2015. Epub 2015 Jun 30

Farzami MR, Aliasgharpour M. Chemiluminescence systems; do all lead to same results in prolactin analysis? J Diabetes Metab Disord. 2017;16:24. https://doi.org/10.1186/s40200-017-0305-7. Published online 2017 June 5. PMCID: PMC5460514

Freeman ME, Kanyicska B, Lerant A, Nagy G. Prolactin: structure, function, and regulation of secretion. Physiol Rev. 2000;80(4):1523–631.

Gillam M, Molitch M. Prolactin. In: Melmed S, editor. The pituitary. 3rd ed. London: Elsevier; 2011a. p. 119–66. https://doi.org/10.1016/B978-0-12-380926-1.10015-X.

Gillam M, Molitch M. Prolactinoma. In: Melmed S, editor. The pituitary. 3rd ed. London: Elsevier; 2011b. p. 475–531. https://doi.org/10.1016/B978-0-12-380926-1.10015-X.

Glezer A, Bronstein MD. Prolactinoma. Endocrinol Metab Clin N Am. 2015;44:71–8.

Gorvin CM. The prolactin receptor: diverse and emerging roles in pathophysiology. J Clin Translational Endocrinol. 2015;2:85e91.

Grattan D. The hypothalamo-prolactin axis. J Endocrinol. 2015;226:T101–22.

Grossman A, Besser GM. Prolactinomas. Br Med J. 1985;20:182–4.

Hilfiker-Kleiner D, Kaminski D, Podewski E, Bonda T, Schaefer A, Silwa K, Foster O, Quint A, Lanmesser U, Doerries C, et al. A cathespin D-cleaved 16kDa form of prolactin mediates postpartum cardiomyopathy. Cell. 2006;128:589–600. https://doi.org/10.1016/j.cell.2016.12.036.

Hilfiker-Kleiner D, Struman I, Hoch M, Podswski E, Silwa K. 16kDa prolactin and bromocriptine in postpartum cardiomyopathy. Curr Heat Fail Rep. 2012;9:174–82. https://doi.org/10.1007/s11897-012-0095-7.

Hoffmann A, Adelmann S, Lohle K, Claviez C, Müller HL. Pediatric prolactinoma: initial presentation, treatment, and long-term prognosis. Eur J Pediatr. 2018;177:125–32. https://doi.org/10.1007/s00431-017-3042-5.

Horseman ND, Gregerson KA. Prolactin actions. J Mol Endocrinol. 2014;52:R95–R106.

Hu Y, Ding Y, Yang M, et al. Serum prolactin levels across pregnancy and the establishment of reference intervals. Clin Chem Lab Med. 2017;56(5):803–7. https://doi.org/10.1515/cclm-2017-0644. Retrieved 19 Jan 2018

Ignacak A, Kasztelnik M, Sliwa T, Korbut RA, Rajda K, Guzik TJ. Prolactin - not only lactotrophin a "new" view of the "old" hormone. J Physiol Pharmacol. 2012;63(5):435–43.

Ikeda H, Watanabeb K, Tominagac T, Yoshimotoc T. Transsphenoidal microsurgical results of female patients with prolactinomas. Clin Neurol Neurosurg. 2013;115:1621–5.

Jankowski PP, Crawford JR, Khanna P, Malicki DM, Ciacci JD, Levy ML. Pituitary tumor apoplexy in adolescents. World Neurosurg. 2015;83(4):644–51.

Jeffcoate SL, Bacon RRA, beastall GH, Diver MJ, Franks S, Seth J. Assays for prolactin: guidelines for the provision of a clinical biochemistry service. Ann Clin Biochem. 1986;23:638–51.

Jethwa PR, Patel TD, Hajart AF, Eloy JA, Couldwell WT, Liu JK. Surgery versus medical therapy in the management of microprolactinoma in the United States. World Neurosurg. 2016;87:65–76.

Johnson MD, Woodburn CJ, Vance ML. Quality of life in patients with a pituitary adenoma. Pituitary. 2003;6(2):81–7.

Kars M, Pereira AM, Smit JW, Romijn JA. Long-term outcome of patients with macroprolactinomas initially treated with dopamine agonists. Eur J Intern Med. 2009;20:387–93.

Kiive E, Maaroos J, Shlik J, Tõru I, Harro J. Growth hormone, cortisol and prolactin responses to physical exercise: higher prolactin response in depressed patients. Prog Neuro-Psychopharmacol Biol Psychiatry. 2004;28(6):1007–13.

Kim Y-M, Seo GH, Kim Y-M, Choi J-H, Yoo H-W. Broad clinical spectrum and diverse outcomes of prolactinoma with pediatric onset: medication-resistant and recurrent cases. Endocrine J [Advance publication]. Released December 27, 2017, Online ISSN 1348-4540, Print ISSN 0918-8959. https://doi.org/10.1507/endocrj.EJ17-0268. https://www.jstage.jst.go.jp/article/endocrj/advpub/0/advpub_EJ17-0268/_article/-char/en

Kleinberg DL, Noel GL, Frantz AG. Galactorrhea: a study of 235 cases, including 48 with pituitary tumors. N Engl J Med. 1977;296(11):589–600.

Klibanski A. Prolactinomas. N Engl J Med. 2010;362(13):1219–26.

Low MJ. Neuroendocrinology. In: Melmed S, Polonsky KS, Larsen PR, Kronenberg HM, editors. Williams textbook of endocrinology. 13th ed. Philadelphia: ScienceDirect Elsevier; 2016. p. 109–75.

Majumdar A, Mangal NS. Hyperprolactinemia. J Hum Reprod Sci. 2013;6(3):168–75. https://doi.org/10.4103/0974-1208.121400.

Marano RJ, Ben-Jonathan N. Minireview: extrapituitary prolactin: an update on the distribution, regulation, and functions. Mol Endocrinol. 2014;28(5):622–33. https://doi.org/10.1210/me.2013-1349.

Medicines and Healthcare Regulatory Agency. WHO International Standard Prolactin, Human. Classification in accordance with Directive 2000/54/EC, Regulation (EC) No 1272/2008: Not applicable or not classified NIBSC code: 83/573 (Version 5.0, Dated 10/11/2016). http://www.nibsc.org/documents/ifu/83-573.pdf. Accessed 28 Feb 2018.

Melmed S, Felipe F, Casanueva FF, Hoffman AR, Kleinberg DL, Montori VM, Schlechte JA, JAH W. Diagnosis and treatment of hyperprolactinemia: an Endocrine Society clinical practice guideline. J Clin Endocrinol Metab. 2011;96(2):273–88. https://doi.org/10.1210/jc.2010-1692.

Mitani S, Amano I, Takatsuru Y. High prolactin concentration during lactation period induced disorders of maternal behavioral in offspring. Psychoneuroendocrinology. 2018;88:129–35.

Molitch M. Medication-induced hyperprolactinemia. Mayo Clin Proc. 2005;80(8):1050–7.

Molitch M. Diagnosis and treatment of pituitary adenomas: a review. JAMA. 2017;317(5):516–24. https://doi.org/10.1001/jama.2016.19699.

Noel GL, Suh HK, Stone JG, Frantz AG. Human prolactin and growth hormone release during surgery and other conditions of stress. J Clin Endocrinol Metab. 1972;35(6):840–51. https://doi.org/10.1210/jcem-35-6-840.

Noel GL, Suh HK, Frantz AG. Prolactin release during nursing and breast stimulation in postpartum and non postpartum subjects. J Clin Endocrinol Metab. 1974;38(3):413–23. https://doi.org/10.1210/jcem-38-3-413.

Noronha S, Stokes V, Karavitaki N, Grossman A. Treating prolactinomas with dopamine agonists: always worth the gamble? Endocrine. 2016;51:205–10. https://doi.org/10.1007/s12020-015-0727-2.

Olukoga AO, Kane JW. Macroprolactinaemia: validation and application of the polyethylene glycol precipitation test and clinical characterization of the condition. Clin Endocrinol. 1999;51:119.

Ranganthan M, Braey G, Pittman B, Cooper T, Perry E, Krystan J, D'Souza DC. The effects of cannabinoids on serum cortisol and prolactin in humans. Psychopharmacology. 2009;203(4):737–944. https://doi.org/10.1007/s00213-008-1422-2.

Rodman EF, Molitch ME, Post KD, Biller BJ, Reichlin S. Long-term follow-up of transsphenoidal selective adenomectomy for prolactinoma. JAMA.

1984;252(7):921–4. https://doi.org/10.1001/jama.1984.03350070039020.

Romijn JA. Hyperprolactinemia and prolactinoma. Handb Clin Neurol. 2014;124:185–95. https://doi.org/10.1016/B978-0-444-59602-4.00013-7. Review. PMID: 25248588

Sairenjia TJ, Ikezawaa J, Kanekob R, Masudaa S, Uchidac K, Takanashia Y, Masudaa H, Sairenjid T, Amanoa I, Takatsurua Y, Sayamae K, Haglundf K, Dikicg K, et al. Maternal prolactin during late pregnancy is important in generating nurturing behavior in the offspring. Proc Natl Acad Sci U S A. 2017;114(49):13042–7.

Salenave S, Ancelle D, Bahougne T, Raverot G, Kamenický P, Bouligand J, Guiochon-Mantel A, Linglart A, Souchon P-F, Nicolino M, Young J, Borson-Chazot F, Delemer B, Chanson P. Macroprolactinomas in children and adolescents: factors associated with the response to treatment in 77 patients. J Clin Endocrinol Metab. 2015;100(3):1177–86. https://doi.org/10.1210/jc.2014-3670.

Sarwar KN, Huda MS, Van de Velde V, Hopkins L, Luck S, Preston R, McGowan BM, Carroll PV, Powrie JK. The prevalence and natural history of pituitary hemorrhage in prolactinoma. J Clin Endocrinol Metab. 2013;98(6):2362–7. https://doi.org/10.1210/jc.2013-1249. Epub 2013 Apr 12

Smith TP, Kavanagh L, Healy ML, McKenna TJ. Technology insight: measuring prolactin in clinical samples. Nat Clin Pract Endocrinol Metab. 2007;3(3):279–89.

Spiegel K, Follenius M, Simon C, Saini J, Ehrhart J, Brandenberger G. Prolactin secretion and sleep. Sleep. 1994;17(1):20–7.

Stewart JK, Clifton DK, DJ K, Rogol AD, Jaffe T, Goodner CJ. Pulsatile release of growth hormone and prolactin from the primate pituitary in vitro. Endocrinology. 1985;116(1):1–5.

Torre DL, Falorni A. Pharmacological causes of hyperprolactinemia. Ther Clin Risk Manag. 2007;3(5):929–51.

Toulis KA, Robbins T, Reddy N, Balachandran K, Gokhale K, Wijesinghe H, Cheng KK, Karavitaki N, Wass J, Nirantharakumar K. Males with prolactinoma are at increased risk of incident cardiovascular disease. Clin Endocrinol. 2018;88:71–6. https://doi.org/10.1111/cen.13498.

Zygourakis CC, Imber BS, Chen R, Han SJ, Blevins L, Molinaro A, Kahn JG, Aghi MK. Cost-effectiveness analysis of surgical versus medical treatment of prolactinomas. J Neurol Surg B Skull Base. 2017;78(2):125–31. https://doi.org/10.1055/s-0036-1592193. Epub 2016 Sep 27

Key Reading

1. Melmed S, Felipe F, Casanueva FF, Hoffman AR, Kleinberg DL, Montori VM, Schlechte JA, JAH W. Diagnosis and treatment of hyperprolactinemia: an Endocrine Society clinical practice guideline. J Clin Endocrinol Metab. 2011;96(2):273–88. https://doi.org/10.1210/jc.2010-1692.
2. Gillam M, Molitch M. Proactin. In: Melmed S, editor. The Pituitary. 3rd ed. London: Elsevier; 2011. p. 119–66. https://doi.org/10.1016/B978-0-12-380926-1.10015-X.
3. Chanson P, Maiter D. Prolactinoma. In: Melmed S, editor. The pituitary. fourth ed. London: Elsevier; 2017. p. 467–514.
4. Glezer A, Bronstein MD. Prolactinoma. Endocrinol Metab Clin N Am. 2015;44:71–8.
5. Romijn JA. Hyperprolactinemia and prolactinoma. Handb Clin Neurol. 2014;124:185–95. https://doi.org/10.1016/B978-0-444-59602-4.00013-7. Review. PMID: 25248588
6. Torre DL, Falorni A. Pharmacological causes of hyperprolactinemia. Ther Clin Risk Manag. 2007;3(5):929–51.

Growth Hormone Producing Adenomas: Acromegaly

20

Karen J. P. Liebert, Daphne T. Adelman, Elisabeth Rutten, and Christine Yedinak

Contents

K. J. P. Liebert (✉)
Neuroendocrine Unit, Massachusetts General
Hospital, Boston, MA, USA
e-mail: kpulaski@partners.org

D. T. Adelman
Division of Endocrinology, Metabolism and
Molecular Medicine, Northwestern University
Feinberg School of Medicine, Chicago, IL, USA
e-mail: d-adelman@northwestern.edu

E. Rutten
Department of Endocrinology, Ghent University
Hospital, Ghent, Belgium
e-mail: els.rutten@uzgent.be

C. Yedinak
Northwest Pituitary Center, Oregon Health and
Sciences University, Portland, OR, USA
e-mail: yedinakc@ohsu.edu

© Springer Nature Switzerland AG 2019
S. Llahana et al. (eds.), *Advanced Practice in Endocrinology Nursing*,
https://doi.org/10.1007/978-3-319-99817-6_20

Abstract

Acromegaly is a rare disorder characterized by overproduction of growth hormone (GH) predominantly by a pituitary adenoma. Clinical features associated with acromegaly are a result of chronic excess GH and insulin-like growth factor-I (IGF-1) effects on tissue, bone, and other organs.

The disease is associated with increased mortality, chiefly from cardiovascular disease, but morbidity from associated comorbidities is also increased. Adequate control of growth hormone excess is paramount to controlling comorbidities.

The diagnosis is made by the biochemical confirmation of elevated GH and IGF-1 levels, the presence of clinical features, and evidence of a pituitary tumor based on MRI imaging. Transsphenoidal surgery, medical therapies, and radiation therapy are all options for disease control. Patients with acromegaly require long-term health surveillance, despite the fact that they may have normal GH and IGF-1 levels. Patients are monitored lifelong for disease recurrence, management of comorbidities and treatments to improve quality of life.

Keywords

Acromegaly · Growth hormone excess · Pituitary · Pituitary tumor · Insulin-like growth factor-1

Abbreviations

BMI	Body Mass Index
CHD	Congestive heart disease
CSF	Cerebrospinal fluid
CVD	Cardiovascular disease
DI	Diabetes insipidus
GH	Growth hormone
GHRH	Growth hormone releasing hormone
IGF-1	Insulin-like growth factor-1
OGTT	Oral glucose tolerance test
OSA	Obstructive sleep apnea
SIADH	Syndrome of inappropriate antidiuretic hormone
SRIF	Somatostatin
SSA	Somatostatin analogue
SSRA	Somatostatin receptor analogue

Key Terms

- **Macroadenoma:** pituitary tumour >1.0 cm in any dimension.
- **Gigantism:** growth hormone excess occurring in childhood prior to the fusing of the long bone growth plates.
- **Somatotroph:** growth hormone secreting cell in the anterior pituitary.
- **Somatostatin:** a peptide hormone secreted by the hypothalamus that inhibits the production of growth hormone.
- **Ectopic Acromegaly:** growth hormone-releasing hormone (GHRH) secretion from neoplastic tissue that stimulates pituitary somatotrophs to inappropriately release growth hormone.

Key Points

- Acromegaly is an insidious disease caused by overproduction of growth hormone and insulin-like growth factor-1 (IGF-1) predominantly from a growth hormone producing adenoma in the pituitary gland.
- Hypersecretion of growth hormone may lead to disturbances in the musculoskeletal, cardiovascular, metabolic system as well as have implications for the development of other neoplasms.
- Early diagnosis and prompt treatment can prevent development of comorbidities and improve mortality and morbidity outcomes.
- Diagnosis is based on clinical and biochemical assessments and should include a screening IGF-1 with confirmation of the disease using an oral glucose tolerance test.
- Treatment of acromegaly includes surgery to remove the adenoma, medical therapy, pituitary irradiation, and/or combinations of each therapy.
- Quality of life may be adversely affected in chronic conditions like acromegaly and should be addressed by all care providers.

20.1   Introduction

Acromegaly is a disorder characterized by the overproduction of growth hormone (GH). Acromegaly comes from the Greek words for "extremities" (acro) and "big" (megaly), as one of the hallmark symptoms of this condition is abnormally large hands (Chanson and Salenave 2008). Growth hormone overproduction is usually from a benign tumor found in the pituitary gland. The pituitary gland is located at the base of the brain and directly below the hypothalamus (See Chap. 1).

GH-secreting pituitary adenomas are thought to arise from abnormal changes to somatotroph cells whose primarily role is to secrete GH. Although the reason GH producing tumors occur is unknown, most are the result of a genetic mutation in the replication of somatotroph cells. When GH hypersecretion occurs before the fusion of long bone growth plates in late adolescence, pituitary gigantism results, characterized primarily by excessive vertical growth (Chanson and Salenave 2008).

GH excess occurring during adulthood does not result in abnormal height, but rather is associated with slow insidious changes to the patient's physical appearance and alterations in body physiology. Hence, acromegaly often goes unrecognized in adults for many years. Many patients complain of non-specific symptoms for many years, seeking consultation from a number of medical specialties.

Early recognition of symptoms and treatment is paramount to limiting the impact of GH excess and subsequent comorbidities. A blood test for IGF-1 is recommended as a screening test when a patient presents with signs and symptoms of acromegaly. If elevated, referral to specialty centers versed in the diagnosis and treatment of pituitary diseases is highly recommended. Comprehensive care and access to health care professionals who are devoted to treating this disease is associated with best patient outcomes.

20.2   Epidemiology

Acromegaly is a slow, progressive disease. It may be up to 10 years (or more) before clear features of the disease emerge and are recognized by health care providers, necessitating a referral to an endocrinologist (Chanson et al. 2014; Nachtigall et al. 2008; Galoiu and Poiana 2015). This delay may largely be the result of the rarity of the disease.

Current population prevalence estimates range from 2.8 to 13.7 cases per 100,000 people with a yearly incidence of 0.2–1.1 cases per 100,000 population (Chanson et al. 2014; Gurel et al. 2014; Knutzen and Ezzat 2006; Lavrentaki et al. 2016). This is a significant increase over historical reports and may represent a true reflection of increased disease, increased awareness of the disease and earlier diagnosis, and/or patients more actively seeking medical attention for symptoms, particularly after internet research (Lavrentaki et al. 2016).

The median age of diagnosis is reported to be in the fifth decade of life, between 40.5 and 47 years of life (men: 36.5–48.5, females: 38–56) (Lavrentaki et al. 2016). Acromegaly generally affects both men and women equally. Over 65% of cases are associated with a pituitary macroadenoma at presentation (Nachtigall et al. 2008). If left untreated, disease comorbidities contribute significantly to increased mortality, which is 2–4 times higher than the general population (Beauregard et al. 2003; Colao et al. 2014a; Melmed 2017; Melmed et al. 2005).

Epidemiologic data is sparse regarding young-onset acromegaly, or gigantism, mainly due to the rarity of the cases. Reports indicate that only 2.4% of all cases of acromegaly were found in children between the ages of 0–19 years old (Daly et al. 2006). GH production from an ectopic source is very rare.

20.3   Pathophysiology

Growth hormone is a peptide hormone manufactured and secreted by somatotroph cells located in the anterior pituitary gland. Women secrete more GH than men, and overall GH production decreases with age. Under normal conditions, growth hormone is secreted in an episodic pulsatile manner and has a half-life of 11–19 min (Faria et al. 1989). GH production during the day is relatively low, but secretion and pulsatility increase at night in association with slow wave sleep (Melmed 2017). Approximately 70% of GH is produced at night, beginning within 2 h of the onset of sleep (Fig. 20.1). This circadian pattern is shifted in jet lag, but is unchanged in shift workers (Fig. 20.1) (Morris et al. 2012).

Episodic or pulsatile GH secretion and release is a complex process influenced by many factors. It is primarily under the central neurogenic control of two hormones released by the hypothalamus, growth hormone releasing hormone (GHRH), and somatostatin. GHRH stimulates (positive action) and somatostatin inhibits GH secretion (negative action) (Fig. 20.2). The alternating action of these hormones is largely responsible for GH pulsatility and the regulation of the appropriate concentration of growth hormone in the body (Bonert and Melmed 2017). Ghrelin is a peptide secreted from the gastrointestinal tract and stomach that modulates the release of GH at the levels of the hypothalamus and pituitary gland. GH and ghrelin have been found to be secreted simultaneously in humans with ghrelin amplifying GH pulses (Melmed et al. 2014). Exercise and stress also influences GH secretion (Melmed et al. 2014).

GHRH (positive stimulation) from hypothalamic neurons is released in response to sex steroids, neuropeptides, neurotransmitters, and opiates (Bonert and Melmed 2017). GHRH travels to the pituitary via the infundibulum and attaches to receptors on somatatroph cells. This process results in the synthesis of GH within these cells. GH is then distributed to receptor sites on target tissues throughout the body to affect nerves, muscles, bones, and other organ functions.

GHRH release and GH synthesis are stimulated by many factors. Leptin regulation of fat mass, food intake, and energy expenditure may provide a metabolic signal in fasting states triggering GH secretion in order to maintain meta-

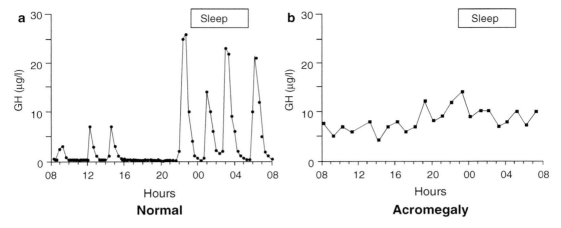

Fig. 20.1 GH circadian pulsatile production. (**a**) Normal subjects circadian pulsatile GH secretion with highest amplitude and frequency of pulses in slow wave sleep. GH levels are undetectable much of the time during the day. (**b**) Acromegaly subjects: Dysregulation of circadian frequency, and amplitude of GH pulses. Elevated baseline GH production. Ref: Chanson P, Salenave S: Acromegaly. Orphanet Journal of Rare Diseases. 3–17 (2008). Reproduced under creative commons license

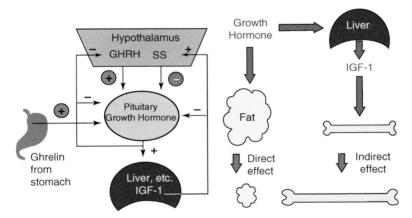

Fig. 20.2 Growth hormone physiology. Growth hormone (GH) or somatotropin secreted by the pituitary gland. Growth hormone releasing hormone (GHRH) stimulates anterior pituitary gland to release GH. The target of growth hormone: adipose tissue, liver, bone, and muscle. GH has direct effects and indirect effects on these targets. Reprinted with permission from http://www.vivo.colo-state.edu/hbooks/pathphys/endocrine/hypopit/gh.html

bolic homeostasis (Bonert and Melmed 2017). Central dopamine and subsequent norepinephrine secretion stimulate GH secretion. Hypoglycemia also increases GH secretion via adrenergic stimulation while cholinergic and serotoninergic neurons have been associated with sleep-induced GH secretion (Bonert and Melmed 2017).

Somatostatin (Somatostatin Receptor Inhibiting Factor or SRIF) is a peptide that blocks GH secretion. SRIF can also inhibit adrenocorticotrophic hormone (ACTH), thyroid stimulating hormone (TSH), insulin, and glucagon secretion. Synthesized in the hypothalamus, SRIF travels down the infundibulum to the anterior pituitary, where it attaches to somatostatin receptors on somatotroph cells, thereby blocking GH secretion. It has similar actions at somatostatin receptors found throughout the body. Somatostatin attaches to five somatostatin subtype membrane receptors (SSTRs), SSTR 1, 2, 3, 4, and 5 (Bonert and

Melmed 2017). These subtypes have varying affinities for coupling with somatostatin (Bonert and Melmed 2017). SSTR 1, 3, and 5 are found on somatotrophs in the pituitary gland, whereas pituitary tumors express SSTR 1, 2, 3, and 5. These receptors provide a target for treatment of GH excess (Bonert and Melmed 2017). Other adrenergic pathways also inhibit GH release.

Once secreted, GH circulates in the blood stream attaching to peripheral receptors inducing specific cellular changes. In the liver, IGF-1 is synthesized via the JAK/STAT signaling pathway (Morris et al. 2012; Burton et al. 2012). IGF-1 is essential for promoting developmental growth activities, but also provides inhibition of GH and GHRH production via negative feedback mechanisms (Melmed et al. 2014).

GH and IGF-1 excess induces multiple downstream physiologic changes. Bone metabolism is increased with periosteal new bone formation and skeletal overgrowth (Bonert and Melmed 2017). Simultaneously, bone resorption is accelerated, increasing the risk of fracture in the presence of GH excess. There is an associated increase in soft tissue growth, adipose tissue, lipolysis, increased muscle and liver uptake of triglycerides (Bonert and Melmed 2017). GH excess antagonizes both insulin action and carbohydrate metabolism, resulting in hyperglycemia.

Pituitary GH producing adenomas are largely thought to be the result of a genetic mutation leading to autonomous GH secretion and proliferation of somatotroph cells. However, some tumors may also result from GHRH synthesis or secretory dysfunction. Most GH adenomas are monoclonal, leading to abnormal proliferation of cells that only produce GH. However, up to 25% of GH producing tumors contain cells that co-secrete GH and prolactin (Melmed et al. 2014). Rare tumors also contain cells that can produce both GH and prolactin from the same cell (Chanson and Salenave 2008). Familial genetic acromegaly syndromes or familial isolated pituitary adenomas (FIPA) associated with acromegaly are rare and include McCune–Albright syndrome, multiple endocrine neoplasia type 1 (MEN-1), and Carney Complex (Melmed et al. 2014). (See Chap. 9).

Histopathology of GH-secreting tumors demonstrates distinct cell cytoplasmic staining for GH granules and may reflect tumor activity (Melmed 2017). These include: sparsely granulated or rapidly growing tumor cells or densely granulated or slowly growing tumor cells (Melmed 2017). Cell proliferation markers Ki67 (a nuclear protein associated with proliferation) and p53 (a tumour antigen and marker of mitotic activity) are usually quantified are considered of concern if elevated. A Ki67 > 3%, mitotic activity in >10% of cells, and positive nuclear staining for p53 (>10 strongly positive nuclei per 10 high power fields) are indicative of more aggressive tumors (Raverot et al. 2017). Higher expression of SSTR2 and p21 (inhibiting cell proliferation) are associated with lower likelihood of tumor aggression and recurrence (Cuevas-Ramos et al. 2015). Two classification systems have been proposed in an effort for early prediction of treatment response, and/or tumor recurrence or progression. Raverot et al. focused primarily on histopathology and tumor invasion, prospectively evaluating a grading system from 1 to 3 for all pituitary adenomas (Raverot et al. 2017) (Table 20.1). Tumors graded as 2b were found to have a 3.7 times higher risk of recurrence or progression than grade 1 tumors. Others examined clinical, radiologic, histopathologic, and outcome characteristics in order to develop a system of risk specifically for patients with acromegaly (Cuevas-Ramos et al. 2015) (Table 20.2). In this tool, level 1 is considered to have minimal risk of recurrence and is most likely to respond to monotherapy, whereas level 3 characteristics carry a significant risk of recurrence and poorer outcomes. This tool is pending further validation.

Table 20.1 Grading system for prediction of tumour recurrence

Grade	Description
1a	Non-invasive, no or low proliferative indicators
1b	Non-invasive but proliferation
2a	Invasive
2b[a]	Invasive with proliferation
3	Malignant

[a]2b had a 3.7 times higher risk of recurrence or progression over 1a (Raverot et al. 2017)

Table 20.2 Characteristics of aggressive GH producing tumors

Type 1	Older age at diagnosis
	Longer disease duration before diagnosis (less symptomatology)
	Nadir GH and IGF-1 lower
	Smaller tumor volumes but both micro- and macroadenomas
	Tumors extend toward sphenoid
	Densely granulated cells on histopathology
	Ki67 < 3%
	p16 low or undetectable
	Highest proportion of cells with SSRT2 staining
	May respond to dopamine agonists as monotherapy
Type 2	Less symptomatology than type 3
	Fewer microadenomas than type 1. Some invasive macroadenomas
	Higher nadir GH and IGF-1
	Invasive macroadenomas
	Similar proportion of densely and sparsely granulated cells on histopathology
	KI67 > 3%
	p16 low or undetectable
	High p21 immunoreactivity
	Lower SSRT2 staining
	More likely to require 2 or more surgeries
Type 3	Younger age at diagnosis
	Macroadenomas all invasive
	Nadir GH and IGF-1 higher than type 1 and 2
	Higher prolactin levels (p = 0.01) than
	Most aggressive tumors
	Sparsely granulated cells
	Ki67 > 3%
	p16 low or undetectable
	Low expression of p21 and alpha subunit
	Negative or low SSRT2 staining
	More likely to require 2 or more surgeries
	More likely to require radiotherapy
	More commonly require combination medical therapy or modalities for control
	More likely to be medication resistant

Adapted from Cuevas-Ramos et al. (2015)

20.4   Clinical Symptoms

The presenting manifestations of acromegaly may be a reflection of disease progression and the time to diagnosis. Since the diagnosis is frequently delayed, it may account for the predominance of macroadenomas (tumors >1 cm) found in the majority of patients with acromegaly and the extent of the observed phenotypic changes (Nachtigall et al. 2008).

The most commonly reported symptoms at presentation are headaches, as well as menstrual disturbances in women and hypogonadism in men (Chanson and Salenave 2008; Chanson et al. 2014). The most prominent physical changes in appearance include acral enlargement (78–85%) and course facial features (70%) (Chanson and Salenave 2008; Melmed 2017).

Excess GH and IGF-1 act at multiple receptor sites on body organs, tissues and bone and muscle that ultimately produce the clinical characteristics and morbidity associated with acromegaly. In bone, high levels of IGF-1 increase chondrocyte and osteocyte activity, stimulating excess skeletal bone and cartilage formation (Chanson et al. 2014). Over time, overgrowth of bone and cartilage results in acral changes (enlargement of the hands and feet) and changes in facial features such as frontal bossing and jaw growth. Joint laxity and remodeling is associated with soft tissue changes and boney overgrowth eventually resulting in arthritis and/or joint deterioration (Chanson et al. 2014). Vertebral fractures occur up to 6.9 times more frequently in patients with acromegaly, particularly in association with hypogonadism (Chanson et al. 2014; Mazziotti et al. 2013). Increases in facial soft tissues result in changes in features, such as a bulbous nose, thickened lips, and enlarged tongue. Increases in peripheral tissue and edema result in enlargement of hands (leading to symptoms of carpal tunnel syndrome) and feet. Skin changes, including oily skin with large pores, excessive hair growth, excessive sweating, and skin hyperpigmentation are observed (Chanson and Salenave 2008; Chanson et al. 2014; Melmed 2017; Melmed et al. 2014). Multiple skin tags may be found under arms and on the trunk (Ben-Shlomo and Melmed 2006; Capatina and Wass 2015). Elevated GH levels are also associated with organ tissue hypertrophy and enlargement. This can promote the development of a goiter and colon polyps. Airway obstruction results from tongue enlargement and hypertrophy of pharyngeal tissue leading to sleep apnea and poor oxygenation (Capatina and Wass 2015). IGF-1 production overstimulates myocyte activity, resulting in ventricular hypertrophy, compounding hypertension, cardiomegaly and congestive heart disease (CHD) (Melmed 2017) (Fig. 20.3).

Other pituitary hormonal changes in acromegaly are common and include hyperprolactinemia, which is seen in about 25–30% of patients with acromegaly (Abreu et al. 2016). In the presence of a large tumor, this may be associated with pituitary stalk compression, but co-secretion of prolactin, either from a single cell type or two different cell types, is possible and may be confirmed on histopathology (Melmed 2017). Patients frequently

present with symptoms or a history of hypogonadism, menstrual abnormalities, and infertility (Melmed 2017). Hypopituitarism can be due to mass effect on the pituitary, or damage of the pituitary gland from surgical tumor excision or radiotherapy.

On presentation, patient reported symptoms include frontal headaches, increase in ring and shoe size, weight gain, excessive sweating, difficulty with speech, snoring and breathlessness, deepening voice, coarse oily skin, multiple joint pains and carpel tunnel symptoms, hirsutism, fatigue, poor endurance, infertility, plus difficulty

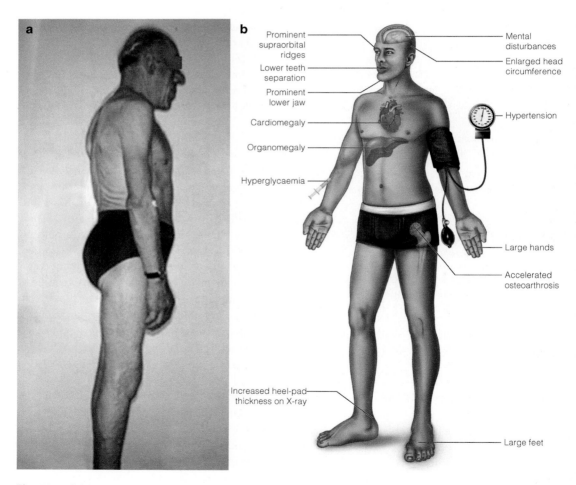

Fig. 20.3 Clinical features of acromegaly. (**a**) Clinical characteristics, (**b**) common morphological changes and comorbities. (**c**) Hand swelling and enlargement (right) (**d**) feet enlargement (left) (**e**) gaps between teeth particu-larly on mandible (**f**) broadening of nose and jaw enlargement (**g**) frontal bossing and jaw enlargement. Adapted from: Chanson P, Salenave S: Acromegaly. Orphanet J Rare Dis 3, 17 (2008)

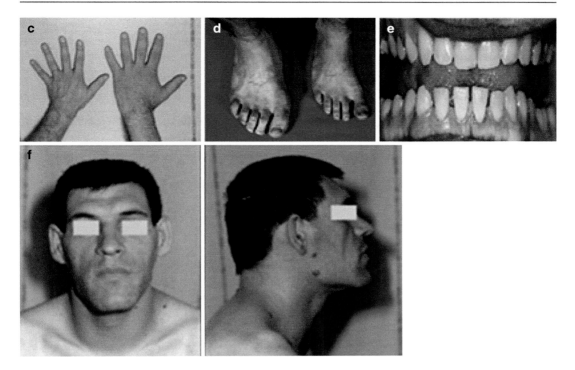

Fig. 20.3 (continued)

with cognition and memory. Patients may also have changes in vision, particularly peripheral vision and acuity when large tumors are present (Chanson and Salenave 2008; Chanson et al. 2014; Melmed 2017).

20.5   Comorbidities

National registries have been created in several countries to track comorbidities and mortality rates and also monitor the effects of treatment. Past reports from registries and other studies have indicated that life expectancy for a patient with untreated acromegaly is reduced by about 10 years compared to the general population. Cardiovascular disease is cited as the leading cause of death. However, in a recent analysis of the French Acromegaly Registry Group, better disease control reduced the incidence of comorbidities, bringing life expectancy close to that of the general population (Maione et al. 2017).

20.5.1 Cardiovascular Comorbidities

Cardiovascular disease (CVD) is the most prevalent comorbidity affecting people with acromegaly. Arrhythmias and sudden cardiac death represent the most common causes of mortality (Colao et al. 1999; Sharma et al. 2017). An increased risk of dilated cardiomyopathy, congestive heart failure (CHF), aortic and mitral valve disease, and coronary artery disease (CAD) are all reported (Sharma et al. 2017). Early studies (published prior to 1995) reported a standardized mortality risk associated with acromegaly of up to 3.31, or over 3 times higher than the general population. However, due to earlier diagnosis and disease control, mortality rates have improved with reported standardized mortality ratio now lower around 2.79 times that of the general population (Esposito et al. 2018). Some studies have found that coronary artery disease (CAD) risk is normalized with disease remission, whereas myocardial fibrosis, valvular dysfunction, and cardiac arrhythmias may be unchanged, despite treatment for acromegaly (Sharma et al. 2017). CAD (stroke and myocardial infarction) risk remains unclear given concomitant risks from diabetes and hyperlipidemia, confounding morbidity and mortality statistics. However, encouraging data from a large German registry study demonstrated no increased risk of myocardial infarction (MI) or stroke in patients with acromegaly (Schöfl et al. 2017). Regardless, early recognition of CVD, treatment in specialty facilities, and pre-surgical treatment with somatostatin analogues have been shown to improve CVD outcomes (Sharma et al. 2017; Schöfl et al. 2017; Colao 2012).

Hypertension plays a significant role in development of cardiac hypertrophy or thickened heart chamber walls. It has been estimated that the incidence of hypertension in acromegaly is 18–60% and is associated with a significant increase in mortality (Pivonello et al. 2017). Pathogenic mechanisms of hypertension are unclear. However, it is postulated that GH and IGF-1 excess also act directly on the kidneys causing antidiuretic and antinatriuretic effects or by indirectly expanding plasma volume, resulting in increased peripheral resistance. Epithelial sodium channels (ENaC) are found in all cells and play a role in extracellular fluid volume and blood pressure. Excess GH stimulates sodium reabsorption in the distal nephrons, resulting in water retention and volume expansion (Kamenicky et al. 2008). Sleep apnea may also play a role (Sharma et al. 2017). Additionally, chronic GH exposure causes myocardial inflammation and fibrosis, hence tissue hypertrophy and loss of tissue elasticity. Using echocardiography, it has been reported that up to 85% of patients with acromegaly have left ventricular hypertrophy (Sharma et al. 2017). Thus, hypertension in acromegaly is multifactorial.

Cardiomyopathy in acromegaly has been described as occurring in progressive stages (Sharma et al. 2017). Early stages involve increased myocardial performance and decreased peripheral vascular resistance progressing to cardiac hypertrophy associated with myocardial inflammation and fibrosis. These early changes can progress to congestive heart failure, primarily through severe systolic and diastolic dysfunc-tion and increased peripheral vascular resistance (Sharma et al. 2017). Dysfunctional changes in the cardiac valves, particularly in the mitral and aortic valves, are also a common feature in cardiomyopathy (Sharma et al. 2017). All patients presenting with acromegaly should be assessed with echocardiography and referred to cardiology as appropriate.

20.5.2 Metabolic Comorbidities

Disorders of glucose metabolism are frequently reported in patients with acromegaly. IGF-1 regulates carbohydrate metabolism and insulin sensitivity, manifesting in a range of comorbidities such as heart disease, hypertension, and diabetes (Galoiu and Poiana 2015; Melmed 2017). Studies have reported variable rates of impaired glucose tolerance (16–46%) and overt diabetes mellitus type II (19–56%) in patients with acromegaly (Alexopoulou et al. 2013). Chronic GH excess is known to lead to insulin resistance in the liver and peripheral tissues. Impaired beta cell function has also been implicated in hyperglycemia. Severity of impairment in this patient population is also influenced by IGF-1 levels, age, and increased BMI (Alexopoulou et al. 2013) (Fig. 20.4). Links have been shown between glucose intolerance, hypertension, and acromegalic cardiomyopathy (Chanson and Salenave 2008).

20.5.3 Respiratory Comorbidities

The most notable respiratory comorbidity in acromegaly is obstructive sleep apnea syndrome (OSA). Risk factors include: anatomical changes in the craniofacial bones, posterior pharyngeal soft tissue thickening, and soft palate hypertrophy and tongue enlargement. These changes lead to airway impairment (Guo et al. 2018).

Sleep apnea affects up to 80% of patients with acromegaly and is a common cause of daytime sleepiness, snoring, sleep hypoxia, headache, and memory dysfunction (Guo et al. 2018; Attal and Chanson 2018; Grunstein 1991). Obesity, particularly in males over 50 years, is a significant risk factor for OSA. Screening for sleep apnea is

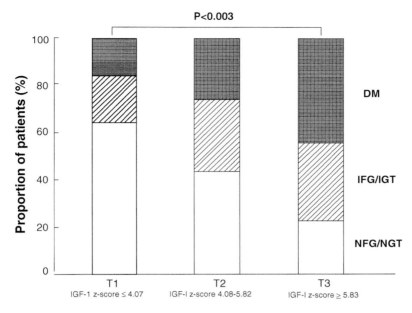

Fig. 20.4 Relationship of acromegaly: Glucose intolerance. Proportion of patients with NFG/NGT, IFG/IGT and DM within groups subdivided according to IGF-I z-score tertiles T1-T3. *NFG* normal fasting glucose, *NGT* normal glucose tolerance, *IFG* impaired fasting glucose, *IGT* impaired glu-cose tolerance, *DM* diabetes mellitus. Ref: Alexopoulou O, Bex M, Kamenicky P et al. Prevalence and risk factors of impaired glucose tolerance and diabetes mellitus at diagnosis of acromegaly: a study in 148 patients. Pituitary 17(1):81–89. Creative commons License with permission

recommended for all patients with active and con-trolled acromegaly.

Lung function changes are also apparent in acromegaly patients, with rib cage remodeling, changes in cartilage and soft tissue that decrease elasticity and shorten inspiratory time (Chanson and Salenave 2008). Although alveolar volume may be increased, subclinical hypoxemia may be present (Chanson and Salenave 2008).

20.5.4 Neoplasia and Malignancies

Higher risk of developing neoplasms and some forms of cancers has been reported in patients with acromegaly. In a large Italian study, renal, thyroid, and colon cancer risk was significantly higher than in the general population (Terzolo et al. 2017). Pre-cancerous adenomatous colorec-tal polyps have been reported in upwards of 28% of acromegaly patients (Chanson and Salenave 2008; Abreu et al. 2016). Overexpression of GH in the colon was shown to increased epithelial cell proliferation and decreased apoptosis rates pre-disposing the development of polyps (Chesnokova

et al. 2016). Thyroid nodules appear to be com-mon and are found in up to 90% of patients with acromegaly. These patients have a greater likeli-hood of developing multinodular goiter when there is a longer interval between onset of symp-toms and diagnosis (Chanson and Salenave 2008). However, some studies report the incidence of thyroid cancer does not appear to be different from the general population. A meta-analysis indicated that the overall cancer incidence for acromegaly patients was only slightly higher than the general population particularly for colorectal, breast, urinary, prostate, and hematologic cancers (Dal et al. 2018). No difference was found with respect to lung or gastric cancers. This empha-sizes the need for ongoing cancer surveillance in patients diagnosed with acromegaly.

20.5.5 Arthropathies

Arthralgias and myalgias are reportedly experi-enced by about 70% of patients with acromegaly. Arthropathies develop after an average of 10 years of excess GH exposure, and can affect all joints, causing progressive pain and dysfunction (Chanson and Salenave 2008; Melmed 2017; Abreu et al. 2016). Carpal tunnel syndrome and hip osteoarthropathy are commonly reported. Range of movement may be limited secondary to mechanical, non-inflammatory etiologies and/or hypermobility and tenderness. On radiographic images, joint spaces are seen to be widened (Melmed 2017). Osteocyte formation and uneven chondrocyte formations are thought to cause joint changes and osteoarthritis. In general, joint degeneration has been found to be irreversible and has been reported to impair activities of daily living and quality of life (Melmed 2017). Neurological conditions in the spine are thought to be associated with neural thickening and nerve entrapment, while disc space widening has been implicated in the development of kyphosis and scoliosis seen in these patients (Melmed 2017). Vertebral fractures have been reported in about 10% of patients (Abreu et al. 2016; Mazziotti et al. 2008).

20.5.6 Other Comorbidities

A higher incidence of asymptomatic cholelithiasis and gallbladder polyps is found in patients with untreated acromegaly (Annamalai et al. 2011; Montini et al. 2010). In addition, the treatment with somatostatins has also been associated with the development of gallstones and gallbladder sludge (Melmed 2017).

20.6 Diagnosis

The diagnosis of acromegaly is made through the clinical assessment of features and the measurement of biochemical parameters. Clinical findings unique to acromegaly, such as changes in facial features, enlarged hands (rings no longer fitting), and an increase in shoe size raise suspicions of acromegaly. Old photographs may be useful in determining changes in facial features (such as a driver's license photograph if taken 5–10 years previously). Other presenting symptoms may include headaches, joint aches or cardiovascular findings and hypogonadism (Chanson and Salenave 2008; Melmed 2017).

Biochemical confirmation of autonomous GH oversecretion is needed to make the diagnosis of acromegaly (Melmed 2017). A screening IGF-1 level should be performed if acromegaly is suspected. An elevated level should prompt a referral to a pituitary specialist or a general endocrinologist if a pituitary specialist is not available. Due to the pulsatile nature of GH secretion, a random GH level to confirm elevated GH is not useful, and is not recommended for diagnosis (Katznelson et al. 2014). According to internationally recognized guidelines, the gold standard test for confirming acromegaly is an oral glucose tolerance test (OGTT/GH suppression test). In this test, an oral glucose load of 75 g is given to the patient and GH levels are monitored every 30 min for 2 h. GH nadir of <1 µg/l (3 mIU/l) at any time point rules out the diagnosis of acromegaly (See Chapter: Provocative Investigations). The diagnosis may be complicated by variability in laboratory assays. Results must be interpreted in the context of the patient's age, BMI, and nutritional status. The presence of diabetes mellitus, renal and liver disease also spuriously alters results (Melmed 2017). Repeat sampling is recommended to confirm biochemical findings (Katznelson et al. 2014).

A pituitary MRI scan should be performed to determine the presence of a pituitary adenoma once an elevated IGF-1/GH is confirmed (Melmed 2017; Katznelson et al. 2014). Given that the majority of GH producing pituitary tumors are macroadenomas (>1 cm) and can impinge on the optic nerves, it is also recommended that these patients undergo ophthalmologic and visual field testing as a component of the initial examination (Katznelson et al. 2014).

20.7 Treatment Options

Treatment goals are to suppress or normalize GH and IGF-1, manage symptoms, and reduce tumor mass without compromising pituitary function (Melmed 2017; Katznelson et al. 2014).

If surgical resection fails to achieve GH control, or if the patient is not a candidate for surgery, medical therapies and/or radiation therapy may be indicated (See Chapter: Pituitary Radiation) (Fig. 20.5).

20.7.1 Transsphenoidal Surgery

First-line treatment where a pituitary tumor is evident on MRI is selective transsphenoidal surgical resection. Success in achieving the aforementioned goals is dependent on a variety of factors, such as tumor size and location and presence of the tumor in the cavernous sinuses (Chanson et al. 2014). If the tumor is a micro-adenoma (<1.0 cm), surgical remission is achieved in approximately 70% of cases versus <50% for those with macroadenomas (>1.0 cm) (Melmed 2017). The best outcomes are achieved by experienced pituitary neurosurgeons. Both microscopic and endoscopic approaches are currently used, along with

sophisticated intraoperative tumor localizing technologies (See Chap. 22).

Post-surgically, new onset hypopituitarism and secondary empty sella may occur (Melmed 2017). Surgical risks and complications include vision loss, cerebral spinal fluid (CSF) leak and epistaxis and hormonal dysfunction. The most common disturbances in hormones following surgery include diabetes insipidus, syndrome of inappropriate antidiuretic hormone (SIADH) and adrenal insufficiency.

Recurrence rates of pituitary tumors postoperatively range from 2 to 8% at 5 years post-op, with reports of up to 10% by 10 years postoperatively (Katznelson et al. 2014; Swearingen et al. 1998). This may be related to residual tumor from incomplete resection with subsequent growth or true recurrence. Re-operation is indicated for patients who experience visual impairment or if there is a high probability for substantial debulking or completely removing

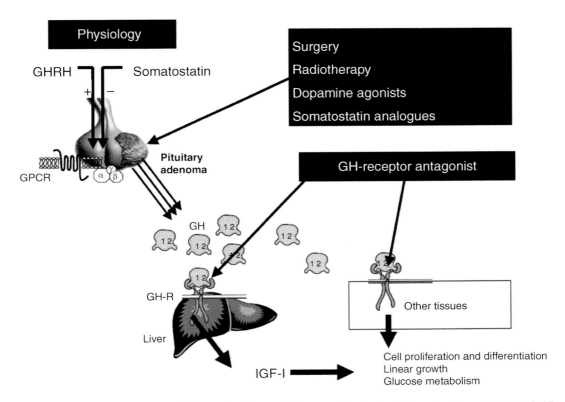

Fig. 20.5 Acromegaly treatments. Chanson P, Salenave S: Acromegaly. Orphanet Journal of Rare Diseases. 3–17 (2008). Reproduced under creative commons license

the tumor. With the potential to either remit disease or lower GH levels, re-operation is thought to be a viable, safe option and may achieve remission in up to 50% of cases (Heringer et al. 2016; Wilson et al. 2013).

20.7.1.1 Nursing Role in Transsphenoidal Surgery (Also See Chap. 23)

Preoperatively, the surgical procedure is reviewed with the patient. Patient needs, tolerance, and desire for specific surgical details vary. An overall description of the procedure itself, the risks, and what is to be expected following surgery are usually included. It is important to review the recommended lifestyle restrictions immediately postoperative, and when it is safe to return work or their previous lifestyle. Depending on the neurosurgeon and the health care system policy, the patient can be expected to stay inpatient for 1–3 days. This may vary based on specific postoperative complications such as CSF leak, diabetes insipidus, or signs of infection.

Immediately postoperatively, patients are monitored for pituitary hormone disturbances, with the most common one being transient diabetes insipidus. Sodium levels will be monitored to detect diabetes insipidus (DI) or syndrome of inappropriate antidiuretic hormone (SIADH). Both conditions are usually transient. Discharge instructions may include activity restrictions for 2–4 weeks, with gradual participation in more strenuous activity over the next several months. Lifting is usually restricted and the use of CPAP for sleep apnea is not recommended for the first 2 or more weeks. Surgical and endocrine follow-up is generally performed 2–12 weeks (practice dependent), at which all the pituitary hormones will be evaluated and MRI is performed.

20.7.1.2 Postoperative Testing

There has been some debate as to the definition of "cure" or disease remission. The Endocrine Society guidelines define postoperative "cure" as a suppressed GH level < 1 ng/ml following a glucose load and normalization of IGF-1 levels (Katznelson et al. 2014). A random GH/IGF-1 and oral glucose for GH suppression (OGTT) is recommended at 12 weeks or later postoperatively. MRI to evaluate any residual tumor is also recommended at 12 weeks postoperatively (Katznelson et al. 2014).

If biochemical testing demonstrates the patient has persistent acromegaly, then further therapy is needed. If the MRI scan shows a residual tumor that is surgically approachable, then re-exploration may be considered. If re-exploration is not an option, then the next line of therapy is medical management.

20.7.2 Medical Management

Medical management should be considered for those patients who did not achieve surgical cure, for whom surgery is contraindicated or in patients who elect not to undergo surgery. There are three classes of medical therapy which may be considered: (1) somatostatin analogues, (2) growth hormone receptor antagonist, and (3) dopamine agonists. These medications are used to decrease the production of growth hormone or block the action of growth hormone on target tissues. Patients with microadenomas are more likely to normalize GH and IGF-1 levels than those with macroadenomas (Melmed 2017).

20.7.2.1 Somatostatin Analogues

The native peptide, somatostatin, circulates throughout the body and attaches to one or more of five somatostatin receptor (SSR) sites found in various central and peripheral tissue. This peptide inhibits growth hormone secretion and regulates a number of gastrointestinal secretions and functions (Melmed 2017). Synthetic somatostatin ligands or analogues (SRL) that mimic the effect of native somatostatins have been developed for clinical use. SSR types 2 and 5 are expressed on somatotroph cells, particularly in GH-secreting adenomas. SRLs octreotide and lanreotide bind to somatostatin receptors, which in turn inhibit the production of growth hormone. Downstream effects include decreasing glucagon, increasing insulin secretion, suppressing pancreatic secretions, and increasing gastrointestinal motility

(Melmed 2017). The latter may lead to a side effect of transient diarrhea in some patients.

Octreotide was the first synthetic somatostatin that suppressed GH and decreased GH and IGF-1 levels in up to 90% of patients in clinical trials. Dosing is by subcutaneous injection every 8 h. Subsequently, somatostatin LAR, a long-acting formulation, given intramuscularly in doses of 20–40 mg every 4 weeks, was found to be safe and effective.

Lanreotide autogel (Somatuline) is another SRL, given as a deep subcutaneous injection in doses of 60, 90, or 120 mg every 28 days. It has been shown to be safely administered at home in some cases, and is approved in the USA for an extended dosing interval of up to 8 weeks (Salvatori et al. 2009).

Most patients will have some response to somatostatin analogues, demonstrated by a drop in GH and IGF-1 levels. However, many patients do not achieve normalization of either marker. Overall, the data suggest that approximately 57% of subjects on octreotide LAR normalize GH levels, and 67% normalize IGF-1 levels, but some studies indicate response rates as low as 41%. Similarly, only 44% of subjects on lanreotide may have normalization of IGF-1 levels (Colao et al. 2015). While the efficacy of somatostatin analogues is sub-optimal, an important characteristic of this class of medication is its effect on tumor shrinkage. About 30% of patients had reduction in tumor size by 20–50% (Colao et al. 2015).

Pasireotide is a somatostatin ligand with a broader affinity to the receptor subtypes over octreotide and lanreotide, and maybe slightly more effective in normalizing GH and IGF-1 levels (Colao et al. 2014a). However, in one head to head study, long-acting formulation of pasireotide achieved biochemical control in 31.3% of the patients compared to 19.2% of the patients treated with octreotide LAR (Colao et al. 2014b). Long-acting pasireotide is given as a once a month, intramuscular injection. One drawback of this medication is its impact on glucose metabolism. New onset diabetes was observed in 19–26% of treated patients, as compared to 4–8% of those treated with long-acting octreotide (Colao et al. 2014b).

Owing to the action of SRLs on pancreatic secretions and gastric motility, the most common side effects in more than 50% of patients are loose stools or diarrhea, nausea and abdominal cramping and gas. These side effects generally occur shortly after initial administration of the medication, and are most often transient in nature and gradually diminish or resolve over time. Biliary tract abnormalities including gallstone formation, biliary sludge and cholelithiasis occur in about 30% of patients, although most patients remain asymptomatic (Freda 2002). Abnormalities in glucose metabolism, hypo- and hyperglycemia, occur in about 2% and 15%, respectively, with up to 26% seen with pasireotide. Other less common side effects include hair loss and hypothyroidism. With the depot preparations, injection site reactions are also common (Freda 2002). Lipodystrophy, sterile abscess, and skin irritations have been reported.

20.7.2.2 Growth Hormone Receptor Antagonist

Pegvisomant is a growth hormone receptor antagonist that blocks the activity of growth hormone. By preventing dimerization at the growth hormone receptor, the critical process of transport of GH into the cell is blocked. Without dimerization, the effect of growth hormone on the cell cannot take place. While systemic GH levels remain elevated in the presence of pegvisomant, due to the nature of the compound's actions, IGF-1 levels are lowered. Initial studies demonstrated normalization of IGF-1 levels in 89% of treated patients (Trainer et al. 2000). There has been some concern that tumor growth may occur in 3–5% of the patients, but it is unclear whether this is due to the nature of the tumor, or due to persistent elevation in systemic GH (Frohman and Bonert 2007).

Pegvisomant is self-administered as a daily injection, and its effectiveness is dependent on patient adherence. It is available in 5 mg incremental doses ranging from 10 to 30 mg. Monitoring of biochemical effects is done through IGF-1 testing, as GH values are expected to be elevated and are therefore not informative (Trainer et al. 2000).

Side effects of pegvisomant can include injection site reactions, including local discomfort and reversible lipoatrophy, abnormal liver function tests, fatigue, and headache.

20.7.2.3 Dopamine Agonist

Dopamine agonists bind to dopamine receptor subtypes, D1 and D2 that are widely found throughout the nervous system and gastrointestinal tract. In healthy individuals, binding will result in stimulation of GH secretion (Jaffe and Barkan 1992). However, in individuals with acromegaly, dopamine agonist binding to these receptors results in an inhibition of GH secretion. The advantage of this class of medication is it's oral administration, and it's relatively lower cost. However, efficacy is low, limiting its use as a monotherapy. Data from several studies show that bromocriptine, the first dopamine agonist to be used in acromegaly, is effective in normalizing IGF-1 in only about 10% of patients (Jaffe and Barkan 1992). Newer dopamine agonists, such as cabergoline and quinagolide, have a greater efficacy rate of between 30 and 44% and are often better tolerated (Abs 1998; Sandret et al. 2011). With such low efficacy rates, dopamine agonists may be used in combination with other medicalx therapies for acromegaly or in those patients with modest elevations in GH or IGF-1 levels. Conversely, dopamine agonists have been used successfully in pituitary tumors which oversecrete prolactin (prolactinomas). Therefore, those patients with acromegaly who have a pituitary tumor that co-secretes GH and prolactin may benefit from medical therapy consisting of combination therapy (dopamine agonist and somatostatin analogue or dopamine agonist and pegvisomant) (Jaffe and Barkan 1992).

Side effects of dopamine agonists include gastrointestinal upset, nausea, headache, postural hypotension, fatigue, nasal congestion, and inhibition of impulse control in some cases. High doses of dopamine agonist used for patients with Parkinson's disease have also resulted in cardiac valve abnormalities (Valassi et al. 2010). However, these abnormalities have not been observed in patients where conservative doses of cabergoline have been used (≤2.0 mg/week) (Valassi et al.

2010). Additionally, no increased risk of valve abnormalities was seen in one study of 42 patients with acromegaly treated with cabergoline for a median of 34 months (Maione et al. 2012).

20.7.2.4 Combination Therapy

Combination therapy, although not FDA approved in the USA, has been used in patients who are not responsive to monotherapy. The combination of somatostatin analogues and dopamine agonists is relatively expensive, and recent studies suggest that IGF-1 levels normalized in about 30–40% of patients (Lim and Fleseriu 2016). This combination therapy is appealing for those patients with mild elevations in IGF-1 levels on somatostatin alone. Additionally, combination of a somatostatin analogue and growth hormone receptor antagonist has been reported to normalize IGF-1 levels in 80–97% of previously uncontrolled patients on monotherapy (Lim and Fleseriu 2016). Although this may achieve biochemical control, the cost of this combination therapy is expensive and requires extra monitoring for elevations in liver function.

20.7.3 Emerging Therapies

New formulations of oral octreotide are currently in clinical trials. One formulation is combined with a transient permeability enhancer (TPE) to allow octreotide absorption by temporarily opening the gap junctions in gut epithelial cells (Melmed et al. 2014). Patients must refrain from eating within 2 h of dosing. The most commonly reported side effect is diarrhea that usually resolves within 2 weeks of starting drug therapy. Efficacy is reported as similar to that of subcutaneous injections of octreotide (Melmed et al. 2014). Additionally, just completed phase 1 clinical trials, CRN00808 is an oral octreotide with a half-life of 42–50 h. Efficacy trials are ongoing (clinical trials.gov).

There are several early stage investigations of molecules designed to block the GH receptors (GHr), resulting in lowering of circulating levels of GH and IGF-1 expression. In recently completed phase 2 clinical trials, ATL1103 administered subcutaneously to two cohorts (once or twice weekly administration) achieved a median fall in IGF-1 of 27.8% from baseline. It was well tolerated in trials with few injection site reactions reported (Trainer et al. 2018). Phase 3 trials are anticipated. Another molecule, ISIS766720 (IONIS GHR-LRX), is an antisense oligonucleotide that also acts to reduce the GHr expression, thus decreasing circulating IGF-1 levels (www.ionispharma.com). Phase 2 studies are planned in patients with acromegaly (clinicaltrials.gov, www.clinicaltrialsregister.eu).

20.7.4 Radiation Therapy

Radiation therapy in acromegaly is primarily used as adjunctive therapy in patients who have not achieved full control through surgical resection, lack of adequate response to medical therapy or with demonstrated tumor growth. Radiation therapy may also be considered to alleviate the burden of lifelong medical therapy (See Chapter: Radiation therapy).

Stereotactic radiotherapy was developed to deliver more focused radiation so as to spare surrounding tissue damage (Minniti et al. 2011). The two types of radiation therapy used to treat acromegaly are conventional fractionated or single dose stereotactic radiosurgery. In conventional fractionated radiation therapy, carefully calculated radiation doses are delivered to a precise area from several angles in divided doses over a period of about 6 weeks (Melmed 2017; Minniti et al. 2011). Patients are usually immobilized in a mask that is placed over the face. GH control is reported in 90% of patients 10 years after treatment. The most rapid decline of around 50% of pre-treatment levels is usually achieved by 2 years after treatment (Minniti et al. 2011). Fractionated treatments are well tolerated and without evidence of cognitive dysfunction, particularly in children after treatment (Minniti et al. 2011). However, there is a risk of optic damage, neurotoxicity, a higher incidence of CVAs, and secondary brain malignancies (2.4% at 20 years) post radiation.

In single dose stereotactic radiosurgery, one high dose is delivered to a single target while the patient is immobilized in a frame. This results in 30–60% of patients achieving remission at 5 years, but may incur a higher risk of radiation-induced side effects (Minniti et al. 2011; Gheorghiu 2017).

It is important to note that patients with active acromegaly continue to require treatment with medical therapy until the radiation takes effect. As GH levels usually fall slowly (over 1–10 years), interim medical therapy is required in over half of post radiation patients (Melmed 2017). Secondary brain neoplasms and radionecrosis may also occur post radiation therapy. Radiation therapy may also be associated with new onset hypopituitarism, requiring ongoing monitoring and initiation of treatment as needed. Regular symptom monitoring, pituitary testing, and MR imaging is indicated post therapy.

20.8 Quality of Life (QoL)

In recent years, the importance of quality of life has become a significant parameter in assessing the overall success in the long-term treatment and management of acromegaly. QoL is recognized by the World Health Organization as one of three patient-related outcome goals along with mortality and morbidity (Geraedts et al. 2017). QoL is multidimensional, comprised of parameters of function such as physical, social, and emotional well-being, and is assessed from the patient perspective. There are multiple general and disease specific tools available for assessment of QOL.

Many studies have demonstrated a decline in QoL in patients with acromegaly despite biochemical disease remission, although results of systematic reviews are inconclusive (Geraedts et al. 2017; Szczesniak et al. 2015; Webb 2006; Webb and Badia 2007). This may be related to factors such as assessments being performed during different stages of the disease, study design, treatment modalities, or differences in parameters assessed. Although drug studies report QoL improvement with currently used medical therapies, significant disease-related decline in QoL compared to the general population persists (Geraedts et al. 2017; Adelman et al. 2013). Significant treatment burdens remain and include: lifestyle restrictions, pain associated with injections, family issues and high economic burden from loss of wages and productivity, medication and health care insurance costs, in some countries (Liu et al. 2017; Yedinak et al. 2018).

Many structural skeletal changes in acromegaly are permanent. Up to 90% of patients with acromegaly report musculoskeletal pain which has a negative correlation on quality of life (Wassenaar et al. 2010). Decreased mobility from increased joint pain and BMI impacts physical functioning and social activities. BMI and boney changes are also associated with changes in body image, contributing to increased anxiety, depression, decreased motivation, and increased social isolation (Biermasz et al. 2004; Conaglen et al. 2015; Crespo et al. 2016; Pantanetti et al. 2002). Osteoarthritic changes and joint space widening may only be partially improved after treatment, contributing to chronic pain and dysfunction (Claessen et al. 2017). Referrals to, and care coordination with, appropriate specialists such as orthopods, counselors and/or psychiatrists and/or rheumatologists should be encouraged.

Cognitive dysfunction is reported to be more prevalent in patients with acromegaly compared to both those with non-functioning pituitary adenomas and the general population. Executive functions of attention, memory, and new learning are affected, particularly when GH and IGF-1

levels are high and may persist, to some extent, despite treatment (Shan et al. 2017; Yedinak and Fleseriu 2013). Cognitive therapy has been demonstrated to improve associated depression, with concomitant improvement in patients perception of QoL (Kunzler et al. 2018). Long-term outcomes and the impact of more specific cognitive training remain unclear.

Comorbidities also play a role in QoL for this patient population. Headaches may improve after treatment but not resolve and may impact many aspects of functioning (Webb and Badia 2007). Screening for other comorbidities such as oncologic diseases, cardiovascular, respiratory (sleep apnea), metabolic (dyslipidemia and diabetes), osteoarticular, and hypopituitarism is recommended pre and post disease remission (Bernabeu et al. 2018). Some studies have suggested that hypopituitarism does not negatively affect QoL (Geraedts et al. 2017). However, other concomitant diseases may all contribute to a decline in QoL (Fig. 20.6).

20.9 Nursing Management Considerations

In addition to medical assessments, nurses must assess physiological, psychological, sociocultural, spiritual, economic, and lifestyle function. As previously discussed, substantial physiologic changes are usually apparent at the time of presentation, with implications for all functional

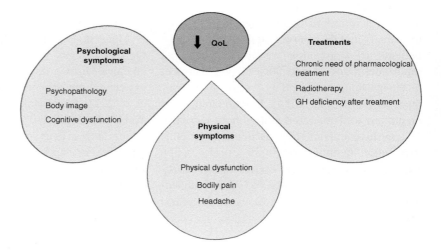

Fig. 20.6 Factors that can affect quality of life (QoL) in patients with acromegaly. From: Crespo, I., Valassi, E. & Webb, S.M. Update on Quality of Life in Patients with Acromegaly. Pituitary (2017) 20: 185. https://doi-org.liboff.ohsu.edu/10.1007/s11102-016-0761-y with permission

domains. Assessment should include family involvement or the patients support structure at diagnosis, as involvement of family/support has shown benefit in treatment adherence and long-term outcomes (Andela et al. 2017; Yedinak 2014). Assessment of memory, coping skills, and mood at baseline can provide direction in the care of these patients. All have been shown to be altered in acromegaly, particularly in the presence of high GH/IGF-1. Baseline assessment alerts the nurse to the potential need for additional resource needs or referrals (Webb and Badia 2007; Yedinak 2014).

Learning styles may also be impacted and require evaluation, although no data was found in the literature in this regard. It is important to note that re-assessment is required as the patient's phase of treatment progresses and life stage needs change.

Medical diagnosis can generate considerable anxiety and relief. Anxiety has been shown to impair memory and patients with acromegaly have also been found to have impaired verbal memory (Crespo et al. 2015). Patients express relief that their symptoms are legitimized with a diagnosis, but the patient may not have realistic posttreatment expectations. Therefore, it is vital to explore the patients' perception of treatment outcomes.

Much disease related information is now freely available on the internet, although not all information is accurate. Determination of the level of patient knowledge and the source of the patient's information can help frame patient and family education needs.

Key issues from patient assessment to address in care planning include: patient and family knowledge regarding acromegaly, the learning style of the patient; how realistic are treatment expectations; resource deficits, particularly with respect to accuracy of information sources; economic and social support; geographic limitations; the patient's level of anxiety and depression; local health care provider availability. Disturbed body image and uncompensated or deficient coping skills will need to be considered in treatment planning.

Care planning is patient centered and goal directed toward self-efficacy. In this model of care, the patient and family are involved in all care decisions. Motivational interviewing is a useful technique when mutually establishing measurable and achievable short- and long-range goals is based on the patient needs assessment. Goals must be meaningful to the patient for best adherence (Hall et al. 2012).

Planning involves multiple phases of care. Beginning with the execution of appropriate testing, preparation for hospitalization progresses through discharge planning and postoperative workup to determine remission versus the need for long-term therapy, medical and or radiologic treatments.

Care planning is complex, requires multidisciplinary collaboration, and must be adaptable. Patient needs change with phase of treatment, age, and life stage, with social and economic changes requiring ongoing adaptation. At each visit it is recommended that the patients' clinical condition, and their geographic, economic, and psychological concerns, treatment expectations and goals be addressed (Plunkett and Barkan 2015). It is estimated that 17–21% of patients with acromegaly are lost to follow-up with around 88% of these patients thought to have uncontrolled disease (Kasuki et al. 2012; Scott et al. 2004). Outcomes must be regularly reviewed and a plan revised to achieve better patient continuity and outcomes.

20.10 Long-Term Management

All patients with a history of acromegaly require periodic evaluations lifelong. The joint European and US Endocrine Societies clinical guidelines recommend a definition of remission as an IGF-1 in normal range for age and gender and a GH of <1 μg/L with glucose suppression. However, an undetectable GH (<0.04 μg/L) along with a normal IGF-1 is thought to be a more rigorous indicator of remission (Katznelson et al. 2014). Using the same GH/IGF-1 assay throughout treatment is advised. Monitoring comorbidities, thyroid studies, and assessment for hypopituitarism is indicated (Katznelson et al. 2014). Follow-up MRI is the suggested imaging modality, but there is no guideline for follow-up imaging beyond 12 weeks postoperatively. Others recommend varying intervals from 20 to 12 months for the first 5 years and then every 5 years lifelong (Fig. 20.7).

Recurrence rates are low, but may be higher in young patients with larger tumors found to be sparsely granulated on pathology (Melmed 2017;

Swearingen et al. 1998). Close and long-term monitoring is necessary. Treatment modalities, particularly transsphenoidal surgery and radiation therapy, may result in damage to the pituitary gland which may lead to the development of hypopituitarism. Hypopituitarism requires frequent biochemical testing and replacement of the missing or decreased pituitary hormones particularly post radiation therapy. Post radiation therapy, ongoing imaging is also recommended for

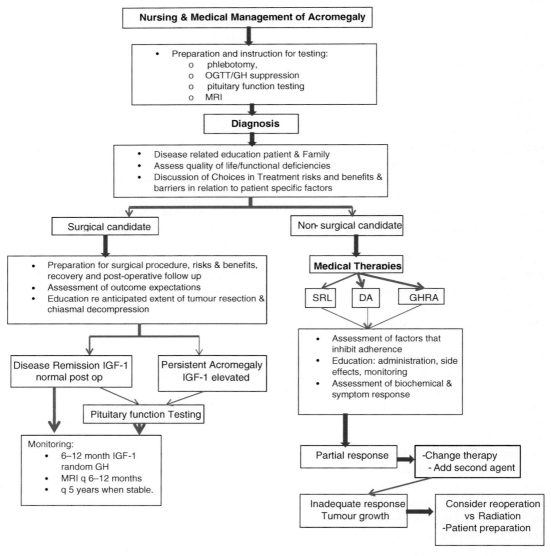

Fig. 20.7 Acromegaly management algorithm. Adapted from: Acromegaly: An Endocrine Society Clinical Practice Guideline J Clin Endocrinol Metab. 2014;99(11):3933–3951. doi:https://doi.org/10.1210/jc.2014-2700. Copyright © 2014 by the Endocrine Society. This article is published under the terms of the Creative Commons Attribution-Non Commercial-No Derivatives License (CC-BY-NC-ND; http://creativecommons.org/licenses/by-nc-nd/4.0/)

secondary tumors that may develop in the field of radiation (Minniti et al. 2011).

Guidelines also recommend monitoring for comorbidities, and for the development or worsening of cardiovascular diseases such as coronary artery disease, cardiomyopathy, and hypertension (Katznelson et al. 2014). Respiratory dysfunction and sleep apnea may persist despite disease remission. Since exposure to elevated IGF-1 levels have been implicated in the development of certain malignancies, routine screening tests for the detection of cancer should be performed on a regular basis and should include colonoscopies for the detection of cancerous colon polyps.

Finally, since there are many clinical features of acromegaly that do not improve with remission of the disease, health care providers should not hesitate to refer a patient to a specialist if needed. Many patients will still have clinical conditions associated with changes to bone and cartilage, such as the development of arthritis or joint issues that require referral to appropriate specialists.

20.11 Home Care Educational Programme

Starting a new medicine solicits many questions about the underlying diagnosis, symptoms, complications, and expected outcomes. A new medicine also means another responsibility for the patient, subcutaneous injections that are to be self administered. Patients have high expectations when a new drug has been introduced. However, they lack confidence in using unfamiliar equipment, substances, and techniques. They are particularly concerned about accuracy in drug preparation, administration, and side effects. The home care educational programme was developed to address these questions and concerns.

20.11.1 Programme Goals

(a) Assist the patient to become confident in self-injection technique.
(b) Provide the support of a trained specialist endocrine nurse.

(c) To improve adherence to drug administration schedules.
(d) To support self-care and improve quality of life.
(e) To provide patient focused education, with an emphasis on self-care, tailored to the specific needs of the individual patient.

20.11.2 Role of the Specialist Endocrine Nurse in Home Care

- Highly valued by patients
- Provides support as needed
- Provides personal contact
- Time to listen
- Knowledgeable about acromegaly
- Respects patient autonomy
- Available to answer questions
- Provide consistent follow-up
- Understand the emotional aspects of disease and diagnosis (Scott et al. 2004).
  - Phase 1: first symptoms, patient worried, feel misunderstood, very eager to find a "cure" or an answer. Risk of being lost to follow-up.
  - Phase 2 Diagnosis: patients are relieved when receiving a correct, final diagnosis.
  - Phase 3 Start of treatment: patients are unaware of the complexity of treatment and the implications of the disease.
  - Phase 4 Follow-up: patients accept the situation as it is, yet are sometimes unaware that follow-up and prevention are needed.

20.11.3 Method: A Home Care Programme

This programme is modeled after successful home care programmes for diabetes and CHD (Scott et al. 2004; Corbett 2003). The key to a successful programme is mutual goal setting.

The programme is divided into four face-to-face visits during the first week (day 1–2–3–7), and after 1 month, there are regular phone calls to

answer questions or titrate dose. Visits are scheduled when needed.

20.11.4 Programme Content

Week 1 (Day 1, 2, 3, and 7).
- Explanation of the disease and the chosen medical therapy.
- Description of the importance of adherence to prescription (dose and frequency).
- Outline of possible side effects
- Demonstration of use of injection technique and patient practice manipulating equipment.
- Description of drug dose and titration protocol.
- Day 7 patient reviewed in autonomous drug administration.
- Questions are answered by specialist endocrine nurse as they arise.
- Observations reported to patient's endocrinologist.

20.11.5 Programme Conclusion

This home care programme assigns one nurse who coaches a group of patients for an introductory week and at regular intervals thereafter. The programme improves patient satisfaction, assists patient adherence to treatment, and improves quality of life by attaining rapid IGF-1/GH normalization.

Patient feedback is positive. They are grateful for the education and training, feel independent and motivated by improved biochemical results, and have a sense of security by establishing direct communication with their endocrine team.

A home care programme for patients with acromegaly was initiated in 2011 at the Ghent University Hospital in Belgium. The protocol was approved by the ethical committee. The programme has since been expanded to 20 hospitals in Flanders, Belgium.

20.12 Conclusions

Patients with acromegaly suffer from physical, social, and psychological challenges related to the disease, many of which can persist during

and after treatment and significantly modify quality of life. The nurses' role is critical in addressing and managing these issues through collaborative medical management, disease-related education, promotion of treatment adherence and lifestyle modifications, coordination of management of comorbidities and more. Multiple studies have shown that assessing and addressing known quality of life indicators in this population should be incorporated into the regular care of patients with acromegaly for best outcomes.

20.13 Patient Case Studies

Case Study 1
A 59-year-old man was referred for further assessment and treatment of suspected acromegaly. Symptoms include aching in his fingers, shoulders, hips, and knees, as well as snoring. On physical examination, his blood pressure is 150/95 mm Hg, he had acromegalic facies, wide fingers and toes, and crepitation on flexion and extension of both knees. His serum IGF-1 level is 753 ng/mL (98.6 nmol/L), (reference range, 41–279 ng/mL [5.4–36.5 nmol/L]) and his fasting blood glucose level is 142 mg/dL (7.9 mmol/L). His baseline GH is 11.7 ng/ml (11.7 µg/L). MRI was obtained and an 11 mm mass on the right side of the sella was visible. Transsphenoidal surgery is recommended. He asks if any of his abnormalities will persist even if the surgery is successful.

Question: what is this patient's morbidity and mortality risk?

Case Study 2
A 23-year-old man is referred for acromegaly. His height is 74 in. (188 cm), and his weight is 210 lb. (95.5 kg). His hands and feet are enlarged, and he has prognathism. A paternal uncle was thought to have had a pituitary adenoma of uncertain type. There is no known family history of calcium disorders or kidney stones. A random GH level is 33 ng/mL (33 µg/L), and his serum IGF-1 concentration is 811 ng/mL (106.2 nmol/L) (reference range, 147–527 ng/mL [19.3–69.0 nmol/L]). His serum calcium level is nor-

mal. MRI shows a 4.3-cm pituitary adenoma with suprasellar extension.

Question: Does this patient have a genetic risk?

20.14   Patient Stories

Patient 1

In 2014, at the age of 36, I had been having irregular periods. I would alternate having one every other month. Since I had always been regular in the past, I tracked my periods for several months and discussed the pattern with my primary doctor at my annual appointment in December, 2014. Lab work found that my prolactin was high at 59.7 ng/mL (normal 3–13 ng/ml).

She scheduled an MRI with contrast in January 2015, and there was a 1.1 cm tumor on my pituitary. It was assumed to be a prolactinoma. I was referred to an endocrinologist, and in March, 2015, my prolactin was still elevated, but my IGF-1 was also high (432 ng/mL) (reference range 128–291 ng/mL). Looking at the MRI, she said that the tumor was pressing against the pituitary stalk, so the elevated prolactin was likely a product of "stalk effect."

A glucose suppression test in April 2015 showed baseline GH was 1.1 ng/mL, which did not suppress to a level of less than 1.0. This confirmed that I had acromegaly.

I was then referred to a neurologist at the University Pituitary Clinic. Surgery was in June 2015, and the neurosurgeon was fairly sure that she had been able to remove the entire tumor. My prolactin levels immediately went back to normal. About a week after surgery, my sodium levels were low (119 mMol/L). I was readmitted to the hospital and placed on a one liter a day fluid restriction. After 2 days, my sodium levels went back to normal, and I was discharged.

At my 1-month follow-up in July 2015, my IGF-1 was still elevated (403 ng/mL). They decided to re-test in a few months. In September 2015, my IGF-1 had decreased to 346 ng/mL, but was still high. Finally, in November 2015, my IGF-1 had fallen into normal range—283 ng/mL!! What a relief! In December 2015, I repeated the glucose suppression test, and my GH level suppressed to 0.3 ng/mL, indicating remission!

I am happy to report that my IGF-1 levels and MRI results have continued to be normal over the last few years since surgery: September 2016/205 ng/mL, and September 2017/150 ng/mL (range 57–241).

I have noticed a decrease in swelling of my face, hands, and tongue as well as less joint pain since surgery. My cholesterol levels have also improved.

Patient 2

I was diagnosed with acromegaly in October of 2010. My condition, like many, if not most of the stories I read and hear about, was missed for many years. In my case, doctors estimated probably around 30 years.

When I look back, it is difficult to isolate many of the symptoms that now clearly were due to the overproduction of growth hormone. Now, hindsight being 20–20, it all makes sense. I am now 63 years old and was diagnosed with acromegaly at age 56. In retrospect, the signs started in my early to mid-30s. My physical characteristics kept changing. I was getting bigger: my hands, my chest, my muscles, my feet, and even my head was growing. I thought it was the process of aging. It never occurred to me that this was not normal. I clearly remember my dentist noticing bottom teeth separation and my primary care physician noticing my blood pressure was consistently higher than normal. I was put on mild hypertension medication in my late 30s to early 40s. By my mid to late 40s my blood sugars started to rise. Sleep apnea was another tail-tell sign. My wife noticed alarming sings of apneas (breathing stops while at sleep). In my early to mid 40s I started noticing marked pain in my leg joints specifically knees, ankles, and hips as well as a noticeable lack of energy.

I met my endocrinologist and neurosurgeon at the Center for Pituitary Disorders on a dreary, grey, drippy November San Francisco morning. "How fitting," I thought, you're going to get bad news on a miserable day! They were amazingly reassuring, particularly to my wife Carol, who was very, very worried. After all, it is not every day you are told you have a tumor in your head. For some strange reason, I was as calm as I've ever been. Finally, knowing exactly what had been bothering me for so many years was like a 5000-pound rock lifted off my back. My first thought, as I was listening to their explanations, the surgery, medical treatment steps, and what the future would hold was: "these guys ooze competence." I was reassured with these two doctors and could not wait to get this thing out of my head.

Three months earlier I had gone to an orthopedic surgeon who recommended a hip replacement and, "by the way, I think you have a condition called Acromegaly." He told me what it was and what caused it. I must have looked at him in horror because immediately, he felt compelled to tell me I was not going to die. He had a colleague with acromegaly and a golf-ball-size pituitary tumor was removed.

At home I "googled" "Acromegaly" and THERE IT WAS!!!. "How is this possible" I thought. The screen was filled with people that looked like me. "I have almost every symptom listed" I screamed loud enough for my wife to hear me three rooms away. "You mean to tell me there are other people running around with this?" "I have most of the physical characteristics!", "Andre the Giant has this?. Don't any of these doctors I've been seeing for 30 years know about this?" "My grandmother could have diagnosed me. I could have diagnosed it," I thought angrily. It was so evident to me!

I felt ignorant, then angry, then depressed. But I also realized that as a patient I should have been more aware and perhaps, if I had been more aware of potential pituitary conditions, I could have asked better questions and help the doctors focus on a diagnosis earlier. I knew things would get better, but growing for 30 years had done irreversible damage to my bones and joints. That was the end of some of my favorite things: tennis, backpacking, hiking, even standing and walking for long periods of time. I was going to have to adjust to all of that.

During transsphenoidal surgery 95% of the pituitary adenoma was removed, but my determination to use my skills to help raise awareness of acromegaly and pituitary disorders so that people could be diagnosed early and properly, was

peaked. The word about acromegaly is not getting out fast or efficiently enough.

I had developed an admiration and great friendship with my endocrinologist. We decided to move forward on a doctor–patient collaborative approach and communicate, not just the medical and scientific knowledge, but also what it is like to live with the chronic conditions associated with acromegaly. The eNews magazine Pituitary World News was the result.

Pituitary World News is a communication and publishing platform designed to encourage collaborations, innovation and creativity between industry experts, the healthcare community and patients and their families. Through awareness and communication strategies its mission is to reduce the time it take to diagnosis, improve knowledge and quality of life.

Published by permission of the author Jorge D Faccinetti.

20.15 Patient Advocacy Groups

The World Alliance of Pituitary Organizations (WAPO) is a self-governed non-profit organization created in order to unite the international pituitary patient community to push for optimal treatment and care for all patients with pituitary and related conditions worldwide. The goal of this organization is to share information, work together, and support all pituitary patients' advocates all around the world. WAPO believes in the strength of a global network of national pituitary patient organizations, which will lead to better outcomes worldwide (Fig. 20.8). The Acromegaly Community is a patient support and advocacy group for people affected by acromegaly patients,

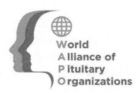

Fig. 20.8 World Association of Pituitary Organization (WAPO)

their families and friends. Presently, the group has over 2000 members worldwide. They provide an emotional and communal support network for people touched by Acromegaly and offer information on issues of interest to people with the disease and provide a network of emotional support for Acromegaly patients, their friends and their family. The Acromegaly Community Website: https://www.acromegalycommunity.org

20.15.1 Best Practice "Bulgarian Association of Patients with Acromegaly"

One WAPO's member organization is the Bulgarian Association of Patients with Acromegaly (ABAB), who has been raising awareness for acromegaly for more than 7 years. For the last 5 years we have been involved in a court trial regarding "access to radiosurgery" and "parallel export or shortage of medicines." Both campaigns were widely spread by the Bulgarian media over a 5-year period. This amounted to an awareness campaign.

One of the most successful ABAB campaigns is the "Shoe Shop project" (Fig. 20.9). The Patient association contacted two Shoe Shop companies in Bulgaria who were already selling "big size shoes." Only one of the two stores accepted to meet and now supports the "Shoe Shop project." The patient advocacy group prepared information brochures, created from validated information on acromegaly. The brochure

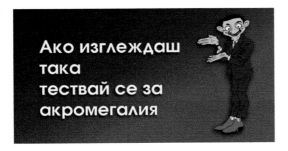

Fig. 20.9 Bulgarian Association of Patients with Acromegaly Email: acromegaly@abv.bgwebsite: http://www.pituitary-bg.com

invited people to be alert for symptoms and encouraged them to be seen by a specialist. The material was translated and approved by a local endocrinology and used in the ABAB campaign (Acromegaly Shoe Shop Awareness). These brochures were distributed by the shoe shop in the boxes of purchased shoes. The shoe company made special boxes for display with a sign to their clients: "**If your feet and hands are growing, check for *acromegaly*.**"

The shoe shop entrepreneur also donated a pair of shoes to ABAB's tallest member and a journalist wrote an article about the support of the shoe shop, as well as highlighting the awareness campaign.

The next awareness campaigns will focus on access to expert diagnostic centers, medications, and reimbursement for treatment. The only center currently is in the capital city Sofia, and not accessible for rural patients.

As in Bulgaria, pituitary patients encounter similar problems in countries worldwide. The most important is late diagnosis. It takes on average 8–10 years to identify the pituitary diseases since their symptoms are not very specific and the cases are so rare. In some countries the situation is even worse and most patients either don't get treatment at all or get to the neurosurgeon when the adenoma is too large to operate. Even when diagnosed, in many countries, patients do not get appropriate treatment on time. Even when treated, patients still suffer from comorbidities, both physical and psychological.

The number or pituitary patients is relatively small but when they join their voices, they become a real power. To this end, patient groups and organizations appear in most countries. The main goals of a patient group are: (1) to represent patients in communication with health care authorities and policy makers, to advocate for patients, (2) to raise awareness about the pituitary diseases among health care professionals and general public, and (3) to empower patients so that they act in order to improve their own situation, either through better adherence, better communication, lifestyle change, or legal action.

Patient organizations are in most cases not-for-profit organizations acting in the best interest of the patients they represent. To make patient organization's activity most efficient, they try to co-operate with health care authorities, doctors, and nurses. Patient advocates are not doctors and cannot make prescriptions. However, patients tend to trust other patients so patient groups can spread the word about the importance of adherence, about patient rights and duties. Patient groups also raise awareness about the disease, thus improving the chances of undiagnosed patients to be diagnosed. These activities require support from all people involved with pituitary patient care including nurses and doctors.

There are patient groups or patient organizations active in most of the countries in the world. In some countries the organizations are well established, like the UK Pituitary Foundation. They have stable financial support from diverse base of sponsors and many fundraising events. In other countries patient groups are just starting their activities and trying to find their way to sustainability. It is not an easy path. In any case they both are ready to support patients and need your support and active involvement.

Some of the many projects in which member organizations are involved include: Acromegaly Community, US, the Vancouver Acromegaly Support Group, Canada are holding Acromegaly Awareness Days; Velikan, the Russian Pituitary Patient Organization, has launched a program for information and legal support for pituitary patients in Russia; The Spanish Association of People Affected by Acromegaly and the Pituitary Alliance of Latin America, jointly enacted a program of awareness of acromegaly; The dental school of Lima, Peru launched a program to educate dentists in signs an symptoms of acromegaly to promote early diagnosis.

To learn more about patient organizations in your region you can address to WAPO, the World Alliance of Pituitary Organizations (www.wapo.org and facebook.com/wapo.org). WAPO was created in 2016 after a series of annual meetings of patient advocacies from all over the world. The WAPO mission is to identify pituitary organizations, to guide the development of their organization, and to create an active global network (Fig. 20.10).

As of May 2017, WAPO membership included 33 organizations from 24 countries (see the map)

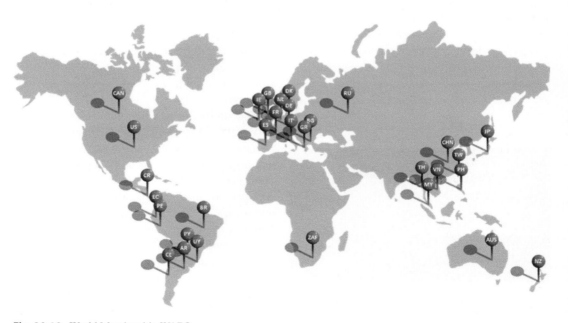

Fig. 20.10 World Membership WAPO

representing 30% of global population of patients with pituitary diseases.

If there is no patient group in your region, maybe you know active people that are ready to create one. Please introduce them to WAPO at mail@wapo.org. In this case WAPO will provide the activists with the best practices collected over the years and all possible support from its members.

Together we can improve the life of pituitary patients worldwide!

Acknowledgement The author acknowledges Shlomo Melmed MB, ChB, FRCP, MACP who is the Professor Cedars-Sinai Medical Center, Dean of the Medical Faculty and Executive Vice President, Chief Academic Officer, Director, Cedars-Sinai Research Institute, Los Angeles, CA, USA.

Special thanks also to Muriël Marks–de Korver, WAPO Executive Director, the World Alliance of Pituitary Organizations (WAPO) (http://www.wapo.org) for her contribution to this chapter with case studies, patient resources, and information on the Patient Advocacy Group

References

Abreu A, Tovar AP, Castellanos R, Valenzuela A, Giraldo CMG, Pinedo AC, et al. Challenges in the diagnosis and management of acromegaly: a focus on comorbidities. Pituitary. 2016;19(4):448–57.

Abs R. Cabergoline in the treatment of acromegaly: a study in 64 patients. J Clin Endocrinol Metab. 1998;83(2):374–8.

Adelman D, Liebert N, Lamerson BB. Acromegaly: the disease, its impact on patients, and managing the burden of long-term treatment. Int J Gen Med. 2013;6:31.

Alexopoulou O, Bex M, Kamenicky P, Mvoula AB, Chanson P, Maiter D. Prevalence and risk factors of impaired glucose tolerance and diabetes mellitus at diagnosis of acromegaly: a study in 148 patients. Pituitary. 2013;17(1):81–9.

Andela CD, Tiemensma J, Kaptein AA, Scharloo M, Pereira AM, Kamminga NGA, et al. The partner's perspective of the impact of pituitary disease: looking beyond the patient. J Health Psychol. 2017:135910531769542.

Annamalai AK, Gayton EL, Webb A, Halsall DJ, Rice C, Ibram F, et al. Increased prevalence of gallbladder polyps in acromegaly. J Clin Endocrinol Metab. 2011;96(7):E1120–E5.

Attal P, Chanson P. Screening of acromegaly in adults with obstructive sleep apnea: is it worthwhile? Endocrine. 2018;61(1):4–6.

Beauregard C, Truong U, Hardy J, Serri O. Long-term outcome and mortality after transsphenoidal adenomectomy for acromegaly. Clin Endocrinol. 2003;58(1):86–91.

Ben-Shlomo A, Melmed S. Skin manifestations in acromegaly. Clin Dermatol. 2006;24(4):256–9.

Bernabeu I, Aller J, Álvarez-Escolá C, Fajardo-Montañana C, Gálvez-Moreno Á, Guillín-Amarelle C, et al. Criteria for diagnosis and postoperative control of acromegaly, and screening and management of its comorbidities: expert consensus. Endocrinol Diabetes Nutr (English ed). 2018;65(5):297–305.

Biermasz NR, van Thiel SW, Pereira AM, Hoftijzer HC, van Hemert AM, Smit JWA, et al. Decreased quality of life in patients with acromegaly despite long-term cure of growth hormone excess. J Clin Endocrinol Metab. 2004;89(11):5369–76.

Bonert VS, Melmed S. Growth hormone. In: Melmed S, editor. The pituitary. London: Elsevier; 2017. p. 85–127.

Burton T, Le Nestour E, Bancroft T, Neary M. Real-world comorbidities and treatment patterns of patients with acromegaly in two large US health plan databases. Pituitary. 2012;16(3):354–62.

Capatina C, Wass JAH. 60 YEARS OF NEUROENDOCRINOLOGY: Acromegaly. J Endocrinol. 2015;226(2):T141–T60.

Chanson P, Salenave S. Acromegaly. Orphanet J Rare Dis. 2008;3(1):17.

Chanson P, Salenave S, Kamenicky P. Acromegaly. Handb Clin Neurol. 2014;124:197–219. https://doi.org/10.1016/B978-0-444-59602-4.00014-9.

Chesnokova V, Zonis S, Zhou C, Recouvreux MV, Ben-Shlomo A, Araki T, et al. Growth hormone is permissive for neoplastic colon growth. Proc Natl Acad Sci. 2016;113(23):E3250–E9.

Claessen KMJA, Canete AN, de Bruin PW, Pereira AM, Kloppenburg M, Kroon HM, et al. Acromegalic arthropathy in various stages of the disease: an MRI study. Eur J Endocrinol. 2017;176(6):779–90.

Colao A. Improvement of cardiac parameters in patients with acromegaly treated with medical therapies. Pituitary. 2012;15(1):50–8.

Colao A, Cuocolo A, Marzullo P, Nicolai E, Ferone D, Morte AMD, et al. Impact of patient's age and disease duration on cardiac performance in acromegaly: a radionuclide angiography study. J Clin Endocrinol Metab. 1999;84(5):1518–23.

Colao A, Vandeva S, Pivonello R, Grasso LFS, Nachev E, Auriemma RS, et al. Could different treatment approaches in acromegaly influence life expectancy? A comparative study between Bulgaria and Campania (Italy). Eur J Endocrinol. 2014a;171(2):263–73.

Colao A, Bronstein MD, Freda P, Gu F, Shen CC, Gadelha M, et al. Pasireotide versus octreotide in acromegaly: a head-to-head superiority study. J Clin Endocrinol Metab. 2014b;99(3):791–9.

Colao A, Auriemma RS, Pivonello R, Kasuki L, Gadelha MR. Interpreting biochemical control response rates with first-generation somatostatin analogues in acromegaly. Pituitary. 2015;19(3):235–47.

Conaglen HM, de Jong D, Crawford V, Elston MS, Conaglen JV. Body image disturbance in acromegaly patients compared to nonfunctioning pituitary adenoma patients and controls. Int J Endocrinol. 2015;2015:1–8.

Corbett CF. A randomized pilot study of improving foot care in home health patients with diabetes. Diabetes Educ. 2003;29(2):273–82.

Crespo I, Santos A, Valassi E, Pires P, Webb SM, Resmini E. Impaired decision making and delayed memory are related with anxiety and depressive symptoms in acromegaly. Endocrine. 2015;50(3):756–63.

Crespo I, Valassi E, Webb SM. Update on quality of life in patients with acromegaly. Pituitary. 2016;20(1):185–8.

Cuevas-Ramos D, Carmichael JD, Cooper O, Bonert VS, Gertych A, Mamelak AN, et al. A structural and functional acromegaly classification. J Clin Endocrinol Metab. 2015;100(1):122–31.

Dal J, Leisner MZ, Hermansen K, Farkas DK, Bengtsen M, Kistorp C, et al. Cancer incidence in patients with acromegaly: a cohort study and meta-analysis of the literature. J Clin Endocrinol Metab. 2018;103(6):2182–8.

Daly AF, Rixhon M, Adam C, Dempegioti A, Tichomirowa MA, Beckers A. High prevalence of pituitary adenomas: a cross-sectional study in the Province of Liège, Belgium. J Clin Endocrinol Metab. 2006;91(12):4769–75.

Esposito D, Ragnarsson O, Granfeldt D, Marlow T, Johannsson G, Olsson DS. Decreasing mortality and changes in treatment patterns in patients with acromegaly from a nationwide study. Eur J Endocrinol. 2018;178(5):459–69.

Faria ACS, Veldhuis JD, Thorner MO, Vance ML. Half-time of endogenous growth hormone (GH) disappearance in normal man after stimulation of GH secretion by GH-releasing hormone and suppression with somatostatin. J Clin Endocrinol Metab. 1989;68(3):535–41.

Freda PU. Somatostatin analogs in acromegaly. J Clin Endocrinol Metab. 2002;87(7):3013–8.

Frohman LA, Bonert V. Pituitary tumor enlargement in two patients with acromegaly during pegvisomant therapy. Pituitary. 2007;10(3):283–9.

Galoiu S, Poiana C. Current therapies and mortality in acromegaly. J Med Life. 2015;8(4):411–5.

Geraedts VJ, Andela CD, Stalla GK, Pereira AM, van Furth WR, Sievers C, et al. Predictors of quality of life in acromegaly: no consensus on biochemical parameters. Front Endocrinol (Lausanne). 2017;8:40.

Gheorghiu ML. Updates in outcomes of stereotactic radiation therapy in acromegaly. Pituitary. 2017;20(1):154–68.

Grunstein RR. Sleep apnea in acromegaly. Ann Intern Med. 1991;115(7):527.

Guo X, Zhao Y, Wang M, Gao L, Wang Z, Zhang Z, et al. The posterior pharyngeal wall thickness is associated with OSAHS in patients with acromegaly and correlates with IGF-1 levels. Endocrine. 2018; https://doi.org/10.1007/s12020-018-1631-3.

Gurel MH, Bruening PR, Rhodes C, Lomax KG. Patient perspectives on the impact of acromegaly: results from individual and group interviews. Patient Prefer Adherence. 2014;8:53–62.

Hall K, Gibbie T, Lubman DI. Motivational interviewing techniques - facilitating behaviour change in the general practice setting. Aust Fam Physician. 2012;41(9):660–7.

Heringer LC, de Oliveira MF, Rotta JM, Botelho RV. Effect of repeated transsphenoidal surgery in recurrent or residual pituitary adenomas: a systematic review and meta-analysis. Surg Neurol Int. 2016;7:14.

Jaffe CA, Barkan AL. Treatment of acromegaly with dopamine agonists. Endocrinol Metab Clin N Am. 1992;21(3):713–35.

Kamenicky P, Viengchareun S, Blanchard A, Meduri G, Zizzari P, Imbert-Teboul M, et al. Epithelial sodium channel is a key mediator of growth hormone-induced sodium retention in acromegaly. Endocrinology. 2008;149(7):3294–305.

Kasuki L, Marques NV, Nuez MJBL, Leal VLG, Chinen RN, Gadelha MR. Acromegalic patients lost to follow-up: a pilot study. Pituitary. 2012;16(2):245–50.

Katznelson L, Laws ER, Melmed S, Molitch ME, Murad MH, Utz A, et al. Acromegaly: an endocrine society clinical practice guideline. J Clin Endocrinol Metab. 2014;99(11):3933–51.

Knutzen R, Ezzat S. The cost of medical care for the acromegalic patient. Neuroendocrinology. 2006;83(3–4):139–44.

Kunzler LS, Naves LA, Casulari LA. Cognitive-behavioral therapy improves the quality of life of patients with acromegaly. Pituitary. 2018;21(3):323–33.

Lavrentaki A, Paluzzi A, Wass JAH, Karavitaki N. Epidemiology of acromegaly: review of population studies. Pituitary. 2016;20(1):4–9.

Lim DST, Fleseriu M. The role of combination medical therapy in the treatment of acromegaly. Pituitary. 2016;20(1):136–48.

Liu S, Adelman DT, Xu Y, Sisco J, Begelman SM, Webb SM, et al. Patient-centered assessment on disease burden, quality of life, and treatment satisfaction associated with acromegaly. J Investig Med. 2017;66(3):653–60.

Maione L, Garcia C, Bouchachi A, Kallel N, Maison P, Salenave S, et al. No evidence of a detrimental effect of cabergoline therapy on cardiac valves in patients with acromegaly. J Clin Endocrinol Metab. 2012;97(9):E1714–E9.

Maione L, Brue T, Beckers A, Delemer B, Petrossians P, Borson-Chazot F, et al. Changes in the management and comorbidities of acromegaly over three decades: the French Acromegaly Registry. Eur J Endocrinol. 2017;176(5):645–55.

Mazziotti G, Bianchi A, Bonadonna S, Cimino V, Patelli I, Fusco A, et al. Prevalence of vertebral fractures in men with acromegaly. J Clin Endocrinol Metab. 2008;93(12):4649–55.

Mazziotti G, Bianchi A, Porcelli T, Mormando M, Maffezzoni F, Cristiano A, et al. Vertebral fractures in patients with acromegaly: a 3-year prospective study. J Clin Endocrinol Metab. 2013;98(8):3402–10.

Melmed S. Acromegaly. In: Melmed S, editor. The pituitary. London: Elsevier; 2017. p. 423–66.

Melmed S, Casanueva F, Cavagnini F, Chanson P, Frohman LA, Gaillard R, et al. Consensus statement: medical management of acromegaly. Eur J Endocrinol. 2005;153(6):737–40.

Melmed S, Kleinberg DL, Bonert V, Fleseriu M. Acromegaly: assessing the disorder and navigating therapeutic options for treatment. Endocr Pract. 2014;20(Suppl 1):7–17; quiz 8–20

Minniti G, Scaringi C, Enrici R. Radiation techniques for acromegaly. Radiat Oncol. 2011;6(1):167.

Montini M, Gianola D, Paganl MD, Pedroncelli A, Caldara R, Gherardi F, et al. Cholelithiasis and acromegaly: therapeutic strategies. Clin Endocrinol. 2010;40(3):401–6.

Morris CJ, Aeschbach D, Scheer FAJL. Circadian system, sleep and endocrinology. Mol Cell Endocrinol. 2012;349(1):91–104.

Nachtigall L, Delgado A, Swearingen B, Lee H, Zerikly R, Klibanski A. Changing patterns in diagnosis and therapy of acromegaly over two decades. J Clin Endocrinol Metab. 2008;93(6):2035–41.

Pantanetti P, Sonino N, Arnaldi G, Boscaro M. Self image and quality of life in acromegaly. Pituitary. 2002;5(1):17–9.

Pivonello R, Auriemma RS, Grasso LFS, Pivonello C, Simeoli C, Patalano R, et al. Complications of acromegaly: cardiovascular, respiratory and metabolic comorbidities. Pituitary. 2017;20(1):46–62.

Plunkett C, Barkan A. The care continuum in acromegaly: how patients, nurses, and physicians can collaborate for successful treatment experiences. Patient Prefer Adherence. 2015;9:1093.

Raverot G, Dantony E, Beauvy J, Vasiljevic A, Mikolasek S, Borson-Chazot F, et al. Risk of recurrence in pituitary neuroendocrine tumors: a prospective study using a five-tiered classification. J Clin Endocrinol Metab. 2017;102(9):3368–74.

Salvatori R, Nachtigall LB, Cook DM, Bonert V, Molitch ME, Blethen S, et al. Effectiveness of self- or partner-administration of an extended-release aqueous-gel formulation of lanreotide in lanreotide-naïve patients with acromegaly. Pituitary. 2009;13(2):115–22.

Sandret L, Maison P, Chanson P. Place of cabergoline in acromegaly: a meta-analysis. J Clin Endocrinol Metab. 2011;96(5):1327–35.

Schöfl C, Petroff D, Tönjes A, Grussendorf M, Droste M, Stalla G, et al. Incidence of myocardial infarction and stroke in acromegaly patients: results from the German Acromegaly Registry. Pituitary. 2017;20(6):635–42.

Scott L, Setterkline K, Britton A. The effects of nursing interventions to enhance mental health and quality of life among individuals with heart failure. Appl Nurs Res. 2004;17(4):248–56.

Shan S, Fang L, Huang J, Chan RCK, Jia G, Wan W. Evidence of dysexecutive syndrome in patients with acromegaly. Pituitary. 2017;20(6):661–7.

Sharma MD, Nguyen AV, Brown S, Robbins RJ. Cardiovascular disease in acromegaly. Methodist Debakey Cardiovasc J. 2017;13(2):64–7.

Swearingen B, Barker FG, Katznelson L, Biller BMK, Grinspoon S, Klibanski A, et al. Long-term mortality after transsphenoidal surgery and adjunctive therapy for acromegaly. J Clin Endocrinol Metab. 1998;83(10):3419–26.

Szczesniak D, Jawiarczyk-Przybylowska A, Rymaszewska J. The quality of life and psychological, social and cognitive functioning of patients with acromegaly. Adv Clin Exp Med. 2015;24(1):167–72.

Terzolo M, Reimondo G, Berchialla P, Ferrante E, Malchiodi E, De Marinis L, et al. Acromegaly is associated with increased cancer risk: a survey in Italy. Endocr Relat Cancer. 2017;24(9):495–504.

Trainer PJ, Drake WM, Katznelson L, Freda PU, Herman-Bonert V, van der Lely AJ, et al. Treatment of acromegaly with the growth hormone-receptor antagonist pegvisomant. N Engl J Med. 2000;342(16):1171–7.

Trainer PJ, Newell-Price J, Ayuk J, Aylwin S, Rees DA, Drake W, et al. A randomised, open-label, parallel group phase 2 study of antisense oligonucleotide therapy in acromegaly. Eur J Endocrinol. 2018:EJE-18-0138.

Valassi E, Klibanski A, Biller BMK. Potential cardiac valve effects of dopamine agonists in hyperprolactinemia. J Clin Endocrinol Metab. 2010;95(3):1025–33.

Wassenaar MJE, Biermasz NR, Kloppenburg M, AAvd K, Tiemensma J, Smit JWA, et al. Clinical osteoarthritis predicts physical and psychological QoL in acromegaly patients. Growth Hormon IGF Res. 2010;20(3):226–33.

Webb SM. Quality of life in acromegaly. Neuroendocrinology. 2006;83(3–4):224–9.

Webb SM, Badia X. Quality of life in growth hormone deficiency and acromegaly. Endocrinol Metab Clin N Am. 2007;36(1):221–32.

Wilson TJ, McKean EL, Barkan AL, Chandler WF, Sullivan SE. Repeat endoscopic transsphenoidal surgery for acromegaly: remission and complications. Pituitary. 2013;16(4):459–64.

Yedinak C, editor Prevalence of depression in patients with pituitary tumors: association of depression with perceived social capital. In Sigma Theta Tau International's 25th International Nursing Research Congress; 2014 July 24–28; Hong Kong, China.

Yedinak CG, Fleseriu M. Self-perception of cognitive function among patients with active acromegaly, controlled acromegaly, and non-functional pituitary adenoma: a pilot study. Endocrine. 2013;46(3):585–93.

Yedinak C, Pulaski Liebert KJ, Adelman DT, Williams J. Acromegaly: current therapies benefits and burdens. Clin Pract. 2018;15(2)

Key Reading

1. Chanson P, Salenave S. Acromegaly. Orphanet J Rare Dis. 2008;3(1):17.
2. Melmed S, Casanueva F, Cavagnini F, Chanson P, et al. Consensus statement: medical management of acromegaly. Eur J Endocrinol. 2005;153(6):737–40.
3. Melmed S, Kleinberg DL, Bonert V, Fleseriu M. Acromegaly: assessing the disorder and navigating therapeutic options for treatment. Endocr Pract. 2014;20(Suppl 1):7–17; quiz 8–20
4. Plunkett C, Barkan A. The care continuum in acromegaly: how patients, nurses, and physicians can collaborate for successful treatment experiences. Patient Prefer Adherence. 2015;9:1093.

ACTH Producing Adenomas: Cushing's Disease

Raven McGlotten

Contents

Abstract

Cushing's syndrome is a rare disorder characterized by prolonged exposure to excessive concentrations of glucocorticoids. Endogenous Cushing's syndrome, which will be the focus of this chapter, is usually divided into adrenocorticotropic hormone (ACTH)-dependent and ACTH-independent causes. ACTH-dependent Cushing's syndrome accounts for approximately 80–85% of all cases and is primarily due to excess ACTH production from a pituitary adenoma. This is also called Cushing's disease. In Cushing's disease, pituitary adrenocorticotropic hormone (ACTH)

R. McGlotten (✉)
National Institutes of Diabetes and Digestive and Kidney Diseases, Bethesda, MD, USA
e-mail: mcglottenr@mail.nih.gov

© Springer Nature Switzerland AG 2019
S. Llahana et al. (eds.), *Advanced Practice in Endocrinology Nursing*,
https://doi.org/10.1007/978-3-319-99817-6_21

oversecretion (from corticotrophs) prompts bilateral adrenocortical hyperplasia, excess production of cortisol, adrenal androgens, and 11-deoxycorticosterone which together cause the clinical and biological features of this disease. The most common clinical features of Cushing's syndrome include central obesity, diabetes, hypertension, moon facies, facial plethora, proximal muscle weakness, and reddish purple striae and in children, impaired growth with concomitant weight gain.

Testing for Cushing's disease first serves to confirm a diagnosis of Cushing's syndrome or hypercortisolemia, then to differentiate the location of the hypersecretory adenoma. Tests used to screen for Cushing's syndrome include measurement of random serum cortisol and ACTH, urine free cortisol, late night salivary cortisol, and a 1 mg dexamethasone suppression test. Tests used to differentiate Cushing's disease from other forms of Cushing's syndrome include an 8 mg high-dose dexamethasone suppression test, a corticotrophin-releasing hormone (CRH) stimulation test, pituitary MRI, and petrosal sinus sampling.

The optimal treatment for Cushing's disease is removal of the culprit pituitary adenoma. However, other treatments exist such as pharmacological therapies. Several medications are available that act at different levels, some on the adenoma itself, others blocking the cortisol receptor sites or inhibiting steroidogenesis at the level of the adrenal glands. In cases of persistent or recurrent Cushing's disease, bilateral adrenalectomy may be performed as a definitive treatment; however, this has long-term implications such as lifelong dependence on replacement glucocorticoids and mineralocorticoids. Pituitary irradiation can be used in cases of recurrent or persistent Cushing's disease.

Cushing's disease is not only associated with increased morbidity and mortality during active disease, but this increased risk may also persist in remission. Cushing's disease is also associated with impaired quality of life, with patients reporting numerous impacts on daily life such as fatigue, interference with family life and relationships with partners, changes in physical appearance, among others. Biochemical remission is typically associated with a small improvement in quality of life impairments when compared to remission of disorders associated with other pituitary adenomas. The nurses' role is vital in the process of patient assessment, postoperative and long-term monitoring and management of these issues.

Keywords

Cushing's syndrome · Cushing's disease · Hypercortisolemia · Adrenocorticotropic hormone · Pituitary adenoma · Glucocorticoid · Cortisol

Abbreviations

ACTH	Adrenocorticotropic hormone
AI	Adrenal insufficiency
CDCS	Cushing's disease
CRH	Corticotrophin-releasing hormone
CS	Cushing's syndrome
CT	Computerized tomography
DST	Dexamethasone suppression test
EAS	Ectopic ACTH syndrome
HPA	Hypothalamic-pituitary-adrenal axis
IPSS	Inferior petrosal sinus sampling
MRI	Magnetic resonance imaging
PCOS	Polycystic ovarian syndrome
PET	Positron emission tomography
TEE	Transsphenoidal endoscopic endonasal surgery
TSS	Transsphenoidal surgery

Key Terms
- **Hypercortisolemia:** A state of excess amount of cortisol in the blood.
- **Cushing's syndrome:** Hallmark symptoms caused by body exposure to high levels of cortisol for an extended period of time. The source of excess cortisol may be iatrogenic, pituitary, adrenal, or ectopic.

- **Cushing's Disease:** Cushing's disease is a type of Cushing's syndrome caused by excess secretion of adrenocorticotropic hormone (ACTH) from tumorous pituitary cells. Cushing's disease is the most common cause of Cushing's syndrome.
- **Hypothalamic-pituitary-adrenal (HPA) axis:** A system of three endocrine glands (hypothalamus, pituitary gland, adrenal glands) that work in a feedback loop to regulate multiple processes within the body.

Key Points

- Cushing's syndrome is a disorder characterized by excess exposure to glucocorticoids. It can be exogenous (from an outside source), or endogenous (from an internal or tumor source).
- Cushing's disease is a type of Cushing's syndrome caused by excess secretion of adrenocorticotropic hormone (ACTH) from tumorous pituitary cells. Cushing's disease is the most common cause of Cushing's syndrome in children >7 years and in adults.
- The optimal treatment of Cushing's disease is removal of the pituitary adenoma producing excess ACTH; however, pituitary adenomas are most often microadenomas (less than 10 mm in size). In 40–60% of cases, the tumor may be so small that it may not be visualized on magnetic resonance imaging (MRI).
- Symptoms of Cushing's disease at patient presentation largely overlap with a variety of other common disorders and present a diagnostic as well as treatment challenge with severe implications related to quality of life. Nursing assessment should include assessment of the multiple comorbidities associated with Cushing's disease, both physical and psychological.

21.1 Introduction to Hypercortisolism

21.1.1 Cushing's Syndrome

Cushing's syndrome is a rare disorder characterized by prolonged exposure to excessive glucocorticoids. The most common cause of Cushing's syndrome is iatrogenic, or exogenous, caused by the use of exogenous glucocorticoids including topical or inhaled corticosteroids in supraphysiologic doses (such as prednisone or hydrocortisone) (Newell-Price et al. 2006; Sharma et al. 2015a). Endogenous Cushing's syndrome, which will be the focus of this chapter, is usually divided into adrenocorticotropic hormone (ACTH)-dependent causes and ACTH-independent causes (Sharma and Nieman 2011; Findling and Raff 2006). ACTH-independent Cushing's, usually characterized by inappropriately low levels of ACTH, accounts for approximately 15–20% of endogenous Cushing's Syndrome in adults, and is primarily caused by unilateral adrenal tumors (Newell-Price et al. 2006) (see adrenal causes of Cushing's syndrome in Part VI).

21.1.2 Cushing's Disease

ACTH-dependent Cushing's syndrome is typically characterized by elevated or inappropriately normal ACTH levels in the setting of hypercortisolism (Sharma and Nieman 2011). In adults, ACTH-dependent Cushing's syndrome, also called Cushing's disease, accounts for approximately 70–80% of all cases and is primarily due to excess ACTH production from a pituitary adenoma (Newell-Price et al. 2006; Sharma and Nieman 2011). Approximately 15–20% of ACTH-dependent Cushing's syndrome cases are from non-pituitary tumors and include ectopic ACTH syndrome (EAS), and the extremely rare corticotrophin-releasing hormone (CRH) producing tumor (<1% of cases). EAS tumors are most often of neuroendocrine origin (bronchial, thymic, pancreatic, etc.). However, EAS tumors can also be derived from other causes such as pulmonary carcinoids, small cell lung carcinoma,

Fig. 21.1 Types and sources of Cushing's syndrome

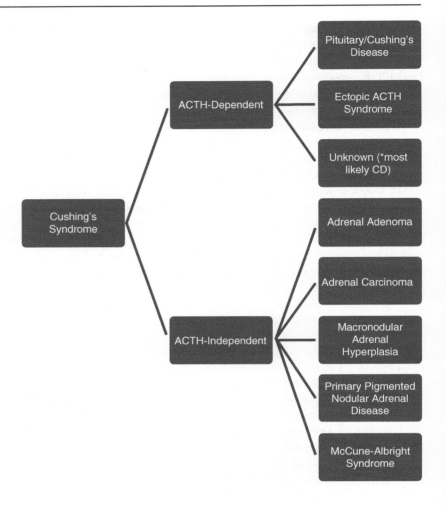

medullary thyroid cancer, pheochromocytomas, and more (Sharma et al. 2015a; Kamp et al. 2016). In children over the age of 7 years, and in adults an ACTH-secreting pituitary adenoma is the most common cause of CS, and adrenal etiology is the most common in children younger than 7 years. Ectopic causes of CS are extremely rare in children (Magiakou et al. 1994) (Fig. 21.1).

21.2 Cushing's Disease

21.2.1 Epidemiology and Pathophysiology

Cushing's disease (CD) is a pituitary disorder marked by pathologic hypercortisolism result-

ing from excess secretion of ACTH by tumorous pituitary corticotrophs (anterior pituitary cells). Cushing's disease is the most common cause of endogenous Cushing's syndrome (~70–80% of cases) (Findling and Raff 2006; Cuevas-Ramos and Fleseriu 2014) In Cushing's disease, pituitary adrenocorticotropic hormone (ACTH) oversecretion prompts bilateral adrenocortical hyperplasia with excess production of cortisol, adrenal androgens, and 11-deoxycorticosterone, which together cause the clinical and biological features of this disease (Lindholm et al. 2001).

Ten to 15% of pituitary tumors secrete ACTH, thus causing CD (Newell-Price et al. 2006) In most cases, the tumors are benign and slow growing. Microadenomas (<10 mm in diameter)

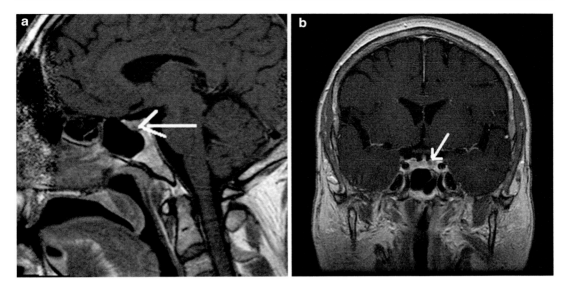

Fig. 21.2 ACTH producing microadenoma of the pituitary. (a) Sagittal T1 view, (b) Coronal T1 view. Used with permission from Mancini T, Porcelli T, Giustina A. Treatment of Cushing disease: overview and recent findings. Ther Clin Risk Manag. 2010;6:505–16

are found in 90% of cases, whereas macroadenomas (>10 mm in diameter) are less common (10% of cases). ACTH producing pituitary adenomas that cause Cushing's disease are usually well-delineated microadenomas, some as small as 1–2 mm, and most often located in the central wedge of the anterior lobe (see Fig. 21.2). Due to their small size, many ACTH producing tumors are undetectable by MRI and difficult to find at surgery. In some cases, the adenomas are localized to the lateral wings of the pituitary, in the pars intermedia or in the neurohypophysis and, rarely, in the pituitary stalk. The size of the tumor can influence treatment outcome (Newell-Price et al. 2006; Syro et al. 2015) (see Chap. 1).

The overall incidence and prevalence of endogenous Cushing's syndrome is 2–3 per million per year and 30–60 patients per million, respectively (Newell-Price et al. 2006; Syro et al. 2015; Graversen et al. 2012). The average age of onset of Cushing's disease in adults is 36 years (mean of 30.5 years in females, 37.1 years in males) (Newell-Price et al. 2006). Severity of presentation varies widely, but a milder clinical phenotype in a patient presenting with Cushing's syndrome, especially if

female, is more likely to be due to Cushing's disease than other etiologies (Sharma and Nieman 2011; Clayton et al. 2011). Cushing's disease also has a definite female preponderance, the female/male ratio ranging between 3:1 and 10:1 (Zilio et al. 2014). Similar to adults, in children there is a female to male predominance that decreases with younger age (see Fig. 21.3) (Magiakou et al. 1994; Nieman et al. 2015).

21.3 Genetics of Cushing's Disease

The majority of ACTH producing pituitary adenomas are the result of sporadic mutations, with most patients reporting no family history of the disease. Since most of these tumors are isolated, this makes hereditary or germ line mutation unlikely. Recent studies have shown that a mutation in a gene known as USP8 is present in approximately one-third of patients with Cushing's disease (Biller et al. 1992; Theodoropoulou et al. 2015). However, the etiology of genetic mutation remains largely unknown.

Fig. 21.3 Patient age at
the time of diagnosis of
Cushing's disease.
Melmed S. The pituitary.
3rd ed.:535. https://doi.
org/10.1016/B978-0-12-
380926-1.10016-1
(Batista et al. 2007)

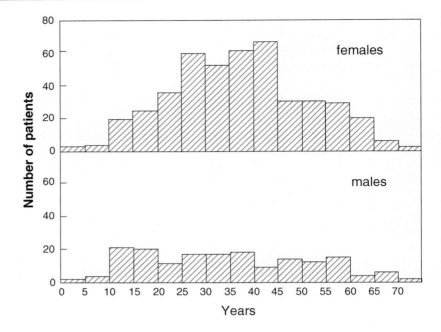

Childhood corticotropinomas, that occur in the familial setting, most commonly occur in the context of multiple endocrine neoplasia type 1 (MEN 1) and rare *AIP* mutations should be considered (Stratakis et al. 2010).

21.4 Morbidity and Mortality

Cushing's disease is a serious condition associated with significant morbidity and severe impacts on patients' quality of life (Syro et al. 2015; Graversen et al. 2012; Dekkers et al. 2013). Morbidity and mortality associated with Cushing's disease is most often related to cardiac and cerebrovascular events, infections due to immunosuppression, osteoporosis, and diabetes. Untreated, CD has a mortality ratio of approximately of 1.9–4.8 (ratio of CD-associated deaths to expected deaths of general population) (Kamp et al. 2016; Lonser et al. 2017). Importantly, mental health disorders, including suicidal ideation, have been reported in children and adults after disease remission (Keil et al. 2016; Dorn et al. 1995). Overall mortality in Cushing's disease is double that of the general population and up to four times higher than in age- and sex-matched controls (Syro et al. 2015; Graversen et al.

2012; Dekkers et al. 2013). In addition, mortality in patients with Cushing's disease is more than twice that of patients with non-functioning pituitary macroadenomas even when previously treated, implying that even transient cortisol over-exposure contributes to the increase in mortality risk (Clayton et al. 2011).

21.5 Patient Presentation and Assessment

Prolonged exposure to excessive cortisol levels results in multiple signs and symptoms affecting various body systems. Although the tumor causing the disease tends to be slow growing, the excess secretion of ACTH means that clinical features can manifest before the tumor has grown large or large enough to be detected. Although Cushing's disease may be more easily identifiable when severe, the signs and symptoms remain broad and may be difficult to distinguish from other disorders such as metabolic syndrome or polycystic ovarian disease (Nieman et al. 2008). The most common clinical features in adults include central obesity, diabetes, hypertension, moon facies, and facial plethora (Lonser et al. 2017; Nieman

Table 21.1 Clinical features of Cushing's syndrome

Clinical features—more specific to Cushing's syndrome	
More common	Less common
Easy bruising	Striae
Facial plethora	
Proximal muscle weakness	
In children, weight gain and decreased linear growth	
Clinical features less discriminatory for Cushing's syndrome or common in the general population	
More common	Less common
Obesity/weight gain	Acne
Depression	Recurrent infections
Lethargy/fatigue	Nephrolithiasis
Hypertension[a]	Female balding
Menstrual changes	Osteopenia or fracture[a]
Hirsutism	
Abnormal glucose tolerance[a]	
Round face	
Decreased libido	
Thin skin[a]	

This table made with data from: Newell-Price et al. (2006), Sharma et al. (2015a), Neiman et al. (2008), Neiman (2015).
[a]Nieman (2015)

et al. 2008) (see Table 21.1). Some symptoms are more unique to Cushing's syndrome and can be helpful in differential diagnosis such as reddish purple striae, proximal muscle weakness, bruising with no obvious trauma, and unexplained osteoporosis, often with a history of one or more fractures (Nieman et al. 2008). In most children, the onset of Cushing's syndrome is somewhat insidious (Magiakou et al. 1994). Lack of height gain concomitant with persistent weight gain is the most common presentation of Cushing's syndrome in childhood, as depicted in a typical growth chart for a child with Cushing's syndrome shown in Fig. 21.4. Other common problems reported in children include facial plethora, headaches, hypertension, hirsutism, amenorrhea, skin fungal infections, and delayed sexual development (Magiakou et al. 1994). Pubertal children may present with virilization. Glucose intolerance and diabetes, fractures, and kidney stones are also associated presenting symptoms. In comparison to adult patients with Cushing's syndrome, symptoms that are less commonly seen in children include sleep disruption, muscular weakness, and problems with memory dysfunction (Magiakou et al. 1994).

Physical characteristics can also include dorsocervical fat pad (buffalo hump), thinning hair, thin skin, striae (most often on the abdomen), purpura, and skin ulcers due to poor wound healing. In addition, other features may manifest, including severe fatigue, hypokalemia, hypertension, depression, cognitive impairment, hyperpigmentation, sexual/menstrual dysfunction, hirsutism, acne, bone fractures, kidney stones, and susceptibility to opportunistic infections (Lonser et al. 2017; Nieman et al. 2008). Patients presenting with pituitary adenomas frequently experience impairment of the gonadotropic axis resulting in amenorrhea in females and impaired fertility (Graversen et al. 2012). Furthermore, the effects of Cushing's disease include cardiovascular complications, as well as metabolic disturbances that can result in fat tissue redistribution and obesity, often most severe in the abdomen (Lonser et al. 2017; Nieman et al. 2008) (see Fig. 21.5).

Although Cushing's disease is less frequent in males, the presentation tends to be more florid with higher cortisol levels and severity of complications (Zilio et al. 2014). Average time from initiation of symptoms to diagnosis ranges from 2 to 3 years in adult males but can be significantly longer in females. Before puberty, the prevalence

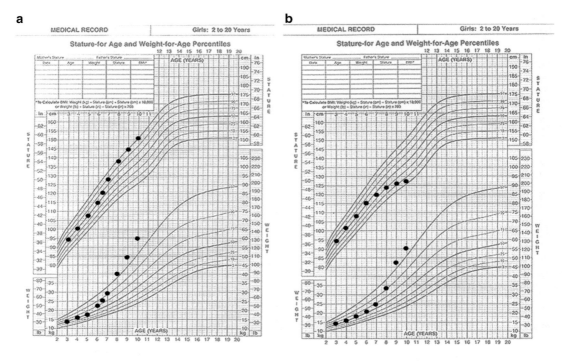

Fig. 21.4 Growth in children with Cushing's disease. (**a**) Obsese child, (**b**) Child with Cushing's disease

of CD is similar in both genders versus in adult cases when females are more frequently affected than males (3:1 vs 5:1, respectively) (Lonser et al. 2017). Few of the symptoms of CD are unique, and many have strong overlap of symptoms with other disorders and in some cases with the general population, presenting challenges in identifying the disorder based on clinical presentation alone (Nieman et al. 2008).

While many physical symptoms of Cushing's syndrome are not completely indicative of the disorder, many other disorders, such as those causing pseudo-Cushing's syndrome (PCS), also present a challenge in the diagnosis of Cushing's syndrome. PCS cases present with a similar clinical phenotype including obesity, diabetes, hypertension, moon face, buffalo hump, striae as well as mild hypercortisolemia. Disorders associated with PCS include chronic alcoholism, psychiatric disorders, severe obesity, poorly controlled diabetes, and extreme physical and psychological stress. Polycystic Ovarian Syndrome (PCOS) can also present with a similar phenotype in women of reproductive age. Metabolic syndrome described in overweight or obese individuals with

comorbidities such as hypertension, diabetes, and dyslipidemia can also mimic Cushing's due to its similar phenotype. Additionally, small elevations in cortisol can contribute to obesity and metabolic syndrome. Treatment of these underlying conditions will lead to resolution of these Cushingoid symptoms, differentiating them from Cushing's syndrome (Alwani et al. 2014; Friedman and Yanovski 1995; Brzana et al. 2014).

21.6 Testing and Diagnostic Procedures

Diagnostic testing for Cushing's disease serves to not only confirm the presence of hypercortisolemia, but to differentiate its cause as ACTH dependent or independent. In ACTH-dependent Cushing's, the next step is to confirm a pituitary source of excess ACTH.

Patients who present with features of Cushing's who are not taking exogenous glucocorticoids (iatrogenic Cushing's syndrome) should first be screened for Cushing's syndrome or the presence of hypercortisolism. The initial screening tests are measurement of urine free cortisol over 24 h, and late night salivary cortisol collected before bedtime to check for inappropriately elevated cortisol (see circadian rhythm, Chap. 1). Multiple measurements should be done to ensure that results are not falsely positive or falsely negative. A 1 mg overnight dexamethasone suppression test (DST)

and the longer 2 day or high-dose DST (over 48 h) are also used. Normal subjects without Cushing's will have suppression of cortisol levels when given one or more dose(s) of exogenous steroids (dexamethasone) due to the HPA axis feedback loop (see Fig. 21.6), but those with Cushing's syndrome and excess cortisol production will not. A longer low-dose DST, over 48 h, is sometimes performed instead of the 1 mg or overnight DST due to increased specificity of this test and may be also be combined with corticotrophin-releasing hormone (CRH) stimulation to increase the test reliability. The normal variability of random serum cortisol or plasma ACTH levels makes these measures unreliable for a diagnosis of Cushing's syndrome (Nieman et al. 2008).

If after screening Cushing's syndrome is confirmed, a basal ACTH level can be used to help differentiate ACTH-dependent from independent Cushing's syndrome. Suppressed plasma ACTH indicates an adrenal or ACTH-independent cause, while inappropriately elevated ACTH levels are consistent with an ACTH-dependent cause (Lonser et al. 2017; Lindsay and Nieman 2005). It is important to measure on several occasions to ensure accuracy.

Multiple dynamic tests are usually conducted to differentiate Cushing's disease from ectopic ACTH-secreting tumors. The high-dose dexamethasone suppression test relies on the concept that pituitary tumor cells retain sensitivity to glucocorticoid feedback effects similar to that of normal pituitary cells. After administration of 8 mg of dexamethasone, if there is a suppression of serum cortisol Cushing's disease should be suspected (Lonser et al. 2017; Lindsay and Nieman 2005). Sensitivity of this test for CD

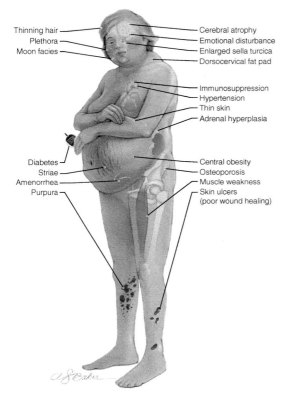

Fig. 21.5 Clinical features of Cushing's syndrome. Used with permission from Lonser RR, Nieman L, Oldfield EH. Cushing's disease: pathobiology, diagnosis, and management. J Neurosurg. 2017;126(2):404–17

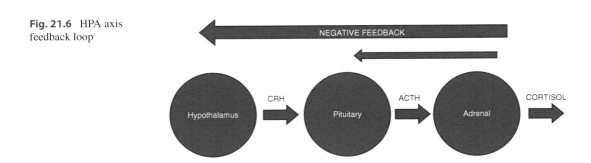

Fig. 21.6 HPA axis feedback loop

varies from 65 to 100%, increasing with degree of cortisol suppression (Lindsay and Nieman 2005). The corticotrophin-releasing hormone (CRH) stimulation test again relies on pituitary tumor cells responding to CRH stimulation. When CRH is given, if cortisol and ACTH rise from basal levels Cushing's disease should be suspected, whereas ectopic tumors generally do not respond to CRH (Lonser et al. 2017; Lindsay and Nieman 2005). A combination of a positive response to CRH and suppression on DST makes CD more likely (Clayton et al. 2011), so the use of multiple biochemical tests is often encouraged.

Less common tests include the metyrapone and desmopressin tests. These have little efficacy when used alone and are not typically recommended for diagnostic purposes (Lindsay and Nieman 2005). It is also important to note that Cushing's syndrome can be cyclic, characterized by fluctuations in, or periods of hypercortisolism, although this is extremely rare (Colao et al. 2014). Because of this, to ensure accuracy of testing, hypercortisolism must be confirmed before undergoing any differential diagnostic testing for Cushing's disease. There is also no widely accepted consensus regarding diagnostic cut-offs related to these tests, therefore ranges may vary by institution and laboratory assays. Specificity among the various diagnostic tests is also variable, and it is recommended that multiple tests are conducted to increase specificity and confirm a diagnosis (Colao et al. 2014).

Diagnosis can be further supported by presence of pituitary adenoma on imaging. However, in 40–60% of cases, microadenomas cannot be detected on MRI (Lonser et al. 2017; Colao et al. 2014). Petrosal sinus sampling, while more invasive, can help with a more definitive diagnosis of Cushing's disease when other results and features are unclear (Colao et al. 2014). Computed tomography (CT) (more preferable than MRI) of the adrenal glands is useful in the distinction between Cushing's disease and adrenal causes of Cushing's syndrome, usually caused by a unilateral adrenal tumor. The distinction is harder in the presence of micronodular forms of bilateral adrenal hyperplasia (BAH) (such as pri-mary pigmented nodular adrenocortical disease (PPNAD)) or the rare case of bilateral adrenal carcinoma. Most patients with Cushing's disease have ACTH-driven bilateral hyperplasia, and both adrenal glands will appear enlarged and nodular on CT or MRI (Tsigos and Chrousos 1996; Batista et al. 2007).

Testing for the differential diagnosis of ectopic ACTH syndrome is similar to the testing for Cushing's disease and is dependent on the correct interpretation of the results. This includes confirmation of hypercortisolism, the high-dose dexamethasone suppression test, pituitary imaging (for absence of pituitary adenoma), and petrosal sinus sampling. Structural (CT and MRI) and functional imaging such as positron emission tomography (PET) scans are also vital in the identification of the source of EAS (Sharma et al. 2015a; Sharma and Nieman 2011; Kamp et al. 2016) (See Fig. 21.7). (See Part VI for detailed information on EAS and ACTH independent Cushing's disease).

For more details on dynamic testing, endocrine testing, and patient instructions, see Chap. 15.

21.7 Treatment Modalities

21.7.1 Surgical Treatment

The optimal treatment for Cushing's disease is the successful removal of the culprit pituitary adenoma by a surgical, selective adenomectomy (removal of the tumor while preserving pituitary tissue). This will immediately eliminate the excess cortisol production with the goal of preserving normal pituitary function (Lonser et al. 2017). Surgical access to the pituitary gland, also known as transsphenoidal surgery (TSS), has multiple approaches. These can be sub-labial, endonasal, endoscopic, and/or microscopic (Lonser et al. 2017). Pituitary adenomectomy generally leads to remission rates of 65–90% of cases in the hands of an experienced neurosurgeon with a higher likelihood of remission for those with microadenomas versus macroadenomas (Lonser et al. 2017; Mancini et al. 2010; Vilar et al. 2015). However, the lifetime recurrence rate after

Fig. 21.7 An algorithm for the assessment and treatment of Cushing's disease. Derived from Neiman et al. 2008; Lonser et al. 2017; Dekkers et al. 2013

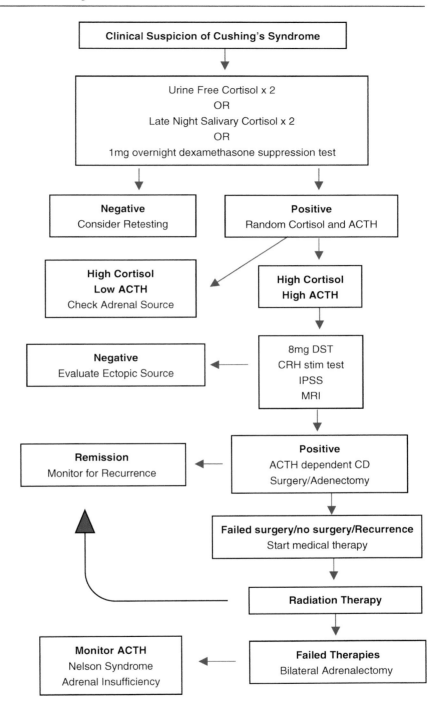

surgical remission is reported as 10–35% (Lonser et al. 2017; Vilar et al. 2015) (See Chap. 11).

Multiple factors influence successful surgical outcome. Magnetic resonance imaging (MRI) is most helpful in localizing the offending tumor; however, 40–60% of microadenomas (diameter of 6 mm or below) will not be clearly detected (Lonser et al. 2017; Mehta and Lonser 2017).

Lateralization of ACTH secretion using IPSS is also helpful to direct the surgeon to the cortico-troph tumor. When the adenoma is seen on MRI, it directs surgical exploration to the adenoma within the gland, increasing chances of identifying the adenoma. Adenomas found to be at least 3 mm are not only easier to identify on MRI, but may develop a histological pseudocapsule, or tissue envelope around its rim. Using this capsule to remove an adenoma can improve remission rates to 97% in adults or 98% in children, again, in the hands of an experienced neurosurgeon (Lonser et al. 2017). Adenomas can also be found to invade the dura or surrounding tissue. Macroadenomas often invade into the cavernous sinus, which makes curative surgery unlikely. In such cases, a portion of the tumor cannot be surgically removed safely without significant risk to structure in the area such as the internal carotid arteries or cranial nerves 11-V1 (Lonser et al. 2017) (See Chap. 22).

While many adenomas not seen on MRI can later be identified during pituitary exploration, some may still be too small to be located. In these cases a portion of the pituitary gland, or a partial hypophysectomy, of the anterior lobe may be performed. Partial and total hypophysectomies have remission rates similar to that of selective adenomectomy (60–80%) but result in significant pituitary hormone deficiencies or panhypopituitarism (Lonser et al. 2017).

The risks of surgery, although not common, include: vision loss, cranial nerve injury, loss of pituitary function, diabetes insipidus, syndrome of inappropriate antidiuretic hormone secretion (SIADH), pituitary apoplexy, delayed hemorrhage, cerebrospinal fluid leakage, infection (meningitis), and very rarely, death (<1%) (Lonser et al. 2017). For more information on pituitary surgery, see Chap. 22. Remission is confirmed by absence of hypercortisolism, and pathologic findings. Typically, biochemical remission is considered achieved when a 24–48 h postsurgical morning serum cortisol level is below 5 mg/dL (90 mmol/L) after glucocorticoids have been withheld for 24 h (Mehta and Lonser 2017).

21.7.1.1 Postsurgical Hypopituitarism and Adrenal Insufficiency

After successful surgery to remove a pituitary adenoma, normal corticotrophs are typically suppressed, causing a temporary secondary adrenal insufficiency. Glucocorticoid replacement is required until the HPA axis recovers, typically for 6–12 months following resection of ACTH producing pituitary tumors or longer. Patients are usually treated with hydrocortisone, prednisone, or dexamethasone using a physiologic dose (usually 15–30 mg of hydrocortisone daily for adults and 10–12 mg/m^2 in children or adults) until laboratory testing reveals a functional HPA axis (via serum cortisol and ACTH level, or dynamic ACTH stimulation test) (Nieman et al. 2015). Higher doses may be required immediately postoperatively to avoid symptoms of adrenal insufficiency. These doses are usually tapered to physiologic dose based on body surface area to avoid acute symptoms of secondary adrenal insufficiency. There is still no general consensus regarding steroid dosing or tapering technique during this time period. Once on a physiologic dose, further dynamic testing to ensure HPA axis is functional is usually undertaken prior to discontinuing glucocorticoids.

It is vital that patients are educated on the signs and symptoms of acute adrenal insufficiency, adrenal crisis, as well as stress dose requirements. An adrenal crisis occurs when a patient with adrenal insufficiency is challenged by severe illness or stressor but unable to meet the demand or increased need of cortisol. Insufficient cortisol coverage during periods of illness (such as infections) is linked to increased morbidity and mortality risk (van der Meij et al. 2016; Johannsson et al. 2015) (see adrenal insufficiency, Chaps. 22, 23, 62, and Part XII).

21.7.2 Medical Therapy

Medical therapy is recommended as a second-line treatment or alternative approach of patients with CD who cannot undergo surgery, who have not achieved remission after surgery, or those who are not candidates for a repeat surgical procedure in the case of recurrence (Mancini et al. 2010; Mehta and Lonser 2017). However, medical therapy can also be used preoperatively to control the metabolic effects of severe hypercortisolism, to reduce surgical and anesthesia risk, or while waiting for the effects of pituitary radiotherapy to manifest (Mancini et al. 2010; Vilar et al. 2015). Types of medical therapy include corticotroph or pituitary directed agents or steroidogenesis (adrenal) inhibitors or glucocorticoid antagonists.

Pituitary directed medical treatments are centrally acting and work to inhibit ACTH secretion from corticotroph tumor cells (Nieman et al. 2015; Vilar et al. 2015; Mehta and Lonser 2017). Somatostatin is a primary neuromodulating hormone that is produced in the hypothalamus and affects the production of ACTH from corticotroph cells. The drug pasireotide binds with four of the five known somatostatin receptor types but with a high affinity for subtype 5 and subsequently inhibits the secretion of ACTH from corticotroph cells and corticotroph tumor cells expressing somatostatin receptors (Johannsson et al. 2015). Dopamine agonists have a similar, but weaker, effect on the dopamine receptors, subsequently inhibiting ACTH.

Although the ideal therapy would be directed at the pituitary adenoma itself, steroidogenesis inhibitors were the first therapies used in the treatment of CD and remain among the most common therapies (Cuevas-Ramos and Fleseriu 2014). Steroidogenesis inhibitors or adrenal enzyme inhibitors, lower serum cortisol levels by blocking one or several steps in the biosynthesis of cortisol from the adrenal cortex (Vilar et al. 2015). Close monitoring of the HPA axis and patient symptoms is required during therapy to avoid the development of adrenal insufficiency.

Glucocorticoid antagonists, such as mifepristone, block systemic effects of hypercortisolism but do not lower serum cortisol (Mehta and Lonser 2017). Therefore, serum cortisol levels and hence urine free cortisol levels will rise but the tissue and end organ effects of cortisol are blocked.

Mitotane, an adrenocorticolytic drug that causes necrosis of adrenocortical cells, is reserved for patients with persistent or recurrent Cushing's disease who cannot undergo bilateral adrenalectomy, due to its severe side effects and high cost (Abdel Mannan et al. 2010). Intravenous etomidate inhibits 11β-hydroxylase and is used for emergent control of severe hypercortisolism, but is used rarely due to its need for intensive care monitoring due to its sedative hypnotic effect and need for airway support (Mehta and Lonser 2017) (Fig. 21.8).

Combination medical therapy with multiple drug classes is a treatment option gaining popularity. While there are still no guidelines or treatment strategies, utilization of multiple therapies may increase efficacy, decrease drug doses, and possibly result in fewer adverse effects (Cuevas-Ramos and Fleseriu 2014) (Table 21.2).

In the USA, only a few medications effective in the medical management of hypercotisolism are FDA approved for use in CS, several are used off-label such as ketoconazole (Vilar et al. 2015). The use and availability of medical therapies for CS varies from country to country.

Each medication comes with multiple side effects, and patients should be closely monitored. With any of the medical therapies, there is a risk of overtreatment that could lead to adrenal insufficiency (Sharma et al. 2015a). Therefore, medical therapy can be used to either block cortisol production to achieve normal levels, or by blocking cortisol production completely, which would require glucocorticoid replacement (Sharma et al. 2015a). Somatostatin analogues also inhibit gut cholecystokinin release affecting gallbladder contractility and may result in gallstone formation. Decreased digestive enzymes result in abdominal bloating and diarrhea (Bertagna et al. 2011). All patients on medical therapy, post-surgery, and post-radiation should be educated regarding therapy side effects and the signs, symptoms, and management of adrenal insufficiency (see Tables 21.2 and 21.3).

Fig. 21.8 Medications and their level of action in Cushing's disease. Fleseriu M. Medical management of persistent and recurrent Cushing disease. Neurosurg Clin N Am. 2012;23(4):653–68. Reproduced with permission from Fleseriu 2012

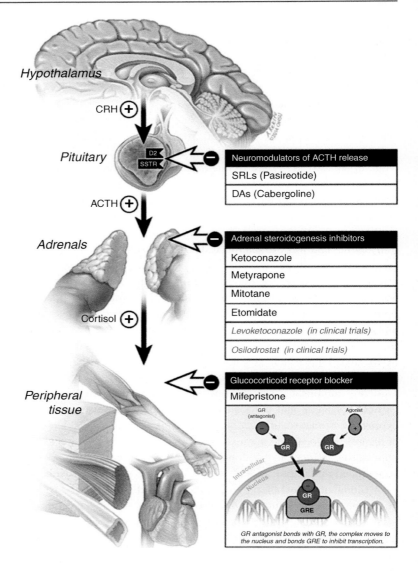

Table 21.2 Medications and side effects

Class	Drug name	Common side effects/considerations
Steroidogenesis inhibitors	Ketoconazole	Hepatitis, gastrointestinal disturbance, gynecomastia, male hypogonadism, adrenal insufficiency
	Fluconazole	Similar to ketoconazole
	Metyrapone	Hypertension, adrenal insufficiency, hirsutism, acne, hypokalemia, edema, gastritis, nausea, accessibility variable across countries
	Etomidate (IV)	Somnolence, nausea, vomiting, adrenal insufficiency (*often require intensive care monitoring—quick onset of action)
	Mitotane	Gastrointestinal disturbance, hepatitis, neurologic disturbance, neutropenia, adrenal insufficiency, slow onset of action
Dopamine agonist	Cabergoline	Headache, nausea, dizziness
Somatostatin receptor binding	Pasireotide	Hyperglycemia, diabetes, diarrhea, nausea, QT prolongation
GR antagonist	Mifepristone	Nausea, fatigue, headache, hypertension, hypokalemia, endometrial thickening, vaginal bleeding, adrenal insufficiency, difficult to titrate (no biomarker)

Table 21.3 Patient education topics

Symptom start/diagnosis	Testing/treatment	Recovery
• Weight management • Fatigue/sleep • Management of comorbidities (diabetes, hypertension, etc.) • Fertility/menstrual cycle/libido • Self-perception/self-esteem	• Dynamic testing • Treatment options • Management of comorbidities (diabetes, hypertension, etc.) • Pre- and postsurgical care and restrictions • Medical therapy	• Fatigue/sleep • Weight management • Returning to work • Self-perception/self-esteem • Support groups • Physical activity/physical therapy • Long-term follow-up

21.7.3 Bilateral Adrenalectomy

As a definitive treatment, a bilateral adrenalectomy (BLA) may be considered. BLA is most often used in cases of refractory Cushing's Disease as last resort (Sharma et al. 2015a; Colao et al. 2014; Mancini et al. 2010). The adrenal glands are the target organs of ACTH and in a hypersecretory state this upregulates the production of cortisol from the adrenal cortex leading to hypercortisolism. Bilateral adrenalectomy leads to immediate resolution of hypercortisolism; however, the patient subsequently will require lifelong glucocorticoid and mineralocorticoid replacement (Sharma et al. 2015a). Education of patients to treat illness and injury by increasing glucocorticoids and in the use and administration of emergency stress doses of intramuscular glucocorticoids may be lifesaving. It is recommended that all patients obtain medic alert jewelry and/or carry a card identifying their surgical absence of adrenal glands, risk of adrenal insufficiency and clearly state their need for IM/IV glucocorticoids, fluid resuscitation, and monitoring of electrolytes in emergent situations (van der Meij et al. 2016).

Long-term clinical, serum ACTH level monitoring, and brain imaging is recommended to evaluate for tumor growth and the development of Nelson's syndrome after BLA. Nelson's syndrome is a potentially life-threatening syndrome that occurs in the presence of residual corticotroph pituitary tumor. ACTH levels may continue to climb secondary to the lack of cortisol opposition and tumor growth (Barber et al. 2010). The incidence of this syndrome is as high as 8–43% in adults and 25–66% in children and has been reported to occur up to 24 years after BLA (Barber et al. 2010). BLA at a younger age is more predictive of the development of Nelson's syndrome with children being at increased risk. Patients may present with compressive symptoms such as visual field deficits, and skin hyperpigmentation that may first become apparent in axillae, hand, and knuckle creases and then become generalized. Treatment with adequate suppressive doses of glucocorticoid may be adequate but first-line therapy is usually redo surgical resection of the pituitary tumor and radiotherapy may be necessary to achieve tumor control (Barber et al. 2010).

21.7.4 Radiation Therapy

In cases of persistent disease post TSS, pituitary radiotherapy can be used to control hypercortisolism. Pituitary irradiation is also an option for those who are poor surgical candidates, patients with residual tumors, and patients with surgically inaccessible tumors (Abdel Mannan et al. 2010). Fractionated external beam radiation and stereotactic radiosurgery have remission rates of approximately 50–60%, but require long-term follow-up to monitor for both initial response and recurrence. Risks of radiation are similar to that of TSS surgery, but also include potential for radiation damage and higher risk of secondary malignancies (Mancini et al., 2010) (see radiotherapy, Chap. 12).

21.7.5 Other Considerations

21.7.5.1 Management of Concomitant Diseases

While it is important to manage the cause of Cushing's disease with surgery or medications, it is also vital to manage comorbidities. After treatment, management of comorbidities remains an important goal as there is a persistently increased cardiovascular risk despite remission (Sharma et al. 2015b). Those patients who experience immediate improvement in comorbidities, such as diabetes and hypertension, require regular monitoring for down-titration of associated medications; however, some comorbidities persist long-term. In many patients, diabetes, hypertension, obesity, hyperlipidemia, osteoporosis or osteopenia, compromised final height (children and adolescents), as well as psychological and cognitive issues can persist after remission. Patients in remission of Cushing's disease overall remain at an increased risk of mortality (Sharma et al. 2015b; Espinosa-de-Los-Monteros et al. 2013; Clayton et al. 2016).

21.8 Quality of Life and Patient Education

Patients with Cushing's disease suffer from multiple health and psychological issues related to the disease, many of which can endure during and after treatment. Health related quality of life (HRQoL) is significantly impaired in patients with active Cushing's disease, and this often remains impaired even after remission is achieved. In a recent analysis of a large cohort of patients treated for CD drawn from a European registry, HRQoL remained lower than patients in remission from adrenal Cushing's syndrome 1 year later (Valassi et al. 2018). All patient scores showed lower HRQoL than normal subjects at baseline. Those patients with CD and baseline depression and patients diagnosed with CD at a younger age also had worse HRQoL scores 1 year after remission (Valassi et al. 2018). In terms of disease impact on daily life, CS patients most commonly report fatigue, weakness, interference with family life and relationships with partners, changes in physical appearance and body image issues, among others. Despite biochemical remission, quality of life measures also remain lower in children when compared to the treatment of other pituitary adenomas (Lonser et al. 2017; Johannsson et al.

2015; Keil et al. 2009). Younger children with CS are also more likely to experience negative cognitive changes (Keil et al. 2009).

Current research using modified glucocorticoid release formulae or delivery methods for glucocorticoid-dependent patients are showing some promise with respect to stabilizing or improving HRQoL, BMI, and blood sugar (Quinkler et al. 2015). Comprehensive education has also been shown to impact HRQoL. A study of 61 Cushing's syndrome patients randomly assigned to a structured nurse directed education program for patients with Cushing's syndrome over a period of 9 months versus no education found statistically significant improvement in physical activity, healthy lifestyle, better sleep patterns, and reduced pain in CS patients (Martinez-Momblan et al. 2016). The program both influenced HRQoL and reduced consumption of health resources.

21.9 Nursing Considerations

The nurses' role is vital in all phases of patient management and in particular patient education. Healthcare programs to address quality of life indicators in this population are lacking. Educational programs and use of support resources can lead to clinical improvement, reduced hospital admissions or visits, and improved overall quality of life (Martinez-Momblan et al. 2016).

Additional quality of life topics that should be addressed include fertility issues, sleep dysfunction, emotional instability, depression, cognitive impairments, among others (Feelders et al. 2012) (Table 21.3).

Advocating for psychological support, family support, and cognitive therapies may be useful to help patients and families negotiate changes during treatment. Referrals and care coordination with other disciplines regarding the assessment and management of comorbidities such as sleep dysfunction, weight management, nutrition, and physical therapies etc. may assist to improve patient outcomes and HRQoL. However, more evidence is needed to support these assumptions. Consideration should be given to the specific needs of the patient's stage of life, functional needs, and economic support.

Patients will require long-term follow-up and monitoring and perhaps a transition plan for all, or a component of, care to be provided at a convenient location in order to ensure ongoing follow-up.

21.10 Conclusions

Hypercortisolemia caused by an ACTH producing pituitary adenoma or Cushing's disease incurs a high mortality risk if not treated. It is a complex disease often with a significant delay in diagnosis. This delay results from the numerous non-specific symptoms that overlap with other disorders such as PCOS and metabolic syndrome. Diagnosis requires multiple test modalities and frequently the resources of a specialty center. The first-line treatment is surgical excision of the causative pituitary adenoma with the best chance of remission achieved by a neurosurgeon who is experienced in removing pituitary tumors.

Although remission rates are higher when surgery is performed in major centers, those patients not in remission with recurrent disease or with large or inaccessible tumors will require medical therapies and/or radiation therapy to control disease. Bilateral adrenalectomy is a definitive cure for CD but risks the development of Nelson's syndrome with high levels of ACTH.

All patients will require long-term management and support from all disciplines. Although quality of life may remain lower than that of the average population, the best patient outcomes are more achievable with collaboration of endocrine physicians and nurses and the involvement and coordination of all axillary services available to meet the patient's needs.

Patient Case Study

Background:

- A 46-year-old female presented to the hospital ER for a non-healing wound on her right foot after an insect bite. She was found to be hypertensive (180/102), hypokalemic (potassium

2.0 nmol/L), and hyperglycemic (300 mg/dL), leading to new diagnoses of diabetes and hypertension. Patient was referred to endocrinology for diabetic management.
- Patient also reported a plethora of symptoms beginning approximately 6 months prior: excessive facial hair, easy bruisability, depression with severe mood swings, weakness, difficulty climbing stairs, and weight gain of approximately 15 lb (6.8 kg).
- On exam the patient was noted to have central obesity purple striae on her abdomen and an unhealed purulent foot wound. A 24 h urine free cortisol was collected due to suspicion for Cushing's syndrome and the patient was referred to specialty center for further diagnostic testing.

Laboratory Results:

24 h urine free cortisol 1505 mcg/24 h (ref 3.5–45)

8 mg DSST pre-dexamethasone dose cortisol: 29.3 mcg/dL, post-dexamethasone dose cortisol: 2 mcg/dL (93.2% suppression)

CRH stimulation test

	−5 min	0	+15 min	+30 min	+45 min	% change?
Cortisol (5–25 mcg/dL)	20.4	20.5	24	28.9	30.8	46%
ACTH (5–46 pg/mL)	97.7	109	294	311	318	193%

MRI pituitary: no clear adenoma identified. Ill-defined area of decreased enhancement in the left half of the pituitary gland, possible adenoma.

With unclear pituitary MRI, IPSS was completed with CRH stimulation.

ACTH (ref 5–46 pg/mL)	Right petrosal	Left petrosal	Peripheral	RP/P ratio	LP/P ratio
−5	850	1148	86.6	9.8	13.3
0	812	1029	83.3	9.7	12.4
+3 min	925	1255	91.7	10.1	13.7
+5 min	865	1211	93.6	9.2	12.9
+10 min	803	1176	113	7.1	10.4

- The samples drawn from the petrosal sinuses, particularly on the left, were significantly higher than those drawn from a peripheral site, supporting a diagnosis of Cushing's disease. Patient underwent a transsphenoidal surgery for resection of a 12 mm × 10 mm × 8 mm pituitary adenoma on the left aspect of the anterior pituitary gland. Pathology showed loss of reticulin fibers, as well as positive staining for ACTH.
- By postoperative day 3, morning serum cortisol level was 1 mcg/dL, ACTH undetectable, and patient was started on 25 mg of hydrocortisone daily, divided into two doses.
- At 6 month follow-up, patient reported a 20 lb (9.1 kg) weight loss, but persistent depressive symptoms. ACTH stim test was conducted with a normal adrenal response (up to 18.7 ug/dL/516 nmol/L), and hydrocortisone was discontinued.
- At 1 year follow-up, patient reports continued improvement in energy levels, as well as continued weight loss. Diabetes and hypertension were also resolved, with patient no longer requiring medical management.

Questions:
1. Outline a potential education programme for this patient.
2. Describe other services that this patient may require to achieve best outcomes.
3. Consider other evidence that may need to be obtained for best practice in the care of this patient.

Acknowledgements The author acknowledges Margaret Keil MSN, CRNP who is the Pediatric Nurse Practitioner of National Institute of Child Health and Human Development (NICHD) and Director of Pediatric Endocrine Clinical Services, Bethesda, MD, USA, and Daphne Adelman BSN, MBA, Division of Endocrinology, Metabolism and Molecular Medicine, Northwestern University, Evanston, IL, USA.

References

Abdel Mannan D, Selman WR, Arafah BM. Peri-operative management of Cushing's disease. Rev Endocr Metab Disord. 2010;11(2):127–34. https://doi.org/10.1007/s11154-010-9140-6.

Alwani RA, et al. Differentiating between Cushing's disease and pseudo-Cushing's syndrome: comparison of four tests. Eur J Endocrinol. 2014;170(4):477–86.

Barber TM, Adams E, Ansorge O, Byrne JV, Karavitaki N, Wass JAH. Nelson's syndrome. Eur J Endocrinol. 2010;163:495–507.

Batista DL, Riar J, Keil M, Stratakis CA. Diagnostic tests for children who are referred for the investigation of Cushing syndrome. Pediatrics. 2007;120(3):e575–86.

Bertagna X, Guignat L, Raux-Demay MC, Guilhaume B, Girad F. Cushings disease. In: Melmed S, editor. The pituitary. 3rd ed. Amsterdam: Elsevier; 2011. https://doi.org/10.1016/B978-0-12-380926-1.10016-1.

Biller BM, Alexander JM, Zervas NT, Hedley-Whyte ET, Arnold A, Klibanski A. Clonal origins of adrenocorticotropin-secreting pituitary tissue in Cushing's disease. J Clin Endocrinol Metab. 1992;75(5):1303–9. https://doi.org/10.1210/jcem.75.5.1358909.

Brzana J, Yedinak CG, Hameed N, Plesiu A, McCartney S, Fleseriu M. Polycystic ovarian syndrome and Cushing's syndrome: a persistent diagnostic quandary. Eur J Obstet Gynecol Reprod Biol. 2014;175:145–8.

Clayton RN, Raskauskiene D, Reulen RC, Jones PW. Mortality and morbidity in Cushing's disease over 50 years in Stoke-on-Trent, UK: audit and meta-analysis of literature. J Clin Endocrinol Metab. 2011;96(3):632–42. https://doi.org/10.1210/jc.2010-1942.

Clayton RN, et al. Mortality in patients with Cushing's disease more than 10 years after remission: a multicentre, multinational, retrospective cohort study. Lancet Diabetes Endocrinol. 2016;4(7):569–76.

Colao A, Boscaro M, Ferone D, Casanueva FF. Managing Cushing's disease: the state of the art. Endocrine. 2014;47(1):9–20. https://doi.org/10.1007/s12020-013-0129-2.

Cuevas-Ramos D, Fleseriu M. Treatment of Cushing's disease: a mechanistic update. J Endocrinol. 2014;223(2):R19–39. https://doi.org/10.1530/JOE-14-0300.

Cuevas-Ramos D, et al. Update on medical treatment for Cushing's disease. Clin Diabetes Endocrinol. 2016;2:16.

Dekkers OM, Horvath-Puho E, Jorgensen JO, Cannegieter SC, Ehrenstein V, Vandenbroucke JP, et al. Multisystem morbidity and mortality in Cushing's syndrome: a cohort study. J Clin Endocrinol Metab. 2013;98(6):2277–84. https://doi.org/10.1210/jc.2012-3582.

Dorn LD, Burgess ES, Dubbert B, et al. Psychopathology in patients with endogenous Cushing's syndrome: 'atypical' or melancholic features. Clin Endocrinol. 1995;43:433–42.

Espinosa-de-Los-Monteros AL, et al. Persistence of Cushing's disease symptoms and comorbidities after surgical cure: a long-term, integral evaluation. Endocr Pract. 2013;19(2):252–8.

Feelders RA, Pulgar SJ, Kempel A, Pereira AM. The burden of Cushing's disease: clinical and health-related quality of life aspects. Eur J Endocrinol. 2012;167(3):311–26. https://doi.org/10.1530/EJE-11-1095.

Findling JW, Raff H. Cushing's syndrome: important issues in diagnosis and management. J Clin Endocrinol Metab. 2006;91(10):3746–53. https://doi.org/10.1210/jc.2006-0997.

Fleseriu M. Medical management of persistent and recurrent Cushing disease. Neurosurg Clin N Am. 2012;23(4):653–68.

Friedman TC, Yanovski JA. Morning plasma free cortisol: inability to distinguish patients with mild Cushing syndrome from patients with pseudo-Cushing states. J Endocrinol Invest. 1995;18(9):696–701.

Graversen D, Vestergaard P, Stochholm K, Gravholt CH, Jorgensen JO. Mortality in Cushing's syndrome: a systematic review and meta-analysis. Eur J Intern Med. 2012;23(3):278–82. https://doi.org/10.1016/j.ejim.2011.10.013.

Johannsson G, et al. Adrenal insufficiency: review of clinical outcomes with current glucocorticoid replacement therapy. Clin Endocrinol. 2015;82(1):2–11.

Kamp K, Alwani RA, Korpershoek E, Franssen GJ, de Herder WW, Feelders RA. Prevalence and clinical features of the ectopic ACTH syndrome in patients with gastroenteropancreatic and thoracic neuroendocrine tumours. Eur J Endocrinol. 2016;174(3):271–80. https://doi.org/10.1530/EJE-15-0968.

Keil MF, Merke DP, Gandhi R, Wiggs EA, Obunse K, Stratakis CA. Quality of life in children and adolescents 1-year after cure of Cushing syndrome: a prospective study. Clin Endocrinol. 2009; 71(3):326–33.

Keil MF, Zametkin A, Ryder C, Lodish M, Stratakis CA. Cases of psychiatric morbidity in pediatric patients after remission of Cushing syndrome. Pediatrics. 2016;137(4). Epub 2016/03/31.

Lindholm J, Juul S, Jorgensen JO, Astrup J, Bjerre P, Feldt-Rasmussen U, et al. Incidence and late prognosis of Cushing's syndrome: a population-based study. J Clin Endocrinol Metab. 2001;86(1):117–23. https://doi.org/10.1210/jcem.86.1.7093.

Lindsay JR, Nieman LK. Differential diagnosis and imaging in Cushing's syndrome. Endocrinol Metab Clin North Am. 2005;34(2):403–21., x. https://doi.org/10.1016/j.ecl.2005.01.009.

Lonser RR, Nieman L, Oldfield EH. Cushing's disease: pathobiology, diagnosis, and management. J Neurosurg. 2017;126(2):404–17. https://doi.org/10.3171/2016.1.JNS152119.

Magiakou MA, Mastorakos G, Oldfield EH, Gomez MT, Doppman JL, Cutler GB Jr, et al. Cushing's syndrome in children and adolescents. Presentation, diagnosis, and therapy. N Engl J Med. 1994;331(10):629–36.

Mancini T, Porcelli T, Giustina A. Treatment of Cushing disease: overview and recent findings. Ther Clin Risk Manag. 2010;6:505–16. https://doi.org/10.2147/TCRM.S12952.

Martinez-Momblan MA, Gomez C, Santos A, Porta N, Esteve J, Ubeda I, Webb S, Resmini E. A specific nurs-

ing educational program in patients with Cushing's syndrome. Endocrine. 2016;53(1):199–209. https://doi.org/10.1007/s12020-015-0737-0.

Mehta GU, Lonser RR. Management of hormone-secreting pituitary adenomas. Neuro Oncol. 2017;19(6):762–73. https://doi.org/10.1093/neuonc/now130.

Newell-Price J, Bertagna X, Grossman AB, Nieman LK. Cushing's syndrome. Lancet. 2006;367(9522):1605–17. https://doi.org/10.1016/S0140-6736(06)68699-6.

Nieman LK, Biller BM, Findling JW, Newell-Price J, Savage MO, Stewart PM, Montori VM. The diagnosis of Cushing's syndrome: an Endocrine Society Clinical Practice Guideline. J Clin Endocrinol Metab. 2008;93(5):1526–40. https://doi.org/10.1210/jc.2008-0125.

Nieman LK, Biller BM, Findling JW, Murad MH, Newell-Price J, Savage MO, et al. Treatment of Cushing's syndrome: an Endocrine Society Clinical Practice Guideline. J Clin Endocrinol Metab. 2015;100(8):2807–31. https://doi.org/10.1210/jc.2015-1818.

Quinkler M, Miodini Nilsen R, Zopf K, Ventz M, Øksnes M. Modified-release hydrocortisone decreases BMI and HbA1c in patients with primary and secondary adrenal insufficiency. Eur J Endocrinol. 2015;172:619–26.

Sharma ST, Nieman LK. Cushing's syndrome: all variants, detection, and treatment. Endocrinol Metab Clin North Am. 2011;40(2):379–91., viii–ix. https://doi.org/10.1016/j.ecl.2011.01.006.

Sharma ST, Nieman LK, Feelders RA. Cushing's syndrome: epidemiology and developments in disease management. Clin Epidemiol. 2015a;7:281–93. https://doi.org/10.2147/CLEP.S44336.

Sharma ST, Nieman LK, Feelders RA. Comorbidities in Cushing's disease. Pituitary. 2015b;18(2):188–94. https://doi.org/10.1007/s11102-015-0645-6.

Stratakis CA, Tichomirowa MA, Boikos S, Azevedo MF, Lodish M, Martari M, et al. The role of germline AIP, MEN1, PRKAR1A, CDKN1B and CDKN2C mutations in causing pituitary adenomas in a large cohort of children, adolescents, and patients with genetic syndromes. Clin Genet. 2010;78(5):457–63.

Syro LV, Rotondo F, Cusimano MD, Di Ieva A, Horvath E, Restrepo LM, et al. Current status on histological classification in Cushing's disease. Pituitary. 2015;18(2):217–24. https://doi.org/10.1007/s11102-014-0619-0.

Theodoropoulou M, Reincke M, Fassnacht M, Komada M. Decoding the genetic basis of Cushing's disease: USP8 in the spotlight. Eur J Endocrinol. 2015;173(4):M73–83. https://doi.org/10.1530/EJE-15-0320.

Tsigos C, Chrousos GP. Differential diagnosis and management of Cushing's syndrome. Annu Rev Med. 1996;47:443–61.

Valassi E, Feelders R, Maiter D, Chanson P, Yaneva M, Reincke M, Krsek M, Tóth M, Webb SM, Santos A,

Paiva I, Komerdus I, Droste M, Tabarin A, Strasburger CJ, Franz H, Trainer PJ, Newell-Price J, Wass JA, Papakokkinou E, Ragnarsson O. Worse health-related quality of life at long-term follow-up in patients with Cushing's disease than patients with cortisol producing adenoma. Data from the ERCUSYN. Clin Endocrinol. 2018;88(6):787–98. https://doi.org/10.1111/cen.13600.

van der Meij NT, et al. Self-management support in patients with adrenal insufficiency. Clin Endocrinol. 2016;85(4):652–9.

Vilar L, Naves LA, Machado MC, Bronstein MD. Medical combination therapies in Cushing's disease. Pituitary. 2015;18(2):253–62. https://doi.org/10.1007/s11102-015-0641-x.

Zilio M, Barbot M, Ceccato F, Camozzi V, Bilora F, Casonato A, et al. Diagnosis and complications of Cushing's disease: gender-related differences. Clin Endocrinol. 2014;80(3):403–10. https://doi.org/10.1111/cen.12299.

Key Reading

1. Lonser RR, Nieman L, Oldfield EH. Cushing's disease: pathobiology, diagnosis, and management. J Neurosurg. 2017;126(2):404–17. https://doi.org/10.3171/2016.1.JNS152119.
2. Feelders RA, Pulgar SJ, Kempel A, Pereira AM. The burden of Cushing's disease: clinical and health-related quality of life aspects. Eur J Endocrinol. 2012;167(3):311–26. https://doi.org/10.1530/EJE-11-1095.
3. Newell-Price J, Bertagna X, Grossman AB, Nieman LK. Cushing's syndrome. Lancet. 2006;367(9522):1605–17. https://doi.org/10.1016/S0140-6736(06)68699-6.
4. Martinez-Momblan MA, Gomez C, Santos A, Porta N, Esteve J, Ubeda I, et al. A specific nursing educational program in patients with Cushing's syndrome. Endocrine. 2016;53(1):199–209. https://doi.org/10.1007/s12020-015-0737-0.

Pituitary Surgery

22

Jürgen Honegger

Contents

J. Honegger (✉)
Department of Neurosurgery, University of
Tuebingen, Tuebingen, Germany
e-mail: Juergen.Honegger@med.uni-tuebingen.de

© Springer Nature Switzerland AG 2019
S. Llahana et al. (eds.), *Advanced Practice in Endocrinology Nursing*,
https://doi.org/10.1007/978-3-319-99817-6_22

Abstract

Today, more than 95% of pituitary adenomas are removed using transsphenoidal surgery. The complication rates both for the traditional microscopic technique and for the more recently introduced endoscopic technique are comparably low. In acromegaly, the overall surgical cure rate of the transsphenoidal operation is approximately 50% in experienced hands. In Cushing's disease, the cure rate is high if an adenoma is visible on MRI. In prolactinomas, surgery should be preferentially offered to patients with microadenomas (<10 mm) as their chance of surgical cure is >90%.

Adequate perioperative endocrinological management is pivotal. Replacement therapy for adrenal insufficiency must be adapted to the perioperative demand. Diabetes insipidus (DI) with impaired ADH secretion is encountered frequently on days 1–5 after surgery while the opposing syndrome of inappropriate antidiuretic hormone secretion (SIADH) with excessive ADH release typically presents on days 3–10. Thorough surveillance of water and electrolyte balance in the postoperative course is paramount for early detection and treatment of these typical postoperative dysregulations of the posterior pituitary lobe. Postoperative endocrine care includes early assessment of remission status and pituitary function. It is recommended that neuro-endocrine and neurosurgical follow-up appointments be scheduled prior to discharge to guarantee professional ongoing follow-up.

For non-functioning pituitary adenomas (NFPA), radiotherapy (RT) may be considered for invasive residual tumour after surgery. The timing of radiotherapy is still a subject of controversy. For functioning adenomas, radiotherapy is indicated if surgery and medical therapy cannot control hormonal oversecretion. Fractionated radiotherapy (fRT) is used for large adenoma volumes to minimize secondary injury to surrounding structures. Stereotactic radiosurgery (SRS) is used for small target volumes with a sufficient distance from the optic apparatus. These two principle techniques have different risk profiles. Both fRT and SRS are highly effective in preventing further adenoma growth. Biochemical cure is less frequent. Reportedly, the biochemical cure rates are slightly higher for Cushing's disease than for acromegaly and are least favourable in prolactinomas. Biochemical remission is often delayed and the cure rates increase over the years after RT.

Keywords

Pituitary surgery · Pituitary adenoma · Transsphenoidal · Microscopic · Endoscopic · Fractionated radiotherapy · Radiosurgery

Abbreviations

ACTH	Adreno-corticotrophic hormone
ADH	Antidiuretic hormone
CD	Cushing's disease
CS	Cushing's syndrome
CSF	Cerebro-spinal fluid
DA	Dopamine-agonist
DI	Diabetes insipidus
fRT	Fractionated radiotherapy
GH	Growth hormone
GKRS	Gamma-knife radiosurgery
Gy	Gray
IGF-1	Insulin-like growth factor 1
LINAC	Linear accelerator based radiosurgery
MRI	Magnetic resonance imaging
NFPA	Non-functioning pituitary adenoma
RT	Radiotherapy
SIADH	Syndrome of inappropriate antidiuretic hormone secretion
SRS	Stereotactic radiosurgery

Key Terms

- **Transsphenoidal:** Surgery is performed through the nose and the sphenoid sinus.
- **Transcranial:** Surgery is performed by removing a piece of skull bone.
- **Microscopic:** The surgeon looks through a microscope during transsphenoidal surgery.
- **Endoscopic:** The surgeon uses an endoscope to visualize during transsphenoidal surgery.

Key Points

- More than 95% of pituitary adenomas are removed through the transsphenoidal route. The complication rates both for the traditional microscopic technique and for the more recently introduced endoscopic technique are comparably low.
- Pituitary surgery is the first line of treatment for large non-functioning adenomas and in functioning adenomas causing Cushing's disease or acromegaly. Prolactinomas, by contrast, are primarily treated with dopamine-agonists (DAs). Transsphenoidal surgery, however, is an accepted alternative for small prolactinomas as cure rates greater than 90% can be achieved.
- Adequate perioperative endocrinological management is pivotal. It includes perioperative hormonal replacement therapy, thorough surveillance of water and electrolyte balance, and assessment of postoperative remission status.
- Radiotherapy is indicated if adenoma growth or hormonal hypersecretion is not controlled by surgery and/or medical therapy. Fractionated radiotherapy (fRT) is used for large adenoma volumes while stereotactic radiosurgery (SRS) is indicated for small target volumes with a sufficient distance from the optic nerves and chiasm.
- Both fRT and SRS are effective in preventing further adenoma growth. Biochemical cure rates are slightly higher for Cushing's disease than for acromegaly and are least favourable in prolactinomas.

22.1 Transsphenoidal Surgery

22.1.1 History of Transsphenoidal Surgery

The first successful operation for a pituitary tumour was performed by Victor Horsley in 1904 at Queen Square in London using a transcranial approach. Only a few years later, Hermann Schloffer, at University Clinic in Innsbruck, performed the very first transsphenoidal operation in 1907 (Schloffer 1907). He approached the sphenoid sinus and sella through an invasive rhinotomy incision along the lateral aspect of the nose (Fig. 22.1a). The nose was reflected to the side and the septum, medial wall of the orbit and portions of the maxillary sinus wall were removed. In the following years,

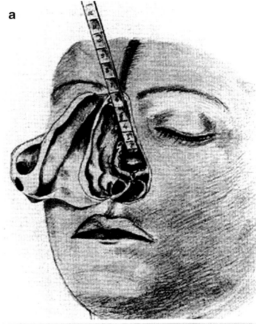

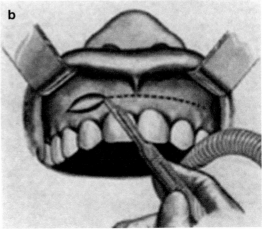

Fig. 22.1 (a) First transsphenoidal surgery using rhinotomy (Courtesy of the National Library of Medicine). (b) Translabial approach (Courtesy of the National Library of Medicine)

transsphenoidal surgery was refined. Inferior nasal approaches were established with the advantage of less disfigurement and a better suprasellar view. The transnasal and sublabial approaches avoided an external incision (Fig. 22.1b). A major pioneer of transsphenoidal surgery was Harvey Cushing who performed 231 transsphenoidal operations in Boston between 1910 and 1925 with a mortality rate of 5.6%. However, he abandoned the transsphenoidal approach in the late 1920s because of the better results of transcranial surgery at that time. One must bear in mind that, at that time, imaging techniques were poor and it was impossible to know the true size and extent of pituitary tumours into the suprasellar space, making transsphenoidal surgery hazardous. Jules Hardy from Montreal who worked together with Gérard Guiot in Paris introduced the operating microscope for transsphenoidal surgery in the late 1960s (Hardy 1969). It offered two major advances that made the approach safer and more effective: First, it allowed better illumination of the operative field in the depth through a narrow approach. Second, selective adenomectomy with preservation of the pituitary gland and identification of small microadenomas became possible with magnification under the microscope. With the introduction of microscopy, the surgical morbidity and mortality of transsphenoidal surgery were significantly reduced and lead to worldwide recognition and adoption.

As early as in 1963, Gérard Guiot suggested the use of the endoscope at the end of a transsphenoidal operation for visualization. In the 1990s, Hae Dong Jho introduced the concept of pure endoscopic transnasal surgery (Jho et al. 1997). In the last two decades, endoscopy has become a generally accepted alternative to microscopy in pituitary surgery.

Today, the transsphenoidal approach is used in 96–99% of the patients for removal of pituitary adenomas (Honegger et al. 2007).

22.1.2 The Microscopic Transsphenoidal Approach

The preferred microscopic approach to the pituitary is the so-called "septum-pushover

technique". This technique is a uninostril-endonasal approach to the sphenoid sinus. The mucosa is incised over the nasal septum in the depth in front of the sphenoid sinus. The nasal septum is disconnected from the rostrum of the sphenoid sinus and displaced to the opposite side with the nasal speculum (Griffith and Veerapen 1987). At the end of the operation, the septum is brought back to the midline. The "septum-pushover technique" is a minimally invasive technique that is performed quickly and causes minimal postoperative discomfort and pain. In particular, the patients appreciate that no nasal packing is required and nasal breathing is possible immediately after surgery.

The microscopic approach (Figs. 22.2a, 22.3) offers the advantage of a 3-dimensional view. A speculum is necessary for visualization of the operative field, because the optic system is outside the nose. On the other hand, surgical manoeuvres are fast and straight-forward because the access to the operative field is held open by the speculum.

22.1.3 The Endoscopic Transsphenoidal Approach

For the endoscopic approach (Figs. 22.2b and 22.4), a binostril or uninostril approach is used to access the sphenoidal sinus (Juraschka et al. 2014). Endoscopic surgery is mostly performed in a "four-hand technique" where one surgeon performs the operation and the other surgeon holds and guides the endoscope. Once the sphenoid sinus is sufficiently opened, the endoscope is positioned in the sphenoid sinus. The position of the optic system inside offers the advantage of a panoramic view. In particular, lateral and suprasellar tumours can be directly visualized which can increase the extent of surgical resection.

One has to bear in mind that the microscope and endoscope are only instruments for visualization. The experience of the surgeon is most important for the success of surgery and not whether a microscopic or endoscopic technique is used.

a

b

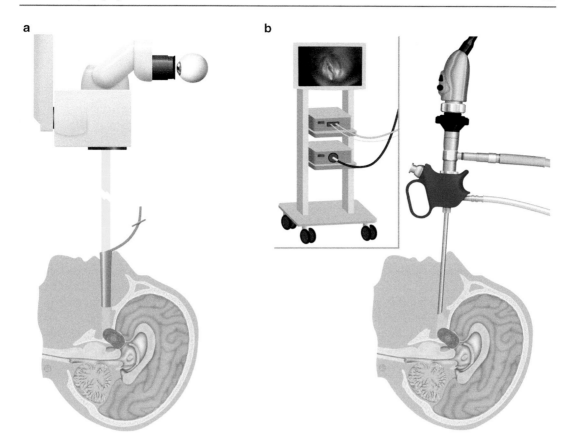

Fig. 22.2 Schematic drawing of the microscopic and endoscopic setting. (**a**) Microscopy. The surgeon visualizes the surgical field through the microscope. The surgical corridor is held open by the nasal speculum. (**b**) Endoscopy. The endoscope is positioned inside the surgical corridor. The surgical field is visualized on the monitor. Copyright: Universitätsklinikum Tübingen

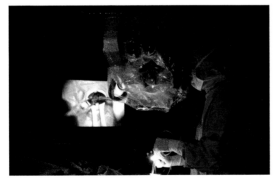

Fig. 22.3 Microscopic transsphenoidal approach. With the microscope, the surgeon has a 3-dimensional view of the surgical field. Additionally, the operation is shown on the screen in the operating theater

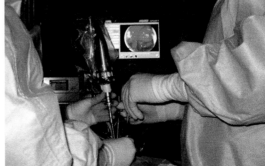

Fig. 22.4 Endoscopic transsphenoidal surgery: four-hand techique of the endoscopic procedure is shown

22.1.4 Tumour Removal
in Transsphenoidal Surgery

Once the anterior wall of the sphenoid sinus has been opened, the pituitary fossa becomes visible. The bony floor of the pituitary fossa is removed. For this surgical step, we use a diamond drill and punches. The next anatomical structure which lines the floor of the sella is the basal dura. Once this is opened in a Y-shaped manner, the pituitary adenoma is exposed. The adenoma is then removed with microinstruments. As adenomas are often soft, curettes are mostly used for adenomectomy. Once the intrasellar tumour is removed, the suprasellar portion can descend into the pituitary fossa and can be resected (Fatemi et al. 2008).

Approximately one-third of surgically treated pituitary adenomas show an invasive character. This means that the adenoma grows into the adjacent anatomical structures. The most frequent site of invasion is the cavernous sinus. Some soft adenomas may be removed from within the cavernous sinus without undue morbidity. However, invasion is clearly an adverse factor for complete resection and incurs risk to cranial nerves III, IV, VI, trigeminal nerve V2 (maxillary branch) and the internal carotid artery that traverse this area.

Under microscopic or endoscopic view, the pituitary gland can be differentiated from the adenoma and then preserved. With large adenomas, the gland has become flattened and displaced and lines the resection cavity.

The diaphragma sellae is the upper border of the pituitary fossa and protects the fossa from the cerebro-spinal fluid (CSF) space. Particularly in large adenomas, the diaphragma is thin and intraoperative CSF rhinorrhea can occur, requiring repair. For closure of a CSF leak, various techniques are used. Repair may be with autologous material from the patient (e.g. fascia late, abdominal fat) or with dural substitutes or both. For large CSF leaks, a vascularized naso-septal flat is often placed over the skull base defect (Hadad et al. 2006). If a large intraoperative leak occurs, an additional prophylactic postoperative lumbar drainage for 5–7 days may be placed to prevent formation of a nasal CSF fistula by lowering the intracranial pressure.

22.1.5 Risk of Transsphenoidal
Surgery

The complication rate in transsphenoidal surgery for pituitary adenomas is relatively low. In a recent meta-analysis (Ammirati et al. 2013), the risk of a CSF leak was 6–7%. Meningitis occurred in 1–2% of cases. The frequency of these typical complications was similar if microscopic and endoscopic series were compared. The risk of death was 0.5% for microscopy and 1.58% for endoscopy. Only for vascular injury, was a significant difference between microscopy (0.23%) and endoscopy (0.49%) found.

Of course, the experience of the surgeons has major influence on the complication rates. In experienced hands, a risk of CSF leak requiring operative repair can be below 1%.

The risk of new postoperative hypopituitarism is about 10%. It is significantly correlated to adenoma size. On the other hand, the chance of postoperative improvement of pituitary function is 30–40%. While transient diabetes insipidus is frequently observed, the rate of permanent diabetes insipidus is only about 1% (Ammirati et al. 2013).

Postoperative deterioration of visual function and visual fields is rare (Fig. 22.5). It can be caused by postoperative bleeding. On the other hand, preoperative visual deficits often recover after surgery. The risk that chiasmal syndrome does not improve postoperatively is particularly high if preoperative deficits were long-standing and pronounced.

22.1.6 Special Considerations
and Outcome in Different
Adenoma Types

Pituitary adenomas are either non-functioning or hormone-secreting. The most frequent types of

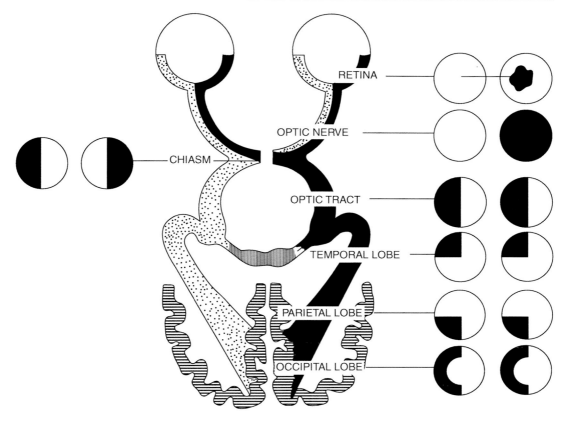

Fig. 22.5 The visual pathway and the visual defects that occur depending on the site of a lesion. A pituitary adenoma typically causes midline compression of the optic chiasm from below that results in bitemporal visual field defects

hormone-secreting adenomas are GH-secreting adenomas causing acromegaly or gigantism, ACTH-secreting adenomas causing Cushing's disease and prolactin-secreting adenomas, which are called prolactinomas. In the following, the special surgical considerations and the surgical outcome of these frequent adenoma types are described.

22.1.6.1   Transsphenoidal Surgery for Non-functioning Pituitary Adenomas (NFPA)

NFPA only become symptomatic if they cause local symptoms due to a space-occupying lesion. Visual deficits and hypopituitarism prevail and represent the indication for surgery. On the other hand, NFPA are often diagnosed incidentally during cranial imaging for other reasons (such as on evaluation of headaches or head injuries). The indication for treatment of asymptomatic adenomas is relative. Surgery is usually performed if the adenoma size is larger than 2 cm or some degree of chiasmal compression is found on MRI.

Despite their large size, more than 90% of NFPA can be removed by a transsphenoidal approach. Figure 22.6 shows the MRI of a large NFPA before and after transsphenoidal removal. If complete removal of a NFPA has been confirmed by MRI, the risk of recurrence is low (Chang et al. 2010). In contrast, residues of NFPA are at high risk for re-growth. Due to the low growth velocity of many pituitary adenomas, re-growth may be detected only after several years of observation.

Fig. 22.6 (**a**) coronal
view and (**b**) sagittal
view: Preoperative MRI
shows a large non-
functioning pituitary
adenoma causing visual
field defects. (**c**) coronal
view and (**d**) sagittal
view: Postoperative MRI
confirms complete
adenoma removal

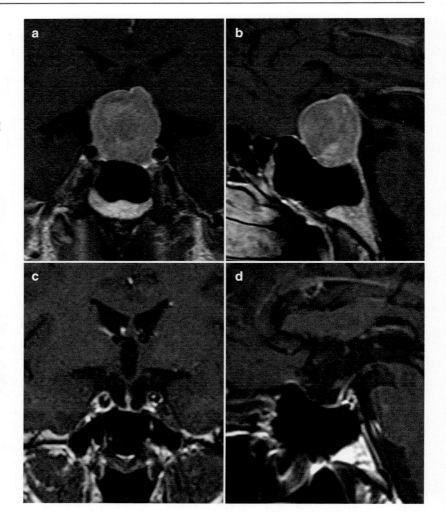

22.1.6.2   Transsphenoidal Surgery and Outcome in Acromegaly

Transsphenoidal surgery is the first choice of treatment in acromegaly.

The anaesthetist must be prepared, as intubation might be difficult. Intubation can be hampered by macroglossia, goitre and spinal kyphosis.

The surgeon must be prepared that the nasal anatomy can be distorted due to overgrowth of the anatomical structures. The nasal septum is often deviated. An extra long nasal speculum may be needed because the approach can be abnormally deep in acromegaly.

Criteria for cure are normalized insulin-like growth factor 1 (IGF-1), normal basal growth hormone (GH) and adequate suppression of GH during an oral glucose tolerance test.

Strong adverse prognostic factors in terms of cure are large adenoma size, invasive character and high preoperative GH and IGF-1 levels. The data of the German Acromegaly Register showed a long-term cure rate of 38.8%, others report lower or similar remission rates (Schöfl et al. 2013; Minniti et al. 2003). In centres with a high case-load of acromegalic patients, the cure rate was 49.8–51% (Mortini et al. 2018). In those patients without complete surgical cure, a significant reduction of GH excess by surgery will improve the success rate of postoperative medical treatment or radiotherapy.

22.1.6.3   Transsphenoidal Surgery and Outcome in Cushing's Disease

Cushing's disease (CD) is a life-threatening disease that is mostly caused by microadenomas. CD is unique in that 30% of microadenomas are so small that they are not detected even with modern MRI of the pituitary.

Endocrinological diagnostics prove the pituitary origin and differentiate CD from ectopic and adrenal Cushing's syndrome (CS). If the pituitary origin is unclear, inferior petrosal sinus sampling (IPSS) is performed as the pituitary blood is drained into the inferior petrosal sinus. Higher ACTH values in the petrosal sinus compared to ACTH in the peripheral vein confirm the pituitary origin. For prediction of the laterality of a microadenoma within the gland, IPSS only has a poor positive predictive value.

Transsphenoidal surgery is the treatment of first choice in CD. If no adenoma is detected by MRI, the pituitary gland is systematically explored by micro-incisions. A special small ultrasound probe for intraoperative detection of minute microadenomas is used in some specialized centres.

In large series with transsphenoidal surgery for microadenomas, postoperative remission rates in the range of 59–98% have been reported (Chandler et al. 2016). The cure rate is clearly superior if a microadenoma has been detected on preoperative MRI.

22.1.6.4   Transsphenoidal Surgery and Outcome in Prolactinomas

In prolactinomas, medical treatment with dopamine-agonists (DAs) is the first choice. However, a re-increase of prolactin occurs in 79% of prolactinomas after withdrawal of DA.

Transsphenoidal surgery is a second choice treatment for prolactinomas. The classical indications for surgery are resistance to DA or intolerable side-effects of DA. Further indications for surgery have emerged: The guidelines of the Pituitary Society from 2006 describe that the possibility of cure by surgery versus long-term DA therapy should be discussed with the

patient, and patient preference is an indication for surgery (Casanueva et al. 2006). Surgery may be preferentially offered in microadenomas where the surgical cure rate is >90% (Casanueva et al. 2006; Kreutzer et al. 2008). The chance of prolactin normalization is still good in circumscribed intrasellar macroprolactinomas. Transsphenoidal surgery is usually not offered in large or invasive prolactinomas because postoperative normoprolactinaemia is unlikely. The risk of cardiac valvulopathy under DA is also a concern. Therefore, young patient age is an argument for surgery in order to avoid long-term DA. If acute visual loss occurs, it should not be hesitated to perform acute surgical decompression instead of awaiting the effect of DA (Kreutzer et al. 2008).

22.1.7   Modern Technologies in Transsphenoidal Surgery

Intraoperative MRI is available in some neurosurgical centres. The completeness of resection can be controlled intraoperatively. Identified residual adenoma can be removed during the same procedure avoiding a second operation.

Today, neuronavigation systems are widely used in neurosurgery and also in pituitary surgery. With neuronavigation, intraoperative tumour and major structure positions can be compared with the preoperative imaging data. With neuronavigation, the location of risk structures (i.e. carotid arteries) and the extent of resection can be verified intraoperatively.

22.2   Perioperative and Postoperative Care

22.2.1   Perioperative and Postoperative Care: Endocrinological

The postoperative endocrine care is demanding. Adequate management of postoperative endocrinological peculiarities is pivotal for the success of surgical treatment.

The details of postoperative management vary between different centres. The practices and therapeutic schemes that are provided in this section only have an exemplary nature.

22.2.1.1 Postoperative Dysregulation of Water and Electrolyte Balance

Disturbances of water and electrolyte balance are frequently encountered during the early postoperative period due to dysregulation of the posterior pituitary lobe. The two major postoperative dysregulations are diabetes insipidus and syndrome of inappropriate antidiuretic hormone secretion (SIADH) which are opposing problems. Diabetes insipidus is caused by impaired secretion of antidiuretic hormone (ADH) from the posterior pituitary lobe. In contrast, SIADH is caused by postoperative degeneration of some ADH-secreting neurons with excessive release of ADH.

Surveillance of water and electrolyte balance plays a central role in postoperative management. (see Chap. 23: Pituitary Surgery: Part 2 Nursing Care) Monitoring incudes:

- Balancing of daily fluid intake and output.
- Specific gravity of every urine portion.
- Daily measurement of serum sodium level.
- Daily measurement of body weight.

22.2.1.2 Diagnosis and Treatment of Postoperative Diabetes Insipidus

Impaired ADH secretion of the posterior lobe results in diabetes insipidus which is frequently encountered in the first days after surgery:

- 40% of patients have polyuria (>2.5 l/24 h) at the first postoperative day after transsphenoidal surgery for a pituitary adenoma.
- 5% suffer from polyuria at the fifth postoperative day.
- Permanent diabetes insipidus is only found in 1% of cases postoperatively.

Algorithm for the Management of Diabetes Insipidus: A Single Centre Protocol

Diagnosis
- Fluid intake and output exceeds 3500 mL in 24 h.
- Urine output exceeds 400 mL within 2 h.
- Serum sodium above upper limit of normal.

Treatment
- Desmopressin 2 µg subcutaneous or intramuscular after transsphenoidal surgery during the first postoperative days (because of reduced nasal uptake following transsphenoidal surgery).
- Nasal application of desmopressin spray 1 puff can be commenced from postoperative day 6 onward.
- Desmopressin tablets are also recommended for cases of mild or partial diabetes insipidus.

22.2.1.3 Diagnosis and Treatment of Postoperative Syndrome of Inappropriate Antidiuretic Hormone Secretion (SIADH)

SIADH usually occurs between postoperative day 3 and day 10 and is a potential life-threatening complication. This is reported in up to 30% of cases. SIADH results in hyponatremia. Therefore, our protocol is to regularly measure serum sodium level until postoperative day 10 but protocols may be site specific.

Asymptomatic SIADH can be treated with restriction of fluid intake to 1 L per day. In symptomatic SIADH, hyperosmolar sodium infusion is often required in addition to fluid restriction. Recently, the vasopressin antagonist tolvaptan became available. It allows efficient treatment of SIADH without fluid restriction. We start with a single dose of tolvaptan 7.5 mg. Mostly, a second dose is necessary 1–2 days later.

It is imperative that an unduly rapid correction of hyponatremia is avoided. A rapid correction can cause damage to the myelin sheath of the nerve cells in the brainstem called central pontine myelinolysis which is a severe neurological disorder with poor prognosis.

Signs and Symptoms of SIADH
- Headache
- Malaise
- Agitation
- Tiredness
- Poor Concentration
- Nausea and vomiting
- Mental state changes and confusion
- Epileptic seizure

22.2.1.4   Perioperative Replacement Therapy of Adrenal Insufficiency

Replacement therapy for adrenal insufficiency is of vital importance. A higher demand of cortisone is required during the stressful event of an operation. Two principle perioperative strategies can be pursued:

(a) Replacement in every patient undergoing pituitary surgery.
(b) Replacement only if:
- Preoperative adrenal insufficiency exists or
- Adrenal function is unknown (for example in emergency cases) or
- New adrenal failure is anticipated based on intraoperative findings.

Table 22.1 shows our regime if glucocorticoid replacement is required during the perioperative period. Physiological doses are continued at discharge as indicated after assessment of HPA axis (Table 22.1).

In some countries, an emergency card is available or provided to the patient if postoperative

Table 22.1 Hydrocortisone Replacement Regime: a single centre protocol

Day of surgery	100 mg hydrocortisone intraoperatively (intravenous) 100 mg hydrocortisone until the next morning (intravenous)
First postop day	50 mg hydrocortisone (oral)
Second postop day	40 mg hydrocortisone (oral)
Third postop day	30 mg hydrocortisone (oral)
Forth postop day	30 mg hydrocortisone (oral)
From fifth postop day onward	20 mg hydrocortisone (oral) (maintenance dose)

adrenal insufficiency is found or if adrenal function is equivocal.

22.2.1.5   Early Postoperative Assessment of Remission Status

In functioning adenomas, postoperative assessment of the oversecreted hormone provides important information about the success of the surgery. Re-assessment should be performed as early as possible because the result is not only important for further treatment but also urgently awaited by the patient.

In *prolactinomas*, prolactin can be assessed on the first postoperative day. In *acromegaly*, we also assess GH on the first postoperative day. However, IGF-1 decline is delayed. Both prolactin and GH are peptide hormones with a short half-life period. Their measurement at the first postoperative day provides valuable information of surgical success regarding correction of the oversecreted hormone (see specific chapters for more information).

In *Cushing's disease*, different methods for early assessment of the remission status are in use: Some centres withhold perioperative hydrocortisone replacement and measure cortisol daily after surgery. A drop in serum cortisol into the hypocortisolemic range indicates remission. As soon as remission is documented or the patient shows clinical signs of adrenal insufficiency, hydrocortisone replacement therapy must be commenced.

This regimen allows for the earliest possible detection of remission. However, continuous clinical surveillance for symptoms of adrenal insufficiency is paramount to avoid adrenal crisis.

Other centres use perioperative hydrocortisone replacement and withdraw hydrocortisone some days after surgery for assessment of the remission status.

22.2.1.6 Early Postoperative Assessment of Anterior Pituitary Function

The regimen of postoperative endocrine reassessment of pituitary function differs between centres. An orienting status of pituitary hormones prior to discharge should be the minimal standard.

22.2.2 Postoperative Care: Neurosurgical

22.2.2.1 Surveillance of Vision

The optic chiasm is in close proximity to the pituitary gland. Patients with pituitary tumours may suffer from chiasmal syndrome preoperatively. Assessment of visual acuity and visual fields is mandatory immediately and regularly postoperatively. Visual fields are tested with finger perimetry.

Knowledge of preoperative vision and visual fields is important for proper judgement of the postoperative state. Furthermore, the nurse must have information from the surgeon about which patients are at risk for visual deterioration.

Visual failure may indicate postoperative bleeding. The risk of bleeding is particularly high during the first postoperative day. On the other hand, improvement of preoperative visual deficits can often be detected immediately after surgery but may also be delayed. Formal ophthalmological re-assessment can be done 1 week after surgery.

Furthermore, optomotor nerves run lateral to the pituitary fossa within the cavernous sinus. Postoperative care includes alertness for double vision and ptosis.

22.2.2.2 Nasal Care After Transsphenoidal Surgery

Regular nasal application of decongestant nose drops enhances nasal breathing and avoids trou-

blesome nasal secretion or painful retention of secretion in the paranasal sinuses. Some centres use xylometazoline 0.1% nasal spray or drops. This shrinks the swollen nasal mucosa via vasoconstriction. It is applied after transnasal surgery until there are minimal secretions and free ventilation is restored which is usually the case after 7–14 days. Other centres use sterile saline spray multiple times daily to achieve a similar outcome.

Medication for nasal pain is not routinely administered. Nonsteroidal anti-inflammatory drugs can be given if required. However, acetylsalicylic acid should be avoided during the first 10 postoperative days because of the anticoagulant effects.

It may be difficult to differentiate nasal secretion from cerebro-spinal fluid (CSF) rhinorrhea. No laboratory test is absolutely reliable. Measurement of glucose in nasal fluid is not helpful after transnasal surgery. Mucosal fluid is a hint for nasal secretion while clear fluid like water is suspicious of CSF. CSF rhinorrhea can be provoked if the patient is brought into a sitting position and the head bend forward.

The nasal conditions must be closely supervised. If CSF rhinorrhea occurs, lumbar drainage or operative repair in a timely fashion is indicated to avoid further complications such as meningitis.

22.2.3 Further Early Postoperative Care

The timing of discharge from the neurosurgical unit varies between centres. The postoperative stay is usually between 3 and 6 days. In some centres, the patients are transferred to the endocrine unit during the postoperative hospital stay. Prior to discharge, the patient is given both verbal and written instructions regarding postoperative home care. After transsphenoidal surgery, an increase of intracranial pressure must be avoided for a period of at least 4 weeks (Knappe et al. 2018). For that time, physical strain, sports activities, steam baths, saunas, and blowing the nose must be avoided. After 4 weeks, physical activities can be slowly resumed. Patients are advised to sneeze with an open mouth to avoid Valsalva pressure. The use of continuous positive airway pressure (CPAP) devices is not recommended immediately postoperatively and patients may need supplemental oxygen. Review with the Ear Nose and Throat (ENT) specialist 2–4 weeks postoperatively is recommended.

The patient's case is booked for the tumour board where decisions of further management (for example requirement of postoperative medical treatment or radiotherapy) are made.

Most importantly, an appointment with the endocrinologist must be arranged prior to postoperative discharge. An exact date for the appointment is strongly recommended to guarantee an endocrinological follow-up. A first re-assessment by the endocrinologist is usually recommended 2–3 weeks after surgery. Some endocrinologists see their patients as early as 1 day after discharge from the neurosurgical unit.

Similarly, a neurosurgical follow-up appointment is mandatory. The first appointment at the neurosurgical outpatient department is usually scheduled 3–6 months postoperatively. The patient is instructed to bring along a recent postoperative MRI or is scheduled the same day for a postoperative MRI. Postoperative endocrine re-assessment may be scheduled simultaneously or independently and these results should be available to the neurosurgery at the time of this appointment. If the adenoma had suprasellar extension or the patient had suffered from chiasmal syndrome, an ophthalmological report should also be presented at the neurosurgical follow-up appointment.

22.3 Transcranial Surgery

22.3.1 Indications for Transcranial Surgery

Transcranial surgery is only required if a pituitary adenoma is not sufficiently accessible by a transsphenoidal operation. The decision for the appropriate approach depends on adenoma size and location. A multilobulated suprasellar extension points to a perforated diaphragm sellae. It means that the adenoma has grown out of the confines of the pituitary fossa into the intracranial (intradural) space. Under these circumstances, the risk of trans-

sphenoidal surgery might be too high because it does not provide adequate control of intracranial neurovascular structures. Transcranial surgery is necessary in some of these adenomas. A predominant suprasellar adenoma with a small pituitary fossa, an eccentric suprasellar extension or a dumbbell shaped adenoma also hamper transsphenoidal resection and are reasons for transcranial surgery (Buchfelder and Kreutzer 2008). Today, less than 5% of pituitary adenomas require a transcranial operation.

22.3.2 Transcranial Approach and Tumour Removal

For a transcranial approach, the skin incision is made fronto-temporal behind the hairline to avoid an externally visible scar. The pterional approach and the fronto-lateral approach are most frequently used. The pterional approach exposes the Sylvian fissure between the frontal and temporal lobes. The arachnoid of the Sylvian fissure is opened for exposure of the adenoma. The adenoma can be visualized and removed through the prechiasmatic space or through the space between the optic nerve and carotid artery (so-called "optico-carotid triangle"). The fronto-lateral approach provides a more anterior view. It is less invasive but the lateral view through the optico-carotid triangle is limited.

22.3.3 Risk of Transcranial Surgery

The reported morbidity and mortality of transcranial surgery is certainly higher than of transsphenoidal surgery. However, one has to keep in mind a selection bias because the difficult adenomas with major intracranial, suprasellar extension require a transcranial operation. The mortality rate of transcranial surgery is approximately 2% (Buchfelder and Kreutzer 2008). Transcranial operations carry a particularly high risk of re-bleeding into the tumour bed. Another specific risk is hypothalamic dysfunction which may be caused by damage to small perforating arteries.

The risk of visual deterioration following transcranial surgery is approximately 15–22%. On the other hand, the chance that a pre-existing visual deficit improves after surgery is 50% (Bulters et al. 2009). In large adenomas with eccentric lateral extension, a significant risk of an oculomotor nerve palsy with ptosis and double vision exists.

The risk of postoperative hypopituitarism and diabetes insipidus is also higher in transcranial surgery than in transsphenoidal surgery and the chance of postoperative recovery of pre-existing endocrine deficits is low (Buchfelder and Kreutzer 2008).

As the adenomas requiring craniotomy are typically large and show invasive character, a gross total resection is mostly not feasible.

22.4 Surgery for Non-adenomatous Pituitary Lesions

22.4.1 Other Pathologies

The vast majority of surgically treated lesions of the pituitary area are adenomas. However, numerous other pathologies of the pituitary, pituitary stalk and hypothalamus are encountered (see Chap. 14). The appropriate surgical approach for other pituitary pathologies also depends on their location.

Among non-adenomatous lesions, tumours of neighbourhood origin that secondarily encroach upon the pituitary such as chordomas, chondosarcomas or perisellar meningiomas must also be considered.

22.4.2 Surgery for Craniopharyngiomas

The second most frequent pathology of pituitary or hypothalamic origin is the craniopharyngioma. In contrast to pituitary adenomas, only 30% of craniopharyngiomas show major intrasellar involvement allowing transsphenoidal surgery (Honegger and Tatagiba 2008). Many craniopharyngiomas are not confined to the pituitary fossa and grow in the suprasellar intradural space above the diaphragm

sellae requiring craniotomy. Various transcranial approaches have to be considered as craniopharyngiomas may involve several intracranial compartments. Large craniopharyngioma cysts can be decompressed by stereotactic cyst puncture.

Recently, extended transsphenoidal operations have been suggested for purely suprasellar craniopharyngiomas (Kim et al. 2011) and other suprasellar tumours. The major disadvantage of such extended approaches is the large defect in the skull base and intraoperative CSF leak which is necessary for tumour exposure. It carries a high risk of a postoperative CSF fistula. Whether purely suprasellar tumours should be operated by craniotomy or extended transsphenoidal surgery is still a matter of debate (Jeswani et al. 2016).

Gross total resection of craniopharyngiomas offers a high chance of recurrence-free long-term survival. Some neurosurgeons recommend an attempt at total removal so long as there is no risk of hypothalamic damage (Honegger and Tatagiba 2008). Other surgeons recommend conservative resection (biopsy or partial resection) followed by radiotherapy. However, the tumour burden remains with this policy and the therapeutic options in the case of re-growth are limited.

22.5 Recommendations for Radiotherapy Postoperatively

22.5.1 Indications for Radiotherapy in Pituitary Tumours

22.5.1.1 Indications for Radiotherapy in Non-functioning Pituitary Adenomas (NFPA)

In NFPA, radiotherapy is indicated for postoperative adenoma remnants with invasive character that are not accessible surgically. The typical indication is a residual adenoma within the cavernous sinus (Fig. 22.7). The timing of radiation for NFPA is a current subject of controversy. Some radiotherapists recommend radiotherapy

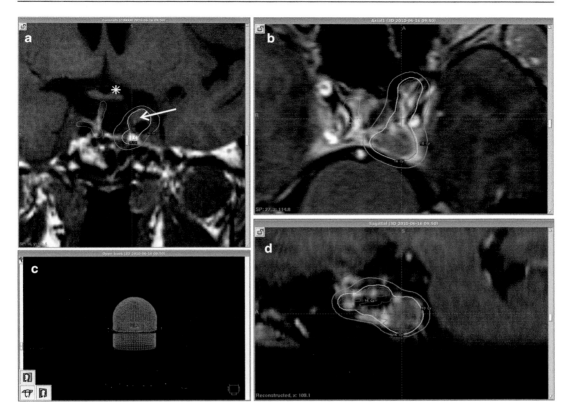

Fig. 22.7 Planning for stereotactic radiosurgery (SRS) with Gamma Knife of a left parasellar residual adenoma (arrow in **a**) within the cavernous sinus following transsphenoidal surgery. (**a**) Coronal view, (**b**) axial view, (**c**) 3D, (**d**) sagittal view. Yellow: 16 Gy isodose of the target volume; Green: 10 Gy isodose of the target volume. Blue: Optic chiasm (asterisk in **a**). Cyan: pituitary stalk and gland. The target volume has a sufficient distance to the optic chiasm to avoid visual compromise. Courtesy by Dr. G.A. Horstmann, Gamma Knife Centre, Krefeld, Germany

after initial surgery. Others use radiotherapy only if further growth of the residual adenoma is observed (Fig. 22.7).

22.5.1.2 Indications for Radiotherapy in Cushing's Disease

Radiotherapy (RT) is a second treatment option in CD. Radiotherapy is indicated if CD persists after pituitary surgery. This can be the case after negative sellar exploration(s) or for non-resectable invasive residual adenoma within the cavernous sinus. RT is also an option for recurrent CD (Estrada et al. 1997).

Other second-line options are medical treatment or bilateral adrenalectomy. The treatment decision in the second-line therapy is usually made on an individual basis. Medical treatment might be required while awaiting the delayed effect of radiotherapy.

22.5.1.3 Indications for Radiotherapy in Acromegaly

In acromegaly, RT competes with medical treatment as the second-line treatment. However, medical treatment is favoured in some countries for second-line treatment and RT is used if GH hypersecretion cannot be controlled by surgery and medical treatment.

22.5.1.4 Indications for Radiotherapy in Prolactinomas

In prolactinomas, RT is used if hyperprolactinaemia persists under dopamine-agonist (DA) treatment and surgery is not successful or not indicated because of invasive adenoma extension. Radiotherapy is rarely used in prolactinomas because of the high efficacy of DAs.

22.5.1.5 Indications for Radiotherapy in Craniopharyngiomas

RT is indicated for residual or recurrent craniopharyngiomas. The ideal timing of RT is yet to be determined. An ongoing study in childhood craniopharyngiomas investigates whether adjunctive RT immediately after incomplete resection or salvage RT upon re-growth is superior.

22.5.2 Tumour Control and Remission Rates with Radiotherapy

Radiation techniques are explained in Chapter 24: Radiotherapy.

22.5.2.1 Tumour Control Rates in Non-functioning Pituitary Adenomas (NFPA)

The goal of radiotherapy in NFPA is tumour control which means that the adenoma remains stable in size or shrinks.

According to the literature, 80–98% of patients with NFPA are recurrence-free after *fRT*. The reported studies of *SRS* for NFPA showed tumour control rates of 83–100% (Sheehan et al. 2012) (Fig. 22.7). On average, the tumour control rate was 96%. However, long-term follow-up was not available in most of the studies on SRS.

22.5.2.2 Remission Rates in Cushing's Disease

With *fRT*, the reported remission rates with complete reversal of ACTH- and cortisol-oversecretion were between 46% and 100% (Estrada et al. 1997).

In published series of *SRS* with more than ten cases, the remission rates were highly variable with a range from 17% to 83%. Recent studies provide evidence that remission rates of 60–80% can be achieved today (Marek et al. 2015).

22.5.2.3 Remission Rates in Acromegaly

In the retrospective data collection of *fRT* for acromegaly from 14 centres throughout the United Kingdom, normalization of IGF-1 was achieved in 63% of the patients at 10 years (Jenkins et al. 2006).

The remission rates of *SRS* in acromegaly reported in the literature are heterogeneous. On average, a remission was achieved in approximately 50% of the patients (Pollock et al. 2008). Recent studies suggest that higher remission rates can be achieved today (Lee et al. 2015).

22.5.2.4 Remission and Control Rates in Prolactinomas

Both with *fRT* and with *SRS*, further tumour growth can be prevented in the vast majority of cases. However, remission with normal prolactin off dopamine-agonist treatment is only achieved in a minority of cases. Evidently, remission in prolactinomas is less frequent than in Cushing's disease and acromegaly (Tanaka et al. 2010).

22.5.2.5 Control Rates in Craniopharyngiomas

In the main published studies on *fRT*, control rates at 10 years after RT were 56.5–100% (Minniti et al. 2009). Long-term results of SRS are still sparse. In the main published studies on *SRS* with mean follow-up periods between 16 months and 17 years, control rates of SRS were 34–88% (Minniti et al. 2009).

Acknowledgement The editors acknowledge manuscript review by Justin Cetas MD who is the Associate Professor of Department of Neurosurgery, Oregon Health & Sciences University, Portland, Oregon, USA.

References

Ammirati M, Wei L, Ciric I. Short-term outcome of endoscopic versus microscopic pituitary adenoma surgery: a systematic review and meta-analysis. J Neurol Neurosurg Psychiatry. 2013;84:843–9.

Buchfelder M, Kreutzer J. Transcranial surgery for pituitary adenomas. Pituitary. 2008;11:375–84.

Bulters DO, Shenouda E, Evans BT, et al. Visual recovery following optic nerve decompression for chronic compressive neuropathy. Acta Neurochir. 2009;151:325.

Casanueva FF, Molitch ME, Schlechte JA, Abs R, Bonert V, Bronstein MD, Brue T, Cappabianca P, Colao A, Fahlbusch R, Fideleff H, Hadani M, Kelly P, Kleinberg D, Laws E, Marek J, Scanlon M, Sobrinho LG, Wass JAH, Giustina A. Guidelines of the Pituitary Society for the diagnosis and management of prolactinomas. Clin Endocrinol. 2006;65:265–73.

Chandler WF, Barkan AL, Hollon T, Sakharova A, Sack J, Brahma B, Schteingart DE. Outcome of transsphenoidal surgery for Cushing disease: a single-center experience over 32 years. Neurosurgery. 2016;78:216–23.

Chang EF, Sughrue ME, Zada G, Wilson CB, Blevins LS, Kunwar S. Long term outcome following repeat transsphenoidal surgery for recurrent endocrine-inactive pituitary adenomas. Pituitary. 2010;13(3):223–9. https://doi.org/10.1007/s11102-010-0221z.

Estrada J, Boronat M, Mielgo M, Magallón R, Millán I, Díez S, Lucas T, Barceló B. The long-term outcome of pituitary irradiation after unsuccessful transsphenoidal surgery in Cushing's disease. N Engl J Med. 1997;336:172–7.

Fatemi N, Dusick JR, de Paiva Neto MA, Kelly DF. The endonasal microscopic approach for pituitary adenomas and other parasellar tumors: a 10-year experience. Neurosurgery. 2008;63(4 Suppl 2):244–56.

Griffith HB, Veerapen R. A direct transnasal approach to the sphenoid sinus. Technical note. J Neurosurg. 1987;66:140–2.

Hadad G, Bassagasteguy L, Carrau RL, Mataza JC, Kassam A, Snyderman CH, Mintz A. A novel reconstructive technique after endoscopic expanded endonasal approaches: vascular pedicle nasoseptal flap. Laryngoscope. 2006;116:1882–6.

Hardy J. Transsphenoidal microsurgery of the normal and pathological pituitary. Clin Neurosurg. 1969;16:185–217.

Honegger J, Tatagiba M. Craniopharyngioma surgery. Pituitary. 2008;11:361–73.

Honegger J, Ernemann U, Psaras T, Will B. Objective criteria for successful transsphenoidal removal of suprasellar nonfunctioning pituitary adenomas. A prospective study. Acta Neurochir. 2007;149:21–9.

Jenkins PJ, Bates P, Carson N, Stewart PM, Wass JAH, On behalf of the UK National Acromegaly Register Study Group. Conventional pituitary irradiation is effective in lowering serum growth hormone and insulin-like growth factor-I in patients with acromegaly. J Clin Endocrinol Metab. 2006;91:1239–45.

Jeswani S, Nuno M, Wu A, Bonert V, Carmichael JD, Black KL, Chu R, King W, Mamelak AN. Comparative analysis of outcomes following craniotomy and expanded endoscopic endonasal transsphenoidal resection of craniopharyngioma and related tumors: a single-institution study. J Neurosurg. 2016;124:627–38.

Jho HD, Carrau RL, Ko Y, Daly MA. Endoscopic pituitary surgery: an early experience. Surg Neurol. 1997;47:213–23.

Juraschka K, Khan OH, Godoy BL, Monsalves E, Kilian A, Krischek B, Ghare A, Vescan A, Gentili F, Zadeh G. Endoscopic endonasal transsphenoidal approach to large and giant pituitary adenomas: institutional experience and predictors of extent of resection. J Neurosurg. 2014;121:75–83.

Kim EH, Ahn JY, Kim SH. Technique and outcome of endoscopy-assisted microscopic extended transsphenoidal surgery for suprasellar craniopharyngiomas. J Neurosurg. 2011;114:1138–349.

Knappe UJ, Moskopp D, Gerlach R, Conrad J, Flitsch J, Honegger JB. Consensus on postoperative recommendations after transsphenoidal surgery. Exp Clin Endocrinol Diabetes 2018 doi: 10.1055/a-0664-7710. [Epub ahead of print].

Kreutzer J, Buslei R, Wallaschofski H, Hofmann B, Nimsky C, Fahlbusch R, Buchfelder M. Operative treatment of prolactinomas: indications and results in a current consecutive series of 212 patients. Eur J Endocrinol. 2008;158:11–8.

Lee CC, Vance ML, Lopes MB, Xu Z, Chen CJ, Sheehan J. Stereotactic radiosurgery for acromegaly: outcomes by adenoma subtype. Pituitary. 2015;18(3):326–34. https://doi.org/10.1007/s11102-014-0578-5.

Marek J, Jezková J, Hána V, Krsek M, Liscák R, Vladyka V, Pecen L. Gamma knife radiosurgery for Cushing's disease and Nelson's syndrome. Pituitary. 2015;18:376–84.

Minniti G, Jaffrain-Rea ML, Esposito V, Santoro A, Tamburrano G, Cantore G. Evolving criteria for postoperative biochemical remission of acromegaly: can we achieve a definitive cure? An audit of surgical results on a large series and a review of the literature. Endocr Relat Cancer. 2003;10(4):611–9. https://doi.org/10.1677/erc.0.0100611.

Minniti G, Esposito V, Amichetti M, Enrici RM. The role of fractionated radiotherapy and radiosurgery in the management of patients with craniopharyngiomas. Neurosurg Rev. 2009;32:125–32.

Mortini P, Barzaghi LR, Albano L, Panni P, Losa M. Microsurgical therapy of pituitary adenomas. Endocrine. 2018;59(1):72–81. https://doi.org/10.1007/s12020-017-1458-3. Epub 2017 Oct 24.

Pollock BE, Brown PD, Nippoldt TB, Young WF. Pituitary tumor type affects the chance of biochemical remission after radiosurgery of hormone-secreting pituitary adenomas. Neurosurgery. 2008;62:1271–8.

Schloffer H. Erfolgreiche Operation eines Hypophysentumors auf nasalem Wege. Wien Klin Wochenschr. 1907;20:621–4.

Schöfl C, Franz H, Grussendorf M, Honegger J, Jaursch-Hancke C, Mayr B, Schopohl J. Long-term outcome in patients with acromegaly: analysis of 1344 patients from the German Acromegaly Register. Eur J Endocrinol. 2013;168:39–47.

Sheehan JP, Xu Z, Lobo MJ. External beam radiation therapy and stereotactic radiosurgery for pituitary adenomas. Neurosurg Clin N Am. 2012;23:571–86.

Tanaka S, Link MJ, Brown PD, Stafford SL, Young WF, Pollock BE. Gamma knife radiosurgery for patients with prolactin-secreting pituitary adenomas. World Neurosurg. 2010;74:147–52.

Key Reading

1. Ammirati M, Wei L, Ciric I. Short-term outcome of endoscopic versus microscopic pituitary adenoma surgery: a systematic review and meta-analysis. J Neurol Neurosurg Psychiatry. 2013;84:843–9.

2. Chandler WF, Barkan AL, Hollon T, Sakharova A, Sack J, Brahma B, Schteingart DE. Outcome of transsphenoidal surgery for Cushing disease: a single-center experience over 32 years. Neurosurgery. 2016;78:216–23.

3. Honegger J, Tatagiba M. Craniopharyngioma surgery. Pituitary. 2008;11:361–73.

4. Sheehan JP, Xu Z, Lobo MJ. External beam radiation therapy and stereotactic radiosurgery for pituitary adenomas. Neurosurg Clin N Am. 2012;23:571–86.

5. Schöfl C, Franz H, Grussendorf M, Honegger J, Jaursch-Hancke C, Mayr B, Schopohl J. Long-term outcome in patients with acromegaly: analysis of 1344 patients from the German Acromegaly Register. Eur J Endocrinol. 2013;168:39–47.

Pituitary Surgery: Nursing Implications

23

Sarah Benzo and Christina Hayes

Contents

Keywords

Pituitary surgery · Postoperative complications · Diabetes insipidus (DI) · SIADH · Adrenal insufficiency · Patient education

Abbreviations

ACTH	Adrenocorticotropic hormone
ADH	Antidiuretic hormone
AI	Adrenal insufficiency

S. Benzo (✉) · C. Hayes
Surgical Neurology Branch, National Institute of Neurologic Disorders and Stroke, National Institutes of Health, Bethesda, MD, USA
e-mail: sarah.benzo@nih.gov; christi.hayes@nih.gov

© Springer Nature Switzerland AG 2019
S. Llahana et al. (eds.), *Advanced Practice in Endocrinology Nursing*,
https://doi.org/10.1007/978-3-319-99817-6_23

CD	Cushing's disease
CRH	Corticotropic releasing hormone
CSF	Cerebrospinal fluid
DDAVP	Desmopressin
DI	Diabetes insipidus
HPA axis	Hypothalamic-pituitary-adrenal axis
IV	Intravenous
SIADH	Syndrome of inappropriate antidiuretic hormone

- **Lumbar Drainage:** Catheter inserted into the lumbar subarachnoid space in order to remove CSF from the body.
- **Transsphenoidal Surgery:** Approach to the pituitary gland for surgery by route of the sphenoid sinus, most commonly through the nose or upper lip.
- **Epistaxis:** Bleeding from the nose, most often originates from the nasal mucosa after transsphenoidal surgery, however may indicate bleeding from more critical structures.

Key Terms

- **Hypothalamic-Pituitary-Adrenal (HPA) Axis:** Complex hormonal interaction between the hypothalamus, pituitary, and adrenal glands that takes place in order to provide hormonal homeostasis.
- **Adrenal Insufficiency:** Inadequate production of cortisol (steroid hormone) from the adrenal glands to support physiologic needs.
- **Antidiuretic Hormone (ADH):** Hormone secreted by the pituitary gland that works at the level of the kidney to regulate fluid and electrolyte balance to maintain appropriate intravascular hydration.
- **Diabetes Insipidus (DI):** Insufficient secretion of ADH results in excessive urinary secretion of dilute urine resulting in intravascular dehydration characterized by elevated serum sodium and decreased urinary specific gravity.
- **Desmopressin (DDAVP):** Medication consisting of a synthetic form of ADH that may be administered to patients with DI.
- **Syndrome of Inappropriate Antidiuretic Hormone (SIADH):** Oversecretion of ADH resulting in excessive retention of free water despite low serum osmolality resulting in intravascular hyponatremia and increased intravascular circulating volume.
- **Cerebrospinal Fluid (CSF):** A clear fluid that circulates in and around the brain and spinal cord.

Key Points

- Nursing considerations in the care of the patient undergoing pituitary surgery include knowledge of patient's preoperative hormone levels, surgical approach, and postoperative monitoring needs.
- Diligent monitoring for disturbances of water and electrolyte balance, and HPA axis dysfunction are essential to the care of pituitary surgery patients.
- The nurse caring for the neurosurgical pituitary patient should monitor for the following potential postoperative complications: infection, CSF leak, visual loss, and epistaxis.
- Key neurologic components in the care of pituitary surgery patients include visual field testing, monitoring for visual changes, CSF leak monitoring, and lumbar drain management, when applicable.
- Thorough patient discharge teaching regarding activity restrictions, prescribed hormone replacement, sign and symptoms of HPA axis dysfunction (with emphasis on signs of adrenal insufficiency), and scheduled follow-up with medical and surgical teams is paramount.

23.1 Introduction

Pituitary surgery is performed to address a variety of pathologies. Surgical technique will vary based upon surgeon preference, tumor location, and any involvement of surrounding structures. Nursing care of the patient undergoing pituitary surgery is founded in a comprehensive understanding of pituitary physiology and pathophysiology. Expert knowledge of the pituitary gland, the hypothalamic-pituitary-adrenal (HPA) axis, underlying pathology, and surgical risks allows for early identification and intervention of postoperative complications. It is important to be aware of hospital specific protocols regarding the routine care of patients undergoing pituitary surgery, as they may vary from institution to institution. Comprehensive, broad based knowledge empowers the nurse to provide diligent, comprehensive care and identify potentially life-threatening complications promptly.

23.2 Review of the Physiology of the Pituitary Gland

Review of the role of the pituitary gland in the endocrine system, each hormonal axis function, and the mechanisms of hormonal homeostasis is recommended (Amar and Weiss 2003; Yuan 2013; Greenberg 2016; Ben-Shlomo and Melmed 2011). For details, refer to Chap. 12.

23.3 Postoperative Nursing Care Considerations

23.3.1 Surgical Approach

The surgical risks for patients undergoing removal of a pituitary adenoma may vary depending on the location of the tumor and the surgical approach as described in Chap. 22. The three standard surgical approaches for pituitary adenomas are transsphenoidal, transethmoidal, and transcranial. Transsphenoidal surgery is often the approach of choice for many surgeons, and this procedure may be performed via a sublabial or trans-nare approach depending upon the tumor

characteristics and surgeon skill set and preferences. There are specific nursing implications associated with the different surgical approaches.

23.3.1.1 Sublabial Approach

Patients who undergo a transsphenoidal procedure with a sublabial approach will have an incision under their lip, and oral care will be essential in preventing infection. Dietary considerations include soft foods and liquid protein supplements until sutures have dissolved. Oral care should be performed after every meal. The use of a straw is usually discouraged (Yuan 2013).

23.3.1.2 Extended Transsphenoidal Skull Base Approach

In this approach, additional cranial base bone is removed to provide better exposure to the parasellar and clival region compared with the standard transsphenoidal approach (Zhao et al. 2010). Both patients who undergo an "extended" transsphenoidal skull base approach and those found to have a CSF leak at the conclusion of a transsphenoidal surgery may require a lumbar drain placement postoperatively (Yuan 2013). Thus, it is important for nurses to be trained in proper care of lumbar drains. The key principle is the drainage is gravity dependent so the amount of drainage will change with the position of the patient (Overstreet 2003). Refer to individual facility lumbar drainage guidelines and physician orders regarding clamping versus opening lumbar drains. Patients with lumbar drainage systems and their family members require education pertaining to lumbar drainage, specifically in regards to patient position and mobilization.

23.4 Key Endocrinological and Neurosurgical Nursing Considerations

The pituitary gland is essential for normal endocrinologic function (See Chap. 1). It is important to know if your patient experienced endocrine dysfunction prior to surgery, and if so what hormones were impacted to determine their level of perioperative risk (Malenković et al. 2011). If hormonal oversecretion was evident, which hormone(s) were biochemically overactive and what disease symptoms was the patient experiencing. These symptoms will need to be monitored postoperatively. Likewise, if there is a deficiency in one or more hormonal axis, it is important to know if these deficiencies were replaced and if they are currently stable. These will also necessitate a monitoring plan postoperatively. Evidence suggests a multidisciplinary team approach to the care of transsphenoidal surgery patient is most effective, inclusive of neurosurgery, neuroendocrinology, and a pituitary nurse specialist (Carminucci et al. 2016). Length of stay was significantly reduced without compromising patient safety or outcomes (Fig. 23.1).

23.4.1 Perioperative Glucocorticoid Replacement

Patients undergoing pituitary surgery are frequently given glucocorticoid replacement therapy during the perioperative period to treat potential cortisol deficiency. However, the practice of glucocorticoid administration post pituitary surgery varies between institutions and remains a controversial practice (Kelly and Domajnko 2013; Glowniak and Loriaux 1997; Pimentel-Filho et al. 2005; Inder and Hunt 2002). There are some data favoring treatment only when the patient is symptomatic of adrenal insufficiency versus protocol driven replacement, and depending on the status of the patient's HPA axis function on preoperative testing. In the event of adrenal insufficiency in the latter circumstance, glucocorticoids must be replaced and continued until postoperative testing indicates normal HPA axis function. In other patients who have an intact HPA function preoperatively, and whom selective adenomectomy is possible, perioperative glucocorticoids may not be necessary. However, most patients with a large adenoma are at risk for cortisol deficiency following surgery. Therefore a stress dose 40–100 mg of IV steroids is frequently given to patients immediately before, during and/or immediately after surgery (Kelly and Domajnko 2013). The recommended replacement dose of glucocor-

ticoid by Endocrine Society Clinical Guidelines is 15–30 mg of oral cortisol daily in divided doses (Nieman et al. 2015). It should be reiterated that the use of glucocorticoid replacement will vary based upon institution protocol, patient pathology, and surgical or endocrine team preference.

Postoperative assessment of glucocorticoid requirement is dependent on clinical assessment and diagnosis of the patient. In cases of Cushing's disease, some centers recommended that all patients in postoperative remission with morning plasma cortisol levels less than 5 µg/dL be treated with glucocorticoids until further testing indicates a normal HPA axis function (Inder and Hunt 2002). Thus, it is important that nurses ensure morning cortisol levels and ACTH levels are drawn postoperatively in order for the physicians to assess HPA axis function and determine if oral hormone replacement after discharge is needed (Yuan 2013). See Box 23.1 for a suggested postoperative glucocorticoid regimen.

If the patient is to be discharged on a glucocorticoid regime, it is essential to provide the patient and family with education regarding: symptoms of adrenal insufficiency (AI); symptoms to report urgently to their physician; administration of emergency glucocorticoid injection for symptoms of AI; to report to the nearest hospital emergency room for evaluation of the etiology of AI. Adrenal insufficiency following surgery may be temporary or permanent. Therefore, it is important for the patient to establish ongoing, follow-up care with a local endocrinologist.

23.4.1.1 HPA Axis Function

Adrenal insufficiency or HPA axis dysfunction may be evident immediately after a successful surgery to remove an ACTH producing tumor or in remitted Cushing's disease. However, manipulation or damage to the pituitary during surgery can also impair ACTH secretion, thus disrupting the HPA axis and secretion of cortisol. Lack of cortisol following surgery can result in adrenal insufficiency (AI). AI can be a life-threatening condition if not identified and treated (Yuan 2013; Nieman et al. 2015) (See clinical indication of AI, Box 23.2).

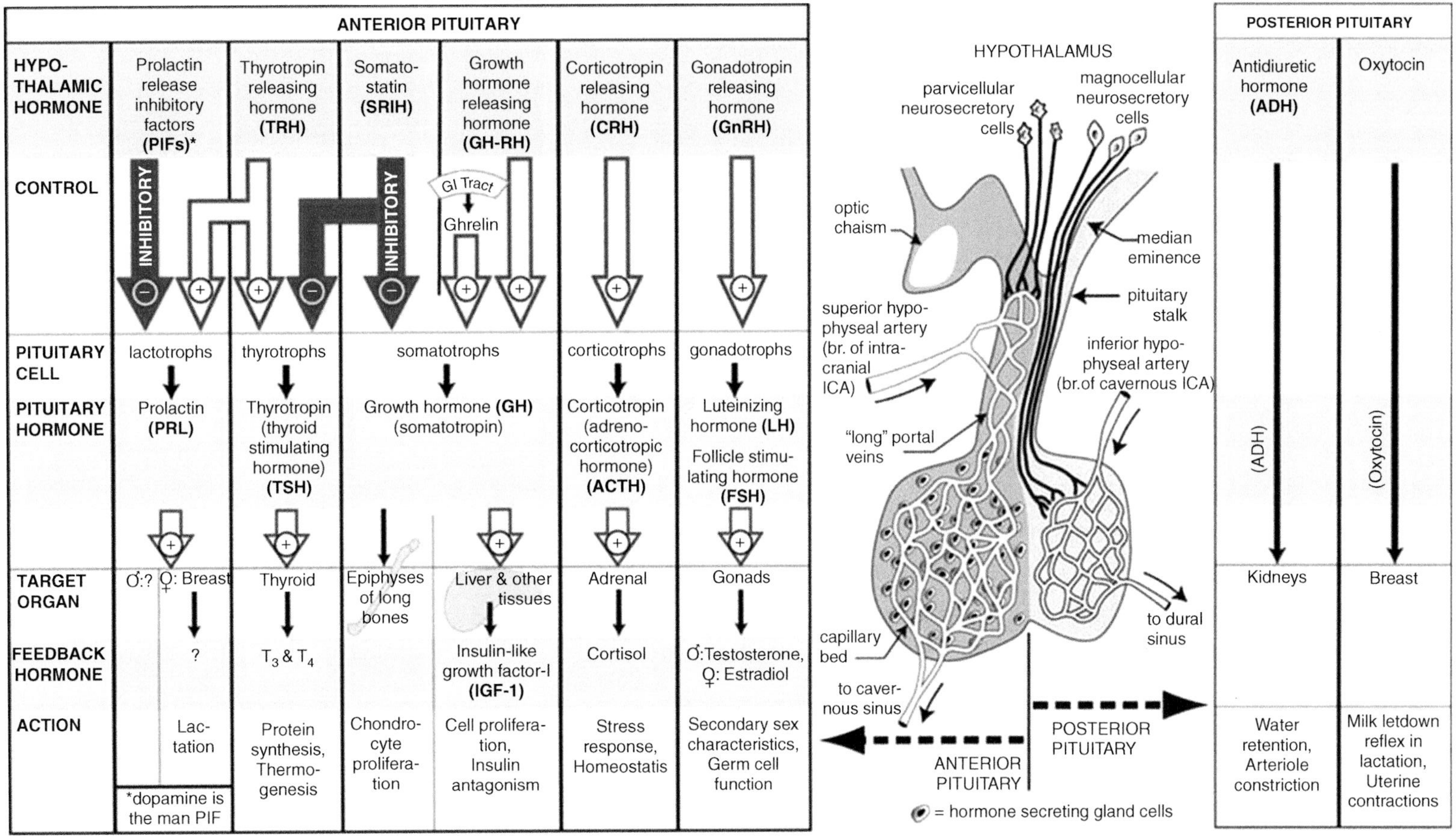

Fig. 23.1 Pituitary neuroendocrinology. Used with permission from Greenberg, M. S. (2016). Handbook of neurosurgery, image 8.1 pg153

The patient may initially complain of worsening headache, dizziness, and fatigue before other symptoms become apparent. Depending on the level of deficiency, symptoms may develop slowly over several hours or become quickly apparent with stressful stimuli such as a blood draw, straining with post-op constipation, or with air travel. If an adrenal crisis is evident, parenteral (intravenous or intramuscular) injection of 100 mg (50 mg/m^2 for children) hydrocortisone must be administered immediately (Naziat and Grossman 2000; Bornstein et al. 2016).

Measurement of serum electrolytes (particularly serum sodium) followed by fluid resuscitation is recommended. Glucocorticoids should be continued every 6 h for 24–48 h (half-life of hydrocortisone is 90–120 min) and until follow-up testing indicates normal function or the patient is stable on a physiologic dose of hydrocortisone (15–30 mg in divided doses daily (Naziat and Grossman 2000; Bornstein et al. 2016)).

23.4.1.2 Cushing Disease: ACTH Hypersecretion

Patients with Cushing Disease have ACTH secreting pituitary adenomas resulting in hypercortisolemia. Oversecretion of ACTH by the pituitary adenoma causes suppression of the normal circadian production of ACTH from surrounding normal corticotrophs and hypersecretion of cortisol from the adrenal glands (Nieman et al. 2015). There may also be a suppressive effect on hypothalamic CRH production that inhibits normal ACTH production. After the ACTH secreting pituitary adenoma is removed, the normal circadian corticotroph production of ACTH may still be absent or suppressed; therefore, ACTH and cortisol levels may be low in remitted disease. The Endocrine Society Guidelines define remission of Cushing's disease as:

> "a morning serum cortisol level < 5 μg/dL (<138 nmol/L) or UFC < 28–56 nmol/day (<10–20 μg/day) within 7 days of selective tumor resection (Nieman et al. 2015)."

There is some controversy around glucocorticoid replacement in patients with CD post remission unless cortisol levels remain low and the patient becomes symptomatic (Pimentel-Filho et al. 2005; Simmons et al. 2001). However, these patients are at increased risk for hypocortisolemia or adrenal insufficiency and, if postoperative cortisol levels indicate remission, most often require glucocorticoid replacement postoperatively. The dose should be adjusted to avoid symptoms of adrenal insufficiency (see Box 23.2 and Part XII; Adrenal Insufficiency). These patients should be monitored closely and require education regarding glucocorticoid taper and adrenal crisis avoidance and management.

23.4.1.3   Hypopituitarism

Postoperative levels of hormones regulated by the anterior pituitary gland will also need to be evaluated to assess for hypopituitarism and perhaps panhypopituitarism which is more common in cases necessitating removal of significant amounts of the anterior gland. The posterior pituitary gland controls Antidiuretic Hormone (ADH) secretion. Manipulation of the posterior pituitary gland and/or pituitary stalk during surgery increases risk for water and electrolyte imbalance.

23.4.1.4   Disturbance of Water Balance

Disturbance in water balance and electrolytes are the most common complication after pituitary surgery with some reports of postoperative water and electrolyte balance occurring in up to 75% of patients (Kristof et al. 2009). Apart from alterations in vasopressin secretion, other factors such as non-atrial natriuretic peptide excess, inappropriate thirst and fluid intake, and low dietary salt intake may contribute (Olson et al. 1997). Although estimates vary between centers, diabetes insipidus (DI) is estimated to occur in between 0.5 and 25% of patients and syndrome of inappropriate antidiuretic hormone (SIADH) 9–25% of cases (Dumont et al. 2005) (See Part XII).

23.4.1.1 Syndrome of Inappropriate Antidiuretic Hormone (SIADH)

Manipulation of the posterior pituitary may trigger excessive release of antidiuretic hormone (ADH), resulting in syndrome of inappropriate antidiuretic hormone (SIADH) and hyponatremia. In this syndrome, under the influence of increased secretion of ADH, despite low serum osmolality, free water intake is in excess of free water excretion, resulting in hyponatremia, increased circulating volume, and increased sodium excretion. SIADH clinically presents as increased extremely concentrated urine output. This is a common condition following hospital discharge or approximately 5–7 days following surgery (Yuan 2013; Dumont et al. 2005).

Although some patients may be asymptomatic, many experience multiple symptoms

> **Box 23.3 Symptoms of SIADH**
> - *Headache*
> - *Lethargy*
> - *Anorexia*
> - *Nausea/vomiting*
> - *Muscle cramps*
> - *Agitation*
> - *Delerium/disorientation*
> - *Seizure*

described in Box 23.3. Laboratory evaluation of SIADH typically displays high urine specific gravity, urine sodium, and urine osmolality; and low serum sodium osmolality (Yuan 2013). Treatment of SIADH is individualized and aimed at correcting sodium and plasma osmolality. In patients with mild and asymptomatic cases of hyponatremia, fluid restriction (typically 1000 cc per day fluid) and daily serum electrolyte monitoring may be the only treatment necessary. Extremely low levels of sodium place the patient at a higher risk for seizures and even death; therefore, a more aggressive treatment may be indicated (Dumont et al. 2005). Patients with severe and symptomatic hyponatremia may require treatment with intravenous hypertonic solution (3% sodium chloride), frequent electrolyte monitoring, and strict fluid restriction (Yuan 2013). It is important for nurses to perform careful monitoring of fluid intake, and electrolyte status when caring for patients with SIADH. Due to the fact that this condition typically presents following hospital discharge, clear and thorough instructions prior to leaving the hospital are essential. Discharge instructions should include information on fluid restrictions, attention to salt intake, and knowledge on the symptoms of hyponatremia (Dumont et al. 2005) (See Part XII).

23.4.1.2 Diabetes Insipidus (DI)

Disturbing the posterior pituitary gland, pituitary stalk, or hypothalamus during surgery may impair the ADH pathway, causing diabetes insipidus (DI). DI occurs when there is an inadequate release of ADH, resulting in the excretion of large amounts of dilute urine. DI is reported to occur in 0.5–25% of cases with most cases of being transient, occurring 24–48 h following surgery, and typically subsiding within 72 h (Dumont et al. 2005) See Symptoms, Box 23.4.

Laboratory values show low urine specific gravity, sodium, and osmolality; and high levels of serum sodium and osmolality (Yuan 2013; Dumont et al. 2005). DI can be very dangerous if not addressed quickly, therefore screening is a very important aspect of postoperative care. It is important for nurses to perform daily weights, thorough intake and output, and assess for thirst, dehydration, hypernatremia, and hypokalemia. Screening should also include monitoring daily serum chemistries, serum and urine osmolality (or more frequently if indicated), as well as urine specific gravities every 4 h (Dumont et al. 2005). Treatment of DI is individualized and based on the severity and duration of the condition. Standard treatment for DI at many institutions consists of monitoring serum electrolytes and urine specific gravity every 4 h, until osmotic homeostasis is restored (Yuan 2013). Specific treatment of DI includes administration of Desmopressin (DDAVP), a synthetic form of ADH, which can be administered orally, subcutaneously, intranasally, or intravenously (Dumont et al. 2005). When caring for a patient following pituitary surgery, it is important to be aware that many patients undergo postoperative diuresis due to intravenous fluid administration during surgery. This is a normal response that does not require treatment. Thus, prior to treatment for DI, it is essential to distinguish between mobilization of postoperative fluids and DI. It is important for nurses to ensure the patient has access to oral fluids and to continue monitoring urine output, urine specific gravity, urine osmolality, serum sodium, serum osmolality, and mental status (Yuan 2013).

23.5 Monitoring Neurosurgical Complications

In addition to the endocrinological complications following surgery, there are also direct neurosurgical complications that may occur following pituitary surgery. These include infection, cerebral spinal fluid (CSF) leak, visual loss, epistaxis, intracranial hematoma, and HPA axis dysfunction.

23.5.1 Infection

As with all surgical patients, the pituitary surgery patient should be monitored for signs of infection with routine labs, vital signs, and incision assessment. Signs of meningitis should also be observed for, particularly in the patient with CSF leak and/or lumbar drain. Signs and symptoms of meningitis (Box 23.5) must be reported urgently so that appropriate antibiotic coverage may be initiated promptly (AANN Clinical Practice Guidelines Series 2011). When the sublabial approach for transsphenoidal pituitary surgery is used, diligent oral care is essential for infection prevention.

23.5.2 CSF Leak

Every patient who undergoes transsphenoidal surgery is at risk for CSF leak. This complication is reported in about 4% of cases (Dumont et al. 2005). There is a layer of dura known as the diaphragma sellae that lies above the pituitary gland. If the pituitary tumor invades the diaphragma sellae, or if the diaphragma sellae is violated intraoperatively, CSF leak will occur. When CSF leak

---

Box 23.4 Symptoms of DI
Polyuria
Polydipsia
Excessive thirst
Hypotension secondary to hypovolemia
Fever

Box 23.5 Signs and Symptoms of Meningitis
- *Fever*
- *Photophobia*
- *Nuchal rigidity*
- *Headache*
- *Vomiting*
- *Change in mental status*

is encountered intraoperatively, CSF diversion with lumbar drainage is generally performed. Nursing care of the patient undergoing lumbar drainage is discussed further below. If CSF leak occurs postoperatively, patients may present with persistent clear, odorless rhinorrhea or complain of a salty, bitter, or metallic taste in their mouth if CSF drains posteriorly (Yuan 2013). Exposure of the meninges to nasopharyngeal flora via CSF leak places the patient at high risk of meningitis. Therefore, signs of CSF leak must be reported to the neurosurgeon immediately and addressed promptly. CSF leak is treated with lumbar drainage, antibiotics, and may require surgery for repair (Yuan 2013). Mucous from rhinorrhea may be sent to the lab to evaluate for presence of beta-2 transferrin, a protein found in CSF but not nasal mucosal secretions; if there is uncertainty, the rhinorrhea is CSF (Naziat and Grossman 2000). It should be noted that availability and turnaround time of this test will vary from institution to institution. Precautions to reduce pressure at the surgical site should be implemented to help reduce the risk of postoperative CSF leak. Precautions should include head of bed elevation per surgeon direction, aggressive postoperative nausea control to avoid vomiting, avoiding use of straws, no sneezing, no nose blowing, no nasal sniffing or bending over such that the head is below the level of the heart (Dumont et al. 2005). Valsalva maneuvers such as in straining with constipation and lifting can cause changes in intracranial pressure and should be avoided

(Prabhakar et al. 2007) Patients using CPAP (continuous positive airway pressure for sleep apnea) may require increased oxygen but CPAP should be withheld until no CSF leak is evident.

23.5.3 Lumbar Drainage

American Association of Neuroscience Nurses, AANN, provides guidelines regarding care of the neurosurgical patient undergoing lumbar drainage (AANN Clinical Practice Guidelines Series 2011). The nurse caring for the pituitary surgery patient must also be familiar with lumbar drain care procedures at their practicing institution.

Lumbar drains are inserted under sterile conditions into the lumbar subarachnoid space at the level of L2-L3 or below so as to avoid injury to the spinal cord, which ends at L1-L2. After insertion, great care should be taken to maintain a sterile lumbar drainage system including monitoring integrity of the insertion site and dressing. Diligent hand hygiene is paramount. Transparent dressings allow for easy visualization of the insertion site and may stay in place so long as they are clean, dry, and intact. Dressings with gauze may require routine dressing changes (AANN Clinical Practice Guidelines Series 2011). The nurse should monitor the insertion site for signs of drainage and notify the neurosurgical provider if drainage is noted. Lumbar drainage may be ordered as continuous or intermittent per surgeon preference and/or institution policy (Lynn 2016) (See Fig. 23.2).

Protocol	Description
Draining at a specific level	• Physician order or hospital policy determins vertical level at which drainage collection device is maintained.
	• Designated level may be at shoulder height or level of catheter insertion
	• Amount of CSF to be drained varies.
Draining to a specific volume	• Physician order and hospital protocol determine amount of drainage desired durine specific period: average drainage is 10-15ml/hour
	• Vertical level of drain is repositioned to achieve desired drainage volume.
	• Attention to drain level is critical to avoid CSF backflow.

Ref: Lynn, S J. Caring for patients with lumbar drains. American Nurse Today. 2016 Vol. 11 No. 3

Fig. 23.2 Lumbar drain management protocols. Ref: Lynn, S J. Caring for patients with lumbar drains. American Nurse Today. 2016 Vol. 11 No. 3 https://www.americannursetoday.com/caring-patients-lumbar-drains/

Fig. 23.3 (**a**) Patient with CSF drain for CSF fistula. The Burton report Jan 2018 Edition http://www.burtonreport.com/. (**b**) Lumbar CSF drain

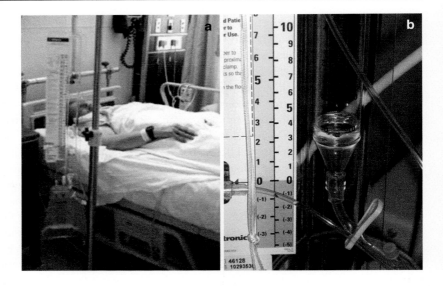

Patients require education regarding their positioning while lumbar drain is in place. Specifically, any changes in bed height, head of bed, or changes in the patient position and mobilization, will require adjustment to the height of the collection chamber and nursing assistance. Any change in patient position while the drainage system is openly draining places the patient at risk for CSF over-drainage (AANN Clinical Practice Guidelines Series 2011; Lynn 2016) (Fig. 23.3a, b).

At the time of insertion, CSF may be collected and sent to the laboratory for analysis. It should be noted that CSF requires prompt delivery to the laboratory for accurate analysis due to rapid decrease in cell counts after collection, 32% decrease after 1 h, and 50% decrease after 2 h. Additionally, bacteria may not survive for long periods of time in the collection tubes (AANN Clinical Practice Guidelines Series 2011).

23.5.4 Visual Loss

The optic chiasm lies directly above the pituitary gland. Therefore, the tumor addressed by pituitary surgery may have caused compression of the optic nerves, causing loss of peripheral vision (Amar and Weiss 2003; Ben-Shlomo and Melmed 2011). Patient will report preoperative visual field deficits or restrictions preoperatively, i.e., when driving. Many surgeons will request formal visual field testing with a neuro-ophthalmologist preoperatively when optic chiasm compression is suspected. Postoperatively the nurse should monitor visual fields and check extraocular movements to evaluate for any changes in vision. Acute postoperative changes in vision should be urgently reported to the surgeon as it may indicate a potential complication such as bleeding at the surgical site.

23.5.5 Epistaxis

Epistaxis may occur in the immediate post-op period or many days delayed postoperatively (Smith et al. 2015). Nasal mucosa is highly vascular and interruption of the nasal mucosa via transsphenoidal approach for resection of pituitary tumors increases risk for epistaxis. Most bleeding originates from the nasal mucosa and resolves quickly by holding pressure and tilting the head forward or nasal packing if bleeding persists. However, proximity of the pituitary gland to the cavernous sinus and internal carotid arteries makes epistaxis a potentially life-threatening symptom that should be taken seri-

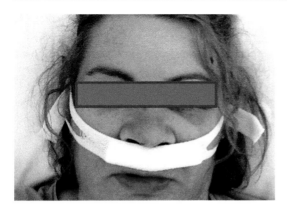

Fig. 23.4 Moustache dressing

ously and reported to the neurosurgeon. Severe epistaxis may require surgical exploration, cautery, or embolization (Smith et al. 2015).

Normal nasal drainage following transsphenoidal surgery is blood tinged mucoid drainage, which is often captured on a nasal drip pad or "moustache" dressing (Fig. 23.4), the first few days following surgery and after the nasal packing is removed. Patients are unable to effectively humidify the air they breathe following transsphenoidal surgery due to disruption of the sinuses and nasal congestion. Humidified air provides comfort to patients recovering from transsphenoidal surgery and should be offered. Additionally, the use of nasal sterile saline spray can help moisturize the nasal mucosa and improve patient comfort after any nasal packing is removed. Use of humidified air and intranasal sterile saline spray should be discussed with the patient's surgeon prior to initiating therapy. It should also be noted that due to the highly vascular nature of the nasal mucosa it is common for patients to ingest blood intraoperatively, which contributes to postoperative nausea.

23.6   Summary of Patient Education

Patient and family education is an important aspect in the management of patients undergoing pituitary surgery. Patient education should be an ongoing process and consideration should be given to education needs during the following phases of surgery.

23.6.1 Perioperative

Patient education should begin as early as possible. Provide the patient with written and verbal information regarding what to expect during the perioperative period (Yuan 2013). This may alleviate anxiety and have a positive impact on patient outcomes.

23.6.1.1 Preoperative

Education should include information pertaining to rationale for surgery, surgical approach, risks of surgery, preoperative medication and food restrictions, and common preoperative routines (i.e., standard preoperative testing and when and where to arrive at the hospital). Prepare the patient for common postoperative complications and treatments. Inform the patient of what to expect through the course of hospitalization and the treatment teams they will encounter in addition to the neurosurgeons such as Ear Nose and Throat (ENT) surgeon(s), anesthesiologists, and endocrinologists.

23.6.1.2 Intraoperative

Education may include information regarding general anesthesia, surgical techniques (possible need for fat graft or lumbar drain), and recovery location immediately following surgery (ICU or PACU).

23.6.1.3 Postoperative

Education should focus on activity. Key aspects may include: elevated head of bed, early ambulation, required assistance when ambulating in the event of a lumbar drain, nasal packing, urinary catheter, monitoring intake and output, monitoring for CSF leak, incision care, and oral care. Oral care is especially important for patients undergoing transsphenoidal surgery. Patients should only brush their teeth using a special ultra-soft toothbrush (for approximately 2 weeks), and special mouthwash and swabs should be utilized to rinse their mouth throughout the day (especially after eating and drinking).

23.6.2 Discharge

Discharge instructions should be provided to the patient in written and verbal format, and be reviewed with the patient prior to leaving the hospital. Clear discharge instructions facilitate a smooth recovery process (Yuan 2013). Specific instructions will vary across hospitals. All discharge instructions should include information on the following:

23.6.2.1 Postoperative Follow-Up Appointment and Testing Needs

Following surgery, patients are typically seen by their neurosurgeon a few weeks after surgery to assess wound healing and by their endocrinologist at approximately 1–6 weeks after surgery to check hormone replacement (Yuan 2013). Patients then typically undergo a magnetic resonance imaging (MRI) and evaluation 3 months following surgery, and then at yearly intervals (or at the discretion of the physician) to follow-up on residual tumor recurrence. Some patients with persistent or recurrent disease may be referred for radiation therapy or radiosurgery (Dumont et al. 2005; Prather et al. 2003).

23.6.2.2 Symptom Management
Upon discharge, patients should be instructed to monitor and report any signs and symptoms of AI, SIADH, DI, and any other neurosurgical complications previously discussed.

23.6.2.3 Activity
It is important for patients to be careful performing certain types of activities following surgery. Specific restrictions may vary depending on the surgical procedure. It is also important to avoid heavy lifting (over 20 lb) for the first 4 weeks following surgery (Yuan 2013). For patients undergoing transsphenoidal surgery, it is important to avoid coughing, blowing or aggressively clean-

ing or picking the nares, sneezing, bending below the knee level, or straining for 1 month following surgery. Patients are instructed to refrain from using CPAP devices for sleep apnea until cleared by ENT clinicians. Patients are typically able to return to work 3–6 weeks following surgery. However, return to work should be discussed with the neurosurgery team.

Case Study
Ms. S is a 38-year-old woman with a 2 year history of excessive weight gain, despite dietary modification and exercise, development of hypertension and diabetes mellitus, thinning skin with easy bruising, and irregular menstruation. Her primary care provider performed blood testing including cortisol and ACTH levels, which were found to be abnormally elevated. She was therefore referred for pituitary imaging which demonstrated a lesion measuring under 10 mm on the left side of her pituitary gland. She was referred to an endocrinologist who identified pituitary source of excess ACTH production therefore confirming Cushing's Disease. Her endocrinologist referred her to neurosurgery for resection of her pituitary microadenoma. She is currently post-op day 1 status post transsphenoidal surgery via sublabial approach and has been assigned to your care today. During your shift you notice an increase in urine output and Ms. S is complaining of excessive thirst. Her serum sodium 8 h ago was 138 mEq/L and now is 146 mEq/L. Her urine specific gravity upon last void is 1.002. She is urinating hourly 300–500 mL/h over the past 3 h.

1. What hormone imbalance do you suspect?
   The increased serum sodium in the setting of decreased urine specific gravity and excessive urine output is characteristic of diabetes insipidus. Diabetes insipidus results when the pituitary gland does not excrete adequate amounts of antidiuretic hormone (ADH).
2. What should you do next?
   Ms. S's medical/surgical providers should be notified of the changes in her fluid balance. Notification to her providers should include most recent intake/output, specifically urine output; laboratory results, specifically serum

sodium, serum osmolality, urine specific gravity; daily weight and updated set of vital signs.

3. What are the nursing considerations of the patient with diabetes insipidus?

   Maintaining diligent intake and output in addition to monitoring daily weights to monitor patient's hydration status is paramount. Understanding that the patient with diabetes insipidus is at risk for dehydration should guide the nurse to monitor vital signs for tachycardia/bradycardia and be cautious during mobilization due to risk for orthostatic hypotension from inadequate intravascular volume. Increased frequency of laboratory testing may be indicated. The nurse should discuss potential need for fluid replacement with the medical/surgical providers.

4. What medication may be ordered for treatment of diabetes insipidus?

   Desmopressin (DDAVP).

5. Ms. S is prescribed hydrocortisone postoperatively for steroid replacement. She will discharge on this medication. What nursing education must occur prior to her discharge?

   Ms. S must receive detailed patient education regarding adrenal insufficiency and the importance of continuing hydrocortisone therapy as prescribed by her providers. She should be taught signs of adrenal insufficiency, what to do and who to contact if she notices any of these signs. The body's steroid needs increase in times of sickness therefore patients require additional steroid medication when they are ill, instructions should be provided to the patient regarding what to do when they are ill. She will require instructions to taper her dose of hydrocortisone if discharged on supraphysiologic doses. Follow-up with endocrinology within approximately 6 weeks postoperatively is important. She will require testing to evaluate HPA axis function to determine her ongoing need for glucocorticoids.

6. What other discharge education should be provided?

Given this patient underwent transsphenoidal surgery via *a sublabial approach, she should be taught about oral care needs and activity restrictions. Specific activity restrictions may vary slightly from institution to institution; however, they are all generally aimed at avoidance of placing pressure on the sphenoid sinus surgical site. General limitations include avoiding nose blowing, sneezing (sneeze with open mouth to diffuse pressure if the patient must sneeze), heavy lifting over 20 lb, or straining. The patient's follow-up plans should be outlined prior to discharge. Follow-up for further endocrinological monitoring is essential.*

References

AANN Clinical Practice Guidelines Series. Care of the patient undergoing intracranial pressure monitoring/external ventricular drainage or lumbar drainage. Chicago: AANN; 2011.

Amar P, Weiss MH. Pituitary anatomy and physiology. Neurosurg Clin N Am. 2003;14(1):11–2.

Ben-Shlomo A, Melmed S. Pituitary development. In: Melmed S, editor. The pituitary. 3rd ed. San Diego: Elsevier; 2011. p. 21–41.

Bornstein SR, Allolio B, Arlt W, Barthel A, Don-Wauchope A, Hammer GD, Husebye ES, Merke DP, Murad MH, Stratakis CA, Torpy DJ. Diagnosis and treatment of primary adrenal insufficiency: an Endocrine Society clinical practice guideline. J Clin Endocrinol Metab. 2016;101(2):364–89. https://doi.org/10.1210/jc.2015-1710.

Carminucci AS, Ausiello JC, Page-Wilson G, Lee M, Good L, Bruce JN, Freda PU. Outcome of implementation of a multidisciplinary team approach to the care of patients after transsphenoidal surgery. Endocr Pract. 2016;22(1):36–44. https://doi.org/10.4158/EP15894.OR. Epub 2015 Oct 5.

Dumont AS, Nemergut EC II, Jane J Jr, Laws ER Jr. Postoperative care following pituitary surgery. J Intensive Care Med. 2005;20:127Y140. https://doi.org/10.1177/0885066605275247.

Glowniak JV, Loriaux DL. A double-blind study of perioperative steroid requirements in secondary adrenal insufficiency. Surgery. 1997;121(2):123–9.

Greenberg MS. Handbook of neurosurgery. 8th ed. New York: Thieme Medical Publishers, Inc; 2016.

Inder WJ, Hunt PJ. Glucocorticoid replacement in pituitary surgery: guidelines for perioperative assessment and management. J Clin Endocrinol Metab. 2002;87(6):2745–50. https://doi.org/10.1210/jc.87.6.2745.

Kelly KN, Domajnko B. Perioperative stress-dose steroids. Clin Colon Rectal Surg. 2013;26(3):163–7. https://doi.org/10.1055/s-0033-1351132.

Kristof RA, Rother M, Neuloh G, Klingmüller D. Incidence, clinical manifestations, and course of water and electrolyte metabolism disturbances following transsphenoidal pituitary adenoma surgery: a prospective observational study. J Neurosurg. 2009;111(3):555–62. https://doi.org/10.3171/2008.9. JNS08191. PubMed PMID: 19199508.

Lynn SJ. Caring for patients with lumbar drains. American Nurse Today 2016;11(3). https://www.americannurse-today.com/caring-patients-lumbar-drains/

Malenković V, Gvozdenović L, Milaković B, Sabljak V, Ladjević N, Zivaljević V. Preoperative preparation of patients with pituitary gland disorders. Acta Chir Iugosl. 2011;58(2):91–6.

Naziat A, Grossman A. Adrenal insufficiency. [Updated 2015 Apr 12]. In: De Groot LJ, Chrousos G, Dungan K, et al., editors. Endotext [Internet]. South Dartmouth: MDText.com, Inc; 2000. https://www-ncbi-nlm-nih-gov.liboff.ohsu.edu/books/NBK279122/.

Nieman LK, Biller BMK, Findling JW, Murad MH, Newell-Price J, Savage MO, Tabarin A. Treatment of Cushing's syndrome: an Endocrine Society clinical practice guideline. J Clin Endocrinol Metab. 2015;100(8):2807–31. https://doi.org/10.1210/jc.2015-1818.

Olson BR, Gumowski J, Rubino D, Oldfield EH. Pathophysiology of hyponatremia after transsphenoidal pituitary surgery. J Neurosurg. 1997;87(4):499–507.

Overstreet M. Clinical Queries: how do I manage a lumbar drain? Nursing. 2003;33(3):74–5.

Pimentel-Filho FR, Silva MER, Nogueira KC, Berger K, Cukiert A, Liberman B. Pituitary-adrenal dynamics after ACTH-secreting pituitary tumor resection in patients receiving no steroids post-operatively. J Endocrinol Invest. 2005;28:502.

Prabhakar H, Bithal PK, Suri A, Rath GP, Dash HH. Intracranial pressure changes during valsalva manoeuvre in patients undergoing a neuroendoscopic procedure. Minim Invasive Neurosurg. 2007;50(2):98–101. https://doi.org/10.1055/s-2007-982505.

Prather SH, Forsyth LW, Russell KD, Wagner VL. Caring for the patient undergoing transsphenoidal surgery in the acute care setting: an alternative to critical care. J Neurosci Nurs. 2003;35(5):270–5. PubMed PMID: 14593938.

Simmons NE, Alden TD, Thorner MO, Laws ER Jr. Serum cortisol response to transsphenoidal surgery for Cushing disease. J Neurosurg. 2001;95(1):1–8.

Smith TR, Hulou M, Huang KT, Nery B, Miranda de Moura S, Cote DJ, Laws ER. Complications after transsphenoidal surgery for patients with Cushing's disease and silent corticotroph adenomas. Neurosurg Focus. 2015;38(2):E12.

Yuan W. Managing the patient with transsphenoidal pituitary tumor resection. J Neurosci Nurs. 2013;45(2):101–7. https://doi.org/10.1097/JNN.0b013e3182828e28. Review. PubMed PMID: 23422696.

Zhao B, Wei Y-K, Li G-L, Li Y-N, Yao Y, Kang J, Ma W-B, Yang Y, Wang R-Z. Extended transsphenoidal approach for pituitary adenomas invading the anterior cranial base, cavernous sinus, and clivus: a single-center experience with 126 consecutive cases. J Neurosurg. 2010;112(1):108–17. https://doi.org/10.3171/2009.3.JNS0929.

Key Reading

1. Ben-Shlomo A, Melmed S. Pituitary development. In: Melmed S, editor. The pituitary. 3rd ed. San Diego: Elsevier; 2011. p. 21–41.

2. Liyanarachchi K, Ross R, Debono M. Human studies on hypothalamo-pituitaryadrenal (HPA) axis. Best Pract Res Clin Endocrinol Metab. 2017;31:459e473.

3. Rollin GAF, Ferreira NP, Junges M, et al. Dynamics of Serum Cortisol Levels after transsphenoidal surgery in a cohort of patients with Cushing's disease. J Clin Endocrinol Metab. 2004;89:1131–9.

4. Barkan AL, Blank H, Chandler WF. Pituitary surgery: peri-operative management. In: Swearingen B, Biller BMK, editors. Diagnosis and management of pituitary disorders. Totowa: Humana Press; 2008. p. 303–19.

5. Eisenberg AA, Redick EL. Transsphenoidal resection of pituitary adenoma: using a critical pathway. Dimens Crit Care Nurs. 1998;17(6):306–12.

Radiotherapy

24

Ahmed Al Sajwani and Mark Sherlock

Contents

A. Al Sajwani
Department of Endocrinology, Tallaght Hospital,
Dublin and Trinity College, Dublin, Ireland

M. Sherlock (✉)
Department of Endocrinology, Beaumont Hospital and
Royal College of Surgeons in Ireland, Dublin, Ireland
e-mail: marksherlock@beaumont.ie

© Springer Nature Switzerland AG 2019
S. Llahana et al. (eds.), *Advanced Practice in Endocrinology Nursing*,
https://doi.org/10.1007/978-3-319-99817-6_24

447

Abstract

Ionizing radiation, discovered in the late nineteenth century, is used to treat pituitary tumors as an adjunctive therapy. Radiotherapy works at a cellular level via a number of mechanisms to cause cell death. This occurs slowly, often taking years to normalize hormone levels. Therefore, adjunctive medical therapies may be required in the interim.

External beam radiation is most commonly used to treat pituitary adenomas with conventional radiotherapy (CRT), the most frequently used method. In CRT, radiation doses are administered in small, fractionated doses, usually for a total of 45–50 Gy. Targeted treatment planning uses CT/MRI and a customized mask is used for head stabilization and precise tumor targeting with each subsequent treatment. Stereotactic radiosurgery (SRS) includes Gamma Knife, and proton beam therapy. These require neuroimaging techniques such as CT/MRI or PET scan mapping for precise targeting of the lesion.

Radiation is delivered using a Linear Accelerator (LINAC), Gamma Knife, Cyberknife, proton beam and, rarely, brachytherapy with the implantation of radioactive seeds. Post treatment progressive hypopituitarism may become apparent in up to 50% of patients, necessitating ongoing monitoring and replacement therapies.

Radiation therapies are used to control tumor growth in persistent or recurrent pituitary tumors or to control excess hormonal production. Radiation has been shown to be effective in a significant proportion of patients to arrest tumor growth and normalize hormonal levels in acromegaly, Cushing's disease, and in large prolactinomas when primary surgical and/or medical therapies fail or when the patient is intolerant or resistant to second line medical therapies. Risk benefit must be considered as in all therapies.

Keywords

Pituitary · Radiation · Hypopituitarism · Adenoma

Abbreviations

ACTH	Adrenocorticotropic hormone
BED	Biological effective dose
CRT	Conventional radiotherapy
CT	Computerized tomography
CVA	Cardiovascular accident
DNA	Deoxyribonucleic acid
FSH	Follicle stimulating hormone
GH	Growth hormone
GHD	Growth hormone deficiency
GK	Gamma Knife radiation therapy
Gy	Gray
HP	Hypothalamic-pituitary axis
HPA	Hypothalamic-pituitary-adrenal axis
IGF-1	Insulin growth factor 1
ITT	Insulin tolerance test
LH	Luteinizing hormone
LINAC	Linear accelerator
MRI	Magnetic resonance imaging
NFA	Non-functioning adenoma
NFPA	Non-functioning pituitary adenoma

PET   Positron emission tomography
RT   Radiotherapy
SRS   Stereotactic radiosurgery
SST   Standard Synacthen Test
TSH   Thyroid stimulating hormone

Key Terms
- **The Gray (Gy)** is the unit used to describe the patient absorbed dose of any form of ionizing radiation (1 Gy = 1 J/kg).
- **Biological effective dose (BED)** is a calculation that aims to quantify the biological effect of any radiotherapy treatment, taking into account changes in dose-per-fraction or dose rate and total dose, over time.
- **Pre-treatment tumor mapping** uses sophisticated coordinated computerized CT/MRI/PET imaging system to construct the shape of the tumor and plan for targeted delivery of radiation.
- **Fractionated conventional radiotherapy** is delivered in the form of small doses of 25–30 fractions over 5–6 weeks.
- **A linear accelerator** is a machine that uses electricity to generate high-energy photons or X-rays.

Key Points
- Radiation therapy is most commonly used as an adjunctive therapy when both surgery and available medical therapies have failed to control the growth or the excess hormonal production from a pituitary adenoma.
- Radiotherapy damages cellular viability by generating highly reactive free radicals and hydrogen reducing species, disrupting plasma membranes, DNA damage and DNA double-strand breakage. Radiation damaged cells die either immediately or more slowly following cell division.
- External beam radiation in the form of fractionated conventional radiotherapy (CRT) is the most commonly used radiation to treat pituitary tumors.
- Stereotactic radiosurgery (SRS) can be divided into Gamma Knife radiation therapy, linear accelerator based and proton beam therapy.
- The efficacy of radiotherapy for different types of pituitary adenomas varies related to factors such as type and dose of radiotherapy; type, size, and position of the pituitary tumor; surgical intervention, prior to irradiation and concurrent use of medical therapy.
- Efficacy for control of hormonal excess may be delayed by many years requiring a patient to continue adjunctive treatment and long-term endocrine monitoring.
- Hormonal deficiencies develop in almost 50% of patients after radiation necessitating close endocrine monitoring and dynamic testing particularly for HPA axis function.
- Other rare complications post radiation therapy include: neural dysfunction; cerebrovascular effects; secondary neoplasms; infertility; memory, cognitive executive function changes.
- Many aspects of planning, patient and family preparation need to be addressed prior to therapy by all members of the care team.

24.1 Introduction

Ionizing radiation, that has sufficient energy to pass through a medium, has been utilized in medicine since the late nineteenth century, soon after the discovery of X-rays by Roentgen in 1895

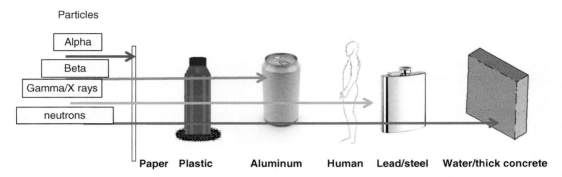

Fig. 24.1 Radiation particles and penetration. Ref: https://www.nrc.gov/about-nrc/radiation/health-effects/radiation-basics.html

and Radium by Marie and Pierre Curie in 1897 (Fig. 24.1). Intracranial tumors are commonly treated with irradiation and approximately 10% of these tumors originate in the pituitary gland. The most common pituitary tumors are adenomas which are benign tumors arising from the adenohypophysis, the anterior part of the pituitary gland. There are a number of other tumors that may arise in the sellar region including: craniopharyngioma, meningioma, optic nerve glioma, osteomas, chordomas, and other rare lesions.

24.2   Pituitary Tumors

Pituitary adenoma are generally classified into functional (secretory) and non-functional (nonsecretory). Functional pituitary adenomas may secrete one (or more) of the following hormones: prolactin, growth hormone, adrenocorticotropic hormone (ACTH), less frequently thyroid stimulating hormone, and gonadotropin secreting adenoma (luteinizing hormone and follicle stimulating hormone).

The first-line management of pituitary tumors, when required, is surgical with the exception of prolactin-secreting tumors, which are primarily treated by medical therapy. Microsurgery in the form of transsphenoidal tumor resection is regarded as one of the most reliable surgical modalities. Open craniotomy is reserved for cases when tumors are not accessible by the endonasal approach (See Chap. 22).

The majority of patients who receive pituitary irradiation do so as an adjuvant therapy following surgery but have a residual tumor (or persistent hormonal hypersecretion) or tumor recurrence. Radiotherapy can be used as the sole therapy in patients not amenable to surgery, when there is little or no medical management to offer, or when tumor has close proximity to sensitive areas particularly in the cavernous sinuses where surgery carries significant morbidity risk. The response to radiotherapy for secretary adenomas is often slow compared to surgery and medical management, the time to endocrine control can be up to 10 years, this is felt to be due to slow rate of division of irradiated cells, which die only after a few divisions. Therefore, patients with functional pituitary adenoma may require medical therapy in the intervening years while waiting for sufficient radiation-induced damage to allow endocrinological control.

24.3   Action of Radiotherapy

At the cellular level, radiotherapy works via a number of mechanisms including the generation of highly reactive free radicals and hydrogen reducing species, plasma membrane disturbance, DNA damage, and DNA double-strand breakage. Radiation damaged cells die either immediately or more slowly following cell division. In general, non-tumorous, normal cells have a better capacity to repair their DNA than abnormal cells (Fig. 24.2).

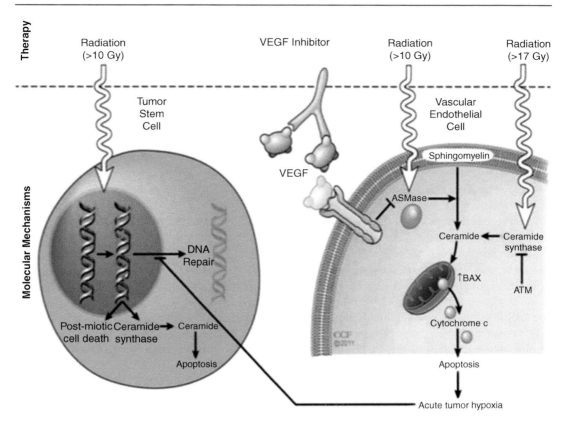

Fig. 24.2 Cell changes with radiation exposure. Used with permission from LAKSHMI DEEPTHI GEDELA, Junior Resident in Radiation Oncology, Postgraduate Institute of Medical Education and Research

Dosing schedules for various conditions can vary between radiotherapy centers with respect to the total radiation dose administered or the number of treatment fractions used. The Gray (Gy) is the unit used for the patient absorbed dose of any form of ionizing radiation (1 Gy = 1 J/kg). It is recognized that the same radiation dose delivered in larger fractions will have a greater biological impact. Another important factor that determines the impact of radiation is the sensitivity of the tissue being exposed: for example, the very rapid cell turnover of intestinal cells make them more sensitive than nervous tissue, which has a much slower turnover rate.

Taking these factors into account, the biological effective dose (BED) can be calculated when considering the impact of different protocols on a tissue. This was pioneered by Barendsen (1982) and Fowler (1989), and makes it possible to standardize the biological effects of a given total radiation dose for any tissue within the body taking into account the fractionation schedule. A key concept in the cell survival theory is that different tissues have different fractionation sensitivities, these tissues have been labelled early and late responding tissues (Schmiegelow et al. 2000).

24.4 Histological Changes in the Pituitary Gland and Pituitary Adenomas Following Radiotherapy

Ionizing radiation is known to affect cell nuclei, the plasma membrane and disturb extracellular as well as intracellular signalling systems (Vincent 1995; Dainiak 1997). Acutely, following radiotherapy, one can visualize pyknosis (irreversible nuclear chromatin changes) or other nuclear changes that indicate imminent cell necrosis or apoptosis. However, long term no apoptotic cells are found as these are quickly cleared by phagocytosis (Vincent 1995).

Two histologic studies comparing tissue samples from patients who underwent anterior pituitary gland irradiation found differences between normal and tumor cells (Nishioka et al. 2001, 2002). Fibrotic changes with thickened connective tissue between glandular structures were found in normal pituitary tissues. This effect was more pronounced the farther the patient was from the original treatment. Fibrosis was found to be absent or mild in pituitary tumor/adenomas cells following conventional fractionated radiotherapy and stereotactic fractionated radiotherapy (Nishioka et al. 2001, 2002). However, diffuse hyaline deposits were found in pituitary adenoma tissue following Gamma Knife radiosurgery (Nishioka et al. 2002). The underlying cellular mechanism of radiation-induced fibrosis has been studied in detail by Rodemann and Bamberg (Rodemann and Bamberg 1995) who have described an altered cytokine and growth factor profile leading to a disturbance in the well-balanced cell type ratio of the interstitial fibroblast/fibrocyte cell system. On immunohistochemical staining of irradiated pituitary tissue, there are stellate-shaped (star shaped) S100 protein positive cells. These stellate-shaped cells are known to synthesize cytokines including interleukin-6 and fibroblast growth factor (Vankelecom et al. 1993) and have been implicated in radiation-induced fibrosis (Nishioka et al. 2001).

Adenohypophyseal (anterior pituitary) necrosis is rare with conventional doses of radiotherapy and it has been reported that doses of greater than 185 Gy are necessary to induce necrosis in the normal adenohypophysis. As one would suspect from the low incidence of cranial diabetes insipidus following cranial irradiation, the neurohypophysis does not show any histological changes (Nishioka et al. 2001, 2002).

24.5 Methods of Delivery of Radiotherapy

Radiotherapy can be administered externally (external beam radiation—teletherapy) or internally (pellets, seeds, etc.—brachytherapy). External beam radiation is the most commonly used to treat pituitary tumors. Radiation can be delivered in the form of photons like X-rays or Gamma rays or in the form of charged particles or protons.

24.5.1 Radiotherapy Techniques

24.5.1.1 Conventional Radiotherapy (CRT)

Conventional radiotherapy (CRT) is the most frequently used method of radiation therapy for pituitary tumors. It is most frequently used in patients who have a tumor remnant with evidence of progression following surgery or if surgery does not lead to normalization of hormone excess. The techniques used for CRT include high-energy CRT with opposed lateral fields, 360° rotational fields, moving arcs, and three field techniques (two lateral fields and a vertex field) (Fig. 24.3a, b) (Suh and Saxton 2000). The lesion anatomy is defined with MRI/CT and 3-D treatment planning with field conformation (Becker et al. 2002). During planning, a custom mask (Fig. 24.4) is made using a thermoplastic mesh, which attaches directly to the radiotherapy treatment machine. This mask limits mobility and minimizes head rotation and chin tilt variation. To account for the larger variation in positioning in 3D-CRT than is seen in stereotactic radiosurgery (SRS), a set up error margin is included in the planned treatment volume that results in a larger radiation target area compared to SRS (Shi et al. 2008).

Radiation doses range from 45 to 50 Gy at 180–200 cGy fractions (Colin et al. 2002; Tran et al. 1991; Tsang et al. 1996). Fractionated conventional radiotherapy is delivered in the form of small doses of 25–30 fractions over 5–6 weeks (Shi et al. 2008). Because stereotactic radiosurgery (SRS) is only a relatively new therapy, the majority of data regarding efficacy and potential adverse effects of radiotherapy is derived from studies assessing the use of CRT. However, there

Fig. 24.3 Conventional radiation techniques. (**a**) Conventional radiation—two opposed lateral fields. (**b**) Conventional radiation 360° rotational fields

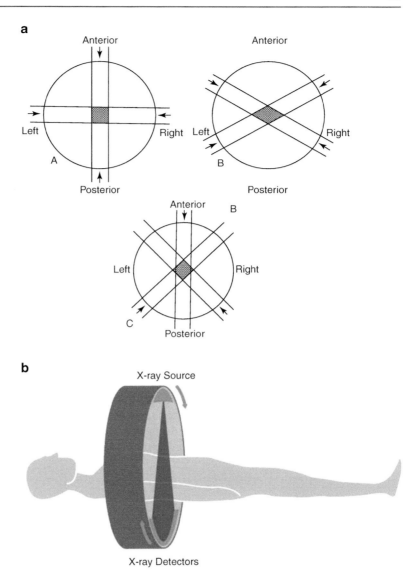

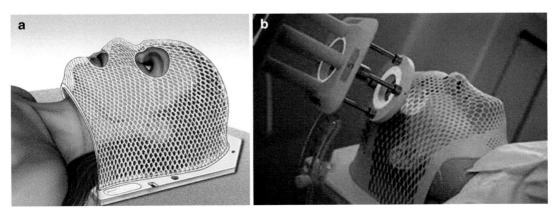

Fig. 24.4 Treatment masks. https://www.cancer.gov/about-cancer/treatment/types/radiation-therapy/radiation-fact-sheet; http://oncocare.co.zw/blog/service/radiation-therapy/

is an increase in the amount of data regarding SRS in recent years.

24.5.1.2 Stereotactic Radiosurgery (SRS)

Stereotactic radiosurgery (SRS) can be divided into Gamma Knife radiation therapy, linear accelerator based and proton beam therapy. Gamma Knife radiation therapy (GK, Elekta, Stockholm, Sweden) uses multiple cobalt-60 gamma radiation emitting sources. Linear accelerator based SRS (LINAC) in which energy is accelerated, shaped and delivered in the form of electrons, or photons. Proton beam therapy uses heavy charged protons and has the added advantage of leading to less excess radiation exposure to surrounding tissue (Shih and Loeffler 2008). SRS is delivered most frequently as a single treatment with the patient immobilized after careful stereotactic imaging planning.

SRS requires accurate mapping of the target tissue (Fig. 24.5) through modern neuroimaging techniques such as CT scan, MRI, and PET/CT. Immobilization of the patient is crucial, allowing radiation to be delivered to a precise location, providing a steep dose gradient that falls off rapidly

leading to limited impact on nearby normal tissues. The SRS delivered via a single dose is biologically more active than the same dose delivered in fractions. It also results in faster response to radiation when compared to fractionated radiotherapy. The dose employed to control tumor growth is usually lower than that required to achieve biochemical remission in secretory pituitary adenoma.

SRS is more convenient for patients but its use depends on patient eligibility, i.e., provided that, the pituitary lesion is not in close proximity to critical brain structures like the optic apparatus and the cranial nerves. Hypothalamic-pituitary dysfunction has been reported to occur less frequently following more focused cranial irradiation delivered via stereotactic radiotherapy.

24.5.2 Forms of Radiotherapy

24.5.2.1 Linear Accelerator (LINAC)

LINAC delivered radiotherapy is the most commonly used form of radiotherapy, and it uses electricity to generate high-energy photons or X-rays. The delivery of radiation is shaped to tumor size

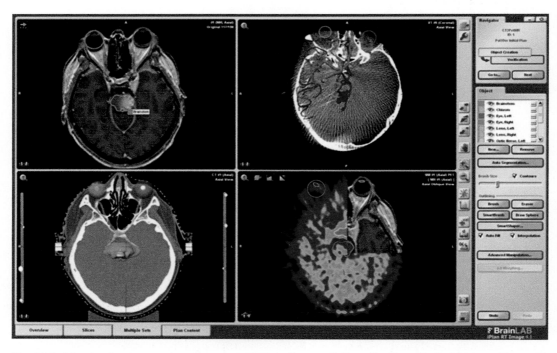

Fig. 24.5 Mapping for stereotactic radiosurgery (SRS) (permission granted). From Epworth Stereotactic radiosurgery and radiotherapy (Australia) Dr. Media enquiries, Contact Colleen Coghlan, Media Manager, Phone: 03 9426 8816, Fax: 03 9426 8997, Mobile: 0423 777 452, colleen.coghlan@epworth.org.au

and location. New devices offer multiple rotating beams and moving arcs, to target desired fields more accurately. The multileaf collimator confers radiation beams shaped automatically to focus on desired locations based on computerized input. The 3-dimensional conformal radiation therapy (3D-CRT) and intensity-modulated radiation therapy (IMRT) are examples of targeted radiotherapy delivery in linear accelerators to confront the shape of the tumor by a coordinated system, aided by sophisticated calculations and computerized imaging techniques (Fig. 24.6).

24.5.2.2 Gamma Knife

Gamma Knife was the first stereotactic radiosurgery (SRS) developed and is widely used to treat pituitary adenomas. Gamma Knife uses radioactive cobalt-60 to deliver photons via numerous sources around the head, which are held by a minimally invasive metal head frame. This results in the emission of low energy beams from numerous sources directed at the center of the tumor, which ultimately receives the maximum dose with great dose heterogeneity between the center and margins of the tumor. This minimizes the radiation exposure to the adjacent tissues. Treatment is usually completed in one session, however; multisession treatment can be extended to deliver a smaller amount of radiation over 2–5 therapeutic sessions, which causes less toxicity to adjacent normal tissues (Fig. 24.7).

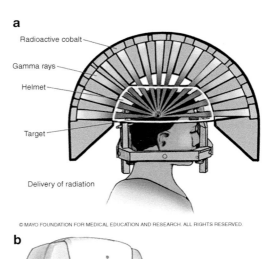

a

Radioactive cobalt

Gamma rays

Helmet

Target

Delivery of radiation

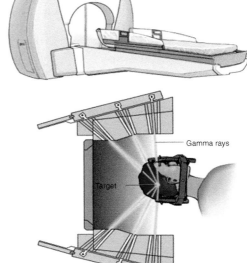

b

Gamma rays

Target

Gamma Knife unit and radiation delivery

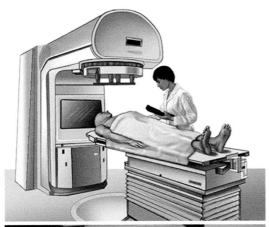

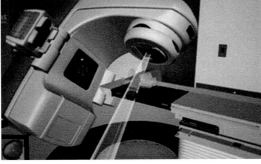

Fig. 24.6 Linear accelerator 3D-CRT. Linear accelerator used for external beam radiation therapy. A LINAC uses electricity to form a stream of fast-moving subatomic particles. This creates high-energy radiation that may be used to treat tumors. www.cancer.gov

Fig. 24.7 Gamma Knife. Mayo foundation for medical education and research

24.5.2.3 CyberKnife

CyberKnife can deliver radiation therapy in a single or multiple sessions, using a robotic arm with mounted radiotherapy source (Linear Accelerator). CyberKnife has an enhanced targeting system for tumors resulting in better accuracy than other radiotherapy modalities. It is also non-invasive allowing for more movement flexibility without the need for head clamps, molds, or frames as the source can adjust itself with patient movement. The length of treatment with CyberKnife, however, is typically longer.

24.5.2.4 Proton Radiation

Proton therapy is available in few centers worldwide and therefore is not widely used at present because of the cost and complexity (Fig. 24.8). The novelty of this method is due to the physical properties and heavy weight of the charged particles used, which result in significantly less damage to the normal tissues and reduce the late side effects of radiation exposure compared with previous methods. The beam is aimed precisely at the tumor and tends not to widen as it reaches the target lesion. Because of dose-distribution characteristics and localized radiation delivery with absent exit dose, increasing radiation dose results in a greater impact on tumor cells and maximizes their damage without increasing risks to the surrounding normal tissues (Fig. 24.9).

24.5.2.5 Brachytherapy

Brachytherapy is rarely practiced now and involves implanting yttrium-90 (Y-90) or gold-198 (AU-198) radioactive seeds into the pituitary gland through a transsphenoidal approach.

24.6 Use of Radiotherapy in Patients with Pituitary Adenoma

In general, radiotherapy is effective in arresting tumor growth or even decreasing tumor size especially if the target lesion is clear and discrete. Hormonal remission is less likely achieved solely by radiotherapy and may take a number of years.

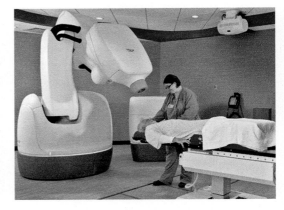

Fig. 24.8 Cyberknife. http://indiamedcare.com/wp-content/uploads/2016/12/Cyberknife-radiosurgery-inindia.jpg

The efficacy of radiotherapy reported in the literature for different types of pituitary adenomas are variable. This may be due to variations in the:

- Type and dose of radiotherapy used
- Type and size of the pituitary tumor
- Rates of surgical intervention prior to irradiation and concurrent use of medical therapy
- Differences in biochemical assays and criteria to define biochemical remission in secretory tumors
- Definition of efficacy used for tumor growth or biochemical control
- Length of follow-up in the study (as these tumors are frequently slow growing and impact on endocrine outcomes may take many years. A long period of follow-up is required for accurate assessment of efficacy)

24.7 Effect of Radiotherapy on Secretory Tumors

24.7.1 Use of Radiotherapy in Patients with Acromegaly

Acromegaly is an excess of growth hormone caused, in the majority of cases, by a pituitary tumor producing excess GH and a subsequently excess IGF-1 from the liver. Acromegaly is associated with increased cardiovascular, respiratory

Fig. 24.9 Proton beam
and no exit dose

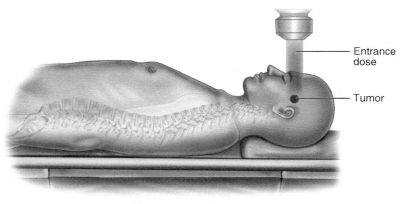

Entrance
dose

Tumor

Targeted proton therapy:
Deposits most energy on target

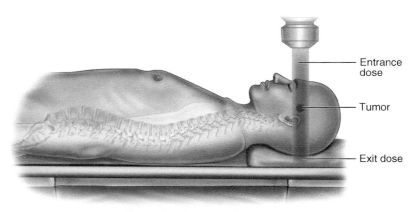

Entrance
dose

Tumor

Exit dose

Conventional radiation therapy:
Deposits most energy before target

and cancer morbidity and increased mortality (Katznelson et al. 2014). Normal life expectancy can be restored by lowering random GH levels to <1.0 μg/L and normalizing IGF-1 concentrations (Katznelson et al. 2014). Surgery remains the first choice therapy for acromegaly; however, adjuvant therapy is often required as surgery renders GH/IGF-1 to safe levels in only 40–80% of patients depending on the tumor size and surgical expertise (Ahmed et al. 1999; Sheaves et al. 1996; Clayton et al. 1999). Medical therapy with long acting somatostatin analogue therapy will lower GH and IGF-1 levels in approximately 90% of patients; however, only ~50% will achieve GH levels <2.5 μg/L and IGF-1 concentrations in

the age-related reference range (Jenkins 2000; Lancranjan and Atkinson 1999; Turner et al. 1999). Other medical therapies include dopamine agonists and GH receptor antagonists.

Conventional radiotherapy has been used in acromegaly for over 30 years and has been shown to be effective in lowering GH levels (Jenkins et al. 2006). GH/IGF-1 physiology is known to be altered following radiotherapy (Peacey et al. 2001). These studies may have been prone to selection bias as patients who followed up regularly and for long duration of time may have also been patients with more active disease. In a study of 884 patients who had received radiotherapy from the UK acromegaly database, a mean

GH level decrease from 13.5 to 5.3 ng/mL was achieved by 2 years, 2.0 ng/mL by 10 years, and 1.1 ng/mL by 20 years after radiotherapy. A GH of <2.5 ng/mL was achieved by 22% of patients at 2 years, 60% by 10 years, and 77% by 20 years after radiotherapy. The IGF-1 levels fell in parallel with GH with 63% of patients having a normal level by 10 years (Jenkins et al. 2006). This is in keeping with other reports (Biermasz et al. 2000a, b; Powell et al. 2000). The single most important factor in eventual success of radiotherapy appears to be the pre-radiotherapy GH/IGF-1 concentration (Jenkins et al. 2006). The higher the baseline lGH/IGF-1 levels the longer to normalization after radiotherapy (Jenkins et al. 2006).

Both fractionated radiotherapy or SRS can be used as an adjunctive modality to surgical and medical therapy in acromegaly, they can be effective in controlling local tumor growth in 95–100% of the cases, but biochemical remission is often more difficult to achieve. The mean time for hormonal normalization is faster with single fraction radiotherapy compared to fractionated therapy. In a recent prospective study of SRS, Hiromitsu et al. (Iwata et al. 2016) reported results using CyberKnife in 52 patients with acromegaly over 5 years duration with 60% of all cases achieving a GH <2.5 ng/mL and normal IGF-1 (age and gender matched) by the end of the study. However, only 17% achieved remission by Cortina consensus criteria (Box 24.1).

> **Box 24.1 Cortina Consensus Criteria**
> Random GH >1 μg/L
> Nadir GH after OGTT ≥0.4 μg/L
> Age and gender adjusted normal IGF-1
> Ref: A. Giustina, P. Chanson, M. D. Bronstein, A. Klibanski, S. Lamberts, F. F. Casanueva, P. Trainer, E. Ghigo, K. Ho, S. Melmed; A Consensus on Criteria for Cure of Acromegaly, The Journal of Clinical Endocrinology & Metabolism, Volume 95, Issue 7, 1 July 2010, Pages 3141–3148, https://doi.org/10.1210/jc.2009-2670

24.7.2 Use of Radiotherapy in Patients with Cushing's Disease

Cushing's disease results from oversecretion of ACTH from a pituitary adenoma which in turn leads to hypercortisolism. Chronic hypercortisolemia can result in significant morbidity such as cardiometabolic conditions, thromboembolic events, muscle weakness, bone loss, skin manifestations, gonadal dysfunction, ophthalmic disorders, neuropsychological changes, infections, and increased mortality. Most of these tumors are microadenomas with only 10% of patients having a macroadenoma. The diagnosis and localization of the lesion in Cushing's disease can be challenging. Transsphenoidal excision remains the cornerstone for management of Cushing's disease.

Radiotherapy in patients with Cushing's disease may be considered after non-curative surgery, recurrence of the tumor or disease invading the cavernous sinuses. Adjuvant medical therapy with agents such as metyrapone or ketoconazole (or newer agents see Chap. 21) is often required to treat hypercortisolemia following non-curative surgery and while awaiting the therapeutic effects of radiotherapy. Conventional radiotherapy is administered in fractions to achieve a cumulative dose between 40 and 50 Gy. SRS has been shown in studies to lead to better tumor control and more efficient hormonal control than conventional fractionated radiotherapy. Because these tumors are often small and well circumscribed, they can be effectively treated with SRS provided that disease is 3–5 mm away from optic chiasm. Sheehan et al. (Sheehan et al. 2013a) followed up in a retrospective trial 96 patients with Cushing's disease receiving a mean dose of 16 Gy through SRS Gamma Knife. During 48 months follow-up, tumor control was achieved in 98% of patients and 70% had biochemical remission. In this study, 5% developed new or worsening optic neuropathy and 36% new or progressive pituitary deficiencies. Wan et al. (Wan et al. 2009) and his colleagues demonstrated biochemical remission in 27.9% of 68 patients who received Gamma Knife for ACTH-producing adenoma, while tumor growth arrested in 89.7% of the patients, only one patient developed hypopituitarism during the period of follow-up.

Nelson's syndrome results from pituitary ACTH-secreting tumor growth following bilateral adrenalectomy for the management of refractory Cushing's disease. Lifelong follow-up is required for patients with Nelson's syndrome that can occur decades after adrenalectomy. Surgery should be the first-line treatment if possible as these tumors are more radioresistant than corticotroph adenomas. Interestingly, there is data suggesting that administration of radiotherapy post adrenalectomy may protect against the development of Nelson syndrome (Gil-Cardenas et al. 2007). In a study with 39 patients assessing the effect of radiotherapy when administered as a neoadjunctive therapy, none of the patients who received radiotherapy developed Nelson's syndrome up to 15 years following surgery compared to 50% in those patients who did not receive prophylactic radiation.

24.7.3 Use of Radiotherapy in Patients with Prolactinoma

Prolactinomas are the most common secretory pituitary adenomas, and they are divided into microprolactinoma and macroprolactinomas. Macroprolactinomas are rarer and can present with tumor mass effects such as headache, visual defects, and neurological manifestations; or symptoms due to prolactin hypersecretion, such as galactorrhea, amenorrhea, infertility, and erectile dysfunction.

Currently, medical therapy with a dopamine agonist is considered first-line treatment. Cabergoline is considered more efficacious than bromocriptine and is better tolerated. In the vast majority of patients dopamine agonist therapy effectively decreases tumor size and leads to normalization of prolactin concentrations (Gillam et al. 2006). Resistance to dopamine agonists can occur (defined as failure to normalize the prolactin or shrink tumor size by less than 50%).

Radiotherapy is reserved for non-responders to medical or surgical treatment. Pan et al. (Pan et al. 2000) have reported results from 128 patients treated with Gamma Knife for prolactinoma with a median follow-up of 33 months at a median dose of 31 Gy. In this study, 99% of patients achieved tumor control and 41% achieved biochemical remission. Wan et al. (2009) reported that 23.3% of 176 patients receiving Gamma Knife for macroprolactinoma achieved biochemical remission without medical therapy after radiosurgery, and tumor volume control was achieved in 90.3%. Repeat Gamma Knife was required in a majority of large tumors. The risk of hypopituitarism over time was estimated at close to 50%, which includes a recognized risk to fertility.

24.7.4 Radiotherapy for Non-functioning Pituitary Adenoma (NFPA)

NFPAs are the most common type of pituitary tumor and may be asymptomatic or present with symptoms secondary to compression of key structures or hypopituitarism. They can compress the optic chiasm and encroach on other vital structures within the cavernous sinuses. These tumors are often managed conservatively but if treatment is required, surgery is the first-line therapy. Radiotherapy may be considered if surgery is not successful or feasible or there is a tumor recurrence which is inoperable.

In the past conventional fractionated radiotherapy was commonly practiced, but due to the high risk of hypopituitarism and other adverse effects this is less frequently used currently. SRS is now gaining popularity and proven to be effective for these adenomas, in a dose range between 14 and 16 Gy. Normally these tumors require less radiation to halt their growth compared to secretory adenomas, as both tumor size and biochemical control are desired in the latter. Sheehan et al. (2013b) reported tumor control following stereotactic radiosurgery with overall tumor control of 93.4%; the actuarial tumor control post radiotherapy were achieved as 98%, 95%, 91%, and 85% in 3 years, 5 years, 8 years, and 10 years, respectively. Better outcomes were observed in patients with smaller size adenoma and tumors without suprasellar extension. New or worsening hypopituitarism was noted in 21% of the patients.

24.8 Complications of Pituitary Radiotherapy

Despite the established effectiveness of radiotherapy for the treatment of both functional and nonfunctional pituitary adenoma, it is rarely regarded as a first-line management for such conditions. In addition to the delay of therapeutic effect following irradiation, the potential irreversible side effects of radiotherapy makes this option less appealing as a first-line therapy. The risk of complications, especially hypothalamic-pituitary axis dysfunction, does not decline with time but rather increases slowly with time and may take years to develop. It is imperative to understand these potential complications and weigh them in relation to any therapeutic benefit.

24.8.1 Short-Term Complications

Nausea, headache, tiredness, hair loss, and skin changes are often reported following radiotherapy. They can be managed symptomatically and are usually self-limiting.

24.8.2 Long-Term Complications

24.8.2.1 Neural Damage
The optic pathway is radiosensitive and more prone to damage compared to other cranial nerves. With increasing understanding of radiation doses and tolerance, this potential risk can be minimized by using fractionated radiotherapy if the optic nerve apparatus is close to the field of radiation. Doses larger than 55 Gy or fractions more than 2 Gy in conventional radiotherapy and single dose exceeding 8 Gy with stereotactic radiosurgery are associated with potential optic nerve injury. If vision deteriorates following radiotherapy, other causes should be considered and excluded such as tumor compression and/or edema.

Cranial nerve palsies can be avoided by careful planning and limiting higher doses of radiation to these nerves, particularly CNIII, IV, V, and VI. These nerves reside in the parasellar (cavernous sinus) and suprasellar regions and can easily be affected by the field of radiation. Brain parenchymal necrosis can manifest with focal neurological deficits, neurocognitive decline, and/or seizures due to changes in vascular permeability, brain edema or even demyelination disorder. Such complications arise within the radiation fields although current modern techniques have reduced these sequelae.

24.8.2.2 Secondary Brain Neoplasms
Secondary oncogenesis following pituitary radiotherapy is controversial. It is impossible to calculate the true incidence of tumors arising following pituitary radiotherapy as patients with pituitary disease in many studies have historically received disproportionate radiation exposure in the form of frequent CT imaging. In recent years, MRI has become the most common form of surveillance imaging for pituitary tumors. In some studies, the incidence of secondary neoplasm is as high as 1–2% occurring with a latency of 8–15 years (Bliss et al. 1994; Brada et al. 1992; Tsang et al. 1993). One study has estimated an incidence of extracranial tumors in NFA patients to be 3.9 fold that of the general population irrespective of whether the patient had radiotherapy or not (Popovic et al. 1998), therefore having a pituitary adenoma may be associated with and underlying increased susceptibility to tumorigenesis. Secondary intracranial tumors (most commonly gliomas or meningioma) due to pituitary irradiation are now relatively rare due to newer techniques which expose a smaller volume of cranial tissue to radiation (Shih and Loeffler 2008). Future studies focusing on patients treated with surgery alone and followed with surveillance MRIs as control subjects rather than using a normal population sample as controls may find different outcomes with respect to secondary neoplasms after radiotherapy (Gittoes 2003).

24.8.2.3 Cerebrovascular Morbidity and Mortality

Increased cerebrovascular disease and death have been reported in a number of studies following conventional pituitary irradiation. In a series of 156 patients with non-functioning pituitary adenoma (NFPA), increased cerebral infarction rates were found in patients administered higher doses of radiotherapy (Flickinger et al. 1989). A relative risk of CVA of 4.1 (CI 3.6–4.7) was found in a study of 331 patients who received pituitary radiotherapy for a number of underlying diagnoses compared with the general population (Brada et al. 1999). On multivariate analysis the authors reported that the main predictors of CVA were older age at diagnosis, prior extensive surgery compared to biopsy or no operation, higher doses of radiotherapy, and an underlying diagnosis of acromegaly (Brada et al. 1999). Brada et al. assessed cerebrovascular mortality in 344 patients who had received radiotherapy (79% also had transcranial or transsphenoidal surgery). Cerebrovascular disease accounted for 26% of all deaths [33 deaths compared to 8 deaths expected (RR 4.11, (CI 2.84–5.75))], with an even further increased risk in female patients [RR 6.9, (CI 4.29–10.6)] compared to males [RR 2.4, (CI 1.24–4.2), $p = 0.002$] (Brada et al. 2002). Surgery also plays a role in the increased cerebrovascular mortality. Patients with prior surgery had an increase RR compared to those with no surgery or biopsy alone [RR 5.19, (CI 3.5–7.42)] vs. [RR 1.33, (CI 0.27–3.88), $p = 0.02$], but there may be several confounders which may have led to this increase such as hypopituitarism (Brada et al. 2002). Data collection was also hampered by variability in reports of cause of death.

24.8.2.4 Hypopituitarism

Over 50% of patients who receive pituitary radiotherapy will develop one or more anterior pituitary hormone deficiency within the following decade (Barrande et al. 2000; Littley et al. 1989a; Tsang et al. 1994). The classic pattern of pituitary hormone deficiency to radiotherapy of GH (100% at 5 years), gonadotrophin (91% at 5 years), ACTH (77% at 5 years) then TSH deficiency (42% at 5 years) (Littley et al. 1989a)

is not always seen and deficiencies may occur in any order. As deficiencies can occur at any time point even up to 20 years later, long-term testing is required (Tsang et al. 1994; al-Mefty et al. 1990; Brada et al. 1993). With conventional RT, the speed of onset of hypopituitarism is related to the total and fractional doses of radiotherapy (Tsang et al. 1994). The rate of hypopituitarism increases with time from irradiation.

24.8.2.4.1 Factors Which Influence the Development of Hypopituitarism Include

- Sensitivity of the hypothalamus compared to the pituitary to irradiation
- Radiation dose
- Length of time since cranial irradiation
- Age of patient at time of cranial irradiation
- The type of radiotherapy administered
- The different radiosensitivities of pituitary hormones

24.8.2.4.2 Sensitivity of the Hypothalamus Compared to the Pituitary to Irradiation

The hypothalamus is more radiosensitive than the pituitary gland (Sklar and Constine 1995) and is therefore more easily damaged by lower doses of radiation (<40 Gy). However, at higher doses of radiation (>50 Gy) there is evidence for both hypothalamic and anterior pituitary damage (Constine et al. 1993; Shalet et al. 1988; Sklar 1991).

The preponderance of early hypothalamic dysfunction following cranial irradiation has been elicited from a number of studies, which have assessed the response of pituitary hormones in subjects using exogenous hypothalamic releasing factors (Chrousos et al. 1982; Samaan et al. 1975; Blacklay et al. 1986; Lam et al. 1986; Darzy et al. 2003) (See Chap. 5).

24.8.2.4.3 Radiation Dose

The dose of radiation delivered to the HP axis is the most important factor in the future development of HP axis dysfunction (Littley et al. 1989b). Low doses of radiation (18–24 Gy) used as prophylactic cranial irradiation for childhood hematological malignancies usually result in only isolated GH deficiency (Brennan et al. 1998; Adan et al. 2001). Patients who receive high dose (60 Gy) cranial irradiation for the treatment of nasopharyngeal carcinoma or non-pituitary intracranial neoplasms are at greater risk of developing multiple hormone deficiencies (Agha et al. 2005), with a small percentage developing panhypopituitarism (Lam et al. 1991).

24.8.2.4.4 Length of Time Since Cranial Irradiation

Hypothalamic-pituitary axis dysfunction may take several years to develop following cranial irradiation. However, in some patients the onset of HP axis dysfunction may be rapid (Duffner et al. 1985) and as such, radiation-induced HP axis dysfunction should be clinically suspected in all patients who develop symptoms early following cranial irradiation. Therefore, the timing of dynamic pituitary testing following cranial irradiation is paramount in the interpretation of a patient's test results and likewise in interpreting the effect of radiation on the HP axis in clinical studies (Littley et al. 1989a). Using stepwise multiple linear regression analysis, Clayton and Shalet (1991) demonstrated that both radiation dose, and time from irradiation, have a significant influence on peak GH response to dynamic testing in children. The late incidence of GH deficiency was similar over the whole dose range, but the speed of onset was dependent on dose. Agha et al. (2005) have shown that in a cohort of patients treated with radiotherapy for non-pituitary brain tumors the development of any degree of hypopituitarism (using multivariate regression models) depended on both the BED and time since irradiation. GH deficiency and ACTH deficiency were associated with the duration since radiotherapy.

It is important to recognize that hypopituitarism develops over a period of years following irradiation and that patients must undergo regular endocrine follow-up with dynamic testing as appropriate. It is for this reason that any patient who has received cranial irradiation is recommended to have up to yearly dynamic pituitary function assessment in order not to miss evolving HPA axis dysfunction or with the development of any symptoms.

24.8.2.4.5 Age of Patient at Time of Cranial Irradiation

Patients who receive cranial irradiation during childhood are more likely to develop HP axis dysfunction than patients receiving cranial irradiation during adult life. Littley et al. (1991) studied 21 adult patients (16–49 years) treated with total body irradiation (10 Gy in 5 fractions or 12–13.2 Gy in 6 fractions) for hematological malignancies. After a mean follow-up of 2.4 years, no patient showed evidence of HPA axis dysfunction. Endocrine abnormalities in these patients were limited to direct radiation-induced damage to either the thyroid gland or gonadal tissue. In contrast, Ogilvy-Stuart et al. (1992) showed that almost 50% of children who received the same total body irradiation protocol developed GH deficiency over a similar time frame.

24.9 The Impact of Radiotherapy on Specific Anterior Pituitary Hormones

24.9.1 Growth Hormone

Growth hormone deficiency is the most common manifestation of HP axis dysfunction following cranial irradiation and often occurs in isolation, with reported incidence between 50 and 100% after radiotherapy for sellar masses. Somatotrophs are reported to be more radiosensitive in children as compared with adults. GHD occurs after low dose radiation with reported cases occurring with doses as low as 18 Gy to the HP axis (Rappaport and Brauner 1989). The development of HP axis dysfunction with single doses of radiation of 9–10 Gy can be explained when the single fraction dose is factored into the equation for the BED. Littley et al. (1989a) reported that GHD occurred in all patients treated for pituitary adenomas 5 years after administration of 37.5–42.5 Gy in 15–16 fractions (Fig. 24.10).

Interestingly, a number of studies using sensitive GH assays have shown that in patients with GHD, GH concentrations never fall to an undetectable level. Darzy et al. (2005) studied

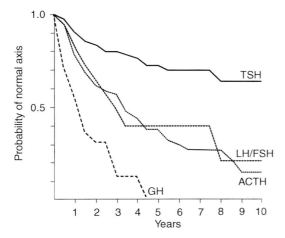

Fig. 24.10 The probability of the anterior pituitary hormone axes remaining normal following radiotherapy for pituitary adenoma. All patients had normal axes before radiotherapy. The presence of underlying pituitary disease increases the speed with which hypopituitarism develops. From Littley et al. Q. J. Med. 70 (1989) 145–160

the dynamics of GH secretion (using a sensitive chemiluminescence GH assay) in GHD adults who received cranial irradiation during childhood for the treatment of non-pituitary brain tumors. GH samples were assessed every 20 min over 24 h. The GH profiles in these patients were compared to GH profiles in 30 gender, age, and BMI matched normal healthy volunteers. This study showed that there was a significant decrease in all amplitude-related measurements of GH secretion (mean GH levels, area under the curve for GH, absolute GH peak height, mean peak GH height, and mean pulse area) for adults post childhood cranial radiation. There was not, however, any difference in frequency-related measurements (GH pulse frequency, GH pulse duration, and inter-pulse interval) compared with control subjects. The authors conclude that the integrity of the HP axis and GH neuroregulation is fundamentally preserved in irradiated GHD patients with a GH secretory pattern similar to that observed in normal subjects and those with GHD secondary to other causes; however, they are rendered GHD due to the decrease in amplitude of GH secretory bursts (Darzy et al. 2005).

24.9.2 FSH/LH

Gonadotropin deficiency is the second commonest pituitary hormone deficiency following cranial irradiation, and it results in estrogen or testosterone deficiency which in turn affects the development of secondary sexual characteristics, fertility, and bone mineralization. In contrast, low dose radiation can induce central precocious puberty in children younger than 7 years old by altering cortical puberty inhibition. Adult patients with pituitary disease develop gonadotropin deficiency more readily after radiation than children with 33% of adults developing gonadotropin deficiency after 20 Gy and 66% after 35–40 Gy (Toogood 2004).

24.9.3 Adrenocorticotropic Hormone

ACTH deficiency is less likely than GH and gonadotropin deficiency following low dose radiation therapy. However, HPA axis dysfunction still occurs and assessment needs to be included in monitoring programs. Lam et al. (1991) have shown that ACTH deficiency is present in 27% of patients 5 years after receiving high-dose radiotherapy (hypothalamus and pituitary were 39.79 +/− .78 (+/− SD) and 61.67 +/− 12.2 Gy, respectively) for nasopharyngeal carcinoma. Agha et al. (2005) have shown that ACTH deficiency occurs in 21% of patients who received cranial irradiation (median BED 54 Gy) for non-pituitary intracranial neoplasms. In this study, development of ACTH deficiency was dependent on time since irradiation and not radiation dose. Schmiegelow et al. (2003) studied the hypothalamic-pituitary-adrenal axis in 73 patients treated with radiotherapy (median dose 73 Gy) for childhood brain tumors. HPA axis insufficiency was noted in 19% using dynamic testing with either the ITT or the SST.

24.9.4 TSH

Central (secondary) hypothyroidism due to pituitary or hypothalamic damage is characterized by a reduced free thyroxine (fT4) level with a normal or reduced TSH level. As with the development of other pituitary hormone deficiencies, the incidence of central hypothyroidism is directly related to the total cranial radiation dose. Primary hypothyroidism as a consequence of direct radiotherapy-induced thyroid gland dysfunction is characterized by a low fT4 and elevated TSH; however, many patients may have elements of both primary and secondary hypothyroidisms due to radiation exposure to both areas (particularly following total body irradiation and craniospinal irradiation). Constine et al. (1993) have shown that at doses <40 Gy to the HP axis in patients with non-pituitary brain tumors central hypothyroidism is rare, but the incidence increases considerably when the dose exceeds 50 Gy. In one study assessing patients with pituitary adenoma who received 40–50 Gy in 25–30 fractions, the incidence of central hypothyroidism after 19 years follow-up was 72% (Brada et al. 1993).

24.9.5 Prolactin

Hyperprolactinemia has been reported to be common following cranial irradiation. Hyperprolactinemia can lead to alterations in the hypothalamic-pituitary gonadal axis by causing alterations in gonadotrophins secretion, which may aggravate the hypogonadotropic hypogonadism that often develops following cranial irradiation. Hyperprolactinemia develops following cranial irradiation due to radiation-induced hypothalamic damage with damage to dopaminergic neurons. As a result, lactotrophs escape from the inhibitory effect of dopamine and prolactin levels subsequently rise.

Following the initial increase in prolactin post cranial irradiation, there is a progressive decline in prolactin levels. This phenomenon is due to a delayed direct radiation effect on the pituitary and was more pronounced in females (Littley et al. 1989a). Mukherjee et al. (2003) have shown that acquired prolactin deficiency following radiotherapy is an indicator of severe pituitary damage with co-existing multiple anterior pituitary hormone deficiencies.

24.9.6 The Long-Term Implications of Pituitary Dysfunction

Hypopituitarism is associated with increased morbidity and mortality. The clinical consequences of GHD, gonadotrophin deficiency, ACTH deficiency, and TSH deficiency have been well described (Vance 1994). A number of studies have described an increased mortality in patients with hypopituitarism compared to age and sex matched controls (Bates et al. 1996; Bulow et al. 1997; Rosen and Bengtsson 1990; Tomlinson et al. 2001). In these studies, the increased mortality was predominantly due to cardiovascular and cerebrovascular mortality. There are conflicting data regarding the impact of radiotherapy on mortality in pituitary patients but it would appear from historic studies that patients with hypopituitarism who have received prior radiotherapy have an increased mortality (Bates et al. 1996; Bulow et al. 1997; Rosen and Bengtsson 1990; Tomlinson et al. 2001; Erfurth et al. 2002).

24.10 The Endocrine Nurse Specialist Role

The endocrine nurse specialist, in conjunction with the radiotherapy team, plays a vital role in counseling and patient education regarding preparation, side effects of radiation, and the importance of hormone monitoring following irradiation. The endocrine nurse specialist is a key member of the multidisciplinary team who performs and interprets the results of dynamic pituitary tests and performs ongoing assessment of pituitary status following cranial irradiation.

24.10.1 Patient Preparation

Patients referred for radiotherapy will usually first consult with the radiation oncologist. Therapy planning and tumor mapping requires CT/MRI to determine the requirements for therapy. The plan will be discussed with the patient in terms of the fractions and length of treatment, risks and benefits as described above.

Patients need to be aware that a thermoplastic mask can be custom made to precisely fit their face. This takes about 15 min. The patient will lie on his/her back on the simulation table while the technician places a warm wet plastic mesh film over their face and neck to create the mask shape. Openings are created for the mouth, eyes, and nose to allow for normal breathing. The patient is asked to bite on a plastic bite block until the mask has hardened and again during each treatment to limit motion. The mask is designed to be secured to a treatment table and gently hold the patients' head in the correct position to ensure accurate and consistent delivery of radiation treatments.

Educating the patient in relaxation breathing and techniques, the use of music or other psychological techniques for distraction that can be employed can help the patient cope with both mask formation and during successive treatments. Extremely anxious patients may require mild sedation.

24.10.2 Short-Term Side Effects of Radiation Therapy

These are usually minimal and include fatigue, lethargy, or a lack of energy, which may persist for some time after radiation is completed.

Local irritation to the skin is rare but may cause some redness, swelling, or a sunburned or tanned appearance. Some hair loss is possible but usually not excessive. Nausea and vomiting is also rare. Many patients return to work or regular activities after each radiation treatment.

24.10.3 Long-Term Side Effects of Radiation Therapy

Some delayed wound healing is possible with a fresh craniotomy scar and a spidery red or purple appearance (similar to telangiectasias) caused by dilated capillary blood vessels on the skin surface. Hormonal deficiencies may develop shortly after radiation as previously discussed or may develop over a number of years and require

ongoing testing and monitoring with the patients endocrinology team.

Some patients may require planning for potential changes. Infertility may occur post radiation and should be discussed with the patient prior to starting treatment. A fertility consult with egg or sperm or embryo preservation should be offered when appropriate. Patients complain of difficulty with short-term memory and alterations to cognitive function such as attention and executive function. Improved tumor targeting techniques limit this effect but it may also be progressive with time. Involvement of occupational therapists and psychologist for psychometric assessment may be helpful in dealing with such changes.

Secondary cancer risks after radiation exposure have been reported, as discussed above, but remain relatively rare. The patient needs to be aware that accurate records are kept of the amount of radiation administered and the area exposure. During treatments health professionals, who deliver radiation, will wear protective equipment to minimize their own exposure.

A patient must determine their own personal risks and benefits in their decision to follow the care team's recommendation for radiation therapy. The nurse can provide guidance in this decision by ensuring all information is available to both the patient and their family members using clear and understandable methods and that all their questions are satisfactorily answered.

24.11 Conclusions

Provider and patient awareness regarding the area of radiation-induced HP axis dysfunction has increased considerably in recent years. The development of "late effects" clinics for adult survivors of childhood cancers has led to an improved multidisciplinary approach to the management of such patients. The number of patients at risk of radiation-induced hypopituitarism will continue to rise as treatment strategies are refined and the number of patients surviving increases. The presence of HP axis dysfunction in this cohort of patients may in itself lead to increased mortality and morbidity, in a group of patients already heavily burdened by significant symptomatology. A multidisciplinary approach in which the endocrine nurse specialist is a key member leads to optimal management of these patients.

References

Adan L, Trivin C, Sainte-Rose C, Zucker JM, Hartmann O, Brauner R. GH deficiency caused by cranial irradiation during childhood: factors and markers in young adults. J Clin Endocrinol Metab. 2001;86:5245–51.

Agha A, Sherlock M, Brennan S, O'Connor SA, O'Sullivan E, Rogers B, Faul C, Rawluk D, Tormey W, Thompson CJ. Hypothalamic-pituitary dysfunction after irradiation of nonpituitary brain tumors in adults. J Clin Endocrinol Metab. 2005;90:6355–60.

Ahmed S, Elsheikh M, Stratton IM, Page RC, Adams CB, Wass JA. Outcome of transphenoidal surgery for acromegaly and its relationship to surgical experience. Clin Endocrinol (Oxf). 1999;50:561–7.

al-Mefty O, Kersh JE, Routh A, Smith RR. The long-term side effects of radiation therapy for benign brain tumors in adults. J Neurosurg. 1990;73:502–12.

Barendsen GW. Dose fractionation, dose rate and iso-effect relationships for normal tissue responses. Int J Radiat Oncol Biol Phys. 1982;8:1981–97.

Barrande G, Pittino-Lungo M, Coste J, Ponvert D, Bertagna X, Luton JP, Bertherat J. Hormonal and metabolic effects of radiotherapy in acromegaly: long-term results in 128 patients followed in a single center. J Clin Endocrinol Metab. 2000;85:3779–85.

Bates AS, Van't HW, Jones PJ, Clayton RN. The effect of hypopituitarism on life expectancy. J Clin Endocrinol Metab. 1996;81:1169–72.

Becker G, Kocher M, Kortmann RD, Paulsen F, Jeremic B, Muller RP, Bamberg M. Radiation therapy in the multimodal treatment approach of pituitary adenoma. Strahlenther Onkol. 2002;178:173–86.

Biermasz NR, Dulken HV, Roelfsema F. Postoperative radiotherapy in acromegaly is effective in reducing GH concentration to safe levels. Clin Endocrinol (Oxf). 2000a;53:321–7.

Biermasz NR, van DH, Roelfsema F. Long-term follow-up results of postoperative radiotherapy in 36 patients with acromegaly. J Clin Endocrinol Metab. 2000b;85:2476–82.

Blacklay A, Grossman A, Ross RJ, Savage MO, Davies PS, Plowman PN, Coy DH, Besser GM. Cranial irradiation for cerebral and nasopharyngeal tumours in children: evidence for the production of a hypothalamic defect in growth hormone release. J Endocrinol. 1986;108:25–9.

Bliss P, Kerr GR, Gregor A. Incidence of second brain tumours after pituitary irradiation in Edinburgh 1962-1990. Clin Oncol (R Coll Radiol). 1994;6:361–3.

Brada M, Ford D, Ashley S, Bliss JM, Crowley S, Mason M, Rajan B, Traish D. Risk of second brain tumour after conservative surgery and radiotherapy for pituitary adenoma. BMJ. 1992;304:1343–6.

Brada M, Rajan B, Traish D, Ashley S, Holmes-Sellors PJ, Nussey S, Uttley D. The long-term efficacy of conservative surgery and radiotherapy in the control of pituitary adenomas. Clin Endocrinol (Oxf). 1993;38:571–8.

Brada M, Burchell L, Ashley S, Traish D. The incidence of cerebrovascular accidents in patients with pituitary adenoma. Int J Radiat Oncol Biol Phys. 1999;45:693–8.

Brada M, Ashley S, Ford D, Traish D, Burchell L, Rajan B. Cerebrovascular mortality in patients with pituitary adenoma. Clin Endocrinol (Oxf). 2002;57:713–7.

Brennan BM, Rahim A, Mackie EM, Eden OB, Shalet SM. Growth hormone status in adults treated for acute lymphoblastic leukaemia in childhood. Clin Endocrinol (Oxf). 1998;48:777–83.

Bulow B, Hagmar L, Mikoczy Z, Nordstrom CH, Erfurth EM. Increased cerebrovascular mortality in patients with hypopituitarism. Clin Endocrinol (Oxf). 1997;46:75–81.

Chrousos GP, Poplack D, Brown T, O'Neill D, Schwade J, Bercu BB. Effects of cranial radiation on hypothalamic-adenohypophyseal function: abnormal growth hormone secretory dynamics. J Clin Endocrinol Metab. 1982;54:1135–9.

Clayton PE, Shalet SM. Dose dependency of time of onset of radiation-induced growth hormone deficiency. J Pediatr. 1991;118:226–8.

Clayton RN, Stewart PM, Shalet SM, Wass JA. Pituitary surgery for acromegaly. Should be done by specialists. BMJ. 1999;319:588–9.

Colin P, Delemer B, Nakib I, Caron J, Bazin A, Bernard MH, Peruzzi P, Scavarda D, Scherpereel B, Longuebray A, Redon C, Petel F, and Rousseaux P. [Unsuccessful surgery of Cushing's disease. Role and efficacy of fractionated stereotactic radiotherapy]. Neurochirurgie. 2002;48:285–93.

Constine LS, Woolf PD, Cann D, Mick G, McCormick K, Raubertas RF, Rubin P. Hypothalamic-pituitary dysfunction after radiation for brain tumors. N Engl J Med. 1993;328:87–94.

Dainiak N. Mechanisms of radiation injury: impact of molecular medicine. Stem Cells. 1997;15(Suppl 2):1–5.

Darzy KH, Aimaretti G, Wieringa G, Gattamaneni HR, Ghigo E, Shalet SM. The usefulness of the combined growth hormone (GH)-releasing hormone and arginine stimulation test in the diagnosis of radiation-induced GH deficiency is dependent on the post-irradiation time interval. J Clin Endocrinol Metab. 2003;88:95–102.

Darzy KH, Pezzoli SS, Thorner MO, Shalet SM. The dynamics of growth hormone (GH) secretion in adult cancer survivors with severe GH deficiency acquired after brain irradiation in childhood for nonpituitary brain tumors: evidence for preserved pulsatility and diurnal variation with increased secretory disorderliness. J Clin Endocrinol Metab. 2005;90:2794–803.

Duffner PK, Cohen ME, Voorhess ML, MacGillivray MH, Brecher ML, Panahon A, Gilani BB. Long-term effects of cranial irradiation on endocrine function in children with brain tumors. A prospective study. Cancer. 1985;56:2189–93.

Erfurth EM, Bulow B, Svahn-Tapper G, Norrving B, Odh K, Mikoczy Z, Bjork J, Hagmar L. Risk factors for cerebrovascular deaths in patients operated and irradiated for pituitary tumors. J Clin Endocrinol Metab. 2002;87:4892–9.

Flickinger JC, Nelson PB, Taylor FH, Robinson A. Incidence of cerebral infarction after radiotherapy for pituitary adenoma. Cancer. 1989;63:2404–8.

Fowler JF. The linear-quadratic formula and progress in fractionated radiotherapy. Br J Radiol. 1989;62:679–94.

Gil-Cardenas A, Herrera MF, Diaz-Polanco A, Rios JM, Pantoja JP. Nelson's syndrome after bilateral adrenalectomy for Cushing's disease. Surgery. 2007;141:147–51; discussion 151–42

Gillam MP, Molitch ME, Lombardi G, Colao A. Advances in the treatment of prolactinomas. Endocr Rev. 2006;27:485–534.

Gittoes NJ. Radiotherapy for non-functioning pituitary tumors—when and under what circumstances? Pituitary. 2003;6:103–8.

Iwata H, Sato K, Nomura R, Tabei Y, Suzuki I, Yokota N, Inoue M, Ohta S, Yamada S, Shibamoto Y. Long-term results of hypofractionated stereotactic radiotherapy with CyberKnife for growth hormone-secreting pituitary adenoma: evaluation by the Cortina consensus. J Neurooncol. 2016;128:267–75.

Jenkins PJ. The use of long-acting somatostatin analogues in acromegaly. Growth Horm IGF Res. 2000;10(Suppl B):S111–4.

Jenkins PJ, Bates P, Carson MN, Stewart PM, Wass JA. Conventional pituitary irradiation is effective in lowering serum growth hormone and insulin-like growth factor-I in patients with acromegaly. J Clin Endocrinol Metab. 2006;91:1239–45.

Katznelson L, Laws RE, Melmed S, Molitch ME, Murad MH, Utz A, Wass JAH. Acromegaly: an endocrine society clinical practice guideline. J Clin Endocrinol Metab. 2014;99(11):3933–51. https://doi.org/10.1210/jc.2014-2700S.

Lam KS, Wang C, Yeung RT, Ma JT, Ho JH, Tse VK, Ling N. Hypothalamic hypopituitarism following cranial irradiation for nasopharyngeal carcinoma. Clin Endocrinol (Oxf). 1986;24:643–51.

Lam KS, Tse VK, Wang C, Yeung RT, Ho JH. Effects of cranial irradiation on hypothalamic-pituitary function—a 5-year longitudinal study in patients with nasopharyngeal carcinoma. Q J Med. 1991;78:165–76.

Lancranjan I, Atkinson AB. Results of a European multicentre study with Sandostatin LAR in acromegalic

patients. Sandostatin LAR Group. Pituitary. 1999;1:105–14.

Littley MD, Shalet SM, Beardwell CG, Ahmed SR, Applegate G, Sutton ML. Hypopituitarism following external radiotherapy for pituitary tumours in adults. Q J Med. 1989a;70:145–60.

Littley MD, Shalet SM, Beardwell CG, Robinson EL, Sutton ML. Radiation-induced hypopituitarism is dose-dependent. Clin Endocrinol (Oxf). 1989b;31:363–73.

Littley MD, Shalet SM, Morgenstern GR, Deakin DP. Endocrine and reproductive dysfunction following fractionated total body irradiation in adults. Q J Med. 1991;78:265–74.

Mukherjee A, Murray RD, Columb B, Gleeson HK, Shalet SM. Acquired prolactin deficiency indicates severe hypopituitarism in patients with disease of the hypothalamic-pituitary axis. Clin Endocrinol (Oxf). 2003;59:743–8.

Nishioka H, Ito H, Haraoka J, Hirano A. Histological changes in the hypofunctional pituitary gland following conventional radiotherapy for adenoma. Histopathology. 2001;38:561–6.

Nishioka H, Hirano A, Haraoka J, Nakajima N. Histological changes in the pituitary gland and adenomas following radiotherapy. Neuropathology. 2002;22:19–25.

Ogilvy-Stuart AL, Clark DJ, Wallace WH, Gibson BE, Stevens RF, Shalet SM, Donaldson MD. Endocrine deficit after fractionated total body irradiation. Arch Dis Child. 1992;67:1107–10.

Pan L, Zhang N, Wang EM, Wang BJ, Dai JZ, Cai PW. Gamma knife radiosurgery as a primary treatment for prolactinomas. J Neurosurg. 2000;93(Suppl 3):10–3.

Peacey SR, Toogood AA, Veldhuis JD, Thorner MO, Shalet SM. The relationship between 24-hour growth hormone secretion and insulin-like growth factor I in patients with successfully treated acromegaly: impact of surgery or radiotherapy. J Clin Endocrinol Metab. 2001;86:259–66.

Popovic V, Damjanovic S, Micic D, Nesovic M, Djurovic M, Petakov M, Obradovic S, Zoric S, Simic M, Penezic Z, Marinkovic J. Increased incidence of neoplasia in patients with pituitary adenomas. The Pituitary Study Group. Clin Endocrinol (Oxf). 1998;49:441–5.

Powell JS, Wardlaw SL, Post KD, Freda PU. Outcome of radiotherapy for acromegaly using normalization of insulin-like growth factor I to define cure. J Clin Endocrinol Metab. 2000;85:2068–71.

Rappaport R, Brauner R. Growth and endocrine disorders secondary to cranial irradiation. Pediatr Res. 1989;25:561–7.

Rodemann HP, Bamberg M. Cellular basis of radiation-induced fibrosis. Radiother Oncol. 1995;35:83–90.

Rosen T, Bengtsson BA. Premature mortality due to cardiovascular disease in hypopituitarism. Lancet. 1990;336:285–8.

Samaan NA, Bakdash MM, Caderao JB, Cangir A, Jesse RH Jr, Ballantyne AJ. Hypopituitarism after external irradiation. Evidence for both hypothalamic and pituitary origin. Ann Intern Med. 1975;83:771–7.

Schmiegelow M, Lassen S, Poulsen HS, Feldt-Rasmussen U, Schmiegelow K, Hertz H, Muller J. Cranial radiotherapy of childhood brain tumours: growth hormone deficiency and its relation to the biological effective dose of irradiation in a large population based study. Clin Endocrinol (Oxf). 2000;53:191–7.

Schmiegelow M, Feldt-Rasmussen U, Rasmussen AK, Lange M, Poulsen HS, Muller J. Assessment of the hypothalamo-pituitary-adrenal axis in patients treated with radiotherapy and chemotherapy for childhood brain tumor. J Clin Endocrinol Metab. 2003;88:3149–54.

Shalet SM, Clayton PE, Price DA. Growth and pituitary function in children treated for brain tumours or acute lymphoblastic leukaemia. Horm Res. 1988;30:53–61.

Sheaves R, Jenkins P, Blackburn P, Huneidi AH, Afshar F, Medbak S, Grossman AB, Besser GM, Wass JA. Outcome of transsphenoidal surgery for acromegaly using strict criteria for surgical cure. Clin Endocrinol (Oxf). 1996;45:407–13.

Sheehan JP, Xu Z, Salvetti DJ, Schmitt PJ, Vance ML. Results of gamma knife surgery for Cushing's disease. J Neurosurg. 2013a;119:1486–92.

Sheehan JP, Starke RM, Mathieu D, Young B, Sneed PK, Chiang VL, Lee JY, Kano H, Park KJ, Niranjan A, Kondziolka D, Barnett GH, Rush S, Golfinos JG, Lunsford LD. Gamma Knife radiosurgery for the management of nonfunctioning pituitary adenomas: a multicenter study. J Neurosurg. 2013b;119:446–56.

Shi XE, Wu B, Fan T, Zhou ZQ, Zhang YL. Craniopharyngioma: surgical experience of 309 cases in China. Clin Neurol Neurosurg. 2008;110:151–9.

Shih HA, Loeffler JS. Radiation therapy in acromegaly. Rev Endocr Metab Disord. 2008;9:59–65.

Sklar CA. Growth and pubertal development in survivors of childhood cancer. Pediatrician. 1991;18:53–60.

Sklar CA, Constine LS. Chronic neuroendocrinological sequelae of radiation therapy. Int J Radiat Oncol Biol Phys. 1995;31:1113–21.

Suh JH, Saxton JP. Conventional radiation therapy for skull base tumors: an overview. Neurosurg Clin N Am. 2000;11:575–86.

Tomlinson JW, Holden N, Hills RK, Wheatley K, Clayton RN, Bates AS, Sheppard MC, Stewart PM. Association between premature mortality and hypopituitarism. West Midlands Prospective Hypopituitary Study Group. Lancet. 2001;357:425–31.

Toogood AA. Endocrine consequences of brain irradiation. Growth Horm IGF Res. 2004;14(Suppl A):S118–24.

Tran LM, Blount L, Horton D, Sadeghi A, Parker RG. Radiation therapy of pituitary tumors: results in 95 cases. Am J Clin Oncol. 1991;14:25–9.

Tsang RW, Laperriere NJ, Simpson WJ, Brierley J, Panzarella T, Smyth HS. Glioma arising after radiation therapy for pituitary adenoma. A report of four patients and estimation of risk. Cancer. 1993;72:2227–33.

Tsang RW, Brierley JD, Panzarella T, Gospodarowicz MK, Sutcliffe SB, Simpson WJ. Radiation therapy for pituitary adenoma: treatment outcome and prognostic factors. Int J Radiat Oncol Biol Phys. 1994;30:557–65.

Tsang RW, Brierley JD, Panzarella T, Gospodarowicz MK, Sutcliffe SB, Simpson WJ. Role of radiation therapy in clinical hormonally-active pituitary adenomas. Radiother Oncol. 1996;41:45–53.

Turner HE, Vadivale A, Keenan J, Wass JA. A comparison of lanreotide and octreotide LAR for treatment of acromegaly. Clin Endocrinol (Oxf). 1999;51:275–80.

Vance ML. Hypopituitarism. N Engl J Med. 1994;330:1651–62.

Vankelecom H, Matthys P, Van Damme J, Heremans H, Billiau A, Denef C. Immunocytochemical evidence that S-100-positive cells of the mouse anterior pituitary contain interleukin-6 immunoreactivity. J Histochem Cytochem. 1993;41:151–6.

Vincent PC. Apoptosis and the assessment of radiation injury. Stem Cells. 1995;13(Suppl 1):153–64.

Wan H, Chihiro O, Yuan S. MASEP gamma knife radiosurgery for secretory pituitary adenomas: experience in 347 consecutive cases. J Exp Clin Cancer Res. 2009;28:36.

Hypopituitarism and Growth Hormone Deficiency in Adults

25

Sofia Llahana, Anne Marland, Mila Pantovic, and Vera Popovic

Contents

S. Llahana (✉)
School of Health Sciences, City, University of
London, London, UK
e-mail: Sofia.Llahana@city.ac.uk

A. Marland
Oxford Centre for Diabetes, Endocrinology and
Metabolism, Radcliffe Department of Medicine,
University of Oxford, Oxford, UK
e-mail: Anne.Marland@ouh.nhs.uk

M. Pantovic
Department of Neuroendocrinology, Clinic for
Endocrinology, Clinical Center Serbia,
Belgrade, Serbia
e-mail: millapantovic@gmail.com

V. Popovic
Medical Faculty, University of Belgrade,
Belgrade, Serbia
e-mail: popver@Eunet.rs

© Springer Nature Switzerland AG 2019
S. Llahana et al. (eds.), *Advanced Practice in Endocrinology Nursing*,
https://doi.org/10.1007/978-3-319-99817-6_25

Abstract

Pituitary conditions are associated with several physical, psychological, and social symptoms. Treatment involves surgery, medical treatment, and/or radiotherapy. Most patients with pituitary conditions have permanent hypopituitarism (congenital or acquired) and require lifelong hormone replacement therapy. Polypharmacy with multiple daily dosing and complex treatment regimens are common and patients may often require more than five different medications daily.

The treatment goal is to achieve normal physiological hormone levels with minimal side effects and to avoid adverse effects associated with deficiency or over-replacement. Growth hormone (GH) deficiency is very common in adults with hypopituitarism and requires replacement with daily subcutaneous injections. A provocative stimulation test is required to establish the diagnosis of GH deficiency in adults with the insulin tolerance test being regarded as the "gold standard". Individualised selection of a suitable injecting device is important in improving adherence to medication and optimal replacement. Treatment with GH in adults improves quality of life, body composition, and bone density. Long-acting GH formulations are in development and aim to improve adherence and convenience with treatment via weekly or monthly injections.

Keywords

Hypopituitarism · Pituitary disorders
Growth hormone deficiency · Hormone
replacement therapy · Daily injections
Quality of life

Abbreviations

ACTH	Adreno-corticotropic hormone
ADH	Antidiuretic hormone
DI	Diabetes insipidus
FSH	Follicle-stimulating hormone
GH	Growth hormone
GHRH	GH-releasing hormone
GST	Glucagon stimulation test
IGF-1	Insulin-like growth factor-1
ITT	Insulin tolerance test
LAGH	Long-acting growth hormone
LH	Luteinising hormone
PRL	Prolactin
QoL	Quality of life
rhGH	Recombinant human growth hormone
TSH	Thyroid-stimulating hormone

Key Terms

- **Anterior pituitary**: The front lobes of the pituitary gland, responsible for secreting TSH, LH, FSH, PRL, GH, and ACTH.
- **Posterior pituitary**: The rear lobes of the pituitary, responsible for producing ADH and oxytocin.
- **Hypopituitarism**: The loss of one or more anterior pituitary hormones leading to deficient hormone production in the corresponding target gland.
- **Panhypopituitarism**: The insufficiency or deficiency of all the pituitary hormones from the anterior and posterior pituitary lobes.
- **Hormone replacement therapy**: Chronic replacement of the hormone produced by the target gland to restore physiological body function and well-being.
- **Growth hormone (GH)**: Produced by the anterior pituitary gland. It has a role throughout lifespan in the regulation of protein, lipid, and carbohydrate metabolism and other important metabolic effects on a variety of target tissues, in addition to linear growth in children.
- **Provocative/dynamic/stimulation testing**: The exposure of patients to a substance or drug to evaluate their bodies' response. This response is compared to average responses from unaffected individuals.
- **Cut-off values** differentiate normal responses from abnormal or dysfunctional responses.

Key Points

- Hypopituitarism refers to the deficiency of one or more hormones secreted by the pituitary gland
- Patients with hypopituitarism have increased mortality and impaired quality of life. They require lifelong hormone replacement therapy with multiple medications and different treatment modalities daily

- Growth hormone deficiency in adults can cause reduced metabolic rate, muscle mass and bone density, and impaired quality of life
- Growth hormone treatment involves daily subcutaneous injections

25.1 Introduction

A tormentor traced *by Simon Neil*
A function is planned for family and friends,
Been absent so many, "I hope he attends",
Sit anxious and quiet, unwilling wall-flower,
Please open up floor, for me to devour,
Embarrassed and saddened with such awkwardness,
My tongue tightly tied, void of loquaciousness.
Impatiently, angrily although they Placate,
Utter intolerance of when they are late,
Anxious, depressed, in total despair,
Will nobody listen, does nobody care,
Apathy of mood, thinning of skin,
Central obesity, "please look further in".
No libido, no interest, no passion, no lust,
"Please join up the pieces, my enthusiasm is trussed",
No strength, no stamina, no staying power,
No concentration, my mind turning sour,
Aches and pains so hard to describe,
Drilling in my head of which I often writhe.
Unexplained tears, no equilibrium of mood,
Cholesterol sky high but it's not down to food,
Weakness of limbs, I feel so unwell,
No end in sight of my enduring hell,
Dull aching pain, disarrayment of sight,
What will it take to discover my blight?
Decrease of muscle, flushing of face,
"Your hormones Sir are all over the place",
No smiling, no banter, no sense of humour,
All above symptoms of my 'Pituitary tumour',
A matter of years for my tormentor to trace,
My Endocrine team, 'My saving grace'….

25.2 Part A: Hypopituitarism

The term *hypopituitarism* refers to the deficiency of one or more hormones of the pituitary gland which is formed of the anterior and posterior lobes (Fig. 25.1). The posterior lobe secretes two hormones: vasopressin (or antidiuretic hormone - ADH) the deficiency of which is called diabetes

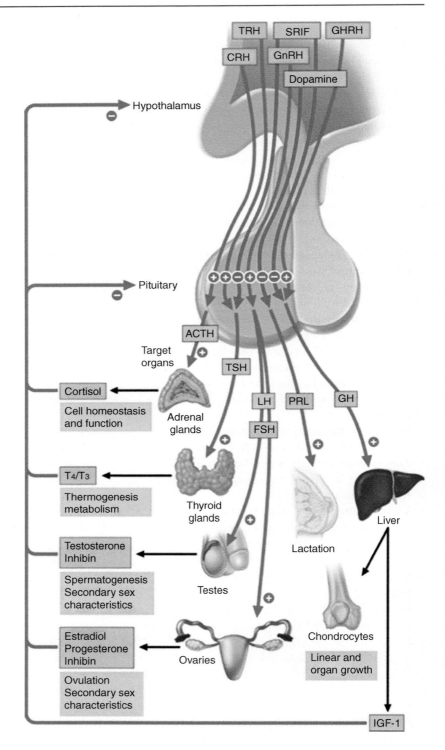

Fig. 25.1 Diagram of anterior pituitary axes and target gland secretion. Used with permission from Melmed, S. & Jameson, J. L. 2017. Anterior pituitary: physiology of pituitary hormones, chapter 3, pages 18–24. In: Jameson, J. L. (ed.) *Harrison's Endocrinology, 4th Edition*. New York: McGraw Hill Education

insipidus (DI), and oxytocin. The term *panhypo-pituitarism,* is used to describe the insufficiency or deficiency of all the pituitary hormones (Toogood and Stewart 2008; Burt and Ho 2016). The pituitary gland is found in the pituitary fossa of the sphenoid bone close to the optic nerves at the base of the skull. It is not part of the brain, but communicates with the hypothalamus via the pituitary stalk which consists of neurones and portal blood vessels. Within the anterior lobe of the pituitary, six hormones are produced: growth hormone (GH), the gonadotropins follicle-stimulating hormone (FSH) and luteinising hormone (LH), adreno-corticotropic hormone (ACTH), thyroid-stimulating hormone (TSH), and prolactin (PRL). Hypothalamic hormones regulate anterior pituitary trophic hormones that in turn determine target gland secretion (Fig. 25.1).

25.3 Prevalence, Mortality, and Morbidity of Hypopituitarism

Hypopituitarism is a rare endocrine condition. Prevalence ranges from 375 to 455 patients per million of the population (Regal et al. 2001; Fernandez-Rodriguez et al. 2013). This, for example, indicates that there are approximately 30,000 patients with hypopituitarism in the UK, although this number is estimated to be significantly higher as these epidemiologic studies only included patients with pituitary adenomas and not the many other causes of hypopituitarism, such as childhood cancer survivors or brain tumours affecting the hypothalamic-pituitary function (Toogood and Stewart 2008).

The standard mortality rate (SMR) for patients with hypopituitarism ranges from 1.10 to 3.6 (95% CI) times higher than the average population (Pappachan et al. 2015; Ntali et al. 2015; Olsson et al. 2015; Burman et al. 2013). Patients also report impaired quality of life (QoL) (Andela et al. 2015) and more than twice health care costs, disability pensions, and sick leave compared to the average population (Ehrnborg et al. 2000; Jonsson and Nilsson 2000; Hahner et al. 2007).

Prevalence of hospitalisations and deaths is high in patients with ACTH-induced adrenal insufficiency; 1 in 12 patients experience at least one hospital admission annually and 0.5 adrenal crisis-related deaths per 100 patient-years occur due to potentially preventable adrenal crisis (Hahner et al. 2015) (please see Chaps. 37 and 62 for more details).

25.4 Causes of Hypopituitarism

Hypopituitarism is the consequence of diseases or treatments that reduce or destroy the secretory function of the pituitary gland leading to stimulating and target gland hormone deficiencies. Hypopituitarism can be congenital (genetic and developmental/structural) or acquired such as tumours involving the hypothalamic-pituitary axis. Causes of hypopituitarism are summarised in Table 25.1 (Burt and Ho 2016; Fleseriu et al. 2016; Melmed and Jameson 2017).

25.5 Clinical Presentation and Diagnosis of Hypopituitarism

Hypopituitarism results from complete or partial deficiency of one or more hormones of the pituitary gland and includes adrenal insufficiency, hypothyroidism, hypogonadism, GH deficiency, and more rarely, diabetes insipidus (Toogood and Stewart 2008; Burt and Ho 2016; Fleseriu et al. 2016; Melmed and Jameson 2017). It is challenging to ascribe specific symptoms to a single hormone deficiency as hypopituitarism presents with similar clinical features such as: weight loss or gain, fatigue, depression, cognitive decline, sexual impairment and infertility, and muscle weakness (except for diabetes insipidus which presents with polyuria, increased thirst). Due to the non-specific symptoms of hypopituitarism, it may often be many years before patients receive the correct diagnosis, as Simon describes in his patient story (Box 25.1) and expressed in his poem earlier.

Table 25.1 Common causes of hypopituitarism

Congenital and developmental/structural
Transcription factor defect
Pituitary dysplasia aplasia
Empty sella syndrome
Congenital hypothalamic disorders (septo-optic dysplasia, Prader-Willi syndrome, Laurence-Moon-Biedl syndrome, Kallmann syndrome)
Midline cerebral and cranial malformations
Genetic: isolated or combined pituitary hormone deficiencies
Idiopathic hypopituitarism
Acquired
Neoplastic
Pituitary adenoma (functioning or non-functioning), craniopharyngioma, meningioma, cysts (e.g. Rathke's cleft), germinoma, glioma, astrocytoma, paraganglioma, teratoma, chordoma, pituitary carcinoma, neoplastic metastases
Surgery for hypothalamic and pituitary tumours
Radiotherapy treatment affecting hypothalamic-pituitary (HP) axis
HP axis tumours, brain tumours, head and neck cancer, acute lymphoblastic leukaemia
Infiltrative/inflammatory disease
Autoimmune (lymphocytic hypophysitis), hemochromatosis, granulomatous hypophysitis, sarcoidosis, Langerhans cell histiocytosis,
Infectious diseases
Bacterial, fungal (histoplasmosis), parasitic (toxoplasmosis), tuberculosis, syphilis
Vascular
Pituitary apoplexy, postpartum Sheehan's syndrome, sickle cell disease, intrasellar carotid artery aneurysm, subarachnoid haemorrhage
Traumatic (head injury)
Medications suppressing pituitary function
E.g. opiates (primarily gonadotropin ACTH, GH), glucocorticoids (ACTH only), Somatostatin analogs (GH, ACTH, TSH)

Note: This table is not inclusive of all causes of hypopituitarism; summarised from Fleseriu et al. (2016), Melmed and Jameson (2017) and Burt and Ho (2016)

Box 25.1 A Patient's Story on Delayed Diagnosis on Hypopituitarism

I have struggled with illness for many years. I struggled to tell people face-to-face how I felt and what the exact symptoms were, and after more than 15 years, I finally got a correct diagnosis last year. I have hypopituitarism including adult-onset growth hormone deficiency due to a small pituitary adenoma. The social isolation of the disease has hit me the hardest; I haven't been able to attend any family or social functions for many years, but until recently didn't know the reason for this. Over the course of the past few months, listening to articles published by your organisation [*The Pituitary Foundation, a UK Patient Advocacy Group, https://www.pituitary. org.uk*], I have come to realise that I am not alone in my disease and that in fact, some of the things I have struggled to describe to doctors are shared by other patients.

This poem [*at the start of the chapter*] is what I have been trying to say about my illness for years but couldn't…

Used with patient consent, contacted by the Pituitary Foundation

The symptoms and treatment of hypopituitarism in adults are summarised in Table 25.2 (Toogood and Stewart 2008; Burt and Ho 2016; Fleseriu et al. 2016; Melmed and Jameson 2017; van Aken and Lamberts 2005).

Table 25.2 Hormone deficiencies, symptoms, and replacement in hypopituitarism (summarised from Bart and Ho 2016; van Aken and Lamberts 2005; Melmed and Jameson 2017; Fleseriu et al. 2016)

Pituitary hormone	Target gland: hormone	Symptoms of hormone deficiency in adults	Treatment (hormone replacement)
ACTH	Adrenals: Cortisol	Hypoadrenalism: weakness, fatigue, dizziness on standing, pallor, hypoglycaemia, hypothermia, shock/coma from adrenal crisis	Tablets 1–3 times daily IM injections when nil by mouth
TSH	Thyroid: Free T4 (thyroxine)	Hypothyroidism: fatigue, constipation, dry skin, hair loss, cold intolerance, weight gain	Tablets once daily
LH & FSH (females)	Ovaries: Oestrogen & Progesterone	Hypogonadism: hot flushes, amenorrhoea, infertility, breast atrophy, osteoporosis, weight gain, fatigue, dyspareunia	Tablets once daily Transdermal patches twice weekly
LH & FSH (males)	Testes: Testosterone	Hypogonadism: impaired libido and sexual function, infertility, osteoporosis, weight gain, fatigue, reduced muscle mass, small soft testes, and reduced body/facial hair	Intramuscular injections monthly or 3-monthly Transdermal gel once daily Subcutaneous implant 6-monthly
Growth Hormone (GH)	All cells and organs in the body	GH deficiency: fatigue, impaired quality of life, depression, weight gain, reduced muscle mass & strength	Daily subcutaneous injections (self-administered)
ADH	Kidneys	Diabetes Insipidus: polydipsia, polyuria, weight loss, dehydration, hypernatremia, renal impairment	Nasal spray 1–3 times daily Tablets 1–4 times daily

ACTH adrenocorticotrophic hormone, *TSH* thyroid-stimulating hormone, *LH* luteinising hormone, *FSH* follicle-stimulating hormone, *GH* growth hormone, *ADH* antidiuretic hormone

The clinical presentation and the cause of hypopituitarism will guide the selection of the diagnostic biochemistry and/or dynamic investigations. Initial investigations with basal hormone measurements will either confirm the diagnosis of hypopituitarism or prompt for further investigations and dynamic tests. The blood tests should be drawn early morning, preferable before 9 am, to reflect diurnal cortisol secretion; testosterone is also higher in the morning. Evaluation of baseline hormones should include the pituitary hormone and target hormone concentrations to assess the appropriateness of both values. In hypopituitarism, the pituitary hormones are generally low which also results in low target gland hormones. This differentiates hypopituitarism (secondary deficiency) from primary gland failure such as Addison's disease or primary adrenal insufficiency, primary hypothyroidism, primary hypogonadism, and primary ovarian insufficiency (please refer to relevant chapters in the textbook for further details). Dynamic testing is required to diagnose

ACTH, ADH, and GH deficiencies for most patients.

It is, however, important to remember that a pituitary mass can lead to the secretion of biologically inactive pituitary hormones, which can present with normal pituitary concentrations but decreased target hormone concentrations (Fleseriu et al. 2016; van Aken and Lamberts 2005). A comprehensive overview of dynamic tests and investigations used to diagnose hypopituitarism is presented in Chap. 15.

25.6 Hormone Replacement Therapy in Hypopituitarism

Polypharmacy is common in hypopituitarism and patients may be taking up to five different medications for replacement therapy in different treatment modalities and multiple daily dosing (Toogood and Stewart 2008; Lee and Ho 2010; Prabhakar and Shalet 2006). Treatment in hypopituitarism includes chronic replacement of the hormone produced by the target gland (Table 25.2) for relevant deficiencies with:

- Cortisol (glucocorticoids);
- Free T4 (thyroxine);
- testosterone for men;
- oestrogen/progesterone for women;
- growth hormone (somatropin)
- desmopressin (DDAVP).

Growth hormone treatment is discussed in details in the next section of this chapter. The reader is also encouraged to refer to relevant chapters in the textbook regarding treatment of other hormone deficiencies: hypothyroidism in Chap. 30; ACTH and cortisol deficiency in Chap. 37; oestrogen deficiency in Chap. 41, and testosterone deficiency in Chap. 46.

The goals of treatment in hypopituitarism are to achieve normal levels of all missing hormones with minimal side effects and to avoid the symptoms and adverse effects associated with deficiency or over-replacement (Toogood and Stewart 2008; Burt and Ho 2016; Filipsson and Johannsson 2009). Full treatment benefit is not achieved unless all missing hormones are optimised.

25.7 Importance of Patient Education and Adherence to Medication in Hypopituitarism

Achieving optimal replacement in hypopituitarism, given the complexity of the treatment regimens, requires the patient to understand and engage with their treatment planning and perceive it as necessary for their condition. Patient education, self-management, and adherence to medication are crucial to achieve optimised well-being and normalise QoL. However, empirical evidence has so far failed to provide a holistic focus on the patients' needs taking into consideration all the hormone replacement therapies found in hypopituitarism. Previous cross-sectional studies looked at patients' adherence to one specific single treatment [cortisol (van Eck et al. 2014; Flemming and Kristensen 1999; Peacey et al.

1993; Forss et al. 2012; Tiemensma et al. 2014; Chapman et al. 2016), GH (Rosenfeld and Bakker 2008; Abdi et al. 2014) and testosterone (Dwyer et al. 2014; Schoenfeld et al. 2013)], even though many patients were on multiple hormone treatments.

This is a significant limitation as treatment benefit is not achieved unless all hormones are assessed as a single treatment. Interactions between replacement hormones means that untreated deficiencies and changes in dose, initiation, discontinuation, or nonadherence to any of the hormones can lead to adverse effects such as impaired well-being and QoL, precipitation of adrenal crisis and hypothyroidism, and medicational side effects (Losa et al. 2008; Cook et al. 1999; Janssen et al. 2000; Wolthers et al. 2001; Omori et al. 2003; Ragnarsson et al. 2014), but also higher cost of the drug. For example, we found that changing the modality for oestrogen treatment to transdermal patches led to significant savings on the cost of GH as patients' daily dose of GH reduced almost by half compared to previous daily dose (Phelan et al. 2012).

Low persistence and high discontinuation rates of 25–65% were reported by patients on GH and testosterone treatment (Abdi et al. 2014; Dwyer et al. 2014; Schoenfeld et al. 2013). GH and testosterone deficiency are associated with risk of osteoporosis, impaired QoL and sexual function (Burt and Ho 2016; Fleseriu et al. 2016). Abdi et al. found that high adherence to GH was closely associated with improvement in QoL (Abdi et al. 2014). Our recent study of 308 patients on GH replacement found that the reported side effects correlated with nonadherence, concerns and dissatisfaction with treatment, impaired QoL, and high or at upper end of reference range for age levels of insulin-like growth factor-1 (IGF-1) (Llahana et al. 2018).

Over-replacement in GC therapy was reported by 25% of patients in a study by Chapman et al. 2016; there is evidence which shows direct association of excessive cortisol treatment with osteoporosis (Schulz et al. 2016) and impaired QoL (Bleicken et al. 2010). Similarly, side effects and long-term complications can result from over- or under-replacement of all hormones in hypopituitarism.

Patients who are adequately informed and engaged in treatment planning are more likely to adhere to their medication and manage possible side effects (Atkinson et al. 2004; Cooper et al. 2015). Similarly, patients' satisfaction with care services and effective clinician-patient communication have been shown to predict adherence and follow-through with treatment plans and appropriate use of care services (Cooper et al. 2015; Ruiz et al. 2008; George et al. 2005; Zolnierek and Dimatteo 2009; Linn et al. 2016).

Evidence from studies in pituitary conditions shows that the patient's engagement with their treatment planning, their satisfaction with the information they receive, and the knowledge of their treatment and condition influence care outcomes (Martinez-Momblan et al. 2016; Llahana and Conway 2006; Repping-Wuts et al. 2013; van der Meij et al. 2016; Gurel et al. 2014; Adelman et al. 2013; Kepicoglu et al. 2014). Assessment of patients' satisfaction with the care and information they receive and their knowledge and understanding of their condition and treatment is, therefore, crucial in identifying and addressing unmet needs. The endocrine nurse should adopt holistic care approach to meet the complex and multiple needs of patients with hypopituitarism and advanced practice skills and competencies are necessary to perform this role adequately.

25.7.1 The Role of Patient Advocacy Groups

Patient advocacy groups (PAGs) play an essential role in raising awareness of the pituitary conditions and providing patients with reassurance that they are not alone. PAGs work closely with health care professionals to develop evidence-based information leaflets and educational resources. The Pituitary Foundation in the UK, as described below, is a great example of a PAG with a vital contribution in the support and self-management of patients with hypopituitarism.

25.7.1.1 The Pituitary Foundation UK

The Pituitary Foundation was launched in 1994 with the support of one of our founders, Professor Stafford Lightman.

We are the UK's leading charity providing support to people affected by conditions such as acromegaly, Cushing's, prolactinoma, diabetes insipidus, and hypopituitarism. Our objectives are:

- To promote the relief and treatment of persons suffering from pituitary conditions, their families, friends, and carers, and to provide information and support.
- To promote and support research and to disseminate for the public benefit the results of any such research.

Our contactable support includes a Patient Support Helpline, a Patient Support email and text service, and an Endocrine Nurse Helpline. We also have trained Telephone Buddies (patients who support other patients via phone or email). We have an extensive library of booklets and fact sheets, plus our magazine, *Pituitary Life,* is produced three times a year for members. Our website is easy to read and access information. We hold National Pituitary Conferences every 18 months. We collaborate with health care professionals through providing clinical resources about pituitary conditions and co-authoring patient information leaflets and booklets. Our members, as described in the patient story below, find the support from the Foundation invaluable:

A patient's story:

I am 42… recently had surgery on a Rathke's Cleft Cyst. The admission to hospital was nerve-wrecking, having never gone under the knife before, to my first operation being brain surgery! … Just prior to discharge, the endocrine nurse specialist discussed hydrocortisone treatment with me and how important it is to take… The nurse discussed sick-day rules and about doubling my dose. If I am truly honest, it went in one ear and straight out the other without even registering. My head and my thoughts were everywhere.

Even as a nurse myself, I was paranoid of everything. Every time I did not feel like myself,

I thought: *"Is this a crisis? Do I need to double my dose? Do I need to give myself an injection?"* I could look at the list of signs and symptoms and say I have every one of those, but did I? The more I sat back and thought, I would start to get palpitations, the nervous feeling right to the pit of your stomach, thinking: *"what is going on with me? What do I need to do?"* One day, I contacted the Foundation using the Helpline email service, saying I didn't feel well, just not myself and really feeling weak. I didn't want to contact the GP *again* in case they thought I was being a pain.

Pat [Head of Patient and Family Services] responded and what can I say, what an inspirational lady! Pat not only responded to my email but also rang me. She provided me with the information I needed. I also then spent some time looking at The Pituitary Foundation website and found it to be an amazing source of simple information which was easily understood. I watched one of the videos which Alison [the Pituitary Foundation Endocrine Nurse] made, and found comfort now knowing, when to give myself a hydrocortisone injection to prevent adrenal crisis…

To contact the Pituitary Foundation, UK:

Website: www.pituitary.org.uk; Email: helpline@pituitary.org.uk

25.8 Part B: Growth Hormone Deficiency in Adults

25.8.1 Clinical Features and Abnormalities of GHD in Adults

Growth hormone (GH) is produced by the anterior pituitary gland. It has a role throughout lifespan in the regulation of protein, lipid and carbohydrate metabolism, and other important metabolic effects on a variety of target tissues, in addition to linear growth in children (Ahmid et al. 2016a) (Fig. 25.2). Its secretion is intermittent and occurs predominantly during deep sleep. Secretion reaches maximal levels during adolescence and then declines with age by approximately 14% per decade (Burt and Ho 2016; Melmed and Jameson 2017).

GH deficiency is adult-onset or childhood-onset and can occur as isolated GH deficiency or as part of multiple pituitary hormone deficiency. Causes of GH deficiency are the same as those of hypopituitarism (Table 25.1). In adult-onset, GH deficiency is commonly due to pituitary or brain tumours and their treatment with surgery or radiotherapy. Childhood-onset GH deficiency is mainly isolated idiopathic which resolves for many children at the end of growth, but it can also be genetic, associated with brain structural defects or with midline facial defect, which are irreversible and GH deficiency continues into adulthood (Molitch et al. 2011). Acquired GH deficiency can also occur in childhood or adulthood in survivors of childhood cancer, because of previous cranial irradiation and/or chemotherapy (Sklar et al. 2018).

Epidemiological studies in hypopituitarism showed that 60 % of patients were GH-deficient (Regal et al. 2001; Fernandez-Rodriguez et al. 2013), giving a prevalence of GH deficiency between 114 and 270 cases per million population and an incidence of approximately 24 patients with GH deficiency per million per year (Burt and Ho 2016).

Adults with GH deficiency have a range of metabolic, body compositional and functional abnormalities and the degree of severity depends on length of diagnosis, childhood- or adult-onset, and the time of GH replacement. GH deficiency is associated with the following adverse symptoms and signs (Burt and Ho 2016):

- Increased body fat, overweight, increased adiposity especially abdominal
- Reduced muscle bulk and poor muscular development
- Reduced muscle strength and physical performance
- Thin dry skin, reduced sweating
- Impaired psychological well-being and QoL
  - Depressed mood
  - Reduced physical stamina
  - Reduced vitality and energy
  - Increased social isolation
  - Reduced focus and concentration
- Hyperlipidaemia: high LDL cholesterol and low HDL cholesterol

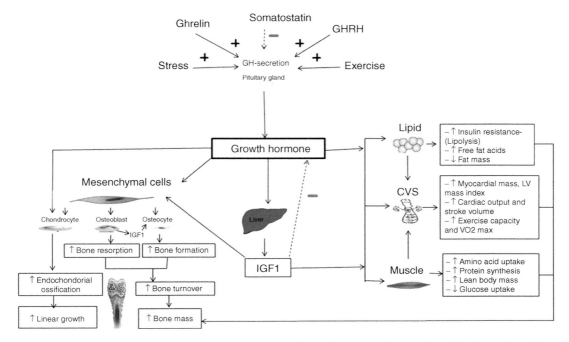

Fig. 25.2 Production of GH and GH-IGF1 actions in bone, muscle, and body metabolism. Key: *GH* growth hormone, *IGF1* insulin-like growth factor-1. GH secretion is regulated by three peptides: GH-releasing hormone (GHRH), ghrelin-stimulating GH release, and somatostatin (SS)-inhibiting GH release. In circulation, GH stimulates the liver and other peripheral tissues to produce IGF1. GH/IGF1 stimulates longitudinal growth, enhances bone mass, and regulates bone metabolism. GH promotes the positive protein balance in skeletal muscle and has lipolytic effects which may play a role in maintaining glucose homeostasis with decreased insulin sensitivity which all promote cardiovascular system (CVS) functional capacity and maximal oxygen consumption (VO₂ max). Used with permission from Ahmid, M., Perry, C. G., Ahmed, S. F. & Shaikh, M. G. 2016b. Growth hormone deficiency during young adulthood and the benefits of growth hormone replacement. *Endocr Connect,* 5, R1-r11

- Insulin resistance and elevated fasting insulin
- Osteopenia or osteoporosis (reduced bone mineral density).

25.8.2 Isolated GH deficiency and Evolving Hypopituitarism

Isolated GH deficiency is the most common pituitary hormone deficiency and can result from congenital or acquired causes; the majority of cases during childhood are idiopathic with no identifiable aetiology and resolve at the end of growth (please refer to Chaps. 1 and 2 on growth and development in childhood). Idiopathic GH deficiency presenting in adulthood is very rare and stringent criteria are necessary with two provocative tests to make the diagnosis. A low insulin-like growth factor-1 (IGF-1) also increases the likelihood of a GH deficiency diagnosis (Molitch

et al. 2011; Melmed 2013). Radiotherapy treatment for tumours lying in the hypothalamic and pituitary axis is also a common cause of hypopituitarism which often starts with isolated GH deficiency. The radiological impact resulting in pituitary deficiencies depends on the dose of radiotherapy, number of fractions, patient age, and duration of follow-up. Somatotropes are the most sensitive and the only pituitary cell types affected by radiation dose below 20 Gy. Radiation dose between 20 and 50 Gy causes more rapid onset of GH deficiency and additional progressive onset of other hormone deficiencies over a period of 10–15 years (Burt and Ho 2016). One of the earlier studies looked at 165 patients who underwent external radiotherapy affecting the hypothalamic-pituitary axis; before radiotherapy, 18% of patients had normal GH secretion, 21% had normal gonadotrophin secretion, 57% had normal corticotrophin reserve, and 80% had normal thyrotrophin secretion. Increasing incidences of progressive hypopituitarism was seen with time; by 8 years post-radiotherapy, all patients were GH-deficient, 96% were gonadotrophin-deficient, 84% were corticotrophin-deficient and 49% were thyrotrophin-deficient (Littley et al. 1989). It is, therefore, important that endocrine testing is performed yearly for the first 10 years and again at 15 years (Burt and Ho 2016). The endocrine nurse should take a detailed history of possible symptoms of hypopituitarism at every consultation and should advise patients and their families to contact the endocrine team should they experience any of these symptoms at any point.

25.9 Diagnosis of Adult GH Deficiency and Provocative Tests

Diagnostic investigations for GH deficiency in adults should be undertaken only in the context of a "probable cause", either a childhood history of GH deficiency or a clinical history making GH deficiency likely (Molitch et al. 2011). The group of adult patients who should be under clinical supervision for developing GH deficiency includes:

- Patients with known or suspected hypothalamic or pituitary disease
- Patients who have received cranial irradiation
- Patients with a deficiency of one or more of the other pituitary hormones
- Patients who have undergone hypophysectomy
- Patients with isolated GH deficiency during childhood

A normal IGF-1 does not exclude the diagnosis of GH deficiency but a low IGF-1, in the absence of poorly controlled diabetes, liver disease, and oral oestrogen therapy, is useful in identifying patients who may potentially be GH-deficient and require further diagnostic investigations (Molitch et al. 2011).

Patients with suspected GH deficiency should undergo pituitary provocative (dynamic) testing to diagnose adult GH deficiency. Several tests are available, with the insulin tolerance test (ITT) being regarded as the 'gold standard' test for adults. The diagnostic criterion for adult GH deficiency (AGHD) is a GH cutoff level between 3 and 5 µg/L in response to insulin-induced hypoglycaemia (glucose <2.2 mmol/L), although this may differ from country to country depending on national guidelines or local assays used for biochemistry analysis (Burt and Ho 2016; Molitch et al. 2011; NICE 2003; Ho 2007).

When the ITT is contraindicated in patients with history of seizure disorders or cardiovascular disease, other tests can be used with equivalent specificity and sensitivity, such as GH-releasing hormone (GHRH)-arginine test or glucagon stimulation test (GST) (Molitch et al. 2011). Please refer to pituitary dynamic testing in Chap. 15.

The endocrine nurse should be vigilant of patients who may develop GH deficiency or require GH replacement for symptom treatment. The following aspects should be included during a patient's routine consultation:

- Ask questions regarding patient's well-being and QoL. Are they feeling more fatigued for no apparent reason? Is the rest of their pituitary profile optimal or adequately replaced?
- If yes to above questions, ask the patient to complete a validated QoL questionnaire such as QoL-AGHDA (Quality of Life Assessment of Growth Hormone Deficiency in Adults) questionnaire (McKenna et al. 1999). An AGHDA-QoL score above 11 indicates impaired QoL and the patient should be investigated for GH deficiency with a provocative test, unless this is not required as discussed earlier. An IGF-1 level should also be checked at every visit.
- Explain to the patient the reason for these tests and what GH treatment involves if the patient is found to be deficient. A number of patients may object to daily injections and it is important to explain the rationale and objectives for treatment and also the simplicity of the GH replacement therapy. If, however, the patient will still object to starting GH replacement, there is no reason to undertake a provocative

testing for GH deficiency (unless indicated for the ACTH-cortisol axis).

For patients younger than 25 years old, continuation or restarting GH is recommended until peak bone mass has been achieved (as indicated by a DEXA bone density scan). If patients report fatigue or impaired well-being after stopping GH, asking them to complete a QoL-AGHDA questionnaire or equivalent is very useful in assessing response to GH treatment with regard to QoL. This also gives an indication that the patient may require GH replacement in the long-term to maintain their well-being.

Criteria for GH treatment in adults may vary from country to country. In the United Kingdom, for example, GH is indicated in adults over the age of 25 years with GH deficiency who report impaired QoL (see Box 25.2) (NICE 2003).

Box 25.2 Criteria for GH Treatment in Adults Set by the National Institute for Clinical Excellence (NICE) in the United Kingdom
The criteria set by NICE in 2003 recommend that an adult older than 25 years of age is treated with GH when:

- Peak GH on an Insulin Tolerance Test or equivalent Dynamic Test such as Glucagon Stimulation Test is less than 9 mU/L (or 3 µg/L);
- Patient has impaired quality of life as measured by an AGHDA_QoL score of 11/25 points or above;
- Patient should be receiving other pituitary replacement and this therapy should be optimised before considering GH start, or in the case of isolated GH deficiency, the pituitary profile should be optimal.
- Assessment of quality of life should be undertaken at 9 months after GH start and continuation of GH replacement long term is determined by an improvement of 7 points on the pretreatment AGHDA_QoL.

Adult patients younger than 25 years of age should continue on GH replacement until this age for achievement of peak bone mass as measured by a DEXA bone mineral density scan. Continuation of treatment past this age will depend on assessment of their quality of life based on above criteria.

AGHDA_QoL: Assessment of Growth Hormone Deficiency in Adults Quality of Life questionnaire

25.9.1 When Is Provocative Testing Not Needed?

Patients in the following two groups do not require a provocative test to establish GH deficiency in adults (Burt and Ho 2016; Molitch et al. 2011), although this may vary between countries or medical insurers:

- Children with GH deficiency following irreversible damage to the hypothalamic-pituitary axis due to structural lesions or proven genetic causes, and a low IGF-1 level at least 1 month off GH therapy at the end of growth;
- Adult patients who have three or more pituitary hormone deficiencies and a low serum IGF-1 level. All pituitary deficiencies must be optimally replaced before GH therapy initiation.

25.10 Transition from Child to Adult and GH Treatment

The transition from paediatric to adult care is an important time to re-evaluate GH status. Once final height is achieved, GH secretion should be retested as a significant percentage of patients with isolated GH deficiency or idiopathic hypopituitarism in childhood recover and have normal GH secretion in adulthood. Patients with confirmed structural damage of the hypothalamic-pituitary axis and low IGF1 do not need to be tested and should continue GH treatment throughout transition. In patients with confirmed GH deficiency, continuation of GH treatment through the late adolescent years into early adulthood (transition phase) is recommenced in order to complete somatic development, structural skeletal maturity, and peak bone mass which is achieved in the mid-twenties (Burt and Ho 2016).

An algorithm for management of patients during transition after treatment with GH during childhood was proposed in a consensus statement from the European Society of Paediatric Endocrinology (ESPE) (Clayton et al. 2005) (Fig. 25.3). When height velocity has decreased to <1.5/2.0 cm/year, GH should be discontinued for 1–3 months. Patients should then be grouped as either high likelihood of continuing to be GH-deficient, with severe deficiency due to genetic or organic causes and particularly with multiple pituitary hormone deficiencies, or low likelihood, including patients with idiopathic GH deficiency that is either isolated or with addi-

tional pituitary hormone deficiencies. Patients with a high likelihood of GH deficiency and an IGF-1 SDS ≤−2 should restart GH without a provocative test. If IGF-1 is >−2 SDS, then a provocative test should be performed, and GH treatment should only be restarted if the stimulated peak GH is below the recommended cutoff value. Patients with low likelihood should have both IGF-1 assessment and a GH provocative test, with GH restarted if both are low indicating continued GH deficiency; if both are normal, then GH deficiency is excluded at that time, and if the results are discordant, then the patient should be followed up in the longterm (Clayton et al. 2005).

The recommended cutoff levels of 3–5 μg/L for peak GH on provocative testing are for measurements in adults, but have not been established for patients in the transition period (Clayton et al. 2005; Aimaretti et al. 2015; Ahmid et al. 2016b).

Fig. 25.3 Algorithm for GH treatment during transition and end of growth. Key: *GH* growth hormone, *IGF-1* insulin like growth factor 1, *SD* standard deviation, *asterisk* value of peak GH level may vary depending on assay—confirm local reference range. Used with permission from Clayton, P. E., Cuneo, R. C., Juul, A., Monson, J. P., Shalet, S. M. & Tauber, M. 2005. Consensus statement on the management of the GH-treated adolescent in the transition to adult care. *Eur J Endocrinol,* 152, 165–70

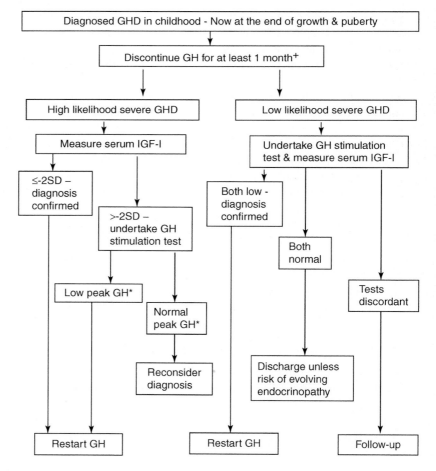

GH dose for patients in the transition period should be adjusted based on IGF-1 levels aiming for upper end of reference range for age. An adequate dose through the transition period is required to attain peak bone mass (Clayton et al. 2005). It is important to remember that young females on oral oestrogen therapy require higher doses of GH, which may be almost a double dose of GH with concomitant ethinylestradiol therapy versus no oestrogen therapy (Wolthers et al. 2001; Phelan et al. 2012). Patients should be advised to inform the endocrine team of any changes to their treatment (e.g. stopping the oral contraceptive pill) as this may lead to potential side effects from over-replacement with GH (see patient case study in Box 25.3).

Box 25.3 Patient Case Study—GH Treatment and Oral Contraceptive Pill

Mary is 24 years old and has a history of isolated idiopathic GH deficiency. She received GH replacement as a child and, following a peak GH level of 1.3 μg/L on insulin tolerance test and low IGF-1 at the end of growth assessment at the age of 18 years, she restarted GH and her daily dose is 1.2 mg. She also takes the oral contraceptive pill (containing ethinylestradiol) for contraception. She reports good adherence to her GH therapy, no side effects, good QoL and her IGF-1 level is stable at the upper end of reference range for age.

She calls the endocrine nurse 4 months after her routine clinic consultation to report joint aches, muscle stiffness, and "aching all over". She stopped running due to severe joint aches. She reports that her relationship with her boyfriend ended recently and she initially attributed these symptoms to her psychological distress. On further questioning, she also reports that she stopped taking the oral contraceptive pill. The endocrine nurse explains that symptoms are most likely due to GH over-replacement and a blood test confirms elevated IGF-1 level.

The dose of GH was halved; a repeat blood test 6 weeks later shows normalised IGF-1 level and Mary's symptoms improve and resolve within 2 months.

The endocrine nurse plays a key role in the seamless and successful transition of children to the adult setting. The patient and their families should be supported and provided with the right information and rationale on the importance of continuation of GH treatment when necessary. Many adolescents and young adults will be reluctant to continue GH injections, especially as they become more independent from their parents, and nonadherence to GH is very prevalent at this age (Rosenfeld and Bakker 2008; Abdi et al. 2014). Patients should be provided with information on the continued effects of GH on lipid metabolism, body composition, achievement of peak bone mass, and maintaining QoL. Peer support and meeting with other young patients who have been through the transition process can be very helpful and the endocrine nurse can organise open events or focus groups to facilitate this.

Transition should not be seen as a simple move from one site to another, but as a multistep process during which the patient's and their families' medical, psychological, social, and educational needs must all be considered. The patient gets to know a new physician and group of health care specialists and, therefore, may experience increased anxiety. Multidisciplinary working between the paediatric and the adult teams is crucial to ensure a smooth transition to the adult clinic. Joint clinics and a "patient passport" that includes all relevant health and treatment information to facilitate the smooth transfer from paediatric to adult service can be useful resources. Many evidence-based health care pathways with specific milestones are available for patients in transition and various models can be adopted depending on organisational and patient needs (please read Chap. 6 for more details on the transition process).

25.11 GH Treatment Initiation and Monitoring in Adults

Each patient should be provided with a comprehensive consultation prior to GH treatment to explain patient with details regarding GH treatment, possible side effects, benefits, dose titration, and long-term monitoring. The checklist in Table 25.3 provides a proposed outline for the consultation which can be used by the endocrine nurse as a guide to ensure that patients receive all the relevant information prior to GH replacement therapy initiation. GH should be initiated only after all other pituitary deficiencies have been fully optimised or after adequate pituitary function is confirmed.

GH replacement is administered by daily subcutaneous injections recommended in the evening to mimic physiological secretion of GH at night. Patients can self-administer and the recommended starting dose of GH in young men is 0.2 mg, in young women 0.3 mg daily and in older individuals 0.1 mg daily. IGF-1 is used as a marker for GH treatment optimisation and the goal for adults with GH deficiency, after peak bone mass has been achieved, is to achieve IGF-1 levels in the middle of the normal reference range appropriate for age and sex. Dose titration by increments of 0.1–0.2 mg should be done every 1–2 months based on IGF-1 and taking into consideration the patient's clinical picture and presence of side effects, but also concomitant use of oestrogen therapy in women. The dose should not be increased while the patient experiences side effects. Once optimal level of IGF-1 is achieved, patients should be monitored every 6–12 months, with a clinical assessment for evaluation of IGF-1, adverse and side effects, adherence to treatment, and other parameters for GH response such as body composition and metabolic parameters, cardiovascular risk factors, and QoL (Burt and Ho 2016; Molitch et al. 2011; Gasco et al. 2013). GH replacement requirements decrease with age, mirroring the physiological production of GH.

The endocrine nurse should explain to the patients that any improvement in QoL post GH start may take up to nine months to notice, as patient's expectations for immediate improvement may have a negative impact on their adherence to GH injections. NICE guidelines in the United Kingdom recommend assessment of QoL at 9 months post-GH initiation, aiming for an improvement of 7 points in the QoL-AGHDA score in order to continue GH treatment in the longterm (NICE 2003). Practical aspects such as injection technique and adherence to medication are also important considerations in the optimisation and monitoring of GH replacement in adults (Box 25.4).

Table 25.3 A checklist to facilitate consultation for GH replacement start

1	Explain results of the provocative test	9	What to do if missing an injection
2	Symptoms of GHD and expected benefits	10	Changes in medication, e.g. starting OCP
3	Possible side effects and what to do	11	When to stop GH, e.g. pregnancy, malignancy
4	Starting dose and further titration	12	Travelling with GH: travel letter, cool bag
5	What is IGF-1 and dose adjustment	13	Cool bag or non-refrigerated GH
6	How to ensure accuracy of IGF-1	14	Choosing a suitable injecting device
7	Long-term monitoring	15	Prescriptions, training for GH injections
8	When to take injections, storage	16	Who to contact for what: telephone numbers

GHD growth hormone deficiency, *IGF-1* insulin like growth factor-1; *OCP* oral contraceptive pill

> ▶ **Box 25.4 Practical Aspects in the Assessment of IGF-1 and GH Treatment in Adults**
>
> If an abnormal IGF-1 is found in a routine clinic follow-up, it should be repeated in 4–6 weeks. It is important to ask the following questions when interpreting an IGF-1:
>
> - Have you taken all your injections in the last 2 weeks or so? Assessment of adherence to medication should be recorded.
> - Is the injection technique correct (ask the patient to demonstrate this in clinic)? Is the injecting device working properly? Is the GH stored properly and used within its time limit?

- Check the patient's injection sites for evidence of nonabsorption.

  If YES to any of the above questions, correct as necessary and repeat IGF-1 in 4–6 weeks; NO dose adjustment should be done at this stage.
  NOTE: IGF-1 can be inaccurate in malnutrition, liver disease, poorly controlled diabetes, and hypothyroidism

Table 25.4 presents a summary of regular clinical and biochemistry assessment. This, however, depends on each individual patient and the clinical setting/country.

A wide range of GH-injecting devices is available making it possible to select an appropriate device based on individual patient needs, such as needle-phobia, need for non-refrigerated GH, etc. Table 25.5 presents a detailed list of available GH detailed list of available GH treatment options and devices and their characteristics. In addition, Fig. 25.4 presents an algorithm which can help the endocrine nurse and the patient to select the most suitable injecting device for the patient's needs without overwhelming them by demonstrating all the available devices.

25.11.1 Safety, Adverse Effects, and Contraindications of GH in Adults

The patient should be advised of the potential side effects and how these can be managed before they start GH treatment. The most common acute side effects arise from the antinatriuretic action of GH, which causes fluid retention (Burt and Ho 2016). Mild ankle oedema following GH start is a normal response for most patients. Similarly, arthralgia (joint pain), myalgia (muscle pain), carpal tunnel syndrome, and paraesthesia can occur. These effects, if they occur, are usually mild and self-limiting and should generally clear within 2–3 weeks post GH start or following GH dose reduction. Hyperglycaemia and hypoglycaemia have also been reported. GH therapy reduces insulin sensitivity in these patients by antagonising the action of insulin—this could increase the risk of diabetes. Caution should be exercised when treating a patient with Diabetes Mellitus with GH; adjustments in the diabetes treatment may be required (Burt and Ho 2016).

Headaches are also common at the start of treatment. Persistent headaches, visual problems, or nausea and vomiting require investigation with fundoscopy for papilledema, which if confirmed benign intracranial hypertension (rare cases reported) should be considered. This is usually recognised shortly after commencement of GH treatment (Burt and Ho 2016). The endocrine nurse should advise patients to stop treatment and report severe and persistent headaches immediately. Other side effects may include mild hypertension, visual problems, and nausea and vomiting.

There is evidence to support no effect of GH replacement on tumour regrowth or recurrence of pituitary tumours, craniopharyngiomas, or other benign brain tumours and published data provide reassurance on the long-term safety profile of GH treatment (Stochholm and Kiess 2018; Pekic and Popovic 2013). GH treatment is contraindicated in active malignancy, proliferative diabetic retinopathy, benign intracranial hypertension, and in

Table 25.4 GH treatment monitoring: what to check and when?

Parameters to check	Pre-GH start	4 weeks	3 M	6 M	9 M	6-monthly	Yearly
IGF-1, TFTs	X	X	X	X	X	X	
Glucose, Lipid, BMI/weight, BP	X			X			X
AGHDA-QoL and well-being	X			X			X
Waist circumference	X			X			X
Response to GH and side effects		X	X	X	X	X	X
BMD—DEXA	X	2–3 yearly thereafter if abnormal depending on T-scores					
MRI pituitary (where needed)	X			X			
IGF-1 & TFTs	**Check 6 weeks after any dose adjustments or regime change**						

IGF-1 insulin-like growth factor-1, *TFTs* thyroid function test, *BMI* body mass index, *BP* blood pressure, *GH* growth hormone, *BMD-DEXA* bone mineral density-dual energy X-ray absorptiometry, *MRI* magnetic resonance imaging

Table 25.5 Available GH injecting devices and their characteristics

GH brand and manufacturer	Device	Device photo	Vial strength/dose increments	Liquid vial	Dose preset	Storage	Stable at room temp (<25 °C)	Auto injector
Omnitrope® Sandoz	SurePal™ Pen 5, 10 & 15 (for use with Omnitrope vials)		5 mg/0.05 mg, 10 mg/0.1 mg, 15 mg/0.1 mg	✓	✓	2–8 °C, use within 28 days once in pen	X	X
Genotropin® Pfizer	Genotropin® Pen 5.3 & 12 (for use with Genotropin® vials, needs reconstitution)		5.3 mg/0.1 mg, 12 mg/0.2 mg	X	X	2–8 °C, use within 28 days once in pen	Up to a month before reconstitution	X
	GoQuick® Pen 5.3 & 12 (prefilled multi-dose disposable pen, needs reconstitution)		5.3 mg/0.05 mg, 12 mg/0.15 mg	X	✓	2–8 °C, use within 28 days once started	Up to a month before reconstitution	X
	MiniQuick® disposable single-use syringe with liquid-powder, needs reconstitution		Set dose 0.2–2.0 mg/0.2 mg increments	X	✓	2–8 °C, use within 24 h post-reconstitution	YES - up to 6 months	X
Norditropin® NovoNordisk	NordiPen® 5, 10 & 15 (for use with Norditropin SimpleXx vials)		5 mg/0.05 mg, 10 mg/0.1 mg, 15 mg/0.1 mg	✓	X	2–8 °C, use within 28 days once in pen	Up to 21 days, can be used for another 7 days if refrigerated	✓ With PenMate
	NordiFlex® 5, 10 & 15 [Norditropin FlexPro® in USA] (prefilled m-dose disposable pen)		5 mg/0.025 mg, 10 mg/0.05 mg, 15 mg/0.075 mg	✓	X	2–8 °C, use within 28 days once in pen	Up to 21 days, can be used for another 7 days if refrigerated	✓ With PenMate

		Vial/dose range*					
Saizen® MerckSerono	EasyPod® digital autoinjector, injects only at skin contact (for use with Saizen Liquid—*specific dose preset for each vial range with min wastage)	6 mg/0.15–0.45 mg 12 mg/0.5–0.7 mg 20 mg/0.75–6.4 mg	✓	✓	2–8 °C, use within 28 days once in device	X	✓
	One.click® autoinjector (for use with ClickEasy 8mg, needs reconstitution)	8 mg/0.12 mg (one click increments)	X	X	2–8 °C, use within 28 days once in pen	X	✓
NutropinAq® Ipsen	NutropinAq® 10 Pen (for use with NutropinAq® vials)	10 mg/0.1 mg	✓	X	2–8 °C, use within 28 days once in pen	X	X
Humatrope® Lilly	HumatroPen® 6, 12 & 24 (for use with Humatrope cartridge and prefilled syringe with diluent for reconstitution)	6 mg/0.025 mg 12 mg/0.05 mg 24 mg/0.1 mg	X	X	2–8 °C, use within 14 days post-reconstitution	X	X
Zomacton® Ferring	ZomaJet VisionX® 4 & 10 NEEDLE FREE pen (for use with Zomacton, needs reconstitution)	4 mg/0.1 mg 10 mg/0.1 mg	X	X	2–8 °C, use within 14 days post-reconstitution	X	✓
TevTropin® USA only Ferring	Tjet® 5 NEEDLE FREE pen (for use with TevTropin, needs reconstitution)	5 mg/0.1 mg	X	X	2–8 °C, use within 14 days post-reconstitution	X	✓

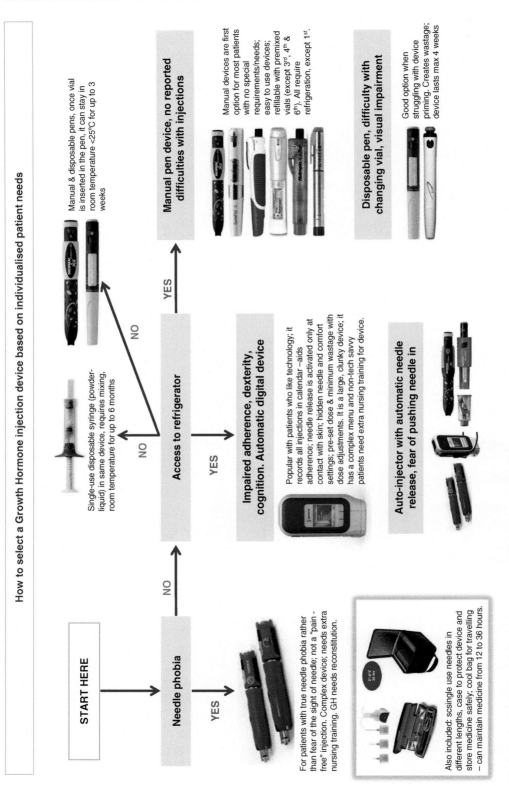

How to select a Growth Hormone injection device based on individualised patient needs

START HERE

Needle phobia

YES

For patients with true needle phobia rather than fear of the sight of needle; not a "pain-free" injection. Complex device; needs extra nursing training. GH needs reconstitution.

Also included: scsingle use needles in different lengths, case to protect device and store medicine safely; cool bag for travelling – can maintain medicine from 12 to 36 hours.

NO

Access to refrigerator

NO

Single-use disposable syringe (powder-liquid) in same device; requires mixing, room temperature for up to 6 months

Manual & disposable pens, once vial is inserted in the pen, it can stay in room temperature <25°C for up to 3 weeks

NO

YES

Manual pen device, no reported difficulties with injections

Manual devices are first option for most patients with no special requirements/needs; easy to use devices; refillable with premixed vials (except 3rd, 4th & 6th). All require refrigeration, except 1st.

YES

Impaired adherence, dexterity, cognition. Automatic digital device

Popular with patients who like technology; it records all injections in calendar –aids adherence; needle release is activated only at contact with skin; hidden needle and comfort settings; pre-set dose & minimum wastage with dose adjustments. It is a large, clunky device; it has a complex menu and non-tech savvy patients need extra nursing training for device.

Auto-injector with automatic needle release, fear of pushing needle in

Disposable pen, difficulty with changing vial, visual impairment

Good option when struggling with device priming. Creates wastage; device lasts max 4 weeks

Fig. 25.4 Algorithm for selecting a suitable GH device for each patient's needs

patients with known hypersensitivity to GH or to any of the excipients. Pregnancy is not a contraindication, but GH becomes unnecessary in the second trimester due to sufficient placental GH production and should be discontinued. Moreover, there is no safety data in the use of GH in pregnancy (Burt and Ho 2016; Molitch et al. 2011).

25.11.2 GH Treatment and Safety in Childhood Cancer Survivors

Concerns have been raised regarding the long-term safety of GH treatment in childhood cancer survivors. Previous data on GH-treated childhood cancer survivors suggest that GH might potentially induce a small increase in the relative risk of developing second neoplasms, particularly meningiomas, compared to survivors not receiving GH treatment (Sklar et al. 2002; Woodmansee et al. 2013). However, recent studies have shown no significant association between GH treatment and the development of a second neoplasm of the central nervous system (CNS) in childhood cancer survivors (Mackenzie et al. 2011; Patterson et al. 2014; Brignardello et al. 2014). The recent guidelines from the Endocrine Society recommend offering GH treatment to childhood cancer survivors with confirmed GH deficiency (Sklar et al. 2018).

25.11.3 Interactions with Other Hormones and Medications

GH affects the action and metabolism of other pituitary hormones and alterations in dose requirements should be anticipated (Filipsson and Johannsson 2009).

GH increases the peripheral conversion of triiodothyronine to thyroxine (T4) and treatment initiation may unmask preexisting central hypothyroidism. Agha et al. looked at 243 patients with severe GH deficiency due to hypothalamic-pituitary disorders, of whom 159 were treated for central hypothyroidism (treated group) and 84 were euthyroid prior to GH commencement (untreated group). Following GH initiation and

dose titration over 3–6 months, 30/84 patients (36%) became hypothyroid and required initiation of T4 therapy. Moreover, 25/159 (16%) of patients in the treated group required increase in T4 dose (Agha et al. 2007). Commencement of T4 replacement is, therefore, recommended in patients with low normal serum T4 concentrations prior to GH initiation to provide a robust baseline from which to judge the clinical effects of GH replacement.

Oestrogen administered by the oral route impairs GH action, leading to higher dose requirements. Physiological non-oral route with transdermal patches or gel is preferable where possible (Wolthers et al. 2001; Phelan et al. 2012). Patients should be advised to update the endocrine clinic on any changes to oestrogen therapy, e.g., starting or stopping the oral contraceptive pill; IGF-1 should be checked for GH dose adjustment.

In adults with GH deficiency, there is an increased 11β-HCD type 1 activity which results in increased cortisol tissue exposure. This is reduced after initiating GH treatment (high GH and IGF-1 levels enhance conversion of cortisol to cortisone, i.e. lower levels of active cortisol), which can unmask central hypoadrenalism and predispose the patient to adrenal insufficiency (AI) and risk of adrenal crisis. Therefore, the assessment of the hypothalamic-pituitary-adrenal (HPA) axis to confirm or exclude AI is mandatory prior to starting GH replacement (Filipsson and Johannsson 2009; Giavoli et al. 2004). For patients on cortisol replacement, an increase in Hydrocortisone dose may be required after starting GH treatment.

25.12 New Developments in GH Treatment (Long-Acting GH)

Currently, treatment with subcutaneous injection of a biosynthetic recombinant human growth hormone (rhGH) requires daily administration. The treatment often enduring for many years increases the risk of poor adherence, i.e. patients admit being lax about taking injections. Long-acting GH (LAGH) preparation aims to improve adherence to treatment by decreasing the inconvenience of daily injections. LAGHs are expected to be as effective, safe, and cost-effective as the currently available rhGH brands. However, the problem of

Table 25.6 Long-acting GH (LAGH) formulations in advanced stages of clinical research

LG Life Sciences	**LB 03002**	GH embedded in sodium hyaluronate microparticles suspended in triglyceride	*Approved but not marketed in Europe Available in South Korea*
Ascendis Pharma A/S	**TransCon GH**	Transiently PEGylated GH prodrug	*Phase 3*
GeneScience	**Jintrolong**	Permanently PEGylated GH	*Available in China*
OPKO Health Inc	**MOD-4023**	GH fused with carboxyterminal peptides	*Phase 3*
Versatis Inc.	**VRS-317**	GH fused to half-life extension technology	*Phase 3*
Novo Nordisk	**NNC0195-0092**	Mutated GH attached to an albumin affinity tag	*Phase 2*
Hanmi Pharm	**LAPS-rhGH/ HM10560A**	GH fused to an Fc fragment	*Phase 3*

big molecules (modified GH) is that this may compromise tissue distribution (penetrance) and direct actions of GH on local IGF-1 production. LAGH should be small enough to permeate all tissues to achieve beneficial effects (for example QoL). Liver is favoured over peripheral tissue via fenestrated hepatic sinusoidal endothelium. There are still many safety considerations unique to LAGHs: (a) supraphysiological GH activity (can LAGH lead to acromegaly?); (b) fluctuating IGF-1 levels; (c) elevated IGF-1 in the absence of GH bioactivity; (d) tissue distribution (local IGF-1 production); (e) GH and LAGH bind to a common receptor, but they might have disparate effects on downstream signalling cascades.

Long action of GH can be achieved utilizing different development approaches (Sprogoe et al. 2017; Christiansen et al. 2016).

(a) **Unmodified GH**: half-life extension is achieved by the slow release of somatotropin from depot, crystal, or prodrug
(b) **Modified GH**: GH analogue has a longer half-life achieved by increasing molecular size

The LAGH formulations which are in advanced stages of clinical research are presented in Table 25.6.

25.12.1 Unmodified GH Superimposed on Inert Prolongation Technology

Sustained-release rhGH (LB03002) is a sustained-release GH formulation consisting of microparticles containing GH incorporated into

sodium hyaluronate and dispersed in an oil base of medium-chain triglycerides. The first study with weekly depot formulation was performed in 155 adults with GH deficiency (Biller et al. 2011). LB03002 dose was adjusted to achieve a serum IGF-1 value between −0.5 and +1.5 SDS at 4 days post-dosing. Final dose of the GH weekly depot preparation was 4.31 ± 1.77 mg/week (men), 4.34 ± 1.64 mg/week (women without oral oestrogen), and 6.45 ± 2.44 mg/week (women on oral oestrogen).

TransCon GH. Sustained-release GH prodrug consisting of recombinant human GH transiently bound to a carrier molecule (methoxy polyethylene glycol-mPEG) via a proprietary TransCon linker. Over a 1-week period, TransCon frees fully active GH via auto-hydrolysis of TransCon linker (nonenzymatic cleavage). This allows PEG elimination from the body via renal filtration. GH-TransCon phase 2 trial in adults with GH deficiency is completed. A dose-dependent increase in GH peak exposure is shown without GH accumulation (Hoybye et al. 2017).

25.12.2 Active GH Analogues: Modified GH Molecule

Permanent pegylation-protein enlargement by attaching polyethylene glycol (PEG) to GH. Many PEGylated pharmacological compounds have been approved by regulatory agencies. Currently, the only available PEGylated-GH is Jintrolong which has been developed and approved in China (Hou et al. 2016). Major drawback is safety concern (PEGylated GH is taken up by reticuloendothelial cells and choroid plexus ependymal cells-vacuolation has been observed within cells with GH receptors). Furthermore, local tolerability issues with permanently PEGylated GH were reported (including lipoatrophy).

MOD-4023 Conjugation of CTP to GH. Carboxy-terminus peptide (CTP) is a natural peptide created during evolution to enhance longevity of hormone hCG. CTP increases protein circulation time. MOD-4023 is a result of conjugation of CTP to GH. High dose of MOD 4023 has low affinity for GH receptor (eightfold). IGF1 was monitored every 2 weeks, 4 days after dose. Single weekly injection of MOD-4023 can replace 7 consecutive daily GH injections (Strasburger et al. 2017). The proposed MOD 4023 dose range is 1.23–5.6 mg/week. Data confirm safety.

GH fusion protein Somavartan (VRS-317) is a fusion protein produced in *Escherihia coli*. GH molecule is fused to two pharmacologically inactive naturally occurring hydrophilic amino acids (XTEN1, XTEN2) with an extended elimination time ($T\frac{1}{2}$ 110 h). Modification of GH reduces the affinity with receptors (for VRS-317 eleven-fold), but the prolonged exposure time achieved a greater potency. In a study in adults with GHD, higher doses of somavartan (VRS-317), male sex, and young age were all associated with greater IGF-1 responses (Yuen et al. 2013). In a phase 3 Velocity trial of somavartan twice monthly at 12 months, height velocity in children was 9.4 cm versus 10.7 cm for Genotropin daily, thus disappointingly missing the endpoint of noninferiority (Versatis press release September 2017).

Other formulations based on modified GH such as TV-1106 (GH fused to albumin) produced by Teva Pharmaceutical, LAPS-rhGH/HM 10560A (GH fused to an Fc fragment) produced by Hanmi Pharmaceutical, NNC0 195-0092 (Somapacitan-mutated GH attached to an albumin affinity tag binding reversibly to albumin) produced by Novo Nordisk are still under evaluation in phase 2 or phase 3 or are discontinued (TV-1106 due to high immunogenic potential).

25.13 Conclusions

This chapter presented an overview of causes and clinical presentation of hypopituitarism and hormone replacement therapy in patients with pituitary conditions. The reader is encouraged to refer to relevant chapters in the textbook regarding hormone deficiencies and replacement therapies. The second part of the chapters focused on GH deficiency and treatment for adult patients. New developments with long-acting GH formulations were also discussed. It is anticipated that long-acting GH compounds will improve adherence to GH replacement therapy. Long-term surveillance registries are needed to confirm the efficacy and address unique safety issues of these formulations. Clinical data are still very limited, and many questions remain to be answered.

Acknowledgments Special thanks to Pat McBride, Head of Patient and Family Services, The Pituitary Foundation (https://www.pituitary.org.uk), for her contribution to this chapter with case studies, patient resources, and information on the Patient Advocacy Group

References

Abdi L, Sahnoun-Fathallah M, Morange I, Albarel F, Castinetti F, Giorgi R, et al. A monocentric experience of growth hormone replacement therapy in adult patients. Ann Endocrinol. 2014;75(3):176.

Adelman DT, Liebert KJ, Nachtigall LB, Lamerson M, Bakker B. Acromegaly: the disease, its impact on patients, and managing the burden of long-term treatment. Int J Gen Med. 2013;6:31–8.

Agha A, Walker D, Perry L, Drake WM, Chew SL, Jenkins PJ, et al. Unmasking of central hypothyroidism following growth hormone replacement in adult hypopituitary patients. Clin Endocrinol (Oxf). 2007;66(1):72–7.

Ahmid M, Perry CG, Ahmed SF, Shaikh MG. Growth hormone deficiency during young adulthood and the benefits of growth hormone replacement. Endocr Connect. 2016a;5(3):R1–r11.

Ahmid M, Fisher V, Graveling AJ, McGeoch S, McNeil E, Roach J, et al. An audit of the management of childhood-onset growth hormone deficiency during young adulthood in Scotland. Int J Pediatr Endocrinol. 2016b;2016:6.

Aimaretti G, Attanasio R, Cannavo S, Nicoletti MC, Castello R, Di Somma C, et al. Growth hormone treatment of adolescents with growth hormone deficiency (GHD) during the transition period: results of a survey among adult and paediatric endocrinologists from Italy. Endorsed by SIEDP/ISPED, AME, SIE, SIMA. J Endocrinol Invest. 2015;38(3):377–82.

van Aken MO, Lamberts SW. Diagnosis and treatment of hypopituitarism: an update. Pituitary. 2005;8(3-4):183–91.

Andela CD, Scharloo M, Pereira AM, Kaptein AA, Biermasz NR. Quality of life (QoL) impairments in patients with a pituitary adenoma: a systematic review of QoL studies. Pituitary. 2015;18(5):752–76.

Atkinson MJ, Sinha A, Hass SL, Colman SS, Kumar RN, Brod M, et al. Validation of a general measure of treatment satisfaction, the Treatment Satisfaction Questionnaire for Medication (TSQM), using a national panel study of chronic disease. Health Qual Life Outcomes. 2004;2:12.

Biller BM, Ji HJ, Ahn H, Savoy C, Siepl EC, Popovic V, et al. Effects of once-weekly sustained-release growth hormone: a double-blind, placebo-controlled study in adult growth hormone deficiency. J Clin Endocrinol Metab. 2011;96(6):1718–26.

Bleicken B, Hahner S, Loeffler M, Ventz M, Decker O, Allolio B, et al. Influence of hydrocortisone dosage scheme on health-related quality of life in patients with adrenal insufficiency. Clin Endocrinol (Oxf). 2010;72(3):297–304.

Brignardello E, Felicetti F, Castiglione A, Fortunati N, Matarazzo P, Biasin E, et al. GH replacement therapy and second neoplasms in adult survivors of childhood cancer: a retrospective study from a single institution. J Endocrinol Invest. 2014;38(2):171–6.

Burman P, Mattsson AF, Johannsson G, Hoybye C, Holmer H, Dahlqvist P, et al. Deaths among adult patients with hypopituitarism: hypocortisolism during acute stress, and de novo malignant brain tumors contribute to an increased mortality. J Clin Endocrinol Metab. 2013;98(4):1466–75.

Burt MG, Ho KKY. Chapter 11 - Hypopituitarism and Growth Hormone Deficiency. In: Jameson JL, De Groot LJ, de Kretser DM, Giudice LC, Grossman AB, Melmed S, et al., editors. Endocrinology: adult and pediatric. 7th ed. Philadelphia: W.B. Saunders; 2016. p. 188–208.e5.

Chapman SC, S L CP, Horne R. Glucocorticoid therapy for adrenal insufficiency: nonadherence, concerns and dissatisfaction with information. Clin Endocrinol (Oxf). 2016;84:664–71.

Christiansen JS, Backeljauw PF, Bidlingmaier M, Biller BM, Boguszewski MC, Casanueva FF, et al. Growth Hormone Research Society perspective on the development of long-acting growth hormone preparations. Eur J Endocrinol. 2016;174(6):C1–8.

Clayton PE, Cuneo RC, Juul A, Monson JP, Shalet SM, Tauber M. Consensus statement on the management of the GH-treated adolescent in the transition to adult care. Eur J Endocrinol. 2005;152(2):165–70.

Cook DM, Ludlam WH, Cook MB. Route of estrogen administration helps to determine growth hormone (GH) replacement dose in GH-deficient adults. J Clin Endocrinol Metab. 1999;84(11):3956–60.

Cooper V, Metcalf L, Versnel J, Upton J, Walker S, Horne R. Patient-reported side effects, concerns and adherence to corticosteroid treatment for asthma, and comparison with physician estimates of side-effect prevalence: a UK-wide, cross-sectional study. NPJ Prim Care Respir Med. 2015;25:15026.

van der Meij N, van Leeuwaarde RS, Vervoort SCJM, Zelissen PMJ. Self-management support in patients with adrenal insufficiency. Clin Endocrinol. 2016; https://doi.org/10.1111/cen.13083.

Dwyer A, Quinton R, Morin D, Pitteloud N. Identifying the unmet health needs of patients with congenital hypogonadotropic hypogonadism using a web-based needs assessment: implications for online interventions and peer-to-peer support. Orphanet J Rare Dis. 2014;9:83.

van Eck JP, Gobbens RJ, Beukers J, Geilvoet W, van der Lely AJ, Neggers SJ. Much to be desired in self-management of patients with adrenal insufficiency. Int J Nurs Pract. 2014; https://doi.org/10.1111/ijn.12368.

Ehrnborg C, Hakkaart-Van Roijen L, Jonsson B, Rutten FF, Bengtsson BA, Rosen T. Cost of illness in adult patients with hypopituitarism. Pharmacoeconomics. 2000;17(6):621–8.

Fernandez-Rodriguez E, Lopez-Raton M, Andujar P, Martinez-Silva IM, Cadarso-Suarez C, Casanueva FF, et al. Epidemiology, mortality rate and survival in a homogeneous population of hypopituitary patients. Clin Endocrinol (Oxf). 2013;78(2):278–84.

Filipsson H, Johannsson G. GH replacement in adults: interactions with other pituitary hormone deficiencies and replacement therapies. Eur J Endocrinol. 2009;161(Suppl 1):S85–95.

Flemming TG, Kristensen LO. Quality of self-care in patients on replacement therapy with hydrocortisone. J Intern Med. 1999;246(5):497–501.

Fleseriu M, Hashim IA, Karavitaki N, Melmed S, Murad MH, Salvatori R, et al. Hormonal replacement in hypopituitarism in adults: an Endocrine Society Clinical Practice Guideline. J Clin Endocrinol Metab. 2016;101(11):3888–921.

Forss M, Batcheller G, Skrtic S, Johannsson G. Current practice of glucocorticoid replacement therapy and patient-perceived health outcomes in adrenal insufficiency - a worldwide patient survey. BMC Endocr Disord. 2012;12:8.

Gasco V, Prodam F, Grottoli S, Marzullo P, Longobardi S, Ghigo E, et al. GH therapy in adult GH deficiency: a review of treatment schedules and the evidence for low starting doses. Eur J Endocrinol. 2013;168(3):R55–66.

George J, Kong DC, Thoman R, Stewart K. Factors associated with medication nonadherence in patients with COPD. Chest. 2005;128(5):3198–204.

Giavoli C, Libé R, Corbetta S, Ferrante E, Lania A, Arosio M, et al. Effect of recombinant human growth hormone (GH) replacement on the hypothalamic-pituitary-adrenal axis in adult GH-deficient patients. J Clin Endocrinol Metabol. 2004;89(11):5397–401.

Gurel MH, Bruening PR, Rhodes C, Lomax KG. Patient perspectives on the impact of acromegaly: results from individual and group interviews. Patient Prefer Adherence. 2014;8:53–62.

Hahner S, Loeffler M, Fassnacht M, Weismann D, Koschker AC, Quinkler M, et al. Impaired subjective health status in 256 patients with adrenal insufficiency on standard therapy based on cross-sectional analysis. J Clin Endocrinol Metab. 2007;92(10):3912–22.

Hahner S, Spinnler C, Fassnacht M, Burger-Stritt S, Lang K, Milovanovic D, et al. High incidence of adrenal crisis in educated patients with chronic adrenal insufficiency: a prospective study. J Clin Endocrinol Metab. 2015;100(2):407–16.

Ho KK. Consensus guidelines for the diagnosis and treatment of adults with GH deficiency II: a statement of the GH Research Society in association with the European Society for Pediatric Endocrinology, Lawson Wilkins Society, European Society of Endocrinology, Japan Endocrine Society, and Endocrine Society of Australia. Eur J Endocrinol. 2007;157(6):695–700.

Hou L, Chen ZH, Liu D, Cheng YG, Luo XP. Comparative pharmacokinetics and pharmacodynamics of a PEGylated recombinant human growth hormone and daily recombinant human growth hormone in growth hormone-deficient children. Drug Des Devel Ther. 2016;10:13–21.

Hoybye C, Pfeiffer AF, Ferone D, Christiansen JS, Gilfoyle D, Christoffersen ED, et al. A phase 2 trial of long-acting TransCon growth hormone in adult GH deficiency. Endocr Connect. 2017;6(3):129–38.

Janssen YJ, Helmerhorst F, Frolich M, Roelfsema F. A switch from oral (2 mg/day) to transdermal (50 microg/day) 17beta-estradiol therapy increases serum insulin-like growth factor-I levels in recombinant human growth hormone (GH)-substituted women with GH deficiency. J Clin Endocrinol Metab. 2000;85(1):464–7.

Jonsson B, Nilsson B. The impact of pituitary adenoma on morbidity. Increased sick leave and disability retirement in a cross-sectional analysis of Swedish national data. Pharmacoeconomics. 2000;18(1):73–81.

Kepicoglu H, Hatipoglu E, Bulut I, Darici E, Hizli N, Kadioglu P. Impact of treatment satisfaction on quality of life of patients with acromegaly. Pituitary. 2014;17(6):557–63.

Lee P, Ho K. Hypopituitarism and growth hormone deficiency. In: Jameson L, De Groot L, editors. Endocrinology: adult and pediatric. Neuroendocrinology and the Pituitary gland. 6th ed. Amsterdam: Elsevier Health Sciences; 2010.

Linn AJ, van Weert JC, van Dijk L, Horne R, Smit EG. The value of nurses' tailored communication when discussing medicines: Exploring the relationship between satisfaction, beliefs and adherence. J Health Psychol. 2016;21:798–807.

Littley MD, Shalet SM, Beardwell CG, Ahmed SR, Applegate G, Sutton ML. Hypopituitarism following external radiotherapy for pituitary tumours in adults. Q J Med. 1989;70(262):145–60.

Llahana S, Conway G. Knowledge of testosterone replacement therapy is significantly correlated with patient satisfaction suggesting greater need for education. 8th European Congress of Endocrinology, Glasgow, UK. Endocrine Abstracts 2006:11 P201.

Llahana S, Conway G, Mumuni A, Baldeweg S, Osz M, Horne R, editors. Patients' beliefs and concerns about growth hormone replacement therapy are associated with their satisfaction with treatment, medication side effects and quality of life. In: 18th International congress of endocrinology, 1–4 Dec 2018, Cape Town, South Africa; 2018.

Losa M, Scavini M, Gatti E, Rossini A, Madaschi S, Formenti I, et al. Long-term effects of growth hormone replacement therapy on thyroid function in adults with growth hormone deficiency. Thyroid. 2008;18(12):1249–54.

Mackenzie S, Craven T, Gattamaneni HR, Swindell R, Shalet SM, Brabant G. Long-term safety of growth hormone replacement after CNS irradiation. J Clin Endocrinol Metabol. 2011;96(9):2756–61.

Martinez-Momblan MA, Gomez C, Santos A, Porta N, Esteve J, Ubeda I, et al. A specific nursing educational program in patients with Cushing's syndrome. Endocrine. 2016;53:199–209.

McKenna SP, Doward LC, Alonso J, Kohlmann T, Niero M, Prieto L, et al. The QoL-AGHDA: an instrument for the assessment of quality of life in adults with growth hormone deficiency. Qual Life Res. 1999;8(4):373–83.

Melmed S. Idiopathic adult growth hormone deficiency. J Clin Endocrinol Metab. 2013;98(6):2187.

Melmed S, Jameson JL. Hypopituitarism, chapter 4. In: Jameson JL, editor. Harrison's endocrinology. 4th ed. New York: McGraw Hill Education; 2017. p. 25–34.

Molitch ME, Clemmons DR, Malozowski S, Merriam GR, Vance ML. Evaluation and treatment of adult growth hormone deficiency: an Endocrine Society clinical practice guideline. J Clin Endocrinol Metab. 2011;96(6):1587–609.

NICE. Human growth hormone (somatropin) in adults with growth hormone deficiency. London: National Institute for Clinical Excellence; 2003.

Ntali G, Capatina C, Fazal-Sanderson V, Byrne JV, Cudlip S, Grossman AB, et al. Mortality in patients with non-functioning pituitary adenoma is increased: systematic analysis of 546 cases with long follow-up. Eur J Endocrinol. 2015;174(2):137–45.

Olsson DS, Nilsson AG, Bryngelsson IL, Trimpou P, Johannsson G, Andersson E. Excess mortality in women and young adults with nonfunctioning pituitary adenoma: a Swedish Nationwide Study. J Clin Endocrinol Metab. 2015;100(7):2651–8.

Omori K, Nomura K, Shimizu S, Omori N, Takano K. Risk factors for adrenal crisis in patients with adrenal insufficiency. Endocr J. 2003;50(6):745–52.

Pappachan JM, Raskauskiene D, Kutty VR, Clayton RN. Excess mortality associated with hypopituitarism in adults: a meta-analysis of observational studies. J Clin Endocrinol Metab. 2015;100(4):1405–11.

Patterson BC, Chen Y, Sklar CA, Neglia J, Yasui Y, Mertens A, et al. Growth hormone exposure as a risk factor for the development of subsequent neoplasms of the central nervous system: a report From the Childhood Cancer Survivor Study. J Clin Endocrinol Metabol. 2014;99(6):2030–7.

Peacey SR, Pope RM, Naik KS, Hardern RD, Page MD, Belchetz PE. Corticosteroid therapy and intercurrent illness: the need for continuing patient education. Postgrad Med J. 1993;69(810):282.

Pekic S, Popovic V. GH therapy and cancer risk in hypopituitarism: what we know from human studies. Eur J Endocrinol. 2013;169:R89–97.

Phelan N, Conway SH, Llahana S, Conway GS. Quantification of the adverse effect of ethinyl-estradiol containing oral contraceptive pills when used in conjunction with growth hormone replacement in routine practice. Clin Endocrinol (Oxf). 2012;76(5):729–33.

Prabhakar VKB, Shalet SM. Aetiology, diagnosis, and management of hypopituitarism in adult life. Postgrad Med J. 2006;82(966):259–66.

Ragnarsson O, Mattsson AF, Monson JP, Filipsson Nystrom H, Akerblad AC, Koltowska-Haggstrom M, et al. The relationship between glucocorticoid replacement and quality of life in 2737 hypopituitary patients. Eur J Endocrinol. 2014;171(5):571–9.

Regal M, Paramo C, Sierra SM, Garcia-Mayor RV. Prevalence and incidence of hypopituitarism in an adult Caucasian population in northwestern Spain. Clin Endocrinol (Oxf). 2001;55(6):735–40.

Repping-Wuts HJWJ, Stikkelbroeck NMML, Noordzij A, Kerstens M, Hermus ARMM. A glucocorticoid education group meeting: an effective strategy for improving self-management to prevent adrenal crisis. Eur J Endocrinol. 2013;169(1):17–22.

Rosenfeld G, Bakker B. Compliance and persistence in pediatric and adult patients receiving growth hormone therapy. Endocr Pract. 2008;14(2):143.

Ruiz MA, Pardo A, Rejas J, Soto J, Villasante F, Aranguren JL. Development and validation of the "Treatment Satisfaction with Medicines Questionnaire" (SATMED-Q). Value Health. 2008;11(5):913–26.

Schoenfeld MJ, Shortridge E, Cui Z, Muram D. Medication adherence and treatment patterns for hypogonadal patients treated with topical testosterone therapy: a retrospective medical claims analysis. J Sex Med. 2013;10(5):1401.

Schulz J, Frey KR, Cooper M, Zopf K, Ventz M, Diederich S, et al. Reduction in daily hydrocortisone dose improves bone health in primary adrenal insufficiency. Eur J Endocrinol. 2016; https://doi.org/10.1530/eje-15-1096.

Sklar CA, Mertens AC, Mitby P, Occhiogrosso G, Qin J, Heller G, et al. Risk of disease recurrence and second neoplasms in survivors of childhood cancer treated with growth hormone: a report from the Childhood Cancer Survivor Study. J Clin Endocrinol Metabol. 2002;87(7):3136–41.

Sklar CA, Antal Z, Chemaitilly W, Cohen LE, Follin C, Meacham LR, et al. Hypothalamic-pituitary and growth disorders in survivors of childhood cancer: an Endocrine Society Clinical Practice Guideline. J Clin Endocrinol Metab. 2018;103:2761–84.

Sprogoe K, Mortensen E, Karpf DB, Leff JA. The rationale and design of TransCon Growth Hormone for the treatment of growth hormone deficiency. Endocr Connect. 2017;6(8):R171–R81.

Stochholm K, Kiess W. Long-term safety of growth hormone-a combined registry analysis. Clin Endocrinol (Oxf). 2018;88(4):515–28.

Strasburger CJ, Vanuga P, Payer J, Pfeifer M, Popovic V, Bajnok L, et al. MOD-4023, a long-acting carboxy-terminal peptide-modified human growth hormone: results of a Phase 2 study in growth hormone-deficient adults. Eur J Endocrinol. 2017;176(3):283–94.

Tiemensma J, Andela D, Pereira M, Romijn A, Biermasz R, Kaptein A. Patients with adrenal insufficiency hate their medication: concerns and stronger beliefs about the necessity of hydrocortisone intake are associated with more negative illness perceptions. J Clin Endocrinol Metab. 2014;99(10):3668.

Toogood AA, Stewart PM. Hypopituitarism: clinical features, diagnosis, and management. Endocrinol Metab Clin North Am. 2008;37(1):235–61. x

Wolthers T, Hoffman DM, Nugent AG, Duncan MW, Umpleby M, Ho KK. Oral estrogen antagonizes the metabolic actions of growth hormone in growth hormone-deficient women. Am J Physiol Endocrinol Metab. 2001;281(6):E1191–6.

Woodmansee WW, Zimmermann AG, Child CJ, Rong Q, Erfurth EM, Beck-Peccoz P, et al. Incidence of second neoplasm in childhood cancer survivors treated with GH: an analysis of GeNeSIS and HypoCCS. Eur J Endocrinol. 2013;168(4):565–73.

Yuen CJ, Conway S, Popovic V, Merriam R, Bailey T, Hamrahian H, et al. A long-acting human growth hormone with delayed clearance (VRS-317): results of a double-blind, placebo-controlled, single ascending dose study in growth hormone-deficient adults. J Clin Endocrinol Metab. 2013;98(6): 2595.

Zolnierek KB, Dimatteo MR. Physician communication and patient adherence to treatment: a meta-analysis. Med Care. 2009;47(8):826–34.

Key Reading

1. Burt MG, Ho KKY. Chapter 11 - Hypopituitarism and growth hormone deficiency. In: Jameson JL, de Groot LJ, de Kretser DM, Giudice LC, Grossman AB, Melmed S, Potts JT, Weir GC, editors. Endocrinology: adult and pediatric. 7th ed. Philadelphia: W.B. Saunders; 2016.

2. Clayton PE, Cuneo RC, Juul A, Monson JP, Shalet SM, Tauber M. Consensus statement on the management of the GH-treated adolescent in the transition to adult care. Eur J Endocrinol. 2005;152:165–70.

3. Fleseriu M, Hashim IA, karavitaki N, Melmed S, Murad MH, Salvatori R, Samuels MH. Hormonal replacement in hypopituitarism in adults: an Endocrine Society Clinical Practice Guideline. J Clin Endocrinol Metab. 2016;101:3888–921.

4. Molitch ME, Clemmons DR, Malozowski S, Merriam GR, Vance ML. Evaluation and treatment of adult growth hormone deficiency: an Endocrine Society clinical practice guideline. J Clin Endocrinol Metab. 2011;96:1587–609.

5. Toogood AA, Stewart PM. Hypopituitarism: clinical features, diagnosis, and management. Endocrinol Metab Clin North Am. 2008;37:235–61.

Part IV

The Thyroid Gland

Violet Fazal-Sanderson

Thyroid Anatomy and Physiology

26

Chloe Broughton and Bushra Ahmad

Contents

Abstract

The term anatomy can be defined as the study of structure and form of an organism including its body parts, while physiology refers to the study of how these structures function and work.

C. Broughton
Specialist Registrar in Endocrinology and Diabetes, Southmead Hospital, North Bristol NHS Trust, Bristol, UK
e-mail: chloebroughton@nhs.net

B. Ahmad (✉)
Consultant Endocrinologist and Senior Honorary Clinical Lecturer, Bristol Royal Infirmary, University of Bristol, Bristol, UK
e-mail: bushra.ahmad@nhs.net

This chapter outlines the anatomy of the thyroid gland, including the embryology and development, location, blood and nerve supply, and histology. It then details thyroid hormone physiology including thyroid hormone synthesis and secretion, transport and metabolism, and mechanism of action. It concludes with discussion of the thyroid hormone axis.

Relevant knowledge and understanding is fundamental to the understanding of thyroid disorders and key to underpinning care in clinical decision-making. Applying accurate knowledge of thyroid anatomy and physiology enables clinical practitioners to care, treat, and manage patients with thyroid disorders more effectively.

© Springer Nature Switzerland AG 2019
S. Llahana et al. (eds.), *Advanced Practice in Endocrinology Nursing*,
https://doi.org/10.1007/978-3-319-99817-6_26

Keywords

Thyroxine (T4) · Triiodothyronine (T3)
Anatomy · Thyroglobulin-iodine

Abbreviations

T3	Triiodothyronine
T4	Thyroxine
TBG	Thyroid-binding globulin
TPO	Thyroperoxidase
TRH	Thyrotropin-releasing hormone
TSH	Thyroid-stimulating hormone
TTR	Transthyretin

Key Terms

- **Calcitonin:** A protein hormone secreted by c cells in the thyroid gland.
- **Deiodinase:** An enzyme involved in the activation or deactivation of thyroid hormones.
- **Enzyme:** A substance that acts as a catalyst of a biochemical reaction.
- **Gland:** A group of cells secreting a particular chemical substance.
- **Hormone:** A chemical messenger that travels in the blood stream to target tissues or organs. It is produced by endocrine glands.
- **Hypothalamus:** A complex region of the brain lying above the pituitary gland.
- **Isthmus:** A small piece of thyroid tissue connecting the right and left lobes of the thyroid gland.
- **Pituitary gland:** A small gland located behind the eyes at the base of the brain. It secretes TSH, as well as other hormones.
- **Thyroglobulin:** A protein produced by the thyroid gland.
- **Thyroid:** An endocrine gland located in the anterior neck that produces thyroid hormones, thyroxine (T4) and triiodothyronine (T3).
- **Thyroid-stimulating hormone:** A hormone produced by the hypothalamus and secreted by the anterior pituitary gland. It stimulates the thyroid gland.
- **Thyroid-binding globulin:** A protein in the blood that binds with thyroxine (T4) and triiodothyronine (T3).

- **Thyroperoxidase:** An enzyme in the thyroid gland that plays an important role in the production of thyroid hormones.
- **Thyrotropin-releasing hormone:** A hormone that stimulates the release of TSH and prolactin by the pituitary gland.
- **Thyroxine:** The main hormone produced by the thyroid gland.
- **Transthyretin:** A protein in the blood that binds with thyroxine (T4) and triiodothyronine (T3).
- **Triiodothyronine:** The second hormone produced by the thyroid gland.

Key Points

- The thyroid gland develops as a diverticulum from the endoderm of the floor of the pharynx.
- The thyroid gland lies in the anterior neck. It is comprised of two lateral lobes joined in the midline by the isthmus. The thyroid gland is highly vascular and receives its arterial blood supply from the right and left superior and inferior thyroid arteries.
- Thyroid follicles are filled with colloid, the main constituent of which is thyroglobulin. Follicular cells surround the follicles and synthesise and secrete thyroid hormones. Parafollicular cells are found in-between follicles and secrete calcitonin.
- The primary function of the thyroid gland is the production of thyroid hormones: thyroxine (T4) and triiodothyronine (T3). The thyroid gland is the only source of T4 and secretes 20% of circulating T3. T4 and T3 act via nuclear receptors inside target cells.
- Thyroid hormones in the blood are tightly controlled by feedback mechanisms involving the hypothalamus-pituitary-thyroid axis.

26.1 Anatomy

The thyroid gland is one of the largest endocrine glands in the body, weighing between 10 and 20 g in adults (Pankow et al. 1985). It is larger in men than women and increases with age and body weight. It is one of the most vascular organs in the body.

26.1.1 Embryology and Development

The thyroid gland is the first endocrine gland to develop, with development occurring from the third week of gestation. It develops as a diverticulum from the endoderm of the floor of the pharynx. The diverticulum becomes bilobed; it descends down the neck and fuses with part of the fourth pharyngeal pouch. It is attached to the floor of the pharynx at this stage by the thyroglossal duct, which is usually obliterated after its decent. In about 55% of individuals, the distal portion persists as the pyramidal lobe. Other portions of the duct may persist as thyroglossal cysts. These present as a mass in the middle and can be excised surgically. By the seventh week of gestation, it has reached its final position anterior to the trachea.

The ultimobranchial body from the fifth pharyngeal pouch becomes infiltrated by neural crest cells and is incorporated into the developing thyroid gland. These cells migrate into the upper third of the thyroid lobes and are the source of the neuroendocrine parafollicular cells (C cells). The C cells make up 0.1% of the thyroid mass and are the source of calcitonin. They give rise to medullary thyroid cancer when they undergo malignant change.

The foetal thyroid begins to concentrate and organifies iodine by 10–12 weeks gestation. The foetal pituitary-thyroid axis is a functional unit distinct from that of the mother by 18–20 weeks gestation. The foetal production of thyroxine (T4) reaches a clinically significant level by 18–20 weeks gestation, but foetal triiodothyronine (T3) production remains low until 30 weeks gestation.

26.1.2 Location

The thyroid gland is located in the anterior neck. It sits just below the larynx and lies against the anterolateral portion of the trachea and oesophagus. It is bordered laterally by the carotid sheath, containing the carotid artery, internal jugular vein, vagus nerve, and deep cervical lymph nodes. Anteriorly, the sternocleidomastoid and the three strap muscles (sternohyoid, sternothyroid, and the superior belly of the omohyoid) overlie the gland.

The thyroid gland is often described as a butterfly-shaped structure. It is comprised of two lateral lobes joined in the midline by the isthmus. Each lobe is about 5 cm long, 3 cm wide, and 2 cm thick (Bliss et al. 2000). The isthmus is a narrow band of thyroid tissue overlying the second and third tracheal rings. A pyramidal lobe is often present (55% of cadaveric specimens (Braun et al. 2007)) projecting upwards from the isthmus.

26.1.3 Blood and Nerve Supply

The thyroid gland secretes thyroid hormones directly into the blood, and therefore, needs to be highly vascular. Each lobe of the thyroid gland receives its arterial blood supply from the right and left superior and inferior thyroid arteries. The superior thyroid artery arises from the external carotid artery and supplies the superior and anterior portions of the gland. The inferior thyroid artery is a branch of the thyrocervical trunk, which arises from the subclavian artery and supplies the posterior and inferior portions of the gland. There are three main veins draining the thyroid gland: superior, middle, and inferior thyroid veins (Fig. 26.1).

The thyroid gland receives parasympathetic nerve innervation from the recurrent laryngeal nerve and the superior laryngeal nerve. However, these nerves do not control endocrine secretion—this is under control of the pituitary gland. It is essential that these nerves are identified during surgery to prevent damage or ligation of the nerves, resulting in paresis or paralysis of the vocal cords.

Fig. 26.1 The thyroid gland with its blood supply. From: Ritchie JE, Balasubramanian SP. Anatomy of the pituitary, thyroid, parathyroid, and adrenal glands. Surgery (Oxford) Volume 32, Issue 10, October 2014, Pages 499–503

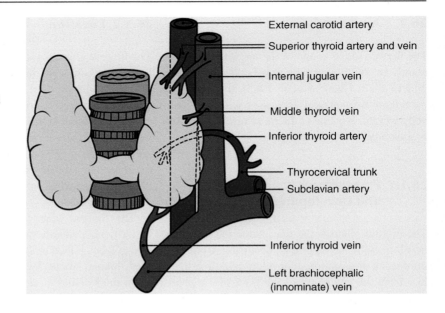

26.2 Histology

Under the microscope, there are three main features of the thyroid gland: follicles, follicular cells, and parafollicular cells (Fawcett and Jensh 2002). Follicles are roughly spherical cavities filled with colloid, a proteinaceous deposit of thyroid hormone precursor. The major constituent of colloid is a large glycoprotein called thyroglobulin. Surrounding the follicles is a single layer of epithelial cells known as follicular cells. These cells are responsible for synthesising and secreting thyroid hormones (T3 and T4). Follicular cells are normally cuboidal in shape, but become columnar when stimulated and squamous when inactive. Parafollicular cells or C cells are found in between follicles and secrete the hormone calcitonin.

Increased thyroid activity over a period of time is usually associated with a decrease in colloid and a reduction in follicular volume. Follicular cells hypertrophy and increase in number; they also become columnar and may proliferate into the colloid. Decreased thyroid activity is associated with a flattening of the follicular cells.

26.3 Physiology

The primary function of the thyroid gland is the production of thyroid hormones. There are two biologically active thyroid hormones: thyroxine (T4) and triiodothyronine (T3).

26.3.1 Thyroid Hormone Synthesis, Storage, and Secretion

The following steps are involved in the synthesis, storage, and secretion of thyroid hormones (Fig. 26.2):

1. Thyroglobulin production by follicular cell and release into colloid by exocytosis.
2. Dietary iodine ingestion, iodine uptake by follicular cell from the blood and transferred to colloid.
3. Oxidation of iodine and iodination of thyroglobulin tyrosine residues (attachments of iodine to tyrosine on the thyroglobulin in colloid).
4. Coupling processes between the iodinated tyrosine molecules to form T4 and T3.

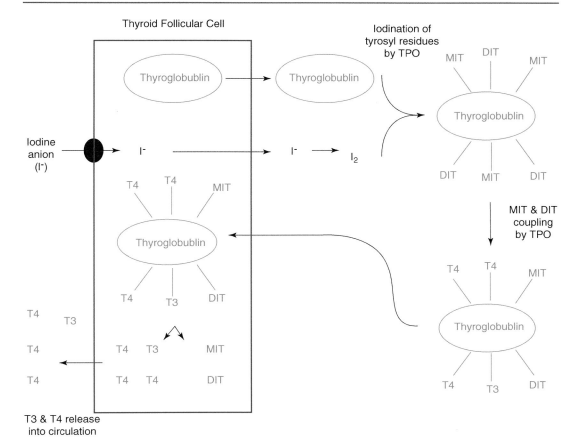

Fig. 26.2 Thyroid hormone synthesis, storage, and secretion

5. Secretion (upon stimulation) of T4 and T3 occurs by endocytosis of a piece of colloid, uncoupling of T4 and T3 and diffusion out of the follicular cell into the blood.

Iodine is essential for normal thyroid function and can be obtained only by consumption of food containing iodine or to which it is added. Iodine is present naturally in soil and seawater. The availability of iodine in food differs in various regions of the world. Iodine is found in seafood, kelp, dairy products and eggs, iodised salt, or dietary supplements as a trace mineral. The recommended minimum intake is 150 μg per day. Dietary iodine reaches the circulation as iodine anion (I−). The thyroid gland transports I− to the site of hormone synthesis. I− accumulation in the thyroid is an active transport process that is stimulated by TSH.

Iodine anion must be oxidised to be able to iodinate tyrosyl residues of thyroglobulin. Iodination of the tyrosyl residues then forms monoiodotyrosine (MIT) and diiodotyrosine (DIT), which are then coupled to form either T3 or T4. Both reactions are catalysed by TPO.

Thyroperoxidase (TPO) catalyses the oxidation steps involved in iodine anion activation, iodination of thyroglobulin tyrosyl residues, and coupling of iodotyrosyl residues. TPO has binding sites for iodine anion and thyroxine. Furthermore, TPO also uses H_2O_2 as the oxidate to activate iodine anion to hypoiodate (OI−), the iodination species.

T3 and T4 are synthesised and stored within the thyroglobulin molecule. Proteolysis is an essential step for releasing the hormones. To liberate T4 and T3, thyroglobulin is resorbed from the follicular cells in the form of colloid droplets, which fuse with lysosomes to form phagolysosomes. Thyroglobulin is hydrolysed to T4 and T3, which are then secreted into the circulation.

26.3.2 Peripheral Conversion of Thyroid Hormone

The thyroid is the only source of T4. The thyroid secretes 20% of circulating T3. The remainder is generated in extra glandular tissues by the conversion of T4 to T3 by deiodinases. There are three iodothyroinine deiodinases (D1-D3) which regulate the availability of T3 to the cells. Type 1 deiodinase is located primarily in the thyroid, liver, and kidneys. This is considered responsible for the production of the majority of circulating T3. Type 2 deiodinase is found primarily in the pituitary gland, brain, brown fat, and thyroid gland. Type 1 and 2 deiodinase result in generation of T3, whereas D3 irreversible inactivates T4 and T3, resulting in production of rT3 and T2. The relative activities of D2 and D3 enzymes in T3 target cells regulate the availability of the active hormone T3 to the nucleus. Type 1 deiodinase has a relatively low affinity for T4, whereas type 2 deiodinase has a much higher affinity.

26.3.3 Thyroid Hormone Transport and Metabolism

About 20 times more T4 is secreted from the thyroid gland than T3. Both T4 and T3 are highly lipophilic, and once in the blood, immediately bind to proteins. 99.98% of T4 and 99.7% of T3 are protein-bound. 70–80% of T4 is bound to thyroid-binding globulin, a thyroid hormone-specific protein. The remainder is bound to transthyretin (TTR) and albumin (Benvenga 2005). T3 is bound 10–20 times less avidly by TBG. T3 is not bound significantly by TTR. Only free T4 and T3 hormones are biologically active and it's the free hormones that produce the effects of thyroid hormones on peripheral tissues and pituitary feedback mechanism. Therefore, free thyroid hormone concentration correlates more closely with the metabolic state rather than the total hormone concentration.

26.3.4 Thyroid Hormone Action

T4 and T3 enter cells by both passive diffusion and active transport via specific transporters, for example, monocarboxylate 8 (MCT8) transporter (Friesema et al. 2003). Once inside the cell, thyroid hormones act via nuclear receptors, thyroid hormone receptors (TR's) α and β (Flamant et al. 2006). The expression of TRα and TRβ varies between tissues, and hence, their roles are tissue-specific. TRα is expressed in the brain, kidneys, gonads, muscle, and heart and mediates effects of T3 in these tissues. TRβ is expressed in the hypothalamus, pituitary, and liver, and therefore, has a role in the feedback control of the hypothalamic pituitary-thyroid axis. The activated receptors can either stimulate or inhibit gene transcription.

26.3.5 Regulation of the Thyroid Axis

The thyroid axis is a classic example of an endocrine feedback loop (Fig. 26.3). Thyroid-releasing hormone (TRH) is secreted by the hypothalamus. This stimulates the pituitary to produce TSH. TSH stimulates the thyroid gland to synthesis and secrete thyroid hormones, mainly T4 but also T3. Thyroid hormones feedback at both the pituitary and hypothalamus to inhibit production of TRH and TSH, respectively, predominantly through thyroid hormone receptor β2. The levels of thyroid hormones in the blood are tightly controlled by these feedback mechanisms in the hypothalamic-pituitary-thyroid axis.

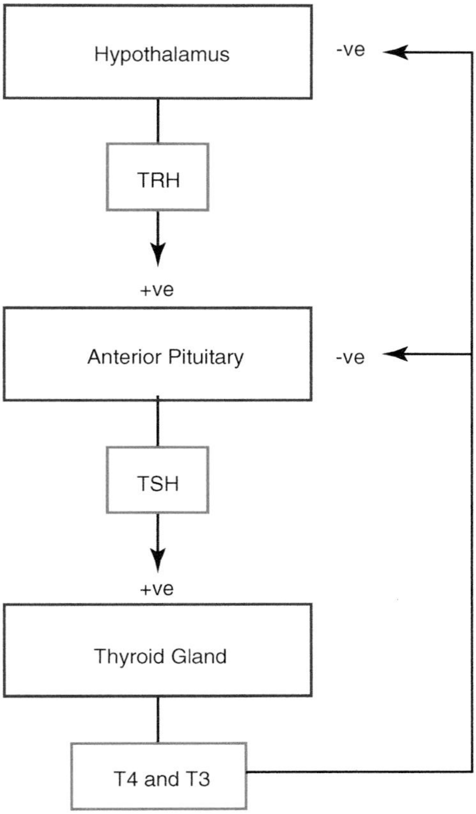

Fig. 26.3 Hypothalamic pituitary-thyroid axis

isthmus and is highly vascular. Thyroid follicular cells synthesise and secrete thyroid hormones. There are two biologically active thyroid hormones: thyroxine (T4) and triiodothyronine (T3). T4 and T3 act via nuclear receptors within target cells to regulate metabolism. The levels of thyroid hormones in the blood are tightly controlled by these feedback mechanisms in the hypothalamic-pituitary-thyroid axis.

References

Benvenga S. Thyroid hormone transport proteins and the physiology of hormone binding. In: Braverman LE, Utiger RD, editors. The thyroid: fundamental and clinical text. 9th ed. Philadelphia: Lippincott Williams and Wilkins; 2005. p. 97.

Bliss RD, Gauger PG, Delbridge LW. Surgeon's approach to the thyroid gland: surgical anatomy and the importance of technique. World J Surg. 2000;24:891.

Braun EM, Windisch G, Wolf G, et al. The pyramidal lobe: clinical anatomy and its importance in thyroid surgery. Surg Radiol Anat. 2007;29:21.

Fawcett D, Jensh R. Bloom & Fawcett's concise histology. New York: Arnold Publishers; 2002. p. 257–8. ISBN 0-340-80677-X.

Flamant F, Baxter JD, Forrest D, Refetoff S, Samuels H, Scanlan TS, Vennstrom B, Samarut J. International Union of Pharmacology. LIX. The pharmacology and classification of the nuclear receptor superfamily: thyroid hormone receptors. Pharmacol Rev. 2006;58(4):705–11.

Friesema EC, Ganguly S, Abdalla A, Manning Fox JE, Halestrap AP, Visser TJ. Identification of monocarboxylate transporter 8 as a specific thyroid hormone transporter. J Biol Chem. 2003;278(41):40128–35.

Pankow BG, Michalak J, McGee MK. Adult human thyroid weight. Health Phys. 1985;49:1097.

26.4   Conclusions

The thyroid gland is a butterfly-shaped gland located in the anterior neck. It is comprised of two lateral lobes joined in the midline by the

Thyroid Investigations

27

Victoria J. Stokes, Rabia Arfan, Theingi Aung,
and Violet Fazal-Sanderson

Contents

V. J. Stokes
Endocrinology and Metabolism, Oxford Radcliffe
Hospitals NHS Foundation Trust, Churchill Hospital,
Oxford, UK
e-mail: victoria.stokes4@nhs.net

R. Arfan
Thames Valley Deanary, Centre for Diabetes and
Endocrinology, Royal Berkshire Hospital NHS
Foundation Trust, Reading, UK

T. Aung · V. Fazal-Sanderson (✉)
Centre for Diabetes and Endocrinology, Royal
Berkshire Hospital NHS Foundation Trust,
Reading, UK
e-mail: Theingi.aung@royalberkshire.nhs.uk;
Violet.sanderson@royalberkshire.nhs.uk

© Springer Nature Switzerland AG 2019
S. Llahana et al. (eds.), *Advanced Practice in Endocrinology Nursing*,
https://doi.org/10.1007/978-3-319-99817-6_27

Abstract

Thyroid dysfunction may result in inappropriate hormone secretion, mass effects, or a combination of both problems. Taking a relevant history and performing a thorough examination is the first step to reaching the correct diagnosis. Investigations should be selected according to the clinical findings and may be used to confirm clinical suspicions, to rule out serious pathology, and to establish the severity of the dysfunction. Blood tests are usually the first line, with biochemistry to confirm the functional status of the gland and, if appropriate, testing for autoantibodies to confirm autoimmunity. Ultrasound is the preferred method for detecting intra-thyroid lesions, with a sensitivity of 2 mm for cystic, and 3 mm for solid lesions. CT and MRI are of limited utility outside of tumour staging. Functional imaging is useful for differentiating thyroiditis and hyperthyroidism due to autoimmunity, toxic nodule, or multinodular goitre. This chapter describes the clinical features of different thyroid disorders; discusses thyroid investigations and their clinical utility; and highlights specific tests used for specific disorders.

Keywords

Thyroid hormone homeostasis · Imaging
Clinical assessment · Thyroid autoantibodies
TSH-oma

Abbreviations

bHCG	Beta human chorionic gonadotropin
CT	Computer tomography
FNA/C	Fine needle aspiration/cytology
fT3	Triiodothyronine
fT4	Thyroxine
MRI	Magnetic resonance imaging
RTSH	Resistance to thyroid stimulating hormone
TG Ab	Antithyroglobulin antibody
TIRADS	Thyroid imaging reporting and data system
TPOAbs	Antithyroid peroxidase antibody
TSH	Thyroid stimulating hormone
TSHoma	Thyroid stimulating hormone secreting pituitary adenoma
TSH receptor antibody	Thyroid stimulating hormone receptor antibody
US	Ultrasound

Key Terms

- **CT:** Computed tomography is a useful imaging technique that is used, for example, to evaluate any thyroid retrosternal or retro-tracheal extension of an enlarged thyroid, and also can be used to look for thyroid cancer spread into distant organs.
- **FNAB:** Fine needle aspiration biopsy is a procedure by which a fine needle is inserted into a mass, for example, a thyroid nodule/s, and is used to draw tissue cells for diagnostic purposes.
- **MRI:** Magnetic resonance is a useful imaging technique that gives a more detailed image of the body's soft tissue, for example, can be used to look for cancer of the thyroid gland and distant spread.
- **TG Ab:** Thyroglobulin antibody blood test. Thyroglobulin is a thyroid glycosylated iodoprotein secreted by the thyroid follicular cells and involved in the production of active thyroid hormone. In the presence of autoimmune disease, antibodies attack the thyroid and disrupt thyroglobulin production, resulting in increased antiTPO antibodies. Also used as a tumour marker in thyroid cancers.
- **TPO Ab:** Thyroid peroxidase antibody. Thyroid peroxidase is an enzyme found in the thyroid gland and involved in thyroid hormone production. A TPO antibody blood test is used to detect antibodies against TPO, and the presence of antibodies usually suggests an autoimmune thyroid disease.
- **TRH:** Thyroid-releasing hormone. A thyrotropin-releasing factor (thyroliberin), a neurohormone produced by the hypothalamus that stimulates the anterior pituitary to release TSH hormone.
- **TSH-oma:** Thyroid stimulating hormone (TSH) or thyrotropinoma. A benign pituitary tumour that secretes excess TSH. Characterized by high levels of circulating TSH, fT4, and fT3.
- **TSH-R ab:** TSH receptor antibody. Thyroid stimulating hormone receptor is a G-protein coupled receptor expressed in the thyroid and important for cell activation. TSH-R abs are associated with thyroid pathogenesis and the cause of autoimmune thyrotoxicosis such as Graves' disease. Antibodies bind to the TSH receptor and cause production of thyroid hormone, growth, and vascularization of the thyroid gland.

Key Points

- Relevant history combined with thorough clinical examination is a important first step for diagnosis of thyroid disorder supported by appropriate investigations. TSH, FT3, and FT4 results must be interpreted with caution taking into account of assay variation and possible interference.
- TSH receptor antibody is a reliable, sensitive, and specific test in diagnosis of Graves disease and if TSH receptor antibody is a positive, uptake scan is not indicated to confirm Graves' disease. TPO Abs is most sensitive test for autoimmune thyroiditis and in post-partum thyroiditis.
- Ultrasound is the most sensitive method for diagnosing thyroid nodule or intrathyroid lesions. Current methods of ultrasonography allow identification of 2 mm cystic lesions and 3 mm solid intra-thyroid lesions. FNAC is indicated for single or multiple nodules for excluding malignancies after the US feature analysis.
- CT scanning is useful in evaluating lymphadenopathy, local tumour extension, extension into the mediastinum and retro-tracheal region and metastasis disease staging.
- Thyroid uptake scan has particular role of functional status of the gland differentiating between hot and cold nodules and Graves' hyperthyroid vs. thyroiditis. Differentiating Graves' disease and thyroiditis is crucial as the management is different.

27.1 Introduction

Thyroid dysfunction may be due to biochemical abnormalities, i.e. dysregulated secretion of thyroid hormones resulting in hyper- or hypothyroidism, changes in the physical characteristics of the gland itself, such as the development of a lump or diffuse enlargement that may produce mass effects or a combination of both biochemical and structural changes. Thyroid investigations can be used as a tool to screen for these problems, i.e. to test for dysfunction in a patient suspected of having thyroid disease or to obtain further information about a known thyroid problem. The information provided from the results of investigations is only as useful as the clinician's interpretation of them. Before ordering a particular test it is important to know what questions are being asked, and how the answers are going to inform the management of the patient. In a patient who is suspected of having thyroid dysfunction it is important to know:

- Is there any hormonal dysfunction, i.e. hyper- or hypothyroidism?
- What is causing the hormonal dysfunction? i.e. autoimmunity? "hot nodules"? or medications?
- Is there a problem due to mass effect from the thyroid itself?
- How severe is the problem?

27.2 Clinical Assessment of a Patient with Thyroid Disease

The thyroid hormones, thyroxine (T4), and triiodothyronine (T3), act on almost every cell in the body to alter the metabolic rate, affect growth, and maturation and to increase sensitivity to catecholamines, therefore over- or under-production of these hormones may result in a vast array of symptoms determined by the history, and signs found on clinical examination.

Symptoms are often highly variable between patients, for example, it is not uncommon for hyperthyroid patients to feel tired (this may be related to poor sleep), and hypothyroid patients may lose weight. Patients may also experience or describe symptoms in different ways, e.g. one person may experience the neurological effects of hypothyroidism as a "fuzzy head", another as "tiredness" and another as "lethargy and depression". The timing and onset of symptoms can also be informative. For example, the onset of hyperthyroid symptoms shortly after delivery suggests post-partum thyroiditis, and the onset of a tender gland and hyperthyroid symptoms shortly after a viral illness suggests De Quervain's thyroiditis. These are important diagnoses to make as they are often self-limiting and are therefore managed differently to Graves' disease. Similarly, a small smooth thyroid nodule that has been present and stable for many years suggests a benign thyroid adenoma, this is far less concerning than a short history of a hard and irregular rapidly enlarging thyroid nodule which may suggest a thyroid carcinoma, and therefore requires more urgent investigation.

The thyroid gland is anatomically close to the larynx, trachea, oesophagus, and jugular veins and an enlarging thyroid gland, or a thyroid nodule, may compress any of these structures and cause local mass effects (Table 27.5), all of which are "red flag" symptoms that indicate the presence of potentially serious pathology (Table 27.1). Most patients are very sensitive to a sense of fullness in the neck, and patients may experience symptoms of a sore throat, dysphagia, or dysphonia with only minimal thyroid gland enlargement on examination. Conversely, occasionally patients with a very large goitre that has been present for many years will be relatively asymptomatic.

27.3 Thyroid Hormones

27.3.1 Thyroid Hormones and Homeostasis

The thyroid gland produces two hormones, thyroxine (T4), which is weakly biologically active, and triiodothyronine (T3), which is 3–5 times

Table 27.1 History and examination findings: Red flag symptoms and signs

System	Symptoms	Signs
Neuro	Anxiety Poor sleep May feel more impatient/angry than usual Difficulty relaxing May experience abnormal thoughts	Appears anxious, tired, agitated Fine peripheral tremor Pressure of speech Occasionally psychosis
CVS	Palpitations Breathlessness Reduced exercise tolerance	Tachycardia Atrial fibrillation Heart failure
GIS	Diarrhoea Borborygmi Weight loss often despite good appetite	Signs of weight loss
Other	Heat intolerance	Dressed inappropriately for the conditions Sweating Warm peripheries Lid retraction Lid lag

Table 27.2 Findings associated with thyroid hormone excess

System	Symptoms	Signs
Neuro	Anxiety Poor sleep May feel more impatient/angry than usual Difficulty relaxing May experience abnormal thoughts	Appears anxious, tired, agitated Fine peripheral tremor Pressure of speech Occasionally psychosis
CVS	Palpitations Breathlessness Reduced exercise tolerance	Tachycardia Atrial fibrillation Heart failure
GIS	Diarrhoea Borborygmi Weight loss often despite good appetite	Signs of weight loss
Other	Heat intolerance	Dressed inappropriately for the conditions Sweating Warm peripheries Lid retraction Lid lag

more potent than T4. T4 and T3 are released into the circulation at a ratio of 14–20:1, and T4 is converted into the more active T3 within cells (Wiersinga 2001) T4 has a much longer half-life than T3, largely due to being strongly bound to plasma thyroid hormone-binding proteins (Schussler 2000), so acts as a "pool" of thyroid hormone to help maintain homeostasis (Table 27.2). As the majority of circulating T4 and T3 is protein-bound, and therefore not biologically active, free T4 (FT4) and free T3 (FT3) are measured in clinical practice. The production of T4 and T3 is maintained within tight limits to maintain normal functioning of the body tissues. This homeostasis is maintained through the hypothalamic-pituitary-thyroid axis. The hypothalamus produces thyrotropin-releasing hormone (TRH) in response to low circulating levels of T4 and T3. TRH stimulates the pituitary to produce thyroid stimulating hormone (TSH), which in turn stimulates the thyroid gland to produce more T4 and T3. TRH is not routinely measured in clinical practice. As the levels of T4 and T3 rise, they exert negative feedback on both the hypothalamus and pituitary, the production of TRH and TSH attenuate, and the thyroid reduces the production of T4 and T3 (Sec.4. Chap. 27).

The vast majority of patients with thyroid hormone dysfunction will have a problem arising in the thyroid gland itself, so the hypothalamus and pituitary can be assumed to be reacting appropriately to the prevailing thyroid hormone levels. Therefore, in most situations, a TSH level within normal limits suggests that the levels of T4 and T3 are normal. For this reason, some laboratories will measure only TSH as a screening test, rather than TSH, FT3, and FT4. If the thyroid gland over-secretes T4 and T3 (e.g. in Graves' disease), the hypothalamus and pituitary detect these high levels and appropriately reduce production of TRH and TSH. Conversely, if the thyroid gland fails to make enough T4 and T3 (e.g. in autoimmune hypothyroidism), these low levels are detected by the hypothalamus and pituitary, TRH secretion increases appropriately and therefore the pituitary increases TSH secretion appropriately.

Table 27.3 Findings associated with thyroid hormone deficit

System	Symptoms	Signs
Neuro	Tiredness Mental fogginess Lethargy Depression	Appears tired Slow speech
CVS	Breathlessness	Bradycardia Signs of heart failure Pleural effusion
GIS	Constipation Weight gain despite constant/reduced food intake	Constipation Ascites
Other	Cold intolerance	Dressed inappropriately for the conditions Cool peripheries Deepening of voice Hypothyroid facies

Rarely, the primary defect is outside of the thyroid gland and the TSH level may be misleading. These conditions are rare but should be considered where the patient's symptoms and signs do not fit with the TSH result, or if there is clinical suspicion of a condition affecting the pituitary or hypothalamus. Central hypothyroidism is usually due to a problem with the pituitary gland that prevents it from responding to TRH, T4 and T3, and from secreting adequate amounts of TSH. Causes include compression of the gland by a tumour, apoplexy, surgery, radiotherapy, autoimmune hypophysitis (primary or drug related), and infection. In this situation, T4 and T3 levels fall and the patient develops symptoms of hypothyroidism, but will have either a low TSH or TSH at the lower end of the normal range that is inappropriate for the circulating low levels of T4 and T3. The pituitary gland is involved in the regulation of many other hormonal axes in addition to the thyroid axis, so patients with pituitary damage may well have symptoms of other hormonal deficits including hypoadrenalism and hypogonadism (Table 27.3). Very rarely, the pituitary may develop an adenoma that autonomously secretes TSH resulting in central hyperthyroidism. These adenomas are called TSH-omas. Dysfunction of the hypothalamus is very rare and is usually apparent before symptoms and signs of thyroid dysfunction develop.

27.3.2 Caution When Interpreting Thyroid Function Tests

When thyroid hormone levels are measured, they are usually reported by the lab with "normal reference ranges". These ranges are derived from a healthy population (i.e. where the hypothalamus, pituitary, and thyroid gland are working normally). Results at the extremes, i.e. the highest and lowest 2.5% of this "normal" population are excluded, so the "normal reference range" is the range of results that can be expected in 95% of healthy individuals. Therefore, 5% of healthy individuals will have an "abnormal result" at any one time (2.5% below the lower limit of the reference range, and 2.5% above the upper limit of the reference range). It should also be noted that occasionally individuals who are developing thyroid dysfunction may have blood test results within the normal range, for example, at the onset of hyperthyroidism, TSH may begin to drop and T4 may begin to rise but still be in the normal range. It is therefore unusual to start treatment based on the results of one abnormal blood test and good practice to have at least one repeat result and to interpret blood test results in the context of the overall clinical picture.

27.3.3 Thyroid Autoantibodies

The presence of thyroid autoantibodies can help to confirm whether the aetiology of thyroid dysfunction is autoimmune. The thyroid autoantibodies most commonly tested for are antithyroid peroxidase antibody (TPO Ab), antithyroglobulin antibody (TG Ab), and TSH receptor antibody (TSH-R Ab).

TPO Abs are the most sensitive antibody for autoimmune thyroiditis. They are elevated in virtually all cases of Hashimoto's thyroiditis and up to 65% of cases of Graves' disease. However, they have a low specificity, with a prevalence of between 8.6 and 11.3% in the normal population (Hollowell et al. 2002; Deshpande et al. 2016). TG Ab may also be elevated in autoimmune thy-

Table 27.4 Findings associated with an autoimmune aetiology

Graves' disease	Hashimoto's
Graves' eye disease—proptosis, difficulty closing eye, periorbital oedema, squint, injected cornea, corneal ulceration, reduced visual acuity	Pretibial myxoedema
Thyroid acropachy	

Table 27.5 Findings associated with mass effects

Laryngeal compression	Change in quality of the voice Stridor
Oesophageal compression	Dysphagia to solids than liquids
SVC obstruction	Flushed face Distended veins on chest and neck Sensation of stuffiness/fullness in head Change in vision/consciousness on bending forwards, coughing, raising arms above head headache
Other	Tethering Rapid growth Irregular surface Hard

roiditis, but also has a low specificity, present in 10.4% of patients without thyroid dysfunction, and it is therefore for not routinely tested for in thyroid hormone dysfunction. TSH Abs are formed against the TSH receptors in the thyroid gland, and activate them abnormally, resulting in an inappropriately elevated TSH secretion. They are both sensitive and specific for Graves' disease (Tozzoli et al. 2012).

Patients with autoimmune thyroid disease may, therefore, have a combination of these auto-antibodies, for example, a patient with Graves' disease may have positive TPO Ab, TSH-R Ab, and TG Ab. As these antibodies are present in the normal healthy population, their presence does not necessarily indicate that the patient has thyroid dysfunction (Table 27.4). Therefore, in practice, they are usually only assessed after thyroid dysfunction has been established to help determine the dysfunction or to guide treatment decisions in the setting of subclinical hypothyroidism (Table 27.5).

27.4 Imaging

The role of plain radiography in the evaluation of thyroid disease is limited. Plain radiographs can show soft tissue masses, tracheal deviation, a retrosternal extension of goitre, calcification in thyroid tumours and metastatic lung disease, but are neither sensitive nor specific. The patterns of calcification from thyroid cancer seen on plain X-ray overlap with those of benign disease, tracheal deviation/stenosis can result from causes other than retrosternal and goitre extension, metastasis in lungs or bone may arise from several primary sites.

27.5 Ultrasound

Ultrasound (US) is the most sensitive method for diagnosing intra-thyroid lesions. Current methods of ultrasonography allow identification of 2 mm cystic lesions and 3 mm solid intra-thyroid lesions (Mandel 2004; Miki et al. 1993). Doppler US helps in estimating overall and regional blood flow to thyroid. However, caution should be taken when relying on the US features alone as results do not correlate perfectly with histopathologic findings. Solid nodules are described as isoechoic if their texture closely resembles that of normal thyroid tissue, hyperechoic if more echogenic and hypoechoic if less echogenic.

The main clinical uses of ultrasonography are:

- To assess the anatomic features of thyroid nodules
- To monitor nodular thyroid disease
- To assist in interventional procedures such as fine needle aspiration (FNA) of thyroid, cervical lymph nodes and thyroid ablation
- To assist in the planning of thyroid cancer surgery
- To assist in surveillance for recurrence in patients with thyroid cancer
- To screen for presence of thyroid nodules in high-risk groups
- To assess fetal goitre

Ultrasound should be performed on all patients with nodules incidentally noted on other imaging studies as non-palpable nodules have approximately the same risk of malignancy as palpable nodules. US may be the only investigation required for haemorrhagic cysts due to their characteristic appearance. Clots may be hyperechoic and after liquefaction may become hypoechoic. A haemorrhagic nodule which looks part cystic and part solid is called a complex nodule.

Ultrasonography also plays an important role in detecting cervical lymphadenopathy in a patient with a thyroid nodule or newly diagnosed thyroid cancer. The US guided aspiration biopsy of enlarged cervical lymph nodes for cytological and immunohistological analysis can differentiate metastasis from thyroid cancer and inflammatory lymphadenopathy. US is also the most frequently used imaging procedure for long-term monitoring of patients with thyroid cancer for recurrence in the thyroid bed after total thyroidectomy or lobectomy. A major advantage of US over functional imaging is that the procedure can be performed without discontinuing thyroxine therapy, therefore, avoiding the risk of hypothyroidism.

27.5.1 Characteristics of Nodules Used for Identifying Cancers

- *Vascularity:* US evidence of vascular invasion may be a most reliable predictor of malignancy but is an uncommon finding.
- *The intensity of echoes:* Malignant thyroid nodules often have a hypoechoic appearance on the US but many benign nodules are less echoic than surrounding normal thyroid tissue. The sensitivity and specificity of a hypoechoic appearance are approximately 53% and 73%, respectively.
- *The sharpness of border:* Typically, 96% benign lesions are well defined and malignant lesions are mostly with irregular margins. However, the sharpness of the nodule border has a lower diagnostic value, and an ill-defined edge of nodule may be a marker of aggressive characteristics of papillary thyroid cancer.

- *Halo:* The "halo" is the name given to the interface between thyroid tissue and nodule which is less echogenic than either of two. The partition could be a capsule, or compressed or atrophied thyroid tissue. An incomplete or absent halo has been reported as a feature of malignancy with poor sensitivity and specificity (Daumerie et al. 1998).
- *Calcifications:* Calcifications are often present in both benign and malignant nodules. Punctate calcifications in the range of 1 mm are uncommonly seen and suggest microscopic psammoma bodies in papillary carcinomas. Peripheral or egg shell calcification is indicative of chronicity and seen in benign lesions (Brunese et al. 2008; Jakobsen 2001; Kwak et al. 2007). Coarse scattered calcification may be seen in haemorrhagic benign or malignant nodules. Large areas of calcification may be a feature of medullary thyroid cancer.
- *Internal structure:* A layered appearance of the echo pattern described as "spongiform" is a useful predictor of benign lesions (Bonavita et al. 2009). The uniformity of internal structure of nodule is not a useful indicator for diagnosis of cancer.
- *The shape of nodule:* Cancers frequently have a tall and narrow shape. An anteroposterior and transverse diameter ratio greater than 1 in combination with other suspicious characteristic has better predictive value (Bonavita et al. 2009; Cappelli et al. 2005).
- *Nodule size:* Large nodule diameter or size and volume may be predictive of the likelihood of thyroid cancer and prognosis (Kiernan and Solórzano 2017; Cavallo et al. 2017).

No single US criterion is reliable in differentiating benign thyroid nodules from malignant ones in isolation (Cappelli et al. 2007; Sipos 2009). The American college of Radiology has proposed a risk stratification system for the ultrasonic appearance of thyroid lesions called Thyroid Imaging Reporting and Data System (TIRADS). Five characteristics of the thyroid mass (composition, echogenicity, shape, margin, and echogenic foci) are graded individually, and then the information is combined to provide an overall score that is predictive for the risk of malignancy. These are TIRADS 1: normal thyroid, TIRADS 2: benign lesions, TIRADS 3: probably benign lesions, TIRADS 4: suspicious lesions, TIRADS 5: probably malignant lesions and TIRADS 6: biopsy proved lesions (Singaporewalla et al. 2017).

27.5.2 The Use of Ultrasound in Assessing for Fetal Thyroid Dysfunction

Ultrasonography is also used to assess the fetal thyroid gland, diagnose fetal goitre, or thyroid dysfunction and to facilitate therapy. Thus, it can reduce obstetric complications and contribute to neonatal health. In mothers with Graves' disease, US by an experienced ultrasonographer is an excellent diagnostic tool which can facilitate assessment of fetal thyroid function (Luton et al. 2005; Cohen et al. 2003). The detection of a fetal goitre on US in conjunction with clinical features such as fetal tachycardia, intrauterine growth retardation, and occasionally cord blood sample showing high levels of free T3, free T4 and suppressed fetal TSH levels indicate fetal thyrotoxicosis. Conversely, fetal goitre without clinical manifestation of fetal thyrotoxicosis may suggest overtreatment of the mother with anti-thyroid drugs and prompt a dose reduction.

27.6 Computed Tomography

CT is not a sensitive technique for demonstrating intra-thyroid lesions. However, it may be useful in evaluating lymphadenopathy, local tumour extension, extension into the mediastinum and retro-tracheal region, and for tumour staging. Thyroid cancer is suggested by certain patterns of calcification within a thyroid mass and when extension into surrounding structures is visualized. Regional lymphadenopathy in association with a thyroid mass is also suggestive of thyroid malignancy. However, thyroid cancers can be missed on CT scans in the presence of multinodular goitre.

27.7 Magnetic Resonance Imaging

MRI is useful in detecting local extension of thyroid neoplasm, spread of disease in the mediastinum or retro-tracheal region, and to assess lymphadenopathy.

Magnetic resonance spectroscopy may be of value in assessing the malignancy of follicular thyroid specimens, taken either through fine needle aspiration or surgery, where differentiation is difficult on basis of cytology. Performing hydrogen spectroscopy at 360 MHz has demonstrated the ratio of peaks at 1.7 and 0.9 ppm, and it can be used to differentiate benign from malignant lesions. Values higher than a ratio of 1.1 is normal and ratios lower than 1.1 indicate malignancy. Normal tissue can be differentiated from papillary and medullary carcinoma with a sensitivity of approximately 95%.

27.8 Nuclear Imaging

Nuclear imaging provides information on both the function and anatomy of the gland. It is contraindicated in patients who are pregnant because of the risk of exposing the fetus to radiation and is not recommended for breast-feeding women. In the past, radionuclide imaging was performed to differentiate malignant from benign lesions; however, 4% of hot nodules are shown to contain tumour compared with 16% of cold nodules (Daumerie et al. 1998). Thus, radionuclide imaging is unreliable in excluding or confirming the presence of cancer.

27.9 Iodine-123 or Iodine-131

Radioactive iodine has many advantages. The short 13.3-h half-life, the 159-keV principal photon and the absence of particulate emission allow for good imaging with modest patient radiation exposure. Metastatic cancer is imaged well because ½ of papillary carcinoma and 2/3 of follicular carcinoma are sufficiently iodine avid to allow their visualization. However, this isotope is cyclotron produced and therefore relatively expensive. In addition, its short half-life necessitates frequent shipment from the producer adding to the cost.

27.10 Technetium-99m Pertechnetate

Technetium-99m is commonly used as it is an inexpensive and readily available isotope which delivers a low dose radiation because of its short 6-h half-life and favourable decay scheme without particulate emission. A gamma camera using a 140-keV photon is used for imaging. However, disadvantages include decreased sensitivity within the mediastinum due to uptake in the oesophagus, poor image quality when uptake is low and, as it is trapped but not organified, it cannot be used to assess organification defects.

27.11 Gallium-67

Gallium-67 may be useful when thyroid lymphoma is suspected, but generally is of limited utility as it does not enable sufficient differentiation between malignant and benign lesions.

27.12 Role of Functional Imaging for Thyroiditis

Subacute thyroiditis is a clinical syndrome that manifests as transient thyrotoxicosis followed by transient hypothyroidism. The thyroid uptake scan reveals markedly decreased glandular activity which helps to differentiate subacute thyroiditis from Graves' disease. Such a distinction is crucial because the management of these thyroid disorders differs significantly. Thyrotoxicosis from subacute thyroiditis will resolve spontaneously and should not be treated with anti-thyroid medication.

27.13 Other Thyroid Investigations in Special Circumstances

27.13.1 Heterophile Antibody Interference

Heterophile antibodies are endogenous antibodies in human serum that may interfere with immunoassays causing a false positive, or falsely elevated, test result. Awareness of the possibility of interference by heterophile antibodies is important to prevent inappropriate management on the basis of erroneous laboratory results.

Heterophile antibodies are common, naturally occurring antibodies with low affinities. Medical researchers have proposed that heterophile antibodies bind and remove foreign antigens from the intestinal tract and help to maintain self-tolerance (Levinson and Miller 2002). They are inherently produced from B cells prior to antigen exposure and are made up of a random combination of genes encoding the heavy and light chain variable regions. These antibodies react with many antigens including a wide variety of chemical structures, self-antigens, and variable regions of other antibodies (anti-idiotypic antibodies) (Warren et al. 2005; Bjerner et al. 2005). Heterophilic antibodies are typically not strong enough to interfere with competitive binding assays (Levinson and Miller 2002; Kaplan and Levinson 1999) clinical practice, if a patient has heterophilic antibodies that are causing interference with one particular type of assay, these same antibodies will only react poorly, if at all, with another type of assay. Therefore, switching the assay kit to one from a different manufacturer, or to a different in-house preparation may reduce or eliminate the interference. The use of nonimmune globulin, serum from several animal species or commercially available preparations, such as heterophile blocking reagents and immunoglobulin inhibiting reagents, can significantly reduce heterophile interference (Levinson and Miller 2002; Preissner et al. 2005). Heterophile antibodies should be suspected in patients that have FT4 and TSH results in which the concentrations together are considered discordant, i.e. an elevated TSH with an elevated FT4, where an alternative cause is statistically unlikely, or does not fit with the clinical picture.

27.13.2 Resistance to Thyrotropin (TSH) and Resistance to Thyrotropin-Releasing Hormone (TRH)

Resistance to TSH (RTSH) is defined as high serum TSH of normal biological activity in the absence of goitre. Affected individuals have normal or hypoplastic thyroid glands, high serum TSH concentrations, and normal or low serum T4 and T3 concentrations. They are often identified at birth through neonatal screening for congenital hypothyroidism. RTSH should be suspected in patients, particularly infants, who have high serum TSH concentrations, normal or low serum-free T4 and T3 concentrations, and a normally located thyroid gland. The differential diagnosis includes all conditions that impair thyroid secretion. TSH is the predominant regulator of thyroid growth and T4 and T3 synthesis and secretion. Because of the important role of TSH in promoting thyroid growth, RTSH is unlikely if the patient has a goitre or ectopically located thyroid tissue.

Three phenotypes of resistance to TSH representing different degrees of resistance to TSH.

1. **Fully Compensated defect:** The impaired response to TSH is compensated by hypersecretion of TSH; this overcomes the resistance, resulting in euthyroid hyperthyrotropinaemia (high TSH). In an individual patient with a genetic mutation causing resistance to TSH, the phenotype tends to be stable over time. This course contrasts to that of acquired subclinical hypothyroidism due to autoimmune thyroiditis, which tends to worsen over time.
2. **Partially compensated defect:** Affected individuals have mild hypothyroidism as the high serum TSH cannot fully compensate for the defect.

3. **Uncompensated defect:** Complete lack of TSH receptor function results in severe hypothyroidism. This most often occurs when both alleles carry mutant TSH receptors with a complete lack of function (Abramowicz et al. 1997; Gagné et al. 1998; Tiosano et al. 1999).

Individuals with fully compensated RTSH are euthyroid and need no treatment. There is no evidence that in the absence of other risk factors, persistent elevation of serum TSH levels produces TSH-secreting pituitary adenomas or thyroid neoplasia. Individuals with partially compensated or uncompensated RTSH should be treated with L-T4, like any other hypothyroid patient. Because these individuals have normal responsiveness to thyroid hormone, the goal is to normalize their serum TSH concentration.

27.13.3 Resistance to Thyrotropin-Releasing Hormone (TRH)

Resistance to thyrotropin-releasing hormone (TRH) is a rare disorder that is transmitted as an autosomal recessive trait. It is due to an inactivating mutation in the TRH receptor.

Patients with resistance to TRH present with findings of central hypothyroidism, i.e. normal serum TSH, low T4 and T3 concentrations, and no serum TSH or prolactin responses to the administration of TRH.

27.14 TSH-oma

The thyrotropin (TSH)-secreting pituitary adenomas (TSH-omas) are a rare cause of hyperthyroidism. It includes autonomous secretion of TSH which is refractory to the negative feedback of thyroid hormones and TSH itself is responsible for the hyper stimulation of the thyroid gland and the consequent hypersecretion of T4 and T3(Beck-Peccoz et al. 1996; Beck-Peccoz et al. 2015). If FT4 and FT3 concentrations are elevated in the presence of measurable TSH levels, it is important to exclude methodological interference first, due to the presence of circulating autoantibodies or heterophilic antibodies. A similar biochemical picture may also be seen in patients on L-T4 replacement therapy. The finding of measurable TSH in the presence of high FT4/FT3 levels may be due to poor compliance or to an incorrect high L-T4 dosage, probably administered before blood sampling.

In patients with a confirmed TSH-oma, clinical features of hyperthyroidism are usually present, but may be milder than expected for the level of thyroid hormones, probably due to their long-standing duration. The presence of a goiter is the rule, even in the patients with previous partial thyroidectomy, since thyroid residue may regrow as a consequence of TSH hyperstimulation. (Abs et al. 1994). The monitoring of the thyroid nodule(s) and the execution of fine needle aspiration biopsy (FNAB) are indicated in TSH-omas since differentiated thyroid carcinomas have been documented in several patients (Beck-Peccoz et al. 1996; Kishida et al. 2000; Nguyen et al. 2010; Gasparoni et al. 1998; Poggi et al. 2009; Perticone et al. 2015).

Patients with TSH-omas may also hypersecrete other pituitary hormones. Hyperthyroid features can be overshadowed by those of acromegaly in the patients with mixed TSH/GH adenomas (Malchiodi et al. 2014; Beck-Peccoz et al. 1986; Losa et al. 1996), thus emphasizing the importance of systematic measurement of TSH and FT4 in patients with pituitary a tumour. Dysfunction of the gonadal axis is not rare and occurs mainly in the mixed TSH/PRL adenomas. As a consequence of tumour suprasellar extension or invasiveness, signs and symptoms of expanding tumour mass predominate in many patients. Partial or total hypopituitarism was seen in about 1/4 cases, headache reported in 20–25% of patients, and visual field defects are present in about 50% of cases.

About 30% of TSH-oma patients with an intact thyroid showed TSH levels within the normal range; TSH levels in patients previously treated with thyroid ablation were sixfold higher than in untreated patients though free thyroid hormone levels were still in the hyperthyroid range (Beck-Peccoz et al. 1996).

27.14.1 Dynamic Testing

Both stimulatory and inhibitory tests have been proposed for the diagnosis of TSH-oma, but neither option is of clear-cut diagnostic value. The tests proposed include T3 suppression test, TRH test, response to native somatostatin and its analogue.

27.14.2 Imaging

MRI is considered the first choice for visualization however when contraindicated, high-resolution computed tomography (HRCT) is an alternative. Pituitary scintigraphy with radiolabeled octreotide (octreoscan) has been shown to successfully localize TSH-omas expressing somatostatin receptors (Brucker-Davis et al. 1999; Losa et al. 1997). However, the specificity of octreoscan is low since positive scans can be seen in other types of pituitary mass, both secreting or non-secreting.

27.14.3 Treatment

Surgical resection is the recommended therapy for TSH-secreting pituitary tumours as stated in a guideline by the European Thyroid Association (Beck-Peccoz et al. 2013). This involves highly invasive, surgical removal or debulking of the tumour by transsphenoidal or subfrontal adenomectomy, depending on the tumour volume and its suprasellar extension.

If surgery is contraindicated or declined, or is unsuccessful, pituitary radiotherapy and/or medical treatment with somatostatin analogues are two valid alternatives (Beck-Peccoz et al. 2013).

27.15 Conclusions

Thyroid investigations are paramount towards reaching a correct diagnosis and thyroid blood tests such as TSH, fT4, and fT3 are usually the first line of investigations, together with biochemistry to confirm the functional status of the gland.

To avoid unnecessary thyroid investigations, a structured approach is required that combines taking relevant patient history and performing a thorough examination with selective investigations according to the clinical findings. This not only serves as cost effective within the health service but more importantly benefits and enhances patient recover.

References

Abramowicz MJ, Duprez L, Parma J, et al. Familial congenital hypothyroidism due to inactivating mutation of the thyrotropin receptor causing profound hypoplasia of the thyroid gland. J Clin Invest. 1997;99:3018.

Abs R, Stevenaert A, Beckers A. Autonomously functioning thyroid nodules in a patient with a thyrotropin-secreting pituitary adenoma: possible cause-effect relationship. Eur J Endocrinol. 1994;131:355–8.

Beck-Peccoz P, Piscitelli G, Amr S, Ballabio M, Bassetti M, Giannattasio G, Spada A, Nissim M, Weintraub BD, Faglia G. Endocrine, biochemical, and morphological studies of a pituitary adenoma secreting growth hormone, thyrotropin (TSH), and a-subunit: evidence for secretion of TSH with increased bioactivity. J Clin Endocrinol Metab. 1986;62:704–11.

Beck-Peccoz P, Brucker-Davis F, Persani L, Smallridge RC, Weintraub BD. Thyrotropin-secreting pituitary tumors. Endocr Rev. 1996;17:610–38.

Beck-Peccoz P, Lania A, Beckers A, Chatterjee K, Wemeau JL. 2013 European thyroid association guidelines for the diagnosis and treatment of thyrotropin-secreting pituitary tumors. Eur Thyroid J. 2013;2(2):76–82.

Beck-Peccoz P, Lania A, Persani L. Chapter 24. TSH-producing adenomas. In: Jameson JL, DeGroot LJ, editors. Endocrinology. 7th ed. Philadelphia: W.B. Saunders; 2015. p. 266–74.

Bjerner J, Olsen KH, Bormer OP, Nustad K. Human heterophilic antibodies display specificity for murine IgG subclasses. Clin Biochem. 2005;38(5):465–72.

Bonavita JA, Mayo J, Babb J, et al. Pattern recognition of benign nodules at ultrasound of the thyroid: which nodules can be left alone? AJR Am J Roentgenol. 2009;193:207.

Brucker-Davis F, Oldfield EH, Skarulis MC, Doppman JL, Weintraub BD. Thyrotropin-secreting pituitary tumors: diagnostic criteria, thyroid hormone sensitivity, and treatment outcome in 25 patients followed at the National Institutes of Health. J Clin Endocrinol Metab. 1999;84:476–86.

Brunese L, Romeo A, Iorio S, et al. A new marker for diagnosis of thyroid papillary cancer: B-flow twinkling sign. J Ultrasound Med. 2008;27:1187.

Cappelli C, Pirola I, Cumetti D, et al. Is the anteroposterior and transverse diameter ratio of nonpalpable thyroid nodules a sonographic criteria for recommending fine-needle aspiration cytology? Clin Endocrinol (Oxf). 2005;63:689.

Cappelli C, Castellano M, Pirola I, et al. The predictive value of ultrasound findings in the management of thyroid nodules. QJM. 2007;100:29.

Cavallo A, Johnson DN, White MG, et al. Thyroid nodule size at ultrasound as a predictor of malignancy and final pathologic size. Thyroid. 2017;27:641.

Cohen O, Pinhas-Hamiel O, Sivan E, et al. Serial in utero ultrasonographic measurements of the fetal thyroid: a new complementary tool in the management of maternal hyperthyroidism in pregnancy. Prenat Diagn. 2003;23:740.

Daumerie C, Ayoubi S, Rahier J, et al. [Prevalence of thyroid cancer in hot nodules]. Ann Chir. 1998;52(5):444–8.

Deshpande P, Lucas M, Brunt S, Lucas A, Hollingsworth P, Bundell C. Low level autoantibodies can be frequently detected in the general Australian population. Pathology. 2016;48(5):483–90.

Gagné N, Parma J, Deal C, et al. Apparent congenital athyreosis contrasting with normal plasma thyroglobulin levels and associated with inactivating mutations in the thyrotropin receptor gene: are athyreosis and ectopic thyroid distinct entities? J Clin Endocrinol Metab. 1998;83:1771.

Gasparoni P, Rubello D, Persani L, Beck-Peccoz P. Unusual association between a thyrotropin-secreting pituitary adenoma and a papillary thyroid carcinoma. Thyroid. 1998;8:181–3.

Hollowell JG, Staehling NW, Flanders WD, Hannon WH, Gunter EW, Spencer CA, et al. Serum TSH, T(4), and thyroid antibodies in the United States population (1988 to 1994): National Health and Nutrition Examination Survey (NHANES III). J Clin Endocrinol Metab. 2002;87(2):489–99.

Jakobsen JA. Ultrasound contrast agents: clinical applications. Eur Radiol. 2001;11:1329.

Kaplan IV, Levinson SS. When is a heterophile antibody not a heterophile antibody? When it is an antibody against a specific immunogen. Clin Chem. 1999;45(5):616–8.

Kiernan CM, Solórzano CC. Bethesda category III, IV, and V thyroid nodules: can nodule size help predict malignancy? J Am Coll Surg. 2017;225:77–82.

Kishida M, Otsuka F, Kataoka H, Yokota K, Oishi T, Yamauchi T, Doihara H, Tamiya T, Mimura Y, Ogura T, Makino H. Hyperthyroidism in a patient with TSH-producing pituitary adenoma coexisting with thyroid papillary adenocarcinoma. Endocr J. 2000;47:731–8.

Kwak JY, Kim EK, Son EJ, et al. Papillary thyroid carcinoma manifested solely as microcalcifications on sonography. AJR Am J Roentgenol. 2007;189:227.

Levinson SS, Miller JJ. Towards a better understanding of heterophile (and the like) antibody interference with modern immunoassays. Clin Chim Acta. 2002;325(1–2):1–15.

Losa M, Giovanelli M, Persani L, Mortini P, Faglia G, Beck-Peccoz P. Criteria of cure and follow-up of central hyperthyroidism due to thyrotropin-secreting pituitary adenomas. J Clin Endocrinol Metab. 1996;81:3086–90.

Losa M, Magnani P, Mortini P, Persani L, Acerno S, Giugni E, Fazio F, Beck-Peccoz P, Giovanelli M. Indium-111 pentetreotide single-photon emission tomography in patients with TSH-secreting pituitary adenomas: correlation with the effect of a single administration of octreotide on serum TSH levels. Eur J Nucl Med. 1997;24:728–31.

Luton D, Le Gac I, Vuillard E, et al. Management of Graves' disease during pregnancy: the key role of fetal thyroid gland monitoring. J Clin Endocrinol Metab. 2005;90:6093.

Malchiodi E, Profka E, Ferrante E, Sala E, Verrua E, Campi I, Lania AG, Arosio M, Locatelli M, Mortini P, Losa M, Beck-Peccoz P, Spada A, Mantovani G. Thyrotropin-secreting pituitary adenomas: outcome of pituitary surgery and irradiation. J Clin Endocrinol Metab. 2014;99(6):2069–76.

Mandel SJ. Diagnostic use of ultrasonography in patients with nodular thyroid disease. Endocr Pract. 2004;10(3):246–52.

Miki H, Oshimo K, Inoue H, et al. Incidence of ultrasonographically-detected thyroid nodules in healthy adults. Tokushima J Exp Med. 1993;40(1-2):43–6.

Nguyen HD, Galitz MS, Mai VQ, Clyde PW, Glister BC, Shakir MK. Management of coexisting thyrotropin/growth-hormone-secreting pituitary adenoma and papillary thyroid carcinoma: a therapeutic challenge. Thyroid. 2010;20(1):99–103.

Perticone F, Pigliaru F, Mariotti S, Deiana L, Furlani L, Mortini P, Losa M. Is the incidence of differentiated thyroid cancer increased in patients with thyrotropin-secreting adenomas? Report of three cases from a large consecutive series. Thyroid. 2015;25(4):417–24.

Poggi M, Monti S, Pascucci C, Toscano V. A rare case of follicular thyroid carcinoma in a patient with thyrotropin-secreting pituitary adenoma. Am J Med Sci. 2009;337(6):462–5.

Preissner CM, Dodge LA, O'Kane DJ, Singh RJ, Grebe SK. Prevalence of heterophilic antibody interference in eight automated tumor marker immunoassays. Clin Chem. 2005;51(1):208–10.

Schussler GC. The thyroxine-binding proteins. Thyroid. 2000;10(2):141–9.

Singaporewalla RM, Hwee J, Lang TU, Desai V. Clinico-pathological correlation of thyroid nodule ultrasound and cytology using the TIRADS and Bethesda Classifications. World J Surg. 2017;41:1807–11.

Sipos JA. Advances in ultrasound for the diagnosis and management of thyroid cancer. Thyroid. 2009;19:1363.

Tiosano D, Pannain S, Vassart G, et al. The hypothyroidism in an inbred kindred with congenital thyroid hormone and glucocorticoid deficiency is due to a mutation producing a truncated thyrotropin receptor. Thyroid. 1999;9:887.

Tozzoli R, Bagnasco M, Giavarina D, Bizzaro N. TSH receptor autoantibody immunoassay in patients with Graves' disease: improvement of diagnostic accuracy over different generations of methods. Systematic review and meta-analysis. Autoimmun Rev. 2012;12(2):107–13.

Warren DJ, Bjerner J, Paus E, Bormer OP, Nustad K. Use of an in vivo biotinylated singlechain antibody as capture reagent in an immunometric assay to decrease the incidence of interference from heterophilic antibodies. Clinl chem. 2005;51(5):830–8.

Wiersinga WM. Thyroid hormone replacement therapy. Hormone Res. 2001;56(Suppl 1):74–81.

Hyperthyroidism in Adults

28

Violet Fazal-Sanderson, Niki Karavitaki,
and Radu Mihai

Contents

V. Fazal-Sanderson (✉)
Department of Endocrinology, Centre for Diabetes
and Endocrinology, Royal Berkshire Hospital NHS
Foundation Trust, Berkshire, UK
e-mail: violet.sanderson@royalberkshire.nhs.uk;
Violetsanderson@royalberkshire.nhs.uk

N. Karavitaki
Institute of Metabolism and Systems Research,
University of Birmingham and Queen Elizabeth
Hospital, Birmingham, UK
e-mail: n.karavitaki@bham.ac.uk

R. Mihai
Department of Endocrine Surgery, Churchill Cancer
Centre, Oxford University Hospitals Foundation
Trust, Oxford, UK
e-mail: Radu.Mihai@ouh.nhs.uk

Abstract

In the UK, the prevalence of hyperthyroidism is estimated to be around 2% in women and 0.2% in men. In Europe, the prevalence of overt hyperthyroidism is in the region of 0.6–16% and in the USA, prevalence is reported to be approximately 1.2%.

Hyperthyroidism refers to conditions that cause increased secretion of thyroid hormones from the thyroid gland leading to thyrotoxicosis. Thyrotoxicosis occurs as a result of elevated circulating thyroid hormones, of either free thyroxine or free triiodothyronine, (or both) and can

© Springer Nature Switzerland AG 2019
S. Llahana et al. (eds.), *Advanced Practice in Endocrinology Nursing*,
https://doi.org/10.1007/978-3-319-99817-6_28

affect almost every organ in the body triggering many symptoms including agitation, rapid weight loss, heat intolerance, and increased heart rate. Left untreated, thyrotoxicosis can have serious health implications on a patient's well being. A specialist clinical practitioners role is to identify the signs and symptoms of thyrotoxicosis through the undertaking of a detailed patient history, assessment, and physical examination in this way a tailored approach for treatment can be implemented safely, efficiently, and cost-effectively with positive outcomes.

The conditions most commonly associated with hyperthyroidism include Graves' disease, multinodular goitre, toxic adenoma, thyroiditis (such as subacute and post-partum), and subclinical thyrotoxicosis. These are briefly outlined in this chapter and provide an overview of related definitions, pathologies, and clinical features including diagnosis and treatments, such as medical therapy, radioiodine, and surgery. Furthermore, it also aims to equip and enhance relevant evidence-based knowledge and understanding of the hyperthyroid disorders seen in the endocrine clinical practice, with a view to provide specialist practitioners useful tips and guidance of how to diagnosis, manage, and treat some of the most common hyperthyroid conditions seen in many endocrinology departments.

Keywords
Hyperthyroidism · Graves' disease · Toxic nodular goitre · Thyroiditis · Anti-thyroid drug therapy · Radioiodine · Thyroid surgery

Abbreviations

ATA	American Thyroid Association
ATDs	Anti-thyroid drugs
BTA	British Thyroid Association
BTF	British Thyroid Foundation
BD	Twice daily
BRLN	Bilateral recurrent laryngeal nerve
CKS	Clinical knowledge summaries
FT3	Free triiodothyronine
FT4	Free thyroxine
HT	Hashimoto's thyroiditis
NICE	National Institution for Health and Care Excellence
OD	Daily
PPT	Post-partum thyroiditis
RAI/RAIU	Radioiodine/Radioiodine uptake
SH	Subclinical hyperthyroidism
TA	Toxic adenoma
TDS	Three times daily
TED	Thyroid eye disease
TFT	Thyroid function test
TMNG	Toxic multinodular goitre
TSH	Thyroid stimulating hormones
TSHRAb	Thyroid stimulating hormone receptor antibody
UK	United Kingdom
USA	United States of America

Key Terms
- **Primary hyperthyroidism**: a disorder of the thyroid gland that causes thyrotoxicosis such as Graves' disease, nodular goitre, or various types of thyroiditis
- **Secondary hyperthyroidism**: is caused by excess extra-thyroidal stimulation of the thyroid by a thyroid stimulating hormone (TSH) secreting pituitary adenoma
- **Thyrotoxicosis:** is caused by an excess of circulating thyroid hormones, either free thyroxine (FT4) or free triiodothyronine (FT3), or both
- **Graves' disease:** is an autoimmune condition in which thyrotropin receptor antibodies stimulate TSH receptors, and as a result, there are increased levels of circulating of thyroid hormone.

Key Points
- Hyperthyroidism refers to conditions that cause increased secretion of thyroid hormones (either free thyroxine or free triiodithyronine, or both), with suppressed thyroid stimulating hormone.
- The classic symptoms of thyrotoxicosis include agitation, palpitations, weight loss, fine hand tremor, heat intolerance, and frequency of bowel movements.

- Common conditions caused by hyperthyroidism include Graves' disease, then toxic adenoma, multinodular goitre and less common, various forms of thyroiditis.
- Investigations such as thyroid radioiodine uptake scan can differentiate thyroid disorders such as Graves' disease by an increased and diffuse uptake, toxic multinodular goitre by focal areas of normal to increased uptake, and thyroiditis by a low uptake.
- Thyroid antibodies are useful indicators for determining thyroid disease, for example, thyroid autoantibodies to thyroglobulin and thyroid peroxidase can show those at risk to developing autoimmune thyroid disease.
- Appropriate diagnosis is critical to formulating a more specific and tailored approach in enhancing patient recovery.
- Thionamides such as Carbimazole and Propylthiouracil are anti-thyroid drugs treatments used in the management of hyperthyroidism, in preparation for thyroidectomy in hyperthyroidism and as prescribed as therapy prior and post-radioiodine treatment.

28.1   Section A: Hyperthyroidism

28.1.1   Introduction

Thyroid hormones are essential for cellular metabolism, normal skeletal growth, and cerebral development (Visser 2011; Harvey et al. 2002). Adequate iodine intake is paramount for normal thyroid function and can be obtained from foods such as white fish, milk, and dairy products (Bath 2016). Deficiency of iodine can lead to impaired thyroid hormone production that can have serious implications on both cognitive function and growth (Vanderpump 2011). The balance of thyroid hormones within the body are controlled through a negative feedback on the hypothalamus and pituitary gland (Visser 2011; Harvey et al. 2002)

> **Box 28.1 Thyrotoxicosis Associated with Hyperthyroidism, Thyroiditis, and Non-thyroidal Disorders**
>
> Thyrotoxicosis and hyperthyroidism in adults
>
> - Graves' disease
> - Toxic adenoma
> - Multinodular goitre
> - Iodine induced
> - TSH secreting tumour
>
> Thyrotoxicosis and thyroiditis
>
> - Subacute thyroiditis
> - Silent thyroiditis
> - Amiodarone induced (type 2)
>
> Thyrotoxicosis of non-thyroidal origin
>
> - Thyroid hormone intoxication
> - Dermoid tumours (Struma ovarii)
> - Metastatic thyroid cancer

Excess circulating thyroid hormones causes thyrotoxicosis and can be associated with hyperthyroidism, thyroiditis, or non-thyroidal disorder (Box 28.1).

28.1.2   Hyperthyroidism

Hyperthyroidism refers to conditions that cause increased secretion of thyroid hormones from the thyroid gland that leads to thyrotoxicosis, whilst **thyrotoxicosis** is termed as a clinical syndrome that results from elevated circulating thyroid hormones, of either free thyroxine (FT4) or free triiodothyronine (FT3), or both (British Thyroid Association-BTA 2006; Franklyn and Boelaert 2012; American Thyroid Association – ATA 2016).

High levels of circulating thyroid hormones can effect almost every organ in the body and trigger numerous unpleasant signs and symptoms including palpitations, weight loss, fine hand tremor, heat intolerance, frequency of bowel movement, etc. (Fig. 28.1), and if left

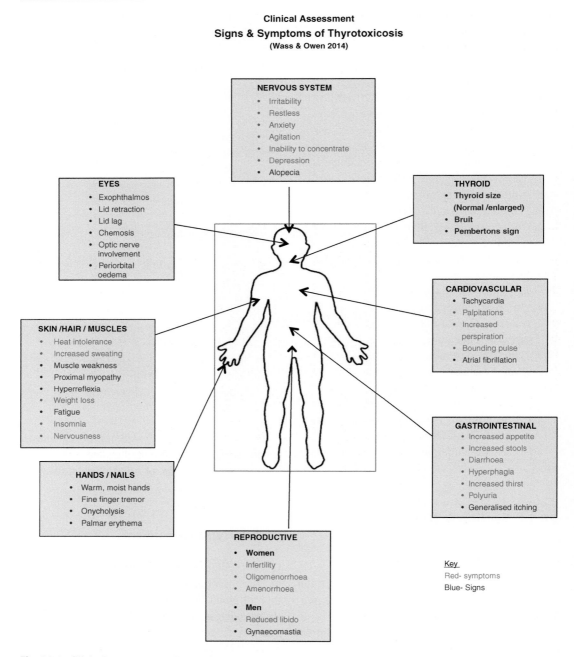

Clinical Assessment
Signs & Symptoms of Thyrotoxicosis
(Wass & Owen 2014)

NERVOUS SYSTEM
- Irritability
- Restless
- Anxiety
- Agitation
- Inability to concentrate
- Depression
- Alopecia

EYES
- Exophthalmos
- Lid retraction
- Lid lag
- Chemosis
- Optic nerve involvement
- Periorbital oedema

THYROID
- **Thyroid size (Normal /enlarged)**
- **Bruit**
- **Pembertons sign**

SKIN /HAIR / MUSCLES
- Heat intolerance
- Increased sweating
- Muscle weakness
- Proximal myopathy
- Hyperreflexia
- Weight loss
- Fatigue
- Insomnia
- Nervousness

CARDIOVASCULAR
- Tachycardia
- Palpitations
- Increased perspiration
- Bounding pulse
- Atrial fibrillation

HANDS / NAILS
- Warm, moist hands
- Fine finger tremor
- Onycholysis
- Palmar erythema

GASTROINTESTINAL
- Increased appetite
- Increased stools
- Diarrhoea
- Hyperphagia
- Increased thirst
- Polyuria
- Generalised itching

REPRODUCTIVE
- **Women**
- Infertility
- Oligomenorrhoea
- Amenorrhoea
- **Men**
- Reduced libido
- Gynaecomastia

Key
Red- symptoms
Blue- Signs

Fig. 28.1 Clinical assessment—signs and symptoms of thyrotoxicosis

untreated, can have serious health implications on a patients' well-being (British Thyroid Association-BTA 2006; Franklyn and Boelaert 2012; American Thyroid Association – ATA 2016; Goichot et al. 2015).

Primary hyperthyroidism refers to disorder of the thyroid gland that causes thyrotoxicosis such as in Graves' disease, nodular goitre, or various types of thyroiditis, whilst **Secondary hyperthyroidism** is caused by extra-thyroidal stimulation of the thyroid gland, for example, a thyroid stimulating hormone (TSH) secreting pituitary adenoma that causes thyrotoxicosis (Weetman 2010).

The prevalence of hyperthyroidism in the United Kingdom (UK) is reported to be around 2% in women and 0.2% in men (Tunbridge et al.

1977; Franklyn and Boelaert 2012). Furthermore, in Europe, the prevalence of endogenous subclinical hyperthyroidism is estimated to be around 0.6–16% (Bondi et al. 2015; Canaris et al. 2000; Bülow Pedersen et al. 2002; Marqusee et al. 1998). The incidence of hyperthyroidism is mostly found in regions of iodine deficiency and in the elderly population. In the United States of America (USA), the prevalence of hyperthyroidism is estimated to be in the region of 1.2% (American Thyroid Association – ATA 2016; Singer et al. 1995).

Overt hyperthyroidism is diagnostic of primary hyperthyroidism, for example, by a low TSH, and high FT4 and FT3 hormone concentrations (British Thyroid Association-BTA 2006; American Thyroid Association – ATA 2016).

In patients with overt Graves' or nodular goitre, serum FT3 levels are often reported to be higher than serum FT4 and termed as FT3-toxicosis (Ross 2016; Laurberg et al. 2007). However, T4-toxicosis can suggest a concurrent non-thyroidal illness demonstrated by a low serum TSH, high serum FT4, and normal serum FT3, due to decreased extra-thyroidal conversion of T4 to T3 (Caplan 1980).

In a TSH secreting pituitary adenoma, the serum TSH is increased as well as serum FT4 and FT3, indicating not only overt hyperthyroid but also diagnostic of secondary hyperthyroidism.

Subclinical hyperthyroidism (SH) is defined by a low biochemical or an undetectable TSH, with both FT4 and FT3 values within the normal reference range, and in the absence of the following diseases (Franklyn 2011; Cooper and Biondi 2012; European Thyroid Association 2015):

- Hypothalamic disease or pituitary disease
- Non-thyroidal illness
- Ingestion of drugs that inhibit TSH secretion, e.g. glucocorticoids and dopamine

SH is frequently found in men and women over the age of 65 years and can give rise to risks for developing osteoporotic fractures from the increased bone turnover as well as coronary heart disease and atrial fibrillation (Cappola et al. 2006; Wirth et al. 2014; Ross 2017a; Blum et al. 2015).

Patients treated with either radioiodine (RAI) or thyroid surgery for underlying hyperthyroid disorders such as Graves' disease or toxic nodular goitre, often require Thyroxine to normalise thyroid function; patients should therefore be warned of the risks associated with SH and aim therefore always to have the thyroid hormones within the normal reference range (Franklyn 2011).

However, there remains an ongoing debate as to whether to treat or not to treat with Thyroxine replacement, for example, there appears to be very little evidence that demonstrate whether there are any related long-term side effects. In these circumstances, a multidisciplinary approach should be practised if treatment is to be considered. However, recurrent guidelines suggest, all patients with SH over the age of 65 are at risk of developing osteoporosis and atrial fibrillation and the use of Thyroxine would benefit such patient (British Thyroid Association-BTA 2006; Franklyn 2011). Furthermore SH can also occur as a result of non-thyroid reasons, for example, major illness, iodine agents, pregnancy, and also drug therapies including Dopamine and Glucocorticosteroids.

A number of risk factors are thought to be associated with hyperthyroidism (Box 28.2).

Box 28.2 Hyperthyroidism Risk Factors (Adapted from BTA 2006; Vaidya and Pearce 2014)

- Age: elderly over the age of 60 and Graves' disease between ages of 40 and 60
- Gender: women more commonly effected
- In recent pregnancy
- In autoimmune diseases such as type 1 diabetes
- Genetics: Family history of thyroid disease
- Iodine deficiency
- Iodine excess
- Ethnicity
- Medical: common viral infections
- Smoking

28.1.3 Causes of Hyperthyroidism

Hyperthyroidism can occur from a variety of thyroidal or non-thyroidal causes, and therefore it is essential that the condition is determined both accurately and promptly.

In-depth knowledge related to thyroid anatomy and physiology is key towards providing appropriate care to patients (Sect. 4, Chap. 26). For example, an astute clinical practitioner will be able to identify the signs and symptoms of thyrotoxicosis through the undertaking of a detailed patient history, assessment, and physical examination. In doing so, this in turn not only provides the pathway for a preliminary diagnosis to be made, but also accelerates a more tailored approach to implementing specific investigations and a treatment plan whilst waiting for a more formal confirmed validated diagnostic test to return (e.g. thyroid receptor antibody or uptake scan results). Moreover, this can benefit the health service in terms of cost-effectiveness as well as enhance patient recovery.

In most endocrinology departments, conditions more commonly associated with hyperthyroidism include Graves' disease, multinodular goitre, toxic adenoma, various types of thyroiditis (subacute and post-partum), and subclinical thyrotoxicosis (British Thyroid Association-BTA 2006; American Thyroid Association – ATA 2016). These common conditions were also evident from a thyroid nurse-led clinic outcomes audit undertaken in Oxford for example the audit showed that out of 134 patients seen over a year, 112 were managed for Graves' disease, 10 with toxic nodular goitre, 10 with thyroiditis (subacute and post-partum), and 2 with subclinical thyrotoxicosis (Fazal-Sanderson et al. 2017).

Other rare hyperthyroid conditions include a TSH secreting adenoma, human chorionic gonadotropin-dependent hyperthyroidism, trophoblastic tumours, hyperemesis gravidarum, familial gestational hyperthyroidism, fetal and neonatal transfer hyperthyroidism, non-autoimmune congenital and familial hyperthyroidism (Latrofa et al. 2011).

Conditions associated with hyperthyroidism and thyrotoxicosis are highlighted below.

28.1.4 Graves' Disease

Graves' disease originally derives its name from an Irish Physician called Joseph Graves (1796–1853) who first associated the disease with thyroid gland enlargement and its association with palpitations (Volpe and Sawin 2011; Smith 2018).

The actual cause of Graves is unknown, although it mostly affects women, often runs in families and thought to be linked to a genetic component, stress, smoking, and pregnancy (Box 28.2). Smoking has also been an associated as a risk factor for developing thyroid eye disease (TED) (Sect. 4, Chap. 31).

In the UK, Graves' disease affects around 75% of patients with overt hyperthyroidism and occurs more frequently in women than in men. Around 30% of these cases are reported to develop Graves' orbitopathy or thyroid eye disease [Vaidya and Pearce 2014; Thyroid Eye Disease Committee Team (TEDct) 2018].

Active TED comprises of an inflammatory process that can lead to eye signs including conjunctival injection, chemosis, visual field defect, double vision, and can ultimately affect the extra-ocular muscle and related cranial nerves (Perros et al. 2015). If left untreated, major eye complications can occur damaging both external and internal orbital soft tissue structures. Body image becomes a huge problem in these patients, as well as depression and low self-esteem (TEDct 2018). Patients with active TED should therefore be referred promptly to a specialist ophthalmologist for appropriate assessment and management (Sect. 4, Chap. 33).

28.1.4.1 Definition

Graves' disease is an autoimmune condition in which thyrotropin receptor antibodies stimulate TSH receptors, and as a result, there are increased levels of circulating of thyroid hormone. The autoantibodies produced mimic the action of thyroid stimulating hormone on follicular cells within the thyroid gland. As a result of continual stimulation of thyroid hormones, fT4 and fT3 are increased in the circulation causing loss of feedback mechanism to the pituitary. Consequently, the TSH becomes suppressed and exerts its effects on the follicular cell of the thyroid causing thyroid enlargement and lymphocytic infiltration (British Thyroid Association-BTA 2006; American Thyroid Association – ATA 2016).

28.1.4.2 Aetiology
Thyroid stimulating immunoglobulin binds to and stimulates the thyroid.

28.1.4.3 Pathogenesis
There is diffuse hyperplasia and hypertrophy of the thyroid follicular cells.

28.1.4.4 Specific Clinical Features
Thyroid gland: The classical hallmarks features of Graves disease includes thyroid gland enlargement, which is usually smooth, soft, diffuse and often symmetrical on palpation, however, a few cases have been diagnosed with accompanying nodules thought to be linked to pre-existing nodule/s or from a longstanding disease (American Thyroid Association – ATA 2016; Berghout et al. 1990).

Signs and symptoms: Patients can present with a range of signs and symptoms relating to overt hyperthyroidism (Fig. 28.1). The severity of symptoms requires a thorough assessment with a full clinical history and physical examination for the purpose of managing symptom effectively and restoration of normal thyroid function.

Graves' ophthalmopathy: All patients with Graves' disease should have a thorough eye assessment as part of the clinical assessment. Eye signs including lid lag and retraction, signs of proptosis, and extraocular movements should be recorded and monitored at every follow-up. Any active signs of TED should prompt a referral to an ophthalmologist for treatment and regular follow-up (Perros et al. 2015) (Sect. 4, Chap. 31).

Smoking: This is considered as a serious risk factor for developing Graves' ophthalmopathy (Perros et al. 2015). Health promotion leaflets should be provided for patients to stop smoking and the consequences for developing TED must be explained (British Thyroid Association-BTA 2006; Thyroid Eye Disease Committee Team 2018; Perros et al. 2015).

Pretibial myxoedema: This is also known as Graves' dermopathy, thyroid dermopathy, or infiltrative dermopathy.

Pretibial myxoedema is a rare condition and can be found in around 5% of cases with Graves' hyperthyroidism. It is also associated with Graves' disease with ophthalmopathy.

Pretibial myxoedema is usually located in the pretibial region just below the knees but also has been associated with ankles, and dorsum of the foot, hands, elbows, upper back, face, and neck (Davis 2017).

The combination of lymphocytic infiltration with cytokines causes pathologic changes that give rise to mucinous oedema within the papillary, reticular dermis and deep beyond into tissue. This results in non-pitting oedema and lesions of the dermis together with high levels of circulating TSHRAb. The lesions are usually raised and the skin appears thick and discoloured often with no pain or symptoms, thus no treatment is required and resolves spontaneously over time. However, in cases where pain and tenderness is experienced, treatment comprises of topical steroids and compression bandages (Schwartz et al. 2002).

28.1.4.5 Biochemical and Imaging Features
A thyroid function test: This is the gold standard diagnostic test for hyperthyroidism and is confirmed by a suppressed TSH, elevated fT4 and fT3.

TSHRAbs: reported to have 98% sensitivity and 99% specificity for testing positive in the diagnosis of Graves' hyperthyroidism (Tozzoli et al. 2012).

Radionuclide thyroid uptake: provides formal confirmation of Graves' disease with increased uptake and when TSHRAb test is inconclusive.

28.1.4.6 Diagnosis
- Thyroid function test shows a supressed serum TSH, increased serum fT3 and fT4.
- Positive TSHRAb test and thyroid peroxidase antibodies (antithyroglobulin and anti-thyroid peroxidase antibodies are markers of autoimmune disease).

- A thyroid uptake scan that shows increased uptake confirms Graves' disease.
- Fine needle aspiration (FNA) thyroid biopsy may be required to exclude thyroid malignancy if a nodule is discovered in presence of Graves' hyperthyroidism.
- Eye signs related to hyperthyroidism that have not settled following normalisation of thyroid hormones should prompt an ophthalmology referral for opinion.

28.1.4.7 Treatment

Hospital policy and protocols vary in countries although guidelines are provided with the most up-to-date evidence-based recommendations (British Thyroid Association-BTA 2006; American Thyroid Association – ATA 2016; Schwartz et al. 2002). Many endocrine centres use the guidelines to form their own policies and care pathways.

Anti-thyroid drugs: In the UK, Europe, China, and Japan, primary treatment for Graves' hyperthyroidism comprises of 6–18 month course of anti-thyroid medications such as Carbimazole. Studies have demonstrated that the duration of treatment in excess of 18 months does not improve remission rates. Furthermore, findings have also suggested that remission is improved if restoration of euthyroid state is achieved independent of drug dose and type. To date, the remission rate in Graves' disease varies in countries and is reported to be around 40–70% (British Thyroid Association-BTA 2006; American Thyroid Association – ATA 2016; National Institute for Health and Care Excellence-NICE 2016; Organzi and Bournard 2011). A thyroid nurse-led clinic audit (Oxford, UK) of long-term follow-up patients with Graves' hyperthyroidism showed the remission rate to be around 33%, and inturn suggesting that definitive treatment could be a future consideration for primary treatment for Graves' disease rather than patients enduring a lengthy course of medical therapy (Sanderson et al. 2012). This not only can have cost-benefits to the health service but also enhances a more rapid restoration of normal thyroid hormone function and patient recovery. In the USA, radioiodine is offered as the first-line treatment for Graves'

hyperthyroidism and thought to be due to the high rate of relapse with anti-thyroid medications.

Definitive treatments radioiodine or thyroid surgery: In the UK, patients who have relapsed following a 12–18 month course of anti-thyroid drugs (ATDs) such as Carbimazole and Propylthiouracil are offered, provided the patients suitability has been assessed (Sect. 4, Chap. 28 B-RAI & C-Thyroid surgery). Both treatments aim to prevent future relapse of Graves' hyperthyroidism (British Thyroid Association-BTA 2006; National Institute for Health and Care Excellence-NICE 2016).

Lifelong thyroxine: is usually required following definitive treatment with either radioiodine or thyroid surgery, and therefore normalisation of thyroid hormones is essential prior to discharge (British Thyroid Association-BTA 2006; National Institute for Health and Care Excellence-NICE 2016).

Following discharge from secondary care: all patients should seek have regular 6–12 monthly thyroid function test, or earlier if thyroid symptoms return (with their assigned General Practitioner (GP), or healthcare provider), to ensure that long-term stability of thyroid status is maintained (British Thyroid Association-BTA 2006; National Institute for Health and Care Excellence-NICE 2016) (Box 28.3).

Thyroid eye disease: Treatment for active TED requires specialist treatment under the care and supervision of an ophthalmologist. Treatment may include steroidal medication, series of eye drops, visual field assessment, orthoptic services, or even orbital surgery (TEDct 2018; Perros et al. 2015) (Sect. 4, Chap. 31).

Box 28.3 Case Study 1. Graves' Disease and a Case of Neutropenia: A Matter of Urgency!

Graves' disease is an autoimmune disorder accounting for about 80% of the cases of hyperthyroidism and affecting predominantly females. In the UK, Carbimazole is the first choice of anti-thyroid medication and is associated with a risk of agranulocytosis (reported in 0.2–0.5% of the patients) and severe infections. In such cases, immediate discontinuation of Carbimazole is needed and alternative management options should be considered. In a Thyroid Nurse-led Clinic in Oxford, most patients opt for an 18-month course of Carbimazole, despite there being only a 30% remission rate. This case study demonstrates the management of Graves' disease and the matter of urgency required for prompt action in cases of neutropenia.

Case study—A 26-year-old female was diagnosed with Graves' disease and opted for an18-months course of Carbimazole. She completed the course of treatment and 1 month after stopping the anti-thyroid medication she was diagnosed with relapse of the Graves'. She responded to treatment well and by month 6, her daily dose was reduced to 5 mg. At this time, she developed a fever and consequently a FBC taken which showed low white cell count of 3.57 and low neutrophil count of 0.84. Carbimazole was stopped and 2 weeks later, the neutrophil count was restored. Swift arrangement was made for an urgent thyroidectomy. She was later discharged on Thyroxine with normal thyroid hormones.

28.1.5 Toxic Adenoma/Toxic Multinodular Goitre

The term goitre refers to an abnormal growth of the thyroid gland that can result either as diffuse or nodular, and effect thyroid hormones production (Ross 2017b). The most common cause of goitre worldwide is reported to be due to iodine deficiency (Vanderpump 2011).

An enlarged goitre usually implies iodine deficiency. It can occur at any age, for example, when iodine intake falls, TSH from the pituitary rises and maximises the availability of iodine from the thyroid gland causing diffuse enlargement. Overtime, and in light of low iodine intake,

nodules develop, the commonest being multinodular goitre, mostly found in the elderly population (Zimmerman 2012).

The incidence of thyroid nodules is reported to be more common in females compared to male population. In the UK, toxic nodular goitre accounts for 15% of hyperthyroid cases and is also reported to be associated with the elderly population in regions of iodine deficiency (Franklyn and Boelaert 2012). Around 5% of nodules are picked up on neck palpation during a clinical assessment (Bomeli et al. 2010).

28.1.5.1 Definition
Toxic adenoma (TA) can be described as a single autonomously functioning nodule within the thyroid gland that secretes thyroid hormones from thyrocyte cells (Latrofa et al. 2011). These are benign tumours that can cause mild to overt hyperthyroidism mostly associated with iodine deficiency (Vaidya and Pearce 2014).

Toxic multinodular goitre (TMG) is usually a heterogeneous disorder of the thyroid gland, comprising of multiple autonomous functioning nodules, also known as Plummer's disease (Weiner and DeVries 1979). Additional nodules may also be present and appear as normal or with reduced uptake on radioiodine uptake imaging.

28.1.5.2 Aetiology
TA comprises of monoclonal autonomously secreting benign tumour, whilst TMG is reported as multiple monoclonal autonomously secreting benign thyroid tumours.

28.1.5.3 Pathogenesis
These nodules are usually benign follicular adenomas. Adenomas are reported to consist of uniform structures containing mitoses that are encompassed by a fibrous capsule formed by the surrounding compressed thyroid tissue. The autonomous function from within the thyroid nodule follicular cells is independent to that regulated by the thyroid stimulating hormone, and in the absence of TSH-receptor stimulating antibodies. The continual autonomous production of thyroid hormones over time can progress from a subclinical state to overt hyperthyroidism.

Unregulated thyroid hormones initially suppress the TSH, and in the presence of overt hyperthyroidism cause tissue atrophy around the adenoma (Fuhrer and Lazarus 2011).

28.1.5.4 Biochemical and Imaging Features

- Measurements of thyroid function tests are essential for diagnosis and confirmed by a suppressed serum TSH, and elevated serum fT4 and fT3.
- T3 toxicosis is often found in TAs (Laurberg et al. 2007).
- A thyroid ultrasonography and scintiscanning identifying nodular activity shows increased uptake with suppression of uptake in the surrounding extranodular thyroid tissue, thus provides a formal diagnosis (Fuhrer and Lazarus 2011).
- Ultrasound scanning of the neck gives information of nodule size and identifies the presence of other existing cold nodules.
- Ultrasound elastography is useful for identifying benign from malignant nodules.

28.1.5.5 Clinical Features

- Signs and symptoms that patients present with are any of those relating to overt hyperthyroidism (Fig. 28.1), and severity of these requires a thorough patient assessment that includes a full clinical history and physical examination for the purpose of symptom relief and management.
- Examination of thyroid anatomy will help to determine the presence of a single or multiple nodules. Furthermore, given that such nodules are commonly found in the elderly population, a thorough assessment of the thyroid is recommended using skills of observation, palpation, auscultation, and percussion. The size, consistency, symmetry, and texture including any tenderness should also be noted. Attention to any signs of obstruction compromising blood flow, or air entry due to thyroid gland enlargement or tracheal deviation should be addressed as a matter of urgency to the medical team.
- Head and neck lymph node examination is also essential noting size, tenderness, consistency,

including whether any are mobile or fixed for the purpose of detecting any associated malignancy (Hogan-Quigley et al. 2012). Although TAs are benign and very rarely malignant, other malignancies can be picked up.

- Ophthalmopathy and other stigmata of Graves' disease, including anti-thyroid antibodies, are usually absent.

28.1.5.6 Diagnosis

- Thyroid function tests confirm hyperthyroidism (low TSH, high fT4, and high fT3) in both TA and in TMNG.
- Thyroid ultrasonography and scintiscanning provides a formal diagnosis of single nodule—TA, or multiple nodules—TMG with increased uptake.
- Thyroid peroxidase Abs are usually absent (TA and TMG).
- Fine needle aspiration biopsy is recommended for nodules greater than 1 cm in diameter or according to local hospital policy. Although the risk of malignancy thought to be low in cases of toxic nodular goitre, occasional cases of malignancy have been reported in TMNG (Cerci et al. 2007).
- Computer tomography (CT) scans or X-ray imaging may be required to assess tracheal compression from a large toxic nodular goitre. However, the use of iodine containing contrasts with CT scanning can exacerbated existing hyperthyroidism, and thus should be avoided; furthermore, caution should be practised with similar agents, for example, barium swallow test to evaluate oesophageal pressure effects.

28.1.5.7 Treatment

The treatment for TA and MNG is aimed to restore normal thyroid function. The treatment options depend on patients' age, severity of hyperthyroidism, size of goitre, and underlying medical illnesses.

28.1.5.7.1 Anti-Thyroid Medication: Carbimazole

In the UK, anti-thyroid drugs (ATDs) such as Carbimazole (CBZ) and Propylthiouracil (PTU) are effective treatments used to control thyroid function in TA or TMNG (CBZ being first choice due to its association with less side effects compared to PTU). Although an ATD is not a curative treatment for an autonomously functioning TA or TMNG, they are used primarily to stabilise thyroid function in preparation for definitive treatment such as radioiodine or thyroid surgery (British Thyroid Association-BTA 2006; American Thyroid Association – ATA 2016; National Institute for Health and Care Excellence-NICE 2016).

Beta blockade drugs: Propranolol is an effective treatment for symptom relief, and can be prescribed in combination with Carbimazole. Once euthyroidism has been achieved, Propranolol should be weaned off gradually as per local hospital policy(British Thyroid Association-BTA 2006; American Thyroid Association – ATA 2016; National Institute for Health and Care Excellence-NICE 2016; British National Formulary 2018a).

TFT monitoring on ATDs: This comprises of 4–6 weekly TFTs monitoring until euthyroidism is achieved on the minimal dose of anti-thyroid medication, for example, a starting dose of Carbimazole 20–40 mg daily is titrated against TFTs, and as TFTs improve every 4–6 weeks, Carbimazole is gradually weaned until maintenance dose of 5 mg daily is achieved in preparation for a definitive treatment(British Thyroid Association-BTA 2006; National Institute for Health and Care Excellence-NICE 2016).

28.1.5.7.2 Definitive Thyroid Surgery

Partial or complete thyroidectomy: surgery aims to remove the entire autonomously functioning nodule. In the case of a large multinodular goitre that compromises a patient's airway, or where surrounding structures cause compression and interfere with swallowing, surgery is usually favourable and often successful in the hands of an expert thyroid surgeon (Sect. 4, Chap. 28 (C) Thyroid Surgery).

Pregnancy: In hyperthyroidism associated with pregnancy, surgery is usually restricted from the first to third trimester(American Thyroid Association – ATA 2016) during which time anti-thyroid medication such as Propylthiouracil is administered to restore normal thyroid function within the safe and specific parameters recommended in pregnancy (American Thyroid Association – ATA 2016) (Sect. 4, Chap. 33).

Monitoring of thyroid function post surgery: TFTs should be monitored 4–6 weekly post-thyroid surgery with the aim to achieve euthyroidism on lifelong Thyroxine replacement.

Checks to ensure thyroidectomy site is adequately healed, calcium level within normal reference range, and importance of taking lifelong Thyroxine replacement are essential prior to discharge from secondary care. Information leaflets can also be made accessible to patients via relevant website (British Thyroid Foundation 2015a).

28.1.5.7.3 Definitive Radioiodine-RAI Treatment

The treatment of TA and TMNG with RAI avoids surgery thus is managed conservatively. In the UK, RAI 131 is prescribed within the safe recommendations of hospital guidelines (British Thyroid Association-BTA 2006; National Institute for Health and Care Excellence-NICE 2016).

It not only ablates hyperthyroidism but has also shown to reduce nodular size. Patients are likely to become hypothyroid and therefore close monitoring of thyroid hormones are paramount in the early stages to avoid the side effects of hypothyroidism.

Monitoring of thyroid function post-RAI: TFTs should be monitored 4–6 weekly to avoid occurrence of hypothyroidism. In this way, ATD can be gradually weaned off until euthyroidism is achieved, with or without Thyroxine replacement.

The effects of RAI for achieving euthyroidism approximates from 6 weeks to 3 month, sometimes even up to 6–8 months (British Thyroid Association-BTA 2006; National Institute for Health and Care Excellence-NICE 2016).

Second dose of RAI: Patients who remain hyperthyroid beyond 6–8 months following first dose of RAI, and still requiring Carbimazole, are usually offered a second dose of RAI, which usually renders the patient euthyroid.

Pregnancy: RAI is contraindicated in pregnancy (see chapter). Females receiving RAI treatment should avoid pregnancy for up to 6 weeks and suggested to seek contraceptive cover.

Long-term monitoring: after successful treatment and restoration of normal thyroid function with or without Thyroxine replacement, long-term monitoring of thyroid function is essential. Healthcare providers such as general practitioners (GPs) should be advised to monitor TFTs 6–12 monthly to avoid potential long-term effects of hypothyroidism. In this way euthyroidism can be maintained with or without Thyroxine replacement (British Thyroid Association-BTA 2006; National Institute for Health and Care Excellence-NICE 2016).

28.1.6 Thyroiditis

The term thyroiditis comes under an umbrella of a variety type of thyroid disorders. It is generally associated with inflammation of the thyroid gland, and often causes transient thyrotoxicosis, followed by temporary hypothyroidism, resulting with either restoration of normal thyroid function or permanent hypothyroidism.

Thyroiditis can also be referred to as painful (Box 28.4) or painless (Box 28.5) thyroiditis, and can occur as a result of drug therapies or through radiation (British Thyroid Association-BTA 2006; American Thyroid Association – ATA 2016).

Acquiring relevant knowledge and understanding of the distinctive features associated with the various types of thyroiditis disorders can contribute significantly towards establishing the correct diagnoses, provide the most appropriate

---

Box 28.4 Thyroiditis with Pain/Tenderness

- Subacute thyroiditis
- Infectious thyroiditis
- Radiation thyroiditis
- Palpation
- Trauma induced thyroiditis

Box 28.5 Thyroiditis with Absence of Pain/Tenderness

- Painless thyroiditis
- Post-partum thyroiditis
- Drug induced thyroiditis
- Chronic Hashimoto's thyroiditis
- Struma Ovarii (Dermoid)

---

treatment and in turn enables the nurse practitioner to manage patients promptly, efficiently and cost-effectively.

Some of the common conditions related to thyroiditis are discussed and include subacute infectious, post-partum, and silent thyroiditis.

28.1.6.1 Subacute Thyroiditis (Infectious)

28.1.6.1.1 Definition

Subacute thyroiditis (or infectious thyroiditis) is a self-limiting inflammatory disorder of the thyroid that can last for several weeks or months. It characterised by transient thyrotoxicosis, followed by hypothyroidism and then returns to normal thyroid function in the majority of patients. It is also known as 'De Quervains' named after Fritz De Quervains, a Swiss surgeon who in 1904 first described granulomatous changes as giant cells in the pathology of thyroiditis (Engkakul et al. 2011; Kaplan et al. 2011; Hennessey 2015).

Subacute thyroiditis is the most common cause of painful thyroiditis in which women, aged 20–50 years, are more frequently affected compared to men.

It is usually triggered by a viral infection, for example, mumps or flu, with highest incidence often occurring around the summer season (Hennessey 2015).

28.1.6.1.2 Aetiology

Inflammation of the thyroid gland (possibly caused by a virus) results with the release of preformed stores of thyroid hormone, including thyroglobulin and iodinated compounds, causing a rise in circulating thyroid hormones fT4 and fT3, and suppression of TSH. This phase lasts for around 1–3 months before going into spontaneous remission as colloid is depleted from the thyroid gland. In the majority of patients this results in hypothyroidism, lasting for around 3–6 months during which time the thyroid follicles begin to regenerate and return to a euthyroid state in the majority of patients.

28.1.6.1.3 Pathogenesis

In subacute thyroiditis there is destruction of follicular epithelium and loss of follicular integrity. These can appear as granulomatous with either partial or complete loss of colloid tissue forming giant cells or granulomatous thyroiditis and consistent in viral infection. On recovery, the inflammation recedes and recovery is generally complete.

28.1.6.1.4 Clinical Features

- Subacute thyroiditis starts with prolonged phase of myalgia, malaise, and fatigue.
- History of frequent upper respiratory infection.
- Fever may be present.
- Moderate to severe pain in the neck, jaw, throat, or ear. Patients can usually localise pain to thyroid region.
- Transient vocal cord paresis.
- Symptoms can be related to transient overt hyperthyroidism (Fig. 28.1) or hypothyroidism (Sect. 4, Chap. 30).
- The thyroid gland is often enlarged, firm to hard on palpation, with tenderness focused in one area spreading to other areas of the thyroid gland.

28.1.6.1.5 Diagnosis

- TFTs usually show transient thyrotoxicosis at onset lasting for around 3–6 weeks (suppressed TSH and elevated fT4 and fT3), followed by hypothyroidism usually lasting for approximately 6 months.
- Clinical features include moderate to severe pain in the neck, jaw, throat, or ear and symptoms at early onset relate to thyrotoxicosis, followed by those related to hypothyroidism.
- Raised erythrocyte sedimentation rate and raised C-reactive protein helps to confirm the diagnosis (usually resolves around 6 months).
- Full blood count may show mild anaemia.
- White blood cell count is usually elevated.
- Radioactive iodine uptake scan RAIU uptake appearance is low or undetectable.
- Thyroid peroxidase and thyroglobulin antibodies are usually low or absent.

28.1.6.1.6 Treatment

Anti-thyroid medication is usually not necessary because no new hormones are being made and due to its transient nature, normal thyroid function is restored return to normal thyroid function.

Beta-blockers such as Propranolol can be prescribed for symptom relief in transient cases of thyrotoxicosis. ATDs are not recommended due to the transient presence associated with subacute thyrotoxicosis and furthermore, Thyroxine therapy is often not required in the short hypothyroid phase; however, it can be prescribed in the very symptomatic patients for up to 3–6 months (British Thyroid Association-BTA 2006; American Thyroid Association – ATA 2016; National Institute for Health and Care Excellence-NICE 2016; British National Formulary 2018a; Shreshtha and Hennessey 2015).

Analgesia: Paracetamol, Aspirin, or nonsteroidal anti-inflammatory including Ibuprofen can all provide effective pain relief (British Thyroid Association-BTA 2006; American Thyroid Association – ATA 2016; National Institute for Health and Care Excellence-NICE 2016; Hennessey 2015; British National Formulary 2018b).

Corticosteroids: If analgesia or non-steroidal anti-inflammatory drugs (NSAID) fail to work, corticosteroids can be used and are effective, for example, prednisolone 15–40 mg daily can be prescribed for 1–2 weeks, followed by reduction of 5 mg over 2–4 weeks (British Thyroid Association-BTA 2006; American Thyroid Association – ATA 2016; National Institute for Health and Care Excellence-NICE 2016; Hennessey 2015; British National Formulary 2018b).

In subacute thyroiditis, the transient phase of thyrotoxicosis is usually 1–3 months, followed by the hypothyroid phase 3–6 months, leading to complete recovery by 12 months from onset. On recov-

Box 28.6 Case 2. A Case of Subacute Thyroiditis

A 27-year-old woman was referred by her GP to the Thyroid Nurse-Led Clinic (TNLC). She presented with a recent history of a swelling and pain of the neck, shortness of breath, feeling flushed, shaky, and anxious. These symptoms developed after an upper respiratory tract infection. Blood tests by the GP showed thyrotoxicosis [TSH <0.01 mU/L (0.35–5.5), fT4 34.6 pmol/L (10.5–20), and fT3 8.6 pmol/L (3.5–6.5)] who started Carbimazole 20 mg od. She was referred to the TNLC at a tertiary centre and assessed. Her symptoms were settling, although on palpating her neck, a very small, non-tender, soft, and symmetrical goitre was noted. Other than mild fine hand tremor, she had no other manifestations of thyrotoxicosis and there were no signs of thyroid eye disease. Investigations showed her TSH receptor Abs to be negative and TFTs: TSH 0.09, fT4 15.2, and fT3 3.5. The thyroid uptake scan showed no uptake. The Carbimazole treatment was then stopped and around 1 month later, her TFTs showed TSH 10.90, fT4 13.9, and fT3 4.3. No Levothyroxine was started and within 3 months she became biochemically euthyroid. She remained stable in the next few weeks and she was discharged back to her GP.

ery, patients should be warned of future repeated relapses that can occur especially following upper respiratory infections, and the possibility of becoming permanently hypothyroid, requiring long-term Thyroxine replacement (Box 28.6).

28.1.6.2 Post-Partum Thyroiditis

Post-partum thyroiditis (PPT) is also referred to as painless thyroiditis. In the USA, the incidence is reported to be around 10% in pregnancies. It usually occurs within the first year following childbirth or within 6 months after pregnancy

(Amino and Kubota 2011; Pearce et al. 2003). The immune system essentially attacks the thyroid gland causing temporary thyrotoxicosis (1–6 months), followed by hypothyroidism (3 months) as the thyroid gland becomes depleted of thyroid hormone, to then becoming fully recovered to euthyroid state within 12 months after childbirth. There are, however, reported cases in which some women fail to recover from the hypothyroid phase and end up requiring Thyroxine replacement (British Thyroid Association-BTA 2006; American Thyroid Association – ATA 2016; National Institute for Health and Care Excellence-NICE 2016; Latrofa et al. 2011).

PPT is often preceded by subclinical autoimmune thyroiditis. For example, immune activation causes transition of subclinical to overt autoimmune thyroid disease. During the post-partum period in patients with previous history of Graves' disease or Hashimoto's thyroiditis, immune activation results in relapse after parturition.

PPT is also seen in women with type 1 diabetes.

28.1.6.2.1 Definition

PPT thyroiditis is defined as an exacerbation of autoimmune thyroiditis during the first post-partum year and characterised by transient hyperthyroidism, transient hypothyroidism, or transient hyperthyroidism followed by transient hypothyroidism after which most women return to a state of euthyroidism at 1-year post-partum (Stagnaro-Green 2002).

28.1.6.2.2 Aetiology

The exacerbation of the underlying autoimmune thyroiditis in PPT is reported to be aggravated by auto-immunological rebound that follows the partial immunosuppression of pregnancy (Stagnaro-Green 2002).

28.1.6.2.3 Pathogenesis

Lymphocytic infiltration into thyroid causes destruction of thyroid gland (similar changes occur in both Hashimoto's and painless thyroiditis). Autoimmune lymphocytic infiltration of the thyroid results in release of stored thyroid hormone (Stagnaro-Green 2002).

28.1.6.2.4 Clinical Features

- Patient may or may not be symptomatic in subclinical thyrotoxicosis. In overt thyrotoxicosis, patients are more likely to experience moderate to severe symptoms such as sweating, palpitations, and fine hand tremor (Fig. 28.1). This phase can occur between 2 and 10 month. Patients entering the hypothyroid phase will experience related symptoms such as cold intolerance, reduced concentration, and constipation (Sect. 4, Chap. 30).
- In some cases, patients may show signs of post-partum depression.
- Graves' eye disease and myxoedema may be present.

28.1.6.2.5 Diagnosis

- Abnormal thyroid dysfunction occurs depending on the phase of PPT, for example, TFTs may indicate subclinical thyrotoxicosis, overt thyrotoxicosis, or hypothyroidism.
- Overt hyperthyroid should be differentiated from post-partum Graves' (e.g. time of onset 2–10 month) and destructive thyrotoxicosis (e.g. onset 1–3 month).
- Elevated (positive) antithyroglobulin antibodies or anti-thyroid peroxidase antibodies.
- RAIU is either low or undetectable.
- Positive TSHRAbs in early pregnancy may indicate risk to developing post-partum Graves' disease and can be confirmed by the presence of a pronounced goitre with bruit, Graves' ophthalmopathy, and increased RAIU.

28.1.6.2.6 Treatment

Untreated hyperthyroidism in post-partum destructive thyrotoxicosis usually resolves spontaneously within 2–3 months, thus the use of anti-thyroid medication is ineffective. However, in patients whose quality of life is disrupted with the burdensome symptoms of hyperthyroidism, use of beta-blockers such as Propranolol or Metoprolol can be prescribed for effective relief. Furthermore, during the hypothyroid phase-related symptoms can be managed with Thyroxine under the guidance of an obstetrician and local hospital policy and guidelines.

Box 28.7 Case 3. Post-Partum Thyroiditis

A 42-year-old mother was referred by her GP feeling unwell with a range of symptoms including tiredness, anxiety, tearfulness, exhaustion, and irritability. Her symptoms started around 6 months after the birth of her baby. Blood tests by her GP showed mild thyrotoxicosis [TSH <0.01 mU/L (0.35–5.5), fT4 24.8 pmol/L (10.5–20), fT3 8.4 pmol/L (3.5–6.9)], and GP commenced anti-thyroid medication. She was referred to the thyroid nurse-led clinic at a tertiary centre 2 months later. Blood tests showed hypothyroidism [TSH 10.99 mU/L (0.35–5.5), fT4 8.7 pmol/L (10.5–20), fT3 4.7 pmol/L (3.5–6.9)] and the medical treatment was stopped. TSH receptor Abs were negative and her anti-TPO Abs were elevated. She was monitored for 6 months, recovered and remained euthyroid and was discharged back to her GP. She was informed that in case of another pregnancy, there was a risk of a future relapse of the post-partum thyroiditis.

In post-partum Graves' disease, if usual course of thyroiditis fails to recover, treatment can be managed with the use of anti-thyroid drugs, radioiodine, or thyroid surgery (Box 28.7).

28.1.6.3 Silent Thyroiditis

Silent thyroiditis is also known as painless thyroiditis. It has a low genetic predisposition and is more common in women than in men.

28.1.6.3.1 Definition

Painless or silent thyroiditis is characterised by an autoimmune-mediated lymphocytic inflammation of the thyroid gland that leads to destructive thyroiditis. This occurs through the release of thyroid hormone, triggering transient thyrotoxicosis that is often followed by a hypothyroid phase, progressing to full recovery by 12–18 months. However, some of these patients will go on to develop early permanent hypothyroidism, whilst in others, long-term hypothyroidism can also occur many years later.

Silent thyroiditis has similarities to post-partum thyroiditis and also to a form of the auto-immune thyroid disorder called Hashimoto's thyroiditis (Sect. 28.1.6.4).

It can also develop from an enlarging existing goitre, or occur as a result of treatments such as radiotherapy, drug induced therapies containing iodine, lithium, interleukin-2 and interferon (British Thyroid Association-BTA 2006; American Thyroid Association – ATA 2016; Latrofa et al. 2011; Kaplan et al. 2011; Pearce et al. 2003).

Hyperthyroidism is an autoimmune disease and in the majority of patients, manifested by positive anti-thyroid peroxidase and antithyro-globulin antibodies.

28.1.6.3.2 Aetiology
Autoimmune lymphocytic infiltration essentially causes release of stored thyroid hormones result-ing in destruction of thyroidal tissue.

28.1.6.3.3 Pathogenesis
Thyroid tissue changes take place as a result of chronic lymphocytic infiltration. For example, the follicular cells within the thyroid gland undergo metaplasia, resulting as larger eosino-philic cells known as Hurthle cells. These contain mitochondria that can progress to fibrosis, and occupy focal regions within the thyroid or affect the entire thyroid gland.

28.1.6.3.4 Clinical Features
- Non-tender goitre, absence of fever, malaise and neck pain
- Asymptomatic although, some patient may experience symptoms-related thyrotoxicosis (Fig. 28.1) or hypothyroidism (Sect. 4, Chap. 30).

28.1.6.3.5 Diagnosis
- Anti-thyroid peroxidase and antithyroglobulin antibodies are usually high (positive)
- Hallmark of silent thyroiditis is the absence of thyroid pain and RAIU of the thyroid is usu-ally low or undetectable.

- A positive TSHRAb test, presence of a goitre, and increased RAIU, is likely to be associated it with a variant of Graves' disease with cyto-toxic properties resulting in a form of Hashimoto's thyroiditis.
- Painless thyroiditis is rarely associated with Graves' ophthalmopathy (Latrofa et al. 2011).
- FNA: may be required if a pre-existing goitre enlarges.

28.1.6.3.6 Treatment
In the initial phase of silent thyroiditis, there is usually transient self-limiting thyrotoxicosis fol-lowed by hypothyroidism that recovers spontane-ously. There is no role for the use of ATDs; however, symptomatic patients can be prescribed beta-blockers such as Propranolol that can be weaned off when the transient phase passes.

If the phase of thyrotoxicosis is so severe, cor-ticosteroids can be administered according to hospital policy.

TFT are usually monitored 4–6 weekly aim-ing to maintain euthyroidism. The recovery period can take 12–18 months; however, few patients may develop permanent hypothyroidism and require long-term treatment with Thyroxine and regular follow-up as per local guidelines.

28.1.6.4 Autoimmune Hashimoto's Thyroiditis

28.1.6.4.1 Definition
Hashimoto's thyroiditis (HT) is an autoimmune condition, named after a Japanese surgeon, Dr. Hakaru Hashimoto, who in 1912 first associated the histology of thyroid with lymphocytic infil-tration, parenchymal atrophy, fibrosis, and eosin-ophilic changes (Pearce et al. 2003; Akamizu and Amino 2018; Hiromatsu et al. 2013).

HT occurs in all ages but mostly seen in young and middle-aged women. The disorder often can run in families and reported to have a genetic pre-disposition. It has also been referred to as pain-less thyroiditis, similar to that associated with silent thyroiditis and post-partum described pre-viously (Pearce et al. 2003; Burman 2017).

In addition, HT can also be associated with other autoimmune conditions including insulin-dependent diabetes mellitus, vitiligo, pernicious anaemia, and Addison's disease.

28.1.6.4.2 Pathology

The follicular tissue is affected within the thyroid gland and becomes occupied by lymphoid tissue. Over time, lymphocytic infiltration and follicular cells changes occur leading to the formation of fibrotic tissue that can effects a local area of the thyroid or occupy the entire gland (Kaplan et al. 2011; Pearce et al. 2003; Akamizu and Amino 2018).

In some patients, lymphoma has been reported in HT although this is extremely rare (Pearce et al. 2003).

28.1.6.4.3 Clinical Features

- HT is mostly seen in middle-aged women and often picked up on routine clinical assessment or incidental finding.
- Patient may report of neck enlargement over years or sudden onset of rapid enlargement.
- There may be signs of local compression, affecting swallowing or compromising airway (this may be accompanied by a vague ache or tenderness).
- On palpation, the goitre is usually symmetrical, can vary in size, and has a soft-to-firm consistency, with an irregular surface (Kaplan et al. 2011).
- Patient may be asymptomatic if euthyroid, or present with symptoms related to hypothyroidism (Sect. 4, Chap. 30) (very occasionally, some patients with HT can present with mild thyrotoxicosis in the very early stage of disease).
- Fine needle aspiration (FNA) may be required in cases where a thyroid nodule may be present.
- Lymph nodes of the head and neck may be enlarged and should be assessed and evaluated accordingly (e.g., noting location, size, mobility) in case of malignancy (Hogan-Quigley et al. 2012).
- Ophthalmology in HT may also be present and evaluated in case an ophthalmology referral is required (Sect. 4, Chap. 31).

28.1.6.4.4 Biochemical and Imaging Features

- Thyroid hormone findings are usually within normal range or may result with permanent hypothyroidism; however, some patients develop mild thyrotoxicosis also known as hashi-toxicosis.
- Imaging in HT usually shows an enlarged thymus.
- RAIU appears low and patchy on uptake and is only useful in identifying a toxic nodule where the uptake will be increased, and then evaluated by an ultrasound.

28.1.6.4.5 Diagnosis

- The hallmark for diagnosis of HT is increased anti-thyroid peroxide and antithyroglobulin antibodies.
- FNA may be required to exclude any nodule malignancy if a goitre presents with a toxic nodule.

28.1.6.4.6 Treatment

Most cases of HT do not require treatment due to the presence of a small goitre and no symptoms (Vickery and Hamlin 1961). Patients who make good recovery are often prone to frequent future relapse and should therefore be made aware of becoming permanently hypothyroid, requiring lifelong Thyroxine replacement.

Patients with hypothyroidism are usually treated with Thyroxine replacement, calculated under medical supervision according to local guidelines or hospital policy.

TFTs are usually monitored 4–6 weekly, and the goal is to achieve normalisation of thyroid hormones. TFTs checks thereafter can be monitored 6–12 monthly in case adjustment is required.

Special attention should be practised when prescribing Thyroxine replacement in any patient over the age of 60 years, for example, gradual incremental doses of 25 μg daily is suggested to avoid any cardiovascular risks.

Thyroxine replacement is also reported to have a beneficial effect on reducing the size of a large goitre; however, in the elderly, reduction in size is thought to be delayed due to the fibrotic changes within the thyroid gland.

28.1.7 Struma Ovarii

Struma ovarii (SO) was first described by Dr. Richard Boettlin who discovered the presence of thyroid follicular tissue in ovaries (Boettlin 1889).

Most of the published data for SO are based on case study findings.

28.1.7.1 Definition
SO is defined as a type of dermoid tumour (germ cell) (Young 1993) and account for 1% of all ovarian tumours and 2–5% of ovarian teratomas (Yoo et al. 2008; Kondi-Parfit et al. 2011).

These tumours comprise over 50% of mature thyroid tissue and although this makes it uniquely termed as struma ovarii, thyrotoxicosis is found in less than 10% of cases making SO often very difficult to diagnose (Yassa et al. 2008; Kraemer et al. 2011).

SO effects women aged between 40 and 60 years (Yoo et al. 2008; Kondi-Parfit et al. 2011). Most cases of SO are benign; however, the potential for malignancy has been found on occasions, the most common being associated with papillary thyroid cancer (Yoo et al. 2008; Kraemer et al. 2011; Makani et al. 2004; DeSimone et al. 2003).

28.1.7.2 Pathogenesis
The histology of SO more often shows the presence of benign thyroid follicular and colloid cells; however, pathological changes can also take place causing hyperfunction of thyroid gland (Szyfelbein et al. 1994; Dunzendorfer et al. 1999). Malignancies can be associated with papillary thyroid carcinoma (Kraemer et al. 2011; Makani et al. 2004).

28.1.7.3 Clinical Features
(Clinical features may or may not be present)

- Hyperthyroid symptoms can occur in less than 10% of cases (Fig. 28.1)
- Lower abdominal pain
- Palpable lower abdominal mass

- Abnormal vaginal bleeding
- Abdominal ascites (Mui et al. 2009)

28.1.7.4 Biochemical and Imaging Investigations
- Hyperthyroidism (although rare): suppressed TSH, raised fT4 and fT3
- Imaging with Radioiodine (I)-whole body scan shows pelvic mass, with thyroid involvement
- Ultrasonography shows ovarian mass
- Antithyroglobulin antibodies usually elevated

28.1.7.5 Diagnosis
- RAIU of thyroid is usually low to undetectable.
- Elevated serum thyroglobulin.
- RAIU in pelvis is increased (not in thyroid gland) and extra-thyroidal struma ovarii suspected.
- Histology and pathology findings reveal thyroid tissue as the major component.

28.1.7.6 Treatment
Surgical resection of mass is the approach for benign disease, including regular serum thyroglobulin level checks used as a marker for recurrence at follow-up.

Surgery with adjuvant radioiodine therapy has been shown to be successful in treating metastatic and recurrent disease (Yoo et al. 2008).

28.1.8 Anti-thyroid Drug Therapy

Thionamides are group of chemically related compounds used as anti-thyroid drug (ATD) treatments for managing hyperthyroidism. They are used in preparation for thyroidectomy in hyperthyroidism or prescribed as therapy prior to and post-radioiodine treatment (British Thyroid Association-BTA 2006; British National Formulary 2018a).

28.1.8.1 Carbimazole and Propylthiouracil
The most commonly used ATD treatment in the UK is Carbimazole (CBZ). Propylthiouracil

(PTU) is also available although this can sometimes be used if patients develop adverse effects to CBZ such as rash, stomach upset, nauseas, and occasionally hair loss (British National Formulary 2018a; Tidy 2014). PTU is usually reserved for pregnancy and is usually administered during the first trimester as it is reported to minimise the potential side effects of fetal malformation that have been associated with Carbimazole in pregnancy (American Thyroid Association – ATA 2016; Cooper and Laurberg 2013; Bowman et al. 2012) (Sect. 4, Chap. 33) (Box 28.8).

CBZ and PTU exert their action on thyroid tissue by inhibiting iodination of thyroglobulin thereby gradually diminishing thyroid hormone secretion, thereby rendering the patient euthyroid and controlling hyperthyroidism in the majority of patients (Laurberg 2006; Cooper 2005). However, the rate of relapse following an 18-month course of ATD treatment is reported to be around 40–60% (Bartelena 2008; Benker et al. 1998; Hedley et al. 1998).

The use and availability of CBZ is known in many parts of Europe. However, in the USA, anti-thyroid treatments used are Methimazole (considered the equivalent of CBZ) and PTU.

The use of healthcare guidelines from reputable organisations often provides an itinerary of recommendations of the most up-to-date evidence-based related research for use in clinical practice. The following governing bodies from the UK, Europe, and the USA have published advice and suggestions for managing patients with hyperthyroidism (Box 28.8).

Anti-thyroid drugs have a number of benefits for managing thyrotoxicosis. The aim of these medications includes:

- Control of symptoms related to hyperthyroidism with the aim to restore normal thyroid function
- To induce remission in Graves' hyperthyroidism
- To achieve euthyroidism in hyperthyroid disorders such as toxic goitre, in preparation for treatment with radioiodine or thyroid surgery

---

Box 28.8 A Consensus of Guideline Recommendations for Managing Hyperthyroidism

- UK guidelines are available for the management of thyroid function tests in thyroid disease published by the Association for Clinical Biochemistry, the British Thyroid Association, and the British Thyroid Foundation (British Thyroid Association-BTA 2006).
- The 2015 European Thyroid Association guidelines on diagnosis and treatment of endogenous subclinical hyperthyroidism (Bondi et al. 2015).
- US evidence-based guidelines on hyperthyroidism and other causes of thyrotoxicosis: management guidelines of the American Thyroid Association and American Association of Clinical Endocrinologists (American Thyroid Association – ATA 2016).

Expert opinion in review articles (Weetman, 2013 & Vaidya and Pearce, 2014). Advice on symptoms suggesting adverse effects (Vaidya and Pearce 2014; Weetman 2013).

- To manage hyperthyroidism in cases of recurrence of Graves' disease
- To maintain normal thyroid function in long-term treatment in the elderly

28.1.8.2 Anti-thyroid Drug Regimes

28.1.8.2.1 Graves' Hyperthyroidism

Titration block regime: In the UK, titration with CBZ is used as primary treatment.

Titration method involves the measurement of thyroid hormones TSH and fT4.

Drug dose regime: This varies according to the severity of hyperthyroidism. In overt hyperthyroidism, many hospital policies adopt a high dose treatment, for example, CBZ 30–40 mg daily for the first 2–3 months (British

Thyroid Association-BTA 2006; National Institute for Health and Care Excellence-NICE 2016).

Thyroid function tests: TSH, fT3, and FT4 monitoring is recommended 4–6 weekly after initiation of ATD (e.g. CBZ or PTU) and during dose titration until euthyroidism is achieved. For example, in Graves' hyperthyroidism, normalisation of thyroid hormones in compliant patients can take around 2–6 months through gradual weaning to a minimal maintenance dose of CBZ 5 mg daily. Thereafter, TFTs can be monitored every 3–4 months until treatment is discontinued at around 18 months or according to local hospital policy (British Thyroid Association-BTA 2006; National Institute for Health and Care Excellence-NICE 2016; Bartelena 2008) (Flow Chart 28.1). The steady weaning process is also thought to decrease thyroid stimulating antibody (TSAb) and TSH-binding inhibitor immunoglobulin (TBII), and furthermore reported to be a reliable predictor of remission in Graves' hyperthyroidism (Takasu et al. 2000).

Duration of treatment for potential remission: The mechanism behind the remission is thought to be due to the immunosuppressive action of the ATD (McGregor et al. 1980). In the UK, treatment for Graves' hyperthyroidism usually comprises an 18 month ATD therapy (British Thyroid Association-BTA 2006; National Institute for Health and Care Excellence-NICE 2016; Bartelena 2008), or according to national or local hospital guidelines. Beyond this time serves no additional benefit (Abraham et al. 2010).

Furthermore, the measurement of TSHRAb levels prior to discontinuation of ATD therapy is thought to be useful in predicting those patients who will have a better chance of achieving remission.

At completion of the 18-month course of ATD treatment, TFTs can be monitored 4–6 weekly. If patient remains euthyroid, the time interval for TFTs monitoring can be extended to 2, 3, and then 6 months. If patient continues to remain euthyroid and in remission by 8–12 months, plans can be made to discharge back to healthcare provider with follow-up instructions (Flow Charts 28.1 and 28.2 Graves').

Block and replace regime: In the UK, this regime is less commonly used compared to the

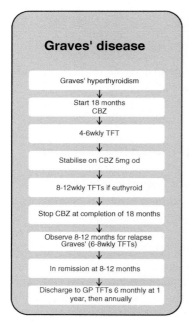
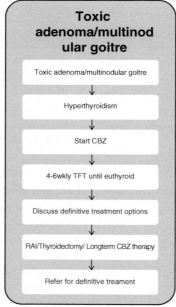
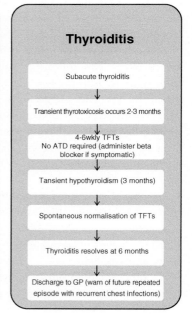

Flow Chart 28.1 Hyperthyroid conditions and ATD summarised

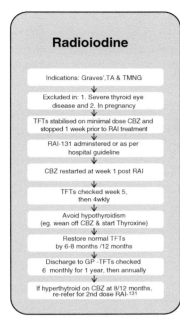

Radioiodine

Indications: Graves', TA & TMNG
↓
Excluded in: 1. Severe thyroid eye disease and 2. In pregnancy
↓
TFTs stabilised on miniimal dose CBZ and stopped 1 week prior to RAI treatment
↓
RAI-131 adminstered or as per hospital guideline
↓
CBZ restarted at week 1 post RAI
↓
TFTs checked week 5, then 4wkly
↓
Avoid hypothyroidism (eg. wean off CBZ & start Thyroxine)
↓
Restore normal TFTs by 6-8 months /12 months
↓
Discharge to GP -TFTs checked 6 monthly for 1 year, then annually
↓
If hyperthyroid on CBZ at 8/12 months, re-refer for 2nd dose RAI-131

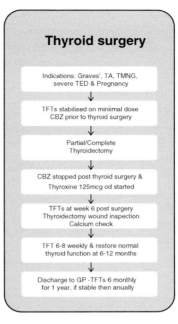

Thyroid surgery

Indications: Graves', TA, TMNG, severe TED & Pregnancy
↓
TFTs stabilised on miniimal dose CBZ prior to thyroid surgery
↓
Partial/Complete Thyroidectomy
↓
CBZ stopped post thyroid surgery & Thyroxine 125mcg od started
↓
TFTs at week 6 post surgery Thyroidectomy wound inspection Calcium check
↓
TFT 6-8 weekly & restore normal thyroid function at 6-12 months
↓
Discharge to GP -TFTs 6 monthly for 1 year, if stable then anually

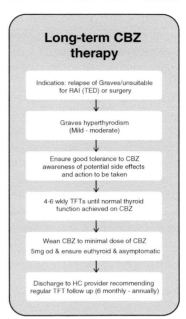

Long-term CBZ therapy

Indicatios: relapse of Graves/unsuitable for RAI (TED) or surgery
↓
Graves hyperthyrodism (Mild - moderate)
↓
Ensure good tolerance to CBZ awareness of potential side effects and action to be taken
↓
4-6 wkly TFTs until normal thyroid function achieved on CBZ
↓
Wean CBZ to minimal dose of CBZ 5mg od & ensure euthyroid & asymptomatic
↓
Discharge to HC provider recommending regular TFT follow up (6 monthly - annually)

Flow Chart 28.2 Definitive (radioiodine and thyroid surgery) and long-term ATD therapy

preferred ATD titration option (Bartelena 2008), and avoided in pregnancy (Cooper 2005; Burch and Cooper 2015; British Thyroid Foundation 2015b). Furthermore, the rate of remission in Graves' hyperthyroidism with this method is no different when compared to dose titration option (Vaidya and Pearce 2014).

Block and replace comprises a combination of CBZ and Thyroxine. CBZ is used to block thyroid hormones synthesis, whilst Thyroxine works by replacing thyroid hormones thought to not only stabilise the thyroid but also minimise the chances of becoming resistant to medication. This regime is used in Graves' disease, and the recommended course of treatment is around 6–12 months (or according to the supervising endocrinologist, national or hospital guidelines). The advantages of this regime is that the patient often requires less frequent patient hospital visits and few drug dose adjustments compared to the titration method; however, poor compliancy to medication may serve as a disadvantage due to the number of tablets the patient has to take on a daily basis (Bartelena 2008), and so caution must be practised when following this regime.

Drug dose regime: This starts with CBZ 20–40 mg daily for the first 4–6 weekly until fT4 has normalised on this dose. Thereafter, Thyroxine 125 μg daily is only then commenced (British Thyroid Association-BTA 2006; National Institute for Health and Care Excellence-NICE 2016).

Thyroid function tests: These should be monitored 4–6 weekly and adjustments only made to the dose of Thyroxine if indicated. When TFTs have normalised, the dose of anti-thyroid drug and Thyroxine usually remains unchanged. TFT monitoring can then be done less frequent as 3–6 monthly or as per local hospital guideline (British Thyroid Association-BTA 2006).

28.1.8.2.2 Toxic Adenoma or Toxic Multinodular Goitre

CBZ or equivalent in TA and TMNG is only used as a short-term measure to control hyperthyroidism, as remission is highly unlikely (Flow Charts 28.1 and 28.2 Nodule/s). When normal thyroid function is achieved, CBZ is continued to maintain control of hyperthyroidism until preparation for a more definitive treatment (radioiodine or thyroid surgery) is arranged (British Thyroid Association-BTA 2006; American Thyroid Association – ATA 2016).

28.1.8.2.3 Thyroiditis

Antithyroid drugs are rarely used in thyroiditis given its transient nature, for example, the temporary spill of thyroid hormones into the circulation results in transient thyrotoxicosis, followed by hypothyroidism, thereafter returning to euthyroid state and fully recovered by 8–12 months (Kaplan et al. 2011) (Flow Chart 28.1 Thyroiditis).

Very occasionally, the use of CBZ can sometimes be indicated in symptomatic cases of postpartum thyroiditis having a previous history of Graves' disease.

28.1.8.2.4 Pregnancy

Treatment of hyperthyroidism in pregnancy reduces the risk for fetal complications, however, following the recommended national or local guidelines can help avoid miscarriage and fetal abnormalities (British Thyroid Association-BTA 2006; American Thyroid Association – ATA 2016) (Sect. 4, Chap. 33).

28.1.8.3 Agranulocytosis

Granulocytes are neutrophils (a type of white cell) that help to fight infection and are manufactured in bone marrow.

One of the rare side effects of ATDs such as CBZ, PTU, and Methimazole is agranulocytosis (Vicente et al. 2017). Agranulocytosis is the term used when the bone marrow fails to produce sufficient amount of granulocytes resulting in decreased neutrophils leading to neutropenia.

Neutropenia in bone marrow suppression can lead to serious life-threatening risk to infection and consequently be detrimental to a patient's well-being.

In the UK, CBZ is the preferred choice of ATD therapy compared to PTU as it has a reduced risk of serious liver damage and reported to be around 1 in 10,000 adults (Cooper and Rivkees 2009).

Healthcare practitioners starting patients on ATDs should always inform and warn patients of the potential side effect of agranulocytosis, and the procedure to take should this occur (Box 28.9).

In circumstances when ATD treatment is discontinued due to low neutrophil count, Propranolol or a similar alternative can be used in place until neutrophils are restored. In addition to this, an urgent referral should be initiated for a

---

Box 28.9 Side Effects of CBZ and PTU (Signs of Bone Marrow Suppression)

Neutropenia

- Sore throat
- Fever or chills
- Bruising
- Mouth ulcers
- Infection
- Sinusitis/otitis
- Swollen or tender gums
- Cough dyspnoea

Agranulocytosis
Sudden onset of:

- Malaise
- Fever (>40 °C) and chills
- Rapid pulse and respiration
- Pharyngitis with difficulty with swallowing
- Painful ulcers and oral cavity

Action taken for any side effects

- **STOP CBZ or PTU**
- Full blood count should be taken straight away.
- Results should be processed and evaluated within 24 h.
- If neutrophils are within normal range, it is safe for CBZ or PTU to be restarted.

If neutrophils are below normal range, patient should remain off CBZ or PTU, and definitive treatment options discussed with an urgent referral for either RAI or thyroid surgery. (Propranolol or alternative can be used in place of CBZ or PTU until neutrophils are restored)

suitable definitive treatment option (radioiodine or thyroid surgery).

28.1.8.4 Thyroid Function Monitoring and Discharge Instructions

28.1.8.4.1 Thyroid Function Monitoring
- Serum FT4 and TSH should be measured in all patients receiving thionamides.
- In most cases, the FT4 result will be the marker of choice to guide therapy.
- 4–6 weekly TFT monitoring is recommended at initiation of ATD until euthyroidism is achieved; then time interval can be extended according to hospital policy guidelines.
- A fall in FT4 to low normal or to below the normal range should prompt reduction in ATD dosage.
- A rise in serum TSH above normal reference range indicates the development of hypothyroidism and the need for dose reduction.
- A persistent suppression of serum TSH may not always indicate a need to increase ATD and should be discussed with senior practitioner for advice.

28.1.8.4.2 Discharge Instructions from Secondary Care to Healthcare Provider
The healthcare provider is recommended to monitor TFTs 6 monthly for the first year, and if the patient remains euthyroid, TFTs can be monitored annually thereafter (or earlier should symptoms of hyperthyroidism re-occur).

If Graves' hyperthyroidism re-occurs, HCP restarts ATD treatment and re-refers the patient back to endocrine services to discuss definitive treatment options (RAI or thyroid surgery).

28.1.8.5 Propranolol and Potassium Iodide

28.1.8.5.1 Propranolol
Propranolol is a beta-adrenoceptor antagonist also known as a beta-blocker (British National Formulary 2018a).

Action
In hyperthyroidism, there is an increased beta-adrenergic activity as a result of the symptoms

caused by high levels of circulating thyroid hormones. For this reason, Propranolol works well to rapidly reduce symptoms such as palpitations, heat intolerance, tachycardia anxiety (British National Formulary 2018a; Marcocci et al. 2011). Furthermore, it also works by inhibiting extrathyroidal conversion of T4 to T3, and although the reduction in T3 is limited, it is considered as an effective short-term treatment for managing thyrotoxicosis especially in the absence of CBZ and PTU (British National Formulary 2018a).

Uses
- When ATD such as CBZ or PTU cannot be used because the patient has developed side effects.
- As a temporary measure until a diagnosis and referral is made for definitive treatment (RAI or thyroid surgery).
- In some cases of thyroiditis where symptom control is required in transient phase of thyrotoxicosis.

Propranolol is effective in reducing many of the clinical features of hyperthyroidism, for example, palpitations, heat intolerance, anxiety, and tremor (Fig. 28.1). Although Propranolol does not completely abolish the symptoms of thyrotoxicosis compared to CBZ or PTU, patients can be relieved of some troublesome symptoms until a suitable treatment pathway is established.

Dosage
- The starting dose of Propranolol for mild to moderate thyrotoxicosis is usually 10 mg/20 mg/40 mg tds.
- In severe cases, Propranolol can be prescribed up to 80–120 mg daily.

Caution
- Beta-blockers should be avoided in patients with history of asthma and chronic obstructive airways disease. In cases of neutropenia due to the use of anti-thyroid drugs such as CBZ or PTU, beta-blockers are often the only available treatment and sometimes can be administered under the close supervision by a senior medical endocrine practitioner (British National Formulary 2018a).

- Dose reduction of Propranolol is required in renal and liver impairment.
- Care should be taken in breastfeeding as small amounts are contained in breast milk.

Contraindicated
- Avoided with Verapamil

Side Effects
- These are rare and can be found in the most up-to-date national guidelines (National Institute for Health and Care Excellence-NICE 2016; British National Formulary 2018a).

Weaning Off Propranolol
- Gradual weaning of Propranolol is recommended according to local hospital/guidelines. This avoids the potential occurrence of myocardial ischaemia.

28.1.8.5.2 Potassium Iodide
Potassium Iodide (KI) is a thyroid-blocking agent (Ross 2017c; Wass and Owen 2014; Electronic Medical Com 2016). It is also known as Lugol's solution, which was discovered in 1829 by a French physician called Jean Guillaume August Lugol. This was used for treating tuberculosis and as a disinfectant for various procedures including dental, histologic preparations, etc.

In around the 1920s, it was being used as a preoperative measure for controlling hyperthyroidism (Callissendorf and Falhammar 2017; Plummer 1924). In the UK, Potassium Iodide is used as a preoperative measure in patients with controlled or uncontrolled hyperthyroidism requiring thyroid surgery (British Thyroid Association-BTA 2006; Wass and Owen 2014).

Mechanism of Action
It works by decreasing thyroidal iodide uptake and blocks the release of thyroid hormones. It also is reported to decrease the thyroidal blood flow by shrinking the thyroid blood vessels, making surgery less risky especially when operating on a very large goitre (American Thyroid Association – ATA 2016; Paul et al. 1988).

Uses and Procedure
- In the UK, ATDs are initially used to achieve euthyroidism prior to thyroid surgery and when RAI is not suitable. In cases where ATDs cannot be used due to agranulocytosis, the use of beta blockade drugs such as Propranolol can be substituted as a temporary measure to stabilise thyroid hormones as best as possible with the necessary precautions in place.
- In patients with uncontrolled hyperthyroidism and when urgent thyroid surgery is required, patients can be prescribed Potassium Iodide 60 mg tds orally that can be given preoperatively for up to 10 days. Thyroid surgery must take place no later than during this time to avoid exacerbation of thyrotoxicosis (Wass and Owen 2014).

Drug information should be thoroughly checked at all times prior to prescribing medications to patients, whilst at the same time ensuring it complies with the most up-to-date, evidence-based recommendations from reputable resources (British Thyroid Association-BTA 2006; American Thyroid Association – ATA 2016; National Institute for Health and Care Excellence-NICE 2016; Electronic Medical Com 2016; British National Formulary 2018c) or local hospital policies and guidelines.

28.1.8.6 Long-Term Anti-Thyroid Drug Therapy
In Graves' hyperthyroidism, ATDs are commonly used to stabilise the thyroid hormones with a view to achieve euthyroid state and remission. However, considering that relapse rate of Graves' hyperthyroidism is high following a 12–18-month course of ATD and remission low (Bartelena 2008; Benker et al. 1998; Hedley et al. 1998), most patients go on to have definitive treatment such as thyroid surgery or radioiodine treatment.

The use of long-term therapy with ATD such as CBZ is considered to be safe and effective in achieving permanent remission (Barrio et al. 2005; Leger et al. 2012).

Therefore, in some patients, it may be appropriate to prescribe long-term control with minimal dose of ATD, for example, Carbimazole 5 mg daily or Propylthiouracil 50 mg equivalent. Caution for safe prescribing of such medications is paramount for example side effects explained and the appropriate action to be taken (Box 28.9), as well as the importance of maintaining normal thyroid function with regular blood checks (Flow Chart 28.2. Long-term Carbimazole therapy). The following principles should therefore be considered carefully for all patients prior to commencing long-term ATD treatment (Organzi and Bournard 2011).

- Suitable in cases with mild–moderate Graves' hyperthyroidism
- Euthyroid state achieved on minimal ATD, e.g. Carbimazole 5 mg daily (or equivalent)
- Has good tolerance to Carbimazole
- In those with a small goitre (absence of a large goitre)
- Patients who are asymptomatic
- Healthcare provider and patients committed to regular annual follow-up to ensure thyroid hormones remain within normal reference range.

Summary of recommendations for the management of hyperthyroidism with antithyroid medication (Box 28.10).

Box 28.10 Specialist Nurse Recommendations on Initial Management of Hyperthyroidism and ATD Therapy

- **Rapport:** is essential between the clinical specialist and the patient. It helps create a climate of trust and cooperation for establishing a successful treatment outcome and positive patient experience.
- **Clear explanation:** patients require clear, understandable explanation of their thyroid condition. Use of diagrams, information leaflets and websites such as BTF (http://www.btf-thyroid.org/), BTA (https://www.british-thyroid-association.org/), and TEDct (http://tedct.org.uk/) are useful sources of evidence-based information.

- **History taking and physical assessment**
  - **O**nset: of neck complaint (e.g. swelling)
  - **L**ocation: of neck swelling (e.g. right or left lobe or both lobes)
  - **D**uration: how long has the swelling been present (e.g over days/months/year/or sudden)
  - **C**haracteristics: of neck swelling (e.g. smooth, irregular, soft, or firm)
  - **A**ssociated characteristics: pain and fever (e.g. sharp/dull/aching or redness/hot)
  - **R**elief strategy: of neck swelling and pain (e.g. Paracetamol for pain relief)
  - **T**reatment: by healthcare provider (e.g. TFTs indicate thyrotoxicosis and referred to endocrinology in secondary care)
  - *Review of systems:* including cardiac, respiratory, renal, abdominal, neuroperipheral.
  - *Eye evaluation for Graves':* ophthalmopathy and plan to refer to ophthalmologist
  - *Past medical and surgical history:* e.g. Asthma and avoiding use of Propranolol
  - *Social:* e.g. smoking and evaluation and health promotion to discourage smoking
  - *Medication history:* noting any potential medications that might interact with anti-thyroid medication
  - **Allergies:** especially if there is a previous history of adverse effects with ATD
- **Females and pregnancy:** Females of childbearing age should avoid pregnancy during ATD. If pregnancy occurs, the Carbimazole should be switched to PTU especially during the first trimester. The doses of PTU should not exceed 200 mg daily. Referral should be made to the endocrine combined obstetrics specialist

services. Specialist nurse monitoring continues after child delivery to manage the thyroid disorder. TFT monitoring 4 weekly or as hospital policy.

- **Baseline blood investigations and vital signs**: This allows to establish diagnosis of hyperthyroidism and any differential diagnosis
  - TFTs, Thyroid TSH receptor, and peroxidase Abs
  - FBC, U & Es, LFT
  - Blood pressure, heart rate, pulse, respiration, weight
- **Side effects of ATD**: Obtain medical history and ensure compatibility with ATD, or if there is a previous history of adverse events with ATD, use of Propranolol or equivalent may be necessary until diagnosis made (such patients would warrant an urgent referral for definitive treatment (e.g. radioiodine or thyroid surgery)
- **Agranulocytosis:** Provide related patient information, e.g. warn patients about the rare side effects of ATD and the importance of stopping CBZ/PTU should a sore throat, fever, mouth ulcers, or any bruising develop. Furthermore to have a FBC followed up within 24 h and to determine whether anti-thyroid drug should be continued or not.
- **Contact details:** Ensure patient has telephone support line and email details of nurse-led clinic/endocrinology services (Benner 1984; BTA 2018; BTF 2018; TEDct 2018; Hogan-Quigley et al. 2012).

28.2 Section B: Radioiodine Therapy (1-131)

28.2.1 Radioactive Iodine Treatment (I-131)

Radioactive iodine has been used in the treatment of hyperthyroidism since the early 1940s. It is offered orally as a capsule or liquid form. The radioactive iodine is taken up by the thyroid and gradually destroys the cells in the gland.

28.2.1.1 Indications for Offering I-131 in Benign Thyroid Disease

- Graves' disease (in the UK, first-line treatment after recurrence)
- Toxic adenoma
- Toxic multinodular goitre

28.2.1.2 Contraindications for Radioiodine 1-131

- Pregnancy
- Breastfeeding
- Planning pregnancy
- Active moderate to severe or sight-threatening Graves' ophthalmopathy
- Inability to comply with radiation safety recommendations
- In patients with thyroid nodules suspicious for or proven (following fine needle aspiration) thyroid cancer

Graves' ophthalmopathy: Patients with mild active Graves' ophthalmopathy, I-131 administration should be followed by prophylactic steroid treatment. Factors related with worsening of the ophthalmopathy after I-131 include smoking, high pre-treatment T3 levels, high TSH-receptor antibody titres, and untreated hypothyroidism after the I-131 (See chapter).

28.2.1.3 Treatment Protocol

Anti-thyroid medication: There is no consensus on the necessity for pre-treating with anti-thyroid medications before the administration of RAI I-131 in terms of protecting against exacerbation of thyrotoxicosis. Nonetheless, anti-thyroid medications would be recommended in the elderly, patients with comorbidities (especially cardiovascular) and cases with severe thyrotoxicosis.

It has also been suggested that pre-treatment with anti-thyroid medications (particularly propylthiouracil) is related with increased risk of treatment failure after the RAI I-131. The anti-thyroid drugs are discontinued 1 week prior to administration of RAI I-131 and are usually restarted 1 week after this. Beta-blocker may be needed if the patient is very symptomatic.

The dose of RAI I-131 can be fixed or calculated based on the radioactive uptake by the thyroid.

Radiation protection rules: Each treatment centre should have relevant detailed information leaflets.

- Advice on transport after the administration of RAI I-131
- Avoid close contact with adults, children. and pregnant women
- Refrain from fathering a child for 4–6 months or conceiving for 6 months
- Recommendations for near future travel plans

Thyroid function: TFTs should be checked 1–2 months after the RAI I-131 and thereafter every 4–6 weeks, until the patient is euthyroid or hypothyroid (off anti-thyroid drugs).

28.2.1.4 Outcomes and Risks of Treatment

Thyroid activity: This will reduce over weeks and the timing of response is variable. Around 60% of the patients will become hypothyroid after 12 months and after this, hypothyroidism can develop at a rate of 3% per year.

Thyroxine replacement: Replacement with Levothyroxine should be offered as soon as hypothyroidism is diagnosed. It should be noted that hypothyroidism might be transient in a small number of patients. Thyroid gland shrinkage may also occur.

Lifelong monitoring: In all patients, lifelong monitoring of the thyroid hormones is required. In cases of treatment failure, a second dose of I-131 can be offered 6–12 months after the previous one.

Factors predicting the outcome of treatment include dose of RAI I-131, size of goitre, female gender, pre-treatment fT4 levels.

RAI 1-131 Risks: These include worsening of thyroid eye disease, acute thyroiditis (in 1% of the patients, lasts a few weeks and is managed with non-steroidal anti-inflammatory drugs and beta-blockers, or, in severe cases, with steroids), acute enlargement in multinodular goitre (caution in severe trachea compression). It has been proposed that cancer incidence is slightly higher in hyperthyroid patients compared with euthyroid people, but is not associated with the type of thyroid treatment.

Summary of recommendations for the management of hyperthyroidism and radioiodine therapy (Box 28.11).

Box 28.11 Specialist Nurse Recommendations for Pre- and Post-radioiodine Management
Pre-radioiodine

- Explanation regarding information of and safety aspect of radioiodine (RAI) therapy is paramount to dispel fear as some patients worry about the effects of radiation and cancer.
- Avoid radioiodine in patients with thyroid eye disease as it may cause progression of the condition (or seek ophthalmology referral for assessment and opinion), and discuss referral for thyroid surgery (Sect. 4, Chap. 28 (C) Thyroid Surgery).
- RAI treatment is contraindicated in pregnancy and in women who are breastfeeding.
- Women should avoid pregnancy for at least 6 months after RAI treatment.
- Men should avoid fathering children for at least 4 months after radioiodine treatment.
- Aim to achieve euthyroidism prior to administering RAI.
- Referral of patient from nurse-led clinic (NLC) services for RAI assessment includes:
  - Interview with endocrinologist
  - RAI procedure explained
  - Consent obtained
  - Protocol provided for post-RAI, NLC, thyroid function test (TFT) monitoring as per hospital protocol
- Assessment with radiologist consultant includes:
  - Detailed RAI protection rules explained

- Leaflets provided with clear instructions as per hospital protocol
- Date provided for RAI treatment

Post-radioiodine considerations for TFT monitoring

- Serum FT4 and TSH should be checked every 4–6 weeks for 6 months after administration of 131 iodine-RAI.
- The frequency of TFT testing may be reduced when the FT4 remains within the reference range, then annually.
- A fall in serum FT4 to below normal, or rise in TSH should prompt a reduction in dose or withdrawal of any thionamide administered post-RAI therapy.
- A more marked or persistent rise in serum TSH (>20 mU/L for more than 1 month), especially if associated with symptoms, should prompt thyroxine prescription.
- Persistent elevation of FT4 at around 6 months after RAI therapy indicates lack of cure and the need for considering a second dose.
- If FT4 is normal (off thionamides) approximately 6 months after radioiodine, the frequency of testing may be reduced to 3 monthly and then 6 monthly.

After an interval of euthyroidism (normal serum FT4) of more than 12 months after RAI therapy, the patient may be transferred to annual testing.

Second dose radioiodine

- Persistent elevation of FT4 6 months after RAI therapy indicates lack of cure and need for consideration of re-dosing.
- Discuss second dose of RAI, and re-refer for assessment with endocrinologist and radio-nuclear physicist (procedure as for first dose of RAI).

- TFT monitoring is required 4 weekly post-RAI treatment until euthyroidism is achieved (off antithyroid drug or on Thyroxine replacement). Then plans to discharge patient from NLC hospital services to healthcare provider or general practitioner.

Discharge Suggestions to Healthcare Provider Following Radioiodine

- Stable TFTs either with or without Thyroxine requires 6 monthly monitoring of TFTs. If stable, for the first year, monitoring can be transferred to annual checks thereafter, or earlier should the patient experience any symptoms related to thyroid dysfunction.
- Patients should be advised to keep up to date with all aspects of thyroid news that may be pertinent to their needs. Access to websites such as British thyroid Association: https://www.british-thyroid-association.org/, British thyroid foundation: http://www.btf-thyroid.org/ and Thyroid eye disease committee: http://tedct.org.uk/ are recommended, as well as attending 'patient information meetings'.
- Healthcare provider may have to adjust Thyroxine dose as required for several months or years following patient discharge.
- Patients previously euthyroid, without Thyroxine, who develop **hypothyroidism** will require Thyroxine replacement with 4–6 weekly TFT monitoring until euthyroidism is achieved, then have less frequent checks at 3, 6, and 12 months monitoring to maintain euthyroidism.
- Patients previously euthyroid, without Thyroxine, who develop recurrence of **hyperthyroidism**, should be re-referred back to endocrinologist for definitive treatment discussion and restoration of normal thyroid function (BTA 2006; NICE 2016; ATA 2016; TEDct 2018).

28.3   Section C: Thyroid Surgery

28.3.1   Preoperative Medical Control of Hyperthyroidism (With Reference at Previous Sections)

28.3.1.1   Length of Treatment

There is significant variation in the length of treatment with anti-thyroid medication before patients are being offered definitive treatment with either thyroid surgery or radioactive iodine ablation. The general consensus is that after 12–18 months of effective blockade with Carbimazole (or Propylthiouracil) medication should be stopped and patients monitored to identify those with recurrent thyrotoxicosis. Recurrence is expected in at least 50% of patients, more likely in smokers and patients with large goitres. If recurrence is suspected clinically and/or demonstrated on biochemical testing, medical control of thyrotoxicosis has to be restarted and patients considered for definitive therapy (i.e. radioactive iodine ablation-RIA or total thyroidectomy).

Despite this expected timeline, in clinical practice most patients who present for thyroid surgery declare that they have been on medical treatment for many years (rather than 12–18 months).

28.3.1.2   Urgent Control of Hyperthyroidism

This can be necessary in patients who develop agranulocytosis whilst on Carbimazole (or PTU) treatment. These patients should be managed through close collaboration between medical and surgical team. A date of the operation should be fixed as soon as feasible and from that date one decides 10 days backwards to start the acute blockade of thyroid function using high iodine intake (e.g. Lugol's drops 10 drops tds or potassium iodide 60 mg tds) and propranolol (40 mg tds, titrating it towards higher doses based on how well tachycardia is controlled). Dexamethasone 1–2 mg daily could be added for 2–3 days prior to surgery.

28.3.1.3   Control of Pre-Op Hyperthyroidism and Post-Op Thyrotoxic Storm

It is imperative to control hyperthyroidism before proceeding with thyroid surgery in order to avoid post-operative thyrotoxic storm. This is a condition rarely seen in today's clinical practice but often discussed in postgraduate exams for anaesthetists and surgeons. It can be triggered by stress (e.g. emergency non-thyroid operations performed on thyrotoxic patients, fractures, road traffic accidents, thyroid surgery) or excessive iodine intake (e.g. use of contrast IV agents for CT scanning). It can be life-threatening hence it requires a low threshold of suspicion. The symptoms and signs of thyroid storm are usually recognisable by the endocrine specialist (6).

28.3.1.3.1 Symptoms and Signs Specific to Thyroid Storm
- Pyrexia (>38.5 °C)
- Tachycardia
- Hypertension
- Tremor
- Confusion
- Nausea and vomiting
- High output cardiac failure

Treatment: Management of hyperthyroidism must be instituted rapidly, with timely involvement of endocrine specialists and critical care physicians. If it occurs after total thyroidectomy, the treatment is supportive and involves cooling, beta blockade (e.g. with propranolol 80 mg), supplemented by dexamethasone. If it occurs in other scenarios, the production of thyroid hormones should be blocked rapidly with Methimazole and Lugol's iodine.

28.3.2 Thyroid Lobectomy for 'Hot' Nodule

A hot nodule (Plummer's adenoma) demonstrated on radioactive uptake scans can be treated with radioactive iodine ablation (if <3 cm and no contraindications for RIA) or offered thyroid lobectomy.

28.3.2.1 Indications
- Large nodules (>3–4 cm)
- Children (in order to avoid exposure to radioactive treatment)
- Patients who need neck exploration for other indications (e.g. parathyroidectomy)
- Patients with ipsilateral or contralateral thyroid nodules with suspicious appearance of ultrasound assessment

Hot nodules should not be assessed with fine needle aspiration (FNA) biopsy because all are follicular adenomas hence FNA would lead to a THY3 cytological appearance (Sect. 4, Chap. 27 and Sect. 4, Chap. 29), which could raise inadvertent concerns/suspicion of malignancy. It is exceedingly rare for a patient presenting with thyrotoxicosis to have a follicular carcinoma.

28.3.3 Total Thyroidectomy for Graves' Disease

28.3.3.1 Indications
Patients have to make an informed decision regarding the choice between RIA and thyroid surgery for Graves' disease.

Definitive indications for thyroid surgery

- Large goitres
- Severe Graves' ophthalmopathy
- Small children
- Patient's fears about radioactive treatment

28.3.3.2 Contraindications
- Patients with pre-existent recurrent laryngeal nerve injury
- Patients with history of neck radiotherapy
- Frail patients who would be better managed on long-term medical therapy

28.3.3.3 Extent of Surgery
In the 1980s, Australian surgeons were the first to demonstrate that total thyroidectomy is the ideal operation for Graves' disease. Subtotal thyroidectomy caries a high risk of recurrent hyperthyroidism and has been abandoned in centres where total thyroidectomy can be performed with low risk of complications (*vide infra*). The only exception from this 'rule' is the treatment of people whose employment does not allow being on thyroxine replacement (e.g. army/air force personnel).

28.3.3.4 Surgical Technique
The 'classical' technique for thyroid surgery has been established in the early twentieth century through the work of famous surgeons like Dr. Theodor Kocker and the principles established in the era are easily recognisable in the way the operation is performed in modern practice.

Around the world there are different degrees of interest in adopting more radical techniques for thyroid surgery and include:

Minimally invasive video-assisted thyroid surgery: This was introduced by Italian surgeons. It relies on the use of a small cervical skin incision (2 cm) through which small instruments and a video camera are introduced to allow dissection of tissue planes under direct vision. The technique is feasible only if the volume of the thyroid is small (so that it can be retrieved through the small skin incision).

Robotic thyroid surgery: This was initially promoted by South Korean surgeons, but in recent years the use of the Da Vinci robot for thyroid surgery has been restricted in many countries (e.g. in the USA insurance companies are not covering the costs of the procedure). The technique avoids an incision in the neck instead access to the thyroid is secured though a long 'tunnel' created from the arm pit in front of the pectoralis major).

Face-lift approach: This relies on a cervical incision away from the thyroid bed, in the hairline, with the dissection under platysma muscle and over the sternocleidomastoidian muscle.

Transoral thyroidectomy: This has been developed by German surgeons by making small incisions on the oral mucosa in front of the mandible and creating a working space for laparoscopic or robotic instruments.

28.3.3.5 Complications

Immediate complications after thyroid surgery can be life-threatening; hence patients have to be looked after on a ward environment where nurses are familiar with such complication and where rigorous protocols are in place for timely recognition of these complications that prompt intervention.

Post-operative bleeding: With the airway compromise, post-operative bleeding is the most dangerous complication that occurs usually in the first 6 h after the operation (though it has been reported up to 24 h post-op). It requires urgent opening of the neck in order to avoid further venous congestion that triggers the mucosal oedema and intraluminal laryngeal obstruction. In extreme situations, the sutures will have to be removed on the ward (i.e. the subcuticular skin sutures and the muscular sutures between the strap muscles so that the haematoma is fully released) before return to theatre for formal neck exploration to identify the source bleeding. The emergency management of neck haematoma could require opening of the neck on the ward. This is freely available as an educational video demonstration using the mnemonic 'SCOOP' (Endocrine Surgery Oxford 2018):-

S: Steristrips - remove

C: Cut - subcuticular suture & push fingers into wound

O: Open - skin to expose strap muscle

O: Open - strap muscle to expose trachea

P: Pack - wound

Bilateral recurrent laryngeal nerve (BRLN) injury: With acute airway compromise is an exceedingly rare complication. Its incidence should be mitigated by the use of intraoperative nerve monitoring that should alert the surgeon if the recurrent laryngeal nerve is injured after completing the first side of the operation hence a decision could be taken to not proceed with bilateral surgery (hence avoiding a BRLN injury) (Table 28.1).

Patients need to be made aware of all these potential complications during the preoperative discussion. Increasingly surgeons are expected to

Table 28.1 Late complications after total thyroidectomy for Graves' disease

Complication	Mechanism	Incidence	Treatment	Prognosis
Hypocalcaemia—hypoparathyroidism	Injury to parathyroid glands (e.g. compromising their vascular supply) or their inadvertent removal. Patients with severe thyrotoxicosis develop hungry bone syndrome and become hypocalcaemic even though their PTH is normal/high.	1:50 Incidence after surgery for Graves' disease is higher (up to 10%) compared with multinodular goitre.	Calcium supplements (e.g. calcichew ii tds) and/or vitamin D replacement (e.g. calcitriol 1 µg od)	Likely to settle within 6–12 months if PTH becomes measurable.
Subtle voice changes (loss of high pitch, loss of projection)	Injury to superior laryngeal nerve	1:10	Possibly the use of voice exercises might be beneficial but it remains unproven.	Likely to improve/settle with 3–6 months
Severe voice changes (hoarse voice)	Injury to recurrent laryngeal nerve (transection, traction, heat injury)	1:100	Voice therapy for those with associated swallowing difficulties is likely to mitigate the difficulties. If symptoms persist over 6–12 months, the paralysed cord could be injected to encourage a more medial position and possible better voice outcome. A clinical trial of reinnervation using ansa cervicalis is being under way.	

Box 28.12 Specialist Nurse Recommendations: Thyroid Surgery
Explanation:

- Surgery indications for Graves' or nodular goitre
- Equip with information leaflets and BTF: website address or local hospital policy and guidelines
- Importance of thyroid hormone control preoperatively with anti-thyroid drug (ATD) or alternative
- Graves' hyperthyroidism usually requiring total thyroidectomy and lifelong Thyroxine replacement
- Toxic nodular goitre often requiring either partial or total thyroidectomy
- Explain rare risks such as vocal cord, laryngeal nerve damage, and transient or permanent calcium deficiency and how these can be managed
- Arrange formal assessment with thyroid surgeon for suitability for surgery and confirmation of surgical date

Preoperative preparation of patient:

- Aim for euthyroidism with ATD or alternative
- Thyroid function test (TFT) 4–6 weekly until euthyroid, then 8 weekly–3 monthly (or as per hospital protocol) when euthyroid until surgery

Post-thyroidectomy monitoring:

- TFTs monitoring 4–6 weekly until euthyroidism achieved either on or off Thyroxine.
- Check surgical site for healing.
- BioOil recommended to be gently massaged over surgical site only when completely healed to minimise scar effects.
- Explain the need for 'lifelong' Thyroxine replacement in Graves' hyperthyroidism and in cases of toxic

nodular goitre where replacement is required.
- When euthyroidism is achieved either on or off Thyroxine replacement, discharge from secondary care back to healthcare provider.

Discharge instruction from secondary care and long-term follow-up:

- Patient will require 'lifelong' Thyroxine replacement.
- TFT monitoring 6 monthly for the first year, if stable then annually thereafter or earlier should symptoms of thyroid dysfunction return.
- Access to websites for further information: BTF http://www.btf-thyroid.org & those with TED: http://tedct.org.uk/

(ATA 2016; BTF 2015a, b; BTA 2006; National Institute for Health and Care Excellence-NICE 2016; Thyroid eye disease committee 2018)

quote the incidence of these complications in their own practice rather than using figures published in large series from centres with large practice.

Summary of recommendations for the management of hyperthyroidism and thyroid surgery (Box 28.12).

28.4 Conclusions

Hyperthyroidism is represented by the presence of supressed thyroid stimulating hormone with increased levels of circulating thyroid hormones, fT4 (thyroxine), and fT3 (triidothyronine).

The most common hyperthyroid condition seen in endocrine clinical practice is firstly Graves' disease, followed by toxic nodular goitre (single adenoma or multinodular) and thyroiditis (subacute).

Pregnancy cases require a prompt obstetrics referral for close specialist monitoring, and patients with signs of thyroid eye disease necessitates a timely ophthalmology referral for monitoring and follow-up.

A number of investigations can be undertaken to diagnose hyperthyroidism and include TFTs, TSHR, TPO antibodies thyroid uptake scan and CT scan. These can be tailored to diagnose Graves' disease, toxic nodular goitre, and thyroiditis. Relevant knowledge and understanding of hyperthyroidisms is therefore paramount to ensure a swift diagnosis can be made without delay so that the appropriate treatment is selected.

The treatment options include anti-thyroid drugs (Carbimazole, Propylthiouracil), B blockers (Propranolol), radioiodine, or thyroid surgery (thyroidectomy).

A multidisciplinary approach is crucial to manage hyperthyroidism appropriately and effectively. This provides an enhanced delivery of efficient, effective and, safe, patient care that ultimately provides optimal outcomes.

Useful Resources

Endocrine Surgery Oxford. SCOOP: how to open the neck quickly and safely to relieve airway pressure in acute post op haemorrhage after thyroid or parathyroid surgery-acute management of post op haemorrhage in thyroid and parathyroid surgery. 2018. Available at: https://www.youtube.com/watch?v=uCM9FuutGbY. Accessed 3 Nov 2018.

References

Abraham P, Avenell A, McGeoch SC, Clark LF, Bevan JS. Antithyroid drug regimen for treating Graves' hyperthyroidism. Primary Review Group-Cochrane. 2010. Available at: http://www.cochrane.org/CD003420/ENDOC_antithyroid-drug-regimen-for-treating-graves-hyperthyroidism. Accessed 22 Oct 2017.

Akamizu T, Amino N. Hashimoto's thyroiditis. Endotext. 2018. Available at: https://www.ncbi.nlm.nih.gov/books/NBK285557/. Accessed 22 Jan 2018.

American Thyroid Association – ATA. Guidelines for diagnosis and management of hyperthyroidism and other causes of thyrotoxicosis. ATA. 2016. Available at: https://www.thyroid.org/professionals/ata-professional-guidelines/. Accessed 24 July 2017.

Amino N, Kubota S. Thyroid disease after pregnancy-3.4.5. In: JAH W, Stewart PM, Amiel SA, Davies MJ, editors. Oxford textbook of endocrinology and diabetes. Oxford: Oxford University Press; 2011.

Barrio R, López-Capapé M, Martinez-Badás I. Graves' disease in children and adolescents: response to long-term treatment. Acta Paediatr. 2005. Available at: https://www.ncbi.nlm.nih.gov/pubmed/16303698. Accessed 20 Oct 2017.

Bartelena. Treatment of hyperthyroidism: block and replace versus titration. Endocrine abstracts. Endocr Connect. 2008. Available at: http://www.endocrine-abstracts.org/ea/0016/ea0016s1.1.htm. Accessed 11 Oct 2017.

Bath S. Food facts-Iodine. The Association of UK Dieticians-BDA; 2016. Available at: https://www.bda.uk.com/foodfacts/Iodine.pdf. Accessed 23 Dec 2017.

Benker G, Reinwein D, Kahaly G, Tegler L, Alexander WD, Fassbinder J, Hirche H. Is there a methimazole dose effect on remission rate in Graves' disease? Results from a long-term prospective study. Clin Endocrinol. 1998. Available at: https://www.ncbi.nlm.nih.gov/pubmed/?term=benker+1998+remission+in+graves. Accessed 22 Dec 2017.

Benner P. From novice to expert: excellence and power in clinical nursing practice. London: Addison-Wesley; 1984.

Berghout A, Wiersinga WM, Smits NJ, Touber JL. Interrelationships between age, thyroid volume, thyroid nodularity, and thyroid function in patients with sporadic nontoxic goiter. Am J Med. 1990. Available at: https://www.ncbi.nlm.nih.gov/pubmed/2239979. Accessed 29 July 2017.

Blum MR, Bauer DC, Collet TH, Fink HA, Cappola AR, Da Costa BR, Wirth CD, Peeters RP, Asvold BO, Den Elzen WP, Luben RN, Imaizumi M, Bremner AP, Gogakos A, Eastell R, Kearney PM, Strotmeyer ES, Wallace ER, Hoff M, Ceresini G, Rivadeneira F, Uitterlinden AG, Stott DJ, Westendorp RG, Khaw KT, Langhammer A, Ferrucci L, Gussekloo J, Williams GR, Walsh JP, Juni P, Aujesky D, Rodondi N. Thyroid Studies Collaboration: subclinical thyroid dysfunction and fracture risk: a meta-analysis. JAMA. 2015. Available at: https://jamanetwork.com/journals/jama/fullarticle/2297170. Accessed 22 Jan 2018.

Boettlin R. Uber zahnentwickelung in dermoid cysten des ovariums. 1889. In: Yoo SC, Chang KH, Lyu MO, Chang SJ, Ryu HS, Kim HS. Clinical characteristics of struma ovarii. J Gynaecol Oncol. 2008. Available at: https://www.ncbi.nlm.nih.gov/pmc/articles/PMC2676458/. Accessed 22 July 2017.

Bomeli SR, LeBeau SO, Ferris RL. Evaluation of a thyroid nodule. 2010. Available at: https://www.ncbi.nlm.nih.gov/pmc/articles/PMC2879398/. Accessed 28 July 2017.

Bondi B, Bartalena L, Cooper DS, Hededus L, Laurberg J, Kahaly GJ. European Thyroid Association guidelines on diagnosis and treatment of endogenous subclinical hyperthyroidism. Eur Thyroid J. 2015. Available at: https://www.ncbi.nlm.nih.gov/pubmed/26558232. Accessed 22 July 2017.

Bowman P, Osborne NJ, Sturley R, Viadya B. Carbimazole embryopathy: implications for the choice of antithyroid drugs in pregnancy. QJM. 2012. Available at: https://www.ncbi.nlm.nih.gov/pubmed/?term=bowman+2012+pregnancy+antithyroid. Accessed 23 July 2017.

British National Formulary. Propranolol hydrochloride/carbimazole/propylthiouracil/thyroxine. BNF-NICE. 2018a. Available at: https://bnf.nice.org.uk/drug/propranolol-hydrochloride.html#medicinalForms. Accessed 22 July 2017.

British National Formulary. Non-steroidal anti-inflammatory drugs/Paracetamol: therapeutic effects. NICE. 2018b. Available at: https://bnf.nice.org.uk/treatment-summary/non-steroidal-anti- inflammatory-drugs.html. Accessed 22 Jan 2018.

British National Formulary. BNF. 2018c. Available: https://www.bnf.org/products/bnf-online/. Accessed 23 May 2017.

British Thyroid Association-BTA. UK guidelines for the use of thyroid function tests: thyrotoxicosis. BTA. 2006. Available at: http://www.british-thyroid-association.org/sandbox/bta2016/uk_guidelines_for_the_use_of_thyroid_function_tests.pdf. Accessed 22 July 2017.

British Thyroid Foundation. Thyroid surgery/radioiodine. BTF. 2015a. Available at: http://www.btf-thyroid.org/information/leaflets/31-thyroid-surgery-guide, http://www.btf-thyroid.org/information/quick-guides/101-hyperthyroidism-radioactive-iodine. Accessed 22 July 2017.

British Thyroid Foundation. Antithyroid drug therapy to treat hyperthyroidism. BTF. 2015b. Available: http://www.btf-thyroid.org/information/leaflets/40-antithyroid-drug-therapy-guide. Accessed 29 June 2017.

Bülow Pedersen I, Knudsen N, Jørgensen T, Perrild H, Ovesen L, Laurberg P. Large differences in incidences of overt hyper- and hypothyroidism asso.ciated with a small difference in iodine intake- a prospective comparative register-based population survey. J Clin Endocrinol Metab. 2002. Available at: https://www.ncbi.nlm.nih.gov/pubmed/12364419. Accessed 23 Oct 2017.

Burch HB, Cooper DS. Management of Graves disease a review. Network-J Am Med Assoc. 2015. Available at: https://jamanetwork.com/journals/jama/article-abstract/2475467. Accessed 10 Jan 2018.

Burman. Overview of thyroiditis. UpToDate. 2017. Available at: https://www.uptodate.com/contents/overview-of-thyroiditis#H5. Accessed 22 Feb 2018.

Callissendorf J, Falhammar H. Lugol's solution and other iodide preparations: perspectives and research directions in Graves' disease. Endocrine. Springer. 2017. Available at: https://www.ncbi.nlm.nih.gov/pmc/articles/PMC5693970/. Accessed 23 March 2018.

Canaris GJ, Manowitz NR, Mayor G, Ridgway EC. The Colorado thyroid disease prevalence study. Arch Intern Med. 2000. Available at: https://www.ncbi.nlm.nih.gov/pubmed/10695693. Accessed 22 Oct 2017.

Caplan RH. Thyroxine toxicosis. A common variant of hyperthyroidism. J Am Assoc. 1980. Available at: https://www.ncbi.nlm.nih.gov/pubmed/6775100. Accessed 22 May 2017.

Cappola AR, Fried LP, Arnold AM, Danese MD, Kuller LH, Burke GL, Tracy RP, Ladenson PW. Thyroid status, cardiovascular risk, and mortality in older adults. JAMA. 2006. Available: https://www.ncbi.nlm.nih.gov/pubmed/16507804. Accessed 23 Oct 2017.

Cerci C, Cerci SS, Eroglu E, Dede M, Kapucouglu N, Yildiz M, Bulbul M, et al. Thyroid cancer in toxic and non-toxic multinodular goiter. J Post Grad Med. 2007. Available at: https://www.ncbi.nlm.nih.gov/pubmed?term=17699987. Accessed 22 May 2017.

Cooper DS. Antithyroid drugs. N Engl J Med. 2005. Available at: http://www.nejm.org/doi/full/10.1056/nejmra042972. Accessed 22 Nov 2017.

Cooper DS, Biondi B. Subclinical thyroid disease. Lancet. 2012. Available at: https://pdfs.semanticscholar.org/49c4/c2df1a7a4470127e09e34aafbae347e4ff6c.pdf. Accessed 22 Oct 2017.

Cooper DS, Laurberg P. Hyperthyroidism in pregnancy. Diab Endocrinol Lancet. 2013. Available at: http://www.thelancet.com/journals/landia/article/PIIS2213-8587(13)70086-X/abstract. Accessed 22 Aug 2017.

Cooper DS, Rivkees SA. Putting Propylthiouracil in perspective. 2009. In Vaidya B, Pearce SHS. Diagnosis and management of thyrotoxicosis-clinical review. Br Med J. 2014. Available at: https://medicinainternaaldia.files.wordpress.com/2014/09/tirotoxicosis.pdf. Accessed 22 Aug 2017.

Davis TF. Pretibial myxedema (thyroid dermopathy) in autoimmune thyroid disease. UpToDate. 2017. Available at: http://www.uptodate.com/contents/pretibial-myxedema-thyroid-dermopathy-in-autoimmune-thyroid-disease. Accessed 22 July 2017.

DeSimone CP, Lele SM, Modesitt SC. Malignant struma ovarii: a case report and analysis of cases reported in the literature with focus on survival and I131 therapy. Gynecol Oncol. 2003. Available at: https://www.ncbi.nlm.nih.gov/pubmed?term=12798728. Accessed 22 Oct 2017.

Dunzendorfer T, DelLas Morenas A, Kalir T, Levin RM. Struma ovarii and hyperthyroidism. Thyroid American Thyroid Association. 1999. Available at: https://www.ncbi.nlm.nih.gov/pubmed/10365682. Accessed 26 Oct 2017.

Electronic Medical Com. Potassium iodide. Elecectronic Medical Compendium. 2016. Available at: https://www.medicines.org.uk/emc/product/3019. Accessed 20 March 2018.

Engkakul P, Mahachoklertwattana P, Poomthavorn P. Eponym: De Quervain thyroiditis. 2011. Available: https://www.ncbi.nlm.nih.gov/pubmed/20886353. Accessed 23 Nov 2017.

European Thyroid Association. Guidelines on diagnosis and treatment of endogenous subclinical hyperthyroidism. Eur Thyroid J. 2015. Available at: http://www.eurothyroid.com/files/download/ETJ-2015-4-149-163-GUIDELINES-SUBCLIN-HYPER-PDF-438750.pdf. Accessed 22 March 2018.

Fazal-Sanderson V, Karavitaki N, Grossman AB, Kalhan A. Abstract: Outcomes of a nurse-led thyroid clinic at a tertiary-care endocrine centre. Endocr Connections. 2017. Available at: http://www.endocrine-abstracts.org/ea/0049/ea0049GP114.htm. Accessed 22 Oct 2017.

Franklyn JA. Subclinical hyperthyroidism:3.3.4. In: Wass JAH, Stewart PM, Amiel SA, Davies MJ, editors. Oxford textbook of endocrinology and diabetes. Oxford: Oxford University Press; 2011.

Franklyn JA, Boelaert K. Thyrotoxicosis. Lancet. 2012. Available at: http://www.thelancet.com/pdfs/journals/lancet/PIIS0140-6736(11)60782-4.pdf. Accessed 28 July 2017.

Fuhrer D, Lazarus JH. Management of toxic multinodular goitre and toxic adenoma-3.3.11. In: JAH W, Stewart PM, Amiel SA, Davies MJ, editors. Oxford textbook of endocrinology and diabetes. Oxford: Oxford University Press; 2011.

Goichot B, Caron P, Landron F, Bouée S. Clinical presentation of hyperthyroidism in a large representative sample of outpatients in France: relationships with age, aetiology and hormonal parameters. Clin Endocrinol. 2015. Available at: https://onlinelibrary.wiley.com/doi/full/10.1111/cen.12816. Accessed 10 Oct 2017.

Harvey CB, O'Shea PJ, Scott AJ, Robson H, Siebler T, Shalet SM, Samarut J, Chassande O, Williams GR. Molecular mechanisms of thyroid hormone effects on bone growth and function. Mol Genet Metab. 2002. Available at: http://www.mgmjournal.com/article/S1096-7192(01)93268-8/pdf. Accessed 22 Oct 2017.

Hedley AJ, Young RE, Jones SJ, Alexander WD, Bewsher PD. Antithyroid drugs in the treatment of hyperthyroidism of Graves' disease: long-term follow-up of 434 patients. Scottish Automated Follow-Up Register Group. Clin Endocrinol – Oxf. 1998. Available at: https://www.ncbi.nlm.nih.gov/pubmed/?term=Hedley+1989+antithyroid. Accessed 22 Dec 2017.

Hennessey JV. Subacute thyroiditis. In DeGroot LJ, Chrousos G, Dungan K, Feingold KR, Grossman A, Hershman JM, Kock C, Korbonitis M, McLachian R, New M, Pumeli J, Rebar R, Singer F, Vinik A, editors. ENDOTEXT. 2015. Available at: https://www.ncbi.nlm.nih.gov/pubmed/25905310, https://www.ncbi.nlm.nih.gov/books/NBK279084/. Accessed 23 Oct 2017.

Hiromatsu Y, Satoh H, Amino N. Hashimoto's thyroiditis: history and future outlook. Hormones (Athens). 2013. In: Tidy C. Hashimoto's thyroiditis. Patient UK. 2015. Available at: https://patient.info/doctor/hashimotos-thyroiditis. Accessed 22 Nov 2017.

Hogan-Quigley B, Palm ML, Bickley L. Bates' Nursing Guide To Physical Examination And History Taking. London: Wolters Kluwer Health/Lippincott Williams & Wilkins; 2012.

Kaplan B, Pearce EN, Farewell AP. Thyroiditis. 3.2.7. In: JAH W, Stewart PM, Amiel SA, Davies MJ, editors. Oxford textbook of endocrinology and diabetes. Oxford: Oxford University Press; 2011.

Kondi-Parfit A, Mavrigigiannaki P, Grigoriadis CH, Kontogianni-Katsarou K, Mellou A, Kleanthis CK, Liapis A. Monodermal teratomas (struma ovarii). Clinicopathological characteristics of 11 cases and literature review. Eur J Gynaecol Oncol. 2011. Available at: https://www.ncbi.nlm.nih.gov/pubmed?term=22335029. Accessed 22 Oct 2017.

Kraemer B, Girschke EM, Staebler A, Hirides P, Rothmund R. Laparoscopic excision of malignant struma ovarii and 1 year follow-up without fur further treatment. Fertil Steril. 2011. Available at: https://www.ncbi.nlm.nih.gov/pubmed?term=21269611. Accessed 22 Oct 2017.

Latrofa F, Vitti P, Pinchera A. Causes and laboratory investigations of thyrotoxicosis-3.3.5. In: Wass JAH, Stewart PM, Amiel SA, Davies MJ, editors. Oxford textbook of endocrinology and diabetes. Oxford: Oxford University Press; 2011.

Laurberg P. Remission of Graves' disease during antithyroid drug therapy. Time to reconsider the mechanism? Eur J Endocrinol. 2006. Available at: https://www.ncbi.nlm.nih.gov/pubmed/17132745. Accessed 12 June 2017.

Laurberg P, Vestergaard H, Neilson S, Christensen SE, Seefeldt, Hellberg K, Pederson KM. Sources of circulating 3,5,3′-triiodothyronine in hyperthyroidism estimated after blocking of type 1 and type 2 iodothyronine deiodinases. 2007. Available at: https://www.ncbi.nlm.nih.gov/pubmed?term=17389703. Accessed 22 May 2017.

Leger J, Gelwane G, Kaguelidou F. Positive impact of long-term antithyroid drug treatment on the outcome of children with Graves' disease: National Long-Term Cohort Study. J Clin Endocrinol Metab. 2012. Available at: https://www.ncbi.nlm.nih.gov/pubmed/22031519. Accessed 20 Dec 2017.

Makani S, Kim W, Gaba AR. Struma Ovarii with a focus of papillary thyroid cancer: a case report and review of the literature. Gynecol Oncol. 2004. Available at: http://www.gynecologiconcology-online.net/article/S0090-8258(04)00414-7/pdf. Accessed 22 Dec 2017.

Marcocci C, Cetani F, Pinchera A. Clinical assessment and systemic manifestations of thyrotoxicosis-3.3.1. In: JAH W, Stewart PM, Amiel SA, Davies MJ, editors. Oxford textbook of endocrinology and diabetes. Oxford: Oxford University Press; 2011.

Marqusee E, Haden ST, Utiger RD. Subclinical thyrotoxicosis. Endocrinol Metab Clin N Am. 1998. Available at: https://www.ncbi.nlm.nih.gov/pubmed/9534026. Accessed 22 Oct 2017.

McGregor AM, Petersen MM, McLachlan SM, Rooke P, Smith BR, Hall R. Carbimazole and the autoimmune response in Graves' disease. N Engl J Med. 1980. Available at: http://www.nejm.org/doi/full/10.1056/NEJM198008073030603. Accessed 23 June 2018.

Mui MP, Tam KF, Tam FK, Ngan HY. Coexistence of struma ovarii with marked ascites and elevated CA-125 levels: case report and literature review. Arch Gynecol Obstet. 2009. Available at: https://www.ncbi.nlm.nih.gov/pubmed/?term=Mui+MP%2C+2009. Accessed 22 Dec 2017.

National Institute for Health and Care Excellence-NICE. Hyperthyroidism. NICE. 2016. Available at: https://cks.nice.org.uk/hyperthyroidism#!management. Accessed 22 Aug 2017.

Organzi, Bournard. Management of graves' hyperthyroidism-3.3.9. In: JAH W, Stewart PM, Amiel SA, Davies MJ, editors. Oxford textbook of endocrinology and diabetes. Oxford: Oxford University Press; 2011.

Paul T, Meyers B, Witorsch RJ, Pino S, Chipkin S, Ingbar SH, Braverman LE. The effect of small increases in dietary iodine on thyroid function in euthyroid subjects. Metabolism. 1988. Available at: https://www.ncbi.nlm.nih.gov/pubmed/3340004. Accessed 24 May 2017.

Pearce EN, Farwell AP, Braverman LE. Thyroiditis-3.2.7. In: JAH W, Stewart PM, Amiel SA, Davies MJ, editors. Oxford textbook of endocrinology and diabetes. Oxford: Oxford University Press; 2003.

Perros P, Dayan CM, Dickinson AJ, et al. Management of patients with Graves' orbitopathy: initial assessment, management outside specialised centres and referral pathways. Clin Med. British Thyroid Foundation. 2015. Available at: http://www.clinmed.rcpjournal.org/content/15/2/173.full.pdf+html. Accessed 03 Aug 2017.

Plummer HS. The value of iodine in exopthalmic goiter. J Iowa Med Soc 1924;14:66–73. In: Calissendorff J, Falhammar H. Rescue pre-operative treatment with Lugol's solution in uncontrolled Graves' disease. Endocr Connect. 2017. Available at: https://www.ncbi.nlm.nih.gov/pmc/articles/PMC5434745/#bib3. Accessed 22 Nov 2017.

Ross D. Treatment of toxic adenoma and toxic multinodular goiter. Up-To-Date. 2016. Available at: https://www.uptodate.com/contents/treatment-of-toxic-adenoma-and-toxic-multinodular-goiter?source=search_result&search=toxic+adenoma&selectedTitle=1%7E150. Accessed 22 May 2016.

Ross DS. Diagnosis of hyperthyroidism. Up-To-Date. 2017a. Available at: https://www.uptodate.com/contents/diagnosis-of-hyperthyroidism. Accessed 22 June 2017.

Ross DS. Clinical presentation and evaluation of goiter in adults. UpToDate. 2017b. Available at: https://www.uptodate.com/contents/clinical-presentation-and-evaluation-of-goiter-in-adults#H1. Accessed 22 June 2017.

Ross DS. Iodine treatment of hyperthyroidism. UpToDate. 2017c. Available at: https://www.uptodate.com/contents/iodine-in-the-treatment-of-hyperthyroidism. Accessed 30 March 2018.

Sanderson V, Alberts B, Grossman AB, Karavitaki, N. Outcome of patients with Graves' disease after long-term follow-up: data from a Nurse-led Clinic. Endocrine Abstracts - Endocr Connect. 2012. Available at: http://www.endocrine-abstracts.org/ea/0028/ea0028P157.htm. Accessed 22 Aug 2017.

Schwartz KM, Fatourechi V, Ahmed DDF, Pond GR. Dermopathy of Graves' disease (Pretibial myxedema): long-term outcome. J Clin Endocrinol Metab. 2002. Available at: https://www.ncbi.nlm.nih.gov/pubmed/?term=schwartz+2002+graves%27+dermopathy. Accessed 22 Oct 2018.

Shreshtha RT, Hennessey J. Acute and subacute thyroiditis. ENDOTEXT. 2015. Available at: http://www.thyroidmanager.org/chapter/acute-and-subacuteand-riedels-thyroiditis/#_ENREF_32. Accessed 24 July 2017.

Singer PA, Cooper DS, Levy EG, Ladenson PW, Braverman LE, Daniels G, Greenspan FS, McDougall IR, Nikolai TF. Treatment guidelines for patients with hyperthyroidism and hypothyroidism. Standards of Care Committee, American Thyroid Association. JAMA. 1995. Available at: https://www.ncbi.nlm.nih.gov/pubmed/7532241. Accessed 22 Oct 2017.

Smith P. Milestone in European thyroidology-Robert James Graves'. European Thyroid Association; 2018. Available at: http://www.eurothyroid.com/about/met/graves.html. Accessed 22 Jan 2018.

Stagnaro-Green. Postpartum thyroiditis. J Clin Endocrinol Metab. Oxford Academic. 2002. Available at: https://academic.oup.com/jcem/article/87/9/4042/2846380. Accessed 22 Dec 2017.

Szyfelbein WM, Young RH, Scully RE. Cystic struma ovarii: a frequently unrecognized tumor. A report of 20 cases. Am J Surg Pathol. 1994. Available at: https://www.ncbi.nlm.nih.gov/pubmed/8037292. Accessed 22 Dec 2017.

Takasu N, Yamashiro K, Komiya I, Ochi Y, Nagata A. Remission of Graves' hyperthyroidism predicted by smooth decreases of thyroid-stimulating antibody and thyrotropin-binding inhibitor immunoglobulin during antithyroid drug treatment. 2000. Available at: https://www.ncbi.nlm.nih.gov/pubmed/11081255. Accessed 22 Nov 2017.

Thyroid Eye Disease Committee Team. Patient information. TEDct. 2018. Available at: http://tedct.org.uk/. Accessed 22 Dec 2017.

Tidy C. Antithyroid medication. Patient UK. 2014. Available at: https://patient.info/health/overactive-thyroid-gland-hyperthyroidism/antithyroid-medicines. Accessed 22 Nov 2017.

Tozzoli R, Bagnasco M, Giavarina D, Bizzaro N. TSH receptor autoantibody immunoassay in patients with Graves' disease: improvement of diagnostic accuracy over different generations of methods. Syst Rev Meta-Analysis. 2012. Available: https://www.ncbi.nlm.nih.gov/pubmed/22776786. Accessed 28 July 2017.

Tunbridge WM, Evered DC, Hall R, Appleton D, Brewis M, Clark F, Grimley Evens J, Young E, Bird T, Smith PA. The spectrum of thyroid disease in a community: the Whickham survey. Clin Endocrinol. 1977. Available at: https://onlinelibrary.wiley.com/doi/full/10.1111/j.1365-2265.1977.tb01340.x. Accessed 22 Sept 2017.

Vaidya B, Pearce SHS. Clinical review: diagnosis & management of thyrotoxicosis. Br Med J. 2014. Available at: https://medicinainternaaldia.files.wordpress.com/2014/09/tirotoxicosis.pdf. Accessed 27 July 2017.

Vanderpump. The epidemiology of thyroid disease. Br Med J-Oxford Academic. 2011. Available at: https://academic.oup.com/bmb/article/99/1/39/298307. Accessed 22 Dec 17.

Vicente N, Cardoso L, Barros L, Carrilho F. Antithyroid drug-induced agranulocytosis: state of the art on diagnosis and management. 2017. Available at: https://www.ncbi.nlm.nih.gov/m/pubmed/28105610/. Accessed 22 Dec 2017.

Vickery AL, Hamlin E. Struma lymphomatosa (Hasimoto's thyroiditis): observations on repeated biopsies in 16 patients. N Engl J Med. 1961. Available at: http://www.nejm.org/doi/pdf/10.1056/NEJM196102022640505. Accessed 22 Dec 2017.

Visser, TJ. (2011) Biosynthesis, transport, metabolism, and actions of thyroid hormones. In, Wass, JAH., Stewart, PM., Amiel, SA. & Davis, MJ. Oxford textbook of endocrinology, diabetes and metabolism (2). Oxford: Oxford University Press.

Volpe R, Sawin C. The history of iconography relating to the thyroid gland-3.1.1. In: JAH W, Stewart PM, Amiel SA, Davies MJ, editors. Oxford textbook of endocrinology and diabetes. Oxford: Oxford University Press; 2011.

Wass JAH, Owen K. Chapter 1. Thyroid. In: Turner HE, editor. Oxford handbook of endocrinology and diabetes. 3rd ed., Advisory Ed. Oxford: Oxford University Press; 2014.

Weetman AP. The thyroid gland and disorders of thyroid function. In: Warrell DA, Cox TM, Firth JD, editors. Oxford textbook of medicine. Oxford: Oxford University Press; 2010.

Weetman AP. Investigating low thyroid stimulating hormone (TSH) level. BMJ. 2013. Available at: http://www.bmj.com/content/347/bmj.f6842. Accessed 22 Nov 2017.

Weiner JD, DeVries AA. On the natural history of Plummer's disease. Clin Nucl Med. 1979. Available at: https://www.ncbi.nlm.nih.gov/pubmed/582300. Accessed 22 July 2017.

Wirth CD, Blum MR, Da Costa BR, Baumgartner C, Collet TH, Medici M, Peeters RP, Aujesky D, Bauer DC, Rodondi N. Subclinical thyroid dysfunction and the risk for fractures: a systematic review and meta-analysis. Annu Intern Med. 2014. Available at: https://www.ncbi.nlm.nih.gov/pubmed/25089863. Accessed 23 Oct 2017.

Yassa L, Sadow P, Marquesee E. Malignant struma ovarii. Nature clinical practice. Endocrinol Metab. 2008. Available at: https://www.ncbi.nlm.nih.gov/pubmed?term=18560398. Accessed 22 Oct 2017.

Yoo SC, Chang KH, Lyu MO, Chang SJ, Ryu HS, Kim HS. Clinical characteristics of struma ovarii. J Gynaecol Oncol. 2008. Available at: https://www.ncbi.nlm.nih.gov/pmc/articles/PMC2676458/. Accessed 22 July 2017.

Young RH. New and unusual aspects of ovarian germ cell tumors. 1993. Available at: https://www.ncbi.nlm.nih.gov/pubmed?term=7694512. Accessed 24 Aug 2017.

Zimmerman MB. Iodine and Iodine deficiency disorders. Wiley Online library. 2012. Available at: https://onlinelibrary.wiley.com/doi/pdf/10.1002/9781119946045.ch36. Accessed 22 Oct 2017.

Key Reading

1. British Thyroid Association-BTA. UK guidelines for the use of thyroid function tests: thyrotoxicosis. BTA. 2006. Available at: http://www.british-thyroid association.org/sandbox/bta2016/uk_guidelines_for_the_use_of_thyroid_function_tests.pdf. Accessed 22 July 2017.

2. American Thyroid Association – ATA. Guidelines for diagnosis and management of hyperthyroidism and other causes of thyrotoxicosis. ATA. 2016. Available at: https://www.thyroid.org/professionals/ata-profes-sional-guidelines/. Accessed 24 July 2017.

3. European Thyroid Association. Guidelines on diagnosis and treatment of endogenous subclinical hyperthyroidism. Eur Thyroid J. 2015. Available at: http://www.eurothyroid.com/files/download/ETJ-2015-4-149-163-GUIDELINES-SUBCLIN-HYPER-PDF-438750.pdf. Accessed 22 March 2018.

4. Stagnaro-Green A. Post-partum thyroiditis. J Clin Endocrinol Metab. Oxford Academic; 2002. Available at: https://academic.oup.com/jcem/article/87/9/4042/2846380. Accessed 22 Nov 2017.

5. Burch HB, Cooper DS. Management of Graves disease: a review. JAMA. 2016. Available at: https://pdfs.semanticscholar.org/fbbd/c83f6b89a-ca96059519b33bbc15a10aae5d5.pdf. Accessed at: 10 Jan 2018.

6. Franklyn JA, Boelaert K. Thyrotoxicosis. Lancet. 2012. Available at: http://www.thelancet.com/pdfs/journals/lancet/PIIS0140-6736(11)60782-4.pdf. Accessed at: 28 July 2017.

7. Vaidya B, Pearce SHS. Clinical review: diagnosis & management of thyrotoxicosis. Br Med J. 2014 Available at: https://medicinainternaaldia.files.word-press.com/2014/09/tirotoxicosis.pdf. Accessed at: 27 July 2017.

8. De Leo S, Lee SY, Braverman LE. Hyperthyroidism. Lancet. 2016. Available at: http://www.thelancet.com/pdfs/journals/lancet/PIIS0140-6736(16)00278-6.pdf. Accessed 22 Dec 2017.

9. Thyroid Eye Disease (committee team). Available at: http://tedct.org.uk/. Accessed 22 Feb 2018.

10. British Thyroid Foundation. Available at: http://www.btf-thyroid.org/. Accessed 22 March 2018.

11. UpToDate: hyperthyroidism. Available at: https://www.uptodate.com/contents/search?search=hyperthyroidism. Accessed 22 March 2018.

12. PubMed: Hyperthyroidism. Available at: https://www.ncbi.nlm.nih.gov/pmc/articles/PMC5014602/. Accessed 22 March 2018.

13. Endotext. Thyroid disease. 2017. Available at: http://www.endotext.org/.

14. Thyroid Disease. Available at: www.thyroidmanager.org. Accessed 22 March 2018.

Thyroid Cancer

29

Ingrid Haupt-Schott, Geraldine Hamilton, and Petros Perros

Contents

I. Haupt-Schott (✉)
Velindre NHS Trust, Velindre Cancer Centre,
Cardiff, UK
e-mail: Ingrid.Haupt-schott@wales.nhs.uk

G. Hamilton
Macmillan Support Line, Macmillan Cancer Support,
Glasgow, UK
e-mail: ghamilton@macmillan.org.uk

P. Perros
Newcastle upon Tyne Hospitals NHS Foundation
Trust and Institute of Genetic Medicine, Newcastle
University, Newcastle upon Tyne, UK
e-mail: petros.perros@ncl.ac.uk

© Springer Nature Switzerland AG 2019
S. Llahana et al. (eds.), *Advanced Practice in Endocrinology Nursing*,
https://doi.org/10.1007/978-3-319-99817-6_29

Abstract

Thyroid cancer is rare and accounts for less than 1% of all cancers, but represents the most common endocrine malignancy. Incidence rates have increased in the past decade in most countries. This is mainly due to an increased use of imaging and subsequent incidental detection of thyroid cancers, but other unidentified factors may also contribute.

The natural history of thyroid cancer, its management and its long-term prognosis are very different to most other solid cancers and therefore warrant specialist support.

The last decade has seen a shift in the management of thyroid cancer with a tendency for less aggressive treatments for the more indolent types and a focus on a more personalised approach to decision-making and management.

The following chapter describes the various types of thyroid cancer, their current management protocols and some developments into future treatments.

Keywords

Thyroid cancer · Papillary · Follicular
Medullary · Anaplastic · Radioiodine
treatment · Thyroid surgery

Abbreviations

ATC	Anaplastic thyroid cancer
CT	Computed tomography
DTC	Differentiated thyroid cancer
FNA	Fine needle aspiration
FTC	Follicular thyroid caner
LN	Lymph node
MRI	Magnetic resonance imaging
MTC	Medullary thyroid cancer
PET	Positron emission tomography
PTC	Papillary thyroid cancer
RAI	Radioactive iodine
RLN	Recurrent laryngeal nerve
Tg	Thyroglobulin
TgAbs	Thyroglobulin antibodies
TKI	Tyrosine kinase inhibitors
US	Ultrasound scan
VC	Vocal cords

Key Terms

- **TNM Staging:** Malignant thyroid tumours are sorted into categories based on size, extension and spread which estimate prognosis.
- **Radioiodine Ablation:** Radioactive iodine is administered orally in order to destroy remnant thyroid tissue and cancer cells.

- **Radioiodine Refractory Disease:** Residual tumour and/or metastatic disease that does not take up radioiodine anymore and therefore cannot be treated with radioiodine any further.
- **Non-invasive follicular thyroid neoplasm with papillary-like nuclear features (NIFTP):** An encapsulated follicular variant of papillary thyroid cancer with a very low risk of an adverse outcome.

Key Points
- The number of thyroid cancer diagnoses is increasing, primarily due to incidental detection of small, biologically indolent tumours.
- The prognosis for most patients with thyroid cancer is good.
- The approach to treatment should be personalised.
- Psychological factors are vital to be considered as patients will remain on monitoring and may experience lifelong physical and emotional consequences.
- An important objective for healthcare professionals managing people with thyroid cancer is remembering to treat the person, not just the disease.

29.1 Introduction

29.1.1 Epidemiology

Thyroid cancers are rare and account for less than 1% of all cancers. They represent however the most common endocrine malignancy. In most countries, thyroid cancer incidence rates have increased in the past decade (Vigneri et al. 2015). In 2012, the global figure for new cases of thyroid cancer was 230,000 and 40,000 deaths (Vecchia et al. 2015). In the UK, there were 3241 cases diagnosed in 2013 (Cancer Research UK n.d.).

In the UK, the increase of incidence amounted to 71% over the last decade (Cancer Research UK n.d.). Incidental detection of small (<1 cm) thyroid cancers due to the widespread use of imaging tech-

niques and pathology reporting of thyroidectomy specimens resected for benign disease is thought to explain most of this increase, but it does not account for all the rises we are seeing. Other factors are thought to be at play such as changes in prevalence of risk factors including obesity, exposure to radiation, dietary iodine levels and hormonal factors (Vigneri et al. 2015). Presently we have very little evidence to back these theories.

While the incidence of thyroid cancers may be on the rise, cure rates are still very high and death rates are declining (Vecchia et al. 2015). Eighty-five to over 95% of people with differentiated thyroid cancer (papillary and follicular) can expect to have a normal life span after treatment.

Thyroid cancer can affect people of all ages from children to the elderly. Of the over 3000 newly diagnosed patients in the UK in 2013, 27% were men and 73% were women (Cancer Research UK n.d.). Incidence in men is strongly related to age, with the highest incidence being in older men. In females, the rates are highest in younger and middle-aged women (Fig. 29.1).

Thyroid cancer is a disease of paradoxes. Most small papillary thyroid cancers (PTCs) are indolent and overdiagnosed in the Western world and potential harm to patients from overtreatment has been highlighted (Brito et al. 2013). The prognosis in young adults (the majority of cases) with differentiated thyroid cancer (DTC) is excellent and the presence of lymph node (LN) metastases in the neck does not appear to influence long-term survival. Unlike many cancers however, late recurrences (sometimes decades after diagnosis) are not uncommon. Some DTCs behave aggressively and are associated with premature death (Reiners 2014; Roman and Sosa 2013). DTC is one among few solid cancers that can be cured even when there are distant metastases (Pawelczak et al. 2010). Many patients with recurrent thyroid cancer still survive for several years. Uncertainty is a companion to many patients with thyroid cancer and although survival overall is very favourable, quality of life is frequently chronically impaired (Sawka et al. 2014; Duan et al. 2015; Banach et al. 2013). Around 10% of patients have refractory disease.

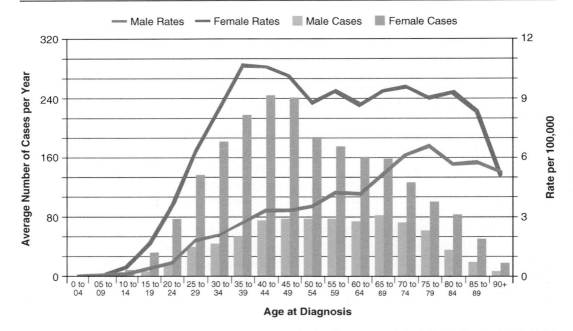

Fig. 29.1 Average Number of New Cases per Year and Age-Specific Incidence Rates per 100,00 Population, UK (2011–2013) (Cancer Research UK n.d.). Content supplied with permission by the world's largest charitable funder of cancer research, © Cancer Research UK [2002] All rights reserved http://www.cancerresearchuk.org/health-professional/cancer-statistics/statistics-by-cancer-type/thyroid-cancer/incidence#heading-One

There are therefore numerous challenges for patients, carers and healthcare professionals associated with the diagnosis of thyroid cancer. The last decade has seen a shift in the management of thyroid cancer with a tendency for less aggressive treatments for the more indolent types and a focus on a more personalised approach to treatment (Perros et al. 2014).

In most cases the cause of thyroid cancer is unknown; however, there are a number of risk factors.

29.1.2 Risk Factors

- **Ionising radiation**: This is known to be the biggest risk factor for thyroid cancer. Studies in childhood cancer survivors have shown an increased risk of thyroid cancer after radiotherapy (Sklar et al. 2012; Veiga et al. 2000). The cancer may not develop until 10–40 years after treatment. Although this risk is highest in children treated with radiotherapy, there is a slightly increased risk for anyone who has had external beam radiotherapy (Schonfeld et al. 2011).

Thyroid cancer is also more common in survivors of atomic explosions or accidents. After the Chernobyl nuclear reactor accident the number of cases in the Ukraine rose in people exposed to radiation, particularly as children or adolescents. Thyroid cancer cases also increased in the USA after nuclear testing in Utah.

- **Familial adenomatous polyposis** (FAP)—a genetic disorder (Triggiani et al. 2012).
- **Family history** of thyroid cancer (Metzger and Milas 2014).
- **Weak associations** (insufficient to justify screening) have been observed with obesity (Pappa and Alevizaki 2014), acromegaly (Wolinski et al. 2014) and diabetes (Schmid et al. 2013).

29.1.3 Overview of the Different Types of Thyroid Cancer

There are four main types of thyroid cancer.

Papillary thyroid cancer is the most common and accounts for around 65–80% of all thyroid cancers. It is a slow growing cancer originating in the follicular cells of the thyroid gland. It is usually well differentiated, may be multifocal and has a good prognosis for most patients. LN spread to the neck is present in up to 60% of papillary tumours (Mazzaferri et al. 2006), but these are often small foci of doubtful significance. LN involvement at diagnosis is associated with a higher risk of recurrence but not a higher mortality. Distant metastases are not common even in patients with neck node involvement. This is an important message for patients as the prospect of a cancer spreading can cause extreme stress. PTC is diagnosed in younger people and the female to male ratio is 2:1. Subtypes and variants of classic PTC include tall cell, columnar, diffuse sclerosing and poorly differentiated PTC (Kazaure et al. 2012). Certain oncogenic mutations are associated with more aggressive clinical behaviour (Xing et al. 2014). These variants generally have a propensity to recur and metastasise, but even then progression can be slow and patients can live for many years with relatively inactive metastases. Noninvasive encapsulated follicular variant PTC (NEFVPTC) has a very low risk of adverse outcome and the classification as 'non-invasive follicular thyroid neoplasms with papillary-like nuclear features '(NITFP) has now been introduced (Lloyd et al. 2017).

Follicular thyroid cancer (FTC) is the second most common type of thyroid cancer and accounts for around 15% of all thyroid cancers. It mostly presents as a solitary, slow growing tumour that is usually well differentiated. It generally has a good prognosis; however, vascular invasion is associated with worse outcomes (Mazzaferri et al. 2006). If more advanced at diagnosis, FTC can metastasise more readily. It has a peak onset between 40 and 60 years of age. People over 55 years often tend to have a more aggressive form of the disease.

There is a distinct subgroup of FTC called Hürthle cell thyroid cancer. One of its characteristics is that it has limited ability to concentrate iodine. It has the highest incidence of metastases among the DTCs with lungs, bones and central nervous system being the most common sites. LNs can also be affected.

Medullary thyroid cancer originates in the C cells of the thyroid gland and accounts for 3–10% of all thyroid cancers. Around 75% are sporadic with the other 25% being familial due to genetic predisposition. It requires genetic testing to establish the specific type.

Families of patients with MTC who carry genetic mutations are offered genetic screening and, if appropriate, assessment and treatment. Disease progression is usually slow and for this reason patients diagnosed with metastases that have spread to LNs or to distant sites can live for many years, but overall prognosis is less favourable than that of DTCs.

Anaplastic thyroid cancer is the rarest form of thyroid cancer and accounts for 1–3% of all thyroid cancers. Its prognosis is poor and its aggressive growth pattern often leads to death within a few months of diagnosis. Anaplastic elements can be found in well-differentiated tumours at diagnosis or at a later stage affecting the progression of these tumour types.

Lymphomas of the thyroid gland such as non-Hodgkin lymphoma are rare and treated as other haematological malignancies.

29.2 Differentiated Thyroid Cancer

29.2.1 Diagnostic Investigations and Staging

The suspicion of a thyroid cancer is raised in several ways and may include one or more of the symptoms listed in Table 29.1.

Increasingly thyroid nodules are found incidentally when imaging of the neck is performed for other clinical reasons. Occasionally patients present with metastases.

29.2.1.1 Pre-operative Investigations and Classification

Thyroid ultrasound (US) with fine needle aspiration (FNA) biopsy: Thyroid ultrasound in expert hands is a valuable investigation and can separate benign nodules (that do not require further investi-

Table 29.1 Clinical presentation (adapted from Hanna et al. (2015))

- Lump in the thyroid area
- Dysphonia (hoarse voice)
- Dysphagia (difficulty in swallowing)
- Stridor or impaired breathing
- Sense of fullness in the neck

gations) and suspicious lesions that merit further assessment with FNA biopsy. This is current advice from the British Thyroid Association (Perros et al. 2014) as performing a FNA of a lump by palpitation might not identify and assess the most suspicious nodules and not yield a reliable diagnostic result.

CT/MRI scan: If there is suspicion of locally advanced disease, a CT or MRI should be performed pre-operatively to facilitate surgical planning. A time interval of 2 months between CT and radioactive iodine (RAI) ablation is required as the CT contrast medium contains iodine and may interfere with the uptake of RAI. Unlike other cancers, extensive pre-operative staging with imaging (e.g. CT, MRI, PET CT) is unnec-

essary in most cases, as in low-risk patients disease outside the neck is highly unlikely, while in intermediate or high risk cases whole-body radioiodine imaging 1–2 weeks after radioiodine ablation provides adequate staging information and the potential presence of metastases will not affect the extent and timing of surgery.

LN involvement is common in PTC, but much less so in FTC. A number of US features are associated with benign or malignant nodules. LN levels are as per Fig. 29.2.

The British Thyroid Association guidelines (Perros et al. 2014) recommend the classification below which will guide the clinician in planning further investigations and treatment (Table 29.2).

Fig. 29.2 The neck and upper mediastinum LN levels, based on surgical compartments. Used with permission from Author/ website owner, accessed via http://www. endocrinesurgery.net.au/ lymph-node-management/

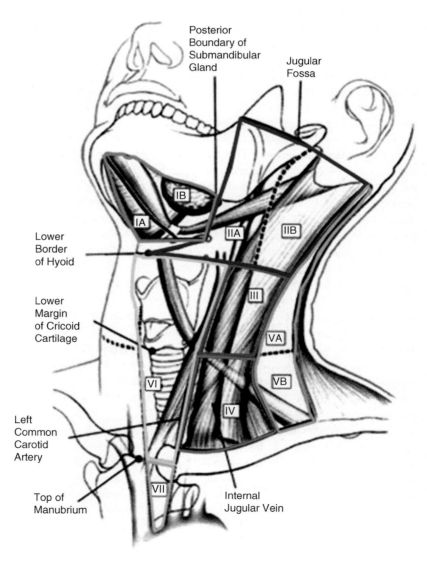

Table 29.2 Thyroid nodules—USS classifications (adapted from Perros et al. (2014))

- U1. Normal
- U2. Benign changes (e.g. cystic changes)
- U3. Indeterminate
- U4. Suspicious (e.g. hypo-echoic area)
- U5. Malignant (solid hypo-echoic nodule, micro-calcification, taller than wide cells)

Table 29.3 Diagnostic classifications of FNA cytology (adapted from Cross et al. (2016))

- THY1—non-diagnostic (e.g. due to poor sampling or only poorly preserved cells)
- THY1c—cystic fluid
- THY2—non-neoplastic (normal thyroid tissue)
- THY2c—non-neoplastic cystic lesion
- THY3—neoplasm possible
  - THY3a—atypical features present, but not enough to categorise
  - THY3f—possible follicular adenoma or carcinoma
- THY4—suspicious of malignancy (usually suspected papillary carcinoma in about 70% of patients)
- THY5—malignant

A U3–U5 finding would be followed by a FNA biopsy to obtain more information about the nature of the nodule. The classification recommended by the Royal College of Pathologists based on the Bethesda system for reporting thyroid cytopathology (www.rcpath.org) is shown below (Table 29.3).

Pre-operatively a vocal cord (VC) check is required to ascertain function. The recurrent laryngeal nerves (RLNs) which innervate the VCs lie very close to the thyroid gland. Any handling of the RLN during surgery can affect VC function (usually temporarily). The incidence of permanent VC damage through surgery in expert surgical hands is low at <1% (Mazzaferri et al. 2006).

29.2.1.2 Thyroid Cancer Staging

Malignant tumours are staged into categories which will allow for treatment planning and risk assessment (Table 29.4). The TNM classification (Tuttle et al. 2017) identifies the tumour size—T, the presence and location of nodules—N and the presence of metastases—M. It is generally used for staging of thyroid cancers.

If the staging categories 1–4 are being used, patients <55 years are either stage 1 (if no metas-

Table 29.4 TNM classification (adapted from Bychkov (2018)) (8th edition)

- T1—Tumour size ≤2 cm in greatest dimension and limited to the thyroid gland
  - T1a—Tumour ≤1 cm in greatest dimension, limited to the thyroid gland
  - T1b—Tumour >1 cm but ≤2 cm in greatest dimension, limited to the thyroid gland
- T2—Tumour size >2 cm but ≤4 cm in greatest dimension, limited to the thyroid gland
- T3—Tumour size >4 cm, limited to the thyroid gland or gross extrathyroidal extension invading only strap muscles
  - T3a—tumour >4 cm limited to the thyroid gland
  - T3b—tumour of any size with gross extrathyroidal extension invading only strap muscles
- T4a—Tumour of any size with gross extrathyroidal extension into subcutaneous soft tissues, larynx, trachea, oesophagus or recurrent laryngeal nerve
- T4b—Tumour of any size invading prevertebral fascia or encasing carotid artery or mediastinal vessels
- N0a—one or more cytologic or histologically confirmed benign lymph nodes
- N0b—no clinical or radiological evidence of locoregional lymph node metastases
- N1a—metastasis to level VI or VII lymph nodes (unilateral or bilateral)
- N1b—metastasis to level I, II, III, IV or V (unilateral, bilateral or contralateral) or retropharyngeal lymph nodes
- M0—no distant metastasis
- M1—distant metastasis

tases) or stage 2 (if metastatic disease present) regardless of TN status. This is because patients <55 years have a slightly better prognosis, so staging is stratified to match outcomes.

For patients ≥55 years Stage 1 equals a T1/2N0/XM0 category and Stage 2 a T1/2N1M0 and a T3N0/1/XM0 category. Stage 3 is defined as T4aN0/1/XM0. Stage IVA disease is T4bN0/1/XM0 and Stage IVb anyT, anyN and M1.

29.2.2 Surgery

Surgery is the most important initial treatment for well-differentiated and medullary thyroid cancer (MTC).

Guidelines recommend that thyroid cancer surgery is performed by experienced surgeons who perform high volumes of thyroid operations (National Cancer Peer Review—National Cancer Action Team n.d.).

The table below lists the types of surgery performed for thyroid cancer (Table 29.5).

A hemithyroidectomy is often performed if the diagnosis is unclear; however, if cancer is confirmed it may be followed by completion thyroidectomy. A hemithyroidectomy is considered adequate treatment for small tumours without adverse factors such as no adverse histological features, no extrathyroidal extension, no multifocal disease, no vascular invasion, no LN involvement, and no distant metastases.

A total thyroidectomy reduces the risk of local recurrence and distant metastases, allows for RAI ablation and facilitates long-term follow-up with serum thyroglobulin (Tg) monitoring.

If there is an underlying symptomatic thyroid disease (like Graves' disease or multinodular goitre), a total thyroidectomy is usually undertaken.

There are two notable recent trends in surgical management of thyroid cancer. Increasingly evidence suggests that hemithyroidectomy is associated with equally good outcomes as total thyroidectomy in carefully selected patients with DTCs up to 4 cm in diameter that are deemed low risk based on well-defined criteria (Kuba et al. 2014). Evidence mainly from Japan suggests that patients with a diagnosis of papillary thyroid microcarcinoma can be followed up safely with US without surgery, with excellent long-term outcomes (Ito et al. 2016).

One of the many paradoxes of PTC is that if sought intensively by pathologists, micrometastases in cervical LNs are found with high frequency, even in patients with microcarcinomas (Qubain et al. 2002). Yet, whether these are resected surgically or not does not seem to make a difference on survival (Randolph et al. 2012). The role of prophylactic neck dissection (i.e. surgery to remove LNs in the neck that are not obviously involved based on palpation and US) is controversial in patients with DTC as such surgery increases the risk of VC palsy and permanent hypopara-

Table 29.5 Types of thyroid cancer surgery

- Hemithyroidectomy
- Total thyroidectomy
- Completion thyroidectomy
- Selective neck dissection
- Isthmusectomy

thyroidism. Therefore prophylactic central LN dissection should only be considered if there are adverse risk factors (age >55 years, tumour size >4 cm, extrathyroidal extension, adverse histological subtype) and be a personalised decision. Equally prophylactic lateral LN dissection should be planned on an individual basis if the central LNs are involved. Radical neck dissection is a mutilating operation, which generally has no role in the surgical management of thyroid cancer. Therapeutic LN removal is indicated if LN involvement is evident pre- or intraoperatively.

29.2.2.1 Surgical Complications

Damage to the RLN can lead to a hoarse/whispery/weak/breathy voice due to compromise or loss of function of one or both of the VCs. Incidental cutting of the RLN or its removal to achieve the best outcome if it is infiltrated by thyroid tumour leads to corresponding VC palsy.

Damage to the superior laryngeal nerve will affect the voice quality, resulting in a lowered voice tone, early voice fatigue and loss of high pitches of the singing voice. This is a more frequent complication than a whispery voice.

The VCs might recover spontaneously during the first few months; therefore active voice rehabilitation is usually commenced only at least 6 months after surgery.

Damage to the hypoglossal nerve will affect the movement of the tongue and eating might be more difficult.

The accessory nerve innervates the sternocleidomastoid and the trapezius muscle and so facilitates the head, arm and shoulder movement. Damage to this nerve during surgery will make it difficult to lift the corresponding shoulder and raise the arm high, and results in neck stiffness. This can in most cases be treated successfully with physiotherapy.

Smaller sensory nerves of the skin can easily be cut during surgery. This can lead to numbness of the skin. For men it is noticeable e.g. during shaving. While sensation can return when nerves grow back together again, it can be lost permanently in certain areas of the face or neck.

Lymphoedema might occur when there is extensive LN removal or surgical removal of the internal jugular vein in neck dissections which will impair the normal lymph drainage. This can occur either immediately or months and even years later.

A chyle leak can occur through damage to the thoracic duct, resulting in leakage of lymphatic fluid (called chyle). It will be seen as a collection under the skin or in the wound drain after the patient has eaten. A strict fat free diet for 2–3 weeks is required until the leak has healed.

Hypocalcaemia results from damage to or removal of one or more of the parathyroid glands. Temporarily reduced functionality of the parathyroid glands due to manipulation during surgery is quite common initially. Permanent damage or loss of all parathyroid function occurs in a minority and requires long-term calcium and vitamin D analogue supplementation supplementation (see 29.2.4.4).

29.2.3 Radioiodine Ablation

29.2.3.1 Indications

Radioiodine ablation has been used in PTC and FTC after total thyroidectomy especially for those patients with an intermediate or high risk of recurrence or death. The potential benefits and problems associated with radioiodine ablation are outlined below (Tables 29.6 and 29.7). The BTA

Table 29.6 Benefits of RAI ablation (adapted from Perros et al. (2014))

- Prolonged survival
- Reduced risk of local and distant tumour recurrence
- Potential detection of distant metastases at diagnosis
- Easier long-term monitoring with undetectable Tg
- Easier detection of possible recurrence or metastases
- Reassurance for patients

Table 29.7 Problems associated with RAI ablation (adapted from Perros et al. (2014) and Hanna et al. (2015))

- Admission to stay in isolation for 1–4 days
- Post RAI ablation contact restrictions
- Having to avoid pregnancy or fathering a child for 6 or 4 months, respectively
- Slight increased risk of miscarriage within the first year
- Effect on salivary glands—sialadenitis (inflammation of the salivary glands) and xerostomia (dry mouth)—short term and possibly long term, even though this is rare
- Second malignancy (low risk)

Table 29.8 RAI Ablation Guidelines for Thyroid Cancer (adapted from Perros et al. (2014))

RAI Ablation Guidelines for Thyroid Cancer	
Definitive indications for RAI ablation	
• Tumour >4 cm	
• Gross extrathyroidal extension	
• Distant metastases at diagnosis	
Indications against RAI ablation	
• Tumour is ≤ 1 cm (unifocal or multifocal) in	– Classical PTC
	– Follicular variant PTC
	– FTC without vascular invasion or extrathyroidal extension

guidelines recommend an individualised approach to RAI ablation as shown in Tables 29.8.

In all other situations, certain risk factors need to be weighed as they might indicate a higher risk of recurrence. These include unfavourable cell type (tall cell, columnar, diffuse sclerosing PTC, poorly differentiated elements), large tumour size, extrathyroidal extension, widespread invasion (capsular and/or vascular invasion), multiple LN involvement, large LN size, high ratio of positive vs negative nodes and/or extracapsular nodal involvement (Table 29.8).

29.2.3.2 Preparation

Withdrawal of thyroid hormones: For optimal iodine transport into thyroid cells TSH levels need to be high (above 30 mU/L). This can be achieved by thyroid hormone withdrawal (2 weeks of withdrawal of liothyronine tablets or—if taking levothyroxine—a change to liothyronine 4 weeks prior to RAI for 2 weeks and then stopping it). However, the symptoms of the occurring hypothyroidism can be debilitating, so in psychiatric conditions, severe ischaemic heart disease or pituitary underfunction this might not be well tolerated or exacerbate comorbidities (adapted from Hanna et al. 2015).

Use of recombinant TSH: The alternative is injecting recombinant TSH 24 h and 48 h prior to RAI administration and continuation of levothyroxine administration. This is currently recommended by the BTA (Perros et al. 2014) for

patients with the following characteristics—
T1–3, N0/X/1, and M0 and R0 (i.e. no residual
disease). It gives a much better quality of life
and patient experience during this time (Hanna
et al. 2015). It also leads to more rapid elimination of the RAI, thus reducing the whole-body
retention, the exposure of healthy tissue to
radiation and possibly the length of the hospital stay while giving very similar ablation
results.

Reduction of dietary iodine: Patients are
advised to reduce their dietary iodine intake
for 1 or 2 weeks prior to RAI ablation to
encourage optimum uptake of RAI (Perros
et al. 2014).

Iodinated contrast medium: An interval of
at least 2 months following scans with iodinated contrast is required to ensure optimal
uptake of RAI.

When to discontinue breastfeeding:
Breastfeeding must be stopped 8 weeks prior
to RAI ablation in order to minimise the radiation uptake into breast tissue and to reduce
any future risk of breast cancer (Perros et al.
2014).

29.2.3.3 Dosage and Scans

Usual doses are between 1.1 GigaBecquerel
(GBq) and 3.7 GBq for ablation (Perros et al.
2014). If RAI administration is repeated for
therapeutic purposes, a dose of 3.7 or 5.5 GBq
is given as there is no scientific evidence of the
optimal dose in persistent or metastatic
disease.

A trend in recent years is to use RAI ablation
less often and in lower doses.

In low-risk DTC, 1.1 GBq is as effective in
ablating thyroid remnant tissue as 3.7 GBq. The
lower dose is recommended (Lamartina et al.
2015; Mallick et al. 2012a). Current clinical trials
are exploring the option of not ablating the remnant thyroid tissue with radioiodine in patients
with low-risk thyroid cancer (Mallick et al.
2012b).

Whole-body radioiodine scans are performed
a few days after RAI administration. This shows
the uptake of RAI into the body. Physiological
uptake is often seen in the thyroid bed, the salivary glands, the digestive tract and in the bladder
(Fig. 29.3). A single-photon emission computed
tomography (SPECT-CT) improves the information obtained through the post-ablation iodine
scan for locating cervical lymph node and any
distant metastases.

29.2.3.4 Potential Side Effects of RAI Ablation

Patients can experience a number of side effects
following RAI ablation (Table 29.9).

Prophylactic steroid cover is recommended
in metastatic disease in the central nervous system, lung and bones (Hanna et al. 2015). Apart
from a slightly increased risk of miscarriage in
the first year after RAI ablation, female fertility
has not been shown to be affected. Male fertility
can be affected if several high doses need to be
given. In such cases, sperm banking should be
discussed.

If repeated doses are required, the long-term
risk of sialadenitis (inflammation of the salivary
glands) and xerostomia (dry mouth) is increased.
The risk of a second cancer is low, but increases
with high cumulative doses (>18.5 GBq as total
dose) and is probably negligible for doses
<3.7 GBq (Clement et al. 2015).

High fluid intake as well as frequent voiding
of bladder and bowels will minimise the exposure of the associated organs to radiation.
Frequent showering and high fluid intake will
help reduce the radiation levels and expedite
discharge.

29.2.3.5 RAI Restrictions

The patient will usually need to stay in isolation
until the radioactivity measures less than
800 MBq. Visiting is restricted to designated
areas close by and to non-pregnant adults only
(Hanna et al. 2015).

Fig. 29.3 Post-radioiodine ablation scan showing physiological uptake in thyroid remnant, nose and salivary glands, colon and bladder. Image from the Author's (Dr. Petros Perros) personal collection

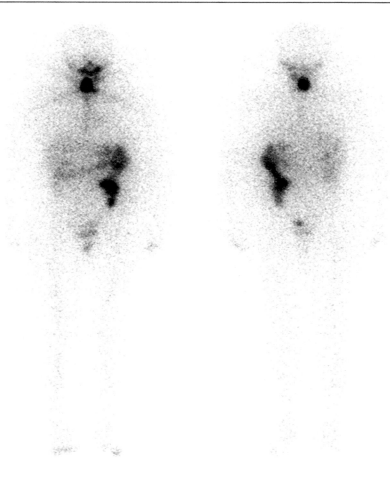

Table 29.9 RAI ablation side effects (adapted from Perros et al. (2014))

- Sensation of tightness in the neck
- Mild nausea
- Inflammation of the salivary glands
- Dry mouth
- Taste changes (usually a week after RAI administration and lasting for 1–2 weeks)
- Radiation cystitis
- Gastritis
- Bleeding/oedema in metastatic disease

After discharge, the patient needs to avoid close and prolonged contact with other people for several days to minimise unnecessary exposure to radiation for others. This restriction period is longer for children and pregnant women due to the higher susceptibility to radiation damage to fast developing cells. Restrictions include sleeping alone for a few days and avoidance of any other close and prolonged contact, including potentially time off work depending on the type of employment. The length of each of these restrictions is decided individually depending on the rate of radiation clearance of the individual patient (Perros et al. 2014). Any personal belongings from the isolation room must either be checked for radiation exposure, left behind or kept separately, e.g. clothes should be washed separately at home on discharge.

Box 29.1 A Letter from Doctor to a GP and a 'Patient's Poem'

Doctor's letter to the GP	A Poem
Multifocal papillary thyroid cancer, 32 mm, encapsulated follicular variant of papillary thyroid cancer with capsular invasion but no vascular invasion, completely excised, left lobe of thyroid, pT2 pNx R0. Single incidental papillary thyroid micro carcinoma, 9 mm, predominantly tall cell variant (TCV) with infiltrative growth, desmoplastic stroma and lymphovascular invasion, minimal extra thyroidal extension, almost reaching the specimen margin, pT3 (on ETE) pNx Rx. Background of Hashimoto's thyroiditis. Left diagnostic hemithyroidectomy followed by completion thyroidectomy and right level 6 dissection (no evidence of malignancy). Background of florid focally fibrotic Hashimoto's thyroiditis's. The MDT recommendation for radioiodine ablation was communicated. She has signed the consent form and I have arranged for her to receive radioiodine	I've had 5 months of tests, of prods and pokes, and probes. Chats about tumours, nodules and nodes. Tubes down my throat, tubes up my nose. Been cut stitched and sliced. Twice! Stapled and diced. Twice! Talked to and talked at, stripped naked and stared at. Handshakes, phone calls, incorrect roll calls, Miss B, Mrs. B, Miss B, Miss B, Who I am doesn't matter. I'm now T3, ETE, PNx, TCV. Papillary, follicular. **I USED TO BE ME.** Uniforms, uniforms, blue, purple and green, stop eating fish, no more iodine. Give up cappucino, change the life I know. So I look really well? So my scar's really great? I'll offer you one, It's not up for debate. I'll hand you my life, do you know what it's worth? Do you know how much impact I have on this earth? Pass my life to the people I've known for no time, relinquish control, you're going to be fine. Drink poison to order, be ill to request. Bleed to be better. To prolong, for how long? Just prolong. For how long?

The text on the left was written by a doctor in a letter to the GP, at the same time as that on the right by the patient in the radioiodine suite who had just received ^{131}I ablation. (*Used with consent from Patient and Dr. Petros Perros*)

29.2.3.6 RAI Refractory Disease

RAI refractory thyroid cancer is defined as any one of the categories listed in Table 29.10.

In metastatic disease thyroid cancer tissue can become completely or partially radioiodine refractory. If there is a partial response to RAI ablation (as evidenced by reduction in serum Tg levels), further treatments might be considered. However, if there is no response, treatment options are limited to conventional palliative measures or tyrosine kinase inhibitors (TKIs) (see under 29.2.5).

29.2.3.7 Follow-Up Assessment

The success of RAI ablation is assessed after 9–12 months with an US of the neck, a stimulated Tg test (if Tg and Thyroglobulin Antibodies (TgAbs) are undetectable), and in some cases iodine scans (Perros et al. 2014). In persistent metastatic or recurrent disease, further RAI treatment can be given.

Table 29.10 RAI refractory disease (adapted from Schlumberger et al. (2014))

1. Patients with metastatic disease that does not take up RAI at the time of initial treatment
2. Patients whose tumours lose the ability to take up RAI after previous evidence of uptake
3. Patients with RAI uptake retained in some lesions but not in others
4. Patients with metastatic disease that progresses despite significant uptake of RAI in the metastases and following a course of adequate radioiodine treatment

29.2.4 Thyroid Stimulating Hormone (TSH) Suppression, Biochemical Monitoring and Dynamic Risk Stratification

29.2.4.1 TSH Suppression

After surgery and RAI ablation, all patients will require thyroid hormone replacement medication in the form of levothyroxine (T4). Patients should have a dose big enough to prevent hypothyroidism and to suppress their blood level of TSH below 0.1 mU/L as this is associated with a reduction in the risk of recurrence of the thyroid cancer in selected cases (Biondi and Cooper 2010). This is called TSH suppression. The level to which each patient will need their TSH suppressed in the long term will be individualised to each patient, and is usually based on their risk of recurrence. Risk of recurrence is generally assessed at two points during treatment. The first point is right after surgery, where people fall into three groups:

- Low risk of recurrence
- Intermediate risk of recurrence
- High risk of recurrence

This is based on histology, tumour size, extent and spread of disease, and extent of surgical resection.

Patients in the high and intermediate categories who go on to have RAI ablation post surgery should have their TSH suppressed to <0.1 mU/L until they are restaged, usually 9–12 months later (Perros et al. 2014).

From this point on TSH suppression will depend on the response to RAI ablation, and patients are stratified according to their risk of recurrence (see under 29.2.4.3).

29.2.4.2 Blood Tests and Thyroid Hormones

The main blood tests done for patients during follow-up are TSH, Free Thyroxine (FT4), Tg and TgAbs.

Tg is a protein secreted by both normal and cancerous thyroid cells. Post total thyroidectomy and RAI ablation, Tg would be expected to be undetectable; however, it can take several months for the levels to reduce.

A persistently raised or rising Tg while on a suppressive dose of T4 is suggestive of persistent or recurrent disease, that warrants further investigation (Evans et al. 2015). Low levels of detectable Tg may be present in patients treated with hemithyroidectomy or total thyroidectomy without RAI ablation.

Around 25–30% of people with thyroid cancer will test positive for the presence of TgAbs, and these antibodies can interfere with the measurement of serum Tg giving misleading results (Hanna et al. 2015). It is essential that patients have blood tests done by the same biochemistry laboratory, as different methods can lead to a variation in results and give misleading interpretation.

A number of assay types are used to measure Tg. Radioimmunoassay (RIA) and Immunometric assay (IMA) are two that are most regularly used. RIA has been used since the 1970s, but in many laboratories it has been superseded by the IMA test which was introduced in the 1990s.

The IMA test is easier to automate, giving quicker results, and is particularly good at picking up very low levels of Tg. Unfortunately, it is more prone to interference from thyroid antibodies than the older RIA test, and therefore the IMA can give falsely low values of Tg. On the other hand, the RIA test can sometimes give falsely raised levels of Tg. Serum Tg results have to be interpreted in the context of the serum TSH concentration, which stimulates secretion of Tg.

Measurement of serum Tg with mass spectrometry was initially reported to be very accurate for detecting Tg in the presence of antibodies; however, investigations have not yet confirmed this (Hoofnagle and Rogh 2013). Its use in the future may be promising, but there is no consensus on its use at present and it is not routinely available.

29.2.4.3 Dynamic Risk Stratification

The follow-up assessment (see above) allows for restaging according to response to RAI and future risk of recurrence—this is called dynamic risk stratification (Table 29.11).

TSH suppression is associated with a risk of atrial fibrillation, cardiovascular disease and osteoporosis and therefore not indicated in low-risk patients whose prognosis is probably unaffected by TSH suppression.

Annual monitoring of serum Tg and thyroid function tests (TFTs) will continue lifelong as thyroid cancer is slow growing and recurrences can occur decades after initial treatment. This monitoring can provide reassurance for patients.

However for some it is an annual reminder of their cancer diagnosis and may provoke anxiety.

If there are detectable or rising Tg and/or TgAbs levels, further investigations are required. As the commonest sites of recurrence are cervical LNs and the thyroid bed, a neck US is the initial recommended imaging test. Neck recurrences are best treated surgically.

29.2.4.4 Hypoparathyroidism and Calcium Supplements

The four parathyroid glands are usually attached to or sit behind the thyroid gland, and are normally no bigger than a grain of rice. The parathyroid glands produce parathyroid hormone (PTH), which helps control calcium levels in the body.

The parathyroid glands can sometimes be removed accidentally or damaged during surgery. An estimated 30% of cases will develop temporary symptoms of low calcium following thyroid surgery, requiring vitamin D analogues and calcium supplements. For most patients this is tran-

sient in that it rights itself very quickly, but for others it can take months. If the parathyroid glands fail to function normally within 6 months post-operatively, the damage is usually permanent. Attempts should therefore be made to gradually wean patients off vitamin D analogues and calcium supplements and to assess whether parathyroid function is restored. The incidence of permanent hypoparathyroidism depends among other factors on the expertise of the surgeon, and in centres where high volume of thyroidectomies are performed by experienced surgeons, the expected rate of permanent hypoparathyroidism is less than 5%. Vitamin D deficiency is common among the general population and it is good practice to screen patients for vitamin D deficiency and correct it pre-operatively.

29.2.5 Metastatic, Recurrent and Radioiodine Refractory DTC

Most patients with DTC have good disease-specific outcomes. However, around 30% of patients are reported to experience persistent or recurrence of disease. Many recurrences occur in the neck while a smaller number of patients can metastasise to the lungs and bones. There are several approaches to recurrent disease (Table 29.12).

Surgery with curative intent is usually the treatment of choice for recurrent disease confined to the thyroid bed or to cervical LNs. However, low volume disease in the neck which is asymptomatic and not progressing may also be managed by active surveillance.

If there is either a rising Tg with an undetectable location of disease, multiple lung metastases or soft tissue metastases that are still responsive to RAI, repeated radioiodine therapy

Table 29.11 Dynamic risk stratification (adapted from Perros et al. (2014))

An excellent response – all of these:
• Suppressed and stimulated Tg of <1 µg/L
• Negative imaging (USS and/or other imaging if performed)
The strict suppression of TSH in this low-risk situation can be lifted to a TSH level in the lower half of normal (0.3–2 mU/L)
In an intermediate response – any of these:
• Suppressed Tg of <1 µg/L and stimulated Tg between ≥1 and <10 µg/L
• Imaging (USS and/or other imaging if performed) with nonspecific changes or stable LNs <1 cm on USS
TSH suppression is recommended for 5–10 years followed by reassessment
Incomplete response – any of these:
• Suppressed Tg of ≥1 µg/L or stimulated Tg of ≥10 µg/L
• Rising Tg levels
• Evidence of disease (newly identified or known) on nuclear medicine and/or other imaging
As thyroid cancer is still present (as evidenced by elevated or rising Tg/TgAbs levels and on imaging), additional treatment may be required and the serum TSH will have to be suppressed lifelong to reduce growth and spread of the disease

Table 29.12 Approaches to recurrent disease (Perros et al. 2014)

• Observation
• Surgery
• RAI
• External beam Radiotherapy (EBRT)
• TKIs

can be considered to increase the possibility of long-term survival. Residual microscopic disease in the neck following surgery for recurrent disease may also be treated with RAI.

Progressive disease in the neck not amenable to surgery with compressive symptoms and/or not responsive to RAI should be considered for other palliative treatments such as external beam radiotherapy. Bone metastases are generally not curable; however, solitary bone metastases may be amenable to EBRT or surgical resection if they are symptomatic.

Recent increasing knowledge about the biology of DTC has led to the use of TKIs (also known as targeted therapies). Targeted therapies are not curative treatment, but studies have demonstrated improved progression free survival for patients.

Sorafenib and lenvatinib are currently licensed for RAI refractory DTC—they have shown a significant increase in progression free survival in trials. They are principally indicated for progressive symptomatic disease; however, access and availability of the drugs differ in various countries. The most problematic side effects of sorafenib include hand and foot skin reaction (palmar plantar), hypertension, diarrhoea and fatigue. Lenvatinib has a similar side effect profile with hypertension being the most common and significant side effect. Side effects of these drugs can be serious and drug-related deaths can occur. The biggest challenge for many clinicians is deciding when to initiate TKI therapy and how to maintain a balance between side effects and benefits for the patient. If side effects are troublesome and both clinical and biochemical benefit are achieved, a dose reduction or 'drug holiday' can be considered. Treatment continues until side effects become intolerable or disease progression occurs. This is an evolving area in thyroid cancer treatment and ongoing studies continue to evaluate new agents.

29.3 Medullary Thyroid Cancer

MTC is the third most common type of thyroid cancer and makes up about 5–10% of all thyroid malignancies. MTCs arise from the calcitonin-secreting para-follicular C cells which are clustered in the upper two-thirds of the thyroid lobes.

Around 75% are known as sporadic MTCs and mostly occur between 50 and 70 years of age.

The incidence rate is 1.5 fold higher in women than in men. Approximately 25% are familial and can present either without any involvement of other glands (in about 55% of patients) or as part of multiple endocrine neoplasia (MEN) type 2 syndromes that comprise a more complex disease pattern such as tumours of the adrenal glands (phaeochromocytomas) and the parathyroid glands as well as other features.

29.3.1 Symptoms/Presentation

The patient with MTC can present with a number of troublesome symptoms including wheezing (Table 29.13). LN involvement at diagnosis is common. About 20% of patients present with locally advanced disease beyond LN involvement. Symptoms indicating metastatic disease include diarrhoea or flushes of the face due to hormone overproduction in large-volume MTC.

29.3.2 Diagnostic Investigations and Staging

Diagnostic procedures in MTC are similar to those for well DTCs (USS and FNA). Serum calcitonin (CTN) and carcinoembryonic antigen (CEA) are useful serum markers. Once the diagnosis of MTC is made, it is important to exclude phaeochromocytoma before surgery. The serum calcium should also be measured as this may be elevated due to hyperparathyroidism in patients with MEN2A. CT scans of the neck, chest, abdomen and pelvis are all part of the pre-operative staging.

Table 29.13 MTC: symptoms and presentation (Hanna et al. 2015)

- A thyroid lump
- Lymphadenopathy
- Diarrhoea and/or flushing

A detailed family history is imperative. All patients with a diagnosis of MTC are offered genetic screening.

The physiological role of calcitonin is unclear. However, in MTC it is a useful tumour marker. A substantial elevation indicates a MTC, possibly with spread to LNs and to distant areas.

The TNM classification is used for staging (Tuttle et al. 2017) (see Table 29.4); however, T4 is described as follows:

- **T4a**: Moderately advanced disease with gross extrathyroidal extension (including into subcutaneous soft tissue, the recurrent laryngeal nerve, larynx, trachea and/or oesophagus), any tumour size
- **T4b**: Very advanced disease which invades the prevertebral fascia, extends towards the spine and/or encases the mediastinal vessels or the carotid artery any tumour size (Bychkov 2018)

If staging I-IV is used, T1N0M0 is a stage I, T2/3N0M0 is stage II and T1-3 N1aM0 is stage III. All other TNM classifications are stage IV.

29.3.3 Treatment

Total thyroidectomy and prophylactic central neck dissection are the standard of care for MTC.

Therapeutic neck dissection in the lateral compartments is also indicated if there is evidence of cervical lymph node involvement. A prophylactic central neck dissection reduces the risk of central LN recurrence (which is common, but difficult to detect with an USS) and the need for repeat surgery.

A prophylactic total thyroidectomy is usually performed in asymptomatic carriers of familial MTC genes, identified by genetic screening. This has revolutionised the outcome and the timing of prophylactic thyroidectomy is dictated largely by the genotype (Wells Jr et al. 2015).

Spread occurs via the lymphatic system and blood circulation. Distant metastases arise commonly in the liver, lung and bones. If they are slow growing and asymptomatic, surveillance may be appropriate. Solitary distant metastases may justify further surgery with curative intent. Palliative surgery to symptomatic resectable metastases may also have a role in some patients.

Palliative radiotherapy may be appropriate for painful bone metastases, impending fracture of a weight bearing bone, airway compromise or lesions causing neurological and functional symptoms (e.g. spinal cord compression).

A MTC is not radioiodine sensitive, so radioiodine ablation is not indicated.

MTC is not TSH dependent, and TSH suppression will not reduce recurrence or improve survival in contrast to PTC and FTC. Therefore thyroid hormone therapy should aim for replacement with a normal TSH level.

29.3.4 Prognosis

Adverse prognostic features include older age at diagnosis, extent of primary tumour, nodal disease and distant metastases.

Patients with distant metastases are viewed as incurable. However, as mentioned above, progression rate is often slow and quality of life maintained for many years. A 10 year survival rate even for Stage III MTC is 71% (Hanna et al. 2015).

The CTN doubling time has prognostic implications with a calcitonin doubling time of <2 years indicating a poor prognosis.

29.3.5 Follow-Up and Monitoring

If surgery can completely remove any cancer and post-operative CTN is undetectable, a biochemical cure has been achieved (with a very good prognosis for the patient).

A rising calcitonin is highly suggestive of recurrent or progressive disease and usually is an indication for restaging.

Asymptomatic patients with known unresectable disease and stable or only slowly rising CTN may be managed with watchful monitoring.

29.3.6 Additional Treatment Options in Advanced MTC

A number of treatments have been reported to be effective in advanced MTC, but have not been evaluated in randomised studies and their role is unclear. They include somatostatin analogues and radiolabelled therapies with MIBG or lutetium.

Targeted therapies with TKIs are increasingly used in the treatment of progressive, metastatic or locally advanced disease. Currently vandetanib and cabozantinib are licensed for use in MTC.

They have a significant side effect profile (hypertension, palmar plantar, skin rashes, diarrhoea, electrolyte disturbances, bleeding, poor wound healing, fatigue, hair loss and loss of appetite). Vandetanib can also cause QT elongation and significant light sensitivity.

Targeted therapies are not curative, but may slow down the progression of the disease and improve quality of life (Dadu et al. 2015). The treatment can be continued until there is no clinical benefit or the side effects become intolerable.

29.4 Anaplastic Thyroid Cancer

The fourth thyroid malignancy is the anaplastic tumour, a rare and aggressive cancer. It accounts for 2–5% of all thyroid tumours. The mean life expectancy at diagnosis is estimated to 6 months or so. Seventy five percent of patients are over the age of 60 at diagnosis and it affects women more so than men.

It can develop spontaneously, but in 20–30% of cases it develops on the background of DTC.

29.4.1 Symptoms/Presentation

ATC presents with a rapidly enlarging tumour, and in some patients growth increase can be seen daily. Symptoms are included in Table 29.14. Most patients have metastatic spread into cervical and mediastinal LNs as well as into the sur-

Table 29.14 ATC: symptoms and presentation (Perros et al. 2014; Mazzaferri et al. 2006)

- Goitre or a rapidly enlarging nodule
- Dyspnoea
- Dysphagia
- Hoarseness
- Cough
- Neck pain
- Less common: haemoptysis, chest pain, bone pain, headache, confusion, abdominal pain
- Weight loss, fatigue, fever of unknown origin

rounding tissue such as muscles, larynx, trachea, oesophagus, blood vessels, sternum or spinal column. Distant metastases are present at diagnosis in 15–50% of patients (mainly in the lung).

29.4.2 Diagnostic Investigations and Staging

The diagnosis is established with a FNA or core biopsy in combination with clinical features. CT or MRI scans are important in staging the disease.

For anaplastic thyroid cancer, the TNM classification is the same as for differentiated thyroid cancer (see Table 29.4). If using staging, intrathyroidal disease is stage IVA, gross extrathyroidal extension or cervical lymph node involvement is stage IVB. If distant metastases are present, the disease is staged as IVC.

29.4.3 Treatment

Aggressive management in selected cases seems to be beneficial. Surgery should only be considered when complete macroscopic resection is feasible. However, this is rare and for most patients the disease is too advanced for surgical intervention at diagnosis. Subtotal resection is rarely justified.

Chemotherapy and radiotherapy are also options to slow down progression, aiming to reduce size and any compressive symptoms. However, the side effects of both treatments can be self-limiting (Hanna et al. 2015).

Palliation of symptoms is usually the main treatment for these patients.

29.4.4 Outcome

Very few patients with ATC survive longer than a year.

Death occurs in 50–60% of patients from upper airway obstruction. In these patients, a tracheostomy may be difficult to justify because of poor survival. Palliative care is considered as a better option.

If a major blood vessel is affected for example through a tumour that invades the wall of a carotid artery, death might come through a catastrophic bleed.

29.5   Genetics

Most people born with inherited faulty genes that can cause MEN2A and MEN2B syndromes develop MTC. Seventy five percent cases of MTC are sporadic (not due to inherited genetic changes), the other 25% are hereditary and caused by genetic changes passed on from parent to child.

For most sporadic non-medullary thyroid cancers, a genetic predisposition has been postulated via multiple low- to moderate-penetrance genes interacting with each other and with the environment, determining individual susceptibility (Landa and Robledo 2011). A number of somatic mutations (changes in genes that are not hereditary) have been identified, which are probably causally related. These are presumed to be acquired as random events and lead to neoplasia (abnormal growth of tissue). Many of these genes are involved in signalling pathways controlling thyroid cell growth. BRAF is a protein produced by the BRAF gene, and is a key player in a number of signalling pathways and a major player in papillary thyroid carcinogenesis. If it has a fault (or a mutation), it can send the gene into overdrive and uncontrolled growth.

We know that somatic mutations are implicated in most cases of DTC. However it is only in the past decade that we have started to understand the role of these molecular drivers, and how they may affect the behaviour of certain cancers. Some studies for example have shown that PTCs with a mutation in the BRAF gene have a higher risk of recurrence. NRAS mutations have been reported in follicular variant thyroid cancers that are more likely to spread.

The clinical behaviour of some thyroid cancers correlates with specific molecular markers (Pak et al. 2015), therefore knowing what mutations are present in a small, otherwise low-risk tumour may change the plan of treatment at the outset. It may also help with the development of new drugs that block these pathways.

Newer biological therapies are treatments that interfere with the signalling pathways. One group of biological therapies (i.e. TKIs) are already being used in the treatment of thyroid cancer.

Molecular profiling of thyroid nodules using FNA material is also being used to diagnose or rule out thyroid cancer in patients with thyroid nodules (Yip 2014).

There is no doubt that genetic profiling is advancing our understanding of the behaviour of thyroid cancers, and opens the possibility of further subclassification of the disease. This gives hope that the future of potential genetic testing will further personalise the management of thyroid cancer.

29.6   Living with Thyroid Cancer

A diagnosis of cancer can be a life-changing experience and can affect all aspects of a patient's life. Focusing on thyroid cancer's excellent survival rate eclipses some of the hardships patients go through in their treatment and lifelong maintenance of the disease. Thyroid cancer is rare, so it is not in the spotlight like other cancers, and the exposure it does get often overlooks some of the other issues that go along with this cancer.

Some of the physical side effects include

- Adverse effects of long-term TSH suppression—possibly atrial fibrillation, cardiovascular disease and osteoporosis
- Long-term voice problems
- Weight gain
- Fatigue

29.6.1 Voice Problems

Permanent VC damage occurs in less than 5% of cases (Perros et al. 2014). Voice quality that is significantly affected can be improved with either a collagen injection (improves the voice quality for a few months) or a thyroplasty for a more permanent outcome (insertion of a small plastic implant that pushes the paralysed fold more centrally, allowing the cords to touch and produce a stronger voice).

Early voice fatigue is a long-standing symptom of VC paralysis. The pitch range or quality of the singing voice may never fully recover to the pre-surgical state.

29.6.2 Weight Gain

A 2014 longitudinal study (Rotondi et al. 2014) has confirmed that thyroidectomy is associated with significant weight gain in many patients, including patients with TSH suppressed to below normal. Underlying mechanisms are not yet fully understood; however, acknowledgment of this combined with healthy eating advice and positive lifestyle changes may help patients to tackle this.

29.6.3 Fatigue

Fatigue is a common problem among different groups of cancer survivors. As expected with a rare cancer, there is very limited data that show studies related to fatigue in thyroid cancer. Some of these patients will experience problems with concentration and memory despite having optimal thyroid hormone dosage. Supportive care is imperative and most oncology teams have allied health professionals who have expertise in providing support and information in managing fatigue.

Patients managed for thyroid cancer can have a number of emotional issues relating to coping with the physical side effects and to coping with lifelong follow-up.

29.6.4 Lifelong Monitoring

Recurrences in thyroid cancer occur in around 10–30% of people (Mazzaferri and Kloos 2001). This can happen decades after the original diagnosis and highlights the importance of lifelong follow-up. This is unlike other survivable or curable cancers, where patients are often discharged after some years. Some patients find this yearly follow-up reassuring, but for many this means living with some uncertainty about the future.

29.7 Future Developments in the Management of Thyroid Cancer

29.7.1 Encapsulated Non-invasive Follicular Variant PTC

A recent review by an international group of pathologists and clinicians focused on redefining encapsulated non-invasive follicular variant of PTC as a neoplasm rather than a carcinoma (Nikiforov et al. 2016).

The classification of PTC is primarily based on characteristic histological nuclear features (Ohori 2015). This variant is known to behave in a non-aggressive manner where when completely excised, neither vascular nor capsular invasion is present. Evidence for showing this is in cases of lobectomy that excludes RAI ablation (Nikiforov et al. 2016). However, rare cases of distant metastases from encapsulated follicular variant PTC have been reported (Baloch et al. 2000 and Rivera et al. 2009 as cited in Ohori (2015)). Suggestions have been made to reclassify this subgroup to a 'non-invasive

follicular thyroid neoplasm with papillary
nuclear features' rather than to classify it as a
cancer due to its benign nature. Specific diagnostic criteria for this subgroup include no
tumour necrosis, a clear demarcation of the
nodule (or encapsulation), no psammoma bodies and no PTC variant like tall cell or diffuse
sclerosing (Nikiforov et al. 2016; Johnson et al.
2016).

While treatment for this subtype is less radical due to the recognition of its low-risk behaviour (e.g. lobectomy), 're-naming' is thought to
have emotional benefits for patients as it will
reduce anxiety associated with a cancer diagnosis. The change in classification was undergoing discussion among thyroid professionals due
to the potential benefits for patients and healthcare providers such as reducing the implications both on finance and insurance issues in
the follow-up care of patients at low risk of
metastases. It has now been given recognition
as non-invasive follicular thyroid neoplasm
with papillary-like nuclear features (NIFTP) in
the latest edition of the WHO classification
(Lloyd et al. 2017).

29.7.2 Role of Radioiodine Ablation in Low-Risk Well-Differentiated Thyroid Cancer

Whether benefits of radioiodine ablation out-
weigh potential harm is unknown in this patient
group of thyroid cancer. Two large randomised
controlled trials are underway in the UK and
France to address this important question
(Mallick et al. 2012b).

29.7.3 Radioiodine Refractory Disease

Selumetinib is another TKI which is currently
being investigated for its ability to re-sensitise
radioiodine refractory disease. Early phase studies have demonstrated increased iodine uptake in
previously radioiodine refractory patients (Ho
et al. 2013). Further trials are underway to add to
this body of research and to establish whether

successful retreatment with RAI might become
feasible for some patients in the future.

29.7.4 Tissue Bank for Anaplastic Thyroid Cancer

Due to the aggressive nature of ATC, very little
research is available. An international tissue bank
has been established to facilitate future studies
through the availability of tissue for research purposes (interNational Anaplastic Thyroid Cancer
Tissue Bank—iNATT: http://www.inatt.org/).

29.8 The Role of the Specialist Nurse

The pathway of patients with suspected or confirmed thyroid cancer can be complex and also at
risk of being disjointed due to the involvement of
the multi-disciplinary professionals involved at
various stages (radiologists, pathologists, head and
neck surgeons, endocrine surgeons, endocrinologists, oncologists, nuclear medicine physicians).
This can be confusing and disorientating for
patients. Specialist nurses play a key role and are
placed in an ideal position to provide continuity of
care, valuable and reliable information and support to patients and their families at all stages of
the disease process (Table 29.15).

Table 29.15 Essential roles of the specialist cancer nurse

- Explanation of investigations for a thyroid nodule
- Support during and after breaking bad news
- Continuous information and communication about planned treatments, investigations and results
- Coordinating and communicating throughout the treatment process
- Support for personalised therapeutic decision-making (e.g. merits and risks of radioiodine ablation)
- Explanation and implications of the outcomes of dynamic risk stratification
- Support for managing temporary and long-term side effects of treatment
- Education and management of thyroid hormone therapy
- Weaning off vitamin D analogues and calcium supplements
- Support for living with and managing chronic symptoms (like fatigue etc.)

29.9 Conclusions

The number of patients with thyroid cancer diagnoses is increasing globally, primarily due to incidental detection of small, biologically indolent tumours. Despite this concerning trend, the prognosis for most patients with thyroid cancer is good. The approach to treatment should be personalised aiming to match the aggressiveness of treatment to the biological nature of the cancer. The psychological impact in the aftermath of diagnosis and treatment of thyroid cancer is significant, and patients may experience lifelong physical and emotional consequences. An important objective for healthcare professionals managing people with thyroid cancer is remembering to treat the person, not just the disease.

References

Baloch et al 2000 and Rivera et al 2009 as cited in Ohori, P. FNA cytopathology and molecular test characteristics in the changing landscape of papillary thyroid carcinoma. J Basic Clin Med. 2015;4(2): 103–9.

Banach R, Bartès B, Farnell K, Rimmele H, Shey J, Singer S, Verburg FA, Luster M. Results of the Thyroid Cancer Alliance international patient/survivor survey: Psychosocial/informational support needs, treatment side effects and international differences in care. Hormones (Athens). 2013;12:428–38.

Biondi B, Cooper DS. Benefits of thyrotropin suppression versus the risks of adverse effects in differentiated thyroid cancer. Thyroid. 2010;20:135–46.

Brito JP, Morris JC, Montori VM. Thyroid cancer: zealous imaging has increased detection and treatment of low risk tumours. BMJ. 2013;347:f4706.

Bychkov A. Thyroid gland. Miscellaneous AJCC/TNM staging. 2018. PathologyOutlines.com. http://www.pathologyoutlines.com/topic/thyroidstaging.html. Accessed 16 Apr 2018.

Cancer Research UK. Thyroid cancer incidence by age. http://www.cancerresearchuk.org/health-professional/cancer-statistics/statistics-by-cancer-type/thyroid-cancer/incidence#heading-One. Accessed Apr 2016.

Clement SC, Peeters RP, Ronckers CM, Links TP, van den Heuvel-Eibrink MM, Nieveen van Dijkum EJ, van Rijn RR, van der Pal HJ, Neggers SJ, Kremer LC, van Eck-Smit BL, van Santen HM. Intermediate and long-term adverse effects of radioiodine therapy for differentiated thyroid carcinoma—a systematic review. Cancer Treat Rev. 2015;41:925–34.

Cross P, Chandra A, Giles T, Johnson S, Kocjan G, Poller D, Stephenson T. Guidance on the reporting of thyroid cytology specimens. Royal College of Pathologists.

2016. http://ukeps.com/docs/thyroidfna.pdf. Accessed 22 March 2018.

Dadu R, Hu MN, Grubbs EG, Gagel RF. Use of tyrosine kinase inhibitors for treatment of medullary thyroid carcinoma. Recent Results Cancer Res. 2015;204:227–49.

Duan H, Gamper E, Becherer A, Hoffmann M. Quality of life aspects in the management of thyroid cancer. Oral Oncol. 2015;51:S1–5.

Evans C, Tennant S, Perros P. Thyroglobulin in differentiated thyroid cancer. Clin Chim Acta. 2015;444:310–7.

Hanna L, Crosby T, Macbeth F, editors. Practical clinical oncology. 2nd ed. Cambridge: Cambridge University Press; 2015.

Ho AL, Grewal RK, Leboeuf R, Sherman EJ, Pfister DG, Deandreis D, Pentlow KS, Zanzonico PB, Haque S, Gavane S, Ghossein RA, Ricarte-Filho JC, Domínguez JM, Shen R, Michael Tuttle R, Larson SM, Fagin JA. Selumetinib-enhanced radioiodine uptake in advanced thyroid cancer. N Engl J Med. 2013;368(7):623–32.

Hoofnagle AN, Rogh MY. Improving the measurement of serum thyroglobulin with mass spectrometry. J Clin Endocrinol Metab. 2013;98:1343–52.

Ito Y, Oda H, Miyauchi A. Insights and clinical questions about the active surveillance of low-risk papillary thyroid microcarcinomas. Endocr J. 2016;63:323–8.

Johnson SJ, Stephenson TJ, Poller DN. NIFTP addendum to the RCPath Dataset for thyroid cancer histopathology reports. London, UK: The Royal College of Pathologists; 2016.

Kazaure HS, Roman SA, Sosa JA. Aggressive variants of papillary thyroid cancer: incidence, characteristics and predictors of survival among 43,738 patients. Ann Surg Oncol. 2012;19:1874–80.

Kuba S, Yamanouchi K, Sakimura C, Kawakami F, Minami S, Fujita F, Takatsuki M, Kobayashi K, Kanetaka K, Kuroki T, Eguchi S. Total versus hemithyroidectomy for well differentiated thyroid cancer. Ann Oncol. 2014;25(suppl 4):iv355.

Lamartina L, Durante C, Filetti S, Cooper DS. Low-risk differentiated thyroid cancer and radioiodine remnant ablation: a systematic review of the literature. Clin Endocrinol Metab. 2015;100:1748–61.

Landa I, Robledo M. Association studies in thyroid cancer susceptibility: are we on the right track? J Mol Endocrinol. 2011;47:R43–58.

Lloyd RV, Osamura RY, Klöppel G, Rosai J. WHO organisation of tumours of endocrine organs. 4th ed. Geneva: WHO; 2017.

Mallick U, Harmer C, Yap B, Wadsley J, Clarke S, Moss L, Nicol A, Clark PM, Farnell K, McCready R, Smellie J, Franklyn JA, John R, Nutting CM, Newbold K, Lemon C, Gerrard G, Abdel-Hamid A, Hardman J, Macias E, Roques T, Whitaker S, Vijayan R, Alvarez P, Beare S, Forsyth S, Kadalayil L, Hackshaw A. Ablation with low-dose radioiodine and thyrotropin alfa in thyroid cancer. N Engl J Med. 2012a;366(18):1674–85.

Mallick U, Harmer C, Hackshaw A, Moss L, IoN Trial Management Group. Iodine or Not (IoN) for low-risk differentiated thyroid cancer: the next UK National

Cancer Research Network randomised trial following HiLo. Clin Oncol (R Coll Radiol). 2012b;24:159–61.

Mazzaferri EL, Kloos RT. Current approaches to primary therapy of papillary and follicular thyroid cancer. J Clin Endocrinol Metab. 2001;86:1447–63.

Mazzaferri E, Harmer C, Mallick U, Kendall-Taylor P, editors. Practical management of thyroid cancer. London: Springer; 2006.

Metzger R, Milas M. Inherited cancer syndromes and the thyroid: an update. Curr Opin Oncol. 2014;26:51–61.

National Cancer Peer Review—National Cancer Action Team. Manual for Cancer Services: Head and Neck Measures Version 3.0. n.d. http://www.mycancertreatment.nhs.uk/wp-content/themes/mct/uploads/2012/09/resources_measures_HeadNeck_April2013.pdf (as cited in BTA 2014).

Nikiforov YE, Seethala RR, Tallini G, Baloch ZW, Basolo F, Thompson LD, Barletta JA, Wenig BM, Al Ghuzlan A, Kakudo K, Giordano TJ, Alves VA, Khanafshar E, Asa SL, El-Naggar AK, Gooding WE, Hodak SP, Lloyd RV, Maytal G, Mete O, Nikiforova MN, Nosé V, Papotti M, Poller DN, Sadow PM, Tischler AS, Tuttle RM, Wall KB, LiVolsi VA, Randolph GW, Ghossein RA. Nomenclature revision for encapsulated follicular variant of papillary thyroid carcinoma: a paradigm shift to reduce overtreatment of indolent tumors. JAMA Oncol. 2016;2(8):1023–9. https://doi.org/10.1001/jamaoncol.2016.0386. [Epub ahead of print].

Ohori P. FNA Cytopathology and Molecular Test Characteristics in the changing Landscape of Papillary Thyroid Carcinoma. J Basic Clin Med. 2015;4(2):103–9.

Pak K, Suh S, Kim SJ, Kim IJ. Prognostic value of genetic mutations in thyroid cancer: a meta-analysis. Thyroid. 2015;25:63–70.

Pappa T, Alevizaki M. Obesity and thyroid cancer: a clinical update. Thyroid. 2014;24:190–9.

Pawelczak M, David R, Franklin B, Kessler M, Lam L, Shah B. Outcomes of children and adolescents with well-differentiated thyroid carcinoma and pulmonary metastases following ^{131}I treatment: a systematic review. Thyroid. 2010;20:1095–101.

Perros P, Colley S, Boelaert K, Evans C, Evans RM, Gerrard GE, Gilbert JA, Harrison B, Johnson SJ, Giles TE, Moss L, Lewington V, Newbold KL, Taylor J, Thakker RV, Watkinson J, Williams GR. Guidelines for the management of thyroid cancer, third edition. Clin Endocrinol. 2014;81(Suppl 1):1–122.

Qubain SW, Nakano S, Baba M, Takao S, Aikou T. Distribution of lymph node micrometastasis in pN0 well-differentiated thyroid carcinoma. Surgery. 2002;131:249–56.

Randolph GW, Duh QY, Heller KS, LiVolsi VA, Mandel SJ, Steward DL, Tufano RP, Tuttle, for the American Thyroid Association Surgical Affairs Committee's Taskforce on Thyroid Cancer Nodal Surgery RM. The prognostic significance of nodal metastases from papillary thyroid carcinoma can be stratified based on the size and number of metastatic lymph nodes, as well as the presence of extranodal extension. Thyroid. 2012;22:1144–52.

Reiners C. Thyroid cancer in 2013: Advances in our understanding of differentiated thyroid cancer. Nat Rev Endocrinol. 2014;10:69–70.

Roman S, Sosa JA. Aggressive variants of papillary thyroid cancer. Curr Opin Oncol. 2013;25:33–8.

Rotondi M, Croce L, et al. Body weight changes in a large cohort of patients subjected to thyroidectomy for a wide spectrum of thyroid diseases. Endocr Pract. 2014;20(11):1151–15.

Sawka AM, Naeem A, Jones J, Lowe J, Segal P, Goguen J, Gilbert J, Zahedi A, Kelly C, Ezzat S. Persistent posttreatment fatigue in thyroid cancer survivors: a scoping review. Endocrinol Metab Clin N Am. 2014;43:475–94.

Schlumberger M, Brose M, Elisei R, et al. Definition and management of radioactive iodine-refractory differentiated thyroid cancer. Lancet Diabetes Endocrinol. 2014;2:356–8.

Schmid D, Behrens G, Jochem C, Keimling M, Leitzmann M. Physical activity, diabetes, and risk of thyroid cancer: a systematic review and meta-analysis. Eur J Epidemiol. 2013;28:945–58.

Schonfeld SJ, Lee C, Berrington de González A. Medical exposure to radiation and thyroid cancer. Clin Oncol (R Coll Radiol). 2011;23:244–50.

Sklar C, Whitton J, Mertens A, Stovall M, Green D, Marina N, Greffe B, Wolden S, Robison L. Abnormalities of the thyroid in survivors of Hodgkin's disease: data from the Childhood Cancer Survivor Study. Radiat Res. 2012;178(4):365–76.

Triggiani V, Angelo Giagulli V, Tafaro A, Resta F, Sabba C, Licchelli B, Guastamacchia E. Differentiated thyroid carcinoma and intestinal polyposis syndromes. Endocr Metab Immune Disord Drug Targets. 2012;12:377–81.

Tuttle M, Morris LF, Haugen B, Shah J, Sosa JA, Rohren E, Subramaniam RM, Hunt JL, Perrier ND. Thyroid-differentiated and anaplastic carcinoma (Chapter 73). In: Amin MB, Edge SB, Greene F, Byrd D, Brookland RK, Washington MK, Gershenwald JE, Compton CC, Hess KR, Sullivan DC, Jessup JM, Brierley J, Gaspar LE, Schilsky RL, Balch CM, Winchester DP, Asare EA, Madera M, Gress DM, Meyer LR, editors. AJCC cancer staging manual. 8th ed. New York: Springer; 2017.

Vecchia C, Malvezzi M, Bosetti C, Garavello W, Bertuccio P, Levi F, Negri E. Thyroid cancer mortality and incidence: a global overview. Int J Cancer. 2015;136:2187–95.

Veiga LH, Lubin JH, Anderson H, de Vathaire F, Tucker M, Bhatti P, Schneider A, Johansson R, Inskip P, Kleinerman R, Shore R, Pottern L, Holmberg E, Hawkins MM, Adams MJ, Sadetzki S, Lundell M, Sakata R, Damber L, Neta G, Ron E. A pooled analysis of thyroid cancer incidence following radiotherapy for childhood cancer. J Clin Endocrinol Metab. 2000;85(9):3227.

Vigneri R, Malandrino P, Vigneri P. The changing epidemiology of thyroid cancer: why is incidence increasing? Curr Opin Oncol. 2015;27:1–7.

Wells SA Jr, Asa SL, Dralle H, Elisei R, Evans DB, Gagel RF, Lee N, Machens A, Moley JF, Pacini F, Raue F, Frank-Raue K, Robinson B, Rosenthal MS, Santoro M, Schlumberger M, Shah M, Waguespack SG, American Thyroid Association Guidelines Task Force on Medullary Thyroid Carcinoma. Revised American Thyroid Association guidelines for the management of medullary thyroid carcinoma. Thyroid. 2015;25:567–610.

Wolinski K, Czarnywojtek A, Ruchala M. Risk of thyroid nodular disease and thyroid cancer in patients with acromegaly—meta-analysis and systematic review. PLoS One. 2014;9:e88787.

Xing M, Liu R, Liu X, Murugan AK, Zhu G, Zeiger MA, Pai S, Bishop J. BRAF V600E and TERT promoter mutations cooperatively identify the most aggressive papillary thyroid cancer with highest recurrence. J Clin Oncol. 2014;32(25):2718–26.

Yip L. Molecular diagnostic testing and the indeterminate thyroid nodule. Curr Opin Oncol. 2014;26:8–13.

Diagnosis and Management of Hypothyroidism in Adults

30

Raluca-Alexandra Trifanescu and Catalina Poiana

Contents

R.-A. Trifanescu (✉)
Department of Endocrinology, "Carol Davila"
University of Medicine and Pharmacy,
Bucharest, Romania

Department of Pituitary and Neuroendocrine
Diseases, "C.I.Parhon" National Institute of
Endocrinology, Bucharest, Romania
e-mail: raluca.trifanescu@umfcd.ro

C. Poiana
Department of Endocrinology, "Carol Davila"
University of Medicine and Pharmacy,
Bucharest, Romania

Department of Pituitary and Neuroendocrine
Diseases, "C.I.Parhon" National Institute of
Endocrinology, Bucharest, Romania
e-mail: catalina.poiana@umfcd.ro

© Springer Nature Switzerland AG 2019
S. Llahana et al. (eds.), *Advanced Practice in Endocrinology Nursing*,
https://doi.org/10.1007/978-3-319-99817-6_30

Abstract

Hypothyroidism is one of the most common endocrine disorders, defined as deficient production of thyroid hormones. In primary hypothyroidism, there is a thyroidal defect in the thyroid gland and decrease in thyroid hormones leads to an increased TSH secretion; in central hypothyroidism, there is either an insufficient thyroid stimulation by TSH (secondary hypothyroidism = pituitary causes) or an insufficient hypothalamic TRH release (tertiary hypothyroidism = hypothalamic causes). The disease is more frequent in women than in men; it affects all ages, but is more frequent in middle-age patients. Incidence varies between 0.6/1000/year in men and up to 4.1/1000/year in women. Primary hypothyroidism is the most frequent, caused by chronic autoimmune thyroiditis, thyroid surgery and radioiodine (^{131}I) ablation, external radiotherapy, thyroid dysgenesis, defects in thyroid hormones biosynthesis, release and action, and drugs. Symptoms include: fatigue, cold intolerance, weight gain, dry skin, constipation, muscle weakness, impaired memory, etc. Signs include: dry skin, carotenemia, puffy facies and loss of eyebrows, edema, bradycardia, diastolic hypertension, bradylalia, bradykinesia, etc. For diagnosis, TSH and free thyroxine (FT_4) are mandatory. TSH is the screening and first-line diagnostic test for primary hypothyroidism; FT_4 is necessary for diagnosis of central hypothyroidism and for diagnosis of overt *versus* subclinical primary hypothyroidism. Treatment consists in administration of levothyroxine (LT_4), orally, once daily, aiming to normalize serum TSH, to restore patients' physical and psychological well-being, and to avoid overtreatment. In first-term pregnant women, TSH should be kept <2.5 mIU/L; in second and third trimesters of pregnancy, TSH should be <3 mIU/L.

Keywords
Adult hypothyroidism · Autoimmune thyroiditis · TSH · Levothyroxine

Abbreviations

^{131}I	Radioiodine
ATA	American Thyroid Association
BTA	British Thyroid Association
CK MB	Isoenzyme MB of the enzyme phosphocreatine kinase
ECG	Electrocardiogram
ETA	European Thyroid Association
FT_4	Free thyroxine
LDL cholesterol	Low-density lipoprotein (LDL) cholesterol
LT_3	Liothyronine
LT_4	Levothyroxine
MCT8	Monocarboxylate transporter 8
MRI	Magnetic resonance imaging
SECISBP2	Selenocystein insertion sequence (SECIS) binding protein 2
T_3	Triiodothyronine
T_4	Thyroxine

TPO	Thyroid peroxidase (thyroperoxidase)
TR	Thyroid hormone receptor
TRH	Thyrotropin-releasing hormone
TSH	Thyroid-stimulating hormone

Key Terms
- **Overt hypothyroidism:** Elevated serum thyroid-stimulating hormone concentration
- **Primary hypothyroidism:** related to thyroid gland failure
- **Central hypothyroidism:** Secondary to hypothalamic or pituitary dysfunction or causes other than primary thyroid gland failure.
- **Overtreatment:** suppression of TSH due to inappropriately high replacement dose of thyroid

---

Key Points
- Hypothyroidism is insufficient thyroid hormone production due to thyroid or central (pituitary or hypothalamic) causes.
- Clinical picture includes fatigue, cold intolerance, weight gain, dry skin, carotenenia, puffy face and loss of eyebrows, constipation, muscle weakness, impaired memory, edema, bfrsdycardia, diastolic hypertension, bradycardia, and bradykinesia.
- Diagnosis is made with TFTs showing, increased TSH, low/normal FT4 in primary hypothyroidism; low-normal/low FT4 with low/inappropriately normal/slightly increased TSH in central hypothyroidism.
- Treatment requires Levothyroxine orally, once daily; in primary hypothyroidism, target TSH in young people is 1–2.5 mlU/L; in the elderly and in patients with ischemic heart disease, target TSH is the upper normal (according to age-specific reference range) and the initial Levothyroxine dose should be low (12.5–25 µg daily) and increase gradually; in pregnancy during first-term, the target TSH is <2.5 mlU/L. In the second and third trimester of pregnancy, the target TSH should be <3 mlU/L.

- In central hypothyroidism, the target FT4 is the upper half of the normal range for young patients, and in the lower half of the normal reference range in the elderly patients.

30.1 Introduction

Hypothyroidism is one of the most frequent endocrine diseases. It is very important to be recognized as early as possible, because overt hypothyroidism could be associated with several complications.

30.2 Definition and Classification

Hypothyroidism is a pathological condition due to insufficient thyroid hormones production.

Myxedema is severe hypothyroidism in adults, characterized by nonpitting edema due to accumulation of glycozaminoglycans in subcutaneous tissue and interstitial tissues.

30.2.1 Primary Hypothyroidism

Primary hypothyroidism refers to deficient thyroid hormones production due to thyroid causes and can result in overt or subclinical hypothyroidism.

Overt hypothyroidism: This happens when the serum thyroid-stimulating hormone concentration is elevated, (for example, TSH > 10 mIU/L) and serum-free thyroxine (FT_4) concentration is low.

In pregnancy, overt hypothyroidism can comprise of a serum TSH > 2.5 mIU/L with decreased FT_4 concentrations during the first trimester of pregnancy or serum TSH > 3 mIU/L with decreased FT_4 concentrations during the second and third trimester of pregnancy (Negro and Stagnaro-Green 2014; Stagnaro-Green et al. 2011). However, recent studies suggest only a modest downward shift (0.5–1 mIU/L) in the first trimester upper normal limit of TSH, typically in weeks 7–12, with significant differences depending on BMI, ethnicity, geography and iodine sta-

Table 30.1 Classification of subclinical hypothyroidism according to TSH levels in different categories of patients (adapted from Biondi and Wartofsky (2014))

Classification of subclinical hypothyroidism	TSH (mIU/L)	FT$_4$
Mild subclinical hypothyroidism	4.5–9.9	Normal
Mild subclinical hypothyroidism in elderly	>7	Normal
Severe subclinical hypothyroidism	≥10	Normal
Subclinical hypothyroidism in pregnancy	2.5–10	Normal

tus, and TPO antibodies positivity. So, overt hypothyroidism will be defined as both elevated TSH and decreased FT$_4$ concentration during gestation as compared with pregnancy trimester-specific reference range values. If pregnancy-specific TSH reference range is not available, upper reference range for TSH should be considered 4 mIU/L (Alexander et al. 2017). Furthermore, overt hypothyroidism can occur in pregnancy, when the serum TSH > 10 mIU/L, irrespective of FT$_4$ concentrations (Negro and Stagnaro-Green 2014; Stagnaro-Green et al. 2011; Alexander et al. 2017).

Subclinical hypothyroidism: refers to a high serum TSH concentration and a normal serum-free thyroxine (FT$_4$) concentration (Cooper and Biondi 2012; Biondi and Wartofsky 2014) (Table 30.1).

30.2.2 Central Hypothyroidism

Central hypothyroidism: also known as secondary hypothyroidism, is referred to deficient thyroid hormone production due to pituitary or hypothalamic causes and characterized by a low serum FT$_4$ concentration and a serum TSH concentration that is not appropriately elevated.

- Secondary hypothyroidism: due to pituitary causes
- Tertiary hypothyroidism: due to hypothalamic causes (Ross and Cooper 2017; Wiersinga 2014)

Hypothyroidism may be persistent or transient. Transient primary hypothyroidism occurs after subacute, painless, or postpartum thyroid-itis, antithyroid drugs, and toxic injury of the thyroid.

30.3 Epidemiology

In the UK, the prevalence of spontaneous overt hypothyroidism is 1–2%, and it is more common in older women and ten times more common in women than in men (Vanderpump 2011; Vanderpump et al. 1995).

The prevalence of subclinical hypothyroidism is higher (5–10%); it is also more frequent in women and its prevalence increases with age (Biondi and Cooper 2008). Factors associated with increased risk of progression from subclinical to overt hypothyroidism are high iodine intake, higher TSH (>10 mU/L), positive thyroid antibodies, low-normal FT$_4$ levels, and adult age (Walsh et al. 2010).

Primary hypothyroidism represents 95–99% of cases, while central hypothyroidism 1–5% (Biondi and Wartofsky 2014).

30.4 Causes of Hypothyroidism

30.4.1 Primary Hypothyroidism with Goiter

- Goitrous chronic autoimmune thyroiditis—the most common etiology in iodine sufficient areas (Tunbridge et al. 1977)

Box 30.1 Case Example 1: Drug-Induced Hypothyroidism

A, 63 year ♂, resident in an iodine deficiency area, treated with Sunitinib for metastatic renal carcinoma, presented with myxedema:

TSH = 75 mIU/L (high)

FT4 = 3.8 pmol/L (low)

Antithyroglobulin antibodies = 11 IU/mL

TPO antibodies = 10 IU/ml

Serum 8 a.m. cortisol = normal

Treatment with Levothyroxine normalized both TSH and FT4.

- Silent and postpartum thyroiditis
- Cytokine-induced thyroiditis
- Iodine deficiency
- Iodine overload (e.g., Amiodarone)
- Drugs: thionamides, lithium carbonate, amiodarone, interferon α, perchlorate, tyrosine kinase inhibitors—sunitinib, sorafenib
- Infiltrative disorders of the thyroid gland (amyloidosis, hemochromatosis, sarcoidosis, Riedl's thyroiditis)
- subacute thyroiditis
- defects in thyroid hormones synthesis

30.4.2 Primary Hypothyroidism Without Goiter

- Atrophic chronic autoimmune thyroiditis
- Iatrogenic: thyroidectomy, radioiodine ablation, external beam radiation therapy for malignant tumors of head and neck (Hodgkin's lymphoma, leukemia, bone marrow transplantation, etc.)
- Congenital thyroid agenesis, dysgenesis.

30.4.3 Central (Secondary and Tertiary) Hypothyoidism: Without Goiter

- Hypopituitarism (pituitary tumors, pituitary surgery or radiotherapy, infiltrative diseases—sarcoidosis, amyloidosis, hemochromatosis), pituitary apoplexy-Sheehan's syndrome, traumatic, genetic, lymphocytic hypophysitis, infectious disorders (tuberculosis), metastases
- Isolated TSH deficiency
- Congenital hypopituitarism (multiple pituitary hormone deficiencies)
- Treatment with somatostatin analogues (octreotide, lanreotide), bexarotene
    Hypothalamic diseases: tumors (craniopharyngioma, germinoma, glioma, meningioma), trauma, infiltrative diseases (sarcoidosis, hemochromatosis, cell hystiocytosis, Langerhans' cell), idiopathic (birth defects)

30.4.4 "Peripheral" (Extrathyroidal) Hypothyroidism

- Mutations in gene encoding TR β, TR α (thyroid hormone resistance), MCT8, SECISBP2
- Massive infantile hemangioma with consumptive hypothyroidism (Ross and Cooper 2017; Wiersinga 2014).

30.5 Clinical Manifestations of Hypothyroidism

Patients with hypothyroidism can present with any of the following signs and symptoms

30.5.1 Symptoms

- Fatigue
- Cold intolerance
- Weight gain
- Dry skin
- Constipation
- Hoarseness
- Muscle weakness and/or cramps, myalgia, and paresthesia
- Impaired memory, slow thinking, decreased concentration, depression, dementia (in elderly people)
- Menstrual disturbances (irregular or heavy menses), infertility, galactorrhoea
- Pleural, pericardial effusions, ascites (Ross and Cooper 2017; Wiersinga 2014).

30.5.2 Signs

- Dry skin, carotenemia
- Puffy facies and loss of eyebrows
- Edema (periorbital)
- Tongue enlargement
- Bradycardia
- Diastolic hypertension
- Slow speech (bradylalia), slow movements (bradykinesia)
- Goiter/thyroid atrophy

- Delayed relaxation phase of the deep tendon reflexes, ataxia
- Loss of hair
- Constipation
- Hypothermia (Ross and Cooper 2017; Wiersinga 2014).

30.6 Patient's Approach

30.6.1 Blood Tests

TSH is the screening and first-line diagnostic test for primary hypothyroidism; third generations assays have detection limit of 0.01 mIU/L and up to 99% sensitivity and specificity. Normal TSH range is usually 0.4–4 mIU/L (Association of Clinical Biochemistry, British Thyroid Association, and British Thyroid Foundation 2006). Note that upper normal limit of TSH range is higher in older people: 97.5th percentile of the upper normal limit of TSH was reported to be: 4.5 mIU/L in people 50–59 years, 5.9 mIU/L in elderly subjects 70–79 years old, and 7.5 mIU/L in those at 80 years and older (Surks and Hollowell 2007). Some studies suggested a much lower cut-off for the upper normal limit of TSH (2–2.5 mIU/L), but there is presently insufficient justification to lower the upper normal limit of TSH (Brabant et al. 2006).

Free T_4–FT_4 is necessary for diagnosis of central hypothyroidism and for diagnosis of overt *versus* subclinical primary hypothyroidism.

Antithyroglobulin antibodies and TPO antibodies are positive in 50–70% and 90–95%, respectively, of cases of hypothyroidism due to autoimmune thyroiditis. They confirm autoimmune etiology and may predict the evolution towards overt hypothyroidism in patients with subclinical hypothyroidism, pregnant women, and in patients treated with amiodarone, lithium, interferon α.

Additional Tests
- Lipids: hypothyroidism is associated with mixed dyslipidemia, for example, increased total cholesterol, low-density lipoprotein (LDL) cholesterol, apolipoprotein B, lipoprotein (a), and triglycerides. Lipid changes

> **Box 30.2 Case Example 2: Increased Creatine Phosphokinase in Severe Hypothyroidism**
>
> 66 year, ♀ resident in an iodine-sufficient area, presented with asthenia, constipation, and depression. Biochemical data showed severe hypothyroidism:
>
> TSH = 71.4 mIU/L (high)
> FT4 = 3.9 pmol/L (low)
> Positive TPO antibodies = 107 IU/mL
> Serum 8 a.m. cortisol = normal
> Patient-associated anemia, and increased creatinine kinase = 1385 IU/L with the upper normal CKMB (28 IU/L)
>
> After 3 months of Levothyroxine treatment, there was significant clinical and biochemical improvement (TSH = 11 mIU/L and creatinine kinase normalized).

are reversible with levothyroxine (LT_4) treatment;
- blood count: anemia (due to blood loss/coexistence of vitamin B_{12} deficiency—pernicious anemia/folic acid deficiency);
- Urea and electrolytes and liver function tests: Hyponatremia (due to hemodilution);
- Increased creatine phosphokinase (CK) or other muscle and liver enzymes;
- prolactin: Hyperprolactinemia: severe, long-standing primary hypothyroidism leads to increased TRH and to hyperprolactinemia (Ross and Cooper 2017; Wiersinga 2014).

30.6.2 Resting ECG (Standard 12-Lead Resting Electrocardiogram)

Sinus bradycardia, low-voltage QRS complexes, flattening or inversion of the T wave, QT prolongation, and increased dispersion of the QT interval may be present. Sometimes, there is prolonged PR interval (first-degree atrioventricular block) or interventricular conduction delays. Premature ventricular beats can also be present. Sustained or non-sustained attacks of ventricular tachycardia and torsades de pointes are seldom reported (Ross and Cooper 2017; Wiersinga 2014).

30.6.3 Thyroid Ultrasound

A thyroid ultrasound is very useful in the diagnostic evaluation of thyroid nodules and can show any of the following features;

- Focal or diffuse thyroid enlargement/thyroid atrophy
- Hypoechogenicity of the thyroid gland in autoimmune thyroiditis (even in 10% patients with negative thyroid antibodies)
- Hypoechoic micronodules (1–6 mm)
- Fine echogenic fibrous septae generating a pseudolobulated pattern
- Doppler colour: increased/decreased/normal vascularization
- Perithyroidal lymph nodes, especially the "Delphian" node may be enlarged (Chaudhary and Bano 2013)

Note: due to higher risk for papillary thyroid carcinoma and thyroid lymphoma, suspected nodules should be referred for fine needle biopsy according to guidelines (British Thyroid Association guidelines for nodules).

30.6.4 Other Tests

Doppler echocardiography: this should be undertaken in patients with severe hypothyroidism.

Chest X rays: in patients with cardiomegaly, pericardial, and/or pleural effusion.

Pituitary MRI: Pituitary enlargement (in primary myxedema, due to thyrotroph and lactotroph hyperplasia (Ross and Cooper 2017; Wiersinga 2014)).

30.7   Biochemical Assessment

30.7.1 Diagnosis

Relies on measurement of thyroid function tests (TFTs): TSH and FT_4 for blood (BTA Guidelines-Table 30.2)

Differential diagnosis of raised TSH: resistance to TSH, TSH-secreting pituitary adenoma, recovery from nonthyroidal illness, presence of heterophilic antibodies against mouse proteins—falsely raise serum TSH.

30.7.2 Algorithm for Hypothyroidism Diagnosis

In the presence of either clinical suspicion or biochemical suspicion (dyslipidemia, hyperprolactinemia, hyponatremia, anemia, and/or elevated creatine phosphokinase), TSH and FT_4 should be measured.

30.7.3 Indications for Screening Patients with Symptoms and Risk Factors for Hypothyroidism

These can include any from the list below:

- Goiter
- Autoimmune diseases (such as type 1 diabetes mellitus, adrenal insufficiency, premature ovarian failure, lymphocytic hypophysitis, vitiligo, celiac disease, pernicious anemia, multiple sclerosis, Sjogren syndrome, primary pulmonary hypertension, etc.)
- Previous history of Graves' disease (with or without radioiodine therapy), subacute thyroiditis, painless thyroiditis
- Head and/or neck irradiation

Table 30.2 Biochemical diagnosis of hypothyroidism (adapted from Cooper and Biondi (2012), Ross and Cooper (2017), Wiersinga (2014), and Association of Clinical Biochemistry, British Thyroid Association and British Thyroid Foundation (2006))

	Serum TSH	Serum FT_4
Overt Primary Hypothyroidism	Increased	Low
Subclinical Primary Hypothyroidism	Increased	Normal
Central hypothyroidism	Low/inappropriately normal/slightly increased	Low-normal/low

- Family history of autoimmune thyroid diseases
- Turner's syndrome
- Down's syndrome

Hypothalamic diseases: tumors, radio-therapy, surgery, infiltrative diseases (sarcoidosis, hemochromatosis, Langerhans' cell histiocytosis)

Pituitary disease: tumors, radiotherapy, surgery, apoplexy (Sheehan's syndrome), metastatic cancer

Pregnant women: from area with iodine deficiency, those who have symptoms of hypothyroidism, a family or personal history of thyroid disease (such as personal history of hemithyroidectomy and/or treatment with radioactive iodine) who are positive for TPO antinodies and antithyroglobulin antibodies, who have type 1 diabetes, head and neck radiation, recurrent miscarriage, morbid obesity, or infertility

On treatment with drugs interfering with thyroid function: lithium carbonate, amiodarone, interferon α, tyrosine kinase inhibitors—sunitinib, sorafenib.

Laboratory test: radiological abnormalities such as: hypercholesterolemia, hyponatremia, hyperprolactinemia, elevated creatine phosphokinase, anemia, hyperhomocysteinemia, pleural and pericardial effusions, pituitary enlargement (Ross and Cooper 2017; Wiersinga 2014)

30.8 Complications

Complications of hypothyroidism can include any of the listed below.

- Dyslipidemia and atherosclerosis
- Coronary heart disease (Rodondi et al. 2010) (especially in patients with TSH > 10 mIU/L)
- Pleural and pericardial effusion
- Heart failure (especially in patients with TSH > 7–10 mIU/L)

30.9 Treatment

30.9.1 Initiation of Therapy Including Doses, Route, and Time of Administration

The aim of treatment is to normalize serum TSH, to restore patients' physical and psychological well-being and to avoid overtreatment, especially in old people (Okosieme et al. 2016).

The exception to this is in the first-term of pregnancy in women where the TSH should be kept <2.5 mIU/L; in second and third trimesters of pregnancy, TSH should be <3 mIU/L (Negro and Stagnaro-Green 2014; Stagnaro-Green et al. 2011).

Methods: Levothyroxine (LT$_4$) as monotherapy, orally, once daily.

Doses:
- 1.6–1.8 µg/kg/day levothyroxine (lean body weight or ideal body weight) in young and middle-age patients for replacement therapy in primary hypothyroidism
- 1.3 µg/kg/day levothyroxine in central hypothyroidism
- 2–2.4 µg/kg/day levothyroxine in pregnant women with overt hypothyroidism
- 2–2.5 µg/kg/day levothyroxine for suppressive therapy

LT$_4$ requirements are higher in young patients than in the elderly, in overt hypothyroidism than in subclinical hypothyroidism, premenopausal women than in postmenopausal, in men, pregnancy (Biondi and Wartofsky 2014) (30–50%), severely obese people—due to increased plasma volume, delayed gastrointestinal absorption, and those with altered T$_4$ to T$_3$ conversion (Michalaki et al. 2011).

Five to ten percent of hypothyroid patients treated with levothyroxine have persistent symptoms, despite TSH normalization. Guidelines recommend against the routine use of combination treatment with LT$_4$ and LT$_3$ (ATA), because of insufficient evidence from randomized controlled trials. However, ETA and ATA guidelines suggested considering combined LT$_4$ and LT$_3$ therapy as an experimental approach in compliant patients treated with LT$_4$, who have persistent symptoms despite serum TSH normalization. Combined LT$_4$ and LT$_3$ are not recommended in pregnancy or in patients with cardiac arrhythmias. If there is no improvement in patient's condition after 3 months, the combined LT$_4$ + LT$_3$ therapy should be stopped (Okosieme et al. 2016).

Oral intake of levothyroxine: this should be taken on fasting in the morning, 30–60 min before breakfast. Some studies suggest some benefits of levothyroxine administration 2 h after the evening meal (Bolk et al. 2007).

Specific situations: *it should be noted that all recommended treatments should adhere to local hospital policy and guidelines*

Subclinical hypothyroidism and indications for treatment:
- Symptomatic patients, depression, goiter, cardiovascular risk factors (high blood pressure, dyslipidemia, diabetes/insulin resistance)
- Patients with positive thyroid antibodies and rising TSH
- Smaller levothyroxine doses are needed compared to patients with overt hypothyroidism.

Suggested levothyroxine starting doses in subclinical hypothyroidism (Teixeira et al. 2008).

- 25 µg LT$_4$ for TSH = 4–8 mIU/L,
- 50 µg LT$_4$ for TSH = 8–12 mIU/L
- 75 µg LT$_4$ for TSH > 12 mIU/L

30.9.1.1 Associated Adrenal Insufficiency (Central or Autoimmune)

Start with hydrocortisone treatment, because full-dose levothyroxine replacement may be associated with exacerbation of adrenal insufficiency (Biondi and Wartofsky 2014).

30.9.1.2 Pregnancy

Both hypothyroidism and maternal hypothyroxinemia are associated with fetal and maternal negative outcomes (miscarriages, preterm delivery,

neurodevelopmental delay, autistic symptoms in the offspring); levothyroxine treatment improves these outcomes in some studies. In hypothyroid women, thyroid hormones requirement increases during pregnancy (Negro and Stagnaro-Green 2014; Stagnaro-Green et al. 2011; Alexander et al. 2017; Biondi and Wartofsky 2014). LT$_4$ dose should, therefore, be increased around 4–6 weeks of pregnancy by 25–30% (Alexander et al. 2017). Oral levothyroxine is the recommended treatment for maternal hypothyroidism.

Overt hypothyroidism diagnosed during pregnancy should be treated with full replacement dose of 2–2.4 µg/kg/day levothyroxine, in order to restore euthyroidism as soon as possible. For women with subclinical hypothyroidism (TSH greater than the pregnancy-specific reference range with positive TPO antibodies and TSH greater than 10 mIU/L with negative TPO antibodies, respectively), a dose of 50 µg levothyroxine/day is usually required (Alexander et al. 2017). Levothyroxine therapy may be also considered in pregnant women with TSH higher than 2.5 mIU/L and below the upper limit of the pregnancy-specific reference range with positive TPO antibodies and in women with TSH levels higher than the upper pregnancy-specific reference range and below 10 mIU/L with negative TPO antibodies (Alexander et al. 2017). T$_3$ or desiccated thyroid should not be used during pregnancy. Targeted TSH during pregnancy is in the lower half of the trimester-specific reference range (when this is not available <2.5 mIU/L). After delivery, LT$_4$ should be reduced to the preconception dose and TSH assessed in about 6 weeks (Alexander et al. 2017).

30.9.1.3 Central Hypothyroidism

The target FT$_4$ should be in the upper half of the normal range for young patients and in the lower half of reference range in older patients.

30.9.2 Monitoring

Serum TSH and FT$_4$: The target TSH in young hypothyroid patients should be 1–2.5 mIU/L (Biondi and Wartofsky 2014)

- 8 weeks after starting levothyroxine
- Every 4–8 weeks after levothyroxine dose adjustment/drug changes (manufacturer)
- Every 6–12 months after establishing the correct dose

Thyroid ultrasound: Recommended annually
ECG, Doppler echocardiography monthly in patients with ischemic heart disease, arrhythmias, and pericardial effusion (Biondi and Wartofsky 2014).

30.9.3 Potential Side Effects of Treatment

Overtreated patients (with suppressed TSH, especially those with TSH < 0.1 mIU/L) are frequent in up to 30–50%. The risks associated with over-treatment include:

- Tachycardia, arrhythmias (atrial fibrillation), increased left ventricular mass, diastolic dysfunction, heart failure
- Loss of bone mass (osteoporosis) and fractures (especially postmenopausal women), and therefore, thyroid hormone excess should be avoided, especially in elderly people and postmenopausal women (Biondi and Wartofsky 2014).

30.9.4 Dose Adjustments

Persistent increased TSH despite levothyroxine treatment should be further investigated. Possible causes are:

- Incorrect LT_4 dose/administration
- Poor patients compliance; for differential diagnosis between poor patient compliance and malabsorption, 1000 µg LT_4 (weekly dose: 1.6 × body weight (kg) × 7) are administered fasting, in the morning, in liquid or tablet form; FT_4 is measured 0, 30, 45, 60 min, 2, 4, 6 h after ingestion; FT_4 above 25 pmol/L or an increment of 20 pmol/L for FT_4 at 2 h suggest poor compliance (Ain et al. 1991).
- Malabsorption (celiac disease, autoimmune gastritis, after gastrointestinal surgery, short

Table 30.3 Drugs interfering with levothyroxine absorption and metabolism (Ross and Cooper 2017; Wiersinga 2014)

Mechanism	Drug
Decrease levothyroxine (LT_4) absorption	Cholestyramine, Colestipol
	Sucralfate
	Aluminum hydroxide
	Ferrous sulfate
	Antiacids, sucralfate, proton pump inhibitors, H2 receptor antagonists
	Laxatives
	Calcium carbonate (allow at least 3–4 h between LT_4 and calcium tablets)
	Food: Soy protein supplements, coffee, grapefruit juice, dietary fibers
Increase metabolic (nondeiodinative) levothyroxine clearance	Rifampicin
	Carbamazepine, Phenobarbital
	± Phenytoin
Block T_4 to T_3 conversion	Amiodarone
	Glucocorticoids
	β blockers
	Selenium deficiency
Increased need for levothyroxine	Estrogens
Precise mechanism unknown	Sertraline, Chloroquine
	Tyrosine kinase inhibitors: Imatinib, Motesanib, Sorafenib

bowel syndrome, lactose intolerance, Helicobacter Pylori infection, cirrhosis, pancreatic diseases)
- Drugs or food that interfere with levothyroxine absorption or thyroid axis (Table 30.3).

30.9.5 Association with Other Comorbidities (for Example: Ischemic Heart Disease)

- Elderly people with or without evidence of cardiac disease: it is advisable to start with low doses, because full-dose levothyroxine replacement is associated with angina, myocardial infarction, and arrhythmias.
- Elderly people (>50–60 years) without evidence of cardiac disease: the starting dose is

usually 25–50 µg/day, increasing the dose with 25–50 µg/day every 3–4 weeks
- Elderly patients over the age of 60 years: the starting dose is lower: 12.5–25 µg/day, increasing the dose with 12.5–25 µg/day every 3–4 weeks
- Patients with ischemic heart disease: the starting dose: 12.5 µg/day, increasing the dose with 12.5 µg/day every 3–4 weeks; in severe ischemic heart disease, increasing dose with 12.5 µg/day every 4–6 weeks
- Coronary revascularization can be necessary in some cases to tolerate levothyroxine treatment (Biondi and Wartofsky 2014).

30.10 Conclusions

Hypothyroidism is one of the most frequent thyroid disorders, of which primary hypothyroidism prevails over secondary hypothyroidism. The causes of primary hypothyroidism include chronic autoimmune thyroiditis (Hashimoto), subacute, silent and postpartum thyroiditis, cytokine-induced thyroiditis, iodine deficiency or iodine overload, drugs-induced hypothyroidism, infiltrative disorders of the thyroid, defects in thyroid hormones synthesis, thyroidectomy, radioiodine ablation, external beam radiation therapy for malignant tumors of head and neck, congenital thyroid agenesis, or dysgenesis.

Central (secondary and tertiary) hypothyoidism is caused by acquired or congenital hypopituitarism, pituitary apoplexy (Sheehan's syndrome), traumatic, genetic, lymphocytic hypophysitis, infectious disorders (tuberculosis), metastases, isolated TSH deficiency, treatment with somatostatin analogues, and hypothalamic disorders. Causes of peripheral hypothyroidism are rare (mutations in gene encoding TR β, TR α—thyroid hormone resistance, MCT8, SECISBP2, massive infantile hemangioma). The screening tools are serum TSH and freeT4. An increased TSH and low FT4 are found in primary overt hypothyroidism. Increased TSH and normal FT4 are found in primary subclinical hypothyroidism. Low-normal/low FT4 with low/inappropriately normal/slightly increased TSH are found in cen-

tral hypothyroidism. Complementary abnormal tests can include mixed dyslipidemia, anemia, hyponatremia, increased creatine phosphokinase (CK) or other muscle and liver enzymes, hyperprolactinemia, ECG (sinus bradycardia, low-voltage QRS complexes, etc.), and chest X rays (cardiomegaly, pericardial, and/or pleural effusion).

The treatment for hypothyroidism is Levothyroxine and is prescribed as monotherapy, orally, once daily (usually in the morning, 30–60 min before breakfast). The dose of levothyroxine in young and middle-age patients for replacement therapy in primary hypothyroidism is 1.6–1.8 mg/kg/day, with lower requirements (1.3 mg/kg/day) in central hypothyroidism and higher doses in pregnancy.

References

Ain KB, Refetoff S, Fein HG, et al. Pseudomalabsorption of levothyroxine. JAMA. 1991;266:2118–20.
Alexander EK, Pearce N, Brent GA, et al. Guidelines of the American Thyroid Association for the Diagnosis and Management of thyroid disease during pregnancy and the postpartum. Thyroid. 2017;27(3):315–89.
Association of Clinical Biochemistry, British Thyroid Association and British Thyroid Foundation. UK guidelines for the use of thyroid function tests. 2006. www.british-thyroid-association.org.
Biondi B, Cooper DS. The clinical significance of subclinical thyroid dysfunction. Endocr Rev. 2008;29(1):76–131.
Biondi B, Wartofsky L. Treatment with thyroid hormone. Endocr Rev. 2014;35(3):433–512. https://doi.org/10.1210/er.2013-1083.
Bolk N, Visser TJ, Kalsbeek A, et al. Effects of evening vs morning thyroxine ingestion on serum thyroid hormone profiles in hypothyroid patients. Clin Endocrinol. 2007;66:43–8.
Brabant G, Beck-Peccoz P, Jarzab B, et al. Is there a need to redefine the upper normal limit of TSH? Eur J Endocrinol. 2006;154(5):633–7.
Chaudhary V, Bano S. Thyroid ultrasound. Indian J Endocrinol Metab. 2013;17(2):219–27. https://doi.org/10.4103/2230-8210.109667.
Cooper DS, Biondi B. Subclinical thyroid disease. Lancet. 2012;379(9821):1142–54. https://doi.org/10.1016/S0140-6736(11)60276-6.
Michalaki MA, Gkotsina MI, Mamali I, et al. Impaired pharmacokinetics of levothyroxine in severely obese volunteers. Thyroid. 2011;21(5):477–81. https://doi.org/10.1089/thy.2010.0149.

Negro R, Stagnaro-Green A. Diagnosis and management of subclinical hypothyroidism in pregnancy. BMJ. 2014;349:g4929. https://doi.org/10.1136/bmj.g4929.

Okosieme O, Gilbert J, Abraham P, et al. Management of primary hypothyroidism: statement by the British Thyroid Association Executive Committee. Clin Endocrinol. 2016;84(6):799–808. https://doi.org/10.1111/cen.12824.

Rodondi N, den Elzen WP, Bauer DC, et al. Subclinical hypothyroidism and the risk of coronary heart disease and mortality. JAMA. 2010;304(12):1365–74. https://doi.org/10.1001/jama.2010.1361.

Ross DS, Cooper DS. Hypothyroidism. UpToDate. 2017. http://www.uptodate.com.

Stagnaro-Green A, Abalovich M, Alexander E, et al. Guidelines of the American Thyroid Association for the diagnosis and management of thyroid disease during pregnancy and postpartum. Thyroid. 2011;21(10):1081–25. https://doi.org/10.1089/thy.2011.0087.

Surks MI, Hollowell JG. Age-specific distribution of serum thyrotropin and antithyroid antibodies in the U.S. population: implications for the prevalence of subclinical hypothyroidism. J Clin Endocrinol Metab. 2007;92(12):4575–82.

Teixeira PF, Reuters VS, Ferreira MM, et al. Treatment of subclinical hypothyroidism reduces atherogenic lipid levels in a placebo-controlled double-blind clinical trial. Horm Metab Res. 2008;40(1):50–5.

Tunbridge WMG, Evered DC, Hall R, et al. The spectrum of thyroid disease in the community: the Whickham survey. Clin Endocrinol. 1977;7:481–93.

Vanderpump MP. The epidemiology of thyroid disease. Br Med Bull. 2011;99:39–51. https://doi.org/10.1093/bmb/ldr030.

Vanderpump MPJ, Tunbridge WMG, French JM, et al. The incidence of thyroid disorders in the community; a twenty-year follow up of the Whickham survey. Clin Endocrinol. 1995;43:55–68.

Walsh JP, Bremner AP, Feddema P, et al. Thyrotropin and thyroid antibodies as predictors of hypothyroidism: a 13-year, longitudinal study of a community-based cohort using current immunoassay techniques. J Clin Endocrinol Metab. 2010;95(3):1095–104. https://doi.org/10.1210/jc.2009-1977.

Wiersinga WM. Adult hypothyroidism. Thyroid manager. 2014. http://www.thyroidmanager.org/chapter/adult-hypothyroidism.

Key Reading

1. Cooper DS, Biondi B. Subclinical thyroid disease. Lancet. 2012;379(9821):1142–54. https://doi.org/10.1016/S0140-6736(11)60276-6.
2. Ross DS, Cooper DS. Hypothyroidism. UpToDate. 2017. http://www.uptodate.com.
3. Wiersinga WM. Adult hypothyroidism. Thyroid manager. 2014. http://www.thyroidmanager.org/chapter/adult-hypothyroidism.
4. Association of Clinical Biochemistry, British Thyroid Association and British Thyroid Foundation. UK guidelines for the use of thyroid function tests. 2006. www.british-thyroid-association.org.
5. Okosieme O, Gilbert J, Abraham P, et al. Management of primary hypothyroidism: statement by the British Thyroid Association Executive Committee. Clin Endocrinol (Oxf). 2016;84(6):799–808. https://doi.org/10.1111/cen.12824.

Thyroid Eye Disease

31

Rebecca Ford and Violet Fazal-Sanderson

Contents

R. Ford
Bristol Eye Hospital, University Hospitals Bristol
NHS Foundation Trust, Bristol, UK
e-mail: Rebecca.ford@uhbristol.nhs.uk

V. Fazal-Sanderson (✉)
Department of Endocrinology, Centre for Diabetes
and Endocrinology, Royal Berkshire Hospital NHS
Foundation Trust, Reading, UK
e-mail: violet.sanderson@royalberkshire.nhs.uk;
Violetsanderson@royalberkshire.nhs.uk

© Springer Nature Switzerland AG 2019
S. Llahana et al. (eds.), *Advanced Practice in Endocrinology Nursing*,
https://doi.org/10.1007/978-3-319-99817-6_31

Abstract

Thyroid eye disease (TED) is an autoimmune condition usually associated with thyroid dysfunction and characterised by inflammatory and fibrotic changes in the periocular tissues. It is most commonly associated with hyperthyroidism, but patients with TED may also be hypothyroid or euthyroid, and it does not always present at the same time as the thyroid dysfunction. Patients may present with inflamed eyes, ocular surface discomfort, double vision, and proptosis and may even progress to optic nerve compression and visual loss.

Risk factors include smoking and radioiodine treatment. Early recognition is important since treatment in the active phase with steroids, immunomodulatory agents, and sometimes radiotherapy can prevent persistent disability and disfigurement. Once the disease is inactive, treatment is focused more on surgical rehabilitation, with orbital decompression, strabismus surgery, and lid surgery. Urgent orbital decompression may be needed if the optic nerve is compressed. People with TED may have significant psychological distress related to hormonal changes, vision problems, changing appearance, and medication side effects, and the psychological care of these patients is often neglected. Future developments may offer the possibility of earlier diagnosis, biologic treatments tailored to the disease to stop its activity, and effective less invasive surgical rehabilitation.

It is imperative that clinical practitioners are familiar with the clinical features of Graves' ophthalmopathy. Furthermore, the thyroid endocrine nurse must be equipped with the relevant knowledge and understanding of eye anatomy and how thyroid eye disease (TED) presents. In this way, any eye signs and symptoms can be identified early, and managed more effectively, potentially reversing GO if referred promptly to an 'endocrine' ophthalmologist who specialises in thyroid eye disease.

Keywords

Graves' ophthalmopathy · Eye anatomy
Signs and symptoms · Extraocular muscles
Proptosis · Management

Abbreviations

CD20 marker	CD20, a transmembrane protein expressed on the surface of pre-B and mature B lymphocytes
CN	Cranial nerve
CT	Computerised tomography
EUGOGO	European Group on Graves' Orbitopathy
FT3	Free total triiodothyronine
fT4	Free thyroid hormone or thyroxine
GP	General practitioner
IGF-IR inhibitor	Insulin-like growth factor-I receptor (inhibits targets of signaling pathways)
MDT	Multidisciplinary team
MRI	Magnetic resonance imaging
NOSPECS	Mnemonic often is used as a scoring system for severity of eye change
RAI	Radioactive iodine
STIR	Short Tau Inversion Recovery (used with MRI)

TED	Thyroid eye disease
TPO antibodies	Thyroid peroxidase antibodies
TSH receptor	Thyroid-stimulating hormone receptor
TSH	Thyroid stimulation hormone
UK	United Kingdom
USA	United States of America
VISA	vision, Inflammation, strabismus, and appearance

Key Terms

- **Proptosis or exophthalmos**: Forward protrusion of the eyeball that can result in failure of the upper and lower eyelids to fully oppose, for example, when patient is asked to close the eyelids the iris or sclera may be visible. This can cause risk of developing corneal ulceration.
- **Keratitis**: Inflammation or infection of the cornea, e.g. due to bacterial, viral, or fungal infection, or associated with autoimmune disease, and can result in blurred vision, eye pain, tearing, photosensitivity, red eyes, or eye discharge.
- **Gritty eyes**: Feeling of sand or grit in the eyes. Occurs in patients with hyperthyroidism as a result of corneal exposure or dry eyes.
- **Excessive tearing of eyes**: Results from impaired tear drainage or excess tear production. In TED, increased tear production can be due to conjunctival inflammation, corneal drying, or corneal exposure due to proptosis.
- **Conjunctiva injection and Chemosis**: Inflammation of the conjunctiva is known as conjunctival injection. It appears similar to the 'pink eye' caused by viral or bacterial infection of the conjunctiva (conjunctivitis). Chemosis is conjunctival oedema- fluid build-up between the inflamed conjunctival layer and the sclera, giving a puffy or gelatinous appearance.
- **Lid retraction**: Visible sclera above the iris when patient looks straight ahead and may be due to stimulation of the levator (lid-lifting) muscle by hyperthyroidism, or direct involvement of the muscle by TED.
- **Lid lag**: When the patient looks down, the eyelid movement lags behind that of the eye. This is a symptom of hyperthyroidism rather than of TED itself.

- **Diplopia**: Also known as double vision. In TED, this is usually 'binocular', i.e. it is due to the two eyes being misaligned and will disappear if one eye is covered. The two images seen may be horizontally or vertically separated, or both. Examination of eye movements is one key way of checking for significant thyroid eye disease.
- **Stare**: The eyes may appear to 'stare' in TED due to proptosis or due to lid retraction.
- **Periorbital oedema**: Puffy upper and lower eyelids and can occur in hypothyroidism myxoedema, but is more often a sign of TED.
- **Corneal ulceration**: Can occur in TED as a result of proptosis or lagophthalmos (incomplete closure of eye) causing exposure of the cornea. Ulcers appear as raw patches on the cornea, which may go densely white if infected. They are usually accompanied by symptoms of pain and red eye.
- **Pain**: Pain in TED may be due to corneal exposure or ulceration; the corneal nerves are very sensitive and corneal pain may be intense. TED patients may also experience a deep-seated orbital pain if there is raised pressure within the orbit, or pain on eye movements if eye muscles are inflamed.
- **Photophobia**: This is painful light sensitivity and usually occurs when the cornea is dry or damaged.

Key Points

- Thyroid eye disease can be bilateral and unilateral. It can occur before, during, or after thyroid dysfunction.
- Knowledge of eye anatomy is paramount to understanding how thyroid eye disease can spotted promptly and managed effectively.
- Smoking is a strong risk factor for TED.
- The active phase of TED lasts 18–24 months on average. Patients may experience red eyes, double vision, proptosis, and visual dysfunction.
- Radioiodine treatment may trigger TED in some patients.
- Stabilising thyroid function may help TED symptoms, but does not in itself treat the condition.

- Early referral to a specialist ophthalmologist enables early treatment and may prevent disabling and disfiguring eye changes. Treatment may involve steroids, radiotherapy, and immunomodulatory drugs.
- Once inactive, patients may need rehabilitative orbital decompression, strabismus, and/or lid surgery.

31.1 Introduction

31.1.1 Overview of the Eye Anatomy

To better understand thyroid eye disease, knowledge of eye anatomy (Fig. 31.1) and physiology is essential.

Structures of the Eye

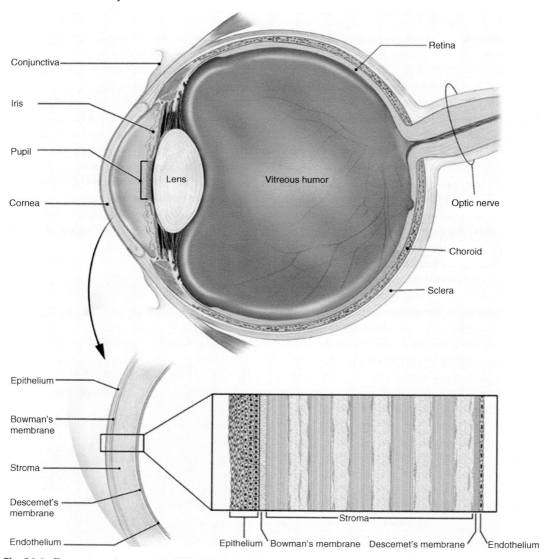

Fig. 31.1 Eye anatomy (accessed via NIH NEI, National Eye Institute, free Images Catalogue- https://nei.nih.gov/photo)

31.1.2 The main Structures of the Eye

Anterior and posterior chambers: The anterior chamber is located behind the cornea, and in front of the iris and lens. It contains clear fluid supplied by the cillary body and provides not only nutrition to local tissue, but also removes any metabolic waste.

The posterior chamber lies behind the iris and in front of the lens. This is filled with a clear gel called vitreous containing small fibres and water. Unlike aqueous fluid, vitreous gel has no consistent formation or drainage process.

Conjunctiva: This is a thin transparent protective membrane that covers the exposed part of the eye (protected by a film of tear fluid) and is continuous to line the under surface of the eye lid.

Cornea: A transparent slightly convex structure located at the anterior of the eye is the cornea. It refracts light as it enters the eye through the pupil. The light is further focussed by the lens as it passes through the vitreous gel, forming an inverted image onto the retina.

The cornea has no blood supply and is composed of three layers

1. The outer epithelial cell layer, continuous with the conjunctiva
2. The central fibrous layer called the stroma.
3. The inner endothelial cell layer, a membrane that lines the anterior chamber of the eye ball

Lens: A transparent biconcave disc located posteriorly to the pupil is the lens surrounded by the ciliary body. The lens helps to refract light passing through the eye to focus an image on the retina. It also changes shape (known as accommodation) to enable the eye to focus on near and distant objects.

Pupil: The circular hole within the iris muscle is the pupil. The size of the pupil depends on the amount of light entering the eyes, controlled by the pupillary muscles of the iris and supplied by the sympathetic and parasympathetic autonomic nervous activity running with the third cranial nerve.

Iris: The coloured part of the eye located in the anterior chamber immediately in front of the lens is the iris. It comprises a ring of muscle at the margins of the iris that controls the size of the pupil, for example, in the presence of bright light the muscles of the iris contract via parasympathetic activity, reducing the size of pupil, whist sympathetic activity in the presence of dim light causes the iris muscles to relax, enlarging the pupils.

Sclera: The outer layer of the eye is composed of tough white fibrous tissue called the sclera and is continuous with the cornea in front of the iris and the pupil.

Choroid: The middle layer of the eye comprises vascular tissue (a dark pigmentation) and is continuous with the ciliary body and the iris. It supplies nourishment to the retina.

Retina: This is located at the inner/ posterior aspect of eye. The retinal vessels have large paired veins and arteries that are usually brighter, red, and narrow compared to veins.

The inner surface retina contains a layer of photosensitive cells on the inner surface of the retina known as cones and rods.

1. **Cones**: There are three types that respond to different parts of the light spectrum and enable colour vision. Cone cells are packed close together in the fovea at the centre of the retina and are also responsible for fine visual detail.
2. **Rods**: these predominate in the peripheral retina enabling vision in dim light and detecting motion.

The images focussed onto the retina are detected by the photoreceptors that pass on information to layers of nerve cells that further process and relay this to the optic nerve and the brain.

Optic disc: this is composed of nerve fibres that converge to form the optic nerve.

The main characteristics of the optic disc

1. Creamy or pinkish in colour
2. Round or oval in shape
3. Sharp demarcated margins mainly at the temporal region
4. A small circular area inside the disc where blood vessels enter and exit giving a cup shape appearance via an ophthalmoscope

Macula and Fovea: the central area of the retina is the macula and fovea that contain cone cells responsible for colour vision and fine detail.

Vitreous humour: this comprises a clear gel that fills the area behind the lens and the retina.

Optic nerve: the optic nerve enters the eyeball posteriorly together with the retinal vessels. It transfers visual information from the retina to the visual area of the brain.

31.1.3 Extraocular Muscles

Six muscles are involved in eye movement and supplied by three different cranial nerves (CN) (Fig. 31.3):

- Superior rectus muscle: CN III (oculomotor)-elevates eye (looks up)
- Inferior oblique muscle: CN III- extorts (outwardly rotates) eye
- Lateral rectus muscle: CN VI (abducens)-abducts eye (moves it laterally)
- Medial rectus muscle: CN III- adducts eye (moves it medially)
- Inferior rectus muscle: CN III- depresses eye (looks down)
- Superior oblique muscle: CN IV (trochlear)-intorts (inwardly rotates) eye

31.2 What Is Thyroid Eye Disease?

Thyroid eye disease (TED) is an autoimmune condition affecting the tissues around the eyes, causing a spectrum of problems from dry, sore, puffy eyes to double vision, proptosis, and even visual loss. It usually occurs in patients with thyroid disorders, most commonly Graves' disease. It is usually self-limiting, but can lead to significant functional impairment, disfigurement, or even loss of vision in severe cases.

31.3 Aetiology of Thyroid Eye Disease

The pathogenesis of thyroid eye disease is far from fully understood. It is an autoimmune disease, and most patients will have detectable autoantibodies against thyroid antigens such as the

TSH receptor (typical in Graves' disease) or thyroid peroxidase at some stage in their disease process. Tests for these antibodies may be helpful in diagnosis of TED, especially in patients with unusual presentations or those without a known history of thyroid dysfunction. However, no single antibody test is diagnostic of the disease and the antibody levels do not correlate well with disease activity.

Autoimmune-activated T lymphocytes circulate into the orbit, where they cause inflammation, stimulate fibroblasts to proliferate and produce more glycosaminoglycans (inter-cellular matrix substances), and trigger adipocytes (fat cells) to mature. This stiffens and enlarges the extraocular muscles and expands the fat in the orbit, leading to congestion and proptosis (bulging eyes).

31.4 Risk Factors for Thyroid Eye Disease

31.4.1 Thyroid Dysfunction

Most people who develop thyroid eye disease have a history of Graves' disease (autoimmune hyperthyroidism), although it may occur in other conditions including Hashimoto's thyroiditis, thyroid cancer, and primary hypothyroidism. About 25% of people with Graves' disease experience some eye symptoms, but only around 2% develop sight-threatening disease. The eye disease does not necessarily start at the same time as the hyperthyroidism—while this is often the case, some patients will develop eye problems years before or after the thyroid disorder. TED disease activity is not directly proportional to thyroid function, which can be a difficult concept for patients and their clinicians to comprehend. While in general controlling the thyroid function is beneficial for eye symptoms, the eye disease may flare or remain active even after thyroid function normalises. Rapid swings from hyperthyroidism to hypothyroidism can risk worsening eye disease, and some treatments of hyperthyroidism carry more risk than others for the eye condition (see later).

31.4.2 Demographics and Genetics

Thyroid eye disease can occur at any age, but is most common in the fifth decade. It is very rare in children but has been reported, and in elderly people, it can take an insidious course with little apparent inflammation, making it challenging to diagnose.

Thyroid eye disease overall is about five times more common in females than males. However, this reflects the female preponderance of thyroid disorders, and when males are affected, they have a relatively higher chance of developing severe disease.

Risk factors for developing TED may be both genetic and environmental. There may be a familial tendency, but no individual genes have been identified as predisposing to TED. All races can be affected. Black Europeans and Americans may have an increased risk of TED, but this is probably not a purely genetic phenomenon; TED is rare in Africa and Korean studies show that while the prevalence of TED is relatively low in Korea, it increases in Koreans living in the USA. Hence, there appears to be an inter-play between genetic and environmental risk factors.

31.4.3 Environment

The most important environmental risk factor for TED is smoking—smokers are about five times more likely to develop TED than non-smokers and also tend to develop more severe disease and respond less well to medical treatment. We don't yet know which chemical(s) in cigarette smoke are responsible for this effect, but support with smoking cessation is critical for people with TED. It is unlikely that nicotine alone is the main driver of TED activity within cigarettes, so switching to nicotine replacement or 'e-cigarettes' is probably a viable option for patients trying to stop smoking after a diagnosis of TED.

Theories of autoimmunity suggest that exposure to pathogens may be a trigger for such disease, though no specific infectious trigger has been identified for TED. Stress also seems to be a risk factor, and research is ongoing into the role of diet and the microbiome in the condition.

31.5 Natural History of Thyroid Eye Disease

Thyroid eye disease has an active phase, in which periocular and orbital tissues are actively inflamed or changing, which on average lasts 18–24 months. Symptoms and signs typically get worse for 3–6 months, before plateauing. As activity reduces, the disease may improve somewhat until around 24 months, by which time some people's eyes will have returned to normal, but most will be left with some degree of residual discomfort, dysfunction, or altered appearance. This can be illustrated as 'Rundle's curve' (Fig. 31.2). Once the active inflammatory phase is over, the disease can be considered to be 'burned out'. The key significance of this is that anti-inflammatory treatment will only work during the active phase. We can use the 'burning house' analogy to explain this to patients and colleagues, i.e. interventions to 'put out the fire' (immunomodulatory treatments to suppress inflammation) will only work before 'the house has burned down' (the eye disease has become inactive and the damage is already done), by which time it is too late for such treatments to be effective. It is likely that the earlier in the disease the treatment is started, the less final burden of disability or disfigurement will result. Once the disease has become 'burned out', signs and symptoms should stabilize, and this is the stage when rehabilitative surgery may be safely considered.

The active phase may be longer in some patients than others; it is likely that factors such as smoking, uncontrolled or unstable thyroid function, and possibly stress can prolong the active phase.

31.6 Symptoms and Signs of Thyroid Eye Disease

It is important that clinical practitioners are familiar with the clinical features of Graves' ophthalmopathy (Fig. 31.3). Furthermore, it is advantageous for endocrine nurses to be equipped with the relevant knowledge and understanding of eye

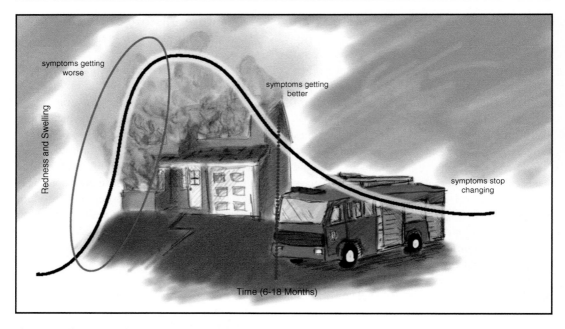

Fig. 31.2 Rundle's curve and the 'burning house' analogy. (Courtesy of Dan Morris, TEDct Newsletter, Spring 2010 edition, Pages 13–16)

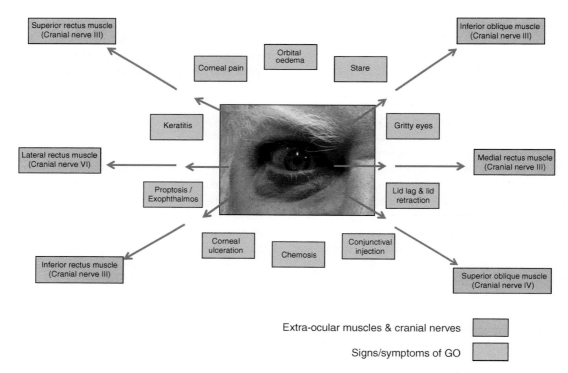

Fig. 31.3 Photo illustration of Graves' Ophthalmopathy and eye muscles at risk. Eye picture provided by Dr. R. Ford from private collection, Illustration by Violet Fazal-Sanderson

anatomy and how thyroid eye disease (TED) presents. Spotting eye signs and symptoms early enables prompt referral to an ophthalmologist who specialises in thyroid eye disease so that early treatment can help prevent the development of distressing or disabling eye problems.

Symptoms and signs of thyroid eye disease can occur in almost any order, and it is worth remembering that one eye may be affected first or more severely than the other, and up to 10% of patients may only ever develop thyroid eye disease in one eye. Those with unilateral signs need early investigation such as scans to ensure that they do not have a serious alternate diagnosis such as an orbital tumour.

31.6.1 Ocular Surface Signs and Symptoms

- **Red eyes**: this can be the earliest sign of active thyroid eye disease, and early disease is often mistaken for conjunctivitis. This is why it is especially important for endocrinologists and endocrine nurse specialists to be aware of TED, since early referral of thyroid patients with eye symptoms to an ophthalmologist can facilitate early diagnosis and treatment, potentially reducing the burden of disease on the patients. Redness in more than one quadrant and redness in the upper quadrant (under the eyelid) are particularly significant as signs of active disease.
- **Dry, sore eyes or watery eyes**: Any can occur or two of these symptoms may alternate or coexist.
- **Chemosis**: This may develop which is oedema beneath the conjunctiva leading to a puffy, jelly-like look to the white of the eye. The caruncle (the pink fleshy part at the inner corner of the eye) may become inflamed, redder, and enlarged.

31.6.2 Eyelid Signs and Symptoms

- **Red and puffy eyelids**: This often occurs in active disease. The redness should resolve with reduced disease activity, but expansion of

tissue matrix can lead to permanently swollen or thickened-looking lids even once the disease has burned out.
- **Upper lid retraction**: This is usually due to overstimulation of the sympathetic nervous system when people are hyperthyroid ('fight-or-flight' type stimulation), but is often due to involvement of the levator palpebrae (eyelid-lifting) muscle in the disease process. This gives the eyes a 'starey' appearance, and patients may be unable to close their eyes (lagophthalmos), leading to sore red eyes and even reduced vision from corneal exposure.

31.6.3 Ocular Motility Signs and Symptoms

- **Double vision**: or diplopia in TED occurs as a result of the impairment of the movements of the extraocular muscles, which can become stiffened or restricted in movement.
- **Painful eye movements**: Eye movements may be painful or feel strained. Scans of the orbit often show enlarged extraocular muscles in TED. Any muscle can be affected, but the inferior rectus and medial rectus are often first to become involved, and restriction of upgaze is common in TED as fibrosis of the inferior rectus tethers the eye down when the affected individual tries to look up. However, virtually any pattern of eye movement abnormality can result from TED. Strabismus surgery may help those with underlying diplopia, though this should not be attempted until the orthoptic measurements (size and type of squint) are stable for 6 months. Those with highly variable orthoptic measurements should be tested for myasthenia gravis, an autoimmune condition of the neuro-muscular junction that may be present in up to 5% of those with TED.

31.6.4 Orbital Signs and Symptoms

- **Eyes bulging forwards**: forwards bulging of the eyes (proptosis) is a common finding in TED and occurs due to the increased volume of tissues inside the orbit. The orbit is contained within solid bony walls, so the only direction in which tissues can move in response to pressure of expanded orbital contents is forwards. Proptosis can be measured with a device called an exophthalmometer.

- **Orbital pressure**: Tissue expansion can also lead to increased pressure within the orbit, causing pain and aching sensations often felt behind the eyes. The intraocular pressure can go up and a minority of patients can develop glaucoma if untreated.

31.6.5 Visual Dysfunction in Thyroid Eye Disease

The vision may be adversely affected in a number of ways in TED.

- **Blurring**: Intermittent blurring is usually caused by ocular surface problems from tear film insufficiency
- **Diplopia**: this can make focusing difficult.
- Proptosis and lid retraction can lead to lagophthalmos and corneal exposure, which can cause serious breakdown of the cornea with ulcers and infections that may need urgent treatment.
- **Optic nerve compression**: Pressure on the optic nerve is perhaps most serious, though fortunately rare, where the pressure within the orbit can become high enough to compress the optic nerve and its vasculature, leading to potentially irreversible visual loss if not treated urgently. Optic nerve involvement (dysthyroid optic neuropathy) may start with subtle signs such as reduced colour vision or red desaturation (red colours looking 'washed out'), so colour vision is typically tested at every eye clinic visit for thyroid eye disease patients. The pupils are also examined for a relative afferent pupillary defect and the optic disc examined for papilloedema. If you suspect dysthyroid optic neuropathy, contact an orbital specialist urgently since early treatment can save vision.

31.7 Grading Thyroid Eye Disease

There are several grading systems in current usage to assess disease activity and severity in TED. The most commonly used grading of disease activity in Europe is the Clinical Activity Score based on that of Mourits, as standardised by the European Group on Graves' Ophthalmopathy (EUGOGO) (Table 31.1).

Other scores in common use include the 'VISA' score, an activity score common in the USA, and the 'NOSPECS' grading, which assesses disease severity rather than activity.

31.8 Investigation of Thyroid Eye Disease

There is no single investigation to diagnose or monitor thyroid eye disease, and the diagnosis is often made clinically; however, the following may be included:

- **An MRI or CT scan**: of the orbits help to confirm the diagnosis by looking at the shape and size of the extraocular muscles. MRI, especially the 'STIR' sequence protocol, examines soft tissue in detail and can help to assess disease activity by revealing the water content of the muscles. CT scans assess the bone structure of the orbit and are useful in

Table 31.1 EUGOGO clinical activity score

Score 1 for each of these 10 findings	
1	Spontaneous orbital pain
2	Gaze-evoked orbital pain
3	Eyelid swelling considered to be due to active TED
4	Eyelid erythema
5	Conjunctival redness considered to be due to active TED
6	Chemosis
7	Inflammation of caruncle OR plica
8	Increase of >2 mm in proptosis
9	Decrease in uniocular ocular excursion in any one direction of >8°
10	Decrease of acuity equivalent to 1 Snellen line or more

NB: Points 1–7 can be measured at the first visit to produce an initial score out of 7; at follow-up visits, all elements can be measured to give a score out of 10

planning bony orbital decompression surgery.

- **Blood tests** such as TSH, T4, and T3 are reviewed in conjunction with the endocrinologists to monitor thyroid function.
- **Auto-antibodies** such as anti-TSH receptor and anti-TPO antibodies can help to reach a diagnosis, and some clinicians believe these may help to monitor disease progress.
- **Other blood** tests may be needed as part of planning and monitoring of immunosuppressive therapy.
- **Orthoptic testing** is essential to assess and objectively monitor ocular motility. Hess charts and field of binocular single vision testing help to quantify eye movements and diplopia.
- **Electro diagnostic tests**: visual-evoked potentials that measure conduction in the optic nerve may sometimes be useful in defining whether visual problems in TED are due to dysthyroid optic neuropathy.

31.9 Treatment of Thyroid Eye Disease

31.9.1 Early and Supportive Treatment

Smoking cessation and thyroid function: Early in the disease process, supportive treatment must include smoking cessation advice and efforts to stabilize thyroid function.

Eye lubricants: Many patients have ocular surface problems and may benefit greatly from provision of tear supplement drops, and those with nocturnal lagophthalmos will benefit particularly from thicker ointment-type lubricants at night. Some will find cold compresses helpful, and raising the head of the bed may reduce the build up of oedema overnight if puffy eyes are problematic on waking.

Selenium: There has recently been some investigation of selenium supplementation for thyroid eye disease. Some studies suggest that thyroid eye disease is more common in those with a relative deficiency of the mineral sele-

nium, and that selenium at a dose of 100 mcg bd may help prevent early disease becoming more severe. Therefore, in the absence of contraindications, patients with early thyroid eye disease may wish to take selenium supplements for 6 months; the level of evidence that this helps is relatively low, but it is unlikely to cause any harm and so many patients and doctors consider it worth trying. Selenium is also present in nuts such as Brazil nuts for those who would prefer to avoid more pills, though this would provide a less consistent dose.

Dark glasses: Patients with photophobia (light sensitivity) may find that dark glasses help, and glasses in general may keep wind out of the eyes and reduce tearing.

Fresnel prisms: For those with double vision, particularly if it affects straight ahead gaze, it may be possible for an orthoptist to fit Fresnel prisms to a pair of spectacles. These stick-on prisms refract the light to compensate for misalignment between the two eyes.

31.9.2 Management of Hyperthyroidism

The therapy chosen to control the hyperthyroidism may have some impact on TED. Firstly, **Normalising thyroid function**: It is important to normalize thyroid function without causing a rapid dip into hypothyroidism. This has led many endocrinologists with an interest in TED to recommend 'block and replace' regimens for Graves with TED; an anti-thyroid drug such as carbimazole is used in a high enough dose to 'block' all the patient's thyroid hormone production, with levothyroxine prescribed alongside from the start to avoid hypothyroidism.

Radioiodine restriction in TED: Radioactive iodine (RAI) therapy can trigger the development or worsening of thyroid eye disease. Around 20% of those treated with RAI develop worsening eye problems compared to 5% of those treated with anti-thyroid drugs, and 7% of those treated with RAI develop severe TED. These figures seem to be higher in smokers. A course of concurrent oral prednisolone started at the time of the RAI much reduces this risk, so a sensible precaution would be to give oral steroid cover for RAI in patients with mild eye signs and consider it in smokers, and to try to avoid RAI wherever possible in those with active or severe eye disease.

Thyroidectomy does not appear to affect thyroid eye disease much, although there is some relatively low-grade evidence that it may be beneficial in controlling TED provided patients are not allowed to become hypothyroid.

31.9.3 Medical Treatment

Medical treatment for thyroid eye disease is based on the strategies of reducing inflammation and suppressing the immune system to treat the underlying autoimmune condition. Many different drugs and regimes have been tried, and thyroid eye disease specialists are far from reaching agreement about the ideal therapy. Patients also have different comorbidities, disease patterns, and needs, so treatments must be selected on an individual basis.

31.9.3.1   Steroid Treatment
Steroid treatment is currently a mainstay of treatment in the active phase. There is some evidence that intravenous therapy is at least as effective as oral, while producing fewer serious side effects. All steroid treatments carry the following risk and require monitoring:

- blood sugar
- hypertension
- gastric ulceration
- mood disturbance
- weight gain
- induction of diabetes
- osteoporosis

Most clinicians aim to keep steroid treatment duration short for TED so that the risks are minimised. A typical protocol would be that recommended by EUGOGO, suggested for patients with active disease and no contraindications to steroid treatments, having a Clinical

Activity Score of 4 or more. This regimen is as follows:

- *500 mg intravenous methylprednisolone* given once weekly for 6 weeks, followed by, *250 mg weekly for a further 6 weeks.*

This may be enough to render the disease inactive in some cases, but bearing in mind that the active phase of the disease may last around 24 months, further therapy is often needed.

31.9.3.2   Immunomodulatory Agents
These can be used to supplement or replace steroid treatment. These drugs work by suppressing the immune system, and hence, the autoimmune activity of the disease. All of these drugs have potential side effects, including increased susceptibility to some infections. However, with proper monitoring they can be safer and more effective in longer term control of inflammation and progress of TED than steroids. No single drug is totally effective for TED, and research studies are ongoing to try to establish which drugs are more effective and how they should be combined with other treatments. Drugs in current use include azathioprine, mycophenolate, ciclosporin, and methotrexate. They would generally be used only for those with more severe or active disease and are continued for a year to 18 months in most cases if tolerated. Active monitoring with blood tests is essential.

31.9.3.3   Orbital Radiotherapy
Orbital radiotherapy has been in use for TED for decades and seems to improve inflammation in some cases. It is not highly effective and is rarely used alone, but usually as a supplementary treatment with steroids or other agents. There is some evidence, though relatively weak, that it may be more effective in patients with extraocular muscle involvement. If radiotherapy is used for TED, it is usually fractionated over 10 days of treatment. Patients should expect to have an initial assessment and fitting for a mask that protects the face outside the treatment area. The treatments

themselves are very short. Side effects are usually minimal, but for some people the inflammatory signs may become temporarily worse before improving, and patients should be warned that there is a theoretical increased risk of tumours in the treated tissues in future (though this has never been demonstrated in reality in patients having the relatively low-dose radiotherapy used for TED).

31.9.3.4 New Drugs in the 'Biologic' Group Are Under Investigation in TED

Biologics are monoclonal antibodies directed against substances involved in the disease to be treated. The most prevalent biologic to be tried in TED so far has been rituximab, which is directed against the CD20 marker on lymphocytes and was originally developed for lymphoma. Use of rituximab results in a long period of B-cell depletion and immunosuppression and knock-on effects on T cell activity, which may be effective for TED if given early enough in the active phase, although studies with this agent have provided conflicting results. TED is not a common enough disease to attract large investment in research funding, so biologic therapies trialled for TED have usually been developed to treat other conditions such as arthritis rather than being designed for TED. There are a few other drugs under investigation, including teprotumumab, an IGF-IR inhibitor, which is showing promise in early studies, though none of these drugs are available in general usage yet.

31.9.4 Surgical Treatment

Surgery for TED can be broadly categorised into orbital decompression, strabismus surgery, and lid surgery. Many patients do not need any surgery, especially if treated early with appropriate medical treatment, but for those left with functional or appearance-related problems once the disease has become inactive, surgery can be a critical part of rehabilitation. Urgent orbital decompression surgery may also be needed to treat dysthyroid optic neuropathy (optic nerve compression).

One surgery can affect the next by affecting the position, pressure, or blood supply to tissues. Hence, the order of surgery is important—any orbital decompression needed should be done first, then strabismus then lid surgery, although many patients do not need all three of these steps. Some researchers are looking into whether it is possible to combine some of these steps.

Orbital Decompression Surgery: This is usually performed to correct proptosis (bulging eyes), but may also be indicated for optic nerve compression or sometimes for other symptoms of raised pressure within the orbit. Other than emergency cases, most surgeons will not recommend this operation until the disease process is inactive. In some cases, orbital congestion and persistently raised intraorbital pressure can mimic active disease (this may be termed 'hydraulic' or 'congestive' disease) and decompression may also help. The surgery aims to make more room for the important orbital structures, either by removing fat to decrease the volume of the orbital contents, or by removing bone from the walls of the orbits to make more space for the tissues, or a combination of the two. The more walls of the orbit that are removed or reduced, the more proptosis is corrected. The exact choice of surgery will depend on the patient's individual situation. Orbital decompression carries a small risk to the vision, as well as a chance of worsening double vision and numbness beneath the eye area if the orbital floor is to be removed. Most patients will stay in hospital overnight and need at least 2 weeks off work.

Strabismus (squint) surgery: is performed for double vision. Eye movement muscles are detached from the sclera of the eyeball and their position is adjusted to change the alignment of the eye. This is usually done under general anaesthetic, but most patients can go home the same day. It is usually safe surgery, with minimal risk to vision, but it is not always possible to correct all double vision in thyroid eye disease and most squint surgery is performed for those who have double vision all the time in straight ahead gaze.

Eyelid surgery: may be done to reduce swelling or excess tissue once the disease is inactive (blepharoplasty). It may also be necessary to surgically lower eyelids that have become retracted. These procedures are often done under local anaesthetic, partly so that the surgeon can check the height and appearance of the lid as the patient looks around with eyes open. They are not always successful, and some patients who have lid lowering will develop an overcorrection (ptosis or drooping of the lid) at some stage and require further surgery, but for many patients this is the final step in achieving a more normal appearance. It is important not to raise expectations too highly, as most patients with TED severe enough to require surgery will not end up looking the same as they did before the disease hit, but the aim is to achieve an acceptable appearance without obvious signs of the disease process. For UK patients in some areas, at the time of writing, lid procedures may unfortunately not be routinely funded on the NHS.

31.10 Multidisciplinary Management of TED

People with thyroid eye disease are often under the care of multiple clinicians, such as an endocrinologist, an oculoplastic surgeon, a GP, and sometimes a thyroid surgeon, an orthoptist, a strabismus specialist, and possibly a radiotherapist (for orbital radiotherapy). Input from scans may be needed from a radiologist, and some centres may have nurse specialists in various roles. It is important that all these professionals work well together, communicate well, and provide consistent information and planning for patients to prevent confusion or conflict. Evidence is growing that working in multidisciplinary teams, such as those based around joint endocrine-oculoplastic clinics, leads to better patient outcomes. Other clinicians should have a low threshold for referral of patients with signs of TED to a specialist MDT clinic, as these are now available in larger centres in most of the UK. The Endocrine Nurse plays a key role as delineated in Box 31.1 below.

Box 31.1 Nursing Recommendations for Graves' Ophthalmopathy Prior to an Ophthalmology Referral

Explanation
- Complications of eye disease
- Importance of ophthalmology referral
- Early referral for effective management of GO

Aim to stabilise thyroid function (TSH, fT4, and fT3)
- In patient with Graves' hyperthyroidism: anti-thyroid medication such as CBZ or equivalent is usually effective; eye disease is a relative contraindication to radioiodine treatment.

Gritty eye and proptosis
- Lubricant eye drops (as per local hospital policy) are useful. Hypromellose is cheap and available over the counter; it may be sufficient for mild to moderate cases. Preservative-free lubricants such as hyaluronate preparations are preferred by many patients and ophthalmologists.
- Sufficient fluids in severely hyperthyroid patients: Frequency of bowel movement and excessive flushing can cause dehydration and thus contribute to dry eyes.
- Dark glasses (sunglasses): Patients with proptosis and corneal dryness may be affected by photophobia.
- Night-time eye ointment according to local hospital policy to prevent corneal exposure
- Cold compresses and raising the head of the bed can help reduce the build up of oedema overnight if puffy eyes are problematic on waking.

Smokers to abstain from smoking

- Smokers have an increased risk for developing TED, and the disease tends to be more severe in those who smoke.
- Leaflets that explain the relevance of *STOPPING SMOKING* should be available to smokers.
- Nicotine patches and referral to smoking cessation services may be an option as per local hospital policy guidelines.

Once referred to the ophthalmologist, a formal assessment will determine the severity of GO. Treatment is aimed at protecting the cornea and relieving symptoms such as photophobia and diplopia in those with active TED (BTA 2015; BTA 2006; NICE 2016).

31.11 Psychological Aspects of Thyroid Eye Disease

A large proportion of people with thyroid eye disease will suffer with psychological distress related to the disease. This is a chronic condition, and many patients will have emotional and psychological symptoms related to hyperthyroidism or fluctuating thyroid hormone levels as they start treatment. They then have to contend with changes in eye and facial appearance that may have far-reaching effects on their self-image, confidence, and relationships with others. Added to this, treatments may have significant side effects, such as steroids causing mood swings, sleep disturbance, and weight loss. Patients may also have functional concerns, such as diplopia or blurred vision affecting driving and reading, which can be enough to stop some people from working and hence contribute to financial worries. Patients with thyroid eye disease, therefore, need attention to their psychological well-being. This is not always easy in a busy clinic setting, but nurse specialists may be particularly well-placed to gently enquire about how a person is coping with their TED. For some patients, it may be enough just to reassure them that their feelings are normal and shared by many others going through the trials of TED. People who placed a high value on their personal appearance before their illness are most at risk from psychological distress related to changes in appearance, and those whose work is affected (either by visual problems or by loss of confidence in facing other people) are another high-risk group. External help may be available for those who are worst affected, such as referral to a psychologist, and others may find benefit from things like patient support groups and meetings, online fora, and online information such as that from Thyroid Eye Disease Charitable Trust (http://www.tedct.org.uk).

31.12 The Future of Thyroid Eye Disease

Research in TED is progressing in a number of areas. The ultimate goal would be to identify the causes and triggers for TED and try to prevent its occurrence. Until that is possible, important areas for development include improving early diagnosis and specialist referral for TED, to allow all patients access to appropriate treatment as soon as possible. This may be achieved by simple methods like education of endocrinologists, general practitioners, and optometrists in how to spot early TED, development of more specialist clinics, and possibly more sophisticated methods like improved diagnostic testing enabling us to predict which patients may become severely affected. Medical therapy is improving all the time, and the aim is to find one or more drugs, possibly from the new biologics category, that can stop TED in its tracks, preventing disease progression and need for surgical interventions. For those whose disease has already left them with problems, improvements in surgical techniques are gradually making the reconstructive surgery safer and less invasive.

31.13 Conclusions

Thyroid eye disease is a complex condition, for which patients require both expert medical care and plenty of psychological and emotional support. Endocrine nurse specialists with a knowledge of thyroid eye disease can be instrumental in spotting the condition early and promoting early specialist referral, as well as being important in long-term care of patients by supplying accurate clinical information and advice, smoking cessation advice, facilitating medical treatment, and providing psychological support.

References

British Thyroid Association (BTA). UK guidelines for the use of thyroid function tests: thyrotoxicosis (online). BTA. 2006. http://www.british-thyroid-association.org/sandbox/bta2016/uk_guidelines_for_the_use_of_thyroid_function_tests.pdf. Accessed 22 Apr 2018.

British Thyroid Foundation. Thyroid eye disease (online). BTF. 2015. http://www.btf-thyroid.org/information/leaflets/36-thyroid-eye-disease-guide. Accessed 22 Apr 2018.

Hogan-Quigley B, Palm ML, Bickley L. Bates' Nursing guide to Physical Examination and History taking. London: Wolters Kluwer Health/Lippincott Williams & Wilkins; 2012.

Khong JJ, McNab AA, Ebeling PR, et al. Pathogenesis of thyroid eye disease: review and update on molecular mechanisms. Br J Ophthalmol. 2016;100:142–50.

National Institute for Health and Care Excellence (NICE). Hyperthyroidism (online). NICE. 2016. https://cks.nice.org.uk/hyperthyroidism#!management. Accessed 22 Apr 2018.

Perros P, Dayan CM, Dickinson AJ, et al. Management of patients with Graves' orbitopathy: initial assessment, management outside specialised centres and referral pathways. Clin Med. 2015;15(2):173–8. https://doi.org/10.7861/clinmedicine.15-2-173.

Perros P, Hegedus L, Bartelena L, Weirsinga WM, et al. Graves' orbitopathy as a rare disease in Europe: a European Group on Graves' Orbitopathy (EUGOGO) position statement. Orphanet J Rare Dis. 2017;12:72. https://doi.org/10.1186/s13023-017-0625-1.

Thyroid Eye Disease Charitable Trust. An introduction to thyroid eye disease (online). TEDct. 2017. http://tedct.org.uk/thyroid-eye-disease. Accessed 22 Aug 2017.

Verity D, Rose GE. Acute thyroid eye disease (TED): principles of medical and surgical management. Eye. 2013;27:308–19.

Weiler DL. Thyroid eye disease: a review. Clin Exp Optom. 2017;100:20–5. https://doi.org/10.1111/cxo.12472.

Wiersinga WM. Graves' ophthalmopathy and dermopathy-3.3.10. In: JAH W, Stewart PM, Amiel SA, Davies MJ, editors. Oxford textbook of endocrinology and diabetes. Oxford: Oxford University Press; 2011.

Key Reading

1. Verity DH, Rose GE. Acute thyroid eye disease (TED): Principles of medical and surgical management. Eye. 2013;27:308–19.
2. Bartelena L, Baldeschi L, et al. on behalf of EUGOGO: The 2016 European Thyroid Association/European Group on Graves' Orbitopathy Guidelines for the Management of Graves' Orbitopathy. Eur Thyroid J. 2016;5:9–26.

Disorders of the Thyroid in Childhood and Adolescence

32

Suma Uday, Christine Davies, and Helena Gleeson

Contents

S. Uday
Birmingham Women's and Children's Hospital NHS
Foundation Trust, Birmingham, UK
e-mail: suma.uday@nhs.net

C. Davies (✉)
Department of Advanced and Integrated Practice,
Children's Hospital for Wales, Cardiff and Vale UHB
University Hospital of Wales (UHW), Cardiff, UK
e-mail: Christine.Davies8@wales.nhs.uk

H. Gleeson
Department of Endocrinology, University Hospitals
Birmingham NHS Foundation Trust,
Birmingham, UK
e-mail: Helena.Gleeson@uhb.nhs.uk

Abstract

Disorders of the thyroid are one of the most common endocrinopathies in childhood and adolescence. The thyroid hormone is not only essential for metabolism and organ function but also plays a key role in the regulation of myelination of the nervous system. It is therefore crucial for normal growth and development in children. Thyroid hormone release is regulated by the hypothalamus and the pituitary gland. Therefore problems in thyroid hormones can occur as a result of disruption in the hypothalamo-pituitary-thyroid axis at any level.

Problems with the thyroid axis usually manifest as an underactive (hypothyroidism) or an overactive (hyperthyroidism) gland. The

© Springer Nature Switzerland AG 2019
S. Llahana et al. (eds.), *Advanced Practice in Endocrinology Nursing*,
https://doi.org/10.1007/978-3-319-99817-6_32

most common cause of an underactive thyroid in children is congenital hypothyroidism (CHT) followed by autoimmune hypothyroidism or Hashimoto's thyroiditis (HT), the incidence of which peaks in adolescence. Introduction of the newborn screening test for CHT has facilitated early diagnosis and treatment of CHT improving outcome related to intellectual disability. Other rare causes of hypothyroidism include TSH deficiency in cases of secondary hypothyroidism which can be part of multiple pituitary hormone deficiency or rarely isolated. Hypothyroidism can also occur following surgical removal of the gland for Graves' disease or damage following radiotherapy for cancer treatment.

The most common cause of hyperthyroidism is Graves' disease which is treated with anti-thyroid drugs (ATDs) in a block and replace or dose titration regimen. The right approach is heavily debated in the medical field. ATD treatment is followed by definitive treatment with surgery or radioactive iodine if the patient relapses after stopping ATD. Another rare but serious cause of hyperthyroidism which carries a significant mortality rate if undiagnosed is neonatal thyrotoxicosis (NT). NT occurs in babies born to mothers with Graves' disease or HT. This is a transient condition which may require treatment with ATDs. Hyperthyroidism can result from thyroid nodules such as toxic adenoma or multinodular goitre or rarely following radiotherapy and in McCune Albright syndrome.

Thyroid nodules can present as underactive or overactive thyroid but most frequently are not associated with thyroid dysfunction. Careful evaluation of nodules is critical due to the higher risk of these being cancerous in children compared with adults. Thyroid cancers can occur independently or as part of multiple endocrine neoplasias or familial neoplasias. Papillary thyroid carcinoma is the most common form of paediatric thyroid cancer. Other rare forms include follicular thyroid carcinoma and medullary thyroid carcinoma. It is important to consider the occurrence of thyroid cancers as part of multiple endocrine neoplasias.

Thyroid disorders are a common endocrinopathy in children and adolescents. Good clinical history and family history are vital in diagnosis, surveillance and planning follow-up in these patients.

Keywords

Thyroid · Hypothyroidism · Thyrotoxicosis · Thyroid nodule · Thyroid cancer

Abbreviations

ATDs	Anti-thyroid drugs
BR	Block and replace
CBZ	Carbimazole
CH	Central hypothyroidism
CHT	Congenital hypothyroidism
DBS	Dried blood spot
DT	Dose titration
ESPE	European Society for Paediatric Endocrinology
FTC	Follicular thyroid carcinoma
GD	Graves' disease
HT	Hashimoto's thyroiditis
L-T4	Levothyroxine
MTC	Medullary thyroid carcinoma
NT	Neonatal thyrotoxicosis
PTC	Papillary thyroid carcinoma
PTU	Propylthiouracil
SOD	Septo-optic dysplasia
T3	Tri-iodothyronine
T4	Tetra-iodothyronine or thyroxine
TFTs	Thyroid function tests
TPO	Thyroid peroxidase
TRAb	Thyroid receptor antibody
TRH	Thyrotrophin releasing hormone or TSH releasing hormone
TSH	Thyroid stimulating hormone
USS	Ultrasound scan

Key Terms

- **Congenital hypothyroidism:** low or inadequate thyroid at birth secondary to an genetic abnormality or error of thyroid metabolism or iodine deficiency
- **Hashimoto's thyroiditis:** an autoimmune form of hypothyroidism

- **Neonatal thyrotoxicosis:** is a rare condition in newborns of mothers with a history of Hashimoto's thyroiditis or Grave's disease
- **Thyroid nodules:** mostly benign masses in the thyroid
- **Multinodular goiter:** multiple benign masses in the thyroid
- **Thyroidectomy:** surgical removal of the thyroid gland
- **Thyroid ablation:** destruction of the thyroid tissue using radioactive iodine or radiofrequency treatment

---

Key Points

- Thyroid hormone is essential for regulation of growth, myelination of the nervous system, metabolism, and organ function.
- Congenital hypothyroidism is the most common condition of the thyroid affecting 1 in 3000 newborn children. It is diagnosed on a newborn blood spot screening test.
- Hashimoto's thyroiditis is the most common cause of autoimmune hypothyroidism in childhood, most common age at presentation is adolescence.
- The most common cause of thyrotoxicosis in children, adolescents, and adults is Graves' disease. Initial treatment is with anti-thyroid drugs with up to 60% requiring definitive treatment with surgery or radioactive iodine due to relapse after stopping anti-thyroid drugs.
- Neonatal thyrotoxicosis is a condition affecting babies born to mothers with Graves' disease or Hashimoto's thyroiditis. It is a rare but serious condition requiring close monitoring of the neonate due to a high mortality rate associated with it.
- Thyroid nodules in children and adolescents are more likely to be malignant and therefore careful evaluation is required.

32.1 Introduction

The thyroid is a butterfly-shaped gland located in the neck in front of the trachea just below the larynx. It comprises two lobes, which are attached by a band of thyroid tissue called the isthmus. Embryologically, the thyroid gland develops from the primitive pharynx and neural crest. Initially, the gland is located at the back of the tongue and during foetal development, migrates to the front of the neck before birth.

The thyroid gland produces two key hormones: tetra-iodothyronine or thyroxine (T4) and tri-iodothyronine (T3) which play a crucial role in the regulation of growth, myelination of the nervous system, metabolism, and organ function.

The thyroid gland uses iodine as its main source to synthesise thyroid hormones. Iodine deficiency can lead to thyroid problems such as underactive gland and enlarged gland (goitre) and is a common problem worldwide. Both T4 and T3 are produced by combining the iodine with the amino acid tyrosine. T4 is the predominant hormone (80%) which is then converted into T3, the more active hormone, in peripheral tissues. Thyroid hormone levels in the blood are regulated by the pituitary gland which is in turn regulated by the hypothalamus; both of which are situated centrally in the nervous system (see Fig. 32.1). Most hormonal axes are based on the negative feedback loop system. Low levels of circulating thyroid hormones stimulate the hypothalamus to release thyrotrophin releasing hormone (TRH) which in turn stimulates the pituitary gland to produce the thyroid stimulating hormone (TSH) which results in increased production of T4 and T3. Similarly high levels of circulating hormones feedback to the hypothalamus to suppress TRH and in turn TSH production.

Thyroid hormone levels vary widely during childhood (see Fig. 32.2). TSH and free T4 values decreased continuously with age, particularly during the first year of life with variance being greatest in the first month of life (Kapelari et al. 2008).

Hyperthyrotropinemia, i.e. raised TSH levels in the context of normal free T4 levels, has been noted in obese individuals. However, it has been heavily debated whether the raised TSH is the cause or effect of obesity.

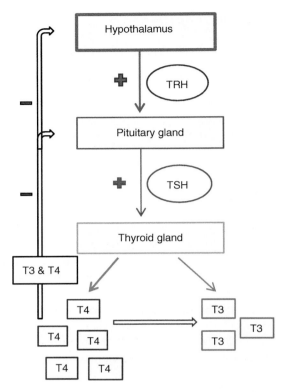

Fig. 32.1 Illustrates the hypothalamo-pituitary-thyroid axis. In response to low circulating levels of thyroid hormone tri-iodothyronine (T3) and tetra-iodothyronine (T4), the hypothalamus releases thyrotrophin-releasing hormone (TRH). The TRH stimulates the pituitary to produce thyroid-stimulating hormone (TSH) which in turn stimulates the thyroid to produce thyroid hormones. In the presence of high circulating levels of thyroid hormones, the T3 and T4 exert negative feedback control over the hypothalamus as well as anterior pituitary, thus controlling the release of both TRH and TSH

Disorders affecting the thyroid gland are common in childhood and adolescence. Early diagnosis and treatment are essential to prevent irreversible and permanent nervous system damage and developmental delay, especially in infants. Problems affecting the thyroid gland often manifest as an underactive gland (hypothyroidism) or an overactive gland (hyperthyroidism) with or without a swelling of the gland (goitre). Conditions affecting the thyroid gland are listed in the table below (Table 32.1).

We now discuss in detail some of the selected common endocrinopathies relating to thyroid dysfunction in children and adolescents using case studies.

32.2 Hypothyroidism

32.2.1 Congenital Hypothyroidism (CHT)

32.2.1.1 Introduction
CHT is a partial or complete loss of function of the thyroid gland (hypothyroidism) that affects infants from birth (congenital). The prevalence of CHT is 1 in 3000 live births.

32.2.1.2 Aetiology
The causes include:

1. Dygenesis (thyroid gland is absent, underdeveloped, or abnormally located)—80%
2. Dyshormonogenesis (abnormal biosynthesis of thyroid hormone)—20%

Commonest cause worldwide is maternal iodine deficiency, which is an essential element in the production of thyroid hormones.

A genetic cause may be present in 15–20% of the cases. Although the cause of thyroid dysgenesis remains unidentified in majority of the cases, 2–5% are said to be due to PAX8 and TSHR gene mutations. Thyroid dyshormonogenesis can occur due to mutation in one of the following genes: DUOX2, SLC5A5, TG, TSHB, and TPO (http://ghr.nlm.nih. gov/condition/congenital-hypothyroidism). Majority of the mutations are sporadic (new); however, a few children inherit it from their parents.

A very small percentage of patients have secondary hypothyroidism where the problem is in the hypothalamus or the pituitary (discussed later).

32.2.1.3 Diagnosis
CHT is diagnosed on dried blood spot (DBS) testing in the newborn. This is employed in all developed countries where blood is collected from a heel prick on all babies around day 5 of life. The diagnosis is mostly made on a raised TSH. The screening is aimed at identifying the more severe forms of primary CHT as early initiation of treatment (<3 months of age) minimises intellectual disability in children with CHT. In the UK, the aim is to start treatment within 21 days of birth. The flowchart (see Fig. 32.3) illustrates the screening and referral criteria and pathway.

Fig. 32.2 Adopted from
Kapelari et al. (2008):
Age-related reference
intervals for TSH (**a**)
and free T4 (**b**). The
central 95% range
(2.5th, 25th, 50th, 75th,
and 97.5th percentiles)
are shown

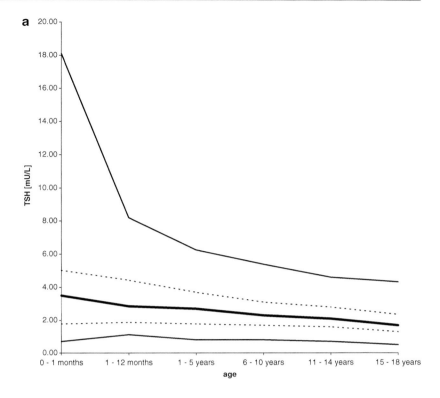

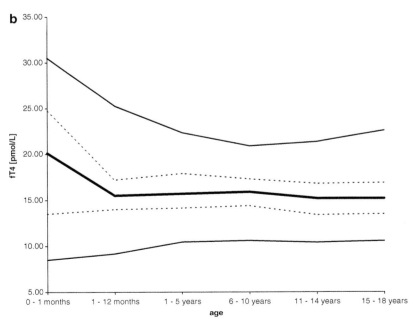

Table 32.1 Conditions affecting the thyroid gland and hormones in the neonatal period, childhood and adolescence are listed below

	Hypothyroidism	Hyperthyroidism
Neonatal period	Congenital hypothyroidism	Neonatal thyrotoxicosis secondary to • Maternal Graves' disease • Maternal Hashimoto's thyroiditis
Childhood and adolescence	• Hashimoto's thyroiditis • Subacute thyroiditis • Following surgical removal of thyroid gland for Graves' disease or for thyroid nodule • Radiation damage to the thyroid gland following cancer treatment	• Graves' disease • Subacute thyroiditis • Hyperfunctioning thyroid nodule (toxic adenoma, toxic multinodular goitre) • McCune Albright syndrome
Rare	• TSH receptor defect causing congenital hypothyroidism • Congenital secondary hypothyroidism due to genetic mutations causing abnormal pituitary gland development	• Thyroid hormone ingestion (factitious or induced) • TSH hypersecretion secondary to pituitary tumours • Pituitary resistance to thyroid hormone • Activating mutation of the TSH receptor • Iodine induced hyperthyroidism

A second test should be considered in pre-term neonates, babies with very low birth weight and in babies who were ill at the time of first sample collection as TSH is known to be elevated.

Neonates may exhibit any of the symptoms and signs of CHT illustrated in the table below (Table 32.2) or may be asymptomatic and detected purely by a raised TSH on screening. A raised TSH on DBS should be confirmed on venous thyroid function tests at referral, prior to initiation of treatment.

The European Society for Paediatric Endocrinology (ESPE) consensus guidelines for CHT (Léger et al. 2014) suggest the following biochemical diagnostic criteria for initiation of treatment:

(a) If DBS reveals TSH of 40 mU/L, await serum results for 1–2 days before initiating treatment.
(b) Start treatment immediately if serum free thyroxine (FT4) concentration is below the normal range for age, regardless of TSH concentration.
(c) Start treatment if venous TSH concentration is persistently greater than 20 mU/L, even if serum FT4 concentration is normal.
(d) If TSH concentration is between 6 and 20 mU/L in a well-baby with normal FT4, consider diagnostic imaging to establish a definitive diagnosis.
(e) If TSH concentration remains high for more than 3–4 weeks, consider starting levothy-

roxine (L-T4) supplementation immediately (in discussion with the family) and retesting, off treatment, at a later stage; or retesting 2 weeks later without treatment.

32.2.1.4 Investigations

Thyroid ultrasound scan (USS) and scintigraphy are the recommended investigations for CHT. Often clinicians choose one of the two investigations; however, both should be considered in those with raised TSH to improve diagnostic accuracy.

An x-ray of the knee may be carried out to assess the severity of intrauterine hypothyroidism by the presence or absence of femoral and tibial epiphyses.

Treatment should not be delayed and can be initiated pending investigations.

Thyroid USS does not detect ectopic thyroid tissue and is user dependent. Thyroid scintigraphy can identify athyreosis (absence of uptake), hypoplasia of a gland, a normal or large gland in situ with or without abnormally high levels of uptake, and an ectopic thyroid at any point along the pathway of the normal embryological descent. It is ideal when performed within 7 days of starting L-T4 treatment.

32.2.1.5 Treatment

Treatment is with L-T4. It should be started before 2 weeks of age or as soon as a diagnosis is

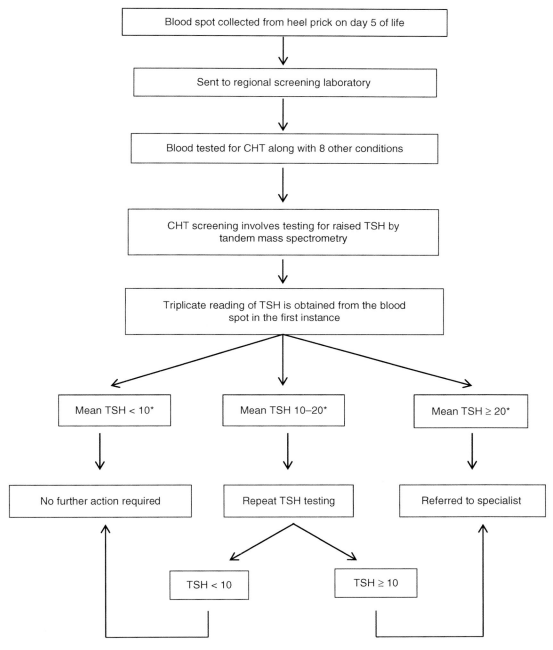

Fig. 32.3 Flowchart representing the screening and referral pathway in the UK. *Please note that different laboratories may have slightly different cut-off values for TSH for further screening and referral

made. The starting dose is 10–15 μg/kg/day. Treatment is monitored by thyroid function tests (TFTs) and tailored to maintain free T4 in the high end of normal range and TSH in the normal range.

32.2.1.6   Nursing Considerations

Levothyroxine is available in different strength solutions or tablets. The absorption is better with tablets. Nurses can be valuable in advising the parents on administering the medication. The

Table 32.2 Symptoms and signs of hypothyroidism in neonates

Symptoms	Signs
• Sleepiness	• Prolonged neonatal jaundice
• Constipation	• Cold extremities
• Not waking for feeds	• Hypotonia
	• Macroglossia
• Poor feeding	• Umbilical hernia
	• Dry skin
	• Coarse and puffy face
	• Large anterior fontanelle
	• Wide sagittal suture

majority of units suggest crushing and dissolving the tablets in milk and giving it via a teaspoon or a syringe. Crushed tablets are not to be added to a whole bottle of milk in case the baby does not complete the full feed. Other centres advise placing the tablet in the side of the baby's cheek at the beginning of a feed, which is then absorbed. Consideration must be given to the strength of tablet available when using the second method.

Parents should be provided with information leaflets. Where unit specific information leaflets are not available, in the UK, one can use generic leaflets available from British Thyroid Association or the UK National Screening Committee. Parents should also be directed towards support groups.

As with any other condition requiring lifelong treatment, it is crucial to emphasise on and ensure compliance at each visit.

32.2.1.7   Follow-Up

Regular 1–2 weekly follow-up is required initially to optimise treatment and achieve a normal TSH. Once TSH normalises, 3 monthly follow-up is recommended to monitor growth and development in the first year of life. More frequent visits may be required if there are clinical concerns.

Re-evaluation of the thyroid axis may be considered at the age of 3 years in those children where the aetiology remains unknown or in those where the presence of CHT is questioned either because treatment was commenced when the

infant was unwell or in the presence of only slightly raised TSH at diagnosis.

32.2.1.8   Outcome

Since the introduction of newborn screening and early initiation of treatment, the neurocognitive outcome for children with CHT has improved (Grosse and Van Vliet 2011). Special measures must be put in place for those children in whom severe CHT affects motor development or school performance.

Case 1

The Paediatric team were notified that a baby girl had had a positive new born screening test result for congenital hypothyroidism with a blood spot TSH of 26.5 mU/L (mean of duplicate results). The family were contacted and the baby was reviewed in the Children's Assessment Unit on the same day.

Parents commented that she was a 'good' baby, and had to be woken up for the majority of her feeds. She was born at 40 weeks gestation by normal vaginal delivery with a birth weight of 2.8 kg. There was no family history of thyroid disease.

On clinical examination there were no dysmorphic features. She had no evidence of a goitre or lesion at the back of her tongue and was not jaundiced. She appeared clinically euthyroid and had no signs of cardiac abnormalities.

Abnormal TFTs with elevated TSH and low normal free T4 were confirmed on venous bloods (table below). Maternal thyroid functions were normal.

The baby was commenced on levothyroxine supplements at a dose of 25 mcgs daily. Thyroid ultrasound and thyroid uptake scan confirmed that the thyroid gland was in situ suggesting dyshormonogenesis as the cause of hypothyroidism.

The patient was seen for follow-up in the paediatric endocrine clinic in 2 weeks. The parents had noted that she was more awake and responsive and feeding well. Thyroid functions had improved.

Treatment	Pre	Post
Day	D9	D23
TSH mU/L (0.35–4.4)	55.2	7.99
Free T4 pmol/L (9–19.1)	13.4	24.2

Discussion: Careful examination of the infant with congenital hypothyroidism (CHT) should be carried out for presence of dysmorphic features and cardiac defects and vice versa. The prevalence of cardiac defects in children with CHT is higher than in the general population. Children

> **Points to Remember**
> - *Congenital hypothyroidism is diagnosed by a raised TSH or low T4 on a heel prick test done as part of the new born screening test.*
> - *Early treatment, within 3 weeks of life, with levothyroxine minimises damage to the central nervous system and improves outcome.*
> - *Close monitoring of growth and development in infants with CHT is essential.*

with certain conditions such as Down's and Pendred syndrome and pseudohypoparathyroidism may have a slightly raised TSH in the neonatal period, which may not be picked up on new born screening test.

32.2.2 Autoimmune Hypothyroidism

32.2.2.1 Introduction

Autoimmune hypothyroidism also known as Hashimoto's thyroiditis (HT) or autoimmune thyroiditis is the commonest cause of acquired hypothyroidism in children and can present at any age but most frequently in adolescence. There are several forms of HT; however, the one in children is referred to as the juvenile form. Females are more affected than males and whites and Asians are more affected than other races. HT can occur in association with other autoimmune diseases such as type 1 diabetes mellitus,

Sjögren syndrome, or other thyroid diseases such as papillary thyroid cancer, and is also more common in conditions associated with autoimmune conditions such as Turner Syndrome.

32.2.2.2 Clinical Features

The most common presenting feature of HT is that of a painless goitre and biochemical euthyroidism (normal thyroid functions). The next most common feature is subclinical hypothyroidism or overt hypothyroidism with clinical features of hypothyroidism (Table 32.3). A small proportion of patients present with features of thyrotoxicosis (Table 32.4) which is transient, known as hashitoxicosis (Htx), before developing permanent hypothyroidism. Htx is believed to result from unregulated release of stored

Table 32.3 Symptoms and signs of hypothyroidism in children and adolescents

Symptoms	Signs
• Muscular weakness	• Low pulse rate and heart rate
• Fatigue	
• Sensitivity to cold	• Thick puffy skin
• Constipation	• Coarse hair
• Slowed mental processes	• Dry skin
• Poor memory	• Goitre (enlarged thyroid)
• Reduced school performance	• Delayed relaxation phase of deep tendon reflexes
• Sleep disturbance	• Decreased growth velocity
• Weight gain	• Precocious (early) puberty
• Menstrual disturbance	• Delayed puberty
	• Raised prolactin levels

Table 32.4 Symptoms and signs of neonatal thyrotoxicosis

Symptoms	Signs
• Irritability	• Goitre
• Jitteriness	• Tachycardia and arrhythmias
• Restlessness	• Cardiac failure
• Voracious appetite	• Sweating and flushing
	• Acrocyanosis
• Diarrhoea	• Eye signs: periorbital oedema, lid retraction, and exophthalmos
• Weight loss	• Hepatosplenomegaly
	• Lymphadenopathy
	• Bruising and petechiae secondary to thrombocytopenia
	• Hyperviscosity
	• Craniosynostosis and microcephaly

thyroid hormones during inflammatory-mediated destruction of the thyroid gland. Children with long-standing hypothyroidism can occasionally present with iso-sexual precocious puberty (same sex early puberty) with delayed bone age and ovarian cysts, a triad referred to as Van Wyk Grumbach syndrome.

32.2.2.3 Diagnosis

The diagnosis of HT is currently established by a combination of clinical features, presence of serum antibodies against thyroid antigens (mainly to thyroperoxidase and thyroglobulin), and reduced echogenicity of the thyroid gland on USS. Antithyroid peroxidase (TPO) and antithyroglobulin (Tg) antibody titres are elevated in 90–95% of children with Hashimoto's thyroiditis (Grosse and Van Vliet 2011). A small proportion of children who are initially negative can become positive later. Around 20% of individuals who have antibody-positive test results do not develop hypothyroidism or hyperthyroidism (Catureglia et al. 2014).

32.2.2.4 Management

Treatment is by supplementation with L-T4 with a starting dose of 5 mcg/kg/day as a single dose. Children and adolescents with long-standing hypothyroidism should be started on a low dose of levothyroxine to prevent rapid overcorrection. Treatment is monitored by regular measurements of thyroid hormones and treatment is tailored to maintain a free T4 at the high end of normal and TSH in the normal range. Surgery is rarely required but must be considered if there are goitre-related pressure effects. It is essential to bear in mind that an increased prevalence of papillary thyroid carcinoma has been reported in patients with HT (Okayasu et al. 1995), although this remains debatable.

Around 20% of patients may return to a euthyroid state after completing puberty, therefore thyroid status should be re-evaluated at this stage by stopping treatment and monitoring using free T4 and TSH levels (De Luca et al. 2013).

Case 2

A 12½-year-old girl was reviewed in the endocrine clinic after recently being diagnosed with autoimmune hypothyroidism. She had first presented 2 months ago to her General Practitioner with a history of tiredness, dry skin, and weight gain. Parents had also reported that her teachers had noticed a decline in her energy levels. There was a family history of hypothyroidism in the maternal aunt.

On examination, the patient looked well and had a pulse of 86 beats per minute. Her height was on the 9th centile and her weight was just above the 50th centile. Previous measurements taken 2 years earlier from a community clinic had placed her height and weight on the 25th centile. There was a small, smooth goitre, not tender and not nodular. She was pre-pubertal.

Her initial TSH was raised with a low free T4 (table below) and TPO antibodies were positive at >1000 U/mL (normal <6.0). The GP had commenced her on levothyroxine 25 mcg daily. Her parents reported that there was a positive noticeable difference in their daughter since starting the medication.

Repeat thyroid function tests showed a reducing TSH and rising free T4. The dose of levothyroxine was increased to achieve a high normal free T4 and normal TSH. She was seen regularly in the endocrine clinic to review her progress and monitor her thyroid function tests.

Treatment	Pre	2 months post
TSH (0.35–4.4) mU/L	53.4	8.6
Free T4 (9–19.1) pmol/L	7.2	12.5

Discussion: Patients with autoimmune hypothyroidism may present with or without goitre. Increasing weight centile and decreasing height centile should always raise the suspicion of hypothyroidism. Treatment is aimed at maintaining a high normal free T4 and a normal TSH. The normal range for free T4 and TSH varies between laboratories and for different ages.

32.2.3 Secondary or Central Hypothyroidism

Central hypothyroidism (CH) is defined as hypothyroidism due to insufficient stimulation by thyroid stimulating hormone (TSH) of an otherwise normal thyroid gland. CH can be congenital (present at birth) or acquired. Congenital CH (CCH) can occur in isolation but most often occurs in association with other pituitary hormone deficiencies. CCH is not identified on newborn screening test as the TSH levels in these neonates are low. The prevalence of CCH is said to be higher than previously known. Countries which use free T4 in the newborn screening report its incidence to be 1 in 16,000 (Schoenmakers et al. 2015). Mutations in transcription factors responsible for normal pituitary development (HESX1, LHX3, LHX4, SOX3, OTX2, PROP1, POU1F1) may cause central hypothyroidism with or without associated extra pituitary abnormalities (Schoenmakers et al. 2015). The other causes of CH in later childhood and adolescence include malignancies such as craniopharyngiomas, previous radiotherapy, previous pituitary surgery, traumatic brain injury, vascular defects, and infiltrative conditions such as histiocytosis.

Case 3

A baby girl born at 37 weeks by normal vaginal delivery was admitted to the neonatal unit due to poor tone (hypotonia) and suspected sepsis. Mum had had a normal pregnancy with normal antenatal scans.

The baby was treated with antibiotics for suspected sepsis. She was screened for prolonged jaundice at 2 weeks of age. Thyroid function tests done as part of screening revealed low TSH (2.9 mU/L) and low FT4 (8 pmol/L) raising suspicion of central hypothyroidism.

She was transferred to a tertiary centre for endocrinology review. Here she was screened for other pituitary hormone deficiencies. A short synacthen test demonstrated suboptimal cortisol response to ACTH revealing cortisol deficiency.

She was commenced on hydrocortisone replacement therapy followed by levothyroxine. Septo-optic dysplasia (SOD) as the cause of multiple pituitary hormone deficiency was suspected and further evaluated. Ophthalmology examination revealed right optic nerve hypoplasia and an MRI of the head showed an absent septum pellucidum, small anterior pituitary, and ectopic posterior pituitary, confirming the diagnosis of SOD.

Discussion: Central hypothyroidism is not diagnosed on new born screening test in countries where the screening programme uses high TSH levels to diagnose CHT. Countries measuring thyroxine levels in screening are more likely to detect babies with secondary hypothyroidism. However, measuring thyroxine is said to be less specific with high frequency of false positives and is therefore not universally practised. Presence of central hypothyroidism necessitates a thorough evaluation for the presence of other pituitary hormone deficiencies. Thyroxine replacement prior to hydrocortisone replacement in children with cortisol deficiency may precipitate an adrenal crisis.

32.3 Hyperthyroidism

32.3.1 Neonatal Thyrotoxicosis

32.3.1.1 Introduction
Neonatal thyrotoxicosis (NT) is the presence of an overactive thyroid (or hyperthyroidism) in the newborn. The prevalence of Graves' disease in pregnancy is 0.2% (Batra 2013). Of those pregnant patients with Graves' disease only 1–12.5% result in neonatal thyrotoxicosis (Batra 2013).

32.3.1.2 Aetiology
NT occurs due to transplacental passage of thyroid stimulating immunoglobulins (TSIs) from mothers with Graves' disease or Hashimoto's thyroiditis. The antibodies can persist despite previous treatment for Graves' disease in the mother. These antibodies which are IgG immunoglobulins cross the placenta and stimulate the foetal thyroid. Although this starts early in pregnancy the effect increases in the last trimester as the placental permeability increases, causing the foetal and maternal antibody levels to be equal.

Another rare cause of NT is an activating mutation of the TSH receptor. NT due to receptor mutation should be suspected if more than two generations in the family are affected by thyrotoxicosis and if there are difficulties in weaning ATDs. Rarely de novo (new) mutations have also been reported to occur. These individuals will need definitive treatment in the long term such as thyroidectomy.

32.3.1.3 Clinical Manifestations
Depending on the antibody levels and maternal control of the disease, the features of thyrotoxicosis may start as early as in the second trimester of pregnancy or not manifest in the neonate at all. Foetal growth can be restricted in utero due to hyperthyroidism and rarely a foetal goitre can be seen on antenatal scans in severe cases. There is an increased incidence of intrauterine death and premature delivery in pregnancies with maternal thyrotoxicosis.

Symptoms and signs (Table 32.3) of thyrotoxicosis may be apparent at birth or may be delayed due to the effect of maternal anti-thyroid drugs or coexistent blocking antibodies. In most cases, features are apparent by day 10 of life. Biochemically the neonate will have a raised free T4 and a suppressed TSH. TSH receptor antibodies (TRAbs) may be in high concentrations.

32.3.1.4 Management
Careful monitoring in pregnancy as detailed in the Endocrine Society Clinical Practice Guideline is essential (De Groot et al. 2012). Foetal thyrotoxicosis is treated by administering anti-thyroid drugs (ATDs), carbimazole or propylthiouracil (PTU) to the mother. These drugs act by preventing the synthesis of thyroid hormone and cross the placenta. Carbimazole is avoided, if possible, in the first trimester due to its association with congenital anomalies. Close monitoring of liver function on PTU is recommended due to its association with liver toxicity.

Neonatal thyrotoxicosis is treated with 0.5–1.5 mg/kg/day of carbimazole in the neonate. A beta blocker such as propranolol is used in a dose of 0.27–0.75 mg/kg 8 hourly in neonates who are symptomatic due to adrenergic stimulation (Ogilvy-Stuart 2002). Thyroid function must be monitored weekly in those on ATD.

In those neonates who are asymptomatic, thyroid function must be checked at birth, day 5–7 and then day 10–14. Parents should be warned of symptoms, as NT has been reported to occur as late as 45 days in certain cases.

32.3.1.5 Prognosis
Most neonates require treatment for no longer than 8–10 weeks. In those who require continued treatment, other causes must be considered. Craniosynostosis, intellectual disability, impaired growth and development have been reported in a small percentage of children with NT, although most of these are neonates with persistent thyrotoxicosis due to a genetic mutation rather than transient due to maternal antibodies.

Case 4
A baby boy was born at term by normal vaginal delivery. Mum had a history of hypothyroidism diagnosed 5 years prior to conception. She developed thyrotoxicosis in pregnancy and was treated with carbimazole. She had high levels of TPO

(2921 Ku/L; normal range 0–51) and thyroid receptor antibodies, TRAb (4.7 U/L; normal range 0–1).

The baby was observed in hospital for 48 h and was discharged home as he was feeding well and did not show any features of thyrotoxicosis such as weight loss, sweating, diarrhoea, tachycardia, or goitre. In an endocrine review on day 5 of life, the baby was tachycardic with a heart rate of 200 beats per minute. His weight was static

and there was no goitre. NT was suspected and confirmed by biochemical tests (table below). Carbimazole (75 mcg/kg/day) treatment commenced. Propranolol (400 mcg/kg/day) was added in view of the tachycardia.

The TRAb (22 U/L; range 0–15) and TPO (675 Ku/L; range 0.0–5.6) antibodies were raised. TFTs were monitored and treatment weaned as below (table).

Treatment	Pre	1 week post	1 month post	3 months post	1 month off treatment	2 months off treatment
TSH (0.4–3.5) mU/L	<0.01	<0.01	0.3	0.3	0.35	0.5
FreeT4 (10.7–21.8) pmol/L	>77.2	18.4	9.8	15	14.5	14.2
Action	CBZ and propranolol	Propranolol stopped and CBZ halved	CBZ halved	CBZ stopped		

Discussion: Women with previous hypothyroidism can develop hyperthyroidism in pregnancy. Close monitoring of neonates with maternal Graves' disease or Hashimoto's thyroiditis is crucial. Treatment with anti-thyroid drugs (ATDs) can eventually be weaned.

Points to Remember
- *Neonatal thyrotoxicosis is caused by transplacental transfer of thyroid stimulating immunoglobulins in maternal Graves' or Hashimoto's thyroiditis.*
- *It is a rare and transient condition in the absence of genetic mutations.*
- *Close monitoring of neonates at risk of developing thyrotoxicosis is essential.*
- *Treatment with anti-thyroid drugs for a brief period may be required.*

32.3.2 Graves' Hyperthyroidism

32.3.2.1 Introduction

Hyperthyroidism is rare in children and adolescents. Majority of the cases are due to Graves' disease (GD). GD is an autoimmune disorder caused by an abnormal thyroid hormone produc-

tion stimulated by thyroid stimulating immunoglobulins, the action of which mimics TSH. Inheritance is polygenic. GD is more common in some families. The production of immunoglobulins is thought to be triggered by certain infections involving the Yersinia series and also viruses. GD is associated with other autoimmune diseases such as diabetes mellitus, Addison disease, vitiligo, immune thrombocytopenic purpura (ITP), and pernicious anaemia. The incidence of GD is around 1 per 100,000 under the age of 15 years (Williamson and Greene 2010).

32.3.2.2 Clinical Features

The triad of GD includes goitre, thyrotoxicosis (Table 32.5), and ophthalmopathy (Table 32.5). However, not all patients present with ophthalmopathy. Fifty percent of patients with eye disease have a mild form and only 2–3% present with severe eye signs (Menconi et al. 2014).

32.3.2.3 Diagnosis

Diagnosis of GD includes elevated levels of serum thyroxine (T4) and tri-iodothyronine (T3), associated with undetectable serum TSH. Antibodies against the TSH receptor (TRAbs) are pathognomonic. They are detectable in the serum of about 98% of untreated GD patients (Menconi et al. 2014). TRAb measure-

Table 32.5 Symptoms and signs of hyperthyroidism and ophthalmopathy in children and adolescents

Symptoms	Signs
Hyperthyroidism	
• Weight loss • Increased appetite • Palpitations • Sweating • Heat intolerance • Tiredness and weak muscles • Nervousness, irritability, and shakiness • Mood swings or aggressive behaviour • Loose stools • Increased thirst and urination • Oligomenorrhoea	• Rapid pulse • Warm • Moist hands • Enlarged thyroid gland with or without a bruit • Tremor
Ophthalmopathy	
• Excess tearing • Irritation • Grittiness • Photophobia • Pain • Redness of the conjunctiva • Diplopia • Blurred vision • Reduced visual acuity	• Soft tissue involvement manifests as Swelling and redness of the eyelids Swelling of the caruncle Chemosis • Proptosis • Extraocular muscle involvement causing limitation of eye movement • Corneal involvement manifests as Stippling and ulceration • Optic nerve involvement • Lid lag

ment is not essential for diagnosing GD; however, it can be used when there is diagnostic uncertainty. Thyroid ultrasound demonstrates a hypoechoic picture with reduced colloid and increased vascularity. USS is also not essential for diagnosis but gives useful information about the size of the gland and detects any thyroid nodules not palpated clinically.

32.3.2.4 Management of GD

The initial management of GD includes antithyroid drugs (ATDs). The most appropriate regimen is highly debated. The goal of therapy is to render the patient euthyroid. This is not a cure and definitive treatment such as thyroidectomy or radioactive iodine is required in the long term in majority of the patients. Only half of the patients go into clinical remission following treatment with ATDs (Cheetham and Bliss 2016).

Anti-thyroid Drugs and Treatment Regimes

The most commonly used ATD in children and adults is carbimazole except in the first trimester of pregnancy or if carbimazole is not tolerated,

when propylthiouracil (PTU) is used. Carbimazole is preferred to PTU, because of the evidence of a lower prevalence of severe side effects, especially idiosyncratic hepatitis and liver failure although this is rare. The other side effects of ATDs include skin rash and, very rarely, hepatitis, agranulocytosis, and vasculitis. It is important that all children and adolescents and their families are counselled about these potential side effects.

A beta blocker such as propranolol may be necessary in the initial stages to control the adrenergic symptoms of thyrotoxicosis. However, beta blockers are contraindicated in children with asthma and are therefore not used.

There are two main approaches to treatment with ATDs:

(a) *Block and replace* where high dose ATD is used to render the patient hypothyroid and levothyroxine is then added to treat hypothyroidism. Some clinicians believe that the side effects of ATDs are more with this regimen; however, others prefer this method as thyroid function is said to be more stable with this regimen and patients need fewer blood tests and clinic follow-up visits initially (Cheetham and Bliss 2016).

(b) *Dose titration* where a titrating dose of ATD is used. This method is preferred by some due to reportedly fewer side effects and a simpler regimen; however, others report the need for frequent blood tests and dose adjustments due to unstable thyroid functions (Cheetham and Bliss 2016).

The relapse rate is reported to be similar with the two regimens, 51% in the block-replace group and 54% in the dose titration group (Abraham et al. 2010). The best approach remains debatable.

Surgery

For those that need definitive treatment, one option is thyroidectomy. Previously subtotal thyroidectomies were performed; however, now total thyroidectomy is increasingly recommended to prevent the recurrence of hyperthyroidism (<3%). The rate of complications with total thyroidectomy when performed by a skilled (high-volume) surgeon is said to be minimal. The most frequent complications include: pain and transient hypocalcaemia secondary to disruption of the parathyroid glands. Less frequent complications include haemorrhage, permanent hypoparathyroidism, and vocal cord paralysis.

Hypothyroidism, requiring levothyroxine replacement, is universal following total thyroidectomy.

Radioactive Iodine

The other option is radioactive iodine (I-131) which is increasingly being used in the treatment of GD and is gaining popularity. Radioiodine is preferably administered after achievement of euthyroidism with ATDs and ATDs are stopped 5–7 days prior to treatment.

The goal of the treatment is to induce hypothyroidism in order to achieve a stable remission. Oral I-131 targets and destroys the follicular cells in the thyroid gland; hence an initial rise in thyroid hormones may be noted. Beta blockers may be used to control symptoms of hyperthyroidism during this time. There is a risk of thyroid storm following I-131 treatment.

The dose of I-131 is calculated based on the gland size and radioiodine uptake by the gland. The reported doses in children and adolescents have ranged from 100–250 mCi/g thyroid tissue (Rivkees 2014). Treatment is less successful in patients with large goitre and high levels of circulating TRAb levels.

Very few short-term side effects are reported and are usually tolerable. Radiation thyroiditis can rarely cause pain and swelling of the neck and may require treatment with simple analgesia. The long-term persistence of hyperthyroidism and occurrence of hypothyroidism post treatment are variably reported and depend on the I-131 dose used. Both hypo- and hyper-parathyroidism have been reported in the long term in a small percentage of patients. There is no evidence of an increased risk of thyroid cancer, other solid tumours, and leukaemia following I-131 therapy in adults with GD. Although the same has been shown in children, the numbers are small (1000 children) and the duration of follow-up (5–15 years) is short to make any definitive conclusions and long-term large studies are still required (Rivkees 2014). No long-term effects on the adult reproductive system in males and females have been described. Recent studies have focused on the association of I-131 therapy with the development or progression of ophthalmopathy, hence its use in patients with active Graves' ophthalmopathy is limited.

Case 5

A 7-year-old girl presented to her General Practitioner with symptoms of anxiety, poor sleep, and weight loss. On examination she was found to have an enlarged thyroid gland (goitre). She was not tachycardic and there were no eye signs.

Hyperthyroidism was suspected based on the history and clinical findings and confirmed on laboratory thyroid function tests. She had a raised FT4 (29 pmol/L) and a suppressed TSH (0.01 mU/L). She was positive for TPO (295 Ku/L; normal range 0–5.6) and TRAb (33 U/L; normal range 0–15) confirming a diagnosis of Graves' hyperthyroidism. Thyroid USS showed multiple hypoechoic nodules and increased vascularity of the thyroid gland in keeping with the diagnosis.

She was treated with carbimazole (1 mg/kg/day in two divided doses). Treatment with propranolol was not indicated. Her free T4 normalised within 8 weeks although the TSH remained suppressed for longer. Following treatment she regained her weight and her sleep pattern was reported to have improved.

Treatment	Pre	2 weeks post	10 weeks post
TSH (0.4–3.5) mU/L	<0.01	0.01	0.03
FreeT4 (10.8–28) pmol/L	69.5	29	15.3

Discussion: Graves' hyperthyroidism is the most common cause of hyperthyroidism in children. Symptoms usually resolve following treatment with anti-thyroid drugs. In patients with increased adrenergic activity, namely increased heart rate and tremor, treatment with a beta blocker such as propranolol is indicated.

Points to Remember
- *GD is the most common cause of thyrotoxicosis in children and adolescents as well as adults.*
- *GD is a triad of thyrotoxicosis, goitre, and ophthalmopathy, although only a small proportion of patients present with all three features.*
- *Although the mainstay of initial treatment is with anti-thyroid drugs, the right regimen is highly debated (block and replace vs dose titration).*
- *In patients who relapse after stopping ATDs, the choice of long-term definitive treatment (surgery or radioactive iodine) depends on several factors such as disease severity, age of the patient, presence of ophthalmopathy, and the size of the goitre.*

32.4 Thyroid Nodules and Cancers

32.4.1 Thyroid Nodules

Thyroid nodules (TNs) are mostly benign and not cancerous, although a higher proportion of them are cancerous in children compared to adults (22–26% vs 5–10%, respectively) (Francis Gary et al. 2015). TN rarely present with clinical features, majority of them are incidentally picked up by physical examination, occasionally patients can present with a painless lump in the neck.

32.4.1.1 Evaluation of the Thyroid Nodule

Careful and thorough evaluation of TNs is essential due to the high risk of malignancy associated with it in childhood. This should include:

History: A detailed history focused on

1. Symptoms of hypothyroidism or hyperthyroidism (Tables 32.3 and 32.5)
2. Disturbance in voice
3. Swallowing difficulty
4. History of malignancy
5. Exposure to radiation
6. Family history of thyroid problems or other malignancies

Examination: A systematic physical examination should assess the thyroid gland, the lateral neck for surrounding lymph nodes, and if indicated, a laryngeal examination and systemic examination for signs of metastatic disease.

Investigations: should include thyroid function tests and ultrasound guided fine needle aspiration (FNA) biopsy.

The American Thyroid Association Guidelines (Rivkees 2014) provide detailed step by step guide on investigation and management of thyroid nodules, discussion of which is beyond the scope of this book.

Case 6

A 14-year-old girl was referred to the endocrine clinic with a 6 month history of feeling hot and shaky. She also had increased appetite and had felt her heart was racing for the past 2–3 months. She had lost weight and experienced irregular menstruation.

There was a family history of Graves' disease in the mother which was diagnosed 5 years ago and was treated with radioactive iodine. Paternal grandmother also had hypothyroidism.

On examination her heart rate was 104 beats per minute and she had mild tremor. She had a smooth, asymmetric, enlarged goitre which was bigger on the right compared to the left. She had no eye signs or lymphadenopathy.

Hyperthyroidism was suspected and confirmed on laboratory investigations. She had a raised FT4 (36 pmol/L) and suppressed TSH (<0.01 mU/L). She was commenced on carbimazole and propranolol to control adrenergic symptoms. Her TPO and TRAb were negative.

A thyroid USS identified a large well-defined solid and cystic lesion with increased vascularity. A fine needle aspiration biopsy was performed which showed normal thyroid tissue. The size of the goitre improved on carbimazole treatment. Technetium scintigraphy showed evidence of increased uptake within the single nodule suggesting a hot nodule amenable to surgery.

Discussion: Thyroid nodules must be evaluated thoroughly in children and adolescents due to the increased risk of cancer. In this case, further evaluation of the nodule with a technetium 99 scan to determine functionality indicated surgery would be the ideal definitive treatment.

32.4.2 Thyroid Cancers

Thyroid cancers are rare in children compared to adolescents. The annual incidence is 1 per million per year in children under 10 years compared to 15.4 cases per million per year in 15–19-year-olds (http://www.thyca.org/pediatric/about/). The two main types of paediatric thyroid cancers include differentiated thyroid cancer and medullary thyroid cancer.

1. **Differentiated Thyroid Cancer**: This includes papillary and follicular thyroid cancer and their variants.
   (a) *Papillary thyroid cancer* (PTC) is the most common type of thyroid cancer in both children, adolescents, and adults. The majority of children with PTC have local spread to the lymph nodes of the neck at the time of diagnosis and up to 20% have distant metastases (http://www.thyca.org/pediatric/about/). Recurrence of PTC is common. However, despite this the prognosis is excellent with appropriate treatment.
   (b) *Follicular thyroid cancer* (FTC) is rare in children, has aggressive characteristics and poorer prognosis.

The mainstay of treatment for both types of cancers is surgery aiming for a total thyroidectomy including resection of the surrounding affected lymph nodes. Radioactive iodine has also been employed followed by doses of L-T4 which suppress TSH levels for a period of time. Long-term follow-up and surveillance to detect recurrence is recommended.

2. **Medullary Thyroid Cancer (MTC)**: MTC is rare in childhood and accounts for 5–10% of all thyroid cancers (http://www.thyca.org/pediatric/about/). MTC comes from the parafollicular C-cells in the thyroid gland that produces a protein called calcitonin. Twenty-five percent of MTC cases are hereditary, the remainder are sporadic. MTC can occur as part of a multiple endocrine neoplasia. A family history of MTC, pheochromocytoma, or hyperparathyroidism may indicate multiple endocrine neoplasia 2A (MEN2A) or multiple endocrine neoplasia 2B (MEN2B), both of which are inherited in an autosomal dominant fashion. All family members should be genetically screened for this mutation. It can also occur by itself in familial medullary thyroid carcinoma (FMTC). MTC is treated with total thyroidectomy if diagnosed before metastatic

spread. Patients are monitored by serum measurement of calcitonin at follow up due to the risk of recurrence in the remnant thyroid tissue.

Case 7

A 14-year-old girl (patient 1) presents with a solitary neck lump. Thyroid function was normal. Ultrasound showed a left sided nodule. Fine needle aspiration (FNA) was inconclusive so she underwent left lobectomy of the thyroid which on histology was medullary thyroid cancer.

Calcitonin levels were checked postoperatively and were raised at 13.1 ng/L (<5 ng/L).

Genetic screening was performed and she had a mutation in the RET gene. This mutation is associated with MEN2. The diagnosis of MEN 2A was made as she had no features like mucosal neuromas suggestive of MEN 2B. Plasma metanephrines were normal. She underwent a total thyroidectomy.

Four other family members were screened and were identified as having the same genetic mutation. One member of the family had been previously diagnosed with a phaeochromocytoma but this had not been followed up. Another two of the family members had biochemical and radiological evidence of medullary thyroid carcinoma and phaeochromocytoma.

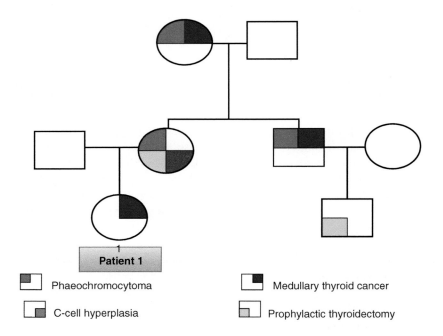

Patient 1

▢ Phaeochromocytoma

▢ C-cell hyperplasia

▢ Medullary thyroid cancer

▢ Prophylactic thyroidectomy

Discussion: Children or adolescents found to have medullary thyroid cancer require genetic screening and if positive family screening. If a mutation is identified in the RET gene early prophylactic thyroidectomy (as medullary thyroid cancer occurs in 95%) is recommended along with ongoing screening for phaeochromocytoma (occurs in 40%) and hyperparathyroidism (occurs in 20%).

Points to Remember
- *Thyroid nodules are mostly benign; however, thorough evaluation is essential as 21–26% of these can be cancerous in children and adolescents.*

- *Papillary thyroid cancer is the most common type of thyroid cancer and has a good prognosis.*
- *Medullary thyroid carcinomas account for 5–10% of childhood cancers and can be inherited as part of multiple endocrine neoplasia or familial medullary thyroid carcinoma.*

32.5   Conclusions

Thyroid disorders of childhood are important endocrinopathies which need prompt investigation and treatment in order to allow for normal growth and development. Although rare, conditions such as foetal and neonatal thyrotoxicosis can be fatal necessitating careful maternal history and close monitoring of the foetus and the neonate. Thorough evaluation of thyroid nodules to exclude neoplasia is crucial. Knowledge of association of thyroid cancers with other endocrine neoplasias and a detailed family history are the key to diagnosing inherited thyroid cancers.

References

Abraham P, Avenell A, McGeoch SC, et al. Antithyroid drug regimen for treating Graves' hyperthyroidism. Cochrane Database Syst Rev. 2010;(1):CD003420. https://doi.org/10.1002/14651858.CD003420.pub4.

Batra CM. Fetal and neonatal thyrotoxicosis. Indian J Endocrinol Metab. 2013;17(Suppl 1):S50–4. https://doi.org/10.4103/2230-8210.119505.

Catureglia P, De Remigisa A, Rose NR. Hashimoto thyroiditis: clinical and diagnostic criteria. Autoimmun Rev. 2014;13:391–7.

Cheetham T, Bliss R. Treatment options in the young patient with Graves' disease. Clin Endocrinol. 2016;85(2):161–4. https://doi.org/10.1111/cen.12871.

De Groot L, Abalovich M, Alexander EK, et al. Management of thyroid dysfunction during pregnancy and postpartum: an Endocrine Society clinical practice guideline. J Clin Endocrinol Metab. 2012;97(8):2543.

De Luca F, Santucci S, Corica D, Pitrolo E, Romeo M, Aversa T. Hashimoto's thyroiditis in childhood: presentation modes and evolution over time. Ital J Pediatr. 2013;39:8.

Francis Gary L, Waguespack Steven G, Bauer Andrew J, et al. Management guidelines for children with thyroid nodules and differentiated thyroid cancer: the American Thyroid Association Guidelines Task Force on Pediatric Thyroid Cancer. Thyroid. 2015;25(7):716–59. https://doi.org/10.1089/thy.2014.0460.

Grosse SD, Van Vliet G. Prevention of intellectual disability through screening for congenital hypothyroidism: how much and at what level? Arch Dis Child. 2011;96:374–9.

http://ghr.nlm.nih.gov/condition/congenital-hypothyroidism.

http://www.thyca.org/pediatric/about/.

Kapelari K, Kirchlechner C, Högler W, Schweitzer K, Virgolini I, Moncayo R. Pediatric reference intervals for thyroid hormone levels from birth to adulthood: a retrospective study. BMC Endocr Disord. 2008;8:15. https://doi.org/10.1186/1472-6823-8-15.

Léger J, Olivieri A, Donaldson M, Torresani T, Krude H, van Vliet G, Polak M, Butler G. European Society for Paediatric Endocrinology consensus guidelines on screening, diagnosis, and management of congenital hypothyroidism. Horm Res Paediatr. 2014;81:80–103.

Menconi F, Marcocci C, Marinòl M. Diagnosis and classification of Graves' disease. Autoimmun Rev. 2014;13:398–402.

Ogilvy-Stuart AL. Neonatal thyroid disorders. Arch Dis Child Fetal Neonatal Ed. 2002;87:F165–71.

Okayasu I, Fujiwara M, Hara Y, Tanaka Y, Rose NR. Association of chronic lymphocytic thyroiditis and thyroid papillary carcinoma. A study of surgical cases among Japanese, and White and African Americans. Cancer. 1995;76:2312–8.

Rivkees S. Pediatric Graves' disease: management in the post-propylthiouracil Era. Int J Pediatr Endocrinol. 2014;2014(1):10. https://doi.org/10.1186/1687-9856-2014-10.

Schoenmakers N, Alatzoglou KS, Chatterjee VK, Dattani MT. Recent advances in central congenital hypothyroidism. J Endocrinol. 2015;227(3):R51–71.

Williamson S, Greene SA. Incidence of thyrotoxicosis in childhood: a national population based study in the UK and Ireland. Clin Endocrinol. 2010;72(3):358–63.

Key Reading

1. Léger J, Olivieri A, Donaldson M, Torresani T, Krude H, van Vliet G, Polak M, Butler G. European Society for Paediatric Endocrinology Consensus Guidelines on screening, diagnosis, and management of congenital hypothyroidism. Horm Res Paediatr. 2014;81:80–103.

2. Cheetham T, Bliss R. Treatment options in the young patient with Graves' disease. Clin Endocrinol. 2016;85(2):161–4. https://doi.org/10.1111/cen.12871.

3. Rivkees S. Pediatric Graves' disease: management in the post-propylthiouracil Era. Int J Pediatr Endocrinol. 2014;2014(1):10. https://doi.org/10.1186/1687-9856-2014-10.

4. Bartalena L, Baldeschi L, Dickinson A, et al. Consensus statement of the European Group on Graves' orbitopathy (EUGOGO) on management of GO. Eur J Endocrinol. 2008;158(3):273–85.

5. Francis Gary L, Waguespack Steven G, Bauer Andrew J, et al. Management guidelines for children with thyroid nodules and differentiated thyroid cancer: the American Thyroid Association Guidelines Task Force on Pediatric Thyroid Cancer. Thyroid. 2015;25(7):716–59. https://doi.org/10.1089/thy.2014.0460.

Thyroid Disease in Pre- and Post-Pregnancy

33

Dev A. Kevat and Lucy Mackillop

Contents

D. A. Kevat
Monash Health and Western Health,
Melbourne, VIC, Australia

Department of Endocrinology, Western Health,
St Albans, VIC, Australia

L. Mackillop (✉)
Oxford University Hospitals NHS Foundation Trust
and Nuffield Department of Women's and
Reproductive Health, University of Oxford, Level 6,
Women's Centre, John Radcliffe Hospital,
Oxford, UK
e-mail: lucy.mackillop@ouh.nhs.uk

Abstract

Thyroid dysfunction affects approximately 3% of pregnant women. Adequate thyroid hormone levels are important for fetal development. Normal physiological changes of pregnancy can contribute to subclinical hypothyroidism which may require treatment with thyroxine during pregnancy. Pre-existing hypothyroidism requires an increase in thyroxine dosage. Pre-existing hyperthyroidism may or may not require continued treatment with anti-thyroid medication, though these medications can rarely cause adverse fetal effects. Gestational

© Springer Nature Switzerland AG 2019
S. Llahana et al. (eds.), *Advanced Practice in Endocrinology Nursing*,
https://doi.org/10.1007/978-3-319-99817-6_33

hyperthyroidism must be distinguished from a new diagnosis of Graves' disease in pregnancy. Gestational hyperthyroidism does not require treatment with anti-thyroid medication. Graves' disease requires additional monitoring of mother and fetus and consideration of anti-thyroid medication. Post-partum thyroiditis is an underdiagnosed condition which can cause transient hyperthyroidism before recovery or hypothyroidism, or hypothyroidism without a hyperthyroid phase. Serial monitoring of thyroid function test is required. The vast majority of women with thyroid conditions can be managed to a successful pregnancy outcome.

Keywords

Pregnancy · Thyroid disease · Prenatal care · Postnatal care · Perinatal care

Abbreviations

bHCG	Beta human chorionic gonadotropin
IQ	Intelligence Quotient is an attempt to measure intelligence
T3	Free triiodothyronine
T4	Free thyroxine
TRAb	Thyroid receptor antibody levels
TSH	Thyroid stimulating hormone

Key Terms

- **Thyroid stimulating hormone (TSH):** a hormone made by the pituitary gland which stimulates the thyroid gland to make thyroxine (T4) and a small amount of tri-iodothyronine (T3).
- **Thyroxine (T4):** a hormone created by thyroid gland which travels in the circulation to the body's tissues.
- **Tri-iodothyronine (T3):** a more biologically active hormone mostly created by conversion of T4 to T3 in the body's tissues. A small amount is created by the thyroid gland itself.
- **Thyroxine-binding globulin:** a globulin protein, mostly created in the liver, that binds to T4 and T3 and carries it in the circulation.

Key Points

- The most common thyroid disorders in pregnancy include pre-existing disorders such as Hashimoto's hypothyroidism and Graves' disease as well as pregnancy-specific conditions such as gestational hyperthyroidism.
- The normal physiological changes of pregnancy play a key role in significant changes in thyroid hormone levels during gestation, including the development of subclinical hypothyroidism.
- Appropriate monitoring and management of thyroid conditions in pregnancy are important for health of both mother and fetus.
- Anti-thyroid medication improves the control of hyperthyroid conditions but may cause fetal adverse effects.
- The vast majority of women with thyroid conditions can be managed to a successful pregnancy outcome.

33.1 Physiology of Changes in Pregnancy Affecting Thyroid Function and Testing

The demands of pregnancy induce a number of significant physiological changes including profound cardiovascular adaptations, a 15% increase in basal metabolic rate, and a symphony of hormonal changes. Human chorionic gonadotropin levels increase greatly during the first trimester; oestrogen, progesterone, cortisol, and prolactin levels also increase, whilst lutenising and follicular stimulating hormone levels decrease. From an immunological perspective, a shift away from cell-mediated immunity (Th1 response) to humoral immunity (Th2 response) can result in some conditions such as Graves' disease improving during pregnancy.

Three key changes drive important changes in thyroid function (Glinoer 1998b)

1. **Increase in thyroid binding globulin levels**
   Thyroid binding globulin levels increase two- to threefold as a result of elevating oes-

trogen levels. As a greater proportion of thyroxine (T4) is bound to thyroid binding globulin, free thyroxine levels tend to decrease. Free triiodothyronine (T3) also tends to decrease. As is the case outside pregnancy, reduced thyroxine levels provide negative feedback to the hypothalamic-pituitary axis (Chap. 1) in order to try to maintain euthyroid equilibrium and steady state via a stimulus to increase in thyroid stimulating hormone (TSH). The increase in thyroid stimulating hormone is evident across trimesters. In women who have sufficient iodine intake, free thyroxine and triiodothyronine levels fall up to 15% during pregnancy.

2. **Action of human chorionic gonadotropin on the thyroid, particularly during the first trimester**

   Human chorionic gonadotropin is an essential hormone for a successful pregnancy. It is produced by the syncytiotrophoblast in the placenta and helps sustain the corpus luteum in the early stages of pregnancy. The corpus luteum produces progesterone which promotes the uterine thickening which allows the successful development of the implanted zygote/embryo.

   Absolute human chorionic gonadotropin levels vary between individuals, but increase exponentially after conception and Week 6 of pregnancy (beta human chorionic gonadotropin (bHCG) levels 1000–55,000 mIU/L), with further large increases to Week 12 (25,000–290,000 mIU/L), before decreasing to less than half the latter concentration by the time of delivery. There is evidence that human chorionic gonadotropin can directly stimulate the thyroid gland in a similar manner to thyroid stimulation hormone due to having a similar chemical structure known as molecular mimicry.

   In some women with bHCG levels greater than 50,000 mIU/L for more than 3 days, the stimulatory effect of human chorionic gonadotropin on the thyroid gland is sufficient to drive thyroxine and triiodothyronine levels high enough to cause symptomatic hyperthyroidism (e.g. with palpitations and tremor). There is a concomitant suppression of thyroid stimulating hormone production. Whilst most women do not suffer from hyperthyroidism in this manner, the effects of human chorionic gonadotropin do still exert a downward or blunting effect on thyroid stimulating hormone levels, particularly during the first trimester. Some research suggests that every 10,000 mIU/L increase in bHCG levels correlates with a 0.6 pmol/L increase in thyroxine levels and a decrease of 0.1 mIU/L in thyroid stimulating hormone level (Glinoer 1999).

3. **The placenta as an active endocrine organ**

   The placenta contains Type II deiodinase and Type III deiodinase. Type II deiodinase converts thyroxine (T4) to triiodothyronine (T3). It is also present in the thyroid gland. Type III deiodinase converts thyroxine and triiodothyronine to biologically inactive reverse triiodothyronine (reverse T3) and diiodothyronine (T2).

   The manner in which placental enzymatic activity regulates the hormonal environment for the developing fetus is not completely understood. It is generally agreed that the placenta plays a role in the need for increased maternal creation and turnover of thyroxine. This increased demand can result in women without sufficient iodine intake becoming hypothyroid.

33.2 An Approach to Abnormal Thyroid Function in Pregnancy

Iodine sufficiency should be ensured in all women, which usually requires supplementation of dietary sources (Box 33.1). Universal thyroid function testing is not currently recommended. Women with a personal history of thyroid disease should be tested when seeking to conceive and in the first trimester with management tailored to the particular condition. Women with a history of autoimmune disease should be considered for testing. Antibody testing is generally a useful adjunct to testing of thyroid function when patients have a history of autoimmune thyroid or other disease. Women who have a diagnosis of any thyroid disorder will require

Box 33.1 Practice Tips: Iodine Requirements in Pregnancy

Iodine is the key component for the biosynthesis of thyroid hormone. Inadequate intake predisposes a woman to hypothyroidism (Glinoer 1997). For both pregnancy and during breastfeeding, 250 μg/day is recommended by the World Health Organization and a number of key bodies, though not yet the United Kingdom Scientific Advisory Committee on Nutrition. This intake recommendation is higher than the 140–150 μg/day suggested for non-pregnant adults. Research has shown that iodine insufficiency does exist in developed countries including the United Kingdom.

Iodine is most often consumed in milk products, seafood, and shellfish. Organic milk contains less iodine. Grains may contain some iodine depending on the soil characteristics of cultivation, though levels vary. In some countries, salt is iodised.

All pregnant and breastfeeding women should be advised to take a supplement to ensure their intake of iodine is at least 250 μg/day. Different formulations of pregnancy vitamins can have different amounts of iodine and this should be scrutinised for adequacy prior to purchase and on clinical review. Consumption of more than 500 μg/day is not recommended.

monitoring throughout pregnancy though most conditions have a tendency to stabilise in the second and third trimesters.

33.3 Thyroid Disorders During Pregnancy

The two most common causes of hyperthyroidism in pregnancy are gestational hyperthyroidism and Graves' disease. Most women with Graves' disease are diagnosed before rather than during pregnancy. Rarer causes of hyperthyroidism can include the hyperthyroid phase of Hashimoto's disease, gestational trophoblastic disease (e.g. molar pregnancy), and exogenous taking of thyroxine tablets inappropriately or at the incorrect dose.

Hypothyroidism and subclinical hypothyroidism is most commonly caused by the physiological changes of pregnancy and is termed gestational (subclinical) hypothyroidism. Women with insufficient iodine intake are at greater risk of becoming hypothyroid. A second important cause is Hashimoto's disease which is an immune condition (See Chap. 30) can be diagnosed prior to or during pregnancy.

33.3.1 Gestational Hyperthyroidism

Gestational hyperthyroidism is due to the direct stimulatory effect of human chorionic gonadotropin on the maternal thyroid gland. It usually occurs during the first trimester and usually resolves by the end of the first half of pregnancy. This is because human chorionic gonadotropin levels are at their highest levels toward the end of the first trimester, and in some women are sustained at high enough levels to drive excess thyroxine (T4) production by the thyroid. Gestational hyperthyroidism is associated in some women with hyperemesis gravidarum which is characterised by severe nausea and vomiting. Both conditions are more common in twin pregnancy (Glinoer 1998a, b, c).

33.3.1.1 Diagnosis
Diagnosis of gestational hyperthyroidism is based on a combination of clinical features and laboratory investigations.

- Women often suffer from classical symptoms and signs of hyperthyroidism including palpitations, tremor, weight loss or lack of weight gain, anxiety and heat intolerance. On examination, they can be tachycardic. They do not have prominent eyes or an eye disease which is associated with Graves' disease. The thyroid gland is usually normal in size.

- On thyroid function testing, thyroxine and tri-iodothyronine levels are elevated beyond the reference range, and thyroid stimulating hormone production are usually less than 0.5 mIU/L and can be undetectably low.
- Thyroid receptor antibody levels (TRAb) are important to perform and are negative.

33.3.1.2 Maternal Concerns

Gestational hyperthyroidism can significantly diminish a women's quality of life (Glinoer 1998b).

Once a diagnosis is made, it is important to ask about symptoms of hyperemesis gravidarum, and seek specialist medical care for that condition if required. Even in the absence of hyperemesis gravidarum, weight loss and lack of weight gain caused by hyperthyroidism can be concerning for the patient, and increased caloric intake to compensate should be encouraged.

33.3.1.3 Fetal Concerns

Women who have gestational hyperthyroidism and hyperemesis gravidarum may not be able to meet nutritional requirements with consequent fetal risk of intrauterine growth retardation. The fetus of a woman with gestational hyperthyroidism only is not at significantly increased risk of adverse outcomes because of the transient nature of the condition.

33.3.1.4 Management

Steps in management include:

- Education and reassurance of the patient that the condition is usually self-limiting and very unlikely to cause any harm to the fetus
- Activate social supports including in cases of anxiety
- Encourage sufficient caloric intake
- Urgent referral to a specialist doctor if hyperemesis gravidarum is suspected
- Consideration of beta-blocker medication in severe cases, e.g. propranolol or labetalol. Side effects and safety in pregnancy should be discussed. Anti-thyroid medication is not required.

- Clinical review of the patient at 3–4 week intervals with repeat thyroid function tests until symptoms and thyroid function tests normalise

33.3.2 Pre-existing Hyperthyroid Conditions

Graves' disease is the most common cause of pre-existing hyperthyroidism. The condition is described fully in Chap. 28. Women of child-bearing age with the condition should be counselled to use contraception until the disease is appropriately managed and disease activity levels are well controlled. Successful pregnancy is certainly possible for women with a history of the condition. Appropriate counselling should occur of the risks the condition poses for pregnancy, including the potential fetal effects of anti-thyroid drugs. Such pregnancies should not be considered "low risk". Women who have had a thyroidectomy to treat Graves' disease can still have circulating thyroid receptor antibodies which can affect a pregnancy. Antibody levels three times the upper limit of the normal reference range denote pregnancies of highest risk. Toxic (hyperfunctioning) nodules (see Chap. 28) can also cause hyperthyroidism in pregnancy.

33.3.2.1 Diagnosis

Diagnosis both in and outside of pregnancy is based on clinical symptoms and supporting investigation results. Women often present with symptoms of hyperthyroidism including weight loss, palpitations, hair loss, difficulty sleeping, and diarrhoea. Graves' disease can cause eye problems including exophthalmos (prominent or bulging eyes), slowed eye movements, and chemosis (swelling of the conjunctivae). Occasionally, women can present reporting that other people have told the patient that their eyes have changed.

- Thyroid receptor antibody (TRAb) levels can be measured in blood. The widely available test is accurate (both sensitive and specific)

tion. The medications can also cause disturbances in liver function, with rare cases of liver failure also reported particularly with propylthiouracil.

33.3.2.3 Fetal Concerns

Graves' disease is associated with intrauterine growth retardation, miscarriage, and pre-term delivery. The fetal thyroid develops from 6 weeks and produces thyroxine during the second half of pregnancy. The thyroid receptor antibodies associated with the Graves' disease can cross the placenta and stimulate the fetal thyroid causing hyperthyroidism. There is some evidence that hyperthyroidism may be associated with an increased risk of later seizure and neurobehavioural disorders.

Anti-thyroid medication reduces thyroxine and triiodothyronine levels in the maternal circulation with transmission to the fetus via the placenta which plays an active role in regulation of these hormones in the intrauterine environment. If such hormone levels are greatly reduced, the fetus can become hypothyroid. In rare cases, the fetus can develop a goitre as a consequence, which can put pressure on its trachea.

Anti-thyroid medication can also directly affect the fetus. Aplasia cutis (absence of a portion of skin, e.g. on scalp) and congenital abnormalities such as oesophageal atresia and dysmorphic facies have been reported with use of carbimazole (Yoshihara 2012). Face or neck cysts and urinary tract abnormalities in male offspring have been reported with propylthiouracil. As these abnormalities are not considered as severe as those with carbimazole, propylthiouracil is usually used during the first trimester, the key period of fetal organogenesis. Specialist medical advice should be sought on medication choice, as guidelines are being revised in a number of countries.

33.3.2.4 Management

Principles of management include:

- Pre-pregnancy counselling and disease control by a specialist physician.
- Regular clinical review with thyroid function tests during pregnancy—e.g. every 4–6 weeks if stable, every 2 weeks if medication changes are being made or the condition is not stable.

and is useful for diagnosis and as a marker of current disease activity.
- Thyroid uptake scans are a nuclear medicine scan which can also be used to diagnosis and assess the activity levels of Graves' disease. However, as the scan requires the use of a radionucleotide tracer which emits radiation, scans are not performed on pregnant women, and are generally avoided in the breastfeeding mother.

33.3.2.2 Maternal Concerns

Even when the condition is adequately treated, Graves' disease is associated with higher rates of miscarriage, pre-eclampsia, placental abruption, preterm delivery, and thyroid storm. Pregnancy carries with it a risk of worsening Graves' eye disease.

The medications used most commonly for Graves' disease in the United Kingdom are carbimazole and propylthiouracil. Methimazole is commonly prescribed in the United States. Both of these anti-thyroid drugs can cause disturbances in the production of red and white blood cells, with consequent anaemia and poor immune func-

- In patients who require medication, use of the lowest dose of anti-thyroid medication required. Propylthiouracil Ideally 250 mg or less (total daily dose) is often used in the first trimester with consideration of patients being changed to Carbimazole Ideally 20 mg or less (total daily dose) in the second and third trimester. Remaining on a single type of medication throughout pregnancy is also appropriate in some cases. Although the potential fetal effects such as intrauterine growth retardation must be considered, beta-blocker medication such as Propranolol can be used to assist with hyperthyroid symptoms.
- Treatment is aimed to keep maternal thyroxine level at the upper limit of the normal range to minimise the risk of fetal hypothyroidism.
- Medication doses can often be reduced or ceased during the second and third trimester due to maternal immune system changes.
- Thyroidectomy can be considered in severe, resistant cases or in cases of allergies to medication.
- Thyroid receptor antibody levels should be performed regularly including at initial review, at 18–22, and at 30–34 weeks gestation to aid in estimating effects on the fetus.
- Post-partum review is essential as women are at risk of disease relapse particularly in the first 2 months after delivery.
- The neonate requires thyroid function tests at day 5 and day 10 and whilst mild abnormalities are often found, they are transient and rarely require treatment. However undiagnosed thyrotoxicosis in the neonate carries a high mortality rate, hence the need to perform these blood tests.
- Use of up to 20 mg of Carbimazole if needed is considered safe for breastfeeding.

Toxic Nodules

Toxic (hyperfunctioning) nodules are a rare cause of hyperthyroidism during pregnancy. Some women will have the nodules ablated using radioactive iodine prior to pregnancy and be euthyroid. Toxic nodules do not produce antibodies. Some women may need anti-thyroid medication

through the pregnancy, usually at low doses. The risks of these medications are described in the previous section. There is no evidence that toxic nodules change their level of activity during pregnancy. Subclinical hyperthyroidism (suppressed thyroid stimulating hormone with thyroxine levels in the normal range) may not need treatment, but overt hyperthyroidism should prompt strong consideration of medication to avoid increased risks of miscarriage and other problems.

33.3.3 Pre-existing Hypothyroidism

Pre-existing hypothyroidism in pregnant women may be due to known Hashimoto's hypothyroidism, or an induced hypothyroid state consequent to the treatment of a hyperthyroid state (e.g. Graves' disease, toxic nodules) with radioactive iodine or thyroidectomy. Thyroidectomy may also have been performed as management for thyroid malignancy or multinodular goitre. Rarer causes of pre-existing hypothyroidism include pituitary dysfunction, previous pituitary surgery, and congenital hypothyroidism. Women with pre-existing hypothyroidism will likely already be on thyroxine replacement. Some will be seeing a specialist physician, though many will be managed at primary care level. The key issue in women with pre-existing hypothyroidism is the need for an increased thyroxine dose due to the physiological changes of pregnancy outlined above.

33.3.3.1 Diagnosis
The original cause of a women's hypothyroidism will usually have been diagnosed prior to pregnancy.

- If thyroxine doses are not increased, some women with pre-existing hypothyroidism will have an increase in their thyroid stimulating hormone levels in the first trimester.
- Women with pituitary dysfunction or previous pituitary surgery will not have such a rise as the pituitary is not able to respond to as

according to usual negative feedback principles (See Chap. 26).

- All women may have free thyroxine levels that reduce to the lower part of below the laboratory reference range. Even in the absence of conclusive evidence that thyroid stimulating hormone levels have risen or thyroxine levels have fallen, it is often the case that a greater dose of thyroxine is required.

33.3.3.2 Maternal Concerns

Women with pre-existing hypothyroidism who become pregnant can be asymptomatic or suffer the symptoms of over hypothyroidism such as tiredness and weight gain. However, symptoms of hypothyroidism may be confused with symptoms of normal pregnancy. Thyroid function testing is therefore essential. Profound untreated hypothyroidism is associated with an increased risk of maternal anaemia, heart failure, muscle weakness, pre-eclampsia, placental abruption, and post-partum haemorrhage.

33.3.3.3 Fetal Concerns

Severe maternal hypothyroidism, usually due to iodine deficiency in developing countries, can cause fetal cognitive, neurological, and developmental abnormalities including a constellation of these effects previously termed "cretinism". Many women with pre-existing hypothyroidism are at risk of milder hypothyroidism in pregnancy, therefore requiring early testing and an increase in the thyroxine dose as indicated. A large cohort study found a 7-point lower IQ in the offspring of undertreated hypothyroid mothers, with delays in motor skill development, language development, and attention at 7–9 years of age (Haddow et al. 1999). Maternal hypothyroidism is associated with an increased risk of a low birthweight baby and prematurity.

33.3.3.4 Management

- Women with pre-existing hypothyroidism should either have thyroid function tested as soon as possible after becoming pregnant with dose titration, or be instructed to increase their dose of Thyroxine by approximately 25% on becoming pregnant. As fetal brain development occurs predominantly in the first trimester, the dose increase should not be delayed whilst awaiting specialist review, or if thyroid function testing will cause undue delay.

- Thyroid function tests should ideally be done early in pregnancy and then 4–6 weekly during the first trimester, and then at least once in each of the second and third trimesters. Titration of Thyroxine dose to keep the thyroid stimulating hormone level at the appropriate trimester-specific range. Some women will need a 50% increase in dose. Rarely, after a significant dose increase, thyroid stimulating hormone levels may depress below the reference range. When this happens, the Thyroxine dose may need to be decreased slightly.

- Women should be re-educated in an ideal manner to take Thyroxine medication, on an empty stomach (usually morning), with a sip of water if required. Milk, including tea or coffee should not be consumed for an hour after taking Thyroxine, and other medication including pregnancy multivitamins should be taken at least an hour later.

- On delivery of the baby, the mother should be instructed to return to her pre-pregnancy dose of Thyroxine. No wean or gradual reduction is required.

- The mother should be asked to have repeat thyroid function testing 6–8 weeks postpartum, ideally with her primary care practitioner who will be managing her ongoing care.

33.3.4 Subclinical Hypothyroidism

Subclinical hypothyroidism is common in pregnancy due to the physiological changes of pregnancy outlined above. Treatment thresholds can vary and are in a state of change. Consequently, it is worthwhile consulting local guidelines and clinical leadership for any established management practices. Gestational subclinical hypothyrodism is a transient condition in which the requirement for treatment with thyroxine ceases on delivery. The condition may reoccur in future pregnancies.

Subclinical hypothyroidism is defined as an elevated thyroid stimulating hormone level with thyroxine and triiodothyronine levels in the normal range. Pregnancy and trimester-specific reference ranges should be used when available. Thyroid peroxidase antibodies should be tested to help determine whether the woman has hitherto undiagnosed hypothyroidism or is likely to develop long-term hypothyroidism due to Hashimoto's disease.

33.3.4.1   Diagnosis

In all cases of subclinical hypothyroidism, thyroxine and triiodothyronine levels should be in the normal range. If these levels are lower than the reference range, the patient has overt hypothyroidism and will also require treatment with Thyroxine.

- Total or free hormone level reference ranges can be used and ideally should be pregnancy specific. Usually, the normal range is defined as being between the 2.5th and 97.5th centiles of the relevant normal population (Table 33.1).

33.3.4.2   Maternal Concerns

Subclinical hypothyroidism has been associated with impaired fertility; with the use of thyroxine in women undergoing treatment with assisted reproductive technology becoming common. An association with miscarriage has also been a concern though more recent data has not supported this finding.

There have been studies and meta-analyses of the relationship between subclinical hypothyroidism and the risks of gestational diabetes, placenta previa, placental abruption, and/or pre-eclampsia. Results have differed consider-

Table 33.1 Thyroid stimulating hormone levels that prompt a diagnosis can vary depending on the guidelines being used

	Trimester			
	1	2	3	
TSH (mIU/L)	Pregnancy/ trimester-specific ranges			
TSH (mIU/L)	>2.5	>3.0	>3.5	European Thyroid Association 2014 (Lazarus et al. 2014)
TSH (mIU/L)	>4.0	>4.0	>4.0	American Thyroid Association 2017 (Alexander et al. 2017)

ably, partly because of variability in inclusion of overtly hypothyroid women.

33.3.4.3   Fetal Concerns

As overt hypothyroidism has been associated with lower IQ in children, there has been concern that the offspring of women with subclinical hypothyroidism may also suffer adverse cognitive effects. Studies have reported conflicting results (Williams 2012). Treating pregnant women to a thyroid stimulating hormone level of <1.0 mIU/L did not improve IQ tested at 3 years of age (Lazarus et al. 2012).

One meta-analysis found an increased risk pre-term delivery and perinatal mortality with subclinical hypothyroidism (Van De Bougard et al. 2011) though many individual studies have not concluded this.

33.3.4.4   Management

- Women should be re-educated in an ideal manner to take Thyroxine medication, on an empty stomach (usually morning), with a sip of water if required. Milk, including tea or coffee should not be consumed for an hour after taking Thyroxine, and other medication including pregnancy multivitamins should be taken at least an hour later.
- On a diagnosis of subclinical hypothyroidism, Thyroxine should be commenced at a dose of 50 mcg. If the thyroid stimulating hormone level is grossly elevated (e.g. >10 mIU/L), and/or the patient is obese or has a high weight, a higher commencement dose can be considered.
- Further thyroid function testing should occur 4–6 weeks after dose commencement or change, at least once a trimester. Dosages can be titrated to achieve the required target thyroid stimulating hormone. In general, the dosage of Thyroxine will be more stable in the second and third trimester.
- Thyroid peroxidase antibody levels should be tested. If they are positive, strong consideration should be given to continuing Thyroxine after delivery with instructions for testing and titration 6 weeks post-partum by the primary care practitioner.
- If thyroid peroxidase antibodies are negative, and the woman thus has uncomplicated sub-

clinical hypothyroidism, the woman should be instructed to return to cease Thyroxine after delivery. No wean or gradual reduction is required (Negro et al. 2011).

Box 33.3 Case Example 2. Anxiety and Explanations

K.P is a 26-year-old lady who is 8 weeks into her second pregnancy. Her first child has Autism Spectrum Disorder. K.P is well and without symptoms. After missing her period, she visited her primary care practice. The GP registrar ordered a number of blood tests including thyroid function tests before referring her to your clinic. K.P is a little anxious about her results. She has no significant past medical history.

Examination is unremarkable. Thyroid function test results are TSH 5.5 mIU/L (NR 0.5-4.0), T4 13 pmol/L (NR 10-20), and T3 5 pmol/L (NR 4-7).

What further test is it important to order? How would you counsel and manage K.P?

Please refer to the end of this chapter for answers related to this case

---

33.3.5 Positive Thyroid Peroxidase Antibodies with Otherwise Normal Thyroid Function

Some women who are seeking to conceive or are pregnant will have positive thyroid peroxidase antibodies but will have thyroid stimulating hormone and thyroxine levels in the normal range. Whilst some research has suggested that commencing such women on Thyroxine will assist with fertility success, a greater number of studies have not supported such a finding. Whilst it is not necessary to cease Thyroxine if it has been commenced by another clinician, it is not desirable to commence Thyroxine in such women. There is a reported association between positive thyroid peroxidase antibodies and spontaneous miscarriage and premature delivery though guidelines do not recommend commencing thyroxine as there is insufficient evidence that this changes outcomes (De Leo and Pearce 2017).

33.3.5.1 Management
- When necessary, counsel women that the majority of the evidence indicates that commencing Thyroxine in their situation is unnecessary and does not change outcomes.
- Inform that the positive antibodies suggest a higher background risk of becoming or developing hypothyroidism in the future
- Monitor the woman's thyroid function tests 4–6 weekly until mid-gestation and then if stable at 30 weeks
- Inform the woman and communicate with her primary care doctor that she should have her thyroid function tested at 6 weeks postpartum, and thereafter 4–6 monthly for at least a year and then as her doctor guides. A woman with positive thyroid peroxidase antibodies is at a higher risk of post-partum thyroiditis and a long-term risk of hypothyroidism

---

33.4 Thyroid Disorders in the Puerperium (Postpartum) Period

33.4.1 Introduction

The most common thyroid disorder during the post-partum period is post-partum thyroiditis which affects approximately 5% of the population (Stagnaro-Green 2015). Unfortunately, this autoimmune condition is underdiagnosed, with symptoms often being attributed to the challenges of caring for a newborn child.

Approximately a quarter of women with postpartum thyroiditis will experience the "classical" course of hyperthyroidism followed by hypothyroidism. Half will develop hypothyroidism without a hyperthyroid phase. The remainder will have isolated hyperthyroidism only. Some women who become hypothyroid will remain so for the long term.

33.4.1.1 Diagnosis

Women can suffer from hyper- or hypothyroid symptoms (Chaps. 3 and 5) depending on the subtype of hypothyroidism.

- Common hyperthyroid symptoms in the condition are palpitations, heat intolerance, irritability, and fatigue.
- Tiredness, cold intolerance, dry skin, and impaired memory are common in those women who become hypothyroid.
- Post-partum thyroiditis is strongly associated with positive thyroid peroxidase antibodies, which is a useful adjunct test together with thyroid function tests. Women who test positive for thyroid peroxidase antibodies have greater than a 30% chance of developing post-partum thyroiditis.
- Thyroid receptor antibodies should also be tested to exclude Graves' disease—there is also an increased risk of the new development of Graves' disease in the post-partum period. The presence of thyroid receptor antibodies is very likely to indicate Graves' disease.
- Thyroglobulin antibodies may also be positive but provide limited further diagnostic value in the modern context.
- A nuclear medicine thyroid uptake scan (I-131, Tc-99m) can be used to help distinguish different types of thyroid disease. Such imaging is possible in the post-partum period provided breast milk is discarded for the required interval (4 days I-131, 1 day Tc-99m), but in practice other diagnostic methods are strongly preferred.
- Given the common nature of post-partum thyroiditis, there should be a low threshold for thyroid function testing during this time. Women are particularly at risk of developing the disorder 6–10 weeks after delivery but it can occur up to 12 months post-partum. Serial thyroid function testing every 2–3 months is often helpful in determining the subtype of disorder.
- Women with autoimmune diseases such as Type 1 diabetes and systemic lupus erythematosus have a two- to threefold increased over-background risk of developing post-partum

thyroiditis. Women with Graves' disease are also at higher risk of developing post-partum thyroiditis. Such women should ideally be reviewed clinically approximately 6 weeks post-partum, with some clinicians reasonably opting to test thyroid function tests in this group regardless of symptomatology.

33.4.1.2 Maternal Concerns

Both the symptoms of hyperthyroidism and hypothyroidism can obviously make caring for a newborn or infant child even more challenging. Given hypothyroidism can cause low mood, particular interest has been focused on the relationship between post-partum thyroiditis and depression. The evidence is conflicting with some studies indicating increased risk whilst other studies have not demonstrated this link. It is prudent to screen women for common depressive symptoms (Table 33.2) and refer appropriately. Research has specifically not shown increased risk of the rarer condition of depression with psychotic features.

33.4.1.3 Neonatal Concerns

There is some evidence that selenium can reduce the risk and severity of post-partum thyroiditis in women who have positive thyroid peroxidase antibodies in pregnancy. However, commencing selenium in this context has yet to become clinical practice, pending further studies to replicate findings.

Table 33.2 Common depressive symptoms in post-partum period

Anhedonia—markedly diminished interest or pleasure in almost all activities
Low mood
Fatigue
Feeling restless or slowed down
Feelings of worthlessness or guilt
Poor sleep—sleeping excessively, difficulty sleeping, and/or early morning wakening
Poor appetite
Thoughts or preoccupation with death or dying including suicide
Irritability
Significant weight loss or weight gain
Difficulty with concentration/memory

Women with autoimmune conditions (e.g. Type 1 diabetes) should receive a clinical review and strong consideration of testing of thyroid function tests and thyroid peroxidase antibodies approximately 6 weeks post-partum.

33.4.1.4 Management

- Management of hyperthyroid phase in affected individuals who are significantly symptomatic is with beta-blocker medication, usually propranolol 10–20 mg three to four times a day.
- Women with post-partum thyroiditis require long-term follow-up to monitor for the emergence of hypothyroidism.

Box 33.4 Case Example 3. Post-partum Struggles

H.O is 5 weeks post-partum, having delivered her first child who was born healthy at term. Her thyroid function tests (thyroid stimulating hormone and thyroxine/T4) during pregnancy were normal though her thyroid peroxidase antibodies were on the upper limit of the normal range. H.O was not started on thyroxine. Her sister and mother have had Hashimoto's hypothyroidism for a number of years.

H.O phones you as you reviewed her during her pregnancy. She says she is struggling to sleep and noticed she is losing hair. H.O says she is often worried about her baby's feeding and sleeping and feels overwhelmed. Her husband works long hours, and her own family are overseas.

How would you manage H.O in this situation?
What tests would you organise and what would you expect to find?

Please refer to the end of this chapter for answers related to this case

---

33.5 Conclusions

Thyroid disease can have a diverse range of causes and presentations during pregnancy. The most common conditions of subclinical hypothyroidism and pre-existing hypothyroidism can be well managed with thyroxine commencement and adjustment, with regular thyroid function test monitoring. Gestational hyperthyroidism is a self-limiting condition which should be distinguished from Graves' disease. Graves' disease requires specialist input throughout pregnancy and surveillance in the post-partum period. Post-partum thyroiditis can cause hypothyroidism or hyperthyroidism. The condition is common and underdiagnosed. Thyroid function tests should be organised if there is clinical suspicion, and patients will require long-term follow-up.

Case Study 2–4. Answers

Case study 2: M.R symptoms of palpitations, difficulty sleeping, and not putting on weight are consistent with hyperthyroidism. Her thyroid function tests support this with an elevated thyroxine/T4 and supressed thyroid stimulating hormone levels. As she is in the first trimester, gestational hyperthyroidism caused by BHCG stimulation of the thyroid is the probable diagnosis. Although the condition is considered "benign" in that it does not cause fetal problems or long-term maternal problems, women can be significantly symptomatic. It is important to test for thyroid receptor antibodies to distinguish from the serious condition of Graves' disease. A positive result for such antibodies should prompt immediate contact with a specialist. M.R should be counselled that the condition is self-limiting and likely to improve in the next 2–6 weeks as BHCGs levels fall in the second trimester. She should be encouraged to eat more and to activate social supports. Beta-blocker medication can be considered in severe cases for short-term use with the involvement of a medical practitioner.

Case study 3: K.P has subclinical hypothyroidism as defined by her thyroid stimulating hormone being marginally elevated and her thyroid stimulating hormone being in the normal range. Most women with this condition are asymptomatic. In the context of having a child with Autism Spectrum Disorder, K.P may be particularly concerned about anything she has read or heard regarding a link between "low thyroid levels" and "intellectual problems". It is important to reassure K.P that this generally occurs in cases much more severe than her situation. K.P should be tested for thyroid peroxidase antibodies, the presence of these may indicate that she would benefit from post-partum monitoring for the development of post-partum thyroiditis or hypothyroidism. During pregnancy, a small dose of thyroxine (e.g. 50mcg daily) should be started with titration to the pregnancy-specific thyroid stimulating hormone targets outlined in this chapter, or as per local guidelines.

Case example 4: H's symptom of losing hair is consistent with hyperthyroidism. Her difficulty in sleeping and concern about her child's welfare may be expected with a newborn child, but may also be due or worsened by hyperthyroidism. It can be difficult to distinguish such a situation clinically, and therefore thyroid function and thyroid antibody tests, especially thyroid peroxidase antibodies, should be requested. Together these results (supressed thyroid stimulating hormone, elevated thyroxine/T4, positive thyroid peroxidase, and thyroglobulin antibodies) may indicate a diagnosis of post-partum thyroiditis. Serial clinical and biochemical monitoring of women with post-partum thyroiditis is required. In the long-term, hypothyroidism may develop and require treatment with thyroxine.

References

Alexander EK, et al. 2017 guidelines of the American Thyroid Association for the diagnosis and management of thyroid disease during pregnancy and the postpartum. Thyroid. 2017;27(3):315–89.

De Leo S, Pearce E. Autoimmune thyroid disease during pregnancy. Lancet Diabetes Endocrinol. 2017. http://www.thelancet.com/pdfs/journals/landia/PIIS2213-8587(17)30402-3.pdf, https://www.ncbi.nlm.nih.gov/pubmed/29246752. Accessed 22 March 2018.

Glinoer D. Maternal and fetal impact of chronic iodine deficiency. Clin Obstet Gynecol. 1997;40(1):102–16.

Glinoer D. Thyroid hyperfunction during pregnancy. Thyroid. 1998a;8(9):859–64.

Glinoer D. The systematic screening and management of hypothyroidism and hyperthyroidism during pregnancy. Trends Endocrinol Metab. 1998b;9(10):403–11.

Glinoer D. Iodine supplementation during pregnancy: importance and biochemical assessment. Exp Clin Endocrinol Diabetes. 1998c;106(Suppl 3):S21.

Glinoer D. What happens to the normal thyroid during pregnancy? Thyroid. 1999;9(7):631–5.

Haddow JE, et al. Maternal thyroid deficiency during pregnancy and subsequent neuropsychological development of the child. N Engl J Med. 1999;341(8):549–55.

Lazarus JH, et al. Antenatal thyroid screening and childhood cognitive function. N Engl J Med. 2012;366(6):493–50.

Lazarus J, et al. 2014 European thyroid association guidelines for the management of subclinical hypothyroidism in pregnancy and in children. Eur Thyroid J. 2014;3(2):76–94.

Negro R, et al. Thyroid antibody positivity in the first trimester of pregnancy is associated with negative pregnancy outcomes. J Clin Endocrinol Metab. 2011;96(6):E920–4.

Stagnaro-Green A. Chapter 4: Approach to the patient with postpartum thyroiditis. In: Wartofsky L, editor. Clinical approach to endocrine & metabolic diseases; 2015.

Van De Bougard E, Vissenburg R, Land JA, Van Wely M, VanDerPost JA, Goddijn M, Bisschop PH. Significance of (sub)clinical thyroid dysfunctionand and thyroid autoimmunity before conception and in early pregnancy: a systematic review. Human Reprod Update. 2011;17(5):605–19.

Williams F, et al. Mild maternal thyroid dysfunction at delivery of infants born ≤34 weeks and neurodevelopmental outcome at 5.5 years. J Clin Endocrinol Metab. 2012;97(6):1977–85.

Yoshihara A, et al. Treatment of graves' disease with antithyroid drugs in the first trimester of pregnancy and the prevalence of congenital malformation. J Clin Endocrinol Metab. 2012;97(7):2396–403.

Key Reading

1. Alexander EK, Pearce EN, Brent GA. Guidelines of the American Thyroid Association for the Diagnosis and Management of Thyroid Disease During Pregnancy and the Postpartum. Thyroid. 2017;27(3):315–89. https://doi.org/10.1089/thy.2016.0457.

2. Lazarus J, Brown RS, Daumerie C, et al. 2014 European thyroid association guidelines for the management of subclinical hypothyroidism in pregnancy and in children. Thyroid J. 2014;3(2):76–94. https://doi.org/10.1159/000362597.

3. Cignini P, et al. Thyroid physiology and common diseases in pregnancy: review of literature. J Prenat Med. 2012;6(4):64–71.

Part V

The Adrenal Gland

Sofia Llahana

Anatomy and Physiology of the Adrenal Gland

34

Phillip Yeoh

Contents

Abstract

The adrenal glands are important endocrine organ that produces corticosteroids including glucocorticoids, mineralocorticoids and androgens. These are important hormones that regulate sodium retention, blood pressure, fluid volume, the immune system, metabolism and behaviour. The adrenals also exert negative feedback mechanism in the hypothalamus and pituitary through the hormone cortisol. High levels of cortisol suppress the pituitary hormone ACTH whereas low cortisol stimulates ACTH secretion by increasing the release of hypothalamic hormones CRH and AVP. The adrenal medulla, which is located in the central part of the adrenal, forms part of the sympathetic nervous system and is referred as the sympatho-adrenomedullary system. It secrets epinephrine (adrenaline), norepinephrine (noradrenaline) and dopamine in response to stimulation by the sympathetic nervous system.

Keywords

Adrenal · Hypothalamic-pituitary axis · Zona glomerulosa · Zona fasciculata · Zona reticularis · Adrenal cortex · Adrenal medulla · Aldosterone · Cortisol · Androgen

P. Yeoh (✉)
The London Clinic, London, UK
e-mail: p.yeoh@thelondonclinic.co.uk

© Springer Nature Switzerland AG 2019
S. Llahana et al. (eds.), *Advanced Practice in Endocrinology Nursing*,
https://doi.org/10.1007/978-3-319-99817-6_34

Abbreviations

ACTH	Adrenocorticotropic hormone
AGP	Adrenogonadal primordium
AngII	Angiotensin II
AR	Androgen receptor
AVP	Arginine vasopressin
CAH	Congenital adrenal hyperplasia
CBG	Corticosteroid-binding globulin
CRH	Corticotropin releasing hormone
DHEA	Dehydroepiandrosterone
DHEAS	Dehydroepiandrosterone sulphate
DHT	Dihydrotestosterone
GC	Glucocorticoid
GR	Glucocorticoid cell receptor
HPA	Hypothalamic pituitary axis
PAPS	3'-phosphoadenosine-5'-phophosulfate
PCOS	Polycystic ovarian syndrome
SCN	Hypothalamic suprachiasmatic nucleus
zF	Zona fasciculata
zG	Zona glomerulosa
zR	Zona reticularis

Key Terms
- **Outer layers of adrenal cortex:** This is made up of the zona glomerulosa (zG), zona fasciculata (zF) and zona reticularis (zR), comprising of 90% of the gland.
- **Inner layer of adrenal cortex:** The adrenal medulla is located in the middle of the adrenal gland beyond the zona reticularis (zR).

Key Points
- The adrenal consist of three outer zones: zona glomerulosa, zona fasciculata and zona reticularis. The inner layer is the adrenal medulla.
- The adrenal is a major endocrine gland in the human body.

34.1 Adrenal Development in Fetal and Postnatal Stage

The embryonic adrenal development derives from neural crest cells and intermediate mesoderm. The early stage of adrenal development appears as an adrenogonadal primordium (AGP) at 28–30 days post-conception in humans. Neural crest cells develop into the adrenal medulla while intermediate mesoderm regresses into the definitive adrenal cortex. During the embryonic stage, the neural crest cells differentiate into neuroblasts (sympathoblasts) and become sympathetic and autonomic ganglion cells as well as phaeochromoblasts, which later become phaeochromocytes or mature chromaffin cells. Phaeochromocytes which form the adrenal medulla are enveloped by mesenchymal primitive adrenal cortex.

During the fetal stage, the zone of adrenal cortex of is called the fetal zone; 80% of it consists of fetal zone cells. These cells produce large quantities of DHEA and DHEAS, which are converted to oestrogen by the placenta for the maintenance of normal pregnancy. Adrenocortical cells emerge by the 8th week of gestation to form the definitive zone that later develops into the adrenal cortex. During the last 6 weeks of gestation, the majority of the prenatal growth is due to the enlargement of the fetal cortex which is the largest zone at birth.

After birth, the fetal zone undergoes changes under the influence of the hormones angiotensin II (AngII) and ACTH, whereby the zona glomerulosa (zG) and zona fasciculata (zF) mature. Unlike the zona glomerulosa and fasciculata, the zona reticularis does not function actively between 6–8 years old in females and 7–9 years old in males. It begins to emerge between the zona fasciculata and the medulla in a process known as 'adrenarche', which involves the proliferation and production of adrenal androgens. Adrenarche is independent of ACTH or gonadotropins. Secondary sexual characteristics also begin to occur at adrenarche. The mechanisms involved in postnatal adrenal formation and the maintenance of these distinct zones remain poorly understood.

34.2   Anatomy of Adrenal Glands

The adrenal glands weigh 4–5 g each in a normal healthy adult and sit on the upper end of the right and left kidneys (Fig. 34.1). The centre of the adrenal gland, the medulla, weighs around 1 g. The outer layer, the zona glomerulosa (zG), is composed of ovoid-shaped cells. The zona fasciculata forms the majority of the adrenal cortex and is organised in fascicles or bundles. There is no anatomical demarcation between medulla and cortex. The medulla is composed of chromaffin cells and contains small vesicles 100–300 nm in diameter in which catecholamines (adrenaline and noradrenaline) are stored and released. In the human, adrenaline accounts for 80% of adrenal catecholamine release into the circulation system and has effects on multiple organs.

The adrenal cortex synthesises corticosteroids, including over 50 distinct steroid hormones. Under normal condition in the absence of stress, the adult adrenal cortex produces approximately 10–15 mg of cortisol per day.

The adrenal glands are highly vascular, with three critical arteries supplying each adrenal gland. The superior suprarenal artery, the superior suprarenal artery and the middle suprarenal artery. Blood flows into the adrenal cortex and drains into the adrenal medulla before entering the inferior vena cava via the central vein on the right adrenal. On the left, the adrenal vein blood drains into the left renal vein. The drainage system of the adrenal gland plays a complex role in steroid synthesis and regulation. The adrenal gland is also well innervated. The nerve supply originates from the coeliac plexus and thoracic splanchnic region of the sympathetic autonomic nervous system, as well as some parasympathetic contributions from the phrenic and vagal nerves. The nerve supply also reaches the chromaffin cells in the medulla, and the innervation has been

Fig. 34.1 Anatomy and hormones secretion of adrenal gland

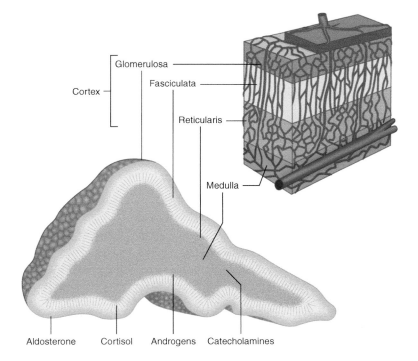

suggested to reach the cortisol arteriolar and capillary bed to regulate cortisol blood flow. Chromaffin cells are also found in the vagus nerve, carotid arteries, bladder, prostate and liver. Besides secreting catecholamine and dopamine, the adrenal medulla also secretes other stress hormones such as enkephalins and neuropeptide Y. One of the most important actions of catecholamine is the fight-or-flight response which leads to an increase in respiration, heart rate, blood pressure and blood vessel constriction (in the skin and gut).

34.3 Functions of the Adrenal Glands

The adrenal cortex is responsible for the production of three major classes of steroid hormones: glucocorticoids, mineralocorticoids and androgens (Fig. 34.2). The zona glomerulosa synthesises the mineralocorticoids aldosterone, the zona fasciculata produces cortisol, while the inner layer zona reticularis secretes androgen steroids such as dehydroepiandrosterone (DHEA), dehydroepiandrosterone sulphate (DHEAS), androstenedione and 1β-hydroxyandrostenedione. Glucocorticoids, such as cortisol, are secreted in high amounts around 10–50 mg/day whereas mineralocorticoids, such as aldosterone, are much less at around 100–200 μg/day. Surprisingly, DHEAS is also secreted in large quantities.

34.3.1 Aldosterone

First isolated in 1953, aldosterone has a plasma half-life of under 20 min and is weakly bound to plasma proteins. The adrenal secretes an average of 100–200 μm of aldosterone in 24 h. Its secretion is mainly stimulated by angiotensin II and an increase of extracellular potassium concentration, compared to other minor modulators such ACTH, stretch receptors in the heart, serum sodium and serotonin. Angiotensin II is converted in the lung from angiotensin I, which is stimulated by the release of the enzyme renin in the kidney

(Fig. 34.3). Aldosterone promotes sodium and water retention and lowers plasma potassium levels by binding to mineralocorticoid receptors in the renal tubules. After binding to the receptor, the complex translocates to genomic DNA which causes gene transcription expression and in turn leads to reabsorption and retention of sodium and excretion of potassium and hydrogen. The sequence also affects blood pressure and extracellular fluid volume. This system is called the renin-angiotensin-aldosterone system and also has a small diurnal rhythm mediated by ACTH.

Aldosterone and corticosterone share the first part of their biosynthesis pathways. They are synthesised from cholesterol catalysed by enzyme of cytochrome P450 family located in the mitochondria (Fig. 34.3). The last part of the aldosterone pathway is mediated by aldosterone synthase, found only in the zona glomerulosa in the adrenal where pregnenolone is transformed to progesterone and then to aldosterone. Aldosterone is catabolised in the liver and kidney and a small amount is excreted in the urine. Aldosterone level in plasma is also affected by the time of the day and posture.

34.3.1.1 Aldosterone Dynamic

Aldosterone excess has a profound impact on blood pressure due to the increase in sodium and fluid retention, including extracellular fluid expansion as well as suppression of plasma renin activity. This chronic hypervolaemic state leads to hypertension. Aldosterone excess is found in primary hyperaldosteronism where excess secretion of aldosterone leads to suppression of renin, hypokalaemia and hypertension. In congenital adrenal hyperplasia (CAH), C21-hydroxylase deficiency caused by 21-hydroxylase gene mutation leads to increased ACTH levels and androgens but loss of major mineralocorticoids. Classic form of CAH presented with salt-losing and virilisation.

Conversely, patients with primary and secondary adrenal failure may present with low blood pressure, low sodium and hyperkalaemia, but only in primary adrenal failure there is loss of mineralocorticoids. Replacement with mineralocorticoid will rectify the electrolyte imbalance in such patients.

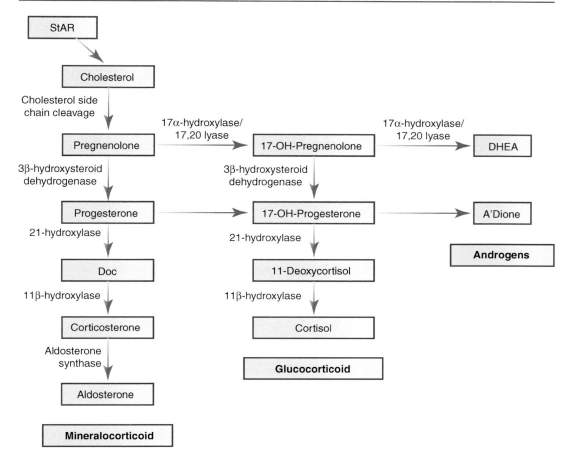

Fig. 34.2 Adrenal steroidogenesis. (Used with permission from Stewart P.M. (2008) The adrenal cortex, chapter 14. In: Kronemberg H.M., Melmed S., Polonsky K.S. and Larsen P.R. (Eds) Williams Textbook of Endocrinology, 11th Edition. Saunders Elsevier, Philadelphia, pages: 445–503)

34.3.2 Cortisol

The 'stress hormone' cortisol plays a major role in the hypothalamic-pituitary-adrenal HPA axis (Fig. 34.4) (please read the Chap. 12 in Part III for more details). Cortisol exerts numerous effects including blood sugar control through gluconeogenesis, affects blood pressure through salt and water regulation and regulates the immune system through its anti-inflammatory effects. It also affects memory, emotion and cognition.

Cortisol production is stimulated by the pituitary hormone ACTH, which itself is regulated by corticotropin releasing hormone (CRH) and arginine vasopressin (AVP) from the hypothalamus.

ACTH is a 39 amino-acid peptide secreted by the anterior pituitary gland. Its secretion also occurs in response to low circulating cortisol, anxiety and stress, as well as the underlying circadian rhythm. It is inhibited by high endogenous and exogenous circulating cortisol or other glucocorticoids, and thus forms a homeostatic loop.

Cortisol is produced in circadian manner (Fig. 34.5), peaking around 8–9 am and at several points throughout the day including following meals. At a cellular level, cortisol binds to the glucocorticoid cell receptor (GR). Once bound to the receptor, it is translocated to the nucleus and leads to changes in metabolism particularly on carbohydrate, fat and protein metabolism. The GR complex also up-regulates the expression of

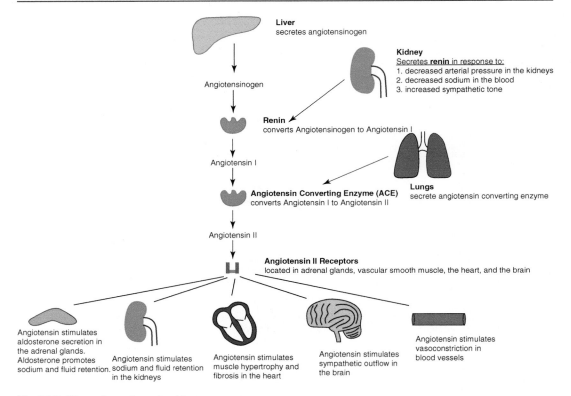

Fig. 34.3 The renin-angiotensin-aldosterone system

anti-inflammatory proteins in which represses the expression of pro-inflammatory proteins.

34.3.2.1 Body Circadian Rhythm of Cortisol Production

The circadian rhythm of cortisol secretion is shown in Fig. 34.5. ACTH is secreted in a pulsatile manner. Peak levels usually occur in the morning coinciding with peak cortisol production with a 30–60 min delay. It has a short life and the response is closely related to physical demands and environmental influences.

This circadian system is controlled by central clock in the hypothalamic—the suprachiasmatic nucleus (SCN)—which synchronises subsidiary cellular peripheral clocks. The SCN is located in the anterior part of the hypothalamus immediately dorsal, or superior (hence supra), to the optic chiasm. The intracellular mechanisms interlock negative and positive transcriptional-

translational feedback loops that oscillate over a 24-h period.

34.3.2.2 Pharmacodynamics of Cortisol

Cortisol is circulated in three forms: protein bound, free cortisol and cortisol metabolites. The largest group is protein-bound cortisol which constitutes approximately 92% of the total cortisol in the circulation. It has a better affinity to corticosteroid-binding globulin (CBG) than to albumin. The free cortisol or unbound fraction is the active hormone that dictates physiological activity. When the cortisol secretion reaches a saturation point with normal CBG secretion, this leads to increased free or unbound cortisol in circulation. Most synthetic glucocorticoids have less affinity to CBG. Prolonged elevation of free or unbound cortisol in circulation adversely produces Cushingoid symptoms.

Fig. 34.4 The
hypothalamic-pituitary-
adrenal (HPA) axis and
regulation of adrenal
glucocorticoid secretion.
(Used with permission
from Arlt W (2017)
Disorders of the adrenal
cortex, chapter 8. In:
Jameson JL (Eds)
Harrison's
Endocrinology, 4th
Edition, McGraw Hill
Education, New York,
pages 107–135)

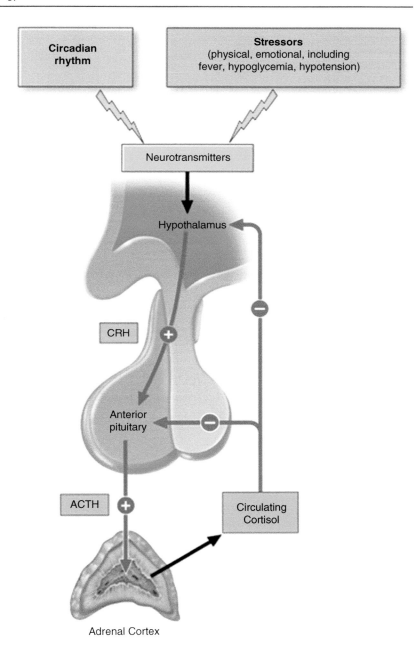

Cortisol is metabolised in the liver and metabolites are excreted via the kidneys.

Standard laboratory assays for serum cortisol
levels include protein-bound and the free or
unbound fractions in order to determine the total
concentration. Cortisol can also be measured in
the saliva and urine. Salivary cortisol reflects the
amount of free unbound cortisol that escapes
binding proteins and enters the tissues throughout the body. Salivary cortisol measures cortisol
collected at that particular time: 24 h urinary free
cortisol (UFC) captures total amount of free and

Fig. 34.5 The circadian rhythm of the cortisol production. (Used with permission from Stewart P.M. (2008) The adrenal cortex, chapter 14. In: Kronemberg H.M., Melmed S., Polonsky K.S. and Larsen P.R. (Eds) Williams Textbook of Endocrinology, 11th Edition. Saunders Elsevier, Philadelphia, pages: 445–503)

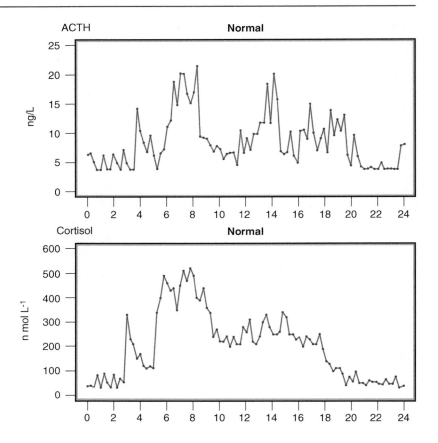

unbound cortisol excreted in urine over 24 h period. It should be emphasised that many cortisol assays will also measure, to some extent, other corticosteroids or their metabolites.

34.3.3 Androgens

Adrenal androgens are synthesised from cholesterol through a series of intracellular and extracellular actions involving oxidases and dehydrogenases. Unlike glucocorticoids, adrenal androgens have little activity at androgen receptors. Instead, they function as precursor molecules ready to be metabolised peripherally to potent androgens such as DHT or aromatised to oestradiol. The C_{19} steroids include DHEA, DHEAS, androstenedione and 11β-hydroxyandrostenedione. They are produced in adrenal gland and gonads in both men and women. Circulating levels of dehydroepiandrosterone (DHEA), DHEA-sulphate (DHEAS), androst-5-ene-3 beta, 17 beta-diol (5-diol), 5-diol-sulphate, 5-diol-fatty acid esters and androstenedione in both men and women were found to decline from the age of 20–80 years old (Labrie et al. 1997). The majority of DHEA and DHEAS comes from the adrenals, including 50% of secreted androstenedione. The conversion to potent androgens such as testosterone or dihydrotestosterone occurs in tissues that express HSD3-B1 and HSD17-B1/5 such as adipose tissue and the skin.

The adrenal gland secretes a small amount of testosterone. In men, testosterone is predominantly produced by Leydig cells in the testes. In women, DHEA can be taken up by ovarian theca cells to synthesise testosterone and may be converted to dihydrotestosterone in peripheral tissues once converted to androstenedione, without requiring transformation to testosterone (Nakamura et al. 2009). In healthy men, circulating testosterone levels are approximately ten times higher than women (Taieb et al. 2003).

DHEA is converted to DHEA-sulphate (DHEAS), an inactive steroid, through the enzyme DHEA sulfotransferase SULTA2-A1. When required, DHEAS is reactivated back to DHEA with the presence of the sulphate donor 3'-phosphoadenosine-5'-phophosulfate (PAPS). PAPS is synthesised by the two isoform of PAPS synthase, PAPSS1 and PAPSS2. The sulphation process is important to prevent excess androgen formation, which could in turn lead to increased androstenedione or testosterone.

However, the regulation of adrenal androgens remain poorly understood. It is thought that ACTH may play a role. This is from data collected from patients with ACTH stimulation during adrenal venous sampling (Rege et al. 2013) where ACTH administration increases DHEAS by fivefold, DHEA by 21-fold, androstenedione by sevenfold and 11β-hydroxyandrostenedione by fivefold. Whether this is physiologically relevant remains unclear.

Androgens play a critical role for the development and maintenance of the male reproductive system. They also influence insulin sensitivity as well as bone and muscle metabolism. It exerts its effects by a genomic mechanism by involving the hormones binding to androgen receptor (AR) resulting in the modulation of gene expression. The androgen receptor is a nuclear receptor that is activated by androgenic hormones such as testosterone or dihydrotestosterone in the cytoplasm, and then translocate into the nucleus. During male sexual development, testosterone is responsible for primary sexual characteristic development, while dihydrotestosterone is responsible for secondary male characteristics, particularly male genital development to form the penis scrotal pouches as well as hair follicle development.

Androgen increases the rate of bone remodelling by prolonging the lifespan of osteoclasts and shortening the lifespan of osteoblasts. This leads to slow the maturation of bone, but the more potent epiphyseal effect comes from oestrogen which is aromatised from androgens.

Androgens also impair adipose tissue to proliferate and differentiate. This in turn induces adipose tissue dysfunction and affects glucose uptake and leads to insulin resistance, intracellular stress and inflammation (Klöting and Blüher 2014). Treatment of androgen excess has been shown to reduce fasting insulin and improve the insulin sensitivity (Banaszewska et al. 2016).

34.3.3.1 Testosterone
Testosterone has a direct impact in body composition of men by increasing lean body mass and this leads to increase insulin sensitivity. Low testosterone independently affects insulin resistance. Androgen replacement therapy improves insulin sensitivity, diabetes and the metabolic syndrome in hypogonadal men (Haider et al. 2014; Traish et al. 2014).

High levels of testosterone correlate with high androstenedione levels in women with polycystic ovary syndrome (O'Reilly et al. 2014) who were found to have an adverse metabolic phenotype. However, Lerchbaum et al. (2014) argued contrarily that high androstenedione and the free testosterone index have a beneficial metabolic effect.

On the other hand, patients with adrenocortical carcinoma often present with Cushing's syndrome and androgen excess including DHEA/DHEAS, androstenedione and testosterone. High testosterone in women may cause hirsutism, acne, deepening of the voice, hair loss and amenorrhoe. However, testosterone excess in men raised haematocrit, seborrhoea, acne and some mood changes.

34.3.3.2 DHEA/DHEAS
Sulphation is an important pathway of DHEA metabolism. Any disruption in this pathway, including patients with PAPSS2 mutations, can lead to high active DHEA and a low DHEAS levels (Oostdijk et al. 2015). A similar pattern was found in two thirds of polycystic ovarian syndrome patients showing an increase in the DHEA/DHEAS ratio with significantly increased excretion of both major androgen metabolites, androsterone and aetiocholanolone (Kempegowda et al. 2016); 20–30% of PCOS women were found to have excess DHEAS levels (Goodarzi et al. 2015). In Asian women with PCOS, high serum

DHEAS is associated with the presence of acne and a significantly reduced risk of abdominal obesity, independent of serum testosterone concentration and insulin resistance (Chen et al. 2011). The study showed that DHEAS and total testosterone have different relationships with body weight, abdominal obesity and dyslipidaemia. A lower prevalence of acne was found in obese PCOS women with lower DHEAS concentrations (Afifi et al. 2017). Asian patients with PCOS have a lower prevalence and severity of hirsutism and obesity which might be attributed to genetic and environmental differences.

34.3.3.3 Conclusions

The adrenals play an important role in the dynamics of the endocrine system. Its complex interactions with hormone pathways, genetic factors, environmental influences and the body's circadian rhythm all play a vital role in its secretion, excretion and homeostasis. Excess and insufficient adrenal secretions underpin the balance between health and disease. Feedback mechanisms are often involved in the synthesis and pathway of the adrenal system.

References

Afifi L, Saeed L, Pasch LA, Huddleston HG, Cedars MI, Zane LT, Shinkai K. Association of ethnicity, Fitzpatrick skin type, and hirsutism: a retrospective cross-sectional study of women with polycystic ovarian syndrome. Int J Womens Dermatol. 2017;3(1):37–43. Published online 2017 Mar 13. https://doi.org/10.1016/j.ijwd.2017.01.006.

Banaszewska B, Wrotyńska-Barczyńska J, Spaczynski RZ, Pawelczyk L, Duleba AJ. Effects of resveratrol on polycystic ovary syndrome: A double-blind, randomized, placebo-controlled trial. J Clin Endocrinol Metab. 2016;101(11):4322–8. Epub 2016 Oct 18.

Chen ML, Chen CD, Yang JH, Chen CL, Ho HN, Yang WS, Yang YS. High serum dehydroepiandrosterone sulfate is associated with phenotypic acne and a reduced risk of abdominal obesity in women with polycystic ovary syndrome. Hum Reprod. 2011;26(1):227–34. https://doi.org/10.1093/humrep/deq308.

Goodarzi MO, Carmina E, Azziz R. DHEA, DHEAS and PCOS. J Steroid Biochem Mol Biol. 2015;145:213–25. https://doi.org/10.1016/j.jsbmb.2014.06.003. Epub 2014 Jul 5.

Haider A, Yassin A, Doros G, Saad F. Effects of long-term testosterone therapy on patients with "Diabesity": results of observational studies of pooled analyses in obese hypogonadal men with type 2 diabetes. Int J Endocrinol. 2014;2014:683515. https://doi.org/10.1155/2014/683515.

Kempegowda P, O'Reilly MW, Hassan-Smith Z, Storbeck KH, Taylor AE, Arlt W. Impaired DHEA sulfation defines androgen excess in women with polycystic ovarian syndrome (PCOS). Endocr Abstr. 2016;41:GP184. https://doi.org/10.1530/endoabs.41.GP184.

Klöting N, Blüher M. Adipocyte dysfunction, inflammation and metabolic syndrome. Rev Endocr Metab Disord. 2014;15(4):277–87. https://doi.org/10.1007/s11154-014-9301-0.

Labrie F, Bélanger A, Cusan L, Gomez JL, Candas B. Marked decline in serum concentrations of adrenal C19 sex steroid precursors and conjugated androgen metabolites during aging. J Clin Endocrinol Metab. 1997;82(8):2396–402.

Lerchbaum E, Schwetz V, Rabe T, Giuliani A, Obermayer-Pietsch B. Hyperandrogenemia in polycystic ovary syndrome: exploration of the role of free testosterone and androstenedione in metabolic phenotype. PLoS One. 2014;9(10):e108263. https://doi.org/10.1371/journal.pone.0108263. eCollection 2014

Nakamura Y, Hornsby PJ, Casson P, Morimoto R, Satoh F, Xing X, Kennedy MR, Sasano H. Rainey WE Type 5 17beta-hydroxysteroid dehydrogenase (AKR1C3) contributes to testosterone production in the adrenal reticularis. J Clin Endocrinol Metab. 2009;94(6):2192–8. https://doi.org/10.1210/jc.2008-2374. Epub 2009 Mar 31.

O'Reilly MW, Taylor AE, Nicola J, Crabtree NJ, Hughes BA, Capper F, Crowley RK, Stewart PM, Tomlinson JW, Arlt W. Hyperandrogenemia predicts metabolic phenotype in polycystic ovary syndrome: the utility of serum androstenedione. J Clin Endocrinol Metab. 2014;99(3):1027–36. Published online 2014 Jan 7. https://doi.org/10.1210/jc.2013-3399.

Oostdijk W, Idkowiak J, Mueller JW, House PJ, Taylor AE, O'Reilly MW, Hughes BA, Mde Vries MC, Kant SG, Santen GWE, Verkerk AJMH, Uitterlinden AG, Wit JM, Losekoot M, Arlt W. PAPSS2 deficiency causes androgen excess via impaired DHEA sulfation—in vitro and in vivo studies in a family harboring two novel PAPSS2 mutations. J Clin Endocrinol Metab. 2015;100(4):E672–80. Published online 2015 Jan 16. https://doi.org/10.1210/jc.2014-3556.

Rege J, Nakamura Y, Fumitoshi S, Morimoto R, Kennedy MR, Layman LC, Honma S, Hironobu S, Rainey WE. Liquid Chromatography-Tandem mass spectrometry analysis of human adrenal vein 19-cardon steroids before and after ACTH stimulation. J Clin Endocrinol Metab. 2013;98(3):1182–8.

Taieb J, Mathian B, Millot F, Patricot MC, Mathieu E, Queyrel N, Lacroix I, Somma-Delpero C, Boulloux

P. Testosterone measured by 10 immunoassays and by isotope-dilution gas chromatography-mass spectrometry in sera from 116 men, women, and children. Clin Chem. 2003;49(8):1381–95.

Traish AM, Haider A, Doros G, Saad F. Long-term testosterone therapy in hypogonadal men ameliorates elements of the metabolic syndrome: an observational, long-term registry study. Int J Clin Pract. 2014;68(3):314–29. https://doi.org/10.1111/ijcp.12319. Epub 2013 Oct 15.

Key Reading

1. Stewart PM. The adrenal cortex, chapter 14. In: Kronemberg HM, Melmed S, Polonsky KS, Larsen PR, editors. Williams textbook of endocrinology. 11th ed. Philadelphia: Saunders Elsevier; 2008. p. 445–503.

Diagnosis and Management of Congenital Adrenal Hyperplasia in Children and Adults

35

Alessandro Prete, Chona Feliciano,
Irene Mitchelhill, and Wiebke Arlt

Contents

A. Prete
Institute of Metabolism and Systems Research,
University of Birmingham and Queen Elizabeth
Hospital Birmingham, University Hospitals
Birmingham NHS Foundation Trust,
Birmingham, UK
e-mail: A.Prete@bham.ac.uk

C. Feliciano
Queen Elizabeth Hospital Birmingham, University
Hospitals Birmingham NHS Foundation Trust,
Birmingham, UK
e-mail: Chona.Feliciano@uhb.nhs.uk

I. Mitchelhill
Department of Endocrinology, Sydney Children's
Hospital (SCHN), Randwick, NSW, Australia
e-mail: Irene.mitchelhill@health.nsw.gov.au

W. Arlt (✉)
Institute of Metabolism and Systems Research
(IMSR), College of Medical and Dental Sciences,
University of Birmingham and Queen Elizabeth
Hospital Birmingham, University Hospitals
Birmingham NHS Foundation Trust,
Birmingham, UK
e-mail: w.arlt@bham.ac.uk

© Springer Nature Switzerland AG 2019
S. Llahana et al. (eds.), *Advanced Practice in Endocrinology Nursing*,
https://doi.org/10.1007/978-3-319-99817-6_35

Abstract

The adrenal cortex produces the steroid hormones, glucocorticoids, mineralocorticoids, and androgens, required for normal metabolic function. They are specifically involved in supporting the stress response, salt and water balance, and sex development. Congenital adrenal hyperplasia (CAH) is a group of genetic disorders caused by enzyme deficiencies in adrenal steroid production. More than 90% of CAH cases are caused by a deficiency of the adrenal steroid enzyme 21-hydroxylase (CYP21A2). Depending on the severity of deficiency, patients can have a variable spectrum of clinical presentation. Classic CAH is the most serious form and is life-threatening, due to severe glucocorticoid and mineralocorticoid deficiency (the so-called salt-wasting classic CAH), or isolated glucocorticoid deficiency but largely preserved mineralocorticoid deficiency (the so-called simple virilising classic CAH). Androgen excess leads to ambiguous genitalia in girls (also termed 46,XX disorder of sex development, 46,XX DSD) and precocious sexual maturation in childhood. Nonclassic CAH is associated with androgen excess and either normal glucocorticoid capacity or borderline glucocorticoid deficiency; it can present as precocious sexual maturation in childhood and hirsutism and irregular menses in adolescents and adult women. Classic CAH requires treatment to correct hormone deficiencies (glucocorticoids and mineralocorticoids) and mitigate androgen excess. In childhood, treatment focuses on issues of gender assignment, genital surgery, and optimisation of growth and pubertal development. Priorities change with increasing age, typically focusing on fertility in early adult life and prevention of metabolic syndrome and bone loss in middle and older age. Prevention of life-threatening adrenal crisis remains paramount throughout the life of these patients. Management of CAH is complex and involves multidisciplinary expertise throughout the life of these patients. This chapter provides endocrine nurses with a synopsis of the approach, evaluation, and management of patients with CAH. Particular emphasis is placed on providing comprehensive coordinated care that includes patient and family education and the understanding of the physical and psychological consequences of the condition.

Keywords

21-hydroxylase deficiency · Adrenal insufficiency · Adrenal crisis · Androgen excess
Ambiguous genitalia

Abbreviations

17OHP	17-hydroxyprogesterone
46,XX DSD	46,XX disorder of sex development
ACTH	Adrenocorticotropic hormone
CAH	Congenital adrenal hyperplasia
FSH	Follicle-stimulating hormone
IM	Intramuscular
IV	Intravenous
LH	Luteinising hormone
SHBG	Sex hormone-binding globulin
TARTs	Testicular adrenal rest tumours

Key Terms

- **ACTH stimulation test:** diagnostic test to assess the adrenal steroid production after the administration of the synthetic ACTH analogue Tetracosactide (Synacthen®, Cortrosyn®, Cosyntropin).
- **Adrenal crisis:** life-threatening emergency caused by inadequate production of the adrenal hormone cortisol in situations of stress.
- **Adrenal insufficiency:** condition in which the adrenal glands do not produce adequate amounts of steroid hormones, primarily the stress hormone cortisol.
- **Ambiguous genitalia:** condition in which an infant's external genitals don't appear to be clearly either male or female.
- **Hirsutism:** excessive terminal hair that appears in a male pattern in women.
- **Virilisation:** abnormal development of male sexual characteristics in females or in pre-pubertal age boys.

Key Points

- Steroid 21-hydroxylase deficiency is the most common cause of congenital adrenal hyperplasia. It accounts for most of the cases of primary adrenal insufficiency in children.
- Severe congenital adrenal hyperplasia causes insufficient production of the adrenal hormones cortisol and aldosterone. Cortisol and aldosterone are necessary for life and patients need lifelong replacement.
- Congenital adrenal hyperplasia causes androgen excess, which can lead to problems in newborns (ambiguous genitalia), children (virilisation and short stature), and adults (hirsutism, infertility, and menstrual irregularities).
- Cortisol deficiency predisposes patients with congenital adrenal hyperplasia to life-threatening adrenal crisis. This is a medical emergency that requires immediate treatment with injectable hydrocortisone (equivalent to the endogenous hormone cortisol).

35.1 Introduction

Congenital adrenal hyperplasia (CAH) is an inherited condition with many physical and psychosocial dimensions. The enzyme deficiency responsible for this condition affects hormone production of the adrenal gland, resulting in a combination of cortisol and aldosterone deficiency and androgen excess, which have detrimental effects both pre- and postnatally (El-Maouche et al. 2017; White and Bachega 2012). In this chapter, we will focus on CAH due to steroid 21-hydroxylase deficiency, which is the most common cause of the condition. We will review pathophysiology, diagnosis, and management, focusing on age-specific challenges associated with this chronic condition.

35.2 Pathophysiology of Congenital Adrenal Hyperplasia

Congenital adrenal hyperplasia (CAH) is a group of autosomal recessive genetic disorders and is the most common cause of primary adrenal insufficiency in children (1:10,000 to 1:20,000 live births) (White and Speiser 2000; Speiser et al. 2010). The most frequent genetic abnormality is a mutation in the *CYP21A2* gene, which encodes the enzyme 21-hydroxylase; this accounts for more than 90% of cases (White and Speiser 2000). CYP21A2 is a key enzyme of adrenal steroidogenesis (Fig. 35.1a).

Adrenal steroidogenesis takes place in the adrenal cortex and leads to the production of **glucocorticoids** (i.e. cortisol, required for normal metabolic function and involved in the response to stress), **mineralocorticoids** (i.e. aldosterone, regulating the level of electrolytes and water in the body), and **adrenal androgens** (serving as sex steroid precursors). Adrenocorticotropic hormone (ACTH) is released by the anterior lobe of the pituitary gland, regulated via negative feedback from circulating glucocorticoids, and is an impor-

tant stimulus of glucocorticoid and adrenal androgen production, promoting uptake and utilisation of cholesterol from the adrenal cortex. Cholesterol is the substrate of all steroid hormones (Fig. 35.1a).

CYP21A2 is crucial for the production of glucocorticoids and mineralocorticoids. As a consequence, the synthesis of cortisol and aldosterone is impaired when this enzyme is defective. A lack of cortisol drives increased ACTH secretion from the pituitary; ACTH then stimulates the adrenal gland to produce excessive amounts of androgens, the only pathway not affected by the lack of CYP21A2 (Fig. 35.1b). Several mutations of *CYP21A2* have been described in CAH. The severity of the condition relates to the degree to which the mutations compromise 21-hydroxylase activity (El-Maouche et al. 2017), reflected by different levels of impairment in cortisol and aldosterone production. The common feature of all

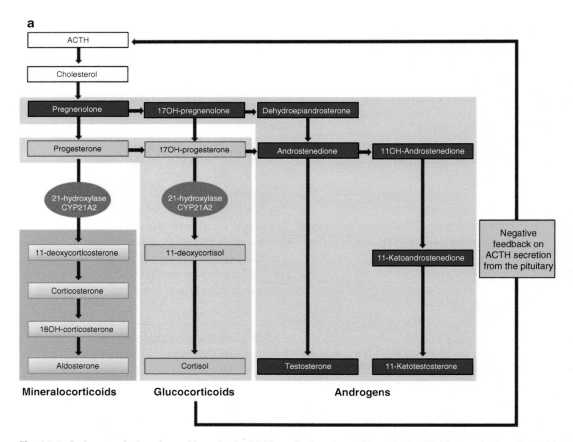

Fig. 35.1 Pathways of adrenal steroid synthesis. (**a**) Normal adrenal steroid synthesis. (**b**) Abnormal adrenal steroid synthesis in classic CAH (see next page); dotted arrows show the pathways affected by the lack of the enzyme 21-hydroxylase

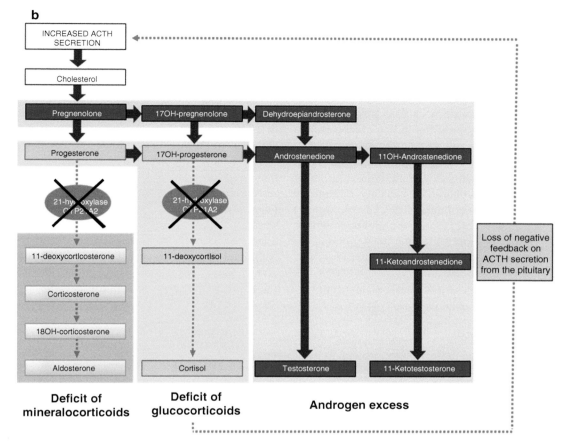

Fig. 35.1 (continued)

forms of CAH due to 21-hydroxylase deficiency is androgen excess.

35.3 Classification and Manifestations of Congenital Adrenal Hyperplasia

Depending upon the degree of cortisol and aldosterone deficiency and androgen excess, CAH can be classified as follows (White and Bachega 2012):

- **Classic CAH**: Severe deficiency of cortisol and androgen excess. Newborn females present with genital ambiguity (=46,XX disorder of sex development, 46,XX DSD). ~75% of newborns who are not identified at birth but harbour the most severe CYP21A2 mutations develop a salt-wasting crisis 7–14 days after birth (="salt-

wasting" CAH—both cortisol and aldosterone deficiency). This is particularly relevant for newborn males, who do not present with genital ambiguity. Children with slightly less severe mutations and therefore largely preserved mineralocorticoid production also present with 46,XX DSD in affected girls at birth. However, affected boys are often only diagnosed in early childhood with signs of increased bone age and virilisation (="simple virilising" CAH—cortisol deficiency only). Children with classic CAH require glucocorticoid replacement (as well as mineralocorticoid replacement in "salt-wasting" genotypes), and this prevents further virilisation through excess androgen production via downregulation of the negative feedback and consequently diminished ACTH stimulation of the adrenal glands.
- **Nonclassic CAH**: It is the most common form of CAH and affects 0.1% of the general

population, with higher rates among Hispanics and Yugoslavs (1–2%) and Ashkenazi Jews (3–4%) (White and Speiser 2000). Patients with nonclassic CAH produce relatively normal amounts of cortisol and aldosterone at the expense of mild-to-moderate androgen excess. However, some patients may have borderline glucocorticoid deficiency and require glucocorticoid replacement during major stress; hence, all nonclassic patients warrant initial assessment of their glucocorticoid capacity through an ACTH stimulation test. They have no signs at birth and present later in childhood, adolescence, or adult life due to symptoms of androgen excess.

Table 35.1 describes the clinical manifestations of classic and nonclassic CAH.

35.4 Assessment, Care, and Management of Patients with Congenital Adrenal Hyperplasia

35.4.1 Diagnosis

In 2010, the Endocrine Society recommended universal newborn screening for CAH, and many countries have implemented this recommendation (Speiser et al. 2010), though there is no screening implemented in the UK at present. In many other countries, screening is done by measuring 17-hydroxyprogesterone (17OHP) in dried blood spots. Abnormal results should be confirmed by a second measurement (White 2009); specificity is increased by additional measurement of 21-deoxycortisol, a steroid only generated in large amounts in 21-hydroxylase

Table 35.1 Manifestations of congenital adrenal hyperplasia

Classic CAH	Nonclassic CAH (late-onset CAH)
Neonates: • Females: ambiguous genitalia (=46,XX DSD) • Males may have subtle findings such as scrotal hyperpigmentation or penile enlargement *~75% of patients present in a salt-wasting adrenal crisis 7–14 days after birth*: • History: failure to thrive; persistent poor feeding; excessive sleepiness; significant weight loss (>10%); vomiting; persistent jaundice • Observations: jaundice; hypothermia; tachypnoea; dyspnoea; dehydration (sunken fontanelle, poor skin turgor) • Hypovolaemic shock, cardiovascular collapse • Laboratory abnormalities: hypoglycaemia; hyponatraemia; hyperkalaemia; metabolic acidosis *Childhood*: • History of rapid growth (crossing centiles) • Advanced bone with reduced height prediction • Early pubic hair development or sexual precocity (typically at 2–4 years of age) • Clitoromegaly • Increased body odour • Oily skin and hair *Adolescence and adulthood*: • Hirsutism • Hair loss and receding hair line (male-patterned baldness in women) • Oily skin and hair • Excessive acne • Menstrual irregularities • Infertility in both men and women	Nonclassic CAH is usually associated with milder signs and symptoms of androgen excess. Patients can be diagnosed anywhere from early childhood to adulthood. Adolescent girls and adult women can have a clinical picture that is indistinguishable from the polycystic ovarian syndrome. Men are often asymptomatic. Affected females do not have ambiguous genitalia. *Late childhood*: • Early pubic hair development or sexual precocity (before the age of 8 years in girls or 9 years in boys) • Clitoromegaly (rare, mild) • Accelerated growth • Advanced bone age • Increased body odour *Adolescence and adulthood*: • Menstrual irregularities • Hirsutism • Hair loss and receding hair line (male-patterned baldness in women) • Excessive acne *Fertility*: Subfertility is milder in comparison to classic CAH. Men usually have a normal testicular function.

deficiency. If 17OHP is elevated, blood sodium, potassium, and glucose must be checked. The measurement of 17OHP after an ACTH stimulation test can be used to confirm the diagnosis (White 2009). Abnormal results should then be complemented with DNA analysis for *CYP21A2* mutations.

In females, the diagnosis of **classic CAH** is most commonly made at birth because of the ambiguity (atypical development) of their genitalia (=46,XX DSD). In males who don't undergo newborn screening and do not develop a salt-wasting crisis in the neonatal period, the diagnosis may be delayed and only present when they develop signs of androgen excess.

Most cases of **nonclassic CAH** are not picked up at neonatal screening (White 2009). The diagnosis of nonclassic CAH can be made at any time from childhood to adulthood, including asymptomatic individuals identified during genetic screening because of affected relatives. The initial assessment is done by measuring early morning 17OHP. Abnormal results should be followed up by an ACTH stimulation test for 17OHP and cortisol (Witchel and Azziz 2010).

35.4.2 Classic Congenital Adrenal Hyperplasia: Medical Treatment

Treatment includes glucocorticoid replacement which aims to normalise hormone balance and reduce excess androgen production from the adrenal glands. Treatment is required lifelong, and adherence to treatment is essential for normal growth and development throughout the lifespan (El-Maouche et al. 2017). It is crucial that families, children, and adult patients with CAH are able to learn the necessary skills to manage the condition and understand why treatment is needed and how it is managed (please refer to Chap. 37 for more information on how to support patients and improve their adherence to treatment in adrenal insufficiency).

The mainstay of treatment of classic CAH are glucocorticoids (**hydrocortisone [=cortisol] or,**

if difficult to control in adulthood, long-acting synthetic glucocorticoids such as prednisolone) and mineralocorticoids (**fludrocortisone**). Glucocorticoids must be given in sufficient doses to replace cortisol deficiency and downregulate excessive production of ACTH from the pituitary and over-secretion of adrenal androgens. Fludrocortisone is given to keep electrolytes and intravascular fluid volume normal. Table 35.2 reports treatment goals and typical regimens in patients with classic CAH (El-Maouche et al. 2017; Speiser et al. 2010; Han et al. 2013a; Joint Lecahwg 2002). These should be seen only as a guide; treatment must be individualised after clinical and laboratory assessment.

Daily treatment in children includes hydrocortisone three to four times daily and fludrocortisone one to two times daily, with additional salt replacement in the newborns:

- For children with CAH, hydrocortisone is the drug of choice. The daily dose per m^2 body surface is higher compared to those children who have other causes of adrenal insufficiency because of the need to downregulate excess ACTH production and mitigate the androgen excess. Daily doses must be prepared from tablets when each dose is due, crushed, and administered in a small quantity of water prior to a feed—the use of oral hydrocortisone suspensions is discouraged, as they are not bioequivalent to the tablets (Speiser et al. 2010). The European Medical Agency has recently granted a paediatric use marketing authorisation for Alkindi® (Diurnal Ltd), a formulation of hydrocortisone granules that allows for more accurate and age-appropriate dosing in children and masks the bitter taste of conventional tablets.
- Fludrocortisone can be administered together with hydrocortisone. Neonates often require higher doses in the first months of life. Blood pressure should be monitored and doses minimised to prevent hypertension.
- Any need to increase treatment to maintain normal sodium and potassium levels can be addressed by the addition of salt (sodium chloride). Solutions of 20% (made by

Table 35.2 Medical treatment of classic congenital adrenal hyperplasia

Treatment goals	**All patients:** • Correct cortisol deficiency and prevent adrenal crisis • In patients with "salt-wasting" CAH: correct aldosterone deficiency to promote normal electrolyte balance • Mitigate androgen excess while avoiding iatrogenic glucocorticoid excess **Children:** • Promote normal growth, development, and final height outcome • Obtain normal sexual maturation **Adolescents and adults:** • Ameliorate hirsutism, acne, and menstrual irregularities in adolescents and women • Preserve fertility • Achieve positive sexual outcomes for females requiring genital reconstructive surgery
Neonates and infants	Medical treatment needs to be adjusted on an individual basis with frequent clinical and biochemical monitoring over the first months of life. Typical doses are initially: • Hydrocortisone: starting dose 20–30 mg/m^2/day in three divided daily doses. Higher doses may be used for initial reduction of markedly elevated androgens, but it is important to very rapidly reduce the dose when target hormone levels are achieved • Fludrocortisone: starting dose 50–100 mcg twice daily • Salt: starting dose 1–2 g/day of sodium chloride divided into several feedings. Salt supplementation can be discontinued as the child begins to eat table food and the taste for salty food increases • Fludrocortisone and salt supplements are balanced carefully with monitoring of blood pressure and electrolytes
Children	Medical treatment needs to be adjusted on an individual basis with frequent clinical and biochemical monitoring over time. Typical maintenance doses are: • Hydrocortisone: maintenance dose 10–15 mg/m^2/day in three divided daily doses • Fludrocortisone: maintenance dose 50–200 mcg/day • Encourage salt intake with exposure to hot weather or with intense exercise

Older adolescents and adults	• Glucocorticoids: hydrocortisone is the treatment of choice. However, long-acting glucocorticoids are often used in adults. Typical glucocorticoid regimens include one of the following:
	  – Hydrocortisone: 15–25 mg/day in two to three daily doses
	  – Prednisolone: 3–7 mg/day in one or two doses
	  – Dexamethasone: 0.25–0.5 mg at bedtime
	• Fludrocortisone: usual maintenance dose 50–200 mcg/day. It is important to reassess mineralocorticoid requirements when the patient transitions from paediatric to adult care because they can differ significantly between these phases
	• Encourage salt intake with exposure to hot weather or with intense exercise
	• Oral contraceptive pills can be considered as an adjunct treatment in women to regularise menses and ameliorate the cosmetic effects of androgen excess (hirsutism and acne). Direct hair removal methods are also an option (e.g. photoepilation, electrolysis, eflornithine cream)

compounding pharmacies for accuracy) can be used to minimise the volume given, with the dose given neat just before a feed or mixed in a small amount of breast milk or formula. Babies adapt fairly quickly to the taste, and simple administration strategies need to be developed to enhance adherence to treatment. Children with classic CAH are salt–losers and therefore have a preference for salty foods. As toddlers, salt should be added to their cooked foods to balance their intake, with older children having the ability to balance their own by "adding salt".

Long-acting glucocorticoids (prednisolone or dexamethasone) are often used in adults instead of hydrocortisone due to convenience of less frequent dosing (Table 35.2). When possible, hydrocortisone should be favoured because of the lower risk of over-replacement; both prednisolone and in particular dexamethasone are long-acting, and activate the glucocorticoid receptor for much longer including evening and night-time when circulating cortisol concentrations in healthy individuals are physiologically low. A novel modified-release formulation of hydrocortisone (Chronocort®, Diurnal Ltd) has been designed to mimic physiological cortisol secretion and improve control of the androgen excess (Mallappa et al. 2015). A phase-III clinical trial is currently evaluating its efficacy in adult patients with classic CAH.

35.4.3 Classic Congenital Adrenal Hyperplasia: Treatment and Prevention of Adrenal Crisis

Patients with classic CAH have primary adrenal insufficiency and do not have the capacity to secrete extra cortisol in situations of stress. If the dose of glucocorticoids is not increased in these situations, a patient with classic CAH can develop a life-threatening adrenal crisis. If not promptly recognised and treated, an adrenal crisis rapidly leads to systemic collapse, hypovolaemic shock, and death (Table 35.3) (Bornstein et al. 2016).

Adrenal crisis is a common occurrence in patients with classic CAH (Hahner et al. 2015;

Reisch et al. 2012). Precipitating factors include intercurrent illness, infections (particularly gastroenteritis and respiratory infections), persistent vomiting or diarrhoea, fever, significant pain, trauma (e.g. fractures), emotional distress, and strenuous physical activity (Hahner et al. 2015). Surgery requiring general anaesthesia, preparation for invasive diagnostic procedures (e.g. colonoscopy), and oral surgery (e.g. dental extractions) are further risk factors. Patients with CAH can also become acutely unwell if they do not have good adherence to medical treatment or do not follow the simple sick day rules outlined below (refer to Chap. 62 for more information on prevention and management of adrenal crisis).

A patient with a suspected adrenal crisis must be promptly treated with lifesaving injectable hydrocortisone (IM as priority pending IV access). Diagnostic measures should never delay treatment. If an adrenal crisis is suspected, act immediately and refer to hospital emergency management guidelines, if available. As a guide (Joint Lecahwg 2002; Bornstein et al. 2016):

- STEP 1: Give hydrocortisone immediately (injection of hydrocortisone IM or IV): 25 mg in those <3 years of age; 50 mg in those

Table 35.3 Adrenal crisis and signs and symptoms of over- and under-replacement

Adrenal crisis	Adrenal crisis is a life-threatening emergency. Patients present with at least two of the following: hypotension (systolic blood pressure <100 mmHg), nausea or vomiting, severe fatigue, fever, somnolence, confusion, and coma. Laboratory evaluation can show hyponatraemia, hyperkalaemia, hypoglycaemia, increased serum creatinine, and metabolic acidosis. Hypoglycaemia is common in children
Glucocorticoid treatment	*Over-replacement*: insomnia, increased appetite, proximal muscle weakness, skin thinning, easy bruising, red stretch marks, weight gain and central obesity, disproportionate supraclavicular and dorsocervical fat pads, facial and upper neck plethora, facial rounding. Reduced growth rates and weight gain in children can be an indication of glucocorticoid over-replacement *Under-replacement*: fatigue, weakness, nausea, lack of appetite, dizziness, hypotension, weight loss, skin hyperpigmentation (due to ACTH excess)
Mineralocorticoid treatment	*Over-replacement*: hypertension, peripheral oedema *Under-replacement*: orthostatic hypotension (e.g. dizziness, lightheadedness, and fainting when standing up); postural blood pressure drop on examination (lying to standing); fatigue, leg cramps, salt craving
Inadequate androgen suppression	*Children*: increased growth rate (before epiphyseal closure); early pubic hair development; early sexual development; clitoromegaly; increased sebaceous secretions; increased body odour *Adolescent and adult women*: hirsutism; excessive acne; oily skin; menstrual irregularities; male-patterned baldness in females

3–12 years of age; 100 mg in those >12 years of age.

- STEP 2: Start rapid rehydration with isotonic saline infusion according to protocols for age and weight.
- STEP 3: Correct hypoglycaemia, if present (IV dextrose). Hypoglycaemia can be common in children with adrenal crisis.
- STEP 4: Start continuous IV infusion of hydrocortisone after the bolus injection: 25–30 mg per 24 h in those ≤3 years of age; 50–60 mg per 24 h in those 3–12 years of age; 100 mg per 24 h in children >12 years of age; 200 mg per 24 h in adults. Alternatively, the total daily dose can be split and administered IM or IV every 6 h.
- STEP 5: Treat the precipitating factor of the crisis, if possible (e.g. infection, trauma).
- STEP 6: Contact an endocrinologist for urgent review of the patient and advice on further tapering of hydrocortisone.

In order to prevent an adrenal crisis, several measures need to be in place (Bornstein et al. 2016). These are simple and are lifesaving:

- Educate parents, patients, and partners regarding correct adjustment of glucocorticoid replacement in case of stress ("sick day rules"):
  - **Sick day rule 1**: double or triple daily oral glucocorticoid dose during illness that requires bed rest and/or antibiotics or is associated with high fever (>38 °C) until recovery. Children should get hydrocortisone in three to four doses and given sweet drinks and salt supplements if off their food. Double or triple the dose on the day of any minor procedure/surgery that do not require fasting (e.g. procedures requiring local anaesthesia and tooth extraction).
  - **Sick day rule 2**: administer hydrocortisone per IM or IV injection during severe illness, prolonged vomiting or diarrhoea, acute trauma and if the patient is confused, drowsy, or unconscious. Hydrocortisone per IM or IV injection must be given in preparation for surgery/procedures requiring general anaesthesia and during pro-

longed fasting (e.g. preparation for colonoscopy). In adults, the recommended dose is 100 mg via bolus injection, followed by 200 mg/24 h.

- Educate patients, parents, and partners regarding symptom awareness and possible precipitating factors of adrenal crisis. They should be advised that "if in doubt" they should give a hydrocortisone emergency injection and seek medical advice.
- Ensure patients have an additional supply of tablets so that they can double/triple their dose for at least 7 days, for example, when travelling abroad. If a patient is unable to tolerate tablets, hydrocortisone should be given IM and medical advice promptly sought.
- Provide patients and caregivers with a hydrocortisone emergency injection kit. Check regularly that their kit is up to date.
- Educate patients, parents, and partners on how to self-administer and inject hydrocortisone IM (for example: www.pituitary.org.uk/information/treating-a-pituitary-condition/hydrocortisone/how-to-give-an-emergency-injection-of-hydrocortisone; www.CAHPepTalk.com).
- Provide the patient with a steroid emergency card (for example: www.endocrinology.org/adrenal-crisis) and encourage them to wear medical alert bracelets or necklaces. Patients must keep the steroid emergency card with them at all times and show it to any health professional they are dealing with.
- Instruct parents of school-aged children affected by CAH to inform school staff about the condition. An emergency letter and response plan can be of use (as an example: www.cah.org.au/products-resources; www.CAHPepTalk.com).
- Provide patients and caregivers with emergency phone numbers for on-call services and the ambulance service (register with their consent onto the red flagged ambulance emergency service, if available locally).
- Instruct patients and caregivers to inform the endocrinologist before surgical procedures so that proper advice can be given to the hospital staff.
- Encourage salt intake with exposure to hot weather or with intense exercise. Before major

physical activity (e.g. long distance running, major sports, or competitive dancing), patients might benefit from taking a small dose of extra hydrocortisone.

- Regular review of the patient by health professionals to reinforce the sick day rules and adherence to treatment.

35.4.4 Classic Congenital Adrenal Hyperplasia: Monitoring

Patients with classic CAH require lifelong care. While the correction of cortisol and aldosterone deficiency and the control of androgen excess are common aims in children and adults, treatment goals do change over time (Table 35.2). In children with CAH prevention of early puberty and achievement of an acceptable final height are paramount. Upon completion of pubertal development and attainment of adult height, continued monitoring of symptoms of androgen excess (menstrual irregularities, hirsutism), quality of life, sexual health, and fertility become increasingly more important. The avoidance of the long-term side effects of excess glucocorticoid treatment is also crucial (e.g. stunted linear growth in children and, in particular in adults, metabolic syndrome, increased cardiovascular risk and osteoporosis) (Reisch et al. 2011; Arlt and Krone 2007).

Medical treatment of CAH can be challenging and is a fine balance between over- and under-treatment (Table 35.3). The goal is achieving the best clinical results with the lowest possible daily glucocorticoid dose. Regular clinical assessment and blood tests are required to monitor the effectiveness of treatment (Table 35.4 and Fig. 35.2) (Escobar-Morreale et al. 2012). The frequency and modalities of monitoring need to be tailored to the individual patient. Management can be complex and should involve multiple heath care professionals including endocrinologist, endocrine nurse specialist, genetic counsellors, gynaecologists, urologists and surgeons, fertility specialists, mental health providers, and social services. The endocrinologist and the specialist endocrine nurse play a pivotal role in coordinat-

ing management to guide the patients and their carers to achieve satisfactory health outcomes.

35.4.5 Classic Congenital Adrenal Hyperplasia: Management in the Neonatal Period

A female newborn with 46,XX DSD requires urgent consultation with the paediatric endocrine team and specific management strategies to provide the family with appropriate information and support to manage the shock and grief process until gender is determined. Placating comments and judgements regarding the gender of the baby should not be made. The focus should be on "your baby" who is "well and beautiful" with positivity expressed about the labour and delivery. Parents are advised that specialist endocrine team will be consulted immediately to explain the situation and assist in ascertaining the gender of their baby.

The paediatric endocrinologist will direct the plan to determine the diagnosis and gender and develop a treatment strategy to manage the glucocorticoid and mineralocorticoid deficiencies. The initial assessment is made on the physical findings, electrolyte and hormone analysis, radiological investigations, and genetic testing. The severity of genital malformation is assessed according to the Prader scale (Fig. 35.3) (White and Speiser 2000).

The surgical management of children born with 46,XX DSD is complex. Patients should be referred to centres with substantial experience and a team of paediatric surgeons, paediatric endocrinologists, mental health professionals, and social work services (Speiser et al. 2010).

Boys with classic CAH who did not undergo neonatal screening can present aged 1–3 weeks of life with a salt-wasting adrenal crisis—a state of systemic collapse which can lead to death if not managed quickly (Table 35.1). Because of the serious state of circulatory collapse, intravenous access may be difficult an intraosseous access may be required. A blood gas will give an immediate indication of the blood glucose, electrolytes, and assess for acidosis. At any stage of concern,

Table 35.4 Monitoring of patients with classic congenital adrenal hyperplasia

Frequency of monitoring	• At least monthly during the first 3 months of life • Every 3 months in the neonate and infant • Every 3–6 months in children and adolescents • Every 6–12 months in adults on stable medical treatment
Clinical assessment	• History taking, including current medications and comorbidities • Assess the adherence to medical treatment • Monitor growth velocity in children • General physical examination • Vital signs and body measurements: height; weight; waist circumference; blood pressure sitting and standing (to look for hypertension and orthostatic hypotension) • Look for signs and symptoms of over- or under-replacement (Table 35.3) • Examination of the genitalia to look for any signs of virilisation in children (e.g. clitoromegaly and precocious pubic hair development) and assess the outcome of reconstructive surgery in girls. It is imperative that such examinations are discussed with the parents and child and are undertaken discretely, particularly as children become older. Testicular examination should be performed periodically in adolescents and adults, looking for palpable masses or testicular atrophy • Assess the menstrual function in adolescents and premenopausal women • Assess women for hirsutism, using the modified Ferriman–Gallwey score (Fig. 35.2) • Assess health-related quality of life. Questionnaires can be used in older children and adults (e.g. PedsQL™ Generic Core Scale, PedsQL™ Fatigue Scale, WHOQoL-BREF scale, MAF scale, SF-36®; EQ-5D™). Investigate psychological, social, and sexual health issues, as well as current health concerns • Ask if the patient had any sick days since the previous visit and needed to increase the dose of glucocorticoids or required hospitalisation • Reinforce the sick day rules and confirm that measures are in place to prevent and treat promptly adrenal crisis (e.g. hydrocortisone emergency injection kit, steroid emergency card, medical alert bracelet) • Investigate family plans in patients of reproductive age
Laboratory assessment	*Hormonal evaluation*: • CHILDREN: morning serum 17-hydroxyprogesterone and androstenedione. Testosterone measurement is sometimes useful in patients whose disease is not well controlled. Adrenal androgen secretion should not be completely suppressed; normal levels of 17-hydroxyprogesterone generally indicate overtreatment • MEN AND WOMEN: morning serum 17-hydroxyprogesterone and androstenedione. The goal is individualised to achieve patient goals, but androstenedione should not be suppressed • MEN: morning serum testosterone, sex hormone-binding globulin (SHBG), and gonadotropins (FSH and LH) • WOMEN: morning follicular-phase progesterone should be checked in those seeking fertility. Testosterone measurement is sometimes useful in patients whose disease is not well controlled *Plasma renin activity or direct renin concentration*: it is used to monitor fludrocortisone replacement. Reference intervals are based on postural state and age, and data should be evaluated accordingly. A suppressed result reflects overtreatment and increases the risk of hypertension *Other tests*: • Blood sodium, potassium, and kidney function • Fasting plasma glucose: in neonates and young children glucose must be monitored because of the risk of hypoglycaemia, particularly if the child is unwell or requiring salt replacement. Conversely, adults are at risk of developing diabetes mellitus • In adults: lipid panel; glycated haemoglobin (HbA1c); vitamin D
Radiological assessment	• Regular bone age assessment in children (X-ray of the hand) • Regular testicular ultrasound in males from adolescence onwards • Monitor adults periodically for low bone density (DEXA scan)

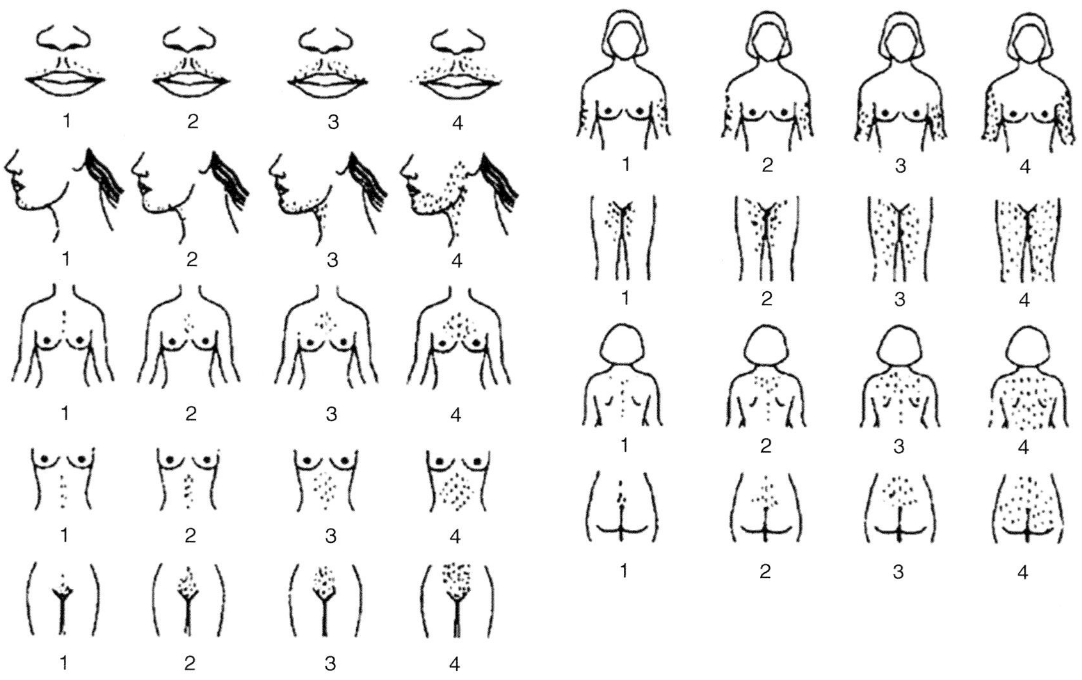

Fig. 35.2 Modified Ferriman–Gallwey score is the gold standard for the evaluation of hirsutism, scoring nine body areas (upper lip, chin, chest, upper and lower abdomen, arm, thigh, upper and lower back). Ferriman–Gallwey total scores that define hirsutism in women of reproductive age are: US and UK black or white women, ≥8; Mediterranean, Hispanic, and Middle Eastern women, ≥9 to 10; South American women, ≥6; Asian women, a range of ≥2 for Han Chinese women to ≥7 for Southern Chinese women. Reproduced with permission from Escobar-Morreale et al. (2012). Copyright Oxford University Press, 2011

or if there is a delay in obtaining intravenous access, hydrocortisone followed by glucagon should be administered IM for suspected adrenal insufficiency and hypoglycaemia. Once intravenous access is established, IV hydrocortisone, dextrose, and normal saline should be administered to correct hypovolaemia, hypoglycaemia, and the electrolyte abnormalities.

35.4.6 Classic Congenital Adrenal Hyperplasia: Management During Infancy and Childhood

The psychosocial adjustment of the parents to the diagnosis of CAH initially, and later for the child, is critical to achieving a positive outcome for the child and the family in the long term. Having a child with a complex chronic condition is a life-altering experience, with the impact on parents and family members depending greatly on individual coping abilities, and also influenced by social background, cultural and family beliefs (Patterson et al. 1990). A family's adjustment to a new diagnosis can be greatly enhanced by a health professionals' approach to the situation through counselling, education, and support (Hatton et al. 1995). By facilitating a process of understanding and adjustment health professionals can increase the likelihood of families having the knowledge, understanding, and confidence to manage difficult situations when they occur, such as a possible adrenal crisis. This education process should be reviewed regularly at clinical follow-up.

Psychological support is important for the parents but also for the children as they grow and adapt to living with a complex condition and its physical and emotional consequences. Managing intercurrent illness in order to prevent serious

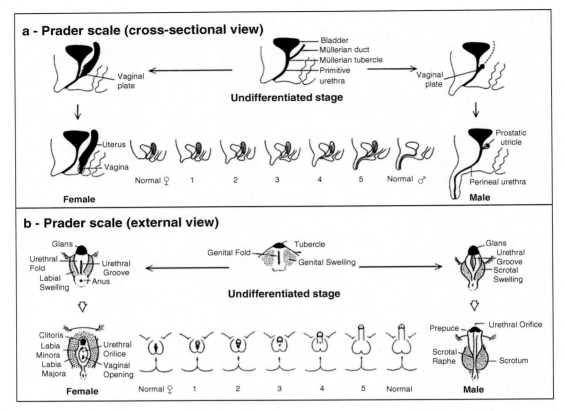

Fig. 35.3 Prader scale. The severity of virilisation is often quantitated using the five-point Prader scale. (**a**) Normal and abnormal differentiation of the urogenital sinus and external genitalia (cross-sectional view). (**b**) Normal and abnormal differentiation of the external genitalia (external view). Reproduced and edited with permission from White et al. (2000). Copyright The Endocrine Society, 2000

deterioration to a possible life-threatening adrenal crisis is a serious concern for parents and always at the forefront of their minds. They have to adapt their daily routine around their child's medication plan, attendance for regular medical reviews, and routine investigations. Health professional should aim to help families adapt the care required for these children into their daily lives in order to ensure positive health outcomes in the long term.

CAH has an element of androgen exposure in utero, which can affect brain development and function (Webb et al. 2018). Girls can have male-typical childhood play and more interest in male-typical activities during childhood and adolescence (Dittmann et al. 1990). Health professionals need to be aware of parental concerns regarding this variation to the norm and guide parents appropriately. Counselling with a psychologist will assist in this process for both the parents and the child. Autism, which is more often found in males than females, has been found to be more prevalent in patients with CAH of both sexes (Knickmeyer et al. 2006).

Support groups are important for parents and extended families, enabling them to share with others their experiences and difficulties in having a child with a diagnosis of CAH. Not all parents are ready to meet other families and will do so in their own time. Support groups can be invaluable in providing families with a sense of normality, and being able to meet other children who have grown up having the diagnosis of CAH. It is important that patients themselves are able to share their experiences in confidence with others with the same diagnosis.

35.4.7 Classic Congenital Adrenal Hyperplasia: Management During Adolescence

Adolescence is the phase of transition from childhood to adulthood. Managing CAH at this stage of development can be challenging, with a rapidly changing body and the impact of the hormonal changes of puberty (Merke and Poppas 2013). Adolescence is also a time of significant emotional change and often adherence to medical treatment is an issue.

Adolescent females can struggle with hormonal control at puberty, which often requires an increase in routine hydrocortisone doses. They may also need the addition of an oral contraceptive pill to regulate their monthly cycle and reduce acne and excess body hair. The outcome of reconstructive genital surgery carried out in infancy should be reviewed in adolescence and discussed with an appropriately skilled surgeon. If (additional) surgery is desired, particular expertise is imperative to ensure comprehensive understanding, appropriate consent by the adolescent and parents for adequate surgical outcomes.

In adolescent males with classic CAH, ACTH hypersecretion can cause hyperplasia of ACTH-sensitive cells present in the testes. This leads to the development of testicular nodules known as "testicular adrenal rest tumours" (TARTs), which can cause infertility (see section on fertility below) (El-Maouche et al. 2017). Poor adherence to hydrocortisone treatment and severe loss-of-function CAH genotypes have been identified as risk factors for the development of TARTs, which should be actively monitored for by ultrasound starting in adolescence, at the latest at the point of transition to adult care.

35.4.8 Classic Congenital Adrenal Hyperplasia: Management in the Adult Care Setting

With adolescence, the patient with CAH must gradually assume primary responsibility for his/her care and eventually transition to adult care. The adolescent's needs and concerns shift to a more adult focus on quality of life, long-term health and eventually relationships, fertility, and family planning (Reisch et al. 2011; Han et al. 2013b; Auchus and Arlt 2013). As patients with classic CAH often require higher doses of glucocorticoids to control the androgen excess, they are at increased risk of obesity, diabetes mellitus, dyslipidaemia, cardiovascular disease, and bone loss during adult life (Auchus and Arlt 2013; Arlt et al. 2010; Han et al. 2014). Consequently, a key priority when managing adults with CAH is to minimise long-term consequences of both the condition itself and its treatment.

The transition of care from a paediatric to an adult care setting remains a major challenge and many patients are lost to follow up (Gleeson et al. 2013). Ideally, patients should be jointly reviewed by the paediatric endocrinologist, the newly introduced adult endocrinologist, a clinical nurse specialist, and a geneticist on their first appointment. Apart from clinical and laboratory assessment, the initial evaluation should also focus on the following:

- Get to know the patient and understand their childhood journey.
- Assess the patient's understanding of the condition, goals of, and adherence to treatment.
- If available medical records are incomplete, these few questions are helpful: "At what age were you diagnosed?" "When did you stop growing?" and "Did you have any genital surgeries?" (Auchus and Arlt 2013).
- If indicated, an external genital examination may be necessary. Discuss sexual health with the patient and consider referral to a gynaecologist or urologist, if appropriate.
- Discuss family plans. Refer the patient to a fertility clinic, if appropriate.
- Consider the need for psychological counselling.

Ongoing follow-up will depend on this baseline assessment. Patients can have both or alternating appointments with their endocrinologist and the clinical nurse specialist, usually on yearly basis if they are on stable medical treatment (Table 35.4). Establishing a good nurse–patient relationship can enhance continued engagement for ongoing care.

35.4.9 Classic Congenital Adrenal Hyperplasia: Fertility

High rates of infertility can occur in patients with classic CAH (Reichman et al. 2014). Fertility correlates with the severity of the condition and can be reduced in both sexes.

Women have low fertility rates mainly due to androgen excess and menstrual irregularities with anovulatory cycles. 46,XX DSD and related surgical outcomes can also impact on sexual relationships and the chance of a positive pregnancy experience. Women seeking a pregnancy often need to intensify glucocorticoid treatment to obtain a more stringent control of the androgen excess and, consequently, promote their ability to ovulate and conceive. They should also be referred for review of the outcomes of previous genital reconstruction surgery; women with complex genital surgery should deliver by Caesarean section.

About 30–50% of men with classic CAH develop TARTs (Auchus and Arlt 2013), hyperplastic adrenal-like tissue, which can compress the surrounding testicular structures and cause oligospermia. Moreover, the adrenal-derived androgens can suppress gonadotropins and cause testicular atrophy. Men should be taught to self-examine their testes and have regular testicular ultrasound examinations to assess atrophy and the presence of TARTs. The term "tumour" should not be interpreted as a neoplasm because these masses actually represent hyperplastic tissue and do not show increased proliferation. It is therefore important not to confuse TARTs with primary testicular tumours when discussing a case with the patient and colleagues from other disciplines (Auchus and Arlt 2013). Poor adherence to glucocorticoid treatment is an important risk factor for the development of TARTs and intensified treatment is sometimes required, but not always effective for decreasing the size of the masses and restore fertility. Adult males with TARTS should be offered semen analysis and counselled on sperm banking.

35.4.10 Classic Congenital Adrenal Hyperplasia: Management of a Genetic Diagnosis

Once a child has been diagnosed with CAH, genetic testing will identify the specific muta-

tion present. This should be arranged following referral for genetic counselling, firstly to determine the mutation in the neonate, and then the carrier status of the family members. This will have an impact on their pregnancy planning in the future.

CAH is autosomal recessive. Parents of a baby with CAH both have one of their two 21-hydroxylase DNA alleles affected and thus have a one-in-four chance of having another baby with CAH and one-in-eight chance of having a female baby with CAH and 46,XX DSD. Treating the mother with dexamethasone before the major period of fetal sexual differentiation (6–8 weeks post-conception) can help to prevent the 46,XX DSD in the female fetus. However, dexamethasone can have adverse effects on the mother receiving treatment during pregnancy and also possible long-term effects on the baby, which require discussion before starting treatment (Speiser et al. 2010). Previously, there was also concern of treating unaffected pregnancies as treatment had to be initiated before the sex of the child was known and before there was clarity about whether or not the child was affected, which previously could only be found out after invasive measures. However, nowadays both the chromosomal sex of the fetus and whether it is affected by 21-hdyroxylase deficiency can be readily detected through analysis of fetal cells circulating in maternal blood, offered by specialist genetic units. A pregnancy undergoing dexamethasone treatment requires frequent monitoring by endocrine and obstetric specialists.

35.4.11 Management of Nonclassic Congenital Adrenal Hyperplasia

Patients with nonclassic CAH do not need continuous glucocorticoid replacement; however, some patients may require glucocorticoid replacement in major stress, such as surgery, trauma, or ICU treatment. If glucocorticoids are needed to control the detrimental effects of androgen excess, they should be given up to the achievement of the treatment goal and then stopped (Auchus and Arlt 2013). Treatment can be considered in:

- Children with progressive signs of virilisation and accelerated growth.
- Women with anovulatory infertility.

If fertility is not desired, glucocorticoids should be avoided in women with bothersome hirsutism and/or menstrual irregularities. In such cases, treatment with oral contraceptives including an anti-androgenic progestin component (e.g. drospirenone or cyproterone) is preferred (Speiser et al. 2010).

35.4.12 Additional Aspects of Optimal Care

Health care professionals have a vital role in assessing and guiding individual and family adjustment to the diagnosis of CAH (Auchus et al. 2010). It is essential that health care professionals understand the need to provide a clear and simple explanation about the diagnosis in a positive way. Information needs to be given in limited amounts at a time, remembering that it may need to be repeated a number of times for it to be retained. Evaluating the information given is understood is an important step in this process. Using a timely approach will ensure that patients and families will acquire the appropriate information they need to manage the condition and assist in allaying any anxieties which may persist (Hatton et al. 1995). Continuous reinforcement of health information is also key.

The nurse–patient relationship is an extremely important factor in achieving effective health education for patients and families (Auchus et al. 2010). The nurse needs to be sensitive to the emotional needs of patients and caregivers, and assess their readiness for learning. For families with a child with a chronic condition such as CAH, the education process takes place over a continuous period of time as the child progresses through the developmental stages of childhood, adolescence, and into adulthood.

Finally, consistency and continuity of care by staff are considered one of the most important factors for patients with CAH, with transition from paediatric to adult care carefully planned (Merke and Poppas 2013; Auchus et al. 2010; Kruse et al. 2004). Adolescence and early adult-hood are crucial times in the life of these patients and associated with significant physical and psychological adjustment. It is important to support the young person in making decisions which build confidence to direct their own care over time. Patient education and assumption of responsibility are critical for adherence to treatment, continuity of care, and successful outcomes.

35.5 Role of Patient Advocacy Groups in Improving Patient Care and Education in CAH

Patient advocacy groups are a highly valuable resource for patients and their families, not just as a clinical and supportive tool, but by also enabling empowerment and enriching the relationship between patients, families, and their health care providers. The advent of social media, with websites and online support groups can add to this, and patients have a reliable and trusted resource for peer support. Most PAGs work very closely with clinical teams to develop evidence-based information and support clinical research; they can form a useful resource and can reach patients and health care teams across the globe especially for rare conditions such as CAH.

35.5.1 The CAH Support Group (Reprinted Permission from CAH Support Group (UK) Patient Advocacy Group)

Robin Brett had CAH and was just 18 years old when he sadly died in 2014. He was taken to hospital with vomiting and unable to keep his medication down; this preceded by constipation which was treated by a large dose of enema. Although an IM injection of hydrocortisone was administered on admittance to hospital, no further medication was given on the ward and few checks were made. Just over 16 h after admittance, he went into an adrenal crisis and subsequently a cardiac arrest from which he could not be revived.

Robin's parents had been members of the CAH Support Group since shortly after he was born and regularly attended conferences so were knowledgeable about his condition but, despite raising concerns about his treatment, were not listened to.

We were very saddened to hear of his death, the cause of which was not originally recorded accurately, which the family found particularly upsetting. However, his brave mother was determined to discover the truth and the support group put her in touch with one of our medical advisors who agreed to view the Coroner's report. After he read this, he issued his own report categorically stating that death was obviously caused by *"acute adrenal insufficiency consequent on a lack of adequate steroid replacement"*. His conclusion was then confirmed by another specialist who was instructed by the Coroner's Office and the death certificate was altered accordingly.

Although nothing could bring Robin back, his mother was determined that her son's death would not be in vain and was keen to work with the support group to try and ensure the mistakes that occurred at the hospital where Robin was admitted would not happen again and cause another family to suffer as they had. We put her in touch with another eminent endocrinologist (who agreed to help) and she tirelessly wrote to the medical director of every hospital trust in the UK, explaining what had happened to her son and asking them to put measures in place to prevent another tragedy. In particular, she asked that a note be added to a patient's medication, requesting to utilise a note function on the current electronic prescribing system, highlighting the importance of administering steroids and also requesting measures are put in place to ensure patients with adrenal insufficiency receive appropriate care, to prevent any more unnecessary deaths.

Mrs. Brett received a fantastic response from these letters, with medical directors promising to make changes as suggested and to better educate staff about adrenal insufficiency/crisis. Robin even featured in a very poignant and moving training video as a result, which we believe helped highlight how fragile life can be for those with CAH and other steroid-dependent conditions.

The primary aims of the CAH group are to support all families affected by CAH and to increase awareness of the condition to the public and the medical profession. We believe the above tragic account of just one of our members is evidence on how we work together with families and the medical profession in order to do this. We provide a variety of information booklets and leaflets, organise conferences, social meetings as well as a regular newsletter to keep our members up to date. We also encourage and contribute to research projects.

| Please contact us for any information: Sue Elford Chair: CAH Support Group E-mail: sue@cah.org.uk | Website: www.livingwithcah.com Sallyann Blackett Treasurer: CAH Support Group E-mail: sallyann@theblacketts.co.uk |

35.5.2 The CARES Foundation (Reprinted Permission from CARES Foundation (USA) Patient Advocacy Group)

The Leight family founded CARES Foundation in 2001 after their daughter was diagnosed with Congenital Adrenal Hyperplasia (CAH), a rare disorder of the adrenal gland. When attempting to learn more about the disorder, they found that there was no support for families and affected individuals and few resources for information. Today, CARES Foundation serves as a global resource for patients and families affected by CAH.

In 2001, only 27 states in the USA were screening newborns for CAH. CARES initiated a grass-roots campaign to advocate for the inclusion of CAH in the newborn screening panel in all 50 states. As of 2008, every state in the USA tests for CAH, saving numerous lives. In 2009, CARES Foundation embarked on another national campaign to establish EMS (emergency medical service) protocols for adrenal crisis which are currently available in nearly 30 states.

CARES Foundation has an extensive support network for patients and families that includes one-on-one support; regional and specialised support groups; regularly scheduled teleconference calls with participation from expert providers, and private support groups on social media. CARES provides referrals to expert physicians and access to online expert via the "Ask the Expert" service.

Education is a key component of our mission. Our educational efforts include:

- Annual education conferences for patients, families, and health care professionals
- A newsletter containing information on new treatments, research studies, and other valuable information
- Guides for educating school and camp personnel
- A guide for travelling with CAH
- Emergency instructions
- Educational packet for school nurses
- Website containing valuable information

Providing patients with access to quality health care is another cornerstone of CARES Foundation. To this end, CARES designated four centres of excellence across the USA where expert care is provided by a multidisciplinary team addressing patient needs throughout their lifecycle. These centres are also conducting research to advance patient care. CARES is also where patients and researchers turn for participation, recruitment, and information on clinical trials.

Since 2001, CARES has established itself as a global resource for not only patients with CAH and their families but also for health care professionals. We encourage all health care professionals to offer CARES as a resource for their patients. Professionals are also encouraged to take advantage of our services.

For more information about CARES Foundation, contact Dina Matos, Executive Director of CARES Foundation, at dina@caresfoundation.org or Tel: 866-227-3737 (USA). You can also visit our website www.caresfoundation.org

35.6 A Patient Perspective (Published with Patient Consent)

I am a 30-year-old woman who is lucky enough to be in a loving relationship but who does have long-term medical conditions to cope with every day. I recently tried to deal with fertility treat-ment and had two unsuccessful rounds of intra-uterine insemination (IUI). Dealing with infertility is emotionally and physically draining. It makes you feel inadequate and alienated from life. I can't express how much I yearn to be called mummy and dream of a future with my own family. I'm having a break from it now and want to share my story with you as this is the most recent in a long series of medical battles in my life.

I was diagnosed with CAH at birth and salt-wasting CAH a few weeks later when I had a salt crisis which nearly put me in a coma. I will always be under the care of an endocrinologist and managed with steroid replacement therapy.

I had surgery at the age of one and then again at four, I remember the later vividly. The surgery for girls with CAH is very painful and sensitive as it involves cosmetic changes to the vagina and clitoris to normalise the genitals. Although cosmetic the extent of these surgeries was enormous and resulted in psychological problems for many years to come, in my case without any professional support. Put simply this isn't something you can speak about freely or easily.

My teens were particularly difficult, not only was I dealing with regular hospital appointments and medication but I also had the underlying problem of knowing I wasn't "normal" and believing there was absolutely no way I could *ever* have sex, which in my young mind equated to *never* being loved (my vaginal entrance was the size of my little finger; need I say more?). I began asking myself if I was asexual and taught myself to avoid all situations which may compromise me and bat away any attention. That way I could ignore the problem and live in denial. I continued with this approach into my early 20s.

My periods started a bit late at age 14 (and have gone on to cause me many problems over the years) and I went into hospital again for vaginal stretching under anaesthetic. The aim: to enable me to use a tampon. The timing: it could not have been worse. Can you imagine experiencing this during puberty in addition to all the usual ups and downs? Constantly being asked by kids at school if you're a lesbian because you're not interested in boys? If only it were that simple. I have never felt as isolated as I did at secondary school. All I can say is I'm pleased I had a happy childhood and loving parents to look back on; it wasn't all bad but it was very challenging!

And the fun didn't stop there. When I was 16 I was diagnosed with Crohn's disease and had surgery a few months later; a right hemicolectomy removing my ascending colon and some of my small intestine all of which had become ulcerated and was causing me incredible pain, nausea, and diarrhoea. Again I was managed with yet more steroids which this time brought along the added frustration of unwanted weight gain and associated difficulties as a teenager. I ended up missing most of year 11 but am pleased to say I did really well in my exams, which I took at home and went on to sixth form college, and later to university. I eventually let my hair down, had a LOT of fun forgetting all that I had been through and enjoying being with people who didn't know me or my past. That said I know now that I was avoiding dealing with my issues by partying all the time rather than seeking help.

In 2005, I moved to another city and finally got up the courage to see a gynaecologist. I desperately wanted to have sex and enjoy my sexuality which I had oppressed for so many years. After an initial period of overdoing "it" I met my partner and we are planning to get married next year…as they say, the rest is history!

Learning points:

- The struggles to live and lead a normal healthy life continue in patients with CAH hence, lifelong monitoring, support, and individualised approach is required.
- Education in the prevention and management of adrenal crisis is paramount for everyone involved in the multispecialty care of patients with CAH.
- The positive patient-health care engagement, empowerment of patients and their families/carers in voicing their concerns, and active involvement of patient support groups will improve all aspects of care being received.

35.7 Conclusions

Classic CAH is a rare and life-threatening chronic condition that needs lifelong adrenal replacement

therapy. Patients and families are required to have a good knowledge and understanding of the condition and its management needs in both the short and long term. Their involvement with the health system will be lifelong and requires regular review and ongoing treatment and medial management. Health professionals have a crucial role in coordinating the care of patients with CAH. Treatment goals must be agreed with family and, as soon as possible, with the patient. The management plan is individualised and needs to be modulated throughout the patient's lifetime. For a patient with CAH, a sense of feeling connected and understood within the health system is one of the most important aspects in achieving positive health outcomes and satisfaction with their life's journey.

Aknowledgments With special thanks to Sue Elford, Chair, and Sallyann Blackett, Treasurer, from *The CAH Support Group*, website: www.livingwithcah.com and Dina Matos, Executive Director, from the CARES Foundation, website www.caresfoundation.org for their contributions with patient case studies and details on information and resources available through their Patient Advocacy Group.

References

Arlt W, Krone N. Adult consequences of congenital adrenal hyperplasia. Horm Res. 2007;68(Suppl 5):158–64. https://doi.org/10.1159/000110615.

Arlt W, Willis DS, Wild SH, Krone N, Doherty EJ, Hahner S, et al. Health status of adults with congenital adrenal hyperplasia: a cohort study of 203 patients. J Clin Endocrinol Metab. 2010;95(11):5110–21. https://doi.org/10.1210/jc.2010-0917.

Auchus RJ, Arlt W. Approach to the patient: the adult with congenital adrenal hyperplasia. J Clin Endocrinol Metab. 2013;98(7):2645–55. https://doi.org/10.1210/jc.2013-1440.

Auchus RJ, Witchel SF, Leight KR, Aisenberg J, Azziz R, Bachega TA, et al. Guidelines for the development of comprehensive care centers for congenital adrenal hyperplasia: guidance from the CARES Foundation Initiative. Int J Pediatr Endocrinol. 2010;2010:275213. https://doi.org/10.1155/2010/275213.

Bornstein SR, Allolio B, Arlt W, Barthel A, Don-Wauchope A, Hammer GD, et al. Diagnosis and treatment of primary adrenal insufficiency: an endocrine society clinical practice guideline. J Clin Endocrinol Metab. 2016;101(2):364–89. https://doi.org/10.1210/jc.2015-1710.

Dittmann RW, Kappes MH, Kappes ME, Borger D, Stegner H, Willig RH, et al. Congenital adrenal hyperplasia. I: gender-related behavior and attitudes in female patients and sisters. Psychoneuroendocrinology. 1990;15(5–6):401–20.

El-Maouche D, Arlt W, Merke DP. Congenital adrenal hyperplasia. Lancet. 2017;390(10108):2194–210. https://doi.org/10.1016/S0140-6736(17)31431-9.

Escobar-Morreale HF, Carmina E, Dewailly D, Gambineri A, Kelestimur F, Moghetti P, et al. Epidemiology, diagnosis and management of hirsutism: a consensus statement by the Androgen Excess and Polycystic Ovary Syndrome Society. Hum Reprod Update. 2012;18(2):146–70. https://doi.org/10.1093/humupd/dmr042.

Gleeson H, Davis J, Jones J, O'Shea E, Clayton PE. The challenge of delivering endocrine care and successful transition to adult services in adolescents with congenital adrenal hyperplasia: experience in a single centre over 18 years. Clin Endocrinol. 2013;78(1):23–8. https://doi.org/10.1111/cen.12053.

Hahner S, Spinnler C, Fassnacht M, Burger-Stritt S, Lang K, Milovanovic D, et al. High incidence of adrenal crisis in educated patients with chronic adrenal insufficiency: a prospective study. J Clin Endocrinol Metab. 2015;100(2):407–16. https://doi.org/10.1210/jc.2014-3191.

Han TS, Stimson RH, Rees DA, Krone N, Willis DS, Conway GS, et al. Glucocorticoid treatment regimen and health outcomes in adults with congenital adrenal hyperplasia. Clin Endocrinol. 2013a;78(2):197–203. https://doi.org/10.1111/cen.12045.

Han TS, Krone N, Willis DS, Conway GS, Hahner S, Rees DA, et al. Quality of life in adults with congenital adrenal hyperplasia relates to glucocorticoid treatment, adiposity and insulin resistance: United Kingdom Congenital adrenal Hyperplasia Adult Study Executive (CaHASE). Eur J Endocrinol. 2013b;168(6):887–93. https://doi.org/10.1530/EJE-13-0128.

Han TS, Conway GS, Willis DS, Krone N, Rees DA, Stimson RH, et al. Relationship between final height and health outcomes in adults with congenital adrenal hyperplasia: United Kingdom congenital adrenal hyperplasia adult study executive (CaHASE). J Clin Endocrinol Metab. 2014;99(8):E1547–55. https://doi.org/10.1210/jc.2014-1486.

Hatton DL, Canam C, Thorne S, Hughes AM. Parents' perceptions of caring for an infant or toddler with diabetes. J Adv Nurs. 1995;22(3):569–77.

Joint Lecahwg. Consensus statement on 21-hydroxylase deficiency from the Lawson Wilkins Pediatric Endocrine Society and the European Society for Paediatric Endocrinology. J Clin Endocrinol Metab. 2002;87(9):4048–53. https://doi.org/10.1210/jc.2002-020611.

Knickmeyer R, Baron-Cohen S, Fane BA, Wheelwright S, Mathews GA, Conway GS, et al. Androgens and autistic traits: a study of individuals with congenital adrenal hyperplasia. Horm Behav. 2006;50(1):148–53. https://doi.org/10.1016/j.yhbeh.2006.02.006.

Kruse B, Riepe FG, Krone N, Bosinski HA, Kloehn S, Partsch CJ, et al. Congenital adrenal hyperplasia—how to improve the transition from adolescence to adult life. Exp Clin Endocrinol Diabetes. 2004;112(7):343–55. https://doi.org/10.1055/s-2004-821013.

Mallappa A, Sinaii N, Kumar P, Whitaker MJ, Daley LA, Digweed D, et al. A phase 2 study of Chronocort, a modified-release formulation of hydrocortisone, in the treatment of adults with classic congenital adrenal hyperplasia. J Clin Endocrinol Metab. 2015;100(3):1137–45. https://doi.org/10.1210/jc.2014-3809.

Merke DP, Poppas DP. Management of adolescents with congenital adrenal hyperplasia. Lancet Diabetes Endocrinol. 2013;1(4):341–52. https://doi.org/10.1016/S2213-8587(13)70138-4.

Patterson JM, McCubbin HI, Warwick WJ. The impact of family functioning on health changes in children with cystic fibrosis. Soc Sci Med. 1990;31(2):159–64.

Reichman DE, White PC, New MI, Rosenwaks Z. Fertility in patients with congenital adrenal hyperplasia. Fertil Steril. 2014;101(2):301–9. https://doi.org/10.1016/j.fertnstert.2013.11.002.

Reisch N, Arlt W, Krone N. Health problems in congenital adrenal hyperplasia due to 21-hydroxylase deficiency. Horm Res Paediatr. 2011;76(2):73–85. https://doi.org/10.1159/000327794.

Reisch N, Willige M, Kohn D, Schwarz HP, Allolio B, Reincke M, et al. Frequency and causes of adrenal crises over lifetime in patients with 21-hydroxylase deficiency. Eur J Endocrinol. 2012;167(1):35–42. https://doi.org/10.1530/EJE-12-0161.

Speiser PW, Azziz R, Baskin LS, Ghizzoni L, Hensle TW, Merke DP, et al. Congenital adrenal hyperplasia due to steroid 21-hydroxylase deficiency: an Endocrine Society clinical practice guideline. J Clin Endocrinol Metab. 2010;95(9):4133–60. https://doi.org/10.1210/jc.2009-2631.

Webb EA, Elliott L, Carlin D, Wilson M, Hall K, Netherton J, et al. Quantitative brain MRI in congenital adrenal hyperplasia: in vivo assessment of the cognitive and structural impact of steroid hormones. J Clin Endocrinol Metab. 2018;103(4):1330–41. https://doi.org/10.1210/jc.2017-01481.

White PC. Neonatal screening for congenital adrenal hyperplasia. Nat Rev Endocrinol. 2009;5(9):490–8. https://doi.org/10.1038/nrendo.2009.148.

White PC, Bachega TA. Congenital adrenal hyperplasia due to 21 hydroxylase deficiency: from birth to adulthood. Semin Reprod Med. 2012;30(5):400–9. https://doi.org/10.1055/s-0032-1324724.

White PC, Speiser PW. Congenital adrenal hyperplasia due to 21-hydroxylase deficiency. Endocr Rev. 2000;21(3):245–91. https://doi.org/10.1210/edrv.21.3.0398.

Witchel SF, Azziz R. Nonclassic congenital adrenal hyperplasia. Int J Pediatr Endocrinol. 2010;2010:625105. https://doi.org/10.1155/2010/625105.

Key Reading

1. Speiser PW, Azziz R, Baskin LS, Ghizzoni L, Hensle TW, Merke DP, et al. Congenital adrenal hyperplasia due to steroid 21-hydroxylase deficiency: an Endocrine Society clinical practice guideline. J Clin Endocrinol Metab. 2010;95(9):4133–60. https://doi.org/10.1210/jc.2009-2631.

2. Auchus RJ, Witchel SF, Leight KR, Aisenberg J, Azziz R, Bachega TA, et al. Guidelines for the Development of Comprehensive Care Centers for Congenital Adrenal Hyperplasia: Guidance from the CARES Foundation Initiative. Int J Pediatr Endocrinol. 2010;2010:275213. https://doi.org/10.1155/2010/275213.

3. Auchus RJ, Arlt W. Approach to the patient: the adult with congenital adrenal hyperplasia. J Clin Endocrinol Metab. 2013;98(7):2645–55. https://doi.org/10.1210/jc.2013-1440.

4. Merke DP, Poppas DP. Management of adolescents with congenital adrenal hyperplasia. Lancet Diabet Endocrinol. 2013;1(4):341–52. https://doi.org/10.1016/S2213-8587(13)70138-4.

5. Kruse B, Riepe FG, Krone N, Bosinski HA, Kloehn S, Partsch CJ, et al. Congenital adrenal hyperplasia—how to improve the transition from adolescence to adult life. Exp Clin Endocrinol Diabet. 2004;112(7):343–55. https://doi.org/10.1055/s-2004-821013.

Adrenal Tumours: Adrenocortical Functioning Adenomas, Pheochromocytomas, Incidentalomas, and Adrenocortical Cancer

36

Andrew P. Demidowich, Miriam Asia, and Jérôme Bertherat

Contents

A. P. Demidowich (✉)
National Institutes of Health, Bethesda, MD, USA
e-mail: andrew.demidowich@nih.gov

M. Asia
Department of Endocrinology, Birmingham
University Hospital, Birmingham, UK
e-mail: Miriam.Asia@uhb.nhs.uk

J. Bertherat
Service d'Endocrinologie, Reference Center for Rare
Adrenal Diseases, Hôpital Cochin, Paris, France
e-mail: jerome.bertherat@cch.ap-hop-paris.fr

© Springer Nature Switzerland AG 2019
S. Llahana et al. (eds.), *Advanced Practice in Endocrinology Nursing*,
https://doi.org/10.1007/978-3-319-99817-6_36

Abstract

This chapter will discuss in detail the background, evaluation, and management of adrenal tumours, with an additional focus on the role of endocrine nursing in the care of these patients. It is divided into three parts, each providing a comprehensive outline of: A) Adrenocortical functioning adenomas and adrenal hyperplasia, B) Pheochromocytomas and Paragangliomas, and C) Adrenal incidentaloma and adrenocortical cancer (ACC).

Evaluation of adrenal tumours and adenomas requires a thorough history and physical examination. Family history is particularly important as adrenocortical disease can be caused by germline mutations passed down from generation to generation. More commonly, however, sporadic somatic mutations are the cause of spontaneous tumour formation and autonomous hormone secretion.

Adrenocortical adenomas, hyperplasia, and incidentalomas are non-cancerous "growths" or proliferation of cells in the adrenal cortex. Adenomas are rare in childhood but become more frequent as humans age. Approximately 20% of adenomas are functional; that is, they produce hormones to some degree in an autonomous or dysregulated manner. Functional adenomas most commonly produce cortisol or aldosterone, whereas androgen-producing tumours are quite rare and may portend a cancerous aetiology. Co-secretion of more than one hormone from adenomas/hyperplasia is also possible.

The biochemical work-up, with screening as well as confirmatory testing, and relevant imaging will be discussed in detail. The treatment, management, and long-term monitoring are also discussed for each of the adrenal tumours, respectively. Discussion in this chapter is illustrated with a rich content of figures, box inserts, and case studies.

Keywords

Adrenal adenoma · Adrenal hyperplasia · Cushing syndrome · Primary aldosteronism · Cortisol · Aldosterone · Adrenocortical cancer · Pheochromocytomas and paraganglioma

Abbreviations

ACC	Adrenocortical cancer
ACE	Angiotensin-converting enzyme
ACTH	Adrenocorticotropic hormone
APA	Aldosterone-producing adenoma
ARR	Aldosterone-to-renin ratio
AVS	Adrenal venous sampling
BMI	Body Mass Index
CAH	Congenital adrenal hyperplasia
CPA	Cortisol-producing adenoma
CRH	Corticotropin releasing hormone
DHEA	Dehydroepiandrosterone
GRA	Glucocorticoid-remediable aldosteronism
HNPGL	Head and neck paraganglioma
IV	Intravenous
L-DOPA	L-dihydroxyphenylalanine
MRA	Mineralocorticoid receptor antagonist
PA	Primary aldosteronism
PAC	Plasma aldosterone concentration
PCC	Pheochromocytomas
PCOS	Polycystic ovarian syndrome
PGL	Paraganglioma
PMNT	Phenylethanolamine N-methyltransferase
RAAS	Renin-angiotensin-aldosterone system
SDHx	Succinate dehydrogenase complex

Key Terms

- **Adrenocortical functioning adenomas:** hypersecreting tumors of the adrenal cortex
- **Adrenal hyperplasia:** enlargement of the adrenal glands
- **Adrenal incidentalomas:** incidentally found benign adenomas on evaluation of unrelated symptoms
- **Co-secretion:** more than one hormone secreted from adrenal adenomas/hyperplasia
- **Cushing Syndrome:** hypersecretion of cortisol from an adrenal adenoma
- **Catecholamines:** are produced in the adrenal medulla and are essential for the stress response
- **Pheochromocytomas:** are tumors arising from the adrenal medulla that produce excess catecholamines

- **Paraganglioma:** are also tumors that produce catecholamines, but they originate in paraganglia along the parasympathetic and sympathetic chains

Key Points
- List the most common hormones produced by adrenal functioning tumours/hyperplasia
- Describe common presenting signs and symptoms of primary aldosteronism, Cushing syndrome, adrenocortical cancer, pheochromocytoma, paraganglioma
- Explain the evaluation for suspected adrenal tumours/hyperplasia
- Discuss the possible treatment and management options for adrenal tumours
- Emphasize and describe the role of the endocrine nurse in the care of these patients

36.1 Part A: Adrenocortical Functioning Adenomas and Adrenal Hyperplasia

36.1.1 Introduction

As described in the anatomy and physiology chapter of this section, the adrenal gland is comprised of two main layers: the cortex and the medulla. The medulla derives from neuroectodermal tissue in early fetal life and is mainly composed of chromaffin cells. The cortex develops from the mesoderm and is organized into three layers: the zona glomerulosa, zona fasciculata, and zona reticularis, responsible for producing the hormones aldosterone, cortisol, and androgens, respectively (Avisse et al. 2000). Part A of this chapter focuses on functional benign adrenal tumours and hyperplasia of the cortex; Part B covers pheochromocytomas and paragangliomas; and Part C covers adrenal incidentalomas and adrenocortical cancer (ACC). Congenital adrenal hyperplasia is covered in a separate chapter in this section.

Tumours and hyperplasia can be thought of as two ends of the same spectrum. A tumour is a proliferation of cells derived from a single progenitor cell. Hyperplasia, in contrast, is a "tissue-wide" proliferation of cells. Patients can develop a single discreet nodule, multiple nodules (in one or both adrenals), or hyperplasia. Additionally, nodules can grow in the background of a hyperplastic gland (Fig. 36.1). Adrenal adenomas and hyperplasia can occur secondary to chronic hormonal stimulation (e.g. ACTH stimulation in CAH or Cushing disease), or due to a somatic or germline mutation (Hsiao et al. 2009).

The imaging characteristics of adrenal tumours and masses are discussed in greater detail in Part B. Briefly, most (~60–90%) benign adrenocortical adenomas are comprised mainly of lipids and are therefore commonly described as "lipid-rich". On CT imaging, they have a lower density than surrounding organs, such as the liver, kidneys, or spleen, and therefore appear darker. The Hounsfield Units (HU; a measure of density) of the adenoma on non-contrast CT is typically less than 10 HU. Additionally, these tumours have a relatively high "washout" of IV contrast, when examined 10–15 min after contrast injection (Zeiger et al. 2009a).

"Lipid poor" adrenal masses, on the other hand, have higher density on non-contrast CT and commonly have low washout. Benign adrenocortical tumours (either functional or nonfunctional) can be lipid poor; however, other types of diseases, such as pheochromocytomas, ACC, adrenal haemorrhage, or metastatic lesions from other organs, can also present as "lipid poor" masses on CT (Zeiger et al. 2009a).

Benign adrenal tumours are extremely rare in childhood, increase to a prevalence of about 3% by age 50, and 10% in elderly adults (Minnaar et al. 2013; Fassnacht et al. 2016). Although 80% of adenomas are non-functional (Zeiger et al. 2009b), the signs and symptoms of a functional adrenal adenoma can be subtle and easily missed for many years, so most adenomas should undergo evaluation for functional status upon initial discovery (Fassnacht et al. 2016; Zeiger et al. 2009b).

The region in which the functional tumour or hyperplasia is located typically determines the hormone produced. In other words, a functional tumour in the zona glomerulosa will typically cause primary aldosteronism, whereas a functional tumour in the zona fasciculata will lead to

Fig. 36.1 Adrenal
adenomas and
hyperplasia

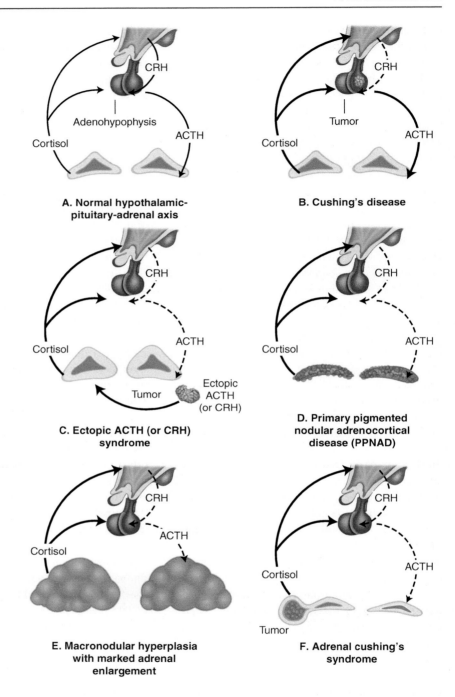

A. Normal hypothalamic-
pituitary-adrenal axis

B. Cushing's disease

C. Ectopic ACTH (or CRH)
syndrome

D. Primary pigmented
nodular adrenocortical
disease (PPNAD)

E. Macronodular hyperplasia
with marked adrenal
enlargement

F. Adrenal cushing's
syndrome

cortisol excess and Cushing syndrome. Functional tumours solely producing androgens are rare and often suggest a malignant, rather than benign, pathology. However, co-secretion of multiple hormones (e.g. cortisol and aldosterone) from benign tumours or hyperplasia can occur (Willenberg et al. 2010; Sakai et al. 1993).

36.1.2 Primary Aldosteronism

Aldosterone, a mineralocorticoid produced by the zona glomerulosa, is a major regulator of blood pressure and intravascular volume status. It exerts its effects primarily by acting on the distal convoluted tubule and collecting duct in the kidney. By binding to its intracellular receptor, aldosterone stimulates production of the ENaC sodium channel, which enables increased sodium and water reabsorption from the urine. To counteract this cationic influx, potassium (and to a lesser degree hydrogen) ions are simultaneously excreted into urine.

Aldosterone synthesis is regulated by several mechanisms. The primary regulator is intravascular volume status via the renin-angiotensin-aldosterone system (RAAS), with hyperkalaemia also being a potent stimulus of aldosterone secretion (please see anatomy and physiology chapter in this section). Adrenocorticotropic hormone (ACTH) can also provoke aldosterone release but plays a minor role overall.

Primary aldosteronism (PA, a.k.a. Conn's syndrome) is the dysregulated hyperproduction of aldosterone from either one or both adrenal glands. Unilateral disease is seen in approximately two-thirds of cases (Mathur et al. 2010) and typically stems from an aldosterone-producing adenoma (APA, a.k.a. Conn's adenoma), frequently caused by a somatic mutation (e.g. *KCNJ5*, *ATP1A1*, *ATP2B3*, *CACNA1D*, or *CACNA1H*). In contrast, bilateral disease most commonly occurs as a result of bilateral adrenal hyperplasia. Heritable forms of PA make up less than 10% of cases; germline mutations include *KCNJ5*, *CLCN2*, *ARMC5*, or a chimeric *CYP11B1/CYP11B2* gene translocation (a.k.a. glucocorticoid-remediable aldosteronism or GRA) (Zilbermint et al. 2015; Dutta et al. 2016).

The most common presenting sign of PA is uncontrolled hypertension. In fact, PA is the leading secondary cause of hypertension, responsible for 5–10% of cases of "presumed" essential hypertension (Funder et al. 2016). Patients may commonly present with symptoms of recurring headache, chest pain, or oedema. More severe cardiovascular sequelae, such as myocardial infarctions, strokes, or congestive heart failure, may manifest at an early age (<40 years). Hypokalaemia is seen only in a minority (~30%) of patients with PA, but can be unmasked when loop diuretics are initiated (Funder et al. 2016).

36.1.2.1 Diagnosis and Treatment of Primary Aldosteronism

In recent years, it has become apparent that other comorbid conditions, including hyperparathyroidism, osteoporosis, nephrolithiasis, renal cysts (Petramala et al. 2014), obstructive sleep apnoea (Di Murro et al. 2010), and insulin resistance, are strongly associated with PA. Moreover, it is important to take a detailed family history, asking specifically about early-onset cardiovascular or cerebrovascular disease in first-degree relatives, as PA can be familial.

Patients should be screened for PA if they have (see Box 36.1 for more details):

1. Blood pressure greater than 150/100 mmHg on more than three occasions
2. Greater than 140/90 mmHg despite using three antihypertensive medications
3. Controlled blood pressure requiring four or more antihypertensive medications
4. Hypertension with adrenal incidentaloma on imaging
5. Hypertension with obstructive sleep apnoea
6. Hypertension with hypokalaemia (even if diuretic-induced)
7. Hypertension with first-degree relative with PA
8. Hypertension with first-degree relative with early-onset hypertension or stroke (age <40) (Funder et al. 2016)

Box 36.1 Principles of Good Clinical Practice for Screening for PA

It is important to follow below instructions when screening for PA, and this is a crucial aspect of the endocrine nurse role. The patient should be appropriately informed and educated about the procedure; supporting patient leaflets to reinforce this information are vital and should be written in an easy to understand language.

Screening consists of measuring a plasma aldosterone concentration (PAC) and plasma renin activity to calculate the aldosterone-to-renin ratio (ARR). Ideally testing should be performed in the morning, after the subject has been out of bed for at least 2 h. Patients should be instructed to be on a liberal salt diet and be volume replete prior to testing. This will suppress the renin level, meaning that most of the circulating aldosterone is probably autonomously produced (i.e. dysregulated), rather than stimulated by the RAAS system. Patients **must** have stopped mineralocorticoid receptor antagonists (e.g. spironolactone, eplerenone) and potassium-wasting diuretics (e.g. furosemide, torsemide) for at least 4 weeks prior to ensure an accurate result. As hypokalaemia can impair aldosterone secretion, patients should also ideally be potassium replete ($[K^+] > 4.0$) prior to testing. Blood should be drawn with the patient in a seated position, rather than recumbent. It should be drawn slowly, ideally into a syringe rather than a vacutainer to avoid haemolysis, transported at room temperature (**not** on ice), and processed within 30 min of collection. An ARR ≥ 750 (SI units) or ≥ 30 (conventional units) with PAC ≥ 280 pmol/L (10 ng/dL) is strongly suggestive of PA (Funder et al. 2016).

Confirmatory testing should be performed, as no diagnosis should depend on a single lab result. Testing options include an oral salt loading test with 24-h urine collection of aldosterone (cut off >33 nmol/day, 12 µg/24 h), saline infusion test (cut off PAC ≥ 280 pmol/L, 10 ng/dL), captopril challenge test, and fludrocortisone suppression test (Funder et al. 2016).

Once confirmed, the patient should undergo CT imaging with IV contrast to better define the adrenal and associated venous anatomy. Because clinicians may be fooled by a non-functional adenoma on imaging, and the disease in fact may be on the contralateral gland or bilateral disease, it is often recommended that patients who are surgi-cal candidates should subsequently undergo adrenal venous sampling (AVS), the current gold standard to confirm the laterality of disease. The rate of success of this technically demanding diagnostic procedure depends on the expertise of the interventional radiologist, so referral to high-volume centre is recommended. Patients younger than 35, with profound aldosterone concentrations (>830 pmol/L or 30 ng/dL), spontaneous hypokalaemia, and an obvious solitary lipid-rich nodule on imaging can forgo AVS and proceed directly to unilateral adrenalectomy (Funder et al. 2016).

Similarly, if AVS lateralizes to one side, it is recommended that the patient proceed to unilateral adrenalectomy (typically performed laparoscopically). Surgery will, in most cases, cure the patient of hypokalaemia and improve hypertension. Hypertension may not improve immediately but may continue to improve even up to 1 year post-operatively (see Box 36.2). Factors that portend a lower rate of hypertension cure include male sex, longer duration of PA (>6 years), multiple antihypertensive medications preoperatively, and overweight or obesity (BMI >25 kg/m^2) (Aronova et al. 2014).

> **Box 36.2 Important Message for Patients for Post-operative Care for PA**
>
> Advise your patient that hypertension may not improve immediately and can continue to improve even up to 1 year post-operatively. Lifestyle factors can influence this so encourage weight loss for your overweight patients.

If the disease is determined to be bilateral by AVS, however, surgery is typically not offered, and medical management with a mineralocorticoid receptor antagonist (MRA) is instituted. Spironolactone is typically cheap (as it is generic), may be the most potent MRA, and is commonly the first-line medication. However, it can have mild off-target anti-androgenic effects leading to gynaecomastia or sexual dysfunction in males. Eplerenone, a newer and more specific MRA, does not cause these side effects and may be a better choice for male patients (Parthasarathy et al. 2011). However, it can also be significantly more costly if not covered by health insurance. If a single medication is unable to control the hypertension, additional agents, such as a calcium channel blocker, ACE inhibitor, or triamterene (ENaC channel blocker) may be added.

36.1.3 Cushing Syndrome

Cortisol, a glucocorticoid produced by the zona fasciculata, has many wide-ranging effects on the body, including regulation of blood pressure, glucose, immune function, metabolism, and bone turnover. Its synthesis and secretion are primarily regulated by ACTH, which is produced in the pituitary.

Among adrenal adenomas, between 5 and 25% have some degree of autonomous cortisol production (Rossi et al. 2000; Mantero et al. 2000). The vast majority of these cortisol-producing adenomas (CPA) do so in small quantities and rarely progress (<1%) to produce overt signs and symptoms typically associated with Cushing syndrome (prevalence 1 per million), such as moon-like face, plethora, dorsal buffalo hump, violaceous abdominal striae, thin skin, easy bruising, frequent infections, fragility fractures, or proximal muscle weakness (Fassnacht et al. 2016; Newell-Price et al. 2006) (Fig. 36.2). Thus, these CPAs have classically been denoted in the literature as causing "Subclinical" Cushing syndrome. In recent years, however, it has been realized that even subclinical Cushing syndrome may have subtle clinical signs such as obesity, acne, or hirsutism and is associated with an increased risk of hypertension, type 2 diabetes, hyperlipidaemia, and osteoporosis (Fassnacht et al. 2016; Rossi et al. 2000). Moreover, as this represents a degree of cortisol excess along a spectrum, the term "autonomous cortisol secretion" is preferred to subclinical Cushing syndrome.

36.1.3.1 Diagnosis of Cushing Syndrome

A thorough history needs to be taken, as effects of hypercortisolaemia may be subtle. Patients may have menstrual irregularities or low testosterone (in men), acanthosis nigricans or skin tags from insulin resistance, acid reflux or peptic ulcer disease from enhanced gastric acid production, and/or silent vertebral compression fractures. Mental disease may be a prominent feature and be very distressing to the patient, manifesting as anxiety, depression, insomnia, mood instability, anger outbursts, fatigue, forgetfulness, or even hallucinations (Rasmussen et al. 2015). Like primary aldosteronism, Cushing syndrome can result from germline (inherited) or somatic (sporadic) mutations (Lodish and Stratakis 2016); therefore, obtaining a good family history is also paramount.

Screening for hypercortisolaemia begins with a 1 mg overnight dexamethasone suppression test (Box. 36.3). Patients are instructed take 1 mg of dexamethasone, a synthetic glucocorticoid that is not recognized by the cortisol laboratory assay, between 11 pm and midnight, and a cortisol level is drawn at 8 am the following morning. Dexamethasone inhibits the hypothalamic production of corticotropin releasing hormone (CRH) and pituitary secretion of ACTH, thereby suppressing normal adrenal cortisol production. A morning cortisol >138 nmol/L (>5 μg/dL) is consistent with autonomous cortisol secretion, whereas a cortisol of ≤50 nmol/L (≤1.8 μg/dL) effectively rules out the disease. A cortisol between these two values is a grey zone and represents "possible" autonomous cortisol secretion (Fassnacht et al. 2016). It is important to note that women on oestrogen (e.g. oral contraceptives) may have a false-positive as oestrogen raises the circulating cortisol binding globulin. Also, some advocate to measure a dexamethasone level simultaneously with the morning cortisol to assess if a) the patient is a "hypermetabolizer" or b) if the patient did not actually take the medication, as both could lead to a false-positive result (Meikle 1982; Nieman et al. 2008).

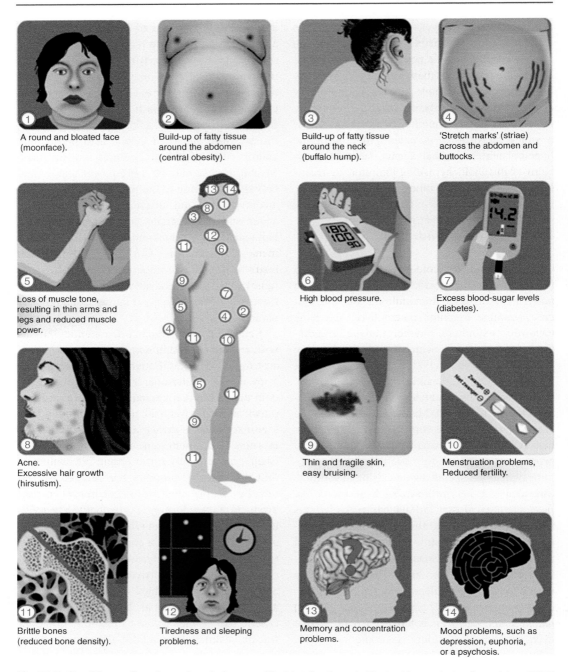

1. A round and bloated face (moonface).

2. Build-up of fatty tissue around the abdomen (central obesity).

3. Build-up of fatty tissue around the neck (buffalo hump).

4. 'Stretch marks' (striae) across the abdomen and buttocks.

5. Loss of muscle tone, resulting in thin arms and legs and reduced muscle power.

6. High blood pressure.

7. Excess blood-sugar levels (diabetes).

8. Acne. Excessive hair growth (hirsutism).

9. Thin and fragile skin, easy bruising.

10. Menstruation problems, Reduced fertility.

11. Brittle bones (reduced bone density).

12. Tiredness and sleeping problems.

13. Memory and concentration problems.

14. Mood problems, such as depression, euphoria, or a psychosis.

Fig. 36.2 Possible manifestations of cortisol excess (Cushing Syndrome). Used with permission from AdrenalNET and accessed via https://adrenals.eu/infographics/cushings-syndrome-infographic/

Patients with signs consistent with overt Cushing syndrome should undergo other screening tests, such as a 24-h urine collection for free cortisol (repeated at least twice), a late-night salivary cortisol (repeated at least twice), or a 48-h low-dose dexamethasone suppression test. Two positive screening tests in the setting of overt signs is consistent with the diagnosis of Cushing syndrome.

It is important to remember that ACTH excess (e.g. functional pituitary adenoma) can cause adrenal hyperplasia ± nodules. A suppressed ACTH level (<1.1 pmol/L, <5 pg/mL) is consistent with an adrenal, rather than an ACTH-dependent (e.g. pituitary or ectopic) source; however, unsuppressed ACTH levels (<3.3 pmol/L, 15 pg/mL) can be seen with adrenal disease as well (Newell-Price et al. 2006). In this case, an 8 mg overnight dexamethasone suppression test or CRH stimulation test may be helpful to distinguish between the two aetiologies.

36.1.3.2 Treatment of CPA Causing Cushing Syndrome

CPA causing Cushing syndrome should be surgically removed, if possible, via laparoscopic resection. If bilateral disease is seen on imaging, the surgical strategy should be thoroughly discussed with the patient. In the past, frequently both adrenal glands were excised leaving the patient cured, but with permanent adrenal insufficiency, requiring lifelong glucocorticoid (e.g. hydrocortisone) and mineralocorticoid (e.g. fludrocortisone) replacement. Recent studies have suggested that simply removing the larger gland on CT/MRI, or the more hypermetabolic gland on FDG PET, may lead to successful remission (Patel et al. 2016; Debillon et al. 2015).

The evidence regarding surgical intervention for autonomous cortisol secretion is less clear. Limited studies suggest that adrenalectomy for individuals who are surgical candidates and who also have related comorbid conditions, such as obesity, hypertension, type 2 diabetes, hypertension, or osteoporosis, may derive benefit (Fassnacht et al. 2016). For non-surgical candidates, medical therapy such as ketoconazole, metyrapone, mitotane, pasireotide, and/or mifepristone can be considered (Sharma and Committee 2017).

36.1.4 Adrenal Androgens

Androgens produced from the zona reticularis include dihydroepiandrostenone (DHEA), DHEA-sulphate (DHEAS), and androstenedione. Regulation of adrenal androgens is a complex system, partially under the control of ACTH. However, numerous other hormones may play a part in regulating the zona reticularis as well, including growth hormone, gonadotropins, oestrogens, and insulin (Parker 1991).

Females suspected of androgen overproduction may present with mild symptoms, such as hirsutism, acne, and menstrual irregularities. These patients should be assessed for non-classical congenital adrenal hyperplasia (see Chap. 35) and PCOS (see Chap. 39). Unlike in NCCAH, PCOS classically has been thought to result from dysregulated ovarian androgen synthesis. However, it has been recently suggested that a subgroup of PCOS patients suffer from mildly hyperactive adrenocortical function and adrenal hyperplasia (Gourgari et al. 2016). Benign androgen-producing adrenal adenomas have been previously described but are exceedingly rare (Ghayee et al. 2011; Goodarzi et al. 2003).

More rapid presentation and severe signs/symptoms of virilization, including deepening of the voice and male-pattern baldness, may signify an androgen-secreting adrenocortical cancer. For this reason, paediatric or female patients with confirmed hyperandrogenism, and particularly those with aggressive disease, should undergo imaging of the adrenals to help establish the aetiology. In instances of ACC or a benign functional adrenal adenoma, surgery is warranted.

Individuals with PCOS may benefit from spironolactone due to its anti-androgenic properties.

36.2 Part B: Pheochromocytomas and Paragangliomas

36.2.1 Anatomy and Physiology

The adrenal medulla is responsible for producing catecholamines (the hormones dopamine, norepinephrine, and epinephrine), which are essential for the stress response, otherwise known as the "fight or flight" response. The catecholamine pathway begins with the conversion of L-tyrosine to L-dihydroxyphenylalanine (L-DOPA) by tyrosine hydroxylase, the rate limiting step. L-DOPA is then converted to dopamine by DOPA decarboxylase, and subsequently to norepinephrine (a.k.a. noradrenaline) by dopamine hydroxylase. The final step is catalysed by phenylethanolamine *N*-methyltransferase (PMNT) to form epinephrine (a.k.a. adrenaline) (Flatmark 2000).

Norepinephrine and epinephrine have potent cardiovascular effects. They can both bind to α1, α2, β1, and β3 adrenergic receptors. α1 binding mediates smooth muscle contraction and increases vascular tone; α2 binding leads to a negative feedback reduction of catecholamine production, decreased gastrointestinal motility, among numerous other actions; β1 binding causes increased heart rate and cardiac contractility; and β3 binding stimulates increased brown adipose tissue thermogenesis. Epinephrine has much greater affinity for the β2 adrenergic receptor than does norepinephrine, leading to increased smooth muscle relaxation in pulmonary bronchi and decreased gastrointestinal motility (Insel 1996, 1989; Sagrada et al. 1987).

For the most part, these hormones are stored in vesicles rather than directly released into circulation. Only upon stimulation do the vesicles fuse with the plasma membrane, thereby releasing the catecholamines in appreciable quantities. In contrast, metabolites of catecholamines (e.g. normetanephrine and metanephrine) are continuously excreted into circulation and are useful for diagnostic purposes (Lenders et al. 2014).

36.2.2 Pheochromocytomas and Paragangliomas

Tumours arising from the adrenal medulla are termed pheochromocytomas (PCC). Paraganglioma (PGL) are similar to PCC in that they can also produce catecholamines, but they originate in paraganglia along the parasympathetic and sympathetic chains. Sympathetic paraganglia are derived from chromaffin cells, are commonly located in the para-axial region from the neck to the pelvis, and secrete catecholamines in response to sympathetic stimulation. Parasympathetic ganglia, on the other hand, are not derived from chromaffin cells and are often found in the head and neck or close to their target organ, such as the carotid body, jugulotympanic ganglion, or along the vagus nerve (Fig. 36.3) (McNichol 2001). Thus, the location of a PGL can clue a clinician to its hormone secretory status; namely, paravertebral PGL often are biochemically active, whereas head and neck PGL (HNPGL) are commonly either non-functional (silent) or only dopamine producing.

PCC/PGL are rare, with an estimated incidence of 1 in 2000–5000 individuals. PCC make up about 80–85% of these cases, with PGL being less common. Sporadic PCC typically presents between ages 40 and 50 although 2–10% of cases are diagnosed in paediatric patients. Both sexes are affected equally (Wyszynska et al. 1992; Lenders et al. 2005; McNeil et al. 2000; Martucci and Pacak 2014).

PCC/PGL classically present with paroxysms of sympathetic excess, including episodic headache/migraines, sweating, and tachycardia. Both blood pressure spikes or sustained hypertension can be seen with PCC/PGL. Hypertensive crises caused by catecholamine surges can present with or lead to heart attacks, strokes, or death (Mazza et al. 2014; Whitelaw et al. 2014). Conversely, patients with predominantly epinephrine-producing PCC can present with orthostatic hypotension or even shock (Bergland 1989; Streeten and Anderson Jr. 1996). Other symptoms can include flushing or facial pallor, palpitations, diz-

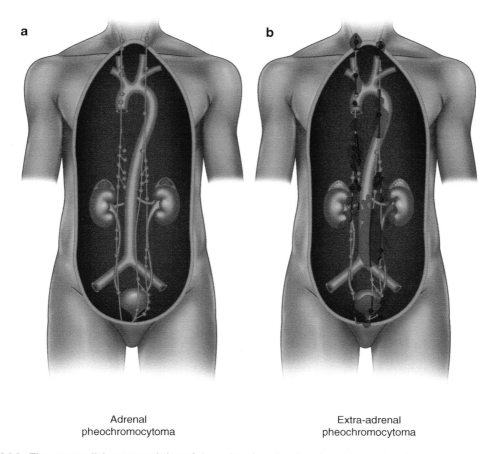

Adrenal
pheochromocytoma

Extra-adrenal
pheochromocytoma

Fig. 36.3 The paraganglial system and sites of shown in red on the adrenals and extra-adrenal

ziness, visual disturbances, and feelings of anxiety or impending doom. Nausea and vomiting can present, particularly after exercise (Martucci and Pacak 2014). Constipation, commonly overlooked, can be severe and significantly impact patient quality of life (Thosani et al. 2015). Lastly, fasting hyperglycaemia or frank diabetes is a rare manifestation of PCC/PGL, particularly in younger patients without other diabetes risk factors (La Batide-Alanore et al. 2003).

The symptoms may occur spontaneously or may be brought on by stimuli, including the ingestion of certain tyramine-containing foods, micturition (in the cases of urinary bladder PCC), or certain medications or illicit drugs (Hodin et al. 2014). Anaesthesia or manipulation of a PCC/PGL during surgery can also lead to a catecholamine surge. PCC/PGL can also be discovered incidentally on

imaging. Indeed, up to 5% of adrenal incidentalomas are found to be PCC (Mantero et al. 2000).

36.2.2.1 Diagnostic Testing

The initial diagnostic test of choice for PCC/PGL is either plasma-free metanephrines or 24-h urine fractionated metanephrines, which have greater than 90% sensitivity and specificity. The plasma or urine metanephrines are typically elevated more than threefold above the upper limit of normal for the reference range. Urine collections should also be measured for creatinine to ensure proper collection (Box. 36.4). These tests have demonstrated superior sensitivity and specificity over plasma or urine catecholamines or vanillyl-mandelic acid (VMA) (Lenders et al. 2002, 2014). HNPGL tend to be biochemically silent, or only secrete methoxytyramine, a dopamine metabolite, for which commercial biochemical testing is not yet widely available (Rao et al. 2017).

Because up to 20% of metanephrine measurements may be false-positives (Yu and Wei 2010), equivocal results (e.g. metanephrine or normetanephrine elevation 1–3× the upper limit of normal) should be repeated, removing any possible offending medications. Patients with persistently equivocal tests or unclear diagnosis can also undergo a clonidine suppression test. The alpha receptor blocker clonidine specifically blocks norepinephrine released from neurons but does not block its release from the adrenal medulla or from PCC tumours. In individuals with PCC, plasma metanephrine levels do not suppress (<40% decrease) at 3 h after clonidine administration. This test has a specificity of 100% with sensitivity of 97%, but has not been validated prospectively. Importantly, the clonidine may cause significant hypotension, so patients should be monitored during this test (Lenders et al. 2014).

Once a diagnosis is established, patients should undergo imaging to locate the PCC/PGL. Typically, a CT of the abdomen and pelvis is pursued since most PCC/PGL are located in the abdomen. Because PCC are typically dense, a lesion with >10 Hounsfield units (HU) on non-contrast CT increases the likelihood, whereas a lesion with <5 HU almost definitively rules out the culprit lesion. To obtain washout values, contrast is injected, and the patient undergoes scanning one and 15 min later. The absolute washout (($(HU_{1\,min} - HU_{15\,min})/(HU_{1\,min} - HU_{baseline})$)) is often less than 60% in PCC/PGL, reflecting their vascular and hypermetabolic nature, and therefore retaining (not "washing out") the IV contrast (Blake et al. 2010; McCarthy et al. 2016).

MRI imaging can be pursued instead, particularly in the paediatric population or in pregnant individuals, as it also has excellent sensitivity. On T1-weighted imaging, PCC/PGL have a signal intensity similar to liver, kidney, and muscle, which distinguishes them from the more common and benign cortical adenomas, which appear bright. Additionally, PCC/PGL do not have "signal drop out" between the in- and out-of-phase images. On T2-weighted images, PCC/PGL have a hyperintense appearance, sometimes nicknamed the "lightbulb" sign (Fig. 36.4) (Blake et al. 2010; McCarthy et al. 2016; Elsayes et al. 2005).

Ultrasound has much poorer sensitivity than CT or MRI, and therefore is not often used in the diagnosis of PCC/PGL, except when bladder PGL or liver metastases are suspected.

If a tumour is not localized on CT/MRI or metastatic disease is suspected, functional imag-

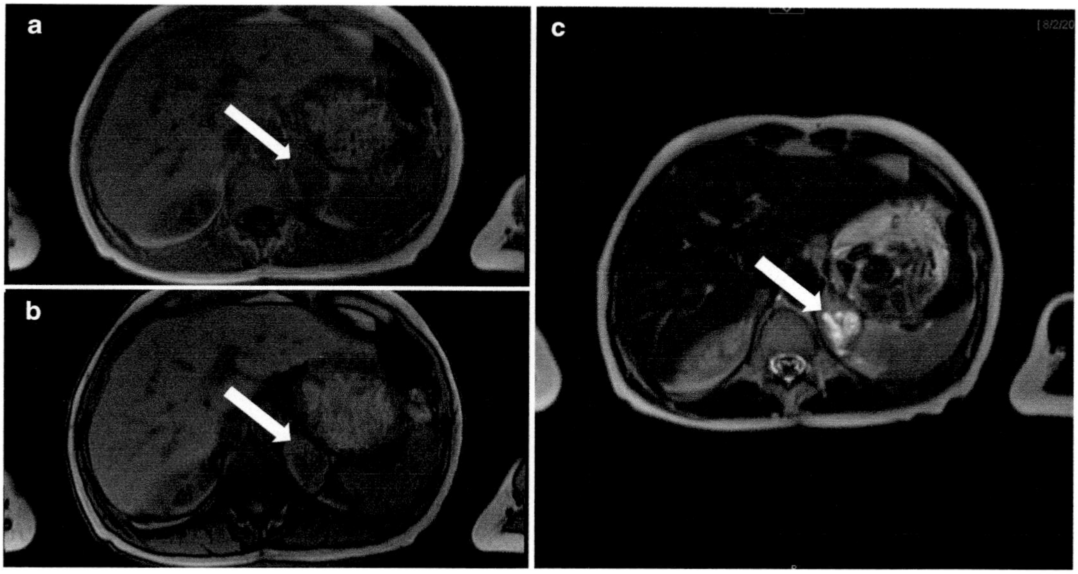

Fig. 36.4 MRI images of a pheochromocytoma (white arrows). Key: (**a**) T1 weighted MRI of the Abdomen In-phase with arrow pointing to pheochromocytoma at the left adrenal gland; (**b**) T1 weighted MRI of the Abdomen Out-phase with arrow pointing to pheochromocytoma at the left adrenal gland; (**c**) T2 weighted MRI of the Abdomen with arrow pointing to a bright pheochromocytoma lesion at the left adrenal gland. **Image provided by and used with permission from Dr Mayank Patel, MD, Special Volunteer, Section on Medical Neuroendocrinology, NICHD/ NIH**

ing should be pursued. MIBG is available at many institutions and has classically been the first-line functional imaging test, as MIBG has high affinity for norepinephrine transporters. ^{131}I-MIBG is less sensitive and emits greater γ radiation than ^{123}I-MIBG and is no longer recommended. However, up to 50% of normal adrenal glands can demonstrate uptake, and false-positivity of MIBG is a significant problem. Conversely, MIBG has poor sensitivity for the detection of malignant, bilateral, or extra-adrenal PCC/PGL, or those related to certain germline PCC/PGL-driver mutations (e.g. *RET*, *VHL*, or *SDHx*) (Lenders et al. 2014; Timmers et al. 2012).

PET imaging is superior to MIBG with respect to PGLs or metastatic disease and is more commonly being used over MIBG in the evaluation of PCC/PGL. ^{18}F-dihydroxyphenylalanine (FDOPA) has been shown to have excellent sensitivity

(>90%) and specificity in metastatic disease but is not commonly available. ^{18}F-fluorodeoxyglucose (FDG) PET is most frequently used and has excellent sensitivity due to the increased metabolic demand PCC/PGL. However, inflammation, infection, benign adrenal adenomas, and other tumours/cancers may also demonstrate positive FDG-PET uptake. Also, if the patient has hyperglycaemia or uncontrolled diabetes mellitus, the elevated circulating glucose may compete with the FDG tracer for uptake, thereby resulting in a false-negative scan (Timmers et al. 2012; Taieb and Pacak 2018).

Lastly, ^{68}Ga-DOTATATE has been shown great promise as a functional imaging modality, particularly in *SDHB* metastatic disease and HNPGL, and has exceptional sensitivity and specificity in abdominal and thoracic PGLs as well (Taieb and Pacak 2018; Janssen et al. 2015, 2016).

As 30–40% of PCC/PGL may arise as part of an inherited syndrome, genetic testing should be offered to all patients diagnosed with PCC/PGL. With improvements and cost reduction in genetic sequencing a plethora of new genes have been linked with PCC/PGL formation, including over 10 major driver genes and 20 minor or rare driver genes (Dahia 2014; Curras-Freixes et al. 2017). Mutations in the succinate dehydrogenase complex (SDHx), a multimer of different protein subunits involved in the electron transport chain, are the most commonly inherited PCC/PGL-driver gene mutations, with *SDHB* and *SDHD* representing 10% and 9% of cases, respectively. Genetic testing is important as it can give prognostic information (e.g. *SDHB* frequently cause metastatic disease), may help with preconception planning or screening of family members, and may guide biochemical and radiologic testing.

36.2.2.2 Treatment for Pheochromocytoma and Paraganglioma

For biochemically active tumours, patients should be started on alpha-blockade immediately (Box. 36.5). For tumours which are very symptomatic (e.g. frequent hypertensive crises, uncontrolled blood pressure) or have very elevated metanephrines, phenoxybenzamine, a powerful non-selective irreversible alpha-blocker, is recommended. Less active tumours may do well with a selective α1-antagonist (e.g. terazosin, doxazosin, prazosin) (Hodin et al. 2014).

Box 36.5 Nursing Considerations for Patients on Alpha-Blockers

The role of the endocrine nurse is crucial in monitoring blood pressure and pulse and titrating alpha-blockers medications. It is important to educate patient about the side effects of these medications and that these can cause postural hypotension. The patient is advised to avoid sudden change of position, i.e. abrupt standing whilst sitting or lying. The patient is advised to increase fluid intake as blood volume is diminished because of excess adrenaline.

Beta-blockers, such as atenolol or metoprolol, can be started at least 3 days after alpha-blockade initiation to help control tachycardia. Beta-blockade prior to alpha-blockade can cause unopposed alpha stimulation and precipitate a pheochromocytoma crisis. Additionally, beta-blockers with both alpha- and beta-adrenergic blocking ability (e.g. labetalol) should be avoided as single or first-line therapy, as the beta-blockade is much more potent than the alpha-blockade and may precipitate a crisis (Lenders et al. 2014). Calcium channel blockers may be used in addition to or instead of alpha-blockers, particularly in those with mild disease or who are intolerant of alpha-blockade (Hodin et al. 2014).

Metyrosine, a tyrosine hydroxylase inhibitor, prevents catecholamine synthesis and can be used in refractory patients. However, it is expensive, difficult to obtain, and poorly tolerated with significant side effects, including depression, fatigue, nausea, and somnolence. Therefore, it should be used as an adjunctive treatment to the above mentioned medications in selected patients (Hodin et al. 2014).

Once medically controlled, most patients should be referred to surgery. Because patients with inherited forms of PCC/PGL may have recurrences and/or bilateral disease, partial cortical-sparing adrenalectomies are preferred when possible to avoid lifelong glucocorticoid and mineralocorticoid replacement. Most surgeries can be performed laparoscopically; however, for large (e.g. >5 cm), invasive, or metastatic tumours, open laparotomies may be required (Lenders et al. 2014). Patients should have intravenous fluids initiated in the immediate preoperative period to ensure adequate intravascular fluid repletion and to help prevent cardiogenic shock from the rapid decline of catecholamine levels post-operatively (Parenti et al. 2012). Patients should be followed up for at least 10 years post-operatively for surveillance (Box. 36.6). Of note, recurrences occur more frequently for patients with familial forms of PCC/PGL or extra-adrenal disease (Lenders et al. 2005).

Tumours greater than 5 cm, *SDHB* carriers, extra-adrenal location, and high Ki-67 on pathology are prognostic markers placing individuals at increased risk for developing metastatic disease. Select patients with malignant PCC/PGL still can be referred to surgery. Although not generally

---

Box 36.6 Important Message for Patients for Post-operative Care for PCC/PGL

Advise your patient that follow-up for at least 10 years post-operatively for surveillance is necessary even if they feel well due to the risk of recurrence for pheochromocytoma and paraganglioma. Recurrences occur more frequently for patients with familial forms of PCC/PGL or extra-adrenal disease.

---

curative, debulking or rending a patient with no evidence of disease may reduce time to recurrence, improve symptoms and quality of life, and may possibly improve response to chemotherapy (Parenti et al. 2012). Radiofrequency ablation may provide benefit for liver or bone metastases. For MIBG-positive tumours, ^{131}I-MIBG therapy may be attempted, although this is rarely curative (Martucci and Pacak 2014). A combination of cyclophosphamide, vincristine, and dacarbazine (CVD) is often used for unresectable metastatic disease (Parenti et al. 2012). Somatostatin analogues (e.g. octreotide, a.k.a "cold" somatostatin) have shown the ability to slow tumour progression in several case reports or small case series although this has not been well studied (van Hulsteijn et al. 2013; Duet et al. 2005). Several new targeted therapies, including radiolabelled DOTA peptides (e.g. ^{177}Lu-DOTATATE) and tyrosine kinase inhibitors, are currently under study (Martucci and Pacak 2014). Patient advocacy groups such as Pheo Para Alliance (USA) (Box. 36.7) provide great support and valuable resources for patients and clinicians and the reader is encouraged to refer to their website.

36.3 Part C: Adrenal Incidentaloma and Adrenocortical Cancer (ACC)

36.3.1 Adrenal Incidentaloma

Adrenal incidentaloma refers to a mass of the adrenal area discovered fortuitously on a medi-

---

Box 36.7 Case Study and Resources Provided by the Pheo Para Alliance (USA) (Published with Consent)

Often called the "Great Mimic", pheochromocytoma and paraganglioma mimic stress-related disorders with symptoms ranging from high blood pressure, flushing, and headaches, to anxiety and panic attacks. Often written off as being overly anxious, it takes the average patient six frustrating years to receive an accurate diagnosis. In some cases, such as mine, a family member makes the diagnosis based on "family history" due to the strong genetic disposition of the disease. My father-in-law had the disease, as do my husband, his siblings, our three adult children, and now two of my young grandchildren have tested positive for the genetic mutation.

Pheochromocytoma and paraganglioma are extremely rare neuroendocrine tumours. Patients with these tumours suffer from the initial challenge of a complicated diagnosis and the difficulty of finding healthcare providers that understand proper diagnosis and treatment. The *Pheo Para Alliance* provides educational support and resources from the time of initial diagnosis through treatment and a lifetime of monitoring. Patients may never meet another patient with their same diagnosis, which is one of the many reasons that the Alliance is so vital to the pheo/para community. We provide an opportunity for members of our community to meet, if not in person, virtually with others who understand what they're going through. Additionally, with a greater understanding of the strong genetic component of the disease, we're helping educate patients and their healthcare providers about the importance of genetic testing for patients and their family members. With the increase in genetic testing, patients are being diagnosed at a younger age, with a lifetime of looking for tumours ahead of them.

Founded in 2007, the Pheo Para Alliance is the longest standing internationally recognized leader in advocacy for and awareness of pheochromocytoma and paraganglioma. Since our inception, the Pheo Para Alliance has dedicated more than $2 million towards research, diagnosis, education, advocacy, and finding a cure for this disease. In August 2017, we consolidated our power and influence by merging with our partner group, the *Pheo Para Troopers*, a true alliance of forces working with a common mission: investing in research to accelerate treatments and cures whilst empowering patients, their families and medical professional through advocacy, education, and a global community of support.

Community support is provided through the following services:

- Website with educational articles and videos for patients and healthcare providers
- Monthly Pheo Para Alliance newsletter with articles on the latest research, educational opportunities, and patients' stories
- Patient forum: An online opportunity for patients and caregivers to reach out for information and support
- Educational brochures provided to medical centres for newly diagnosed patients
- Facebook page
- Annual Pheochromocytoma and Paraganglioma Patient Conference
- Support for patients and families to attend regional patient education forums
- Funding grants for research
- Doctor tracker: The Alliance assists patients from all over the world in finding healthcare providers and facilities equipped to handle their unique requirements
- Pheo Para Alliance medical advisors are on three continents, helping us keep patients advised of medical treatments

that are available in their part of the world.

Once referred to the Pheo Para Alliance, patients are able to connect with a global community that understands the unique healthcare challenges they face. Advocacy, education, research, and a community of support form the core of the Alliance's work on behalf of those with these rare neuroendocrine cancers.

Emily Collins
President, Pheo Para Alliance
Pheo Para Alliance
9721 Whitley Park Place
Bethesda MD 20814
Website: www.pheopara.org
E-mail: pheoalliance@gmail.com

cal imaging indicated initially to explore a "non-adrenal" disease or symptom (Fassnacht et al. 2016; Grumbach et al. 2003; NIH 2002; Terzolo et al. 2011; Tabarin et al. 2008). The frequency of these masses of more than one centimetre varies from 1 to 8.7% on autopsy series. In the radiological series, the prevalence is between 0.3 and 4.4% and increases with age to reach 7% from 60 years. Five to ten percent of adrenal incidentaloma are bilateral. The etiologies are multiple and summarized in Table 36.1. Among these lesions some must be operated (primary malignant tumours of the adrenal or secreting tumours), others treated medically

Table 36.1 Adrenal incidentalomas—frequency of the different causes [adapted from Fassnacht et al. (2016)]

Type of adrenal mass	Median % (range %)
Benign adenomas	80
Non-functioning	75 (71–84)
Autonomously cortisol-secreting	12 (1.0–29)
Aldosterone-secreting	2.5 (1.6–3.3)
Pheochromocytoma	7.0 (1.5–14)
Adrenocortical cancer	8.0 (1.2–11)
Metastasis	5.0 (0–18)

(lymphoma) and most simply monitored (non-secreting benign adenoma).

36.3.1.1 Diagnostic Testing

In fact, most incidentalomas are benign non-secreting adenomas, but it is important to rule out first other diagnosis. This highlights the importance of a rigorous diagnostic approach to define the management of an incidentaloma (Box. 36.8). This approach is based on the analysis of imagery and biological investigations. Several consensus conferences or guidelines, the most recent being released by the European Society of Endocrinology, have defined this diagnostic procedure and patients management (Fassnacht et al. 2016).

nant tumour). CT-scan with spontaneous density measurement can provide very reliable parameters (Figs. 36.5 and 36.6). A spontaneous density of less than 10 HU is specific of a benign adenoma (Hamrahian et al. 2005). The washout after injection of the contrast medium with a signal drop of more than 50% is also a very specific element for a benign adenoma. The MRI study with chemical shift analysis can be used as an alternative or in addition to CT-scan for the diagnosis of benign adenoma. In practice, a well-conducted CT-scan may be sufficient for imaging of an incidentaloma if it classifies it as a benign adenoma. When the mass cannot be classified with this imaging, MRI and eventually FDG-PET scan can be done.

> **Box 36.8 Important Message for Patients Diagnosed with Adrenal Incidentaloma**
> Advise your patient that most adrenal masses cause no health problems and usually are asymptomatic (there are no symptoms or signs of the disease). The majority are non-functioning, benign tumours but a small number can cause serious disease. Consult and prepare the patient that they may have to undergo several investigations to set the diagnosis and to define the management of an incidentaloma.

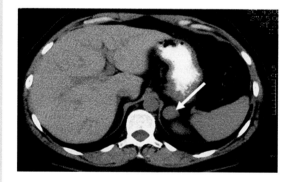

Fig. 36.5 CT-scan of a left adrenal adenoma (white arrow) incidentally discovered

Radiological investigations are by definition the initial step. It gives essential data and must focus on providing a certain amount of information to clarify the nature of the lesion and its risk of malignancy. This sometimes requires to repeat the initial imaging to have a specific and rigorous analysis of the adrenal mass. CT-scan or MRI are the methods of choice for this initial investigation. Some lesions (pure cysts, myelolipomas, haematoma) have specific imaging characteristics that allow an accurate diagnosis. In addition to these particular situations, the first step is to define whether the lesion can be formally classified as a benign adenoma (the most common case) or not (leaving the possibility of a malig-

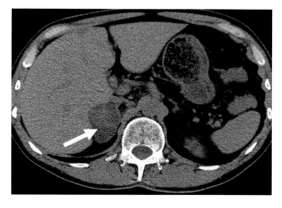

Fig. 36.6 CT-scan of a right adrenocortical cancer (white arrow) incidentally discovered

Adrenal tumours found in the investigation of an adrenal incidentaloma can cause excess secretion of steroid or catecholamine. It is important to identify the lesions responsible for hypersecretion that may warrant therapeutic intervention. The detection of a hormonal alteration is also an important step in the initial investigation for the diagnosis of an incidentaloma. Secreting tumours can be diagnosed after hormonal investigations in patients whose clinical signs are absent, modest, or non-specific, justifying a minimal systematic biological search whatever the clinical presentation. Bilateral lesions caused by infiltrative process or metastatic tumours can cause adrenal insufficiency, which should also be investigated by systematic biological investigations (Tabarin et al. 2008). Hormonal investigations will therefore be more complete in the context of bilateral lesions to explore this possibility. The initial reading stage of the imagery and the clinical data can obviously guide the hormonal work-up; however, a systematic minimal hormonal investigation is recommended by most consensus or guidelines (Fassnacht et al. 2016; Grumbach et al. 2003; NIH 2002; Terzolo et al. 2011; Tabarin et al. 2008).

It is recommended to systematically search hypersecretion of catecholamine and cortisol to look for hypokalaemia and hyperglycaemia. The systematic search for a pheochromocytoma is justified by the frequency of this tumour in the operated incidentalomas (about 10%), and the potential risk represented by hypersecretion of catecholamine, mostly cardiovascular complications. Screening for pheochromocytoma can be done on 24-h urine metanephrine derivatives with simultaneous measurement of urinary creatinine or on plasma assay when available. Urinary assays have a very good sensitivity and acceptable specificity and have been most often used in published series. The chromogranin A assay, by its lack of sensitivity and specificity, is not recommended systematically in the incidentaloma. The investigation of a potential hypersecretion of cortisol should detect tumours of the adrenal cortex responsible for Cushing syndrome.

A significant part of the incidentalomas is represented by the benign adenomas responsible for a more modest hypersecretion of cortisol, called "subclinical" or "autonomous cortisol secretion".

Although the consequences of this cortisol excess are still a matter of debate, it is admitted that it should be screened systematically as 10–20% of patients with adrenal incidentaloma might have benign adenoma responsible for autonomous cortisol secretion. The biological investigations used for the diagnosis of clinical Cushing syndrome (cortisoluria, midnight cortisol) have a good specificity but are not sensitive enough in this situation. The 1 mg dexamethasone suppression test is more sensitive (Box. 36.9), using a stringent cut-off (Fassnacht et al. 2016).

> **Box 36.9 The 1 mg Dexamethasone Suppression Test**
> It is recommended to detect cortisol autonomous secretion by an overnight 1 mg dexamethasone suppression test with a threshold of cortisolaemia at 18 ng/mL (50 nmol/L) (Fassnacht et al. 2016). It is important to remember that this is a very sensitive threshold (>98%), but not very specific (<80%). For this reason, a patient with a cortisol level above this threshold should be further investigated and the test might have to be repeated few months later. In this situation, cortisoluria, blood or salivary midnight cortisol, and ACTH can be added to the diagnostic work-up.

Screening for aldosterone excess will be done in patients with hypertension and/or hypokalaemia. It is then suggested to carry out as a first screening blood assay of aldosterone and renin (or renin activity) (Fassnacht et al. 2016; Tabarin et al. 2008). The assay of androgens (testosterone, DHA or SDHA) or precursors (17 hydroxyprogesterone, compound S, DOC) will not be systematic but may be performed according to the radiological or clinical data, or preoperatively in a suspected adrenocortical cancer.

In the bilateral incidentalomas, an ACTH-stimulation test (250 μg) with 9 am cortisol and 17-hydroxyprogestrone assays, as well as an ACTH measurement will be added to this hormonal workout. This aim at the screening of adrenal insufficiency requiring substitutive steroid treatment and it is also interesting for the etiological diagnosis. The purpose of the 17-hydroxyprogesterone assay is to search for 21-hydroxylase deficiency (congenital adrenal hyperplasia). The aim of the ACTH assay is to demonstrate the primary origin of the adrenal failure when present. Conversely, in situations of bilateral adrenocortical lesions such as macronodular hyperplasia, which is nowadays more often diagnosed in patients with incidentaloma causing cortisol autonomous secretion, the dosage of ACTH can help to refine the assessment of adrenal autonomy; ACTH being suppressed in this cause of Cushing syndrome.

36.3.1.2   Monitoring and Treatment of Adrenal Incidentalomas

The majority of adrenal incidentalomas are benign adenomas. If the hormonal investigations exclude cortisol autonomy, a simple monitoring will be offered. In the case of hypersecretion of steroids or catecholamine surgery is the rule. In patients with a "subclinical" Cushing due to a benign adenoma surgery will be discussed on an individual basis depending on potential complications of cortisol excess (diabetes, hypertension, obesity, osteoporosis). When imaging investiga-

tions suggest malignancy or if there is a remaining doubt about a malignant lesion, surgical removal is indicated (Fig. 36.7).

36.3.1.3   Nursing Role in the Diagnosis of Adrenal Incidentalomas

During the diagnostic phase, the endocrine nurse meets the patient for review to get a complete history, organize, and coordinate baseline adrenal biochemistry work-up to be completed and to ensure the patient understand the rationale of the tests. More specifically, the nurse will consult the patient in the following diagnostic aspects of the work-up:

1. *Metanephrine levels*
   Plasma normetanephrine and metanephrine test can have false-positive results, and it is important to consult the patient appropriately. Antidepressants, caffeine, and nicotine could potentially induce an elevation in the results. The endocrine nurse may organize for a fasting supine plasma metanephrines to ensure that there's no interference with the results.
2. *Overnight dexamethasone suppression test with 24 h urinary-free cortisol collection*
   Overnight dexamethasone involves taking a 1 mg of dexamethasone tablet between 11 pm

Fig. 36.7 Management of adrenal masses considered for surgery [reproduced from Fassnacht et al. (2016)]

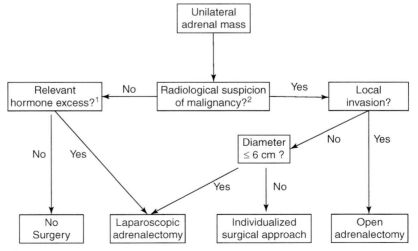

[1] Autonomous cortisol secretion is not automatically judged as clinically relevant

[2] In tumors with benign radiological features and a tumor size >4 cm, surgery might also be individually considered

and 12 mn, the cortisol level the following morning by 9 am should be suppressed in patients who do NOT secrete excess steroids.

The 24 h urinary-free cortisol collection involves a collection of urine in a plain bottle for 24 h, usually starts in the morning with the first void discarded to ensure that the bladder is empty thereby ensuring an accurate collection, then collects all urine for the next 24 h including the first void the next morning. This test will determine the total cortisol excretion within a 24 h period which is usually <130 nmL/24 h.

It is important to advise the patient the importance of proper timing of the test and the rationale behind the test, i.e. to complete the urine collection first before the dexamethasone test. The patient does not need to fast and can take their usual medications as prescribed. However, there are factors that need to be considered which can cause false-positive and false-negative results.

False-positive can occur in female patients taking oestrogen which increases the cortisol binding globulin leading to increase in total cortisol. The patient should be advised to discontinue oestrogen for 6 weeks before testing. Patients on medications that induce the enzyme CYP3A4 (e.g. antiepileptic, rifampicin, alcohol) can increase hepatic clearance of dexamethasone.

False-negative can occur on patients with renal failure because of the drop in albumin and cortisol binding globulin, patients with liver failure and patients on medication that inhibits the enzyme CYP3A4 (e.g. fluoxetine, cimetidine) decreasing hepatic clearance.

If required, salivary cortisol can be completed. This involves the patient to chew a salivette (swab) for at least 2–3 min, ensuring that the swab is saturated with saliva. The salivette comes in a plastic container to put the sample back after. The patient is advised not to eat, drink, or brush teeth for at least 30 min before collection. The patient can rinse mouth with water at least 15 min before collection. The sample needs to be put in the fridge if not delivered within 2–3 days.

3. *Plasma aldosterone and renin levels*
   It is very important to identify any medications that can interfere with the renin-angiotensin system (e.g. angiotensin-converting enzyme (ACE) inhibitors and angiotensin II receptor blockers (ARBs)) before performing the tests. The endocrine nurse will review the medication history of the patient and identify and replace medications that can interfere. Once initial blood test suggests hyperaldosteronism, a saline suppression test is performed. The patient should be advised that test will require a day admission for minimum of 5 h. The patient will receive saline infusion of 500 mL/h for 4 h whilst the patient is lying in bed. Aldosterone and renin will be checked before and after the procedure. The patient needs to be potassium replete. Normal response shows a suppressed aldosterone as a response to the high plasma sodium. Failure to suppress suggests hormone aldosterone excess secretion.

36.3.2 Adrenocortical Cancer (ACC)

Cancer of the adrenal cortex (adrenocortical cancer, ACC) is a rare tumour, the annual incidence being estimated between 1 and 2 per million. In the USA, the Surveillance, Epidemiology and End-Results Study (SEER) studying deaths from 1975 to 1992 estimates the incidence of ACC at 1.8 cases/million/year. The Norwegian cancer registry from 1970 to 1980 reports a rather similar incidence of 1.5 cases/million/year. In children, ACC is considered ten times rarer than in adults. In southern Brazil, however, the incidence of ACC is very high in children, close to that of adults. Children's ACC in Brazil are due in almost all cases to the existence of a specific germline mutation of the *TP53* tumour suppressor gene (R337H) (Else et al. 2014; Libe et al. 2007; Fassnacht et al. 2009).

36.3.2.1 Diagnosing ACC

ACC can cause adrenal steroid excess in about three quarter of the cases. Signs of hypersecretion are mainly related to androgens in women and cortisol in both sexes (Libe et al. 2007). Androgen excess causes hirsutism, acne, and menstrual disorders (spaniomenorrhoea or amenorrhoea). In man, a tumour-secreting oestrogen can lead to the development of gynaecomastia. Excess glucocorticoid causes all the clinical signs of Cushing syndrome. When the tumour secretes aldosterone or steroid precursors with mineralocorticoid activity, arterial hypertension with hypokalaemia and oedema can be observed. When referred to an endocrine clinic, most patients are diagnosed by the presence of these endocrine signs and clinical symptoms. In some patients, ACC is diagnosed in the presence of clinical symptoms due to tumour mass or growth. It is primarily pain, more rarely venous thrombosis. In recent years, it is becoming more evident that some ACCs, previously considered as non-secreting, in fact secrete some urine steroid metabolites and recently urine steroid metabolomic analysis have been introduced in routine use (Arlt et al. 2011).

Adrenal incidentaloma has become an increasingly common mode of discovery. This mode of discovery often reveals a localized tumour whose prognosis after surgery is much better. Although the frequency of the adrenal cortex among the incidentalomas is low (3–10% of the operated tumours), this diagnosis must obviously be systematically considered. Recent advances in the survival of patients with adrenocortical carcinomas are certainly largely related to this earlier mode of diagnosis, allowing resection at a stage where the probability of complete remission is better (Libe et al. 2007; Fassnacht et al. 2009).

36.3.2.2 Management of ACC

The management of ACC requires a multidisciplinary expertise, which can be difficult to assemble in the case of a rare tumour. Complete surgical excision is without any discussion currently the best treatment of ACC (Gaujoux and Brennan 2012). If it is possible in stages 1 and 2 that are localized to the adrenal, it remains difficult in stages 3 (loco-regional extension), sometimes justifying sacrifice of adjacent organs. Half a century after its first use, mitotane (O, p'-DDD) remains to date the first-line medical treatment (De Francia et al. 2012). Although the place of mitotane is recognized by most teams in non-operable ACC (stage 4 mainly as seen in Fig. 36.8), there is currently no consensus on its place in adjuvant treatment after complete surgical resection. The side effects of mitotane are mostly digestive (nausea, vomiting) but also neurologic (confusion, somnolence, ataxia). By its adrenolytic action, mitotane also induces adrenal insufficiency requiring a steroid coverage, whose dosage adjustment is not always simple.

The assay of mitotane blood level is a valuable indicator to adjust the treatment. In fact, the severe adverse effects, in particular neurologic signs, are most often observed for mitotane blood levels higher than 20 mg/L. Different studies have showed that mitotane is more effective on tumour progression when its blood levels are higher than 14 mg/L. The therapeutic range (14–20 mg/L) is therefore narrow, which requires regular monitoring and frequent dose adjustment. In patients whose tumour disease progresses after surgery and under mitotane, various cytotoxic chemotherapies have been used (Berruti et al. 2012). Cisplatin is the most consistently successful drug. The first international randomized trial (FIRM-ACT) has established the association of Cisplatin, Etoposide, and Doxorubicin (Fassnacht et al. 2012) as the first-line cytotoxic chemotherapy in progressive ACC.

36.3.2.3 Nursing Role Considerations for Mitotane Treatment of ACC

Mitotane treatment should be performed only after the patient has received detailed information on the expected toxicity and its treatment. The main role of the endocrine nurse once patient is on adjuvant mitotane therapy is to counsel the patient about the medication, its mode of action, side effects and how to lessen its side effects, follow-up, and monitoring of the mitotane level. Patients are at risk of adrenal insufficiency and should be initiated on hydrocortisone replace-

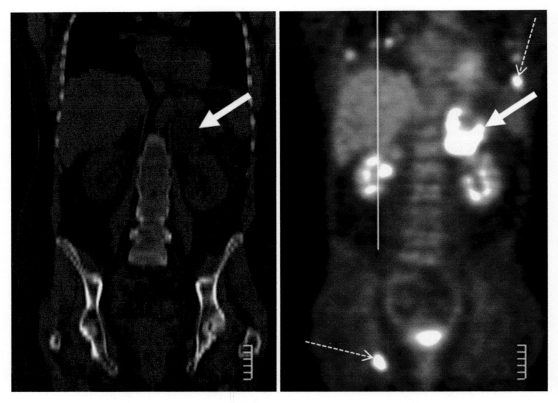

Fig. 36.8 FDG-PET scan of a left stage 4 adrenocortical cancer (white arrow) with distant metastasis (dotted thin arrows) (right image: CT-scan; left: FDG-scintigraphy)

ment concurrently with mitotane treatment to avoid potential adrenal crisis. High doses of hydrocortisone are needed (e.g. 20-10-10 mg or 20 mg three times daily) due to a substantial, mitotane-induced increase in cortisol binding globulin.

Patients should be consulted and be provided with comprehensive advice and education on management of adrenal insufficiency, sick day rules and prevention of adrenal crisis (please refer to Chaps. 37 and 62 for details). The endocrine nurse plays a vital role in this aspect.

Mitotane is lipophilic, accumulates in adipose tissue, from where it is slowly released back in to the blood stream. This means that plasma mitotane levels may substantially increase during ongoing treatment with the same dose. Thus, doses easily tolerated at the beginning may later cause significant side effects. The endocrine nurse should make patients aware of this poten-

tial adverse event and emphasize the need for regular follow-ups and monitoring of plasma mitotane levels.

Patient Case Study and Key Learning Points
A 46-year-old male patient, with no previous medical history or health issues, was diagnosed with hypertension in 2011. In the second half of 2012, he complained of being increasingly unwell, abdominal bloating, discomfort, and dyspepsia and was diagnosed with type 2 diabetes. A CT abdomen was done in December 2012 and showed a large adrenal mass. The patient was referred to his local hospital and was reviewed by the surgeons who subsequently referred him to the GI surgeons at the local tertiary specialist hospital. He was reviewed at the sarcoma MDT and as protocol; all patients with retroperitoneal masses, undergo biopsy. The patient was scheduled for CT-guided adrenal biopsy after a 24-h urine collection for catechol-

amines was sent for analysis. Prior to receiving the results, the patient was admitted for a CT-guided adrenal biopsy and had a large venous bleed as a result.

Key Learning Points:

- Biopsy should not be done for adrenal masses without prior confirmation of ALL these distinct criteria: history of malignancy, CT pre-contrast tumour density >20 HU, exclusion of pheochromocytoma with plasma metanephrines. Outcome of these test will dictate the therapeutic strategy.
- The cells obtained by a needle biopsy of an adrenal tumour cannot confirm whether the tumour is a benign adrenal mass or a rare adrenal carcinoma. It will only help in determining a primary adrenal tumour versus metastatic tumour. Most commonly, a biopsy is done if there is evidence of cancer outside the adrenal gland, or a patient with a known cancer has a suspicious adrenal mass. It is important to exclude a pheochromocytoma with biochemical testing prior to a biopsy.

36.4 Conclusions

The role of the endocrine nurse in the patient's journey following the incidental finding of an adrenal adenoma starts from diagnosis to follow-up. It involves coordinating the tests accurately and in timely manner, support in the diagnosis and management in close collaboration with the core members of the adrenal multidisciplinary team, education and training, follow-up of patients, and counselling. During this time, it is also important to take into consideration the possible psychological impact of the diagnosis to the patient and their families.

Acknowledgments With special thanks to Diane Silverman, Interim Executive Director, and Emily Collins, President, of the Pheo Para Alliance (Pheochromocytoma and Paraganglioma) www.pheopara.org for their contribution to this chapter with a case study and information on the Patient Advocacy Group. Also special thanks to Dr. Mayank Patel, MD, Special Volunteer, Section on Medical Neuroendocrinology, NICHD/NIH for providing the MRI image on pheochromocytoma.

References

Arlt W, Biehl M, Taylor AE, Hahner S, Libe R, Hughes BA, et al. Urine steroid metabolomics as a biomarker tool for detecting malignancy in adrenal tumors. J Clin Endocrinol Metab. 2011;96(12):3775–84.

Aronova A, Gordon BL, Finnerty BM, Zarnegar R, Fahey TJ 3rd. Aldosteronoma resolution score predicts long-term resolution of hypertension. Surgery. 2014;156(6):1387–92; discussion 92–3.

Avisse C, Marcus C, Patey M, Ladam-Marcus V, Delattre JF, Flament JB. Surgical anatomy and embryology of the adrenal glands. Surg Clin North Am. 2000;80(1):403–15.

Bergland BE. Pheochromocytoma presenting as shock. Am J Emerg Med. 1989;7(1):44–8.

Berruti A, Baudin E, Gelderblom H, Haak HR, Porpiglia F, Fassnacht M, et al. Adrenal cancer: ESMO Clinical Practice Guidelines for diagnosis, treatment and follow-up. Ann Oncol. 2012;23(Suppl 7):vii131–8.

Blake MA, Cronin CG, Boland GW. Adrenal imaging. AJR Am J Roentgenol. 2010;194(6):1450–60.

Curras-Freixes M, Pineiro-Yanez E, Montero-Conde C, Apellaniz-Ruiz M, Calsina B, Mancikova V, et al. PheoSeq: a targeted next-generation sequencing assay for pheochromocytoma and paraganglioma diagnostics. J Mol Diagn. 2017;19(4):575–88.

Dahia PL. Pheochromocytoma and paraganglioma pathogenesis: learning from genetic heterogeneity. Nat Rev Cancer. 2014;14(2):108–19.

De Francia S, Ardito A, Daffara F, Zaggia B, Germano A, Berruti A, et al. Mitotane treatment for adrenocortical carcinoma: an overview. Minerva Endocrinol. 2012;37(1):9–23.

Debillon E, Velayoudom-Cephise FL, Salenave S, Caron P, Chaffanjon P, Wagner T, et al. Unilateral adrenalectomy as a first-line treatment of Cushing's syndrome in patients with primary bilateral macronodular adrenal hyperplasia. J Clin Endocrinol Metab. 2015;100(12):4417–24.

Di Murro A, Petramala L, Cotesta D, Zinnamosca L, Crescenzi E, Marinelli C, et al. Renin-angiotensin-aldosterone system in patients with sleep apnoea: prevalence of primary aldosteronism. J Renin-Angiotensin-Aldosterone Syst. 2010;11(3):165–72.

Duet M, Guichard JP, Rizzo N, Boudiaf M, Herman P, Tran Ba Huy P. Are somatostatin analogs therapeutic alternatives in the management of head and neck paragangliomas? Laryngoscope. 2005;115(8):1381–4.

Dutta RK, Soderkvist P, Gimm O. Genetics of primary hyperaldosteronism. Endocr Relat Cancer. 2016;23(10):R437–54.

Elsayes KM, Narra VR, Leyendecker JR, Francis IR, Lewis JS Jr, Brown JJ. MRI of adrenal and extraadrenal pheochromocytoma. AJR Am J Roentgenol. 2005;184(3):860–7.

Else T, Kim AC, Sabolch A, Raymond VM, Kandathil A, Caoili EM, et al. Adrenocortical carcinoma. Endocr Rev. 2014;35(2):282–326.

Fassnacht M, Johanssen S, Quinkler M, Bucsky P, Willenberg HS, Beuschlein F, et al. Limited prognostic value of the 2004 International Union Against Cancer staging classification for adrenocortical carcinoma: proposal for a revised TNM classification. Cancer. 2009;115(2):243–50.

Fassnacht M, Terzolo M, Allolio B, Baudin E, Haak H, Berruti A, et al. Combination chemotherapy in advanced adrenocortical carcinoma. N Engl J Med. 2012;366(23):2189–97.

Fassnacht M, Arlt W, Bancos I, Dralle H, Newell-Price J, Sahdev A, et al. Management of adrenal incidentalomas: European Society of Endocrinology Clinical Practice Guideline in collaboration with the European Network for the Study of Adrenal Tumors. Eur J Endocrinol. 2016;175(2):G1–g34.

Flatmark T. Catecholamine biosynthesis and physiological regulation in neuroendocrine cells. Acta Physiol Scand. 2000;168(1):1–17.

Funder JW, Carey RM, Mantero F, Murad MH, Reincke M, Shibata H, et al. The management of primary aldosteronism: case detection, diagnosis, and treatment: an endocrine society clinical practice guideline. J Clin Endocrinol Metab. 2016;101(5):1889–916.

Gaujoux S, Brennan MF. Recommendation for standardized surgical management of primary adrenocortical carcinoma. Surgery. 2012;152(1):123–32.

Ghayee HK, Rege J, Watumull LM, Nwariaku FE, Carrick KS, Rainey WE, et al. Clinical, biochemical, and molecular characterization of macronodular adrenocortical hyperplasia of the zona reticularis: a new syndrome. J Clin Endocrinol Metab. 2011;96(2):E243–50.

Goodarzi MO, Dawson DW, Li X, Lei Z, Shintaku P, Rao CV, et al. Virilization in bilateral macronodular adrenal hyperplasia controlled by luteinizing hormone. J Clin Endocrinol Metab. 2003;88(1):73–7.

Gourgari E, Lodish M, Keil M, Sinaii N, Turkbey E, Lyssikatos C, et al. Bilateral adrenal hyperplasia as a possible mechanism for hyperandrogenism in women with polycystic ovary syndrome. J Clin Endocrinol Metab. 2016;101(9):3353–60.

Grumbach MM, Biller BM, Braunstein GD, Campbell KK, Carney JA, Godley PA, et al. Management of the clinically inapparent adrenal mass ("incidentaloma"). Ann Intern Med. 2003;138(5):424–9.

Hamrahian AH, Ioachimescu AG, Remer EM, Motta-Ramirez G, Bogabathina H, Levin HS, et al. Clinical utility of noncontrast computed tomography attenuation value (hounsfield units) to differentiate adrenal adenomas/hyperplasias from nonadenomas: Cleveland Clinic experience. J Clin Endocrinol Metab. 2005;90(2):871–7.

Hodin R, Lubitz C, Phitayakorn R, Stephen A. Diagnosis and management of pheochromocytoma. Curr Probl Surg. 2014;51(4):151–87.

Hsiao HP, Kirschner LS, Bourdeau I, Keil MF, Boikos SA, Verma S, et al. Clinical and genetic heterogeneity, overlap with other tumor syndromes, and atypical glucocorticoid hormone secretion in adrenocorticotropin-independent macronodular adrenal hyperplasia compared with other adrenocortical tumors. J Clin Endocrinol Metab. 2009;94(8):2930–7.

Insel PA. Adrenergic receptors. Evolving concepts on structure and function. Am J Hypertens. 1989;2(3 Pt 2):112S–8S.

Insel PA. Seminars in medicine of the Beth Israel Hospital, Boston. Adrenergic receptors—evolving concepts and clinical implications. N Engl J Med. 1996;334(9):580–5.

Janssen I, Blanchet EM, Adams K, Chen CC, Millo CM, Herscovitch P, et al. Superiority of [68Ga]-DOTATATE PET/CT to other functional imaging modalities in the localization of SDHB-associated metastatic pheochromocytoma and paraganglioma. Clin Cancer Res. 2015;21(17):3888–95.

Janssen I, Chen CC, Taieb D, Patronas NJ, Millo CM, Adams KT, et al. 68Ga-DOTATATE PET/CT in the localization of head and neck paragangliomas compared with other functional imaging modalities and CT/MRI. J Nucl Med. 2016;57(2):186–91.

La Batide-Alanore A, Chatellier G, Plouin PF. Diabetes as a marker of pheochromocytoma in hypertensive patients. J Hypertens. 2003;21(9):1703–7.

Lenders JW, Pacak K, Walther MM, Linehan WM, Mannelli M, Friberg P, et al. Biochemical diagnosis of pheochromocytoma: which test is best? JAMA. 2002;287(11):1427–34.

Lenders JW, Eisenhofer G, Mannelli M, Pacak K. Phaeochromocytoma. Lancet (London, England). 2005;366(9486):665–75.

Lenders JW, Duh QY, Eisenhofer G, Gimenez-Roqueplo AP, Grebe SK, Murad MH, et al. Pheochromocytoma and paraganglioma: an endocrine society clinical practice guideline. J Clin Endocrinol Metab. 2014;99(6):1915–42.

Libe R, Fratticci A, Bertherat J. Adrenocortical cancer: pathophysiology and clinical management. Endocr Relat Cancer. 2007;14(1):13–28.

Lodish M, Stratakis CA. A genetic and molecular update on adrenocortical causes of Cushing syndrome. Nat Rev Endocrinol. 2016;12(5):255–62.

Mantero F, Terzolo M, Arnaldi G, Osella G, Masini AM, Ali A, et al. A survey on adrenal incidentaloma in Italy. Study Group on Adrenal Tumors of the Italian Society of Endocrinology. J Clin Endocrinol Metab. 2000;85(2):637–44.

Martucci VL, Pacak K. Pheochromocytoma and paraganglioma: diagnosis, genetics, management, and treatment. Curr Probl Cancer. 2014;38(1):7–41.

Mathur A, Kemp CD, Dutta U, Baid S, Ayala A, Chang RE, et al. Consequences of adrenal venous sampling in primary hyperaldosteronism and predictors of unilateral adrenal disease. J Am Coll Surg. 2010;211(3):384–90.

Mazza A, Armigliato M, Marzola MC, Schiavon L, Montemurro D, Vescovo G, et al. Anti-hypertensive treatment in pheochromocytoma and paraganglioma: current management and therapeutic features. Endocrine. 2014;45(3):469–78.

McCarthy CJ, McDermott S, Blake MA. Adrenal imaging: magnetic resonance imaging and computed tomography. Front Horm Res. 2016;45:55–69.

McNeil AR, Blok BH, Koelmeyer TD, Burke MP, Hilton JM. Phaeochromocytomas discovered during coronial autopsies in Sydney, Melbourne and Auckland. Aust NZ J Med. 2000;30(6):648–52.

McNichol AM. Differential diagnosis of pheochromocytomas and paragangliomas. Endocr Pathol. 2001;12(4):407–15.

Meikle AW. Dexamethasone suppression tests: usefulness of simultaneous measurement of plasma cortisol and dexamethasone. Clin Endocrinol. 1982;16(4):401–8.

Minnaar EM, Human KE, Henneman D, Nio CY, Bisschop PH, Nieveen van Dijkum EJ. An adrenal incidentaloma: how often is it detected and what are the consequences? ISRN Radiol. 2013;2013:871959.

Newell-Price J, Bertagna X, Grossman AB, Nieman LK. Cushing's syndrome. Lancet (London, England). 2006;367(9522):1605–17.

Nieman LK, Biller BM, Findling JW, Newell-Price J, Savage MO, Stewart PM, et al. The diagnosis of Cushing's syndrome: an Endocrine Society Clinical Practice guideline. J Clin Endocrinol Metab. 2008;93(5):1526–40.

NIH. NIH state-of-the-science statement on management of the clinically inapparent adrenal mass ("incidentaloma"). NIH Consens State Sci Statements. 2002;19(2):1–25.

Parenti G, Zampetti B, Rapizzi E, Ercolino T, Giache V, Mannelli M. Updated and new perspectives on diagnosis, prognosis, and therapy of malignant pheochromocytoma/paraganglioma. J Oncol. 2012;2012:872713.

Parker LN. Control of adrenal androgen secretion. Endocrinol Metab Clin N Am. 1991;20(2):401–21.

Parthasarathy HK, Menard J, White WB, Young WF Jr, Williams GH, Williams B, et al. A double-blind, randomized study comparing the antihypertensive effect of eplerenone and spironolactone in patients with hypertension and evidence of primary aldosteronism. J Hypertens. 2011;29(5):980–90.

Patel D, Gara SK, Ellis RJ, Boufraqech M, Nilubol N, Millo C, et al. FDG PET/CT scan and functional adrenal tumors: a pilot study for lateralization. World J Surg. 2016;40(3):683–9.

Petramala L, Zinnamosca L, Settevendemmie A, Marinelli C, Nardi M, Concistre A, et al. Bone and mineral metabolism in patients with primary aldosteronism. Int J Endocrinol. 2014;2014:836529.

Rao D, Peitzsch M, Prejbisz A, Hanus K, Fassnacht M, Beuschlein F, et al. Plasma methoxytyramine: clinical utility with metanephrines for diagnosis of pheochromocytoma and paraganglioma. Eur J Endocrinol. 2017;177(2):103–13.

Rasmussen SA, Rosebush PI, Smyth HS, Mazurek MF. Cushing disease presenting as primary psychiatric illness: a case report and literature review. J Psychiatr Pract. 2015;21(6):449–57.

Rossi R, Tauchmanova L, Luciano A, Di Martino M, Battista C, Del Viscovo L, et al. Subclinical Cushing's syndrome in patients with adrenal incidentaloma: clinical and biochemical features. J Clin Endocrinol Metab. 2000;85(4):1440–8.

Sagrada A, Fargeas MJ, Bueno L. Involvement of alpha-1 and alpha-2 adrenoceptors in the postlaparotomy intestinal motor disturbances in the rat. Gut. 1987;28(8):955–9.

Sakai Y, Yanase T, Takayanagi R, Nakao R, Nishi Y, Haji M, et al. High expression of cytochrome b5 in adrenocortical adenomas from patients with Cushing's syndrome associated with high secretion of adrenal androgens. J Clin Endocrinol Metab. 1993;76(5):1286–90.

Sharma ST, Committee AAS. An Individualized approach to the evaluation of cushing syndrome. Endocr Pract. 2017;23(6):726–37.

Streeten DH, Anderson GH Jr. Mechanisms of orthostatic hypotension and tachycardia in patients with pheochromocytoma. Am J Hypertens. 1996;9(8):760–9.

Tabarin A, Bardet S, Bertherat J, Dupas B, Chabre O, Hamoir E, et al. Exploration and management of adrenal incidentalomas. French Society of Endocrinology Consensus. Ann Endocrinol. 2008;69(6):487–500.

Taieb D, Pacak K. Molecular imaging and theranostic approaches in pheochromocytoma and paraganglioma. Cell Tissue Res. 2018;372(2):393–401.

Terzolo M, Stigliano A, Chiodini I, Loli P, Furlani L, Arnaldi G, et al. AME position statement on adrenal incidentaloma. Eur J Endocrinol. 2011;164(6):851–70.

Thosani S, Ayala-Ramirez M, Roman-Gonzalez A, Zhou S, Thosani N, Bisanz A, et al. Constipation: an overlooked, unmanaged symptom of patients with pheochromocytoma and sympathetic paraganglioma. Eur J Endocrinol. 2015;173(3):377–87.

Timmers HJ, Taieb D, Pacak K. Current and future anatomical and functional imaging approaches to pheochromocytoma and paraganglioma. Horm Metab Res. 2012;44(5):367–72.

van Hulsteijn LT, van Duinen N, Verbist BM, Jansen JC, van der Klaauw AA, Smit JW, et al. Effects of octreotide therapy in progressive head and neck paragangliomas: case series. Head Neck. 2013;35(12):E391–6.

Whitelaw BC, Prague JK, Mustafa OG, Schulte KM, Hopkins PA, Gilbert JA, et al. Phaeochromocytoma [corrected] crisis. Clin Endocrinol. 2014;80(1):13–22.

Willenberg HS, Spath M, Maser-Gluth C, Engers R, Anlauf M, Dekomien G, et al. Sporadic solitary aldosterone- and cortisol-co-secreting adenomas: endocrine, histological and genetic findings in a subtype of primary aldosteronism. Hypertens Res. 2010;33(5):467–72.

Wyszynska T, Cichocka E, Wieteska-Klimczak A, Jobs K, Januszewicz P. A single pediatric center experience with 1025 children with hypertension. Acta Paediatr. 1992;81(3):244–6.

Yu R, Wei M. False positive test results for pheochromocytoma from 2000 to 2008. Exp Clin Endocrinol Diabetes. 2010;118(9):577–85.

Zeiger MA, Thompson GB, Duh QY, Hamrahian AH, Angelos P, Elaraj D, et al. The American Association of Clinical Endocrinologists and American Association of Endocrine Surgeons medical guidelines for the management of adrenal incidentalomas. Endocr Pract. 2009a;15(Suppl 1):1–20.

Zeiger MA, Thompson GB, Duh QY, Hamrahian AH, Angelos P, Elaraj D, et al. American Association of Clinical Endocrinologists and American Association of Endocrine Surgeons Medical Guidelines for the Management of Adrenal Incidentalomas: executive summary of recommendations. Endocr Pract. 2009b;15(5):450–3.

Zilbermint M, Xekouki P, Faucz FR, Berthon A, Gkourogianni A, Schernthaner-Reiter MH, et al. Primary Aldosteronism and ARMC5 Variants. J Clin Endocrinol Metab. 2015;100(6):E900–9.

Key Reading

1. Fassnacht M, Arlt W, Bancos I, Dralle H, Newell-Price J, Sahdev A, et al. Management of adrenal incidentalomas: European Society of Endocrinology Clinical Practice Guideline in collaboration with the European Network for the Study of Adrenal Tumors. Eur J Endocrinol. 2016;175(2):G1–g34.
2. Funder JW, Carey RM, Mantero F, Murad MH, Reincke M, Shibata H, et al. The Management of Primary Aldosteronism: Case Detection, Diagnosis, and Treatment: An Endocrine Society Clinical Practice Guideline. J Clin Endocrinol Metab. 2016;101(5):1889–916.
3. NIH. NIH state-of-the-science statement on management of the clinically inapparent adrenal mass ("incidentaloma"). NIH Consens State Sci Statements. 2002;19(2):1–25.
4. Sharma ST, Committee AAS. An individualized approach to the evaluation of cushing syndrome. Endocr Pract. 2017;23(6):726–37.
5. Zeiger MA, Thompson GB, Duh QY, Hamrahian AH, Angelos P, Elaraj D, et al. The American Association of Clinical Endocrinologists and American Association of Endocrine Surgeons medical guidelines for the management of adrenal incidentalomas. Endocr Pract. 2009;15(Suppl 1):1–20.

Diagnosis and Management of Adrenal Insufficiency in Children and Adults

37

Sofia Llahana, Irene Mitchelhill, Phillip Yeoh, and Marcus Quinkler

Contents

S. Llahana (✉)
School of Health Sciences,
City, University of London, London, UK
e-mail: Sofia.Llahana@city.ac.uk

I. Mitchehill
Department of Endocrinology, Sydney Children's
Hospital (SCHN), Randwick, NSW, Australia
e-mail: Irene.mitchelhill@health.nsw.gov.au

P. Yeoh
The London Clinic, London, UK
e-mail: p.yeoh@thelondonclinic.co.uk

M. Quinkler
Endocrinology in Charlottenburg Stuttgarter Platz 1,
Berlin, Germany

© Springer Nature Switzerland AG 2019
S. Llahana et al. (eds.), *Advanced Practice in Endocrinology Nursing*,
https://doi.org/10.1007/978-3-319-99817-6_37

Abstract

Adrenal insufficiency (AI) is a common life-threatening endocrine condition. It is caused by the inability of the adrenal glands to produce cortisol, a hormone essential for life, either due to failure of the adrenals (primary AI), or due to diseases affecting the hypothalamus or the pituitary which control the adrenals (secondary AI). Patients with AI require lifelong glucocorticoid (GC) replacement therapy and increased GC doses during periods of intercurrent illness or other major psychological and physical stress to mimic the normal increase in physiological cortisol response to such situations. Inadequate GC replacement for daily   maintenance and increased doses during illness, can precipitate an adrenal crisis (AC) an adrenal crisis which can be fatal if the immediate administration of parenteral hydrocortisone is delayed.

The prevalence of primary AI is 93–140 patients/million population and of secondary AI is 150–280/per million. Standard mortality rate for patients with AI is more than twofold compared to the general population according to retrospective hospital data. AI has significant impact on patients' quality of life, and suboptimal GC replacement (over- or under-replacement) can lead to acute and long term complications such as osteoporosis and type 2 diabetes.

AI encompasses a wide variety of medical diagnoses and can be an unrecognised underlying condition masked by another diagnosis in both paediatrics and adults. There should be a heightened sense of suspicion in the presentation of any seriously unwell neonate, child or adult where an unexplained presentation, deterioration of an intercurrent illness or other stress (e.g. surgery or significant trauma) may have precipitate an AC.

The diagnosis of AI brings many challenges for children, parents, adult patients and their families with the impact of a multiple daily medication routine, and the need for sick day surveillance and management, and for vigilance to detect potential illness and possible events which may be life threatening. Health professionals need to provide adequate ongoing psychological support and education for patients and families long term as they adapt to their health needs of their condition and incorporate treatment plans into their daily lives. Understanding of the education process is crucial and one of the most one important aspects of the role of the endocrine nurse.

Keywords

Adrenal insufficiency · Adrenal crisis · Hydrocortisone · Glucocorticoids · Fludrocortisone · Patient education · Primary adrenal insufficiency · Secondary adrenal insufficiency · Quality of life

Abbreviations

AC	Adrenal crisis
ACTH	Adrenocorticotropic hormone
AD	Addison's disease
AI	Adrenal insufficiency
CA	Cortisone acetate
CAH	Congenital adrenal hyperplasia
CRH	Corticotropin-releasing hormone
CSHI	Continuous subcutaneous hydrocortisone infusion
DHEA	Dehydroepiandrosterone
GC	Glucocorticoids
HPA	Hypothalamic-pituitary-adrenal axis
ITT	Insulin tolerance test
PAI	Primary adrenal insufficiency
QoL	Quality of life
SAI	Secondary adrenal insufficiency
SST	Short synacthen test

Key Terms

- Adrenocorticotropic hormone (ACTH) is the hormone responsible for stimulating cortisol production from the adrenal glands, which is essential for life.
- Adrenal insufficiency (AI) refers to the failure or impairment of the adrenal glands which can be primary adrenal insufficiency (PAI) most commonly autoimmune or Addison's disease, or secondary adrenal insufficiency (SAI) due to hypothalamic-pituitary diseases, resulting in cortisol deficiency.
- ACTH stimulation test is a diagnostic test to assess the adrenal steroid production after the administration of the synthetic ACTH analogue Tetracosactide.
- Adrenal crisis is life-threatening emergency caused by inadequate production of the adrenal hormone cortisol in situations of stress.

Key Points

- Patients with adrenal insufficiency need to have adequate steroid replacement in order to have a better outcome in quality of life, reduce their risk of adrenal crisis, and preventable hospital admissions and fatalities.
- GC replacement needs to take in account a patient's needs, the daily dosage variation and timing, and consideration of the most effective delivery options for effective absorption in order to maximise the benefit of therapy.
- Endocrine nurses play a key role in the care of patients with adrenal insufficiency. They provide education and support in order to engage with these patients life-long to ensure they achieve positive health outcomes for life.

37.1 Introduction

Adrenal insufficiency (AI) is a common life-threatening endocrine condition. It refers to the failure or impairment of the adrenal glands which can be primary adrenal insufficiency (PAI) most commonly autoimmune or Addison's disease, or secondary adrenal insufficiency (SAI) due to hypothalamic-pituitary diseases. In children, the most common cause is Congenital Adrenal Hyperplasia (see Chap. 35). Long-term corticosteroid treatment which can lead to adrenal gland atrophy can also result in AI, and is often referred to as tertiary adrenal insufficiency. The adrenal glands produce glucocorticoids (GC) (cortisol in humans, but e.g. corticosterone in rats), mineralocorticoids (aldosterone), and androgens. Cortisol secretion exhibits a distinct circadian rhythm reaching peak levels in the early morning prior to awakening and low levels in the evening with lowest levels at midnight (Arlt 2017). In the case of neonates, their circadian rhythm is not established until later in their first year of life (Miller et al. 2008; Mendoza-Cruz et al. 2013); hence cortisol levels are difficult to interpret and can be confusing. Please read Chap. 34 for more details on anatomy and physiology of adrenal glands. It is important to have a clear understanding of the circadian rhythm as it plays a crucial role in the planning of GC replacement therapy.

The prevalence of primary AI is 93–140 patients/million population and of secondary AI is 150–280/per million (Arlt and Allolio 2003). AI arising from prolonged administration of corticosteroid treatment leading to suppression of the hypothalamic-pituitary-adrenal axis (HPA) is much more common, occurring in 0.5–2% of the population in developed countries (Arlt 2017); in the UK for example an average of 0.75% of the population was prescribed long-term oral corticosteroid therapy (e.g. prednisolone, dexamethasone) at any time point (Fardet et al. 2011).

37.2 Causes and Clinical Presentation of Adrenal Insufficiency in Children and Adults

Primary adrenal insufficiency (PAI) refers to glucocorticoid deficiency in the context of adrenal failure or disease in the gland itself, whereas secondary adrenal insufficiency (SAI) arises because of ACTH deficiency due to causes affecting the hypothalamic or pituitary function (Fig. 37.1). A major distinction between PAI and SAI is that PAI is invariably accompanied by deficiency of mineralocorticoids which are regulated by the renin-angiotensin-aldosterone (RAA) system (please see chap. 34 for anatomy and physiology of the adrenal gland); this does not occur in SAI because only ACTH is deficient, and the RAA system is intact (Arlt and Allolio 2003; Stewart 2008). A summary of the most common causes and associated features of AI is presented in Table 37.1 (Arlt 2017; Arlt and Allolio 2003; Stewart 2008; Barthel et al. 2016; Bancos et al. 2015).

37.2.1 Primary Adrenal Insufficiency

Thomas Addison was the first physician to describe the clinical phenotype of PAI in 1855 hence the name Addison's disease. PAI is most commonly caused by autoimmune-mediated adrenalitis accounting for 68–94% of cases in adults. It can occur in isolation (30–40% of cases) or in combination with other autoimmune diseases as part of the autoimmune polyglandular syndrome type 1 (APS1) in 10–15% of cases, and type 2 (APS2) in

50–60% of cases (Table 37.1). In children, most frequent monogenic cause of AI is congenital adrenal hyperplasia (CAH) which is caused by mutations in enzymes involved in steroid hormone synthesis, most commonly mutations in CYP21A2 encoding 21-hydroxylase, with an incidence of 1 in 12,000–15,000 people (Arlt and Allolio 2003; Bancos et al. 2015) (please see Chap. 35). Worldwide, infectious diseases such as tuberculosis fungal infections, HIV and cytomegalovirus, are common causes of AI (Stewart 2008).

37.2.2 Secondary Adrenal Insufficiency

SAI is the consequence of the dysfunction of the HPA axis. The most frequent causes of SAI are tumours involving the hypothalamic-pituitary region associated with ACTH deficiency caused by tumour growth leading to suppression of the pituitary function, or treatment with surgery or radiotherapy resulting in hypopituitarism (Table 37.1) (please see chapters in Section 3, the Pituitary Gland). In children, SAI is due to mal-development of the hypothalamus and pituitary gland: aplasia, hypoplasia or ectopic placement of the pituitary are most common and lead to multiple pituitary hormone deficiency (MPHD). In neonates and infants, birth trauma, and in childhood head injury and brain tumours are other causes of SAI (Migeon and Lanes 2009; Miller et al. 2008).

37.2.3 Iatrogenic Adrenal Insufficiency

An underestimated and significant cause of AI is the suppression of the HPA axis by exogenous long-term GC treatment leading to atrophy of adrenal cortex. This becomes apparent when patients cease treatment and HPA axis is not restored for endogenous production of ACTH and hence cortisol. Two recent systematic reviews demonstrated that the risk of AI after cessation of GC therapy varied significantly and there is no administration form, dosing, treatment duration, or underlying disease for which AI can be excluded with certainty (Joseph et al. 2016; Broersen et al. 2015). This risk increases with a

Physiological situation

Primary adrenal insufficiency

Secondary adrenal insufficiency

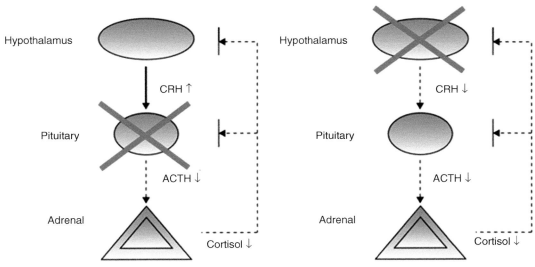

Pituitary disease   **Hypothalamic disease**

Fig. 37.1 Differentiation between primary and secondary adrenal insufficiency. Key: *ACTH* adrenocorticotropic hormone, *CRH* corticotropin-releasing hormone. Used with permission from Arlt, W. & Allolio, B. 2003. Adrenal insufficiency. *Lancet,* 361, 1881–93

dose equivalent of 5 mg of prednisolone or higher for longer than 4 weeks, irrespective of route of administration, i.e. topical, inhaled, oral, or injected (Bancos et al. 2015; Joseph et al. 2016). The risk of AI is difficult to predict hence all patients must be generally considered at risk of developing AI and consulted regarding prevention and management of adrenal crisis (Joseph et al. 2016; Broersen et al. 2015; Quinkler et al. 2013) (see Chap. 62). Administration of exogenous opioids, e.g. in pain therapy, may also cause suppression of plasma ACTH and serum cortisol, leading to AI, particularly in susceptible individuals (Policola et al. 2014; Lee and Twigg 2015).

Table 37.1 Common causes and associated features of adrenal insufficiency [adapted from Arlt (2017), Arlt and Allolio (2003), Stewart (2008), Barthel et al. (2016), and Bancos et al. (2015)]

Primary Adrenal Insufficiency (PAI)
Autoimmune adrenalitis (Addison's disease)
Isolated autoimmune adrenalitis
Adrenalitis as part of autoimmune polyglandular syndrome
Type 1 (APS1 or APECED): hypoparathyroidism, chronic mucocutaneous, candidiasis, other autoimmune disorders
Type 2 (APS2): thyroid disease, type 1 diabetes mellitus, other autoimmune diseases
Type 4 (APS4): Other autoimmune diseases, excluding thyroid disease or diabetes
Adrenalitis caused by infections
Tuberculosis, HIV, systemic fungal infections occurring mostly in immunosuppressed patients (histoplasmosis, blastomycosis, cryptococcosis, coccidioidomycosis), cytomegalovirus
Genetic disorders leading to adrenal insufficiency
Adrenoleukodystrophy, adrenomyeloneuropathy
Demyelination of CNS (cerebral adrenoleukodystrophy), spinal cord, or peripheral nerves (adrenomyeloneuropathy)
Congenital adrenal hyperplasia (see Chap. 35)
Ambiguous genitalia, salt wasting
ACTH insensitivity syndromes (familial glucocorticoid deficiency)
Glucocorticoid deficiency, but no impairment of mineralocorticoid synthesis
Triple A syndrome (Allgrove's syndrome)
Alacrima achalasia, neurological impairment, deafness, mental retardation, hyperkeratosis
Bilateral adrenal haemorrhage
Meningococcal sepsis, primary antiphospholipid syndrome
Adrenal infiltration
Amyloidosis, hemochromatosis, adrenal metastasis, lymphomas, sarcoidosis
Bilateral adrenalectomy
For management of Cushing's or other adrenal disease, after bilateral nephrectomy
Drug-induced adrenal insufficiency
Treatment with mitotane, aminoglutethimide, etomidate, abiraterone, trilostane, ketoconazole, suramin, mifepristone
Secondary Adrenal Insufficiency (SAI)
Pituitary adenomas (see Part III)
Adrenal insufficiency caused by ACTH deficiency from tumour growth or post-surgery or radiotherapy.
Idiopathic hypopituitarism (see Chap. 25) or isolated idiopathic ACTH deficiency
Other tumours of the hypothalamic-pituitary region
Craniopharyngioma, meningioma, ependymoma, and intrasellar or suprasellar metastases
Pituitary irradiation for tumours outside the hypothalamic-pituitary axis, e.g. leukaemia
Lymphocytic hypophysitis
Autoimmune hypophysitis
Often associated with pregnancy; may present with isolated ACTH deficiency or panhypopituitarism; can also be associated with autoimmune thyroid disease, vitiligo, premature ovarian failure, type 1 diabetes, pernicious anaemia
Pituitary apoplexy or Sheehan's syndrome (see Chap. 64)
Pituitary infiltration or granulomatous disease
Tuberculosis, actinomycosis, sarcoidosis, histiocytosis X, Wegener's granulomatosis
Head trauma
Iatrogenic Adrenal Insufficiency
Prolonged treatment with exogenous glucocorticoids
Treatment with opioids leading to ACTH suppression

37.3 Clinical Presentation of Adrenal Insufficiency in Adults

Table 37.2 presents a summary of the clinical manifestations of AI (Arlt 2017; Arlt and Allolio 2003; Stewart 2008; Bornstein et al. 2016). Presenting symptoms of AI are often non-specific such as fatigue, loss of energy, loss of appetite, nausea, or weight loss which often result in a delayed or missed diagnosis, for example, depression or anorexia (Arlt 2017; Bancos et al. 2015). In a study by Bleicken et al., less than 30% of women and 50% of men with AI were diagnosed within the first 6 months after onset of symptoms

Table 37.2 Clinical manifestations of adrenal insufficiency [adapted from Arlt (2017), Arlt and Allolio (2003), Stewart (2008), and Bornstein et al. (2016)]

Common sign and symptoms in PAI and SAI (caused by glucocorticoid and androgen deficiency)
Fatigue, lack of energy or stamina, reduced strength
Anorexia, weight loss (in children failure to thrive)
Gastric pain, nausea, vomiting (more frequent in PAI)
Myalgia, joint pain
Dizziness
Fever
Low blood pressure, postural hypotension, and dizziness (pronounced in PAI)
Hyponatraemia (more common in PAI)
Hypoglycaemia
Symptoms specific to adrenal androgen deficiency
 In women: dry and itchy skin, impaired libido loss of axillary or pubic hair
 In girls: absence of adrenarche or pubarche

Sign and symptoms specific in PAI (caused by mineralocorticoid deficiency)
Salt craving
Skin hyperpigmentation
Raised serum creatinine
Hypercalcaemia
Hyperkalaemia
Increased thyroid stimulating hormone

Additional sign and symptoms in SAI
Related to pituitary adenomas, such as acromegaly, Cushing's, prolactinoma (see relevant chapters in Part III), hormone deficiencies in hypopituitarism (see Chap. 25), and visual-field impairment from compression of the optic chiasm.

POMC stimulation, the precursor peptide of ACTH and melanocortin-1, the latter stimulating melanocytes. This is mostly seen in sun-exposed areas, pressure points, axillae, nipples, genitalia, and mucous membranes. Vitiligo and other autoimmune endocrinopathies (hypothyroidism) can often present in patients with autoimmune Addison's disease (Stewart 2008) (Fig. 37.2). A high biochemical measure of ACTH will also distinguish between PAI (being excessively raised) from SAI where the level will be low.

The clinical features of PAI in adults (Addison's disease) result from the loss of both glucocorticoid and mineralocorticoid and tend to be more acute in the onset. Hyponatraemia and hyperkalaemia are found in 80% and 40%, respectively, of patients with PAI at diagnosis. Acute AI presents with postural hypotension which can progress to hypovolaemic shock; it can also present with acute gastrointestinal symptoms of abdominal tenderness, nausea vomiting, and fever. Symptoms can often be mistaken as episodes of isolated gastroenteritis or appendicitis and if misdiagnosed can lead to a potentially life threatening AC. Autoimmune causes are rare in childhood, but the occurrence increases in the second decade of life into adolescence and onto adulthood (Arlt 2017; Kwok et al. 2005; Rushworth et al. 2017).

37.3.1 Clinical Presentation of Adrenal Insufficiency in Children

Similar to adults, undiagnosed AI in children can often be overlooked when another more significant diagnosis arises with symptoms often masking the underlying cortisol deficiency and which can mislead or confuse the diagnostic process. A new diagnosis of AI can reveal itself with either an acute presentation or have a prolonged insidious onset with a history of evolving features and concerns by parents with failure to thrive, poor weight gain and growth failure, and prolonged recovery from illnesses. An acute presentation occurs with the presentation of a infant or child in a state of systemic collapse, often precipitated by a significant intercurrent illness, when their adrenal function is no longer adequate to support their

and 20% suffered for longer than 5 years before being diagnosed. Almost 70% of patients were given a false diagnosis and had consulted at least three physicians in the process (Bleicken et al. 2010a). This is more common in PAI as a history of pituitary conditions affecting the HPA axis with an increased risk of SAI prompts for further investigations to confirm ACTH deficiency. Hypothalamic-pituitary conditions can also manifest with other symptoms such as visual impairment caused by chiasmal compression suggesting a possible pituitary or brain tumour. It is important to remember that AI resulting from cessation of exogenous GC therapy can present with all the symptoms associated with GC deficiency even though these patients appear clinically Cushingoid from previous long-term exposure to GC therapy (Arlt 2017).

The most obvious clinical feature that distinguishes PAI from SAI, which is often present in PAI, is skin pigmentation caused by excess

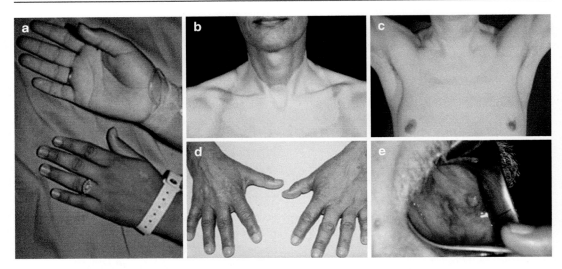

Fig. 37.2 Skin pigmentation and vitiligo in Addison's disease. Key: (**a**) hands of an 18-year-old woman with autoimmune polyendocrine syndrome and Addison's disease. (**b**) Pigmentation and vitiligo in a patient before and (**c**) after treatment with hydrocortisone and fludrocortisone. (**d**) Change in skin pigmentation of the hands of a 60-year-old man with tuberculous PAI before and after GC replacement, and (**e**) buccal pigmentation in the same man before treatment. Used with permission from Stewart P.M. (2008) The adrenal cortex, Chapter 14. In: Kronemberg H.M., Melmed S., Polonsky K.S. and Larsen P.R. (Eds) Williams Textbook of Endocrinology, 11th Edition. Saunders Elsevier, Philadelphia, pages: 445–503

metabolic needs in response to stressful situation (Migeon and Lanes 2009; Miller et al. 2008).

37.3.1.1 Acute Clinical Presentation of AI in Children and Neonates

In acute presentation of AI, examination will reveal a pale and lethargic child, with progressive signs of deterioration of a listless and floppy demeanour and a reduced level of consciousness due to hypoglycaemia. The child will be cool to touch and has hypothermia due to, hypovolaemia and peripheral shutdown (evident with poor skin turgor, delayed capillary return), dry mucous membranes and a history of minimal urine output indicating significant dehydration. Background history may reveal a period of intercurrent illness, poor oral intake, maybe a period of persistent diarrhoea and/or vomiting. Observations reveal tachycardia, dyspnoea, hypotension, and hypoglycaemia. A blood gas and peripheral blood is needed to confirm or rule out any biochemical cause, and a septic workup to determine a bacterial or viral cause for the presentation (Migeon and Lanes 2009; Miller et al. 2008).

An acute presentation in a neonate or infant is life threatening. It may occur following a history of persistently poor feeding, excessive sleepiness, persistent jaundice, and failure to regain birth weight, with significant weight loss of >10% of their total body weight. Acute episodes of AI require to be managed immediately, guided by standard emergency protocol guidelines, to prevent otherwise a fatal outcome due to AC (see Chap. 62 for more details).

37.4 Diagnosis of Adrenal Insufficiency in Adults

The diagnosis of AI is based on the patient's medical history, clinical sign and symptoms suggestive of AI, adrenal and/or pituitary imaging, and diagnostic biochemistry provocative tests. Figure 37.3 presents the diagnostic algorithm for adults with clinical sign and symptoms suggestive of AI and diagnostic test which can set the differential diagnosis (Bancos et al. 2015).

The diagnosis of AI is established by the ACTH stimulation test, also known as the short

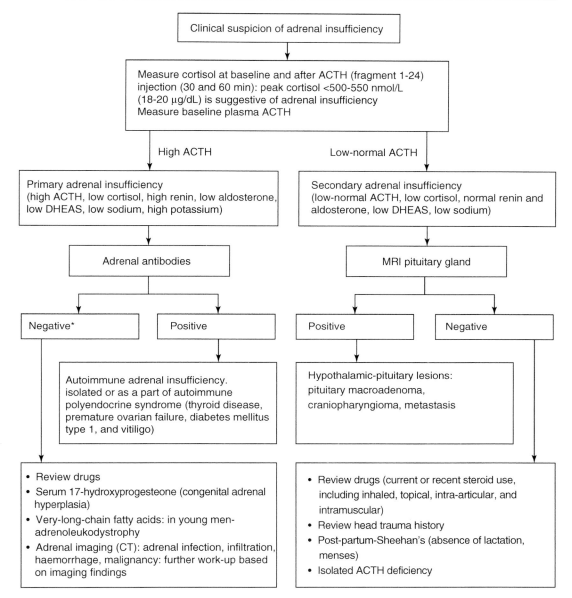

Fig. 37.3 Diagnostic algorithm for adults with clinical signs and symptoms suggestive of adrenal insufficiency. Key: *ACTH* adrenocorticotropic hormone, *DHEAS* dehydroepiandrosterone. Important to remember: Diagnostic measures must never delay the start of hydrocortisone treatment in suspected adrenal crisis and should be done when the patient is better. Cut-off values to exclude AI vary depending on the assay uses; always check local reference ranges. Used with permission from Bancos, I., Hahner, S., Tomlinson, J. & Arlt, W. 2015. Diagnosis and management of adrenal insufficiency. *Lancet Diabetes Endocrinol*, 3, 216–26

cosyntropin or short synacthen test (SST), through assessment of cortisol at baseline, 30 min and 60 min post administration of synthetic ACTH hormone of 250 µg for adults and children ≥2 years of age, 125 µg for children <2 years of age, and 15 µg/kg for infants (Bornstein et al. 2016). Cortisol response tends to be slightly higher at 60 min but there are no documented advantages in specificity and sensitivity for either time point (Bancos et al. 2015).

The cut-off values for cortisol for exclusion of AI are recommended at 500 nmol/L (18 μg/dL) (Bornstein et al. 2016), but this may vary according to the assay used. For example, a study reported that the low reference limit for cortisol 30 min after ACTH stimulation ranged from 420 to 574 nmol/L (15.2–20.8 μg) depending on the assay used (El-Farhan et al. 2013); cut-off values for cortisol may differ significantly between measurements using immunoassays or mass spectrometry assays and therefore specific local reference ranges must always be confirmed before setting the diagnosis.

The ACTH stimulation test is a test of adrenal function and therefore should not be used to diagnose SAI before adrenal gland atrophy has occurred, which takes approx. 3–4 months. Therefore, testing with the SST for SAI, for example, within a month after a pituitary insult and suspected ACTH deficiency, may not detect SAI. It has also been suggested that ACTH stimulation testing could lack sensitivity in chronic SAI due to the 250 μg supraphysiological dose and the 1 μg was advocated as an alternative (Dorin et al. 2003). However, later evidence found that significant proportion of patients fail the 1 μg test using the agreed cut-off cortisol limit, and this could lead to unnecessary life-long GC replacement (Neary and Nieman 2010); therefore, it is not recommended to use as a diagnostic test. In addition, diluting a 250 mg ampoule in 1 mg portions is not recommended. The insulin tolerance test (ITT) is an alternative, but it is more invasive and contraindicated in patients with a history of seizures, cardiovascular disease, untreated hypothyroidism, and elderly patients, and in particular it is contraindicated in children owing to the dangers of significant hypoglycaemia and risk of an AC (Miller et al. 2008). (please refer to Chap. 15, in Part III for more details on provocative diagnostic testing). In addition, ITT should be avoided in SAI when random morning cortisol concentrations are lower than 80 nmol/L (3 mg/dL) which are strongly predictive of AI (Bancos et al. 2015). Suspected AI presenting with acute AC must be treated promptly with parenteral hydrocortisone (Bancos et al. 2015; Bornstein et al. 2016; Wass and Arlt 2012) (Box 37.1). In

the paediatric population the IV synacthen test has been useful in determining suspected cortisol deficiency and utilised in determining recovery of the adrenal gland function following adrenal suppression following iatrogenic use of steroids (Mendoza-Cruz et al. 2013).

> **Box 37.1 *Treat first, diagnose later!* Management of Acute AI**
>
> For patients admitted with adrenal crisis where AI is suspected, hydrocortisone must be given without delay along with intravenous fluid resuscitation. Blood samples for paired cortisol and ACTH should be taken if there is an opportunity but it is crucially important to promptly treat the AC and undertake diagnostic investigations later when the patient is better (please see Chap. 62 for more details on management of AC).

It is also important to remember that oral oestrogen preparations increase total cortisol concentration (which is measured in current assays) by increasing circulating cortisol-binding globulin (CBG) and therefore should be discontinued for at least 6 weeks prior to evaluating cortisol levels although one study showed that these effects were not seen in patients using transdermal oestrogen replacement (Qureshi et al. 2007).

37.4.1 Diagnosis of Adrenal Insufficiency in Children

Specific considerations need to be given making the diagnosis of AI in children and neonates in addition to those discussed earlier in the diagnosis of adults with AI. In addition to clinical manifestations of AI described earlier, observations confirm **hypothermia** (temperature less than 36 °C), **hypoglycaemia** (<2.6 mmol/L) via peripheral blood glucose analysis or blood gas, and **hypotension** with unmeasurable blood pressure. Table 37.3 presents a summary of the relevant biochemistry and microcytic investigations

Table 37.3 Investigations in the differential diagnosis of AI in children

Investigation	Biochemical features and results
Venous blood gas	Immediate assessment of BGL, EUC metabolic status/acidosis
EUC	Hyponatraemia and high serum potasium indicating aldosterone deficiency
Urea and creatinine	Assess for dehydration Elevated levels confirm dehydration
Blood glucose	Confirms hypoglycaemia Lack of glucocorticoid and gluconeogenesis (fasting and vomiting)
Insulin	Normal insulin level in presence of hypoglycaemia rules out hyperinsulinism as cause of low BGL
Cortisol, growth hormone	Low levels in view of hypoglycaemia, confirms—multiple pituitary hormone deficiency (MPHD) and cortisol deficiency
Thyroid function tests	Low TSH/T4 confirms MPHD
17 OHP, androgen profile	Raised levels indicate possible CAH
ACTH	Raised level ++ Indicates—primary adrenal insufficiency
Lactate/pyruvate, free fatty acid, ammonia, carnitine	Assess metabolic acidosis as cause of hypoglycaemia—rule out metabolic diagnosis Rule out deficiency—causes hypoketotic hypoglycaemia
Aldosterone and renin	Low levels of aldosterone with high levels of renin indicate PAI, e.g. salt losing CAH—deficiency
Urinary keto-steroids	Positive levels determine CAH Minimise multiple blood tests requiring large amounts of blood (not done if acutely unwell)
Blood culture	Rule out sepsis
Urine culture	Rule out urinary tract infection

undertaken in the differential diagnosis of AI in children.

The most common cause of AI in childhood is Congenital Adrenal Hyperplasia (PAI) with mineralocorticoid deficiency or associated with multiple pituitary hormone deficiency (SAI). The distinguishing feature between PAI and SAI is the presence or absence of a significantly raised ACTH, 17OHP level and significant electrolyte imbalance in PAI. The synacthen test and a urine steroid profile (Miller et al. 2008; Koyama et al. 2014) are useful in diagnosing PAI. In SAI, determining diurnal variations in serum cortisol (8 am and 4 pm) and understanding normal secretion rates in neonates, infants and childhood can be helpful in interpreting the results (Migeon and Lanes 2009; Miller et al. 2008; Koyama et al. 2014). Other investigations for SAI include a closely monitored brief fasting study in a neonate or infant to measure the response of counter-regulatory hormones (cortisol & growth hormone) along with insulin to rule out hyperinsulinism in response to hypoglycaemia. A glucagon stimulation test (GST) can be useful in place of an ITT (contraindicated in childhood) to determine a child's cortisol response to hypoglycaemia along with possible growth hormone deficiency in children (Miller et al. 2008).

37.4.1.1 Psychological Impact of Diagnosis of AI on Children and Parents

The diagnosis of AI in the child can have a significant psychological impact on the parents. The parental role to nurture and protect is challenged by a medical condition which has life-long implications. The distress and shock following the diagnosis impacts greatly on the parents' ability to rationalize the situation which is out of their control. As such the effectiveness of information which the medical and nursing staff impart can be diminished (Betman 2006). As health professionals, we have no control over this process, other than to provide emotional support and explanation in a timely manner in an initial and ongoing process. The significance of a potentially life-threatening condition, challenges parental strengths and weaknesses and puts many relationships under extreme pressure. They need to grieve for the loss of their expected healthy child and fear the limitations such a diagnosis will have on their child's future life. Eventually, rationalising their fears and worries about the future will see subsequent resolution with final acceptance to move forward and manage the care required for their child. The endocrine nurse needs to understand the grief process that parents experience following a significant diagnosis in order to provide the support they need to move forward with their child's journey in life (Betman 2006).

37.5 Treatment of Adrenal Insufficiency

Treatment of AI is multifaceted and, although it is primarily focused on replacement therapy, it should not be considered in isolation from the self-management and psychological well-being of patients and their families. A holistic overview of the patient's psychosocial environment, quality of life (QoL), well-being, other health needs and comorbidities, as well as their priorities, beliefs on and expectations from their treatment, is necessary. In addition, patient/family empowerment and shared decision-making are crucial in achieving an individualised treatment regimen and improved patient adherence. The objectives for treatment in AI are summarised in Box 37.2 [summarised from Arlt and Allolio (2003), Barthel et al. (2016), Bancos et al. (2015), Bornstein et al. (2016), Fleseriu et al. (2016), Grossman (2010), and Chapman et al. (2016)].

37.5.1 Mineralocorticoid Replacement Therapy

Mineralocorticoids are vital for maintaining water and electrolyte homeostasis, and thereby blood pressure. Only patients with PAI have mineralocorticoid deficiency as this is controlled by the RAA system and not the HPA axis. Fludrocortisone is a synthetic mineralocorticoid used to replace aldosterone in patients with PAI. It is recommended that all patients with confirmed aldosterone deficiency should be on fludrocortisone replacement starting at 50–100 µg and taken on waking up together with GC. In childhood, fludocortisone doses may be required

> **Box 37.2 Objectives for Treatment Optimisation in Adrenal Insufficiency**
>
> The following objectives should be taken into consideration when planning and monitoring the treatment regimen for patients with AI:
> - To provide optimal replacement for GC, androgens and, specifically for patients with PAI, mineralocorticoids
> - To involve patients and families in planning a treatment regimen which is tailored to each patient's individual needs in order to minimise or avoid where possible complications and symptoms from over- or under-replacement
> - To restore normal well-being, quality of life, sexual function, weight balance, normal growth for children, and social, family, and professional activity
> - To ensure patients and families are well informed of their condition and can recognise the symptoms of over- or under-replacement
> - To ensure patients and families receive support and education on their treatment so they can self-manage their daily replacement, adjust GC appropriately during intercurrent illness, and know how to prevent an adrenal crisis
> - To ensure that the education provided translates to behavioural change for patients and families; any potential detrimental medication behaviours need to be identified and patients should be supported to address these factors
> - To develop an infrastructure and health service that supports the needs of patients with AI and ensures prompt management of AC to minimise or avoid hospitalisations and to eradicate preventable deaths from AC

twice daily in the first few years of life, owing to mineralocorticoid pathway resistance. The addition of salt supplements is essential in neonates and infants as dietary sodium is inadequate in this age group (Migeon and Lanes 2009; Miller et al. 2008). Fludrocortisone is primarily monitored based on clinical assessment of salt cravings, postural hypotension, or presence of peripheral oedema alongside blood pressure, blood electrolytes (sodium and potassium) and renin (Quinkler et al. 2015); salt intake should not be restricted (Bornstein et al. 2016). For patients who develop hypertension, a reduction in the dose of fludrocortisone is recommended alongside monitoring of electrolytes but antihypertensive treatment can be initiated whilst continuing fludrocortisone if blood pressure remains uncontrolled (see also Box 37.3). During pregnancy fludrocortisone doses often need to be increased due to the anti-mineralocorticoid effect of progesterone (Quinkler et al. 2015). Also during episodes with hot weather fludrocortisone dose increases of 50 mg/day often lead to better physical performance. Hydrocortisone also exerts a mineralocorticoid activity and a 20 mg dose is equivalent of 50 µg of fludrocortisone (Arlt 2017; Bornstein et al. 2016) hence with increasing the dose of hydrocortisone during illness or managment of an AC, there is no need to increase the dose of fludrocortisone.

Box 37.3 Key Points in the Assessment of Mineralocorticoid Replacement

Does your patient crave salt, feel light-headed, have low blood pressure, postural hypotension, low blood sodium, high potassium and reports a general feeling of being unwell? If the answer is YES, replacement is inadequate, and the dose of fludrocortisone should be increased. Advise your patient that temporary dose increments of fludrocortisone by 50–100% or increase in salt intake are also needed in a hot climate or situations that promote excessive sweating.

37.5.2 Adrenal Androgen Replacement Therapy in Women

Dehydroepiandrosterone (DHEA) is the main source of androgen production in women and plays important role in maintaining sexual function, energy, and libido. DHEA replacement in women with AI also leads to development or restoration of pubic hair and may therefore have a role in pubertal females (Neary and Nieman 2010). DHEA replacement at 25–50 mg as a single dose should be considered for women with PAI complaining of low libido, depressive symptoms, dry skin, and fatigue when GC and mineralocorticoids are optimised (Bornstein et al. 2016). This can be on a 6-month trial and can be discontinued if there is no benefit. Women should be monitored for possible androgenic side effects of hirsutism or hair thinning. Small studies found that patients with SAI also reported improvement in psychological well-being on DHEA replacement (Brooke et al. 2006). However, evidence in this patient group population is controversial regarding QoL outcomes and recent guidelines recommend against routine use of androgens for women with SAI (Fleseriu et al. 2016).

37.5.3 Glucocorticoid Replacement Therapy in Adult Patients with AI

As already discussed, cortisol secretion exhibits a circadian rhythm and the objective for GC replacement therapy is to mimic this rhythm in an as closest as possible manner although this has so far been a challenge. A crucial step to understand is the regulation of cortisol metabolism by interconversion of cortisol to cortisone, governed by the intracellular 11β-hydroxysteroid dehydrogenase (11β-HSD) enzymes; type 1 (11β-HSD1) modulates local tissue cortisol levels by converting cortisone (*inactive* GC) to cortisol (*active* GC) and type 2 (11β-HSD2) converts cortisol to cortisone which functions as a systemic glucocorticoid reservoir (Oksnes et al. 2015; Aulinas et al. 2013). Box 37.4 lists the three aspects which should be considered for optimal GC replacement.

Box 37.4 The Three Important Aspects of Optimal GC Replacement Therapy

Consult and educate the patient and their families on the following three aspects of GC replacement therapy:

1. **Circadian rhythm daily dosing for oral GC**

   Objective: to optimise well-being, improve adherence and minimise or avoid negative effects of over- or under-replacement

   Action plan:

   - work with patient and family to select an individualised treatment regime and the correct dose and type of GC
   - advise patient of special situations such as travelling, shift working, extreme physical or emotional stress

2. **GC replacement during intercurrent illness—"sick day rules"**

   Objective: to support the patient and aid recovery from illness by increasing GC dose as needed

   Action plan:

   - advise your patient and family on the different situations which require "sick

day rules" and how to adjust the dose of their GC

   - patients are often on different GC regimens so a blanket rule of "double or triple" dose will not be applicable to everyone
   - provide supporting information, e.g. leaflets, emergency ID card, and an emergency GC injection kit, smartphone applications, as well as education on how to recognise and prevent AC

3. **Prevention and management of adrenal crisis**

Objective: recognise and manage AC in a timely manner to avoid hospitalisation

Action plan:

   - ensure patients and their families are aware of the symptoms of AC and able to take immediate action
   - check that patents wear emergency ID card and have access to GC injection which can be administered promptly
   - advise patients on supporting services which they can call upon in case of AC, e.g. ambulance service, inform family and friends about risks of AC

There are several GC formulations used to treat AI (Table 37.4). The most commonly used GC is hydrocortisone (cortisol) given in two or three divided oral doses daily (total daily dose of 15–25 mg for patients with PAI (Bornstein et al. 2016) and 15–20 mg for patients with SAI (Fleseriu et al. 2016)). Cortisone acetate two to three times daily to a total of 20–35 mg is also used although not available in some countries such as the UK or Germany. Contrary to hydrocortisone, cortisone acetate (*inactive*) requires activation via hepatic 11β-HSD1 before it becomes biologically *active* cortisol. This may result in broader interindividual variability of cortisol which can make it difficult to obtain a precise profile. However, it has been suggested

that the slower onset and offset of cortisol levels may be advantageous in smoothing fluctuations in levels (Grossman 2010), and this would be a good option for patients complaining of "energy dips" between doses.

The first and largest dose of hydrocortisone should be given on waking up on empty stomach, for faster absorption and as early in the morning as possible. The second dose is given at lunch time and the third dose, if required, given late afternoon but no more than 4–6 h before sleep (with a 5–6-h gap between doses). Generally, patients with PAI require higher and more frequent doses of hydrocortisone compared to patients with SAI who may have some residual cortisol reserve. Caution is required in patients

Table 37.4 Formulations, characteristics, and dose equivalent for GCs

GC name	Equivalent GC dose (mg)	Potency relative to hydrocortisone	Half-life plasma (min)	Duration of action (h)
Hydrocortisone	20	1	90	8–12
Cortisone acetate	25	0.8	30	8–12
Prednisone	4–5	4–5	60	12–36
Prednisolone	3–4	5–6	60	12–36
Dexamethasone	0.5	30–50	200	36–54

with SAI to avoid over-replacement (Grossman 2010). The general aim is to give the lowest possible dose of hydrocortisone without compromising the patient's well-being or put them at risk of AC. Two large studies including more than 1000 patients with AI, showed that most patients take hydrocortisone, i.e. 75% (Forss et al. 2012) and 87.4% (Murray et al. 2017), respectively, at either twice or thrice daily. The most common regimen of hydrocortisone was 10 mg on waking up, 5 mg at lunch time, and 5 mg late afternoon or evening (Murray et al. 2017), which is generally the most accepted regimens we use in clinical practice. Interestingly, both studies showed a large variation of daily regimens, regarding total daily dose and number of divided doses; Murray et al. reported that 25 different regimens were being used by patients to deliver a total daily hydrocortisone dose of 20 mg (Murray et al. 2017). This emphasises that requirements for GC replacement are individual to each patient's needs. Endocrine nurses have a pivotal role in identifying and addressing these needs to plan an optimal GC replacement regimen for patients. A small study concluded that hydrocortisone dosing and regimen should be adjusted according to the patient's weight (Mah et al. 2004), but there is no robust evidence to support this approach over current practice, and this would add to the already very complex regimen for patients with AI.

Prednisolone 3–5 mg once or twice daily, which is a long-acting GC, can be considered as an alternative treatment option for patients who continue to report impaired QoL or poor adherence to the twice or thrice daily regimen (Bornstein et al. 2016). It is however not a preferred choice, as it

has been associated with an increased tendency to adverse metabolic complications including weight gain, dyslipidaemia, and type 2 diabetes (Filipsson et al. 2006; Quinkler et al. 2016), and osteoporosis (Frey et al. 2018). Dexamethasone should not be used as GC replacement in AI due to the Cushingoid side effects and difficulties in dose titration (Bornstein et al. 2016) although there is a rare indication for use in certain patients with CAH (please see Chap. 35).

The modified dual-release hydrocortisone (Plenadren®) is an alternative option for GC replacement. It comes in tablets of 20 mg and 5 mg taken once daily on waking up. It has an immediate release coating combined with an extended-release core and provides physiological levels and a smoother cortisol profile during the day when compared to immediate release thrice daily hydrocortisone (Aulinas et al. 2013; Johannsson et al. 2009) (Fig. 37.4). It is important to note that the bioavailability of Plenadren is 20% less than hydrocortisone which may require a dose adjustment. In addition, cortisol levels during the evening decrease by up to 58% (Johannsson et al. 2009) and some patients may experience fatigue in the last part of the day especially if they are active. Two randomised studies showed that after switching from conventional thrice daily to once daily modified-release hydrocortisone, patients have a more circadian-based cortisol profile during the day, improved QoL scores, and a reduction in body weight, blood pressure, and glucose metabolism over 12 and 24 weeks (Isidori et al. 2018; Johannsson et al. 2012).

Infacort® (licenced for use in children with AI and CAH) is an immediate-release, granule

S. Llahana et al.

Fig. 37.4 Comparison of cortisol profiles between thrice daily immediate release and once daily modified-release hydrocortisone. Used with permission from: Aulinas, A., Casanueva, F., Goni, F., Monereo, S., Moreno, B., Pico, A., Puig-Domingo, M., Salvador, J., Tinahones, F. J. & Webb, S. M. 2013. Adrenal insufficiency and adrenal replacement therapy. Current status in Spain. *Endocrinol Nutr,* 60, 136–43

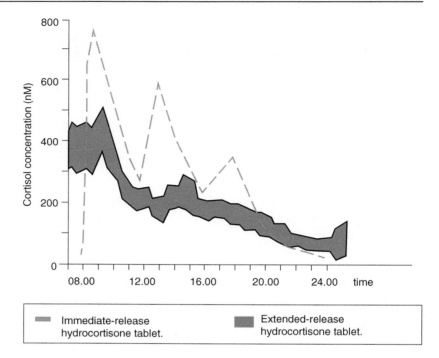

Immediate-release hydrocortisone tablet.

Extended-release hydrocortisone tablet.

formulation of hydrocortisone with taste masking for a dose-appropriate formulation of hydrocortisone for children with adrenal insufficiency (Neumann et al. 2018; Uta et al. 2018). Chronocort® (developed for adults with CAH) is a modified-release hydrocortisone formulation based on a multi-layered multi-particulate technology where the sustained release and enteric coats are varied to provide differing release profiles (release of hydrocortisone 4–5 h after intake). Taken twice daily, 20 mg before sleep and 10 mg on waking up, it can mimic circadian rhythm of cortisol with a release of hydrocortisone in the early hours of the morning providing a pre-waking cortisol rise, which is not provided with other oral GCs (Whitaker et al. 2014).

Up to now, there has been no robust evidence to inform us whether one GC formulation is superior to the others regarding short term and long term goals (Grossman et al. 2013); therefore more research is needed in this area. It is important however to remember that every patient has different needs, and treatment should be individualised. The endocrine nurse has a crucial role in identifying and addressing these needs by adopting a holistic care approach.

37.5.3.1 Continuous Subcutaneous Hydrocortisone Infusion (CSHI)

Continuous subcutaneous hydrocortisone infusion (CSHI), using an insulin pump (Fig. 37.5), can mimic the physiological cortisol rhythm and is suggested as a potential alternative treatment option for patients with difficult to control AI and those in whom oral GC are not absorbed (Oksnes et al. 2015), as also demonstrated by our patient in the case study (Box 37.5). Preliminary evidence suggests that CSHI improves health-related QoL scores and improves fatigue in patients with AI (Oksnes et al. 2014) although it can be quite a cumbersome regimen for patients. Further studies are however needed to investigate long-term outcomes of CSHI treatment and to refine the infusion regimen.

37.5.3.2 GC Dose Adjustment During Intercurrent Illness in Adults

Patients with AI need to increase the dose of their GC replacement in order to mirror the physiological increase in serum cortisol levels during major stress and illness. This is normally referred to as "sick day rules". There is no

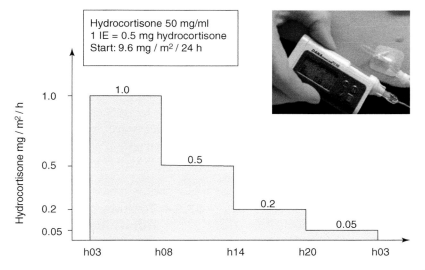

Fig. 37.5 Starting doses for continuous subcutaneous hydrocortisone infusion. The insulin pump reservoir is filled with hydrocortisone 50 mg/mL. Doses are adjusted to body surface area (BSA/m2). The daily dose is divided into four dosing intervals, with the highest dose during the last part of the night, half that dose during the first part of the day, and further decreasing doses in the afternoon and early part of the night. **Used with permission from:** Oksnes, M., Ross, R. & Lovas, K. 2015. Optimal glucocorticoid replacement in adrenal insufficiency. *Best Pract Res Clin Endocrinol Metab,* 29, 3–15. [Figure 4, page 11]

Box 37.5 Case Study of a Patient Using Continuous Subcutaneous Hydrocortisone Infusion (CSHI) for GC Replacement

What being on the CSHI Pump means to me

I was diagnosed with severe adrenal insufficiency in September 2016 even with oral hydrocortisone my blood cortisol levels were virtually non-existent.

I also have several pre-existing gastric issues—I have gastroparesis so reliably taking oral hydrocortisone was impossible as I was vomiting several times daily... Secondly, as I have Crohn's disease which is refractory and always active to some degree I was having diarrhoea several times daily so was burning through the hydrocortisone...

Between the end of March and beginning of May I had 6 back-to-back infections including a life-threatening sepsis and pneumonia. Since being on the pump I have been infection free...

I had heart palpitations due to tachycardia, constant terrible headaches which are so painful that I couldn't sleep, extreme fatigue—I had no energy and even sitting zapped me of my resources, every day I fainted up to five times daily as my blood pressure was persistently low... Since being on the pump I now have energy, my life is much more predictable and whilst I have a life-threatening condition I am much more in control of it rather than it controlling me. ... my quality of life is exponentially better, and I no longer feel like death warmed up. The gastric and duodenal ulcers are now a thing of the past...

The other great thing is I am now on 21 mg of hydrocortisone daily... This means my chances of getting long-term side effects from excess steroid treatment, e.g. diabetes, heart disease, are drastically reduced ... Some people may think being on a pump is restrictive but in all honesty most of the time I forget I am even wearing it...

(published with patient consent)

evidence on the optimal replacement during illness, but general consensus is to double or triple the dose of GC tablets for minor to moderate illness were oral intake is possible. For more severe illness and when the patient is unable to take oral tables in situations such as vomiting, diarrhoea or nil by mouth procedures, hydrocortisone needs to be administered immediately intramuscularly or intravenously at 50–100 mg starting dose followed by 50–100 mg every 6 h or 100–200 mg/24 h by continuous intravenous infusion (Arlt and Allolio 2003; Bornstein et al. 2016; Husebye et al. 2014). Patient education is crucial to ensure that patients and their families are familiar with the sick day rules. The endocrine nurse should take a detailed history of the patient's treatment, how and when they take their medication. A blanket rule of "double the dose" as reflected in the case study presented in Box 37.6, is not always applicable to every patient and patient education needs to take an individualised approach. Please read Chap. 62 for a comprehensive overview of the management of intercurrent illness and the diagnosis, prevention and timely management of AC. Chapter 62 also provides details on best approaches to patient education in AI.

> **Box 37.6 Case Study of GC Dose Adjustment During Intercurrent Illness**
>
> John is a 49-year-old man with SAI. He calls for an urgent consultation and is seen in the nurse-led clinic. He tells me he has not been feeling well and has had a lingering nasty cold for over 3 weeks, even though he doubled the dose of his hydrocortisone. His prescribed daily dose is 10 + 5 + 5 mg three times daily, but on further questioning, he tells me he has been taking 20 mg first thing in the morning. He also takes the double dose of 40 mg as single dose on waking up. Following an education session, John understands the rationale for thrice daily regimen based on

his insulin tolerance test results. A blood test when we met, taken 9 h after 40 mg of hydrocortisone, also shows a very low level of cortisol 68 nmol/L. We discuss ways to help him remember his second and third doses. He calls me a month later to say he has recovered and energy levels have "picked up".

37.5.4 Treatment of AI and GC Adjustment for Intercurrent Illness in Children

The treatment objective in children is to find a balance between under- or over-replacement with GC, to minimise acute and long-term complications and to minimise the risk of AC with a dose that allows normal growth and pubertal development (Bornstein et al. 2016; Salprietro et al. 2014; Kwok et al. 2005). The Endocrine Society guidelines recommend treatment with hydrocortisone in three or four divided doses (starting daily dose of 6–8 mg/m^2 in children with SAI and 12–16 mg/m^2 in children with PAI. For its short acting properties, hydrocortisone is used in preference) over other GC replacement therapies in children (Migeon and Lanes 2009; Bornstein et al. 2016; Fleseriu et al. 2016). Children with PAI and confirmed aldosterone deficiency should be treated with fludrocortisone (starting dose of 100 μg daily); it does not require adjustment by body surface and generally remains the same throughout early life. However, in neonates and infants, mineralocorticoid pathway resistance requires higher fludrocortisone doses of 50–200 μg daily in order to maintain sodium levels in PAI (Migeon and Lanes 2009; Miller et al. 2008). Many of these patients also require sodium chloride supplementation of 1–2 g daily divided in several feedings (Bornstein et al. 2016).

Treatment of inter-current illness requires increasing the dose of oral hydrocortisone to at least 45–50 mgs/M2/day in divided doses 6 hourly until well again. In children with SAI, where there is a lower maintenance replacement dose, doubling or tripling the daily dose maybe inadequate (Miller et al. 2008). Regular clinical review and monitoring of growth and development are essential long term. Blood tests and a yearly bone age X-ray are included in this process to ensure hormonal and biochemical parameters are stable. The endocrine nurse should support parents to manage their child's condition and treatment and ensure there is an understanding of the importance of adherence with medication administration and attendance for clinical reviews to monitor growth and development. Patient and parent education is a critical component in the care of these children as parents integrate managing their child's care into their daily lives and in the future empower their children to gain independence as adolescents and adults.

Understanding the importance of managing health issues with stress hydrocortisone is imperative. All patients need stress hydrocortisone along with consideration of a sweet drink to prevent hypoglycaemia. Children with PAI require the addition of a salt supplement when unwell because of the risk of possible hyponatraemia and failure or absorption of their oral medication. At home this may be administered using salt tablets/sachets in water, rock salt, or with high salt containing foods. Table 37.5 presents a summary of daily and stress treatment for children with AI. Please refer to Chap. 62 for more details on management of adrenal crisis.

37.6 The Importance of Patient Education in AI

Patient education is paramount in optimising replacement therapy and minimising complications of over- and under-replacement. Endocrine nurses play a crucial role in educating patients and their families on day-to-day self-management, intercurrent illness, or special situations and how to prevent AC. Their role is also vital in educating other healthcare professionals and raising awareness of the life-threatening nature of AI. This is especially important in the care of children as parents can be in a state of shock. Endocrine nurses begin their patient education by assessing

Table 37.5 Maintenance and stress dosing for children with AI

Two different dosing plans for children with AI	
Primary Adrenal Insufficiency (PAI)	12–16 mgs/m²/day hydrocortisone 0.05–0.2 mgs per day Fludrocortisone *(Note: in CAH patients doses need not only to replace but also to suppress excess androgen secretion to prevent virilisation)*
Secondary adrenal insufficiency (SAI)	6–8 mgs/m²/day *(Exact replacement dosing)*
Stress doses for hydrocortisone doses are the same in PAI and SAI	
Stress dosing—oral *Moderate illness*	45–50 mgs/m²/day divided into 4 doses 6-hourly
Stress dosing—Intramuscular injection or intravenous *Significant illness, vomiting, diarrhoea, reduced consciousness*	45–100 mgs/m² stat Followed by: 45–100 mg/m²/day divided in 4 doses 6-hourly 6-hourly or Hydrocortisone infusion with 100–200 mg/24 h

parental grief, understanding and coping strategies in adapting to their child's diagnosis. It is important to instil confidence into parents' coping abilities and to reassure them that there is advice and support available to guide them through any difficulties they may encounter in managing the day-to-day care of their child. At each consultation, it is crucial to check the patient's knowledge on management of intercurrent illness and prevention of AC, and provide relevant education if gaps are identified. The process of patient education is described in more detail in Chap. 62.

37.7 Role of Adherence to Medication in Optimising GC Replacement

Current treatment options, although not yet perfected, can offer an individualised approach that can meet the needs of most patients with AI, especially with the new formulations developed recently. However, *"drugs don't work in patients who don't take them*" (C.Everett Koop, MD, US Surgeon General, 1985). Nonadherence has been recognised as a significant challenge by the World Health Organisation suggesting that only 50% of patients with chronic conditions take their medications as recommended (Nunes et al. 2009). More specifically in AI, adherence to GC replacement encompasses the three aspects of appropriate dosing of daily GC to avoid over- or under-replacement, dose adjustment during intercurrent illness and prevention of adrenal crisis (AC).

Adherence to medication is defined as the extent to which a patient's behaviour matches agreed recommendations from their healthcare professional (Nunes et al. 2009). It is also important to understand that adherence to medication is not always in the patient's control. To understand this, Professor Robert Horne uses a simple analogy of *"patients don't want or cannot take their medications"* (quote from personal communication, November 2016). His *Perceptions and Practicalities Approach* provides a theoretical framework to understand the complex human behaviour nature of nonadherence (Horne et al. 2005; Horne 2006) which can be:

- Unintentional where the patient wants to adhere but is prevented from doing so by **practical barriers** or resources beyond their control (*ability*). These include barriers such as forgetfulness, complexity of regimen, difficulty with prescriptions, poor recall or lack of information about the medication, and side effects.
- Intentional where the patient decides not to follow the prescribed treatment regime whether this is conscious or subconscious. **Perceptual barriers** such as beliefs about medicines or fear of side effects can influence patient's *motivation* to start and continue treatment.

37.7.1 Evidence of Nonadherence to GC Replacement

Tailoring the GC dose to patients' needs and achieving optimal adherence are two of the main challenges reported by endocrine clinicians (Grossman et al. 2013). Forss et al. found that

23% of patients with AI ($N = 1245$) report dissatisfaction with treatment, 38% find multiple daily dosing problematic, over 50% perceive that GC interferes with life aspects such as work, travel, or sex life, and many missed tablets or took them before sleep which resulted in fatigue or insomnia (Forss et al. 2012). Chapman et al. found that 25% of patients took higher doses than advised (Chapman et al. 2016) which can lead to complications. Both studies found that over 50% of patients report concerns about side effects and long-term complications (Chapman et al. 2016; Forss et al. 2012); concerns were strongly associated with nonadherence (Chapman et al. 2016). About 1 in 25 patients reported prolonged treatment interruptions (Chapman et al. 2016); GC dose reduction or cessation was a significant factor to trigger AC for 3.9% (Smans et al. 2016) and 5.5% (Hahner et al. 2010) of patients with AI.

37.7.2 How to Identify and Address Nonadherence to GC Replacement

The endocrine nurse is the best placed person in the multidisciplinary team to identify nonadherence factors and to support patients, their families, and other healthcare professionals to improve adherence to GC replacement; Box 37.7 summarises the key steps in this process adapted from (Horne 2006).

Box 37.7 Key Steps in Improving Adherence to GC Replacement Therapy

1. **Provide a rationale for the need to take GC replacement and the various treatment adaptations**

   Provide patients and their families with a clear rationale for why they should take GC daily, emphasise the difference between a hormone replacement therapy and a steroid pharmacotherapy, and explain the need for dose adjustment in intercurrent illness and prevention of adrenal crisis. Explain what diagnostic tests mean. Illustrations or other patient stories often help patients to understand and to recall the information received.

2. **Elicit and address concern about GC replacement and potential side effects**
   GC treatment in high doses is associated with a high prevalence of side effects, and these can affect patients' adherence as they increase their concerns and beliefs of harm from taking the medicine. Similarly, some patients may take more than the prescribed dose believing that more is better which can lead to adverse effects and treatment nonadherence. Advise patients of potential side effects from the start, how to recognise and deal with them. Emphasise that GC replacement is individualised and not a "one size fits all" treatment.

3. **Identify and address the practical barriers**
   Adopt a shared decision-making approach when planning GC replacement and develop an easy-to-follow managed care plan which can guide patients, their families, or parents of children with AI, on how to manage the daily GC regimen. Identify and address any barriers which may potentially prevent the patient from following this regimen, such as: Can they remember or are they able (external barriers) to take their tablets? What hours do they work? How do they get their prescriptions? Will the school teachers/nurses help? These are some of the factors that can inhibit adherence and are not always within the patient's control.

4. **Patient and family beliefs**
   Nonadherence may also be associated with concerns arising from more abstract beliefs about medications.

They may come with preconceived misconceptions about steroid treatment. Some of my patients tell me they *"don't want to take hydrocortisone and get fat"*. Adopt an empathetic and non-judgmental approach when eliciting and addressing these beliefs and emphasise that with appropriate monitoring and correct GC dose, complications can be minimised.

37.8 Glucocorticoid Replacement in Special Therapeutic Situations

37.8.1 Fertility and Pregnancy

Total cortisol concentrations start to rise in pregnancy and free cortisol also increases substantially in the third trimester from the 22nd week of gestation onwards. Hydrocortisone is recommended over cortisone acetate, prednisolone, or prednisone during pregnancy; dexamethasone should not be used because it is not inactivated in the placenta (Bornstein et al. 2016). Common AI symptoms (fatigue, nausea, hyponatraemia, vomiting) are difficult to differentiate in pregnancy, and it is recommended that hydrocortisone doses are increased based on individual patient assessment. It is also recommended that hydrocortisone dose should be increased by 50% in the third trimester (Arlt and Allolio 2003; Bancos et al. 2015; Bornstein et al. 2016).

In addition, the increased levels of serum progesterone in pregnancy exert an anti-mineralocorticoid action, but clinical assessment can be difficult due to overlapping unspecific symptoms of oedema and postural hypotension. Fludrocortisone should be adjusted if necessary according to blood pressure and serum sodium and potassium; while plasma renin is not accurate as it is physiologically increased during pregnancy. During delivery (active phase of labour) parenteral hydrocortisone should be administered at doses similar to that used in major surgical stress (refer to Chap. 62 for more details) and after delivery hydrocortisone can be tapered back to pre-pregnancy doses within 2–4 days (Bancos et al. 2015; Bornstein et al. 2016).

37.8.2 Thyroid Dysfunction

Hyperthyroidism increases cortisol clearance and therefore in patients with AI and unresolved hyperthyroidism, GC doses should be doubled or tripled. In addition, thyroxine treatment should only be initiated once GC deficiency has been excluded or confirmed and GC replacement has been established (Arlt and Allolio 2003). Thyroxine can precipitate adrenal crisis in untreated hypocortisolism and the patient needs to be advised appropriately when reviewing their treatment regimen and adherence to medication.

37.8.3 Growth Hormone Deficiency in Adults

In growth hormone (GH) deficiency in adults, there is an increased 11β-HSD type 1 activity which results in increased cortisol tissue exposure (see Sect. 37.5.3). This is reduced after initiating GH treatment (high GH and IGF-1 levels enhance conversion of cortisol to cortisone, i.e. lower levels of active cortisol) which can unmask central hypoadrenalism and predispose the patient to AI and risk of AC. Therefore, the assessment of the HPA axis to confirm or exclude AI is mandatory prior to starting GH replacement (Filipsson and Johannsson 2009; Giavoli et al. 2004).

37.8.4 Increased Physical and Emotional Stress

In healthy subjects, in addition to the circadian profile, cortisol levels increase in response to

stressful daily stimuli such extreme physical extortion or emotional distress. Patients with AI should take an extra dose of 5–10 mg prior to being exposed to the stressful situation (Grossman 2010; Quinkler and Hahner 2012). It is often difficult to define "stress" for individual patients and a detailed history would reveal fatigue, feeling unwell and light-headed, the same or the next day after exerting increased levels of stress. Examples include training and running a marathon, mountain biking, triathlon, moving to a new house, long flights, bereavement, or acute depression episodes. Short lasting stressor, such as exams, house work, or work-related meetings, do not normally require dose adaptation.

37.8.5 Prolonged Fasting or Shift Working

During the month of Ramadan, Muslims tend to fast, i.e. abstain from eating, drinking, and use of oral medication from predawn to sunset. This can put patients with AI at risk of dehydration, fainting, hypotension, or low glucose levels which can precipitate AC. A cross-sectional study of 180 patients with AI found that of the 91 patients who did fast, 67% developed complications such as asthenia, intense thirst, dehydration, and symptoms of hypoglycaemia; one patient was hospitalised with AC (Chihaoui et al. 2017). It is important that patients wanting to fast during Ramadan are well educated on the risks of fasting and given the option for alternative treatment. A longer acting formulations such as immediate-sustained release hydrocortisone (Plenadren® 20 mg) or prednisolone 4–5 mg at dawn before starting the fast is a preferred option during the fasting period.

Similarly, the cortisol circadian rhythm is misaligned in people who sleep outside a normal sleep cycle such as shift workers or during jet lag. Patients with AI who work shifts or travel between wide timezones should adapt their GC intake to their wake-sleep pattern (Quinkler and Hahner 2012), i.e. take first dose of hydrocortisone on waking up and the last dose no later than

5–6 h before sleep. Short acting hydrocortisone versus long-acting formulations is advisable to avoid exposure to cortisol during the sleep periods which can result in increased risk of glucose intolerance or impaired quality of sleep. The case study in Box 37.8 delineates the importance of adapting hydrocortisone intake during night working.

> **Box 37.8 Case Study of a Patient on Emergency Night Shifts**
>
> Richard is 54 and has SAI following pituitary surgery. He takes hydrocortisone 10 + 5 mg twice daily on waking up at 7 am and at 3 pm. He volunteers as coast guard and often is called on emergencies in the middle of the night. This can be quite stressful physically and emotionally. He described feeling exhausted the next day of such events and on one occasion he developed adrenal crisis for which he needed a hospital admission. We advised him to take 10 mg of hydrocortisone as soon as he is being called for duty and another 10 mg if he is out at sea for longer than 5 h. This helped him significantly to overcome fatigue post emergency duty he did not experience any further AC episodes.

37.8.6 Medications and Food Interactions with Glucocorticoids

Table 37.6 presents a list of drugs and food types that interact with GC and mineralocorticoids in AI (Arlt and Allolio 2003; Liu et al. 2013; Methlie et al. 2011). It is important to take a detailed history from patients on prescribed medication, including oral contraceptive pill, over the counter medications, supplements, herbal remedies, and foods that can decrease or increase concentrations of bioavailable cortisol.

37.9 Morbidity and Mortality Related to Glucocorticoid Replacement Therapy

AI was a fatal condition until cortisone was synthesised and used as life-saving treatment in 1949 by Kendall, Reichtein, and Sarrett (Arlt and Allolio 2003). Even though GC treatment has been available for over half a century, optimal replacement therapy in AI, negative acute and long-term health outcomes, including hospitalisations from AC, GC-induced morbidities, and impaired QoL, are still presenting major challenges.

37.9.1 Mortality and Risk of Adrenal Crisis

The standard mortality rate (SMR) for patients with AI is more than twofold compared to the general population (Tomlinson et al. 2001; Bergthorsdottir et al. 2006). AC is a factor that increases the mortality rate in patients with AI. SMR was significantly elevated in patients diagnosed before the age of 40 years; this was more pronounced in males with SMR 2.03 (CI 1.19–2.86) and younger patients were at higher risk of sudden death from AC (Erichsen et al. 2009). Approximately 1 in 100 patients with AI are expected to die from a potentially preventable AC (Hahner et al. 2015). One in 12 patients report at least one hospital admission per year related to AC (Forss et al. 2012; Hahner et al. 2015; White and Arlt 2010) and about 10% of patients with PAI who reported AC, had this on four or more occasions (Hahner et al. 2015) indicating that there is a subgroup of patients at high risk, and we need to identify and support them with relevant individualised treatment planning and education. AC is mainly precipitated by gastrointestinal infection and fever but also other stressful physical or emotional events (more details on AC mortality are discussed in Chap. 62).

Table 37.6 Common food and drug interactions with glucocorticoids

Interacting drug class (drug example) or food type	Interaction mechanisms (key: ↓-reduces; ↑-increases; GC-glucocorticoids)	Suggested management
Anticonvulsants (phenytoin, carbamazepine, phenobarbital)	Enhanced GC metabolism ↓ Efficacy of GC may persist for weeks following discontinuation of anticonvulsant	Monitor outcomes, may need GC dose adjustment (increase)
Anti-Tuberculosis (rifampicin, rifabutin)	Increases cortisol clearance ↓ Efficacy of GC which may persist for weeks following discontinuation of anti-tuberculosis drugs	Monitor outcomes, increase GC dose during rifampicin
Antifungal drugs (ketoconazole, itraconazole)	↑ GC bioavailability	May need antifungals or GC adjustment if show signs of GC overdose
Anticoagulants (warfarin)	May ↑ effects of anticoagulant and ↑ risk of GI bleeding	Monitor INR within 3–7 days, may need significant warfarin dose adjustment
Antibiotics (erythromycin, telithromycin, and clarithromycin)	May inhibit the metabolism of corticosteroids ↑ GC bioavailability	Monitor signs of GC over-replacement, may need to change antibacterial or adjust GC dose
Antidiabetic agents (insulins)	Antagonism of hypoglycaemic effect ↓ Efficacy of GC	↑ frequency of blood glucose monitoring adjust antidiabetic therapy
Antivirals (atazanavir, indinavir, ritonavir, saquinavir)	↑ GC bioavailability	Monitor signs of GC over-replacement
Oral oestrogen replacement and oral contraceptive pill	Increases circulating cortisol-binding globulin False high plasma cortisol levels	Oestrogen needs to be discontinued for diagnostic investigations
Mitotane	↓ concentration and increased metabolism and efficacy of bioavailable GC	Usual GC doses need to be at least doubled or tripled
Herbal remedies (St John's wort)	↑ GC bioavailability	Avoid or take at least 2–3 h later
Grapefruit, grapefruit juice, Liquorice	↑ GC bioavailability	Avoid or take at least 2–3 h later

37.9.2 Bone Metabolism

GCs affect the rate of bone remodelling; they impair the replication, differentiation, and function of osteoblasts, induce the apoptosis of mature osteoblasts and osteocytes, and increase osteoclastogenesis. Supraphysiological doses of GC are associated with a decrease in markers for bone formation and resorption, leading to osteoporosis (Canalis et al. 2007). Several studies found that patients with AI on GC replacement have lower bone mineral density (BMD) scores compared to the average population and that BMD decreases with increasing doses of hydrocortisone over 30 mg daily (Zelissen et al. 1994; Lovas et al. 2009; Schulz et al. 2016; Bjornsdottir et al. 2011). A population-based cohort study identified

hip fractures in 6.9% of patients with PAI compared with 2.7% of controls although authors did not investigate association of fractures with GC dose (Bjornsdottir et al. 2011). Schulz et al. found that by reducing the total daily dose of hydrocortisone equivalent to 20–25 mg from 30 to 35 mg, values of BMD significantly improved 2 years later, and the risk of AC did not increase (Schulz et al. 2016). It is therefore important to remember that high doses of GCs have a detrimental effect on bone health (Johannsson et al. 2015) and replacement doses of hydrocortisone should be maintained generally to a total daily dose below 20–25 mg, where indicated. Patients should be reassured that the risk of AC will not increase if they adjust GC doses appropriately during increased stress and illness.

37.9.3 Blood Pressure, Glucose/Lipid Metabolism, and Body Composition

The physiologic circadian rhythm of cortisol affects fluctuations in glucose tolerance throughout the day. Abnormal glucose tolerance is therefore more common in patients with AI. This is especially important to keep in mind for patients with PAI and concomitant type 1 diabetes as insulin requirements, especially in the afternoon, are higher compared to patients with type 1 diabetes alone (Johannsson et al. 2015).

Patients with hypopituitarism and SAI are at higher risk of developing metabolic syndrome with a combination of hypertension, dyslipidaemia, central obesity, and insulin insensitivity (Johannsson et al. 2015). A large pharmacovigilance study of patients with hypopituitarism ($N = 2424$) treated with growth hormone, compared patients with and without ACTH deficiency. Patients with ACTH deficiency treated with a total daily dose of hydrocortisone-equivalent of 20 mg or more had an unfavourable metabolic profile with greater body mass index, waist circumference, serum levels of total cholesterol, triglycerides, and low-density lipoprotein; this was not observed in patients taking doses lower than 20 mg (Filipsson et al. 2006). Changes in body weight and blood pressure may also be a contributing risk factor to the increased prevalence of premature cardiovascular deaths in patients with AI (Tomlinson et al. 2001; Bergthorsdottir et al. 2006). Detrimental effects of over-replacement can be more significant in patients with SAI as there is often residual cortisol production and it is very important to plan for an individualised GC replacement regimen. The modified-release hydrocortisone also has a favourable profile with regard to body weight, glucose metabolism, and insulin insensitivity at equivalent total daily doses of hydrocortisone (Muller and Quinkler 2018; Johannsson et al. 2012).

37.9.4 Quality of Life (QoL) and Subjective Well-Being

AI has significant impact on patients' lives with 64% of them reporting impaired QoL, 40% absence from work/school every 3 months, and 38% at least one hospital admission annually (Forss et al. 2012). Almost a quarter of patients with AI receive disability pension compared to 4–10% of the general population (Lovas et al. 2002; Hahner et al. 2007). Delay in the diagnosis of AI has a negative impact on QoL; Bleicken found that patients who received a correct diagnosis within 3 months reported significantly better subjective health status compared to those for whom diagnosis was delayed (Bleicken et al. 2010b). Higher GC replacement doses are associated with a negative effect on the patient's QoL, although it is unclear if the increased dose itself diminishes QoL, or if the dose was increased by the clinician due to an impaired QoL. Two studies found that QoL decreased with increasing dose of GC and the worst QoL was reported by patients who took hydrocortisone-equivalent doses of more than 25 mg daily (Filipsson et al. 2006) and 30 mg daily (Bleicken et al. 2010a), respectively. This was more significant in patients with SAI. Additional hormone deficiencies in SAI may also impact on QoL and often patients increase the dose of GC to compensate for impaired QoL and fatigue caused by unoptimised concomitant deficiencies.

It is also important to remember that current conventional GC replacement therapy in patients with PAI does not restore the unphysiologically low cortisol levels in the night, particularly the last part of the night, which may reduce early morning glucose levels (Oksnes et al. 2015). Patients may complain of impaired quality of sleep and waking up with nausea, dizziness fatigue, and headaches, and it is important to discuss a GC therapy regimen that can combat these symptoms.

Validated questionnaires are useful in clinical practice to assess patient's QoL and agree on a relevant care plan to respond to individualised needs. In addition, they can be used to track improvement or deterioration of QoL over time or post changes in the management of patient's care. The AddiQoL is a validated Likert scale questionnaire of 36 items with high internal validity and psychometric properties which make it a useful tool for use in clinical practice (Lovas et al. 2010).

37.10 Long-Term Monitoring of Patients with AI

The goal of treatment and follow-up for patients with AI is to restore normal well-being by optimising replacement therapy, to minimise or avoid complications from over- or under-replacement, and to minimise episodes of AC and avoid hospital admissions due to AC. Monitoring of replacement is mainly based on clinical symptoms but cortisol day curve may be useful and indicated when symptoms persist or when malabsorption of hydrocortisone is suspected (see case study in Box 37.5). Similarly, random cortisol levels are helpful to obtain evidence of adequate cortisol uptake (Bornstein et al. 2016) and to establish peak and trough levels, but they must only be interpreted with an accurate history of timing and dose of hydrocortisone and are not needed routinely.

Routine laboratory analyses and imaging are requested depending on diagnosis and cause of AI; these should include blood serum sodium and potassium levels for patients with PAI. In addition, surveillance for other autoimmune disorders, such as thyroid disease or type 1 diabetes, is necessary in patients with PAI given the increased prevalence of concomitant autoimmune disorders; genetic counselling should also be provided to patients with PAI due to monogenic disorders (Bornstein et al. 2016). Patients should be made aware and educated on possible symptoms related to other autoimmune disorders.

It is recommended that adults and children with PAI are seen by an endocrinologist or a healthcare provider, including nurses, with expertise in endocrinology at least annually. Infants should be seen at least every 3–4 months (Bornstein et al. 2016). There is no consensus regarding frequency of monitoring for patients with SAI as this depends on other concomitant comorbidities, but patients should be seen at a minimum 6–12 monthly (Fleseriu et al. 2016).

Patients should be examined and asked questions to evaluate physical and psychological (QoL, subjective health status) condition in relation to possible over-replacement or under-replacement and adverse effects from the GC therapy. A UK-wide study of patients with asthma showed a dissociation between patient-reported concerns and side effects about corticosteroid treatment and those perceived by physicians (Cooper et al. 2015). Medication side effects are strongly associated with nonadherence and treatment discontinuation. It is therefore important to take a detailed history of any possible side effects to the AI medication and address them accordingly; this should also include possible interactions with other concomitant medications, food and over-the-counter supplements and hormone deficiencies.

A holistic assessment will identify and support patients with medical but also psychosocial and educational needs. It is crucial to ensure that patients are familiar with and are provided with education on management of intercurrent illness and prevention of AC. Exploring and addressing all potential needs in a single consultation can however be time consuming for the nurse. It is also difficult to remember all relevant points relating to AI and GC treatment which need addressing, particularly if patients have other comorbidities or treatments. Consultation checklists are often useful toolkits which nurses can use to ensure a productive and effective consultation. On the other hand, there is a risk of "information overload" for patients or repeating what they already know to the detriment of missing out on information which patients really need.

It is useful to advise patients to come with a list of questions and concerns which can be addressed during each consultation and are pertinent to each individual's needs. There is however evidence to suggest that patients often do not know what to ask, believe that concerns are not relevant to their condition or treatment, feel there is too little time to address everything, or feel embarrassed to disclose information such as nonadherence to medication or sexual dysfunction (Henselmans et al. 2015). To facilitate the process of consultations and to provide support for self-management, our research team developed a one-page questionnaire based on behavioural medicine, which can help patients identify concerns about their AI and GC replacement therapy (Box 37.9), adopting this way an individualised approach to patient care and treatment planning. The questionnaire is accompanied by a comprehensive patient information booklet designed to address the concerns identified in the questionnaire which patients can read before attending clinic. This is also used as an aid to stimulate further questions or help the patient to identify more needs. An online survey involving 100 patients with AI, members of the Pituitary Foundation in the UK, showed good acceptability of this consultation aid and booklet as a resource to support self-management in AI (Llahana et al. 2016).

Box 37.9 A Questionnaire to Identify and Address Individualised Patient Needs in the Treatment and Management of AI

This questionnaire was developed specifically to help with the management of cortisol replacement therapy for patients with adrenal insufficiency (AI). The questionnaire aims to get you thinking about the things that matter most to you about your AI and your cortisol replacement therapy. You may also be taking additional medications for AI and other conditions. However, please ONLY take into account your cortisol replacement therapy when answering these questions.

There are no right or wrong answers—simply answer the questions by ticking the relevant box if it applies to you. Use the answers to guide you to the most relevant sections of the accompanying booklet, specific to you and your needs. You can also

use this questionnaire during your consultation with your doctor or nurse to focus your discussion on areas which you identified as a concern.

Section A: Managing Adrenal Insufficiency

A1	I know how to adjust my cortisol replacement dose during illness	Yes No
A2	I need help in managing an adrenal crisis	Yes No
A3	I often feel tired during the day	Yes No
A4	The quality of my sleep is impaired (I don't sleep well)	Yes No

Section B: Medication (managing cortisol replacement therapy)

B1	I am not sure why I need to take cortisol replacement therapy every day	Yes No
B2	I am concerned about the side effects of my cortisol replacement therapy	Yes No
B3	Having to take cortisol replacement therapy affects aspects of my life:	
	Travel	Yes No
	Physical activities	Yes No
	Family	Yes No
	Social	Yes No
	Work	Yes No
	Other—please specify	Yes No
B4	Having to take more than one dose every day is an inconvenience for me	Yes No

Section C: Your way of taking cortisol replacement therapy

C1	I sometimes/often miss my doses for a day or more	Yes No
C2	I sometimes/often miss my second or third dose	Yes No
C3	I sometimes/often take an extra dose just to feel better	Yes No
C4	I don't take extra doses when I'm ill or have "sick days"	Yes No
C5	I don't always take my dose(s) at the recommended times	Yes No

Please include any additional information here

Original version of the questionnaire and the patient booklet are available by request from Spoonful of Sugar, a behaviour-change consultancy in London, http://sos-adherence.co.uk/

37.11 The Role of Patient Advocacy Groups in Improving Patient Care and Education

Patient advocacy groups (PAGs) are a highly valuable resource for patients and their families, not just as a clinical and supportive tool, but by also enabling empowerment and enriching the relationship between patients, families, and their healthcare providers. The advent of social media, with websites and online support groups can add to this, and patients have a reliable and trusted resource for peer support. Most PAGs work very closely with clinical teams to develop evidence-based information and support clinical research. As seen in the example below, PAGs can form a useful resource and can reach patients and healthcare teams across the globe especially for rare conditions such as AI.

37.11.1 The Australian Addison's Disease Association Inc (AADAI)

Through an amazing amount of volunteer work by people across the nation, the Association has grown from just a handful of members to over 300 spread across this vast country. The goal of the AADAI is to:

- Educate the medical profession and the general public to have a higher awareness of Addison's disease and AI
- Supply up-to-date information to people living with Addison's disease/AI
- Create a caring network to give support for people with Addison's disease/AI

To provide the best possible information and support to people living with adrenal insufficiency, the association works closely with healthcare professionals, especially endocrine nurses and endocrinologists. All our online and print educational and resource materials are thoroughly reviewed before publication by our medical advisor; seminars are presented each year for people living with AI and these are strongly supported by key healthcare professionals.

Our quarterly member newsletter focuses on a range of support and medical information issues.

These are written by people with medical expertise including our medical advisor and our pharmacy advisor. The website provides detailed information about materials we produce. These include new member packs: online and print information material and the regular newsletter. A telephone support service to help members find specific information is also offered by the AADAI President and the Secretary. To find out more about the AADAI, please visit our website at http://addisons.org.au.

37.12 Conclusions

AI is a life-threatening condition if not managed appropriately but with correct and individualised replacement therapy and adequate support and education, patients can lead a normal life. This is a chronic condition and the initial diagnosis will have a significant impact on how the condition is perceived by the patient and their families and especially for parents and their young children. Patients and their families require sensible day-to-day management plans, careful dosing regimens, and an action plan for times of illness, injury, or procedures. The endocrine nurse is a key person in supporting patients and families in the process of acceptance, understanding, and confidence to manage situations as they arise.

AI is a condition where mortality rate is high and a team approach and interdisciplinary collaboration in key to offering the best treatment options to improve patients' health outcomes and QoL. Patients with AI and their families need to gain an understanding about their condition and treatment, which can be very complex especially when dose titration is required during stress, intercurrent illness, and prevention of AC. Having an endocrine service with sound and knowledgeable endocrine nursing team can offer best treatment options in chronic disease condition such as AI. Endocrine nurses with advanced practice skills can utilise their specialist knowledge and excellent communication skills to tailor treatment options to meet individual needs of their patients.

Acknowledgments With special thanks to our patients for their case studies and to Grahame Collier from the Australian Addison's Disease Association Inc (http://addisons.org.au; email: secretary@addisons.org.au) for the information on their Patient Advocacy Group.

References

Arlt W. Chapter 8: Disorders of the adrenal cortex. In: Jameson JL, editor. Harrison's endocrinology. 4th ed. New York: McGraw Hill Education; 2017. p. 107–35.

Arlt W, Allolio B. Adrenal insufficiency. Lancet (London, England). 2003;361(9372):1881–93.

Aulinas A, Casanueva F, Goni F, Monereo S, Moreno B, Pico A, et al. Adrenal insufficiency and adrenal replacement therapy. Current status in Spain. Endocrinol Nutr. 2013;60(3):136–43.

Bancos I, Hahner S, Tomlinson J, Arlt W. Diagnosis and management of adrenal insufficiency. Lancet Diabetes Endocrinol. 2015;3(3):216–26.

Barthel A, Willenberg HS, Gruber M, Bornstein SR. Chapter 102—Adrenal insufficiency. In: Jameson JL, De Groot LJ, de Kretser DM, Giudice LC, Grossman AB, Melmed S, et al., editors. Endocrinology: adult and pediatric. 7th ed. Philadelphia: W.B. Saunders; 2016. p. 1763–74.e4.

Bergthorsdottir R, Leonsson-Zachrisson M, Oden A, Johannsson G. Premature mortality in patients with Addison's disease: a population-based study. J Clin Endocrinol Metab. 2006;91(12):4849–53.

Betman JEM. Parental grief when a child is diagnosed with a life threatening chronic illness: impact of gender, perceptions and coping strategies. University of Canterbury NZ. Thesis submitted for Doctor of Philosophy degree; 2006.

Bjornsdottir S, Saaf M, Bensing S, Kampe O, Michaelsson K, Ludvigsson JF. Risk of hip fracture in Addison's disease: a population-based cohort study. J Intern Med. 2011;270(2):187–95.

Bleicken B, Hahner S, Loeffler M, Ventz M, Decker O, Allolio B, et al. Influence of hydrocortisone dosage scheme on health-related quality of life in patients with adrenal insufficiency. Clin Endocrinol. 2010a;72(3):297–304.

Bleicken B, Hahner S, Ventz M, Quinkler M. Delayed diagnosis of adrenal insufficiency is common: a cross-sectional study in 216 patients. Am J Med Sci. 2010b;339(6):525–31.

Bornstein SR, Allolio B, Arlt W, Barthel A, Don-Wauchope A, Hammer GD, et al. Diagnosis and treatment of primary adrenal insufficiency: an endocrine society clinical practice guideline. J Clin Endocrinol Metab. 2016;101(2):364–89.

Broersen LHA, Pereira AM, Jørgensen JOL, Dekkers OM. Adrenal insufficiency in corticosteroids use: systematic review and meta-analysis. J Clin Endocrinol Metabol. 2015;100(6):2171–80.

Brooke AM, Kalingag LA, Miraki-Moud F, Camacho-Hubner C, Maher KT, Walker DM, et al. Dehydroepiandrosterone improves psychological well-being in male and female hypopituitary patients on maintenance growth hormone replacement. J Clin Endocrinol Metab. 2006;91(10):3773–9.

Canalis E, Mazziotti G, Giustina A, Bilezikian JP. Glucocorticoid-induced osteoporosis: pathophysiology and therapy. Osteoporos Int. 2007;18(10):1319–28.

Chapman SC, Llahana S, Carroll P, Horne R. Glucocorticoid therapy for adrenal insufficiency: nonadherence, concerns and dissatisfaction with information. Clin Endocrinol. 2016;84(5):664–71.

Chihaoui M, Chaker F, Yazidi M, Grira W, Ben Amor Z, Rejeb O, et al. Ramadan fasting in patients with adrenal insufficiency. Endocrine. 2017;55(1):289–95.

Cooper V, Metcalf L, Versnel J, Upton J, Walker S, Horne R. Patient-reported side effects, concerns and adherence to corticosteroid treatment for asthma, and comparison with physician estimates of side-effect prevalence: a UK-wide, cross-sectional study. NPJ Prim Care Res Med. 2015;25:15026.

Dorin RI, Qualls CR, Crapo LM. Diagnosis of adrenal insufficiency. Ann Intern Med. 2003;139(3):194–204.

El-Farhan N, Pickett A, Ducroq D, Bailey C, Mitchem K, Morgan N, et al. Method-specific serum cortisol responses to the adrenocorticotrophin test: comparison of gas chromatography-mass spectrometry and five automated immunoassays. Clin Endocrinol. 2013;78(5):673–80.

Erichsen MM, Lovas K, Fougner KJ, Svartberg J, Hauge ER, Bollerslev J, et al. Normal overall mortality rate in Addison's disease, but young patients are at risk of premature death. Eur J Endocrinol. 2009;160(2):233–7.

Fardet L, Petersen I, Nazareth I. Prevalence of long-term oral glucocorticoid prescriptions in the UK over the past 20 years. Rheumatology (Oxford, England). 2011;50(11):1982–90.

Filipsson H, Johannsson G. GH replacement in adults: interactions with other pituitary hormone deficiencies and replacement therapies. Eur J Endocrinol. 2009;161(Suppl 1):S85–95.

Filipsson H, Monson JP, Koltowska-Haggstrom M, Mattsson A, Johannsson G. The impact of glucocorticoid replacement regimens on metabolic outcome and comorbidity in hypopituitary patients. J Clin Endocrinol Metab. 2006;91(10):3954–61.

Fleseriu M, Hashim IA, Karavitaki N, Melmed S, Murad MH, Salvatori R, et al. Hormonal replacement in hypopituitarism in adults: an endocrine society clinical practice guideline. J Clin Endocrinol Metab. 2016;101(11):3888–921.

Forss M, Batcheller G, Skrtic S, Johannsson G. Current practice of glucocorticoid replacement therapy and patient-perceived health outcomes in adrenal insufficiency—a worldwide patient survey. BMC Endocr Disord. 2012;12:8.

Frey KR, Kienitz T, Schulz J, Ventz M, Zopf K, Quinkler M. Prednisolone is associated with a worse bone mineral density in primary adrenal insufficiency. Endocr Connect. 2018;7(6):811–8.

Giavoli C, Libé R, Corbetta S, Ferrante E, Lania A, Arosio M, et al. Effect of recombinant human growth hormone (GH) replacement on the hypothalamic-pituitary-adrenal axis in adult GH-deficient patients. J Clin Endocrinol Metabol. 2004;89(11):5397–401.

Grossman AB. Clinical review: the diagnosis and management of central hypoadrenalism. J Clin Endocrinol Metab. 2010;95(11):4855–63.

Grossman A, Johannsson G, Quinkler M, Zelissen P. Therapy of endocrine disease: perspectives on the management of adrenal insufficiency: clinical insights from across Europe. Eur J Endocrinol. 2013;169(6):R165–75.

Hahner S, Loeffler M, Fassnacht M, Weismann D, Koschker AC, Quinkler M, et al. Impaired subjective health status in 256 patients with adrenal insufficiency on standard therapy based on cross-sectional analysis. J Clin Endocrinol Metab. 2007;92(10):3912–22.

Hahner S, Loeffler M, Bleicken B, Drechsler C, Milovanovic D, Fassnacht M, et al. Epidemiology of adrenal crisis in chronic adrenal insufficiency: the need for new prevention strategies. Eur J Endocrinol. 2010;162(3):597–602.

Hahner S, Spinnler C, Fassnacht M, Burger-Stritt S, Lang K, Milovanovic D, et al. High incidence of adrenal crisis in educated patients with chronic adrenal insufficiency: a prospective study. J Clin Endocrinol Metab. 2015;100(2):407–16.

Henselmans I, Heijmans M, Rademakers J, van Dulmen S. Participation of chronic patients in medical consultations: patients' perceived efficacy, barriers and interest in support. Health Expect. 2015;18(6):2375–88.

Horne R. Compliance, adherence, and concordance: implications for asthma treatment. Chest J. 2006;130(Suppl 1):65S–72S.

Horne R, Weinman J, Barber N, Elliot R, Morgan M. Concordance, adherence and compliance in medicine taking: a conceptual map and research priorities. London: National Institute for Health Research (NIHR) Service Delivery and Organisation (SDO) Programme; 2005.

Husebye ES, Allolio B, Arlt W, Badenhoop K, Bensing S, Betterle C, et al. Consensus statement on the diagnosis, treatment and follow-up of patients with primary adrenal insufficiency. J Intern Med. 2014;275(2):104–15.

Isidori AM, Venneri MA, Graziadio C, Simeoli C, Fiore D, Hasenmajer V, et al. Effect of once-daily, modified-release hydrocortisone versus standard glucocorticoid therapy on metabolism and innate immunity in patients with adrenal insufficiency (DREAM): a single-blind, randomised controlled trial. Lancet Diabetes Endocrinol. 2018;6(3):173–85.

Johannsson G, Bergthorsdottir R, Nilsson AG, Lennernas H, Hedner T, Skrtic S. Improving glucocorticoid replacement therapy using a novel modified-release hydrocortisone tablet: a pharmacokinetic study. Eur J Endocrinol. 2009;161(1):119–30.

Johannsson G, Nilsson AG, Bergthorsdottir R, Burman P, Dahlqvist P, Ekman B, et al. Improved cortisol exposure-time profile and outcome in patients with adrenal insufficiency: a prospective randomized trial of a novel hydrocortisone dual-release formulation. J Clin Endocrinol Metabol. 2012;97(2):473–81.

Johannsson G, Falorni A, Skrtic S, Lennernas H, Quinkler M, Monson JP, et al. Adrenal insufficiency: review of clinical outcomes with current glucocorticoid replacement therapy. Clin Endocrinol. 2015;82(1):2–11.

Joseph RM, Hunter AL, Ray DW, Dixon WG. Systemic glucocorticoid therapy and adrenal insufficiency in adults: a systematic review. Semin Arthritis Rheum. 2016;46(1):133–41.

Koyama Y, Homma K, Hasegawa T. Urinary steroid profiling: a powerful method for the diagnosis of abnormal steroidogenesis. Endocrinol Metab. 2014;9(3):273–82.

Kwok MY, Scanlon MC, Slyper AH. Atypical presentation of shock from acute adrenal insufficiency in an adolescent male. Paediatr Emerg Care. 2005;21(6):380–3.

Lee AS, Twigg SM. Opioid-induced secondary adrenal insufficiency presenting as hypercalcaemia. Endocrinol Diabetes Metab Case Rep. 2015;2015:150035.

Liu D, Ahmet A, Ward L, Krishnamoorthy P, Mandelcorn ED, Leigh R, et al. A practical guide to the monitoring and management of the complications of systemic corticosteroid therapy. Allergy Asthma Clin Immunol. 2013;9(1):30.

Llahana S, Philips D, Webber J, Chapman S, Carroll P, McBride P, et al., editors. Development and evaluation of the acceptability of new materials to address individualised needs to support self-management for patients with adrenal insufficiency Society for Endocrinology. Brighton: BES; 2016.

Lovas K, Loge JH, Husebye ES. Subjective health status in Norwegian patients with Addison's disease. Clin Endocrinol. 2002;56(5):581–8.

Lovas K, Gjesdal CG, Christensen M, Wolff AB, Almas B, Svartberg J, et al. Glucocorticoid replacement therapy and pharmacogenetics in Addison's disease: effects on bone. Eur J Endocrinol. 2009;160(6):993–1002.

Lovas K, Curran S, Oksnes M, Husebye ES, Huppert FA, Chatterjee VK. Development of a disease-specific quality of life questionnaire in Addison's disease. J Clin Endocrinol Metab. 2010;95(2):545–51.

Mah PM, Jenkins RC, Rostami-Hodjegan A, Newell-Price J, Doane A, Ibbotson V, et al. Weight-related dosing, timing and monitoring hydrocortisone replacement therapy in patients with adrenal insufficiency. Clin Endocrinol. 2004;61(3):367–75.

Mendoza-Cruz AC, Wargon O, Adams S, Tran H, Verge CF. HPA axis recovered within 6-12 weeks of infant prednisolone therapy. J Clin Endocrinol Metab. 2013;98(12):E1936–40. https://doi.org/10.1210/jc.2013-2649.

Methlie P, Husebye EE, Hustad S, Lien EA, Lovas K. Grapefruit juice and licorice increase cortisol availability in patients with Addison's disease. Eur J Endocrinol. 2011;165(5):761–9.

Migeon CJ, Lanes R. Adrenal cortex: hypofunction and hyperfunction (Chpater 8). In: Lifshitz F, editor. Pediatric endocrinology. Growth, adrenal, sexual, thyroid, calcium and fluid balance disorders, vol. 2. 5th ed. New York: Informa Healthcare; 2009.

Miller W, Achermann JC, Fluck CE. The adrenal cortex and its disorders (Chapter 12). In: Sperling MA, editor. Pediatric Endocrinology. 3rd ed. Philadelphia, PA: Saunders Elsevier; 2008.

Muller L, Quinkler M. Adrenal disease: imitating the cortisol profile improves the immune system. Nat Rev Endocrinol. 2018;14(3):137–9.

Murray RD, Ekman B, Uddin S, Marelli C, Quinkler M, Zelissen PM. Management of glucocorticoid replacement in adrenal insufficiency shows notable heterogeneity—data from the EU-AIR. Clin Endocrinol. 2017;86(3):340–6.

Neary N, Nieman L. Adrenal insufficiency: etiology, diagnosis and treatment. Curr Opin Endocrinol Diabetes Obes. 2010;17(3):217–23.

Neumann U, Whitaker MJ, Wiegand S, Krude H, Porter J, Davies M, et al. Absorption and tolerability of taste-masked hydrocortisone granules in neonates, infants and children under 6 years of age with adrenal insufficiency. Clin Endocrinol. 2018;88(1):21–9.

Nunes V, Neilson J, O'Flynn N, Calvert N, Kuntze S, Smithson H, et al. Clinical Guidelines and Evidence Review for Medicines Adherence: involving patients in decisions about prescribed medicines and supporting adherence. London: National Collaborating Centre for Primary Care and Royal College of General Practitioners; 2009.

Oksnes M, Bjornsdottir S, Isaksson M, Methlie P, Carlsen S, Nilsen RM, et al. Continuous subcutaneous hydrocortisone infusion versus oral hydrocortisone replacement for treatment of Addison's disease: a randomized clinical trial. J Clin Endocrinol Metab. 2014;99(5):1665–74.

Oksnes M, Ross R, Lovas K. Optimal glucocorticoid replacement in adrenal insufficiency. Best Pract Res Clin Endocrinol Metab. 2015;29(1):3–15.

Policola C, Stokes V, Karavitaki N, Grossman A. Adrenal insufficiency in acute oral opiate therapy. Endocrinol Diabetes Metab Case Rep. 2014;2014:130071.

Quinkler M, Hahner S. What is the best long-term management strategy for patients with primary adrenal insufficiency? Clin Endocrinol. 2012;76(1):21–5.

Quinkler M, Beuschlein F, Hahner S, Meyer G, Schofl C, Stalla GK. Adrenal cortical insufficiency—a life threatening illness with multiple etiologies. Dtsch Arztebl Int. 2013;110(51–52):882–8.

Quinkler M, Oelkers W, Remde H, Allolio B. Mineralocorticoid substitution and monitoring in primary adrenal insufficiency. Best Pract Res Clin Endocrinol Metab. 2015;29(1):17–24.

Quinkler M, Ekman B, Marelli C, Uddin S, Zelissen P, Murray RD, et al. Prednisolone is associated with a worse lipid profile than hydrocortisone in patients with adrenal insufficiency. Endocr Connect. 2016;6(1):1–8.

Qureshi AC, Bahri A, Breen LA, Barnes SC, Powrie JK, Thomas SM, et al. The influence of the route of oestrogen administration on serum levels of cortisol-binding globulin and total cortisol. Clin Endocrinol. 2007;66(5):632–5.

Rushworth RL, Chrisp GL, Dean B, Falhammar H, Thorpy DJ. Hospitalisation in children with adrenal insufficiency and hypopituitarism: is there a differential burden between boys and girls and between age groups? Horm Res Paediatr. 2017;88(5):339–46. https://doi.org/10.1159/000479370.

Salprietro V, Polizzi A, Di Rosa G, Romeo AC, Dipasqualw V, Morabito P, Chirico V, Arrigo T, Ruffieri M. Adrenal disorders and the paediatric brain: pathophysiological considerations and clinical implications. Int J Endocrinol. 2014. https://doi.org/10.1155/2014/282489. 15 pages.

Schulz J, Frey KR, Cooper M, Zopf K, Ventz M, Diederich S, et al. Reduction in daily hydrocortisone dose improves bone health in primary adrenal insufficiency. Eur J Endocrinol. 2016;174(4):531–8. https://doi.org/10.1530/eje-15-1096.

Smans LC, Van der Valk ES, Hermus AR, Zelissen PM. Incidence of adrenal crisis in patients with adrenal insufficiency. Clin Endocrinol. 2016;84(1):17–22.

Stewart PM. Chapter 14: The adrenal cortex. In: Kronemberg HM, Melmed S, Polonsky KS, Larsen PR, editors. Williams textbook of endocrinology. 11th ed. Philadelphia: Saunders Elsevier; 2008. p. 445–503.

Tomlinson JW, Holden N, Hills RK, Wheatley K, Clayton RN, Bates AS, et al. Association between premature mortality and hypopituitarism. Lancet (London, England). 2001;357(9254):425–31.

Uta N, WM J, Susanna W, Heiko K, John P, Madhu D, et al. Absorption and tolerability of taste-masked hydrocortisone granules in neonates, infants and children under 6 years of age with adrenal insufficiency. Clin Endocrinol. 2018;88(1):21–9.

Wass JA, Arlt W. How to avoid precipitating an acute adrenal crisis. BMJ (Clin Res Ed). 2012;345:e6333.

Whitaker M, Digweed D, Huatan H, Eckland D, Spielmann S, Johnson T, et al. Infacort, oral hydrocortisone granules with taste masking for the treatment of neonates and infants with adrenal insufficiency. Endocr Rev. 2014;35.

White K, Arlt W. Adrenal crisis in treated Addison's disease: a predictable but under-managed event. Eur J Endocrinol. 2010;162(1):115–20.

Zelissen PM, Croughs RJ, van Rijk PP, Raymakers JA. Effect of glucocorticoid replacement therapy on bone mineral density in patients with Addison disease. Ann Intern Med. 1994;120(3):207–10.

Key Reading

1. Bancos I, Hahner S, Tomlinson J, Arlt W. Diagnosis and management of adrenal insufficiency. Lancet Diabetes Endocrinol. 2015;3(3):216–26.

2. Bornstein SR, Allolio B, Arlt W, Barthel A, Don-Wauchope A, Hammer GD, et al. Diagnosis and treatment of primary adrenal insufficiency: an endocrine society clinical practice guideline. J Clin Endocrinol Metab. 2016;101(2):364–89.

3. Grossman AB. Clinical review: the diagnosis and management of central hypoadrenalism. J Clin Endocrinol Metab. 2010;95(11):4855–63.

4. Migeon CJ, Lanes R. Adrenal cortex: hypofunction and hyperfunction (Chapter 8). In: Lifshitz F, editor. Pediatric endocrinology. Growth, adrenal, sexual, thyroid, calcium and fluid balance disorders, vol. 2. 5th ed. New York: Informa Healthcare; 2009.

5. Arlt W. Disorders of the adrenal cortex (Chapter 8). In: Jameson JL, editor. Harrison's endocrinology. 4th ed. New York: McGraw Hill Education; 2017. p. 107–35.

6. Arlt W, Allolio B. Adrenal insufficiency. Lancet. 2003;361(9372):1881–93.

Printed by Printforce, the Netherlands